# CARDIOLOGY IN PRIMARY CARE

# CARDIOLOGY IN PRIMARY CARE

## EDITORS

**William T. Branch, Jr., M.D.**
Carter Smith, Sr., Professor of Medicine
Vice Chairman for Primary Care
Director, Division of General Medicine
Department of Medicine
Emory University School of Medicine
Atlanta, Georgia

**R. Wayne Alexander, M.D., Ph.D.**
R. Bruce Logue Professor and Chair
Department of Medicine
Emory University School of Medicine
Atlanta, Georgia

**Robert C. Schlant, M.D.**
Professor of Medicine
Division of Cardiology
Department of Medicine
Emory University School of Medicine
Atlanta, Georgia

**J. Willis Hurst, M.D.**
Consultant to the Division of Cardiology
Former Professor and Chairman of the
    Department of Medicine (1957–1986)
Emory University School of Medicine
Atlanta, Georgia

## McGraw-Hill
### MEDICAL PUBLISHING DIVISION

New York  St. Louis  San Francisco  Auckland  Bogotá  Caracas  Lisbon  London  Madrid
Mexico City  Milan  Montreal  New Delhi  San Juan  Singapore  Sydney  Tokyo  Toronto

# McGraw-Hill

*A Division of The* **McGraw·Hill** *Companies*

**CARDIOLOGY IN PRIMARY CARE**

1234567890 DOCDOC 09876543210

ISBN 0-07-007162-4

This book was set in Times Roman by TCSystems, Inc.
The editors were Joseph Hefta, Darlene B. Cooke, Mariapaz Ramos Englis, and Lester A. Sheinis.
The production supervisor was Catherine H. Saggese.
The text designer was Marsha Cohen/Parallelogram.
The cover designer was Kelly Parr.
The indexer was Barbara Littlewood.
R.R. Donnelley & Sons Company was the printer and binder.

This book is printed on acid-free paper.

Library of Congress cataloging-in-publication data for this book are on file with the Library of Congress.

# CONTENTS

# CONTRIBUTORS

**R. Wayne Alexander, M.D., Ph.D.**
R. Bruce Logue Professor and Chair
Department of Medicine
Emory University School of Medicine
Atlanta, Georgia
Chapters 2, 3, 26

**Joseph Ansley, M.D.**
Associate Professor, Vascular Surgery
Emory University School of Medicine
Atlanta, Georgia
Chapter 10

**Wilbert S. Aronow, M.D.**
Adjunct Professor of Geriatrics and Adult
  Development
Mount Sinai School of Medicine
Bronx, New York
Corporate Medical Director
Hebrew Hospital Home
Bronx, New York
Chapter 48

**Michael A. Balk, M.D., F.A.C.C.**
Director of Nuclear Cardiology
Northside Hospital
Atlanta, Georgia
Chapter 47

**April Barbour, M.D.**
Assistant Professor
Department of Medicine
Primary Care
Emory University School of Medicine
Atlanta, Georgia
Chapter 6

**Louis L. Battey, M.D.**
Assistant Professor
Department of Medicine
Emory University School of Medicine
Atlanta, Georgia
Chapter 32

**Wendy M. Book, M.D.**
Assistant Professor

Division of Cardiology
Emory University School of Medicine
Atlanta, Georgia
Chapter 33

**William T. Branch, Jr., M.D.**
Carter Smith, Sr., Professor of Medicine
Vice Chairman for Primary Care
Director, Division of General Medicine
Department of Medicine
Emory University School of Medicine
Atlanta, Georgia
Chapters 2, 4, 5, 7, 11, 12, 17

**W. Virgil Brown, M.D.**
Charles Howard Candler Professor of Internal
  Medicine
Chief of the Medical Services
Atlanta VA Hospital
Emory University School of Medicine
Atlanta, Georgia
Chapter 18

**Elliot L. Chaikof, M.D., Ph.D.**
Associate Professor of Surgery
Division of Vascular Surgery
Emory University School of Medicine
Atlanta, Georgia
Chapters 9, 13

**Nicolas A. F. Chronos, M.D.**
Private Practice
Atlanta, Georgia
Chapter 53

**Stephen D. Clements, M.D.**
Division of Cardiology
Emory Clinic
Atlanta, Georgia
Chapter 24

**Donald C. Davis, M.D., Ph.D.**
Associate Professor of Medicine
Associate Director, Division of General Medicine

Department of Medicine
Emory University School of Medicine
Associate Medical Director
Emory University Hospital
Atlanta, Georgia
Chapter 52

**David B. De Lurgio, M.D.**
Division of Cardiology
Emory Clinic
Atlanta, Georgia
Chapter 6

**Mario Di Girolamo, M.D.**
Professor of Medicine and Physiology
Emory University School of Medicine
Atlanta, Georgia
Chapter 23

**Thomas F. Dodson, M.D.**
Associate Professor of Surgery
Program Director
Vice Chairman for Education
Department of Surgery
Emory University Hospital
Atlanta, Georgia
Chapter 35

**Joyce P. Doyle, M.D.**
Assistant Professor of Medicine
ASH Specialist in Clinical Hypertension
Emory University School of Medicine
Atlanta, Georgia
Chapters 30, 31

**James G. Drougas, M.D.**
Fellow in Vascular Surgery
Division of Vascular Surgery
Emory University School of Medicine
Atlanta, Georgia
Chapter 13

**Joel M. Felner, M.D.**
Associate Dean of Clinical Education
Professor of Medicine in Cardiology
Emory University School of Medicine
Atlanta, Georgia
Chapter 40

**Jacqueline B. Fine, Ph.D.**
Assistant Professor of Medicine
Emory University School of Medicine
Atlanta, Georgia
Chapter 23

**Gerald F. Fletcher, M.D.**
Professor of Medicine
Cardiovascular Diseases
Mayo Medical School
Mayo Clinic, Jacksonville
Jacksonville, Florida
Chapter 20

**Harry R. Foster, Jr., M.D.**
Assistant Clinical Professor of Pediatrics
Emory University School of Medicine
Atlanta, Georgia
Chapter 38

**Robert H. Franch, M.D.**
Division of Cardiology
Emory Clinic
Atlanta, Georgia
Chapter 33

**Stephen C. Frohwein, M.D.**
Division of Cardiology
Emory Clinic
Atlanta, Georgia
Chapter 34

**Ziyad Ghazzal, M.D.**
Associate Professor of Medicine
Department of Cardiology
Emory Hospital
Atlanta, Georgia
Chapter 52

**Thomas M. Guest, M.D.**
Emory University School of Medicine
Atlanta, Georgia
Chapter 21

**W. Dallas Hall, M.D.**
Emeritus Professor of Medicine
Emory University School of Medicine
Atlanta, Georgia
Chapters 30, 31

**William Z. H'Doubler, M.D.**
Fellow in Vascular Surgery
Division of Vascular Surgery
Emory University School of Medicine
Atlanta, Georgia
Chapter 9

**J. Willis Hurst, M.D.**
Consultant to the Division of Cardiology
Former Professor and Chairman of the Department
  of Medicine (1957–1986)
Emory University School of Medicine
Atlanta, Georgia
Chapters 1, 7

**Halit M. Isiklar, M.D.**
Division of Vascular Surgery
Emory University School of Medicine
Atlanta, Georgia
Chapter 11

**Kara L. Jacobson, M.P.H., C.H.E.S.**
Health Behavior and Education Specialist
USQA Center for Health Care Research
Aetna U.S. Healthcare
Atlanta, Georgia
Chapter 54

**Terry A. Jacobson, M.D.**
Associate Professor of Medicine
Director, Office of Health Promotion and Disease
  Prevention
Emory University School of Medicine
Atlanta, Georgia
Chapters 18, 19, 54

**Thomas S. Johnston, M.D.**
Private Practice
Nashville, Tennessee
Chapters 8, 49

**Jennifer Kleinbart, M.D.**
Assistant Professor of Medicine
Division of General Medicine
Emory University School of Medicine
Atlanta, Georgia
Chapter 5

**Stephen Konigsberg**
Physician's Assistant—Certified

Vascular Surgery
Emory Clinic
Atlanta, Georgia
Chapter 12

**Phyllis E. Kozarsky, M.D.**
Associate Professor of Medicine, Infectious Diseases
Adjunct Professor of International Health
Emory University School of Medicine
Atlanta, Georgia
Chapter 50

**Sunil Kripalani, M.D.**
Senior Associate
Department of Medicine
Emory University School of Medicine
Atlanta, Georgia
Chapter 19

**Angel R. León, M.D.**
Emory Clinic
Atlanta, Georgia
Chapters 36, 37

**James L. Levenson, M.D.**
Professor of Psychiatry, Medicine, and Surgery
Chairman
Division of Consultation, Psychiatry
Vice-Chairman
Department of Psychiatry
Medical College of Virginia, Commonwealth University
Richmond, Virginia
Chapter 51

**Alan B. Lumsden, M.D.**
Associate Professor, Vascular Surgery
Emory University School of Medicine
Atlanta, Georgia
Chapters 11, 12

**Jerre F. Lutz, M.D.**
Associate Professor of Medicine
Division of Cardiology
Emory Clinic
Emory University School of Medicine
Atlanta, Georgia
Chapters 28, 29

**Steven V. Manoukian, M.D.**
Division of Cardiology

Emory Clinic
Atlanta, Georgia
Chapter 39

**Barry J. Maron, M.D.**
Director, Cardiovascular Research Division
Minneapolis Heart Institute Foundation
Minneapolis, Minnesota
Chapter 45

**J. Jeffrey Marshall, M.D.**
Division of Cardiology
Department of Medicine
Emory University School of Medicine
Atlanta, Georgia
Chapter 25

**Jonathan J. Masor, M.D.**
Associate Professor of Medicine
Emory University School of Medicine
Atlanta, Georgia
Chapter 42

**Sally E. McNagny, M.D.**
Associate Professor of Medicine
Division of General Internal Medicine
Department of Medicine
Emory University School of Medicine
Atlanta, Georgia
Chapter 22

**Michael Mollod, M.D.**
Fellow, Division of Cardiology
Emory University School of Medicine
Atlanta, Georgia
Chapter 40

**Joseph G. Ouslander, M.D.**
Vice President for Professional Services
Wesley Woods Center of Emory University
Professor and Director
Division of Geriatric Medicine and Gerontology
Emory University School of Medicine
Atlanta, Georgia
Chapter 48

**Clyde Partin, M.D.**
Assistant Professor of Medicine
Emory University School of Medicine
Atlanta, Georgia
Chapter 27

**William H. Plauth, Jr., M.D.**
Professor Emeritus of Pediatrics
Emory University School of Medicine
Atlanta, Georgia
Chapter 38

**Kimberly Rask, M.D.**
Assistant Professor of Medicine
Division of General Medicine
Emory University School of Medicine
Atlanta, Georgia
Chapter 44

**Larry G. Ray, Jr., M.D.**
Assistant Professor of Medicine
General Internal Medicine
Emory University School of Medicine
Atlanta, Georgia
Chapter 24

**David L. Roberts, M.D.**
Assistant Professor
Department of Medicine
Emory University School of Medicine
Atlanta, Georgia
Chapter 26

**Paul H. Robinson, M.D.**
Associate Professor of Medicine
Emory University School of Medicine
Atlanta, Georgia
Chapters 43, 50

**Donald St. Claire, Jr., M.D.**
Division of Cardiology
Emory Clinic
Atlanta, Georgia
Chapter 32

**Atef A. Salam, M.D.**
Professor, Vascular Surgery
Emory University School of Medicine
Atlanta, Georgia
Chapter 16

**Tarek AbdelAzim Salam, M.D.**
Assistant Professor of General Vascular Surgery
Ein-Shams University School of Medicine
Cairo, Egypt
Chapter 16

**Mahomed Y. Salame, B.Sc. (Hons), M.B. B.S., M.R.C.P.**
Fellow in Interventional Cardiology
Andreas Gruentzig Cardiovascular Center
Emory University Hospital
Atlanta, Georgia
Chapter 53

**Owen B. Samuels, M.D.**
Department of Neurosurgery
Emory University School of Medicine
Atlanta, Georgia
Chapter 15

**Robert C. Schlant, M.D.**
Professor of Medicine
Division of Cardiology
Department of Medicine
Emory University School of Medicine
Atlanta, Georgia
Chapters 17, 41

**David P. Schroeder, M.D.**
Private Practice
Asheville, North Carolina
Chapter 54

**Charles D. Searles, M.D.**
Assistant Professor of Medicine
Department of Medicine
Division of Cardiology
Emory University School of Medicine
Atlanta, Georgia
Chapter 43

**Laura C. Seeff, M.D.**
Formerly Assistant Professor of Medicine
Department of Medicine
Division of General Medicine
Emory University School of Medicine
Atlanta, Georgia
Chapter 43

**Andrew L. Smith, M.D.**
Division of Cardiology
Emory Clinic
Atlanta, Georgia
Chapter 27

**Barney J. Stern, M.D.**
Professor of Neurology
Emory University School of Medicine
Atlanta, Georgia
Chapter 15

**James L. Sutherland, M.D.**
Assistant Professor of Pediatrics
Emory University School of Medicine
Atlanta, Georgia
Chapter 46

**W. Robert Taylor, M.D., Ph.D.**
Associate Professor of Medicine
Emory University School of Medicine
Atlanta, Georgia
Chapter 21

**Clyde Watkins, Jr., M.D.**
Assistant Director
General Medical Clinics
Grady Health System
Assistant Professor of Medicine
Division of General Medicine
Emory University School of Medicine
Atlanta, Georgia
Chapter 47

**William S. Weintraub, M.D.**
Division of Cardiology
Emory Clinic
Atlanta, Georgia
Chapter 44

**Victor J. Weiss, M.D.**
Assistant Professor of Medicine
Division of Vascular Surgery
Emory University School of Medicine
Atlanta, Georgia
Chapter 10

**Nanette K. Wenger, M.D.**
Professor
Division of Cardiology
Emory University School of Medicine
Atlanta, Georgia
Chapter 22

**Byron R. Williams, Jr., M.D.**
Division of Cardiac Radiology
Emory Clinic
Atlanta, Georgia
Chapters 14, 42

# PREFACE

This book is for *primary care physicians* and all others who participate in the general care of patients with cardiovascular disease.

Internists, family physicians, physician assistants, and nurse clinicians participate in the care of millions of individuals in this and other countries. They are of prime importance in the delivery of health care because they are the professionals patients and potential patients contact initially. They guide the system of health care.

Primary care physicians and those who work with them do not specialize in the diseases that involve a specific body system. Rather, they focus and specialize in the *care of the individual as a person*. They manage the medical problems they are trained to manage and consult with and refer their patients to other more specialized physicians when the need arises. They prevent disease when it is possible to do so. They care deeply about the person who is sick and enjoy dealing with the small and large problems they encounter. Accordingly, the primary care physicians and those who work with them have always been among the mainstays in the broad scheme of health care in this country.

This book deals exclusively with cardiovascular problems. One can properly ask why should primary care physicians, who are interested in all health problems, need a book on a single organ system. The answer is because cardiovascular problems are common and preventive care is of crucial importance. For example, if you are a 40-year-old male, you have one chance in two of having a "coronary event" sometime during your life. If you are a 40-year-old female you have one chance in three of having a coronary event during your life.

A potential reader might ask, "Since there are many types of cardiovascular diseases and there are several 2000-page books on the subject, how can a book be created that would meet the needs of those individuals who are involved in primary care?" Another potential reader might ask, "How does this book differ from the section on cardiovascular disease provided by a textbook of general medicine?" These questions lead to an explanation of the evolution of the creation of this book that separates it from other books. Simply stated, this is why this book is unique. *The subjects that are discussed were selected by primary care physicians who appreciate the type of information that primary care physicians need to "get through a day" of dealing with many types of health problems.* Such a book would not, and should not, attempt to present all the information that is known about all cardiovascular subjects but should assist primary care physicians in determining which cardiovascular problems they can, and should, manage and which conditions should be referred to others for consultation or more specialized care. This effort was abetted by having both the cardiologists and primary care physicians write many of the same chapters in the book while other chapters were written separately by cardiologists and by primary care physicians. The editors, including one primary care physician and three cardiologists, reviewed and edited all of the chapters in order to make certain that the needs of the primary care physicians and those who work with them are met.

Much effort and thought were expended in an endeavor to meet the stated goals for the book. The editors thank the authors for their willingness to try to implement a new idea. We also thank Lynda Prickett Mathews for her ability to keep order. We also appreciate the interest of Joseph Hefta of McGraw-Hill who had faith in the project as well as Darlene Cooke, Mariapaz Englis, Catherine Saggese, and Lester A. Sheinis who shepherded the book through to publication. We wish to thank our assistants for their invaluable help in carrying the book to fruition—Kim Gardner, Mary Glenn Costley, Nell McDonald, and Sharon Hailey.

*The Editors:*
*William T. Branch, Jr., M.D.*
*R. Wayne Alexander, M.D., Ph.D.*
*Robert C. Schlant, M.D.*
*J. Willis Hurst, M.D.*

J. WILLIS HURST

CHAPTER

1

# THE PREVALENCE OF CARDIOVASCULAR DISEASE IN THE GENERAL POPULATION AND THE ROLE OF THE PRIMARY CARE PHYSICIAN

The service offered by the competent primary care physician is central to the panoply of services offered by the medical profession. The compassionate primary care physician who is skilled in the analysis of symptoms, the performance of a defined physical examination, and the interpretation of routine laboratory tests, including the electrocardiogram and chest x-ray film, is able to make a diagnosis of cardiovascular disease or to create a differential diagnosis that lists the cardiovascular diseases that could be present. The ordering of other procedures is done in order to gain further insight about the patient's diagnosis or to identify the diagnosis when there is a list of possibilities.[1] Foremost in the minds of primary care physicians is the welfare of their patients. Accordingly, all of their actions, including the use of high technology, must benefit the patients they serve.

Physicians who provide primary care to the population at large face many challenges. They must identify and treat illnesses that affect every age group; recognize those conditions that are troublesome, but not life-threatening, as well as those conditions that are of a more serious nature; know when high-technology procedures are indicated but perform none of them themselves; be highly skilled in determining which patients should be referred to specific specialists for another opinion or for the performance of procedures; be constantly aware of the current methods of preventing diseases; be skilled in dealing with the emotional problems exhibited by most patients at some time in their lives; be available for counseling and advice on a wide range of subjects; and accomplish all of this within the framework of reasonable cost.

The cardiovascular system usually performs its important duties in a most remarkable way. The cardiovascular system, however, is commonly affected by diseases that may lead to death or disability. This latter fact led to the choice of subjects discussed in this book. An effort was made by the authors and editors to discuss conditions that primary physicians are likely to face as they go about their daily work seeing patients of all ages.

The cardiovascular diseases that primary care physicians encounter include the following:

- A small number of newborn infants will have congenital heart disease. The primary care physician must recognize the presence of congenital heart diseases but, as a general rule, should refer the patient to a pediatric cardiologist for further care.

  For the prevention of congenital heart disease, the primary care physician must ensure that all nonimmune women are vaccinated for rubella prior to childbearing.
- As children grow older, they engage in vigorous athletics. The primary care physician must be able to screen young adults for cardiovascular diseases known to occur in that age group and to specifically search for conditions that may cause unexpected death during vigorous exercise.
- The pregnant female may have heart disease or may develop heart disease or pulmonary emboli.
- Essential hypertension is one of the most common problems seen in young and old adults. All of the recent evidence emphasizes that the normal range of blood pressure is lower than was formerly believed. All recent studies indicate that physicians must make a major effort to normalize even the slightest elevation of blood pressure in an attempt to decrease the likelihood of strokes, heart failure, renal failure, atherosclerotic vascular disease, and dementia. Evidence is also available indicating that, despite an array of effective drugs, the maintenance of normal blood pressure in patients with essential hypertension is still inadequate. In addition, the primary care physician must be able to identify those patients with hypertension who might have a secondary cause for the serious abnormality.

  The level of blood pressure considered to be desirable has changed over the years, and treatment guidelines stress a more aggressive approach in patients with additional cardiovascular risk factors, especially diabetes mellitus. All physicians must be aware of the latest recommendations for treatment of hypertension. In addition, many new drugs have become available, so that, with careful monitoring, it is possible to normalize the pressure in nearly all individuals.
- Atherosclerotic coronary heart disease and peripheral vascular disease are likely to affect most individuals as they move through the decades of their lives.

For example, at age 40 the male should realize that the chances are *one in two* that he will develop atherosclerotic coronary heart disease during his lifetime.[2] The female at age 40 should realize that during her lifetime her chances of having atherosclerotic coronary heart disease are *one in three*. This disease is responsible for most of the deaths in the United States, and the gender differences must be understood. For example, for women who experience a myocardial infarction under the age of 50, the risk of dying is about 6 percent, compared to about 3 percent for men of that age. The mortality of women and men with myocardial infarction becomes higher each decade, with the mortality always being higher in women until the age of 80, when the mortality of infarction is 20 to 25 percent and is almost equal in the sexes.[3]

Strokes are the most common cause of disability. Many strokes are potentially preventable by treatment that may modify the outcome of intracranial or extracranial atherosclerotic arterial disease, hypertension, and emboli in patients with atrial fibrillation or mitral thrombi.

Most observers of the medical scene recognize that primary care physicians as well as cardiologists have failed to expand their knowledge of peripheral vascular disease, including that of the carotid arteries, aorta, and arteries in the legs. This, of course, must be corrected. Accordingly, this common problem is discussed in this book.

The primary care physician must be expert in the prevention of atherosclerotic disease and must be obsessed with implementing his or her knowledge of the subject.

Modern therapy is not used by everyone. For example, not every physician who treats patients with myocardial infarction utilizes thrombolytic therapy. This issue is addressed in this book.

- Valvular heart disease is less common than it was formerly. Years ago, rheumatic fever and syphilis were major causes of valvular heart disease. Effective preventive measures have almost eliminated these causes of heart disease.

    The most common cause of mitral valve regurgitation today is cardiac enlargement due to dilated cardiomyopathy, including ischemic cardiomyopathy. The most common cause of primary mitral valve regurgitation is mitral valve prolapse. The prevalence of mitral valve prolapse is less now than it was 5 years ago because the criteria used to diagnose the condition have been refined.[4] This, plus new information that establishes that the risk of complications from the condition is less than previously thought, will decrease the anxiety of many patients.[4]

    Mitral valve regurgitation in an elderly woman may be caused by mitral valve annulus calcification, which can be seen on the lateral x-ray film of the chest.

    Mitral stenosis due to rheumatic heart disease is still with us, and new causes for the condition have been identified.[5]

    The murmur of aortic valve sclerosis, without left ventricular outflow tract obstruction, is common in patients beyond the age of 60.[6] This condition marks a patient as one who is highly likely to have signs of atherosclerotic coronary heart disease in the years ahead. Such a condition is also the forerunner of aortic valve stenosis in the elderly, which is associated with an increased prevalence of atherosclerotic coronary heart disease, as well as causing syncope, sudden death, and heart failure. Many experts believe that aortic sclerosis and aortic stenosis of the elderly are actually due to the atherosclerotic process itself. Infective endocarditis as a cause of valve disease must never be missed; to overlook it will result in the death of the patient. Measures to prevent infection of the heart valves must be implemented.

- Lung disease due to smoking is common. With advanced lung disease, cor pulmonale is common. Heart failure due to lung disease is commonly overlooked.

    The prevention of pulmonary heart disease must be implemented.

- Dilated cardiomyopathy following multiple infarcts due to atherosclerotic coronary heart disease or myocarditis, or appearing without apparent cause, is common. The indications for cardiac transplantation must be appreciated.

    Restrictive cardiomyopathy due to amyloid infiltration of the myocardium or other causes is uncommon but must be recognized.

    Hypertrophic cardiomyopathy is genetically determined and occurs in all age groups. It is one of the causes of sudden death in athletes.

    Myocarditis can occur in any age group and can be prevented in patients who are at high risk of contracting Lyme disease.

- Neoplastic disease of the heart is not rare. A primary left atrial myxoma is curable with surgical removal and must never be overlooked.

    Metastatic disease to the myocardium is common in patients with cancer of the lung, breast, and esophagus.

- Heart failure is common. It is not a disease. It is the consequence—a complication—of heart disease. The recognition and treatment of heart failure have improved during the recent past. Unfortunately, the known therapeutic approaches to treatment are not all uniformly prescribed.

- Cardiac arrhythmias are common. Atrial fibrillation is likely to occur in most patients as they grow older. It occurs with greater frequency in patients with heart disease, especially those with mitral valve stenosis or regurgitation. A number of extracardiac conditions may increase the likelihood of atrial fibrillation. The point to emphasize, however, is that lone atrial fibrillation in older people occurs most commonly when there is no other evidence of heart disease. This serious rhythm disturbance may be the cause of embolic stroke, produce troublesome palpitations, and aggravate heart failure. The treatment of atrial fibrillation today is very different from that of a decade ago. Warfarin to prevent embolic strokes and emboli to other organs must be prescribed in most patients with persistent atrial fibrillation unless there is a contraindication to its use.

- Most of the drugs used in cardiovascular medicine have unwanted, and sometimes serious, side effects on the heart and other organs. These toxic findings must be sought in all patients taking such drugs.

    Noncardiac drugs may cause serious cardiac disease. For example, some of the drugs used to treat neoplastic disease and psychiatric problems may damage the heart. The physician must be aware of this possibility when treating a patient with noncardiac drugs. Primary care physicians are in the best position to detect harmful effects of drugs on the heart and other organs.

Many other conditions could be discussed here, but the foregoing are sufficient to indicate why a book of this sort seems justified. In it we have tried to discuss the recognition, treatment, and prevention of the common cardiovascular problems that primary care physicians encounter. In addition, we have tried to indicate the clues that signal that the cardiovascular system is functioning improperly so that appropriate consultation and procedures not done by the primary care physician will be obtained.

---

## REFERENCES

1.  Hurst JW: *Cardiac Diagnosis: The Initial Examination of the Heart.* St. Louis, Mosby, 1993.
2.  Lloyd-Jones DM, Larson MG, Beiser A, Levy D: Lifetime risk of developing coronary heart disease. *Lancet* 1999; 353:89–92.
3.  Vaccarino V, Parsons L, Every NR, et al: Sex-based differences in early mortality after myocardial infarction. *N Engl J Med* 1999; 341:217–225.
4.  Freed LA, Levy D, Levine RA, et al: Prevalence and clinical outcome of mitral-valve prolapse. *N Engl J Med* 1999; 341:1–7.
5.  Duffy J, Rodeheffer RJ: The heart and lyme disease. In: Hurst JW (ed): *New Types of Cardiovascular Diseases.* New York, Igaku Shoin, 1994:164–174.
6.  Otto CM, Lind BK, Kitzman DW, et al: Association of aortic-valve sclerosis with cardiovascular mortality and morbidity in the elderly. *N Engl J Med* 1999; 341:142–147.

# EVALUATION OF SYMPTOMS AND SIGNS OF CARDIOVASCULAR DISORDERS

R. WAYNE ALEXANDER /
WILLIAM T. BRANCH, JR.

CHAPTER

# 2

# EPISODIC CHEST DISCOMFORT

The evaluation of chest pain is, at once, one of the most difficult and one of the most important of the situations presenting to the practicing generalist. The causes range from the trivial to the potentially catastrophic.[1] *A careful, probing history is the one absolutely essential element in assessing chest pain. Overreliance on stress or invasive testing as a substitute for a diligently taken history can be misleading, is potentially risky, and will certainly be expensive.* Patients will frequently seek care and advice for pains in the chest that they would ignore in other locations because of their anxiety about having a "heart attack." The practitioner should approach all patients with chest pain with a high index of suspicion that the complaint may represent serious cardiopulmonary disease, in particular ischemic heart disease. In general, the focus is on excluding the possibility that the symptom complex represents pain associated with inadequate myocardial oxygen delivery or angina pectoris. Pain associated with dysfunction of the cardiovascular system in the chest is virtually always episodic rather than chronic and unremitting. This chapter will focus on the causes of episodic chest pain with emphasis upon coronary ischemia.

## DIFFERENTIAL DIAGNOSIS

The differential diagnosis of chest pain is extensive, and the clinician must consider not only angina pectoris but other cardiovascular diseases, pulmonary and pleural processes, certain gastrointestinal diseases, cutaneous and musculoskeletal disorders of the chest wall, and neural and psychogenic factors. The differential diagnosis of chest pain is summarized in Table 2-1.[1]

## ANGINA PECTORIS

In many ways the original description of angina pectoris by Heberden in 1772 is more graphic and compelling than any of those that have followed.[2] He wrote:

**TABLE 2-1.   Differential Diagnosis of Chest Pain**

1. Angina pectoris/myocardial infarction
2. Other cardiovascular causes
    a. Likely ischemic in origin
        (1) Aortic stenosis
        (2) Hypertrophic cardiomyopathy
        (3) Severe systemic hypertension
        (4) Severe right ventricular hypertension
        (5) Aortic regurgitation
        (6) Severe anemia/hypoxia
    b. Nonischemic in origin
        (1) Aortic dissection
        (2) Pericarditis
        (3) Mitral valve prolapse
3. Gastrointestinal
    a. Esophageal spasm
    b. Esophageal reflux
    c. Esophageal rupture
    d. Peptic ulcer disease
4. Psychogenic
    a. Anxiety
    b. Depression
    c. Cardiac psychosis
    d. Self-gain
5. Neuromusculoskeletal
    a. Thoracic outlet syndrome
    b. Degenerative joint disease of cervical/thoracic spine
    c. Costochondritis (Tietze's syndrome)
    d. Herpes zoster
    e. Chest wall pain and tenderness
6. Pulmonary
    a. Pulmonary embolus with or without pulmonary infarction
    b. Pneumothorax
    c. Pneumonia with pleural involvement
7. Pleurisy

*Source:* O'Rourke RA, Shaver JA, Salerni R, et al: The history, physical examination, and cardiac auscultation. In: Alexander RW, Schlant RC, Fuster V, et al (eds): *Hurst's The Heart,* 9th ed. New York, McGraw-Hill, 1998: 231.

But there is a disorder of the breast marked with strong and peculiar symptoms, considerable for the kind of danger belonging to it and not extremely rare, which deserves to be mentioned more at length. The seat of it and sense of strangling and anxiety with which it is attended make it not improperly called angina pectoris. They who are afflicted with it are seized while they are walking (more especially if it be up a hill and soon after eating) with a painful and most disagreeable sensation in the breast, which seems as if would extinguish life if it were to increase or to continue; but the moment they stand still, all this uneasiness vanishes.

Heberden's description incorporates some of the key elements that are used by the skilled clinician in differentiating angina pectoris from noncoronary chest discomfort: character; location; and precipitating events, including reproducibility, duration, and associated symptoms. Other important features to be considered include the quality of the pain, its mode of onset, and its pattern of disappearance or relief.

Understanding the physiology of myocardial ischemia is necessary for understanding of its clinical manifestations.[3] Fundamentally, it develops in any situation in which oxygen delivery is inadequate to meet the needs of the myocardium. The most clinically relevant circumstance in which this occurs is when coronary blood flow is restricted by an atherosclerotic plaque encroaching upon the coronary artery lumen and/or when the diseased artery is hypercontractile and vasospasm occurs. In either instance, the heart responds in a predictable manner to inadequate oxygen delivery. The initial manifestation is electrical, with ST-segment elevation or depression. Subsequently, diastolic and systolic dysfunction occur, with resulting increasing pressure that is reflected in the lungs and may result in the patient's feeling dyspneic. Finally, in this sequence, pain (angina) may be perceived. The important point for the clinician to remember is that angina pectoris and its associated symptoms are crescendo in nature and "build up" rather than reaching peak intensity instantaneously. Furthermore, coronary myocardial ischemia [as opposed to myocardial infarction (MI)] is, by definition, transient in nature and does not persist unabated for hours or days.

Another key point is that the patient may use any of a number of expressions to describe an unpleasant sensation in the chest. The clinician should not simply ask if the patient has chest pain but should inquire whether he or she has had any sensation in the chest that is new to his or her experience. A list of terms that patients may use in describing angina pectoris is given in Table 2-2. In general, these terms connote sustained discomfort rather than transient, lancing-type pains, although oc-

**TABLE 2-2.   Common Terms Used to Describe Angina Pectoris**

| | | |
|---|---|---|
| Pressure | Uncomfortable | Ache |
| Tightness | Swelling | Weight |
| Heaviness | Burning | Heartburn |
| Constricting | Dull | Soreness |
| Compressing | Searing | Bursting |
| Fullness | Hard | Like a toothache |
| Choking | Strangling | Like a vise |
| Discomfort | Indigestion | |

*Source:* Schlant RC, Alexander RW: Diagnosis and management of chronic ischemic heart disease. In Schlant RC, Alexander RW (eds): *Hurst's The Heart,* 8th ed. McGraw-Hill, New York, 1994: 1056.

casionally patients will use terms such as "knife-like" or "stabbing" to describe coronary ischemic pain. An important fact for the clinician to remember is that patient and physician may use different terms in describing chest pain. It is the physician's responsibility to put the patient's language into the appropriate clinical context, as will be discussed below.

Chest pain should be considered in the context of the patient's overall risk for coronary disease, but a complaint should never be prejudged on the basis of presumed low risk. For example, exertionally induced chest pain in a 50-year old male smoker would certainly create a high index of suspicion for angina in most clinicians, but it is important to take a disciplined, thorough, and systematic approach to *all* patients with chest pain. Coronary ischemic pain can and does occur in even very young patients from a variety of causes, including, occasionally, coronary artery disease. It is particularly important to remember that cardiovascular disease overall is by far the leading cause of death in women and that the protection provided by female gender is only relative, not absolute, and is rapidly dissipated by age and/or the presence of risk factors such as diabetes, smoking, and hyperlipidemia.

The key elements in the chest pain history should be sought through a systematic, organized approach.[1,4] The location of the discomfort is usually readily volunteered by the patient. Angina pectoris can manifest virtually anywhere in the thorax, although most commonly it is located anteriorly and substernally or precordially. It can present as pain in the shoulder or on the right side of the chest (less commonly). It is common for patients to describe a "band-like" tightness around the chest. Pain localized to the cardiac apical area frequently is not ischemic in origin. Angina occasionally manifests as pain in the posterior chest, and in this case esophageal causes or aortic dissection would also be higher than normal in one's index of suspicion. Relatively unusually, angina can manifest as epigastric pain. Pain can also radiate from the chest to the neck, mandible, or arm (in particular, the upper left arm), and radiation to the antecubital fossa or wrist is also sometimes seen. Interestingly, coronary ischemic pain may sometimes be seen exclusively in the referral area. In this case, the setting, reproducibility, and duration of the discomfort and a high index of suspicion by the clinician are key to making the correct diagnosis.

The *character* of the pain or discomfort is essential to building a case for or against a coronary origin. As mentioned, angina pectoris is crescendo in nature. It is useful to ask the patient whether the pain is as severe as it is going to get within several seconds or whether it "builds up." Shooting or lancing pain of short duration usually suggests musculoskeletal or neural pain. The terms that patients commonly use to describe angina pectoris were discussed previously and frequently include "pressure" or "tightness."

The *setting* in which chest pain occurs, including the *precipitating events, pattern, and reproducibility,* is perhaps the most important feature leading to the clinical diagnosis of the presence or absence of angina pectoris. It can be especially useful to ask such questions as: "Can you predict when the pain is likely to occur?"; "If I asked you to bring the pain on, could you?"; or "Does becoming angry bring on the pain?" If, for example, the patient says that the pain is brought on or made worse by deep breathing or moving in a certain way, coronary ischemia is unlikely to be the cause of the pain. It is important to remember that the threshold for eliciting angina by any activity is usually variable, which probably reflects variability in coronary tone and the extent of contraction or spasm of a coronary artery at a lesion site at any given time.[5] Typically, for example, angina associated with activities of daily living is more likely to occur in the morning and may not recur with similar activities during the rest of the day. Similarly, a golfer may have angina on the first hole and not have a recurrence for the rest of the round. Furthermore, activity after smoking or after a meal may be more likely to be associated with angina than the same level of activity at another time. The presence of such patterns of precipitation of chest pain increases the likelihood that the etiology is coronary artery disease (CAD).

It is important to establish whether other symptoms are associated with the chest pain. Some associated symptoms are characteristic, and their consistent presence can be helpful in arriving at a diagnosis. *Shortness of breath* that may be somewhat paroxysmal in onset and closely related temporally to the chest pain is frequently observed. *Diaphoresis* is also seen commonly with angina pectoris; in severe cases, it may be associated with nausea, reflecting vagal activation. Angina pectoris can also precipitate anxiety attacks, which must be distinguished from the symptoms associated with the coronary ischemic episode.

As noted, *duration* is a critically important element in characterizing angina pectoris. Attacks usually last from 1 to 10 min. Also, as noted, sharp shooting pains lasting a few seconds with complete relief between episodes usually are nonanginal. Angina pectoris does not last for hours at a time. It is important, as mentioned, to distinguish an anginal episode from an attack of anxiety or a full-blown panic attack that may be precipitated by the episode of coronary ischemia. In this setting, for example, the characteristic chest discomfort of angina may disappear, to be followed by anxiety and hyperventilation, which may be associated with chest pressure of a clearly different type. A carefully taken history is essential in establishing that the initiating event in a prolonged episode of discomfort was, in fact, a typical anginal episode.

The manner and mechanism by which a patient achieves *relief* from an episode of chest discomfort is also very important in the clinical assessment. If pain abates rapidly in 1 to 5 min after stopping activity, angina pectoris should be strongly considered. If, on the other hand, the discomfort just gradually disappears over 30 min to 1 h, angina is less likely, and this is also the case if the pain is promptly relieved by a change in position. The clinician should keep in mind that patients with angina pectoris may modify their activity by decreasing the intensity of exercise or avoiding certain endeavors altogether in order to minimize their chances of precipitating discomfort. Patients should be asked if they are engaging in their usual level of activity. This is most important in assessing the effects of therapy and clinical stability, as discussed in Chap. 25. It is also important to realize that nitroglycerin can be used diagnostically as well as therapeutically. Prompt (1 to 5 min) and reproducible relief of chest pain by sublingual or buccal nitroglycerin is very strong evidence that the pain being evaluated is angina pectoris.

## Classification of Angina Pectoris

**STABLE AND UNSTABLE ANGINA.**    All patients with angina pectoris should be classified, primarily on clinical grounds, as "stable" or "unstable." This classification infers information about the biologic state of atherosclerotic plaques in coronary arteries. Stable angina pectoris is defined as a chest pain pattern that has not changed within the previous 60 days in frequency, intensity (duration and severity), setting in which it occurs, or mechanisms of relief (number of nitroglycerin tablets required, for example). This stability of the pain pattern suggests that culprit plaques limiting coronary blood flow are not in a state in which the underlying inflammatory disease is "active" and that the physical integrity is intact. Conversely, unstable angina is defined as a worsening of angina pectoris in the terms utilized above within the prior 60 days. Patients with unstable angina may have "active" plaques with an exacerbation of the inflammatory state of a lesion resulting in propensity to rupture or erode and cause thrombosis and/or spasm. Unstable angina represents a clinical urgency or emergency depending upon the setting. Unstable angina should also be diagnosed when stable angina increases in frequency, lasts longer than usual, occurs upon less exertion, or occurs with rest during the last 60 days prior to episode.

*STABLE ANGINA.*    Patients with stable angina pectoris are classified most commonly functionally according to the Canadian Cardiovascular Society criteria (Table 2-3).[6] It is important to classify patients for several reasons. The level of impairment is quantified, which can guide therapeutic decision making and which can facilitate recognition of worsening of angina, sometimes a hallmark of developing instability. The establishment of a class for a patient with angina can also guide recommendations for level of exercise.

**TABLE 2-3.   Canadian Cardiovascular Society Functional Classification of Angina Pectoris**

| | |
|---|---|
| I. | Ordinary physical activity, such as walking and climbing stairs, does not cause angina. Angina results from strenuous or rapid or prolonged exertion at work or recreation. |
| II. | Slight limitation of ordinary activity. Walking or climbing stairs rapidly, walking uphill, walking or stair climbing after meals, in cold, in wind, or when under emotional stress, or only during the few hours after awakening. Walking more than two blocks on the level or climbing more than one flight of ordinary stairs at a normal pace and under normal conditions. |
| III. | Marked limitations of ordinary physical activity. Walking one to two blocks on the level or climbing one flight under normal conditions. |
| IV. | Inability to carry on any physical activity without discomfort—anginal syndrome may be present at rest. |

*Source:* Modified from Campeau L: Letter to the editor. *Circulation* 1976; 54:522. Reproduced with permission from the American Heart Association, Inc., and the author.

*UNSTABLE ANGINA.*   As inferred above, unstable angina can represent a spectrum of clinical situations, which has led to a variety of classification schemes to guide clinical decision making.[7] The basic goal is to ascertain the level of risk for having an acute coronary event. An early clinical objective is to gain insight into whether, in fact, exacerbation of symptoms could be due to conditions other than worsening of the inflammatory state of an atherosclerotic plaque. Worsening of angina pectoris can occur in the setting of a stable plaque if severe anemia develops (for example, with acute gastrointestinal bleeding) that results in myocardial ischemia because of decreased oxygen-carrying capacity of the blood. Alternatively, increased myocardial oxygen demand caused by poorly controlled hypertension or tachycardia could cause worsening of angina symptoms in absence of plaque instability. Unstable angina in these cases is classified as "secondary" and usually is defined in retrospect after treatment of the underlying, exacerbating condition.

Primary unstable angina connotes an unstable lesion. This category, however, also represents a clinical spectrum that dictates varying clinical responses. Classification of severity depends upon: the presence or absence of rest pain; duration of pain episodes; whether or not pain has occurred within the last 48 h; and whether or not the pain develops within 2 weeks of a prior acute myocardial infarction (AMI). These points are summarized in the classification of Braunwald[8] (Table 2-4). Patients may be further characterized in this scheme by whether or not there has been prior treatment for stable angina, and whether ST-segment changes are present during pain. Thus, a patient on minimal or no antianginal medication with primary angina pectoris and with no rest pain and who had the last episode of exertional pain more than 48 h previously (Class IB) possibly could be managed and evaluated safely as an outpatient. On the other hand Class III patients should generally be hospitalized acutely. Given the wide spectrum of clinical circumstances and the gravity of the implications, the general physician should have a low threshold for seeking consultation in the case of suspected unstable angina. The management of acute coronary syndromes is discussed in Chap. 26.

## New-Onset Angina Pectoris

It is essential to recognize angina pectoris of recent onset because such angina has virtually the same implications as established angina that has suddenly worsened—that is, that a coronary atherosclerotic lesion is in an active inflammatory state with the potential to rupture and to cause occlusive thrombosis. Unfortunately, in patients with an initial AMI, it is common to find that in the days preceding their event they had experienced one or more episodes of chest discomfort that, in retrospect, were clearly angina pectoris. *Failure on the part of patient or clinician to recognize these warning symptoms obviously can have catastrophic consequences.*

TABLE 2-4.   Braunwald's Classification of Unstable Angina

**Severity**

Class I.   New-onset, severe, or accelerated angina
Patients with angina of less than 2 months' duration, severe or occurring three or more times per day, or angina that is distinctly more frequent and precipitated by distinctly less exertion, no rest pain in the last 2 months

Class II.   Angina at rest, subacute
Patients with one or more episodes of angina at rest during the preceding month but not within the preceding 48 h

Class III.   Angina at rest, acute
Patients with one or more episodes at rest with the preceding 48 h

Clinical circumstances
Class A:   Secondary unstable angina
A clearly identified condition extrinsic to the coronary vascular bed that has intensified myocardial ischemia, e.g., anemia, infection, fever, hypotension, tachyarrhythmia, thyrotoxicosis, hypoxemia secondary to respiratory failure

Class B:   Primary unstable angina

Class C:   Postinfarction unstable angina (within 2 weeks of documented myocardial infarction)

Intensity of treatment
1.   Absence of treatment or minimal treatment
2.   Occurring in presence of standard therapy for chronic stable angina (conventional doses of oral beta blockers, nitrates, and calcium antagonists)
3.   Occurring despite maximally tolerated doses of all three categories of oral therapy, including intravenous nitroglycerin

*Source:* Reproduced with permission from Braunwald E: Unstable angina: A classification. *Circulation* 1989; 80:410. Copyright © 1989 American Heart Association.

# CARDIAC CHEST PAIN NOT RESULTING FROM CORONARY ATHEROSCLEROSIS

## Coronary Ischemia in the Absence of Coronary Artery Disease

Ischemic cardiac pain can occur in any situation in which myocardial oxygen demands are so high that even normal epicardial coronary arteries may be incapable of delivering sufficient oxygenated blood. Such situations, which have the common feature of left ventricular hypertrophy, may exist in any of the conditions listed in section 2a of Table 2-1, such as aortic stenosis and hypertension. Angina in these conditions is usually exertional, but the clinical picture may exhibit some unique features. Pain or discomfort may be more prolonged and more likely to extend into (or begin during) the rest period than is the case in angina pectoris associated with coronary artery disease. Persistent, as opposed to episodic, dyspnea and shortness of breath are more commonly a significant component of the symptom complex associated with hypertrophic disease because of the associated high left ventricular filling pressures. High ventricular diastolic pressures impair endocardial blood flow, which can also cause the prolonged episodes of chest pain associated with hypertrophic heart disease such as that associated with hypertension.

## Evaluation and Management of Angina-like Chest Pain

The management of chest pain is discussed in detail in Chap. 25, as is its evaluation. The initial course of action after deciding that a patient's history is compatible with angina pectoris is dictated by the strength of the evidence from the history and the perceived likelihood that the patient has angina.[9] A very typical story of angina of recent onset (appearing within the prior 6 weeks) in a 50-year old hypertensive male smoker, for example, should lead to possible hospital admission and referral for cardiac catheterization. A very atypical (but possible) anginal history in a 25-year old woman with no cardiovascular risk factors should usually be dealt with expectantly with further observation and a search for other causes, before proceeding to noninvasive cardiac assessment. The rationale for this approach is that in the first case, the pretest probability for a positive result from a noninvasive test (exercise treadmill with or without nuclear or ultrasound imaging) is so high that a negative test result should not dissuade one from the course of action outlined. In the second case, the pretest probability of coronary artery disease is so low that a false-positive test is more likely than a true positive and thus could lead to unnecessary invasive testing. The true utility of noninvasive cardiac testing is in the case of intermediate pretest likelihood of CAD. For example, a 42-year old woman who is a moderately hypertensive smoker and has a less than typical, but suspicious, story for angina pectoris would be an ideal candidate for noninvasive testing.

## Nonischemic Cardiovascular Chest Pain

As shown in section 2b of Table 2-1, there are three causes of cardiovascular chest pain that are nonischemic in origin: aortic dissection, pericarditis, and mitral valve prolapse.

Aortic dissection is a cause of acute, excruciating pain that most commonly is seen in emergency rooms and can be confused with AMI. The pain is characteristically extremely severe and tearing, may migrate from the anterior chest to the back, and may radiate widely, including to the neck, arms, and legs, depending on its location and progression. Clinical manifestations are determined in part by the branch arteries that are occluded by the dissection and by the extent of residual lumen in the aorta. Cerebral or spinal cord neurologic complications as well as AMI can occur. Dissection should be considered in the setting of severe hypertension or Marfan syndrome. Transesophageal echocardiography or magnetic resonance imaging is usually diagnostic. Urgent referral should be made to experts in the condition.

Pericarditis is a cause of prolonged chest pain that is frequently precordial and may be sharp and stabbing. Pain may radiate to the neck, shoulders, and back. Worsening of the pain by changing position, deep breathing, or swallowing is a characteristic feature. Patients frequently find relief by leaning forward while sitting. Pericarditis has multiple etiologies, including infections (viral and bacterial), malignancies, metabolic disorders (uremia), post-AMI, and post-cardiac surgery. In the latter two instances, the pain must be distinguished from recurrent infarction. A careful history and the presence of the characteristic friction rub and electrocardiographic changes are key elements in suggesting the diagnosis. Echocardiography, magnetic resonance imaging, or computed tomography (CT) can confirm the diagnosis. Management consists of providing symptomatic relief with anti-inflammatory agents and, where appropriate, treating the underlying condition.

Mitral valve prolapse can present with chest pain, which in many cases represents palpitations from premature ventricular beats. Chest pain syndromes have been described in association with prolapsed mitral valves that are of undetermined etiology.

# CHEST PAIN CAUSED BY GASTROINTESTINAL DISORDERS

Esophageal pain is the most common gastrointestinal cause of chest pain mimicking angina pectoris.[1] Two pathologic processes are involved: spasm and gastroesophageal reflux. Esophageal spasm, which is most common from middle age onward, is the condition most commonly confused with angina pectoris. The pain is retrosternal and may go directly through to the back. It is squeezing, burning, or aching in quality and may radiate to the arm, jaw, or neck. It may be precipitated by exercise and may even be relieved by nitroglycerin. Thus, the pain of esophageal spasm sometimes may be indistinguishable from angina pectoris clinically, and this may account for the fact that the most common discharge diagnosis of patients admitted to rule out ischemic chest pain is gastrointestinal pain. Gastroesophageal reflux mimics angina pectoris less closely than does esophageal spasm but still can create a diagnostic dilemma. A history of "heart burn" can usually be elicited: a burning sensation after eating, with recumbency, and with bending over, especially after a meal. Both entities are usually diagnosed by gastrointestinal evaluation after coronary ischemia has been evaluated and ruled out. Peptic ulcer disease and biliary colic less commonly are confused with angina pectoris.

## CHEST PAIN CAUSED BY PSYCHOGENIC FACTORS

Many chest pain syndromes are caused by anxiety states, including panic attacks. The chest pains frequently are "shooting" or "stabbing" and are more likely to be near the cardiac apex rather than substernal as in angina pectoris. On the other hand, the pains may be very prolonged and not related to exertion. Patients may feel free-floating anxiety and have associated symptoms of hyperventilation, such as shortness of breath, blurred vision, and circumoral and digital paresthesias. They may have a depressive, anxious affect. It is frequently useful to determine whether forced, voluntary ventilation will reproduce the symptoms. It is often necessary to perform a noninvasive cardiac stress test to provide evidence against myocardial ischemia. Pharmacologic therapy for the underlying psychiatric disorder/psychological state frequently is helpful in managing these sometimes difficult patients.

## CHEST WALL PAIN

Patients presenting with complaints of chest pain often will be found to have discomfort in the chest wall itself. The clinician should always consider this possibility early in the visit by inquiring as to whether the area of discomfort is sore to the touch or whether it is affected by position or movement. Inquiry should be made about whether the pain began after unusual activity or injury. These pains are usually prolonged, at least for a few days, and are not episodic. During the physical examination, the patient's chest wall should be palpated, and pressure should be applied to the area in question. If pain is elicited in this manner, the clinician should ascertain that it is exactly the same pain about which the patient is concerned (it is possible to have both chest wall pain and angina). Costochondritis or Tietze's syndrome is a specific form of chest wall pain associated with inflammation of one or more of the costochondral junctions. Most of the conditions associated with local inflammation may be treated with oral anti-inflammatory/analgesic agents and reassurance. Local injection of steroids and analgesics sometimes is helpful. The persistence of a local swelling or lump should be investigated further to rule out more serious disease. The preeruptive phase of herpes zoster will occasionally cause a diagnostic challenge. Very localized pain along a specific dermatome is the key finding suggesting the diagnosis. The appearance of skin vesicles in the eruptive phase is confirmatory.

## PULMONARY/PLEURAL CAUSES OF CHEST PAIN

Large pulmonary emboli can cause acute onset of chest pain that may mimic AMI. The severe dyspnea, hypotension, arterial hypoxemia as determined by blood gases or observation, and absence of diagnostic electrocardiographic changes of ischemia will suggest the diagnosis. Additionally, a clinical setting of prior immobilization with bed rest, prolonged travel, or deep venous thrombosis should increase suspicion of pulmonary embolus. The occurrence of pulmonary infarction after a pulmonary embolus of any size can cause a local pleuritic response associated with chest pain (pleurisy) that is accentuated by inspiration and usually is associated with a pleural rub heard over the painful area upon auscultation. Pneumonia or malignancy involving the pleural surfaces can also cause pleurisy. Pneumothorax can also cause acute chest pain and is associated with dyspnea, decreased breath sounds, and hyperresonance on the affected side.

## REFERENCES

1.  O'Rourke RA, Shaver JA, Salerni R, et al: The history, physical examination, and cardiac auscultation. In: Alexander RW, Schlant RC, Fuster V, et al, (eds): *Hurst's The Heart,* 9th ed. New York, McGraw-Hill, 1998; 229–342.
2.  Heberden W: Some accounts of a disorder of the breast. *Med Trans* 1772; 2:59.
3.  Malliani AM: The elusive link between transient myocardial ischemia and pain. *Circulation* 1986; 73:201–204.
4.  Christie LG Jr, Conti CR: Systemic approach to evaluation of angina-like chest pain: pathophysiology and clinical testing with emphasis on objective documentation of myocardial ischemia. *Am Heart J* 1981; 102:897–912.
5.  Epstein SE, Talbot TL: Dynamic coronary tone in precipitation, exacerbation and relief of angina pectoris. *Am J Cardiol* 1981; 48:797–803.
6.  Campeau L: Letter to the editor. *Circulation* 1976; 54:522.
7.  Theroux P, Waters D: Diagnosis and management of patients with unstable angina. In: Alexander RW, Schlant RC, Fuster V, et al (eds): *Hurst's The Heart,* 9th ed. New York, McGraw-Hill, 1998; 1307.
8.  Braunwald E: Unstable angina: A classification. *Circulation* 1989; 80:410.
9.  O'Rourke RA: Diagnostic approach to the patient with chest pain compatible with definite or suspected angina pectoris. In: Sobel BE (ed): *Medical Management of Heart Disease.* New York, Marcel Dekker, 1996; 4–22.

R. WAYNE ALEXANDER

# DYSPNEA AND FATIGUE

Dyspnea and fatigue are the most common symptoms of a number of cardiovascular diseases that are associated with abnormal ventricular function and/or decreased oxygen delivery to the periphery. Fatigue is the most common symptom limiting exercise in congestive heart failure (CHF), whereas normal persons and, for example, patients with mitral stenosis appear to be limited equally by dyspnea and fatigue.

## FATIGUE

The term *fatigue* as commonly used is rather nonspecific. Patients may use this term to refer to the malaise associated with, for example, the systemic symptoms of an infection. Fatigue has also been used to describe the premonitory symptoms of malaise or exhaustion that can be precursors of myocardial infarction or sudden death.[1] In a prospective study of risk factors for myocardial infarction (MI), exhaustion, over the relatively short term, was a less powerful predictor than age, smoking, or cholesterol but was more powerful than hypertension.[2] The data do not lend themselves to mechanistic interpretation but do confirm the importance of the symptom of fatigue as a risk factor for MI that should be evaluated during routine history taking. It is possible that the general malaise that may be an antecedent to MI may reflect the inflammatory nature of atherosclerosis in its active stages and thus might be analogous to the systemic symptoms seen in other inflammatory diseases.

Fatigue is also used to describe the feeling of tiredness or weakness in skeletal muscle that may limit exercise in normal people as well as in those with disease. In cardiovascular disease, the symptom refers to relatively premature exercise-limiting muscle weakness. Unusual fatigue at low levels of exertion is characteristic of any cardiac disease with decreased myocardial reserve and limited capability to increase cardiac output appropriately. In the particular case of CHF, hypoperfusion of large muscle groups during exercise has been demonstrated and would presumably result in the early onset of anaerobic metabolism.[3] It is likely that the biochemical consequences of these metabolic changes are associated with the development of neural signals that are interpreted by the patient as fatigue.

Fatigue is among the most nonspecific of symptoms. It can be a manifestation of any acute or chronic infection or of other inflammatory diseases, such as collagen vascular disease, or "active" atherosclerotic disease, such as unstable angina. Other conditions as diverse as depression, insomnia and sleep deprivation, obesity, and physical deconditioning can be associated with complaints of fatigue. The most important lesson for the clinician to remember is that complaints of fatigue of recent onset can represent serious and sometimes life-threatening illness and should not be ignored or minimized.

# DYSPNEA

Dyspnea or a feeling of breathlessness occurs when there is higher demand for ventilation than can be met by comfortable breathing. It is frequently described as air hunger or as having to breathe too much or not being able to breathe enough. Everyone, during vigorous exercise, has experienced the sensation, which is unpleasant but not painful in the usual sense.

It has frequently been assumed that dyspnea refers to a single sensation or symptom. It has become clear, however, that "dyspnea" is used to denote a number of sensations that patients may describe as shortness of breath or breathlessness. In normal subjects, dyspnea represents a number of different stimuli and is not explainable by a single physiologic mechanism.

Studies of the sensations associated with breathlessness in patients with a spectrum of diseases causing dyspnea, including CHF, chronic obstructive pulmonary disease, asthma, pulmonary hypertension, chest wall and neuromuscular disease, interstitial lung disease, and pregnancy, indicate that there are different types of dyspnea in patients with a variety of cardiorespiratory abnormalities and suggest that the symptoms may be mediated by several mechanisms.[4]

## Clinical Manifestations of Dyspnea

Dyspnea occurring during the usual activities of daily life is one of the most common manifestations of cardiac or pulmonary disease. The appreciation of breathlessness is usually dependent on the level of activity involved in a given patient's lifestyle.[5] Sedentary patients may reach an advanced state of cardiorespiratory compromise before experiencing dyspnea. On the other hand, an athlete may experience unusual dyspnea with mild dysfunction. Distinguishing cardiac causes of dyspnea—most commonly congestive heart failure—from pulmonary causes, in fact, can sometimes be a major clinical problem. The differential diagnoses for the causes of acute and chronic dyspnea are shown in Tables 3-1 and 3-2.[5]

## Approach to the Evaluation of Chronic Dyspnea

**HISTORY.**   A detailed history is essential in assessing chronic dyspnea and in attempting to distinguish among potential cardiac or pulmonic causes or to determine

TABLE 3-1.   Differential Diagnosis of Acute Dyspnea

| |
|---|
| Anxiety/hyperventilation |
| Asthma |
| Chest trauma<br>    Pneumothorax<br>    Fractured ribs<br>    Pulmonary contusion |
| Pulmonary edema |
| Pulmonary embolism |
| Spontaneous pneumothorax |

*Source:* From Mahler DA: Dyspnea: diagnosis and management. *Clin Chest Med* 1987; 8:215–230. Reprinted with permission of publisher and author.

that the etiology is marked deconditioning or even psychogenic. In many ways the approach is similar to that for evaluating chest pain. The frequency, duration, severity, precipitating events, and exercise threshold should be determined. Whether or not the dyspnea is associated with chest pain, exertion, wheezing, cough, anxiety, or sputum production should be established.

**PHYSICAL EXAMINATION.**   A detailed physical examination should be performed to assess the cardiovascular and respiratory systems, as outlined by Hurst and Branch.[6]

**LABORATORY EVALUATION.**   Laboratory evaluation of chronic dyspnea should be guided by the history and physical examination. A chest x-ray is indicated in most patients and will provide information on heart size, specific chamber enlargement, pulmonary vascularity, and the presence of pulmonary edema, pleural effusion, pneumothorax, chest wall abnormalities, or evidence of pulmonary parenchymal disease. Distinguishing among various potential causes of dyspnea may require pulmonary function measurements and/or exercise testing. The pathophysiology of various disorders causing dyspnea and tests designed to identify them are summarized in Table 3-3.

# DYSPNEA IN CHRONIC CONGESTIVE HEART FAILURE

Although fatigue is the most common symptom in CHF, dyspnea occurs during daily living. Dyspnea may occur with both isotonic and isometric exercise, and extensive aerobic exercise is not necessary for it to be induced. The traditional view has been that increased pulmonary capillary wedge pressure is an important

## TABLE 3-2. Differential Diagnosis of Chronic Dyspnea

Cardiovascular
  Decreased cardiac output
    Cardiomyopathy
      Dilated
      Hypertrophic
      Infiltrative
      Ischemic
      Valvular disease
      Pericardial disease
      Congenital disease

  Increased pulmonary venous pressure
    Diastolic dysfunction
      Hypertrophic disease
      Ischemia
    Mitral stenosis
    Pulmonary venous occlusive disease
    Right-to-left shunt

Respiratory
  Airway disease
   Upper airway obstruction
   Asthma
   Chronic bronchitis
   Emphysema
   Cystic fibrosis
  Parenchymal lung disease
   Interstitial lung disease
   Malignancy—primary or metastatic
   Pneumonia
  Pulmonary vascular disease
   Arteriovenous malformations
   Intravascular obstruction
   Vasculitis
   Venous occlusive disease
  Pleural disease
   Effusion
   Fibrosis
   Malignancy
  Chest wall disease
   Deformities (e.g., kyphoscoliosis)
   Abdominal "loading" (e.g., ascites, pregnancy, obesity)
  Respiratory muscle disease
   Neuromuscular disorders (e.g., myasthenia gravis, polio)
   Phrenic nerve dysfunction
   Weakness
Anemia

Anxiety/psychological

Deconditioning

*Source:* Modified from Mahler DA: Dyspnea: diagnosis and management. *Clin Chest Med* 1987; 8:215–230. Reprinted with permission of publisher and author.

**TABLE 3-3.  Causes of Dyspnea, Pathophysiology, and Discriminating Clinical Measurements**

| Disorder | Pathophysiology | Discriminating Measurements |
|---|---|---|
| Anemia | $O_2$ carrying capacity | HB, $\downarrow V_{O2max}$; $\downarrow$ AT |
| Cardiac | | |
|    Coronary artery | Ischemia | ECG changes; BP changes: $\downarrow V_{O2max}$; |
|    Valvular | Limited cardiac output | $\downarrow$ AT; $\downarrow O_2$-pulse |
|    Myopathy | Limited cardiac output | |
| Deconditioning | Detraining | $\downarrow V_{O2max}$; $\downarrow$ AT; $\downarrow O_2$-pulse |
| Malingering | Hyper- and hypoventilation | Breathing pattern; $P_{aCO_2}$ |
| Obesity | $\uparrow$ work to move body weight; if severe, respiratory restriction | $\uparrow V_{O_2}$—work relationship; $\downarrow V_{O2max}$ |
| Pulmonary | | |
|    Airway obstruction | Diminished ventilatory capacity $\dot{V}/\dot{Q}$ mismatching | $\uparrow V_{Emax}$/MVV; expiratory flow limitation |
|    Interstitial disease | $\dot{V}/\dot{Q}$ mismatching | $\uparrow V_D/V_T$; $O_2$ desaturation; $\downarrow V_{O2max}$ |
| | Diffusion impairment during exercise | $\uparrow O_2$ desaturation during exercise; $\downarrow V_T$ and respiratory frequency; $\downarrow V_{O2max}$ |
| Pulmonary vascular | Physiological $V_D$ | $\uparrow V_D/V_T$; $\uparrow O_2$ desaturation during exercise<br>$\uparrow V_E/V_{O_2}$; $\downarrow V_{O2max}$ |
| Psychogenic | Hyperventilation with regular respiratory rate | Breathing pattern; $\downarrow Pa_{CO_2}$ |

*Note:* Hb = hemoglobin value; $V_{0_{2max}}$ = maximal oxygen consumption; AT = anaerobic threshold; ECG = electrocardiogram; BP = blood pressure; $Pa_{CO_2}$ = arterial carbon dioxide tension; $V_{Emax}$ = maximal exercise ventilation; MVV = maximal voluntary ventilation; $V_D$ = dead space volume; $V_T$ = tidal volume; $\dot{V}_E$ = ventilation.

*Source:* Adapted from Wasserman K, Whipp BJ: Exercise physiology in health and disease. *Am Rev Respir Dis* 1975; 112:219–249, with permission.

contributor to dyspnea in CHF. While this is probably true to some significant extent in acute pulmonary edema, recent work has failed to substantiate this view in the case of chronic ambulatory heart failure.[7,8] In fact, poor correlation exists between pulmonary capillary wedge pressure and the feeling of dyspnea (Fig. 3-1[9]). Similarly, there is no evidence of sufficient changes in arterial blood gases during exercise in patients with heart failure to account for dyspnea by stimulation of arterial chemoreceptors.[7] Recent evidence suggests that ventilatory abnormalities may be centrally important in contributing to ventilatory drive in chronic CHF.[7] Although ventilatory control mechanisms regulated by, for example, $CO_2$ are normal in patients with CHF, there are demonstrable abnormalities in pulmonary mechanics. The feeling of dyspnea likely results from neural impulses generated in atrophic, underperfused, and metabolically abnormal respiratory muscles.

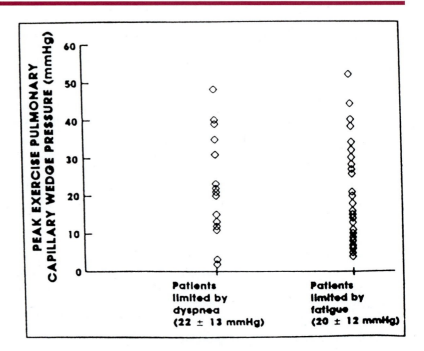

Figure 3-1   Peak exercise pulmonary capillary wedge pressure in patients limited to dyspnea versus those limited by fatigue. (From Sullivan MJ: Exertional dyspnea and ventilatory control mechanisms in chronic heart failure. *Heart Failure* 1992; 8:190–201. Reprinted with permission of publisher, editor, and author.)

## Special Types of Dyspnea in Congestive Heart Failure

**ORTHOPNEA.**   This term refers to the dyspnea that occurs in the supine but not in the upright position. It is characteristic of heart failure, although it may occur in patients with lung disease or with weakness or paralysis of the diaphragm. In heart failure, it is thought to result from the shift of blood volume from the periphery to the pulmonary circulation. Since pulmonary venous pressures are already elevated, mild pulmonary edema may develop, and pulmonary mechanoreceptors are thought to be stimulated.

**PAROXYSMAL NOCTURNAL DYSPNEA.**   In a patient with CHF, this symptom complex manifests as a sudden awakening from sleep with marked dyspnea that may take 5 to 15 min to clear after the patient assumes the upright posture. The mechanisms are thought to be similar to those for orthopnea. Paroxysmal nocturnal dyspnea, like orthopnea, can occur in heart diseases of diverse etiologies ranging from dilated cardiomyopathy to valvular and coronary artery disease.

# DYSPNEA IN OTHER CARDIOVASCULAR DISEASES

The mechanism of dyspnea in cardiovascular diseases other than CHF has not been studied extensively. It is likely that the mechanisms defined for chronic congestive heart failure also apply to the conditions listed in Table 3-2 that are characterized by limited ability to increase cardiac output in response to exercise.

## REFERENCES

1. Alonzo AA, Simon AB, Feinleib M: Prodromata of myocardial infarction and sudden death. *Circulation* 1975; 52:1056–1062.
2. Appels A, Mulder P: Excess fatigue as a precursor of myocardial infarction. *Eur Heart J* 1988; 9:758–764.
3. Sullivan MJ, Knight JD, Higgenbotham MB, Cobb FR: Relation between central and peripheral hemodynamics during exercise in patients with chronic heart failure. *Circulation* 1989; 80:769–781.
4. Simon PM, Schwartzstein RM, Weiss JW, et al: Distinguishable types of dyspnea in patients with shortness of breath. *Am Rev Respir Dis* 1990; 142:1009–1014.
5. Mahler DA: Dyspnea: diagnosis and management. *Clin Chest Med* 1987; 8:215–230.
6. Hurst JW, Branch WT Jr: Physical examination of the heart, arteries, and jugular veins. In: Branch WT Jr, Alexander RW, Schlant RC, Hurst JW (eds): *Cardiology in Primary Care.* New York, McGraw-Hill, 2000.
7. Sullivan M, Higginbotham M, Cobb F: Increased exercise ventilation in patients with chronic heart failure: intact ventilatory control despite hemodynamic and pulmonary abnormalities. *Circulation* 1988; 77:552–559.
8. Fink L, Wilson JR, Ferraro N: Exercise ventilation and pulmonary artery wedge pressure in chronic stable congestive heart failure. *Am J Cardiol* 1986; 57:249–253.
9. Sullivan MJ: Exertional dyspnea and ventilatory control mechanisms in chronic heart failure. *Heart Failure* 1992; 8:190–201.

WILLIAM T. BRANCH, JR.

# SYNCOPE

**CHAPTER**

**4**

## CAUSES OF SYNCOPE

A number of prospective and retrospective studies suggest that the most common cause of syncope is neurally mediated or vasovagal syncope (Table 4-1).[1-3] Up to 40 percent of patients with syncope appear to have this etiology. Of the remaining patients, about 10 percent have cardiac and neurologic causes of syncope. Syncope of unknown cause may range from 13 to 41 percent of cases. The wide variation in the proportion of reported cases of syncope of unknown cause and of neurally mediated syncope reflects the selection of patients to be included in various series and varying definitions of neurally mediated or vasovagal syncope.

Currently the term *neurally mediated syncope* is preferred for syncope induced by a reflex resulting in withdrawing of sympathetic tone and vagal predominance. A variety of terms have been used to describe this entity, including not only *vasovagal syncope* but also *neurocardiogenic syncope, vasodepressor syncope, cardioinhibitory syncope,* and *benign situational syncope.*[4] Some additional categories of neurally induced syncope also include cough syncope, micturition syncope, and carotid sinus syncope. In these latter cases, a specific maneuver induces inappropriate vasodilatation, generally leading to brief loss of consciousness. Pregnancy in the third trimester also predisposes to syncope (presumably by aortocaval compression from an enlarged uterus), that may be considered benign if there is no evidence of heart disease, dysrhythmias, pulmonary embolism or other serious causes.[3] The more general form of neurally mediated or vasovagal syncope probably results when pooling of blood in the venous system of the lower extremities causes a sympathetic response, with tachycardia and forceful left ventricular contraction. Mechanoreceptors in the wall of the left ventricle and possibly the atria and pulmonary vasculature are stimulated, producing a reflex-induced withdrawal of sympathetic tone and increased vagal tone, causing hypotension and bradycardia. If sufficiently severe, the bradycardia and/or hypotension produce syncope. This sequence explains the clinical features of vasovagal syncope, which include premonitory symptoms of weakness, tachycardia, diaphoresis, and nausea. Recovery follows restitution of blood

TABLE 4-1.   Summary of the Causes of Syncope[1-3]

| Cause | Approximate Percent | |
| --- | --- | --- |
| | Mean | (Range) |
| Neurally mediated (vasovagal) | 18 | 8–37 |
| Cardiac syncope<br>    Structural abnormalities<br>    Dysrhythmias | 14 | 4–38 |
| Neurologic syncope<br>    Seizures<br>    Transient ischemia, stroke, brain tumor, migraines | 10 | 3–32 |
| Orthostatic hypotension | 8 | 4–10 |
| Medications | 3 | 2–4 |
| Psychogenic<br>    Panic attack<br>    Major depression<br>    Somatization disorder<br>    Generalized anxiety disorder | 2 | 1–7 |
| Neurally induced<br>    Carotid sinus sensitivity<br>    Micturition syncope<br>    Cough syncope<br>    Defecation<br>    Swallow | 5 | 1–8 |
| Syncope of unknown cause | 34 | 13–41 |

pressure and heart rate of the unconscious or semiconscious patient in the recumbent position. Though it is now thought that all of the terms listed above refer to syncope by a single mechanism, some authors use the term *vasovagal syncope* for patients whose loss of consciousness is apparently related to an event, such as receiving bad news. *Benign situational syncope* may likewise refer to that in healthy young people who are exposed to certain events or settings that induce the neurally mediated reflex. The term *neurocardiogenic syncope* has been employed by some authors to refer to more unpredictable episodes in somewhat older patients that may more often be associated with injury or accident.

Table 4-1 also shows a limited number of other causes of syncope that are commonly encountered. These include orthostasis due to volume depletion, adrenal insufficiency, autonomic neuropathy, and other causes, as well as syncope as a side effect of medication. Psychogenic syncope is associated with panic attacks, depression, somatization, and anxiety disorders. The category of cardiac syncope includes a variety of dysrhythmias, plus structural heart diseases associated with syncope. The category of neurogenic syncope includes seizures as well as transient neurologic events associated with altered consciousness. Overall, syncope and presyncope probably account for 1 to 2 percent of patients seen in a general medical practice or an emergency room. Presyncope, defined as near loss of consciousness, occurs more often than syncope, defined as transient loss of consciousness with loss of postural tone and full recovery after a brief time. In fact, syncope and presyncope are highly prevalent in the population. Informal estimates suggest that up to half of all individuals have experienced these symptoms at some time or another, but the majority recognize the spell as situational or benign and do not consult their physician.

## DIFFERENTIAL DIAGNOSIS

The practitioner's approach to the patient with syncope or presyncope follows a sequence of several steps. First, syncope must be separated from other categories of symptoms causing dizziness or altered consciousness. In contrast to syncope, defined above, *coma* consists of a prolonged period of unconsciousness, such as that seen with profound hypoglycemia or hepatic insufficiency. *Confusional state* consists of confusion, disorientation, and sometimes agitation, without loss of consciousness. *Vertigo* consists of an illusory sense of motion, which can be a spinning or tilting sensation, with a clear sensorium and no loss of consciousness. *Dizziness* includes several categories of symptoms described by patients. The most common is disequilibrium, which means unsteadiness of gait generally caused by peripheral neuropathy, parkinsonism, or other gait disorders; whereas "giddiness" or "light-headedness" is sometimes difficult to distinguish from presyncope, but generally refers to patients who experience a vague instability or "giddy" feeling induced by anxiety and/or hyperventilation. History taking generally separates these categories of symptoms from syncope and presyncope, but several maneuvers that can be performed in the office may be helpful. Transient vertigo and nystagmus may be reproduced by movement of the head, including the Barany maneuver (Chap. 5). The physician may instruct patients with vague waxing and waning "giddiness" to hyperventilate purposefully; this may reproduce their symptom exactly, thereby establishing its cause. The careful separation of these categories of symptoms is essential in order to direct the physician's evaluation appropriately.

Once syncope or presyncope has been recognized, it seems logical that the next step in evaluation involves separating benign neurally mediated syncope from other causes. In primary care practice, it is expected that a large number of patients will have benign situational syncope of the neurally mediated type, which may require little workup in addition to the history and physical examination. The physician may form the hypothesis that the patient has benign neurally mediated syncope from the detailed description of the event. Table 4-2 contrasts the clinical features of benign syncope with those of cardiac syncope and seizures. Data collected from patients with these disorders suggest that features implying neurally mediated syncope include some combination of the following: (1) an event or setting that typically induces syncope (bad news, painful stimulus, prolonged standing); (2) premonitory

TABLE 4-2.   Clinical Features of Common Causes of Loss of Consciousness

|  | Neurally Induced | Dysrhythmia | Seizure |
| --- | --- | --- | --- |
| Precipitant | Prolonged standing<br>Pain<br>Psychological shock | Generally none | Flashing lights<br>Repetitive sounds |
| Premonitory symptoms | Sweatiness<br>Weakness<br>Nausea<br>Palpitations | Generally none<br>Abrupt onset<br>Palpitations | None or déjà vu,<br>numbness, or<br>other aura |
| Appearance and findings | Pale<br>Weak pulse | Tachycardia or<br>bradycardia | "Blue"<br>Bounding pulse |
| Recovery period | Weakness on<br>standing | May be normal | Postictal confusion |

symptoms, including awareness of heartbeat, weakness, sweatiness, and nausea, lasting up to several minutes; and (3) rapid recovery of clear sensorium once recumbent but persistent weakness on attempting to arise shortly after the event.[5] Cardiac syncope, in contrast, often occurs abruptly with no warning, and the patient may recover rapidly.[5] Exceptions include some cases due to angina equivalent or aortic stenosis when diaphoresis, weakness, and sometimes dyspnea precede the event, and some cases of ventricular fibrillation or prolonged asystole in which seizure-like activity and some postevent confusion prolong the recovery period.

Seizures generally occur abruptly or are preceded by a specific aura, such as déjà vu, or visual, sensory, or motor phenomena. Seizures are followed by prolonged postictal confusion. Syncope, even when there are convulsive movements, produces little or no postictal confusion. Akinetic spells and drop attacks that produce brief alterations of consciousness and little or no confusion may also rarely occur. Difficulty distinguishing seizure from syncope may arise when syncopal patients are incontinent of urine—as they may be with a full bladder—or have hypoxic convulsive movements. Such movements typically consist of opisthotonos and short, jerky arm movements, whereas the convulsive movements of a seizure generally follow a sequence of increasing and decreasing amplitude. Syncopal patients are "never" incontinent of feces.

Transient ischemic attacks due to interruption of blood flow in a cerebral vessel cause neurologic symptoms such as transient monocular blindness or weakness or numbness on one side, rather than global loss of consciousness. When the posterior cerebral circulation is interrupted, loss of consciousness or drop attacks may occur, but most are preceded or followed by other neurologic symptoms, such as vertigo, dysarthria, visual loss, bilateral weakness or numbness, and/or memory loss and confusion.

Patients with benign neurally mediated syncope have an excellent prognosis, whereas those with cardiac or neurologically induced syncope experience a much higher than expected death rate.[6] Hence, it is important to separate these causes of syncope.[7] Those suspected of cardiac and/or neurologically induced syncope require more extensive evaluation and possibly treatment. In addition to the clinical features outlined in Table 4-2, cardiac syncope is more likely in persons over the age of 50 years, and much more likely in those with known underlying heart disease. Likewise, altered consciousness due to transient ischemic attack of the posterior cerebral circulation will generally occur in patients with risk factors for stroke, including hypertension, cigarette smoking, and advanced age.

Some relatively rare causes of syncope will be missed if they are not suggested by the patient's history and physical examination. These include many of the structural heart diseases. Valvular aortic stenosis and hypertrophic cardiomyopathy with or without dynamic stenosis as well as other valvular and structural diseases of the heart are detected on cardiac examination by finding a murmur or other characteristic features. Postural hypotension should be sought routinely by comparing the patient's pulse rate and blood pressure supine and on standing. Some experts recommend testing for carotid sinus sensitivity in all patients over 60 years of age with syncope of unknown cause, but this recommendation needs to be tempered by the awareness of false-positive responses in many elderly patients and potential hazards in patients with bruits. Pulmonary embolism is a rare cause of syncope. Generally, massive pulmonary embolism produces syncope by significant obstruction of right ventricular outflow. Thus, any feature of massive pulmonary embolism should be sought. These include tachycardia, tachypnea, hypotension, right ventricular strain on electrocardiogram, history of predisposing factors, and/or any sign of phlebitis. Interestingly, some patients with syncope due to massive pulmonary embolism experienced diaphoresis prior to the syncope and were attempting to move their bowels or otherwise performing Valsalva maneuvers. This probably reflects a drop in left ventricular filling pressure exacerbated by the maneuver in a patient already compromised. Further unusual causes of syncope such as subclavian steal syndrome or aortic dissection may be detected by finding a bruit or other clinical features. Features of panic attack, depression, anxiety, or somatization disorder may point toward psychogenically induced syncope.

A further subcategory of syncope appears in the very elderly, patients in their late seventies, eighties, and nineties.[8] The very elderly patient may have one recognizable cause, but often has a combination of factors inducing syncope, which may include polypharmacy, sluggish baroreceptor responses to postural changes and other stresses, hypovolemia, mild aortic stenosis, and transient arrhythmias. In many very elderly persons, the proper approach is to identify all contributing causes and eliminate those that are reversible. An interesting subcategory of elderly patients includes those in nursing homes who commonly faint after breakfast. These patients have sluggish baroreceptor responses to the tendency of blood pressure to fall after a meal. The condition can be rectified in some cases by having the patient drink coffee with breakfast, which apparently stimulates the baroreceptor or other vasoconstrictor mechanisms.

Evaluation of syncope is further complicated by the need to separate benign neurally mediated syncope from neurally mediated syncope that endangers or impairs the patient. The mechanism may be the same in both groups of patients, but the latter may experience recurrent episodes, sometimes with no apparent precipitating event or with little or no warning, which are more likely to cause injury or accident. These latter patients may have a relatively abrupt fall in blood pressure (vasodepressor spell) or may experience profound slowing of the heart or transient asystole (cardioinhibitory spell). Such patients now are generally identified by tilt table testing. In the past, many of these patients were probably classified as having sick sinus syndrome, which might produce similar findings on electrocardiographic monitoring. An additional subcategory of neurally mediated syncope includes patients with dysautonomia. These are generally elderly patients with autonomic neuropathy. Unlike patients with neurally mediated syncope, these patients experience a slow fall in blood pressure when tilted upright that culminates in loss of consciousness.

Figure 4-1 illustrates the initial approach to the patient with syncope. The first step involves determining that the symptom truly represents a transient loss of consciousness. The second step involves meticulous history and physical examination to identify patients with structural abnormalities and other specific causes of syncope or presyncope, which can be confirmed by directed testing. The third step is required with those patients whose history and physical examination are unrevealing at the time they are seen. These are the majority. This step separates patients with benign neurally mediated and other recognizable forms of benign syncope, who require little or no further evaluation, from patients who require more extensive evaluation or follow-up because they are suspected of having cardiac syncope, neurologically induced syncope, or neurally mediated syncope causing disability or injury, especially if recurrent. Most effort in evaluating patients with syncope is directed at this third step. About 50 percent of patients with syncope can be diagnosed by history, physical examination, and surface electrocardiogram as having either a benign form of syncope or a suspected specific cause that can be confirmed by directed testing.[3] The remaining patients include those with possible cardiac, seizure-induced, unrecognized neurally mediated, psychiatric, and unknown syncope, who may require additional testing.[3]

## EVALUATION

### General Tests

An electrocardiogram (ECG) is indicated in most patients with syncope. A diagnosis obtained from a positive ECG has been reported in only 3 to 4 percent of patients, but this small yield would seem worthwhile.[5] In addition to major dysrhythmias, if the ECG reveals multiple ventricular or atrial ectopic activity, marked first-degree heart block, and/or bifascicular block, further testing might be considered. Ambulatory (Holter) monitoring or an event recorder could also be considered. Suspicion of a cardiac etiology of the symptoms should also be considered if the ECG shows evidence of left ventricular hypertrophy. No other general tests have been shown to be useful in patients with syncope, but should the patient have symptoms or the appearance of anemia or have postural hypotension, a hematocrit

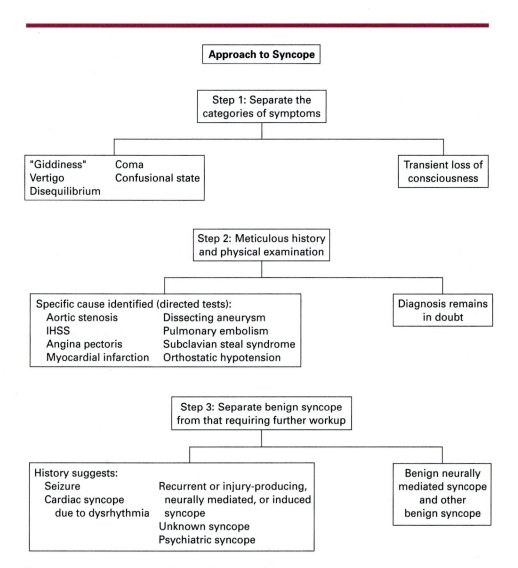

Figure 4-1   Summary of the steps in the clinical evaluation of patients suspected of syncope or presyncope.

should be obtained. If there are features of encephalopathy, confusional state, or altered mental status, then blood sugar, electrolytes, and kidney and liver function tests are indicated.

## Directed Tests

Certain tests should be performed when specific clinical features are present in patients with syncope. *Echocardiography* should be performed when a murmur, enlarged heart, or other findings suggesting organic heart disease are present or when the history suggests the presence of heart disease. *Exercise testing* with or without nuclear imaging should be performed when the history and other findings suggest the possibility of ischemic heart disease. The Persantine thallium test or dobutamine stress echocardiography might be indicated for individuals with syncope suspected of having ischemic heart disease who cannot exercise on a treadmill. Studies suggest that brain imaging with computed tomography (CT) or magnetic resonance imaging (MRI) scanning or neurovascular studies with carotid or transcranial Doppler ultrasonography are not indicated in patients with syncope unless there are features suggesting a neurologic etiology. Likewise, electroencephalography (EEG) is indicated in individuals who have a history suggesting seizure disorder. Clinical features that indicate a need to perform MRI or CT scanning, Doppler ultrasonography, and/or EEG include altered mental status, abnormal findings on neurologic examination, evidence of cerebrovascular disease, or features on history taking suggesting a seizure or transient neurologic event. Lung scanning is indicated when there are clinical features of pulmonary embolism.

## Additional Evaluation

**ELECTROPHYSIOLOGIC TESTING.**    Electrophysiologic testing is an invasive procedure, performed on an inpatient or outpatient basis, consisting of a series of studies obtained by right heart catheterization. Studies include atrial and ventricular pacing to induce tachyarrhythmias, measuring the sinus node recovery time, testing the refractoriness of the atrioventricular node, and measuring the A–H and H–V intervals. These studies are designed to detect a propensity for heart block, sick sinus syndrome, or atrial and/or ventricular arrhythmias. Electrophysiologic testing is indicated when syncope is strongly suspected of being caused by cardiac dysrhythmia. The indication is generally a patient with syncope who has known or suspected serious underlying heart disease.[9,10] Commonly, these are patients with syncope and known congestive heart failure (CHF) or ischemic heart disease, whose syncope does not occur in the setting of an acute myocardial infarction (AMI) or ischemic event but is suspected of being caused by a transient dysrhythmia. Electrophysiologic testing is performed less often in patients with syncope and structurally normal hearts, but such individuals would be candidates for testing should multiple syncopal episodes or unexplained syncope that places the patient at significant risk for injury or accident have features of cardiac syncope (abrupt onset, cluster of spells, evidence of conduction disease on electrocardiography, evidence of cardiac arrest). For individuals with features of cardiac syncope whose occupations place them or others at risk, such as airline pilots or heavy machinery operators, the threshold for recommending electrophysiologic testing may be diminished.

Published results of electrophysiologic testing reflect the highly selective nature of the study population. Over half of patients tested had a dysrhythmia documented.[2] In a "normal" control population, the comparable rate of significant dysrhythmias on electrophysiologic testing is 1 to 2 percent. The number of false-positive tests, however, depends somewhat on the protocol of the investigators. For example, more aggressive ventricular stimulation produces more false-positive runs of ventricular tachycardia, but also enhances the sensitivity of the test for detecting true positives. In general, the reported results include approximately equal numbers of ventricular tachycardias, bradyarrhythmias, and atrial tachyarrhythmias. In some reports concentrating on patients with ischemic heart disease, the predominant dysrhythmia has been ventricular tachycardia.

**TILT TABLE TESTING.**  Tilt table testing performed by a cardiologist is indicated for recurrent syncope suspected of being neurally mediated.[4,11] Performed on an outpatient basis, the tilt table test consists of having the patient lie with feet on a footboard, followed by tilting to about 60 degrees for a variable time, generally 45 min.[12] A positive test consists of a significant decrease in blood pressure and/or pulse rate, reproducing symptoms identical to those that the patient has previously experienced. If the test is not positive, it may be repeated with isoproterenol infusion.[13] The isoproterenol infusion presumably reproduces the forceful ventricular contractions that are thought to stimulate mechanoreceptors, and thus induce reflexes causing syncope. Generally, 30 to 40 percent of patients who are thought to have neurally mediated syncope have a true positive test without isoproterenol, and up to 80 percent if isoproterenol is added. The rate of false-positive tests in normal individuals who have never experienced neurally mediated syncope averages 15 to 20 percent in most literature, but increases with longer durations of tilting and higher doses of isoproterenol and has been reported to be as high as 40 percent in one study.[14] Young, healthy individuals with presumably active reflexes appear to have more false-positive tests than the somewhat older population that may be subject to evaluation for syncope. In elderly patients, tilt table testing sometimes promotes a gradual decline in blood pressure, culminating in symptoms attributable to dysautonomia. Treatment for this response is different, so it should be distinguished from the usual positive response.

Tilt table testing is indicated specifically for patients with recurrent syncope suspected of being neurally mediated, as opposed to cardiac, that is causing sufficient disability to warrant evaluation and treatment. The test is usually indicated for recurring spells, but may be indicated after a single episode of syncope suspected to be neurally mediated when the individual has an occupation that places him or her or others at risk should syncope recur, or if accident or injury has occurred or is likely. Tilt testing may also be indicated as part of an evaluation when two or more causes are suspected, one of which is neurally mediated syncope. The test is not indicated after isolated, benign episodes of vasovagal syncope that have not endangered the patient, nor is it indicated as an ancillary test when syncope can be attributed solely to another cause. The test is relatively contraindicated in patients with significant left ventricular outflow obstruction and/or unstable ischemic heart disease.[4] Some authorities suggest pregnancy testing in women of childbearing age, and exercise stress testing in men and women older than 45 years and 55 years, respectively, be performed prior to tilt testing.[12]

Tilt testing has elucidated the etiology of syncope in a number of patients in whom it previously would have been called unknown. Variations of clinical presentations of neurally mediated syncope have been documented. Some patients have profound bradycardia and/or transient asystole. Others have a profound drop in blood pressure, or both bradycardia and hypotension. There appears to be no difference in response to therapy depending on whether the predominant mechanism is bradycardia or hypotension. Some individuals with transient asystole reproducible by tilt table testing might in the past have been thought to have sick sinus syndrome. Some of these patients have relatively abrupt onset of syncope. In these cases, the clinical features also are similar to carotid sinus hypersensitivity, though initiated by a different sequence of events. Individuals with fully developed seizures, apparently caused by hypoxia due to hypotension, have also been identified as having neurally mediated syncope on tilt table testing. Some of these patients have been treated with various antiseizure medications without benefit, but cease to have spells once treated for neurally mediated syncope. Tilt table testing may also be helpful in assessing treatment of neurally mediated syncope, as discussed further on.

**PROLONGED MONITORING.**   Formerly, *24-h Holter monitoring* was the standard test for patients suspected of cardiac syncope. Nowadays, electrophysiologic testing would be performed promptly in patients with suspected cardiac syncope and known heart disease. The role of 24-h Holter monitoring is less clear. The test is less invasive than electrophysiologic testing and may be indicated in some patients as a follow-up test for unknown syncope where the suspicion of cardiac syncope is too low to indicate electrophysiologic testing and the clinical features do not suggest neurally mediated syncope. It is well known, however, that the 24-h Holter monitor has numerous false-positive and false-negative findings. The overall true positive rate of three 24-h monitors in patients suspected of cardiac syncope averages about 15 percent, in the majority of which patients experienced spells recorded in their diaries while remaining in normal sinus rhythm, thus positively ruling out a cardiac arrhythmia as the cause of the symptoms. A minority had significant dysrhythmia while experiencing symptoms, thus documenting a cardiac cause. In elderly patients, nonsustained ventricular tachycardia, brief runs of supraventricular tachycardia or atrial fibrillation, and multiple ventricular or atrial ectopic activity are quite common in the absence of symptoms. Thus, it is difficult to determine if these findings are important in a patient with syncope when the patient experiences no symptoms while being monitored. Some dysrhythmias are sufficiently unusual to be considered important or virtually diagnostic if detected on monitoring (or on the standard ECG), even in the absence of symptoms. These include Mobitz type 2 and complete heart block, sustained vertricular tachycardia, and torsades de pointes.

The *event recorder* represents an advance in the ability to detect cardiac syncope. These recorders are worn by the patient. Some may be triggered by the patient, whereas others require recording via telephone. Because they do not record the heart rate over long periods of time, but record it only during the brief time that symptoms occur, they are cheaper to interpret, and may be worn over a longer period of time by the patient. If triggered, the memory loop in the recorder is activated usually for 2 to 5 min pre- and 60 s postsymptoms. This should enable the recording of rhythm during symptoms, thus definitively establishing or excluding the diagnosis of cardiac syncope. Published studies in patients suspected of cardiac syncope—probably representing problematic patients, whose diagnosis had not been established by other tests—revealed 24 to 47 percent accurate diagnoses, about half due to cardiac syncope, mostly bradyarrhythmias, and the other half to syncope with sinus rhythm, thus positively excluding cardiac dysrhythmia.[12] Other studies suggest that the event recorder may have best utility as the initial diagnostic test in patients with frequent episodes of suspected cardiac syncope but no detectable heart disease.[15] A major limitation of the test is many patients' inability to trigger the recorder at the time of the event. Carefully done education of these generally elderly patients is warranted to prevent an unacceptably high failure rate with the device.

## Summary of the Evaluation

A large number of patients seen in primary care practice will have benign neurally mediated or other benign types of situational syncope. Varieties of situational syncope such as cough syncope or micturition syncope can also be identified by history taking. These patients may need no further evaluation if they are otherwise young and healthy. The remaining patients include some suspected of cardiac syncope whose event occurred recently. These patients are often seen in an emergency room setting. They generally require admission for monitoring, because of the danger of recurrent events. If the patient has known serious heart disease and there is reason to suspect cardiac syncope, a cardiologist should be consulted, and electrophysiologic testing should probably be included in the evaluation. Electrophysiologic testing can be performed in some of these patients electively as outpatients if their suspected cardiac syncope occurred remotely, so that the danger of an immediate recurrence is unlikely. If cardiac syncope is suspected but uncertain, one may confirm the presence of heart disease by exercise stress testing and echocardiography prior to proceeding to further testing.[3] Another group of patients have recurrent syncope or syncope possibly causing accident or injury that is suspected of being neurally mediated. If these patients are suffering sufficient disability, they should have tilt table testing to document the diagnosis and establish a treatment. If patients are over the age of 60 years with no carotid bruit, history of ventricular tachycardia, recent stroke or myocardial infarction (MI), testing for carotid sinus sensitivity should be added.[3]

It should be emphasized that many specific etiologies of syncope are suspected on the initial history and physical examination and baseline tests. These suspected causes should lead to performing directed tests, such as exercise tolerance testing for ischemic heart disease or echocardiography for suspected structural heart disease; CT or MRI scanning and/or electroencephalography for suspected seizure or neurologic event; or evaluation for disorders such as pulmonary embolism. Other patients have documented postural hypotension that needs to be evaluated to determine if the patient is hypovolemic, taking medications that induce postural hypotension, or has an endocrine insufficiency or an autonomic neuropathy. Specific features of a psychiatric disorder such as panic attacks or major depression may direct the evaluation toward therapy with psychotropic agents and/or psychotherapy.

Psychiatric conditions associated with syncope or altered consciousness include generalized anxiety disorder, panic attacks, depression, alcoholism, and conversion disorder.[12] Syncope associated with dizziness is sometimes induced by anxiety plus hyperventilation. The hyperventilation maneuver described in Chap. 5 and screening with psychiatric instruments may be indicated in these patients.

There may be patients who do not fall into any of the above categories, but must be classed as syncope of unknown cause.[12] These would be individuals who do not have recognizable clinical features of benign neurally mediated or vasovagal syncope, but who also lack features of cardiac syncope that would lead to electrophysiologic testing or prolonged monitoring, and also do not fit the category of recurrent or complicated neurally mediated syncope, which would indicate tilt table testing. We lack an evidence-based approach to this subgroup of patients. Some physicians might perform a single 24-h monitoring in such patients with low suspicion of cardiac syncope, with further evaluation if frequent dysrhythmias are discovered. Some physicians might simply follow individuals in this category closely, with further evaluation should syncope or presyncope recur. For frequently recurrent episodes of syncope of unknown cause, the event or loop recorder may have utility.[15] Psychogenic causes should also be considered, especially in young persons with frequent episodes.[3] Tilt testing is usually performed prior to prolonged monitoring when recurrences are infrequent.

A rare but serious cause of syncope is the long QT syndrome. This hereditary disorder may occur in young adults. The patient may develop ventricular fibrillation and lose consciousness abruptly at any time, but events such as major emotional stress or exercise sometimes induce the syncope. A prolonged QT interval should be identifiable on baseline electrocardiography. A family history of sudden death may also be helpful in directing attention to this possibility. Syncope during exercise also raises the possibility of aortic stenosis or other valvular heart disease or ischemic heart disease. However, neurally mediated syncope can also occur during exercise. More likely, the onset of neurally mediated syncope occurs after pausing from exercise, but the evaluation of any patient fainting during or immediately after exercise should exclude cardiac etiologies.[16]

## TREATMENT

The most important treatment for the majority of patients who have benign neurally mediated syncope is patient education. The patient must be taught to assume the recumbent position whenever premonitory symptoms are experienced. Patients may also be taught to avoid situations likely to induce vasovagal syncope. These include prolonged standing, standing after a warm bath, prolonged sauna bath, and other stress. Rapidly getting one's head down when experiencing presyncopal symptoms generally aborts the loss of consciousness.

Recurrent or injury-producing neurally mediated syncope can be treated in several ways. The most popular treatment currently is metoprolol.[17] This drug diminishes ventricular contractivity, thereby preventing attacks. It may also work by blocking venous dilatation and pooling of blood in the lower extremities. Several other drugs with beta-blocking or anticholinergic effects may work, including disopyramide and clonidine. Metoprolol has been effective in patients whose symptoms correlated with bradycardia as well as hypotension. If a patient is preloaded with metoprolol for several days or weeks prior to tilt table testing, the positive response to tilt may be blocked. However, there is no good randomized trial proving that tilt table testing accurately predicts clinical response.[18,19] If the patient fails medical management, a pacemaker may be indicated for recurrent neurally mediated syncope chiefly produced by transient asystole or profound bradyarrhythmia.[20]

For dysautonomia, where the blood pressure gradually falls on tilt table testing, management may be aimed at preventing hypotension. Treatments include Florinef or increased salt intake to increase intravascular volume, adrenergic drugs aimed at maintaining blood pressure, and pressure gradient stockings to prevent pooling of blood in the legs.

Treatment of cardiac syncope is essentially the treatment of the underlying disease, or of arrhythmias (Chap. 37). Outcomes of treatment based on electrophysiologic testing suggest that antiarrhythmic drugs selected to suppress arrhythmias induced at testing are effective in preventing arrhythmias on follow-up. However, the subsequent mortality of patients so treated has been high, so that the benefits of this approach are not documented. It has not been proved that treatment with antiarrhythmic drugs, though successful in suppressing arrhythmias, prolongs life. It is conceivable that such treatment may have net detrimental effects on survival. Modern treatment for patients who survive ventricular fibrillation often entails an implantable cardioverter-defibrillator.[21] It is also important to recognize syncope in the setting of an ischemic event, which may be treatable with a revascularization procedure. This treatment would differ from that of syncope due to an arrhythmia in a patient with underlying ischemic heart disease who is not experiencing ischemia at the time of the syncope. The latter may not respond to revascularization.

## REFERENCES

1. Branch WT Jr: Syncope and dizziness. In: *Office Practice of Medicine.* Philadelphia, Saunders, 1987:323–327.
2. Kapoor WN: Diagnostic evaluation of syncope. *Am J Med* 1991; 90:91–106.
3. Linzer M, Yang EH, Estes M, et al: Clinical guideline diagnosing syncope: Part 1. Value of history, physical examination, and electrocardiography. *Ann Intern Med* 1997; 126:989–996.
4. Benditt DG, Ferguson DW, Grubb BP, et al: ACC Expert Consensus Document. Tilt table testing for assessing syncope. *J Am Coll Cardiol* 1996; 28:263–275.
5. Calkins H, Shyr Y, Frumin H, et al: The value of the clinical history in the differentiation of syncope due to ventricular tachycardia, atrial ventricular block, and neurocardiogenic syncope. *Am J Med* 1995; 98:365–373.
6. Kapoor WN, Hanusa BH: Is syncope a risk factor for poor outcomes? Comparison of patients with and without syncope. *Am J Med* 1996; 100:646–655.

7. Day SC, Cook EF, Funkenstein H, Goldman L: Evaluation and outcomes of emergency room patients with transient loss of consciousness. *Am J Med* 1982; 73:15–23.

8. Lipsitz LA: Syncope in the elderly. *Ann Intern Med* 1983; 99:92–105.

9. California Chapter of the American College of Cardiology: *Guidelines for Referral to a Cardiovascular Specialist.* Task Force Report, July 1995, p. 3.

10. Zipes DP, DiMarco JP, Gillette PC, et al: ACC/AHA Task Force Report. *J Am Coll Cardiol* 1995; 26:555–573.

11. Grubb BP, Kosinski D: Current trends and etiology, diagnosis, and management of neurocardiogenic syncope. *Curr Opin Cardiol* 1996; 11:32–41.

12. Linzer M, Yang EH, Estes M, et al: Clinical guideline diagnosing syncope: Part 2. Unexplained syncope. *Ann Intern Med* 1997; 127:76–86.

13. Tonnessen GE, Haft JI, Fulton J, Rubenstein DG: The value of tilt-table testing with isoproterenol in determining therapy in adults with syncope and presyncope of unexplained origin. *Arch Intern Med* 1994; 154:1613–1617.

14. Kapoor WN, Brant NL: Evaluation of syncope by upright tilt testing with isoproterenol: a non-specific test. *Ann Intern Med* 1992; 116:358–363.

15. Fogel RI, Evans JJ, Prystowsky EN: Utility and cost of event recorders in the diagnosis of palpitations, presyncope and syncope. *Am J Cardiol* 1997; 79:207–208.

16. Calkins H, Seifert M, Morady F: Clinical presentation and long term follow-up of athletes with exercise induced vasodepressor syncope. *Am Heart J* 1995; 129:1159–1164.

17. Biffi M, Boriani G, Sabbatani P, et al: Malignant vasovagal syncope: a randomized trial of metoprolol and clonidine. *Heart* 1997; 77:268–272.

18. Sheldon R, Rose S, Flanagan P, et al: Effect of beta blockers on the time to first syncope recurrence in patients after a positive isoproterenol tilt table test. *Am J Cardiol* 1996; 78:536–539.

19. Morillo CA, Klein GJ, Gersh BJ: Can serial tilt testing be used to evaluate therapy in neurally-mediated syncope? *Am J Cardiol* 1996; 77:521–523.

20. Connolly SJ, Sheldon R, Roberts RS: The North American Vasovagal Pacemaker Study (VPS): A randomized trial of permanent cardiac pacing for the prevention of vasovagal syncope. *J Am Coll Cardiol* 1999; 33:16–20.

21. Link MS, Costeas XF, Griffith JL, et al: High incidence of appropriate implantible cardioverter-defibrillator therapy in patients with syncope of unknown etiology and inducible ventricular arrhythmias. *J Am Coll Cardiol* 1997; 29:370–375.

JENNIFER KLEINBART

WILLIAM T. BRANCH, JR.

# DIZZINESS

Dizziness is one of the complaints most frequently encountered in general medical practice. It is common in the young, in whom the cause is most often benign, such as benign paroxysmal positional vertigo or hyperventilation. It is even more common in older persons, who frequently have gait disorders and are also more likely than young persons to have a vascular etiology such as transient cerebral ischemia. A complaint of dizziness presents the classic dilemma for the physician of separating the numerous benign causes, which may require little evaluation beyond the history and physical examination, from the smaller number of serious etiologies that require more extensive testing and treatment. When patients use the nonspecific term *dizziness,* they are often referring to one of four specific symptoms:

- *Vertigo.* An illusory sense of motion, vertigo accounts for almost half of patients seen in an outpatient setting with complaints of dizziness.[1] Though commonly described as a spinning sensation, vertigo may also be experienced as "tilting," "moving," "whirling," or momentary imbalance.
- *Nonspecific dizziness* or *lightheadedness.* It is always difficult for the patient to describe this symptom in precise terms. Given a choice of terms, many patients choose the word *giddiness* to describe this sensation, which seems to feel more subjective than a true loss of balance or alteration of consciousness. Often the benign, recurrent nature of this symptom, its gradual onset and offset, and its relatively prolonged duration of 20 min to 1 h allow clinicians to recognize nonspecific dizziness.
- *Presyncope* is also sometimes described as lightheadedness. It may be difficult to distinguish from the above, but it consists of "almost blacking out." Since this is an aborted attack of syncope, which otherwise would lead to loss of consciousness, this form of dizziness is generally brief in duration.
- *Disequilibrium* refers to loss of balance. It is therefore generally present when the patient is upright and walking, and is associated with gait disorders and disorders of the central nervous system, especially in elderly persons.

## HISTORY

The history is most valuable in determining the category of dizziness, since most patients are not experiencing symptoms at the time they are evaluated. Asking an open-ended question followed by requests for the patient to elaborate by describing the symptoms generally leads to the correct category. Patients who have the most difficulty describing their symptoms most often have nonspecific dizziness. Those with vertigo may be asked if they felt that they were moving or that the room was in motion, and will usually describe a clear sensorium. Those with presyncope generally do experience "nearly blacking out or passing out." Other important historical information includes the duration of the episodes; precipitating factors, such as turning over in bed; associated symptoms, such as tinnitus, headache, dysarthria, diplopia, or focal weakness; and recent illness or trauma.

## PHYSICAL EXAMINATION

Physical examination should include a thorough neurologic examination that includes testing vision and hearing. The next most likely means for ascertaining the category of dizziness is provocative testing, which includes moving the patient's head (Hallpike-Dix or Bárány maneuver) to produce vertigo, having the patient purposely hyperventilate to produce nonspecific dizziness, measuring the blood pressure both lying and standing to detect postural hypotension, and observing gait such as by tandem walking to detect disequilibrium.

Some patients have more than one cause of dizziness. In one series, the history identified those with vertigo in 87 percent of cases, those with presyncope in 74 percent, those with psychiatric disorders in 55 percent, and those with disequilibrium in 33 percent.[2] Physical examination was more likely to confirm than to establish the diagnosis.[2] In this series, virtually no patient volunteered the likelihood of a psychiatric cause of dizziness, but a number of cases were attributed to psychiatric disorders detected by standardized psychological testing using the diagnostic interview schedule (DIS).[2]

## VERTIGO

Vertigo is the most common cause of dizziness in unselected outpatients.[1-4] More than 90 percent of cases are caused by a peripheral disorder of the vestibular system, usually benign and self-limited; central nervous system disorders or abnormalities of the eighth cranial nerve account for the remainder. The most common causes of vertigo are benign paroxysmal positional vertigo, vestibular neuronitis (acute labyrinthitis), and Ménière's disease, although chronic labyrinthine imbalance (a "wastebasket" term for unexplained chronic or recurrent vertigo) also accounts for many cases (Table 5-1).[1] Acoustic neuroma is a rare but treatable condition involv-

**TABLE 5-1. Common Causes of Vertigo**

**Peripheral**

Benign paroxysmal positional vertigo

Acute vestibular neuronitis

Recurrent vestibular neuronitis

Ménière's disease

Head trauma

Arteriosclerosis

Herpes zoster oticus

Cholesteatoma

Perilymph fistula

Aminoglycoside ototoxicity

Chronic labyrinthine imbalance

**Central or Eighth Nerve**

Acoustic neuroma

Brainstem cerebrovascular accidents

Vertebrobasilar transient ischemic attacks

Cerebellar stroke

Brain tumors

Multiple sclerosis

Vertebrobasilar migraine

*Source:* Adapted with permission from Branch WT: Vertigo. In: Branch WT (ed): *Office Practice of Medicine*, 3d ed. Philadelphia, W. B. Saunders, 1994: 716, and Froehling D, Silverstein M, Mohr D, Beatty C: Does this dizzy patient have a serious form of vertigo? *JAMA* 1994; 271:385–388.

ing the eighth cranial nerve that physicians should consider to be in the "cannot miss" category. Central nervous system disorders causing vertigo include trauma, brain tumor, stroke, transient ischemic event, drug toxicity, and multiple sclerosis.

## Benign Paroxysmal Positional Vertigo

Benign paroxysmal positional vertigo (BPPV) may be caused by calcium crystals or otoliths that dislodge from the utricle and become embedded in the most dependent portion of the inner ear, the posterior semicircular canal.[5,6] The condition may result from ear trauma or infection in 15 to 50 percent of patients[7]; however, there is often no identifiable precipitant. The symptoms of vertigo occur when turning the head to one side. The vertigo is typically moderately severe, lasts seconds to several minutes, and is usually associated with nausea and vomiting.[8,9]

Physical examination reveals nystagmus elicited with provocative head-hanging maneuvers such as the Hallpike-Dix (Bárány) maneuver (Fig. 5-1).[10] In this maneuver, the head is moved in a plane parallel to the posterior semicircular canal, resulting in stimulation of those cells irritated by the presence of otoliths. Because the semicircular canals are involved with angular acceleration, the nystagmus that occurs is horizontorotatory, with the last phase to the affected side. Vertigo and nystagmus occur after a latency of several seconds, and there is fatigability, meaning that with repetition of the maneuver, vertigo and nystagmus become less pro-

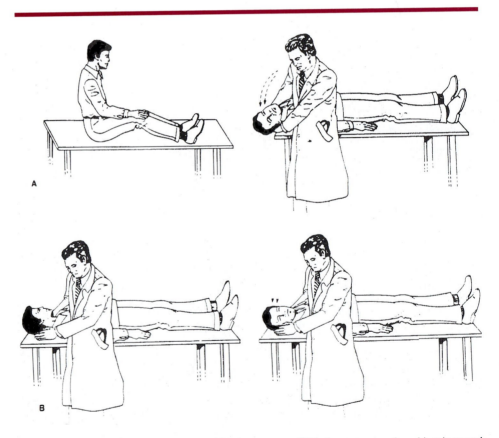

Figure 5-1   Benign positional vertigo. *A.* The Bárány response. With the eyes open, the subject is moved rapidly from the sitting position to the lying position. Nystagmus develops that is maximal with one ear down, has a quick component in one direction only, and is brief in duration with fatigue of the response. *B.* The head is moved from side to side while the patient is lying down. Positional vertigo and nystagmus may be produced. No specific diagnosis is implied, although positional vertigo with transient nystagmus is usually peripheral, indicating vestibular pathology. [From Branch WT: Vertigo. In: Branch WT (ed): *Office Practice of Medicine,* 3d ed. Philadelphia, W. B. Saunders, 1994:719, with permission.

nounced. The sensitivity of this maneuver is only 50 to 78 percent in terms of elicit-ing a positive response consisting of vertigo and nystagmus, so that a negative test does not exclude BPPV. Some 30 percent of patients with a negative test on initial examination may have a positive test if the maneuver is repeated at a later time.[11,12] In BPPV, hearing loss, resting nystagmus, and other neurologic abnormalities are absent.

The clinical course of BPPV is self-limited, although attacks may persist for months and later recur. Some 75 percent of patients have spontaneous resolution or improvement of symptoms at 1 year.[13] Treatment consists of head positioning or canalith repositioning maneuvers, which are exercises that move the head through a series of positions in an attempt to dislodge particles settled in the posterior semi-circle canal. One of these, the Epley maneuver, resulted in improvement in 85 or more percent of patients.[14] Several sessions may be necessary for resolution of symptoms.

In another positioning maneuver that is somewhat simpler, the patient is seated with eyes closed and tilted to the side that precipitates symptoms, with the side of the head against the bed. This position is maintained until vertigo subsides. The pa-tient is then returned to a seated position for 30 s and the procedure is repeated on the other side for 30 s. These maneuvers result in relief of symptoms in almost all patients within 3 to 14 days.[15] Other smaller studies using various positioning ma-neuvers have shown improvement or resolution of symptoms in the majority of pa-tients.[16,17] Occasionally, patients with intracranial tumors may present with symp-toms that mimic those of BPPV. Therefore, some advise that patients who do not respond to head positioning maneuvers undergo magnetic resonance imaging (MRI) to exclude intracranial pathology.[8] Medical treatment with antivertigo drugs such as scopolamine and meclizine may be utilized; however, this is less effective than head positioning maneuvers.[16,17]

## Vestibular Neuronitis

Vestibular neuronitis results from inflammation of the vestibular nerve to the labyrinth with at most mild involvement of the cochlea and hence minimal if any loss of hearing. A viral etiology has been postulated, as some patients report a pre-ceding febrile illness or upper respiratory illness,[9] and histologic studies are consis-tent with postinfectious inflammation of the vestibular system.[18]

Vertigo in this condition generally occurs suddenly and, especially as the condi-tion begins to resolve, may be positional, worsened by rapid changes in head posi-tion. The vertigo is moderately severe and sustained, and is often associated with nausea and vomiting. Physical examination shows spontaneous horizontorotary nys-tagmus, with the fast component away from the affected side when looking away from that side. When looking toward the affected side, the nystagmus is reduced.[5,6]

In most cases vestibular neuronitis resolves spontaneously, usually within 6 weeks, with the most severe symptoms lasting only several days.[5,6] Antivertigo drugs such as meclizine may produce some relief of symptoms.

## Ménière's Disease

Ménière's disease is thought to result from a disturbance of the endolymphatic sac or obstruction of a narrow endolymphatic duct, resulting in decreased absorption of endolymph and therefore an increased volume of fluid, causing rupture of the membranous labyrinth.[9,19] Because of the continuity of the vestibular and cochlear labyrinths, patients experience a triad of vertigo, tinnitus, and sensorineural hearing loss. Attacks of vertigo are severe enough to require bed rest, may last from hours to days, and are associated with nausea, vomiting, and diaphoresis.[18] Over half of patients complain of headache and may describe falling during attacks of vertigo.[18] Nystagmus occurs only during the episodes of vertigo. At the beginning of the attack, the nystagmus occurs with the fast component toward the side of the lesion, but it later occurs with the fast component away from the affected side, representing irritative and paralytic phases.[9]

Vertigo attacks may occur in clusters or with intervals of up to years between attacks. Tinnitus and loss of hearing often persist between attacks.[5,6] The hearing loss may occasionally improve as the ruptured labyrinth heals; however, it usually becomes more severe as the disease progresses.

The disease may generally be diagnosed from its typical features, but when unilateral progressive sensorineural hearing loss is a prominent feature, MRI may be necessary to rule out acoustic neuroma.

Medical treatment has two goals. The first is to relieve symptoms during acute attacks; treatment consists of an antiemetic such as prochlorperazine, an antivertigo agent such as meclizine, and bed rest. The second is to modify symptoms and attempt to widen the intervals between attacks; for this purpose, a diuretic such as hydrochlorothiazide may be instituted along with a low-salt diet.

For disease unresponsive to medical therapy, surgery may be indicated. Several procedures are used, including destruction of the labyrinth, decompression using an endolymphatic-subarachnoid or endolymphatic-mastoid shunt, and sectioning of the vestibular nerve. These procedures are generally effective in relieving vertigo; however, hearing may be sacrificed.[9] Chemical destruction of the labyrinth using gentamicin is a nonsurgical procedure that has been found to eliminate or improve vertigo in more than 90 percent of patients with Ménière's disease, but it also entails a reduction in hearing.[20,21]

## Central Vestibular Disorders

Central causes of vertigo are encountered less often than peripheral vestibular causes. The etiologies of central vertigo most commonly seen in a general medical practice include vertebrobasilar disease and cerebellopontine angle tumor (acoustic neuroma).

**VERTEBROBASILAR DISEASE.** The blood supply to the eighth cranial nerve and vestibular nuclei comes from the basilar artery, most commonly via branches of the anterior inferior cerebellar artery. Vertigo is a complaint in 75 to 100 percent of patients with strokes of the posterior circulation; however, only rarely, if ever, does vertigo accompany anterior circulatory ischemia.[22,23] With vertebrobasilar ischemia, associated symptoms of dysarthria, diplopia, ataxia, facial numbness, and weakness make the diagnosis clear in more than two-thirds of patients.[22] In the remaining patients, dizziness alone is the presenting symptom.[22,23] In these patients, other neurologic findings generally occur within 6 weeks, so that isolated dizziness of greater than 6 weeks' duration is rarely due to cerebrovascular disease.[22] Vertebrobasilar thrombosis characteristically has a stuttering onset, with transient ischemic attacks occurring during several weeks prior to the onset of the stroke.[24]

With basilar ischemia, findings on physical examination may include coarse nystagmus between dizzy spells, vertical nystagmus, ataxia, dysarthria, visual impairment, unilateral or bilateral weakness, sensory deficits of the face or limbs, and Horner's syndrome.

Ischemia of the internal auditory artery is a less common occurrence. In 90 percent of the cases it produces dizziness, and it is associated with the sudden onset of unilateral deafness in all patients.[22]

Cerebellar ischemia due to disease of the distal posterior inferior cerebellar artery may mimic peripheral vertigo. There is acute onset of vertigo, nausea, and vomiting. Associated findings include swaying, mild dysarthria, vertical nystagmus, and dysmetria in only one arm. When ischemia involves the more proximal posterior inferior cerebellar artery, other signs of brainstem ischemia will be found.

Ischemia of the posterior circulation may be transient or persistent. Transient symptoms may result not only from transient ischemic attack but also from mechanical disruption resulting from rotation of the neck and from the subclavian steal syndrome, in which blood is diverted from the brainstem to one arm during the use of that arm.[6] Physical examination revealing a subclavian artery bruit and decreased blood pressure in the affected arm are consistent with this syndrome. Persistent symptoms with an abrupt onset are consistent with brainstem or cerebellar infarction.

**ACOUSTIC NEUROMA (CEREBELLOPONTINE ANGLE TUMOR).**
Acoustic neuromas, arising from the Schwann cells covering the vestibular division of the eighth cranial nerve, are the most common tumors of the cerebellopontine angle. Because destruction of the vestibular nerve occurs slowly, vestibular symptoms, if present early, are not prominent and may be transient.[25] Attacks of vertigo may last from minutes to hours, may be mild to modest in intensity, and may occur only infrequently (3 to 12 times a year in one study).[7,18] Tinnitus is usually the presenting symptom, caused by compression of the acoustic branch of cranial nerve VIII, which precedes sensorineural hearing loss and vertigo by months to years.[5,6] Some 95 percent of patients note hearing loss for 1 to 4 years prior to the time the diagnosis is made.[18] Diagnosis is best made by MRI using gadolinium. Computed tomography (CT) using contrast is less sensitive but is a second choice of diagnostic procedure in patients unable to tolerate MRI. Treatment is surgical resection.

## Tests Used for Evaluation of Vertigo

**NYSTAGMUS.**   Although nystagmus is always present during vertigo, it may not be visible, but may be elicited only by provocative maneuvers or electronystagmography (see below). Physiologic (normal) nystagmus consists of a few horizontal beats, present symmetrically when looking in either direction. Abnormally pronounced nystagmus of this type may indicate a central nervous system disorder, such as drug toxicity. Nystagmus due to peripheral etiologies is generally horizontorotatory, horizontal, or rotary, with its quick component in one direction only (Table 5-2). It may cease with fixation of vision. Central lesions may produce more pronounced and prolonged nystagmus, which can be vertical or oblique in addition to horizontal, rotatory, or horizontorotatory in direction.[26]

**OFFICE TESTING OF HEARING.**   Patients can usually identify whether they have hearing loss, and if so, whether in one ear or both. One may confirm the presence of unilateral hearing loss by testing with whispered voice or finger rubbing. When an asymmetric loss is suspected, it can be further confirmed using the Weber test, where the tuning fork is placed in the middle of the forehead and the patient is asked in which ear the sound is loudest. For sensorineural loss the sound is louder in the unaffected ear, and for conductive loss, in the affected ear. Further confirmation by the Rinne test consists of placing the tuning fork on the mastoid bone fol-

**TABLE 5-2.   Characteristic Features of Vertigo and Nystagmus**

| Feature | Vestibular Lesions | Central Lesions |
|---------|--------------------|-----------------|
| Vertigo | Abrupt onset of whirling or spinning <br> Severe <br> Paroxysmal <br> Seconds to weeks in duration <br> Usually positional | Less clear onset of disequilibrium <br> Less severe <br> May be continuous <br> Often prolonged <br> Somewhat less likely to be positional |
| Tinnitus | Common | Less common |
| Nystagmus | Horizontal, rotatory, or horizontorotatory <br><br> Accompanied by vertigo <br> Turning eyes toward quick component increases its amplitude but does not alter its direction <br><br> Always in both eyes <br><br> May cease with fixation of vision; more pronounced with eyes closed <br> Gradually diminishes | Vertical, oblique (also rotatory, horizontal, or horizontorotatory) <br> Of long duration or present without vertigo <br> Direction of nystagmus may change with changes in gaze. May resemble exaggerated physiologic nystagmus (especially in drug toxicity) <br> May be in one eye only (internuclear ophthalmoplegia) <br> Not suppressed by fixating; equally pronounced with eyes open <br> May wax and wane or begin spontaneously after ceasing |

*Source:* From Branch WT: Vertigo. In: Branch WT (ed): *Office Practice of Medicine*, 3d ed. Philadelphia, W. B Saunders, 1994: 722, with permission.

lowed by holding it next to the ear. In sensorineural hearing loss, the patient hears the sound louder when the fork is held near the ear, and in conductive hearing loss, the patient hears the sound louder when the fork is placed on the mastoid bone.

**AUDIOMETRY.**   Audiologic tests may be utilized to aid in differentiating several causes of vertigo. BPPV and vestibular neuronitis are not associated with hearing impairment. In Ménière's disease, low-frequency hearing loss occurs, whereas with an acoustic neuroma, high-frequency hearing loss is more often present, but these features are not sufficiently characteristic to secure the diagnosis.[5] Middle ear disorders will show conductive rather than sensorineural hearing loss. The majority of acoustic neuromas may be suspected by detecting unilateral sensorineural hearing loss on audiometry.

**CALORIC TESTING.**   The patient is seated with the head tipped back at 60° or supine with the head at 30° to align the horizontal semicircular canal. One milliliter of ice water is introduced into the external ear canal, and nystagmus is observed. Normally the fast component will be toward the opposite ear. With the use of warm water (44°), nystagmus should occur with the rapid phase toward the stimulated ear. Abnormal responses indicate dysfunction of the vestibular system but are not diagnostically specific.[5]

**ELECTRONYSTAGMOGRAPHY (ENG).**   This test records nystagmus while the eyes are open or closed by measuring changes in the electrical potential between the cornea and the retina. It provides a more precise, objective measure of nystagmus than either direct observation or caloric testing. Caloric testing can be done during ENG. The combination of features of nystagmus observed during ENG testing, such as whether it is horizontorotatory or vertical, positional or present spontaneously, or persistent or diminished when gaze is fixed, and features of the caloric response may help to suggest whether a peripheral or a central etiology is causing vertigo.[5]

**BRAINSTEM-EVOKED AUDIOMETRY.**   This test measures the electrical response of the brainstem to a sound and is highly sensitive for detecting acoustic neuroma. More than 90 percent of patients with neuromas have an abnormal response,[22] but the abnormality is nonspecific and may result from any other condition causing sensorineural hearing loss.[25]

## Drugs Used to Treat Vertigo

Meclizine and dimenhydrinate are drugs with histamine-1 receptor blocking properties, which depress labyrinthine excitability and vestibular stimulation. These drugs may also have antiemetic effects, possibly as a result of inhibition of the medullary chemoreceptor trigger zone. Side effects include drowsiness; this is more prominent with dimenhydrinate. Anticholinergic side effects may also occur.

Scopolamine is used for treatment of vertigo associated with motion sickness. Its antimuscarinic action may block pathways from the vestibular nuclei in the inner ear to the brainstem and from the reticular formation to the medullary chemore-ceptor trigger zone. Scopolamine is effective for nausea and vomiting related to motion sickness or vestibulopathies, but does not treat nausea and vomiting caused by other disorders.

## NONSPECIFIC DIZZINESS

A patient may complain that he or she is dizzy but be unable to describe the symptom. If offered a choice of words, he or she will generally choose *giddiness* or *lightheadedness* over *spinning* or *blacking out*. For the most part, nonspecific dizziness develops gradually, wanes away gradually, and persists for about 20 min. Nonspecific dizziness may be associated with psychiatric disorders. In one study, one-fourth of individuals whose nonspecific dizziness was attributable to psychiatric disorders had major depression, one-fourth had generalized anxiety disorder, and one-fourth had panic disorder.[2] The remaining individuals had somatization disorder, alcohol dependency, and/or personality disorders.[2] Certain other conditions, such as fibromyalgia, have been associated with nonspecific dizziness.[27] Because persons with nonspecific dizziness may have dizziness of more than one etiology, a psychiatric disorder should be diagnosed from its typical features, with treatment given if indicated based on these features, and other causes of dizziness should be excluded.

In young individuals, nonspecific dizziness is commonly related to hyperventilation. In these cases, the diagnosis can be confirmed by a provocative maneuver. This consists of having the patient hyperventilate until he or she becomes dizzy, then ascertaining if this is the exact same sensation. This maneuver may be therapeutic if the patient becomes reassured that the cause is benign. Other disorders may produce a nonspecific lightheadedness or sensation of weakness related to presyncope that may at times be indistinguishable from nonspecific dizziness. These include cardiac dysrhythmias, episodes of coronary ischemia, worsening congestive heart failure, and pulmonary embolism.[28] Such persons may also present with dyspnea, palpitations, or chest discomfort. Trauma, including whiplash injuries, can produce a nonspecific dizziness (as well as vertigo).

## PRESYNCOPE

Presyncope results from decreased cardiac output that leads to cerebral hypoperfusion. The causes of presyncope are identical to those of syncope (see Chap. 4). It is somewhat less likely that an individual who has experienced only episodes of presyncope without losing consciousness will have a serious disorder, such as a life-threatening cardiac dysrhythmia, than that an individual presenting with syncope will have such a disorder. However, one must generally perform the same evaluation (see Chap. 4). The true challenge for the clinician evaluating a patient with "dizziness" is to recognize that presyncope is present; as mentioned above, its features typically include the sensation of "almost blacking out," the short duration of symptoms prior to recovery or to proceeding to syncope, sometimes typical premonitory symptoms of neurocardiogenic or vasovagal syncope (nausea, diaphoresis, weakness, typical setting such as stressful event or prolonged standing), and being able to abort the episode by assuming recumbency. After a clear sensorium has been restored in a supine position, patients with neurocardiogenic or vasovagally induced presyncope typically experience recurrence of weakness on attempting to stand.

## DISEQUILIBRIUM

Disequilibrium is a sense of imbalance, which many patients refer to as "dizziness." They generally feel as though they are losing balance while standing or walking. This symptom is more common in the elderly. It may result from diseases of the cerebellum that cause ataxia, from the combination of a proprioceptive abnormality caused by peripheral neuropathy plus visual impairment due to conditions such as cataracts, from weakness of the lower extremities, or from progressive neurologic disorders such as Parkinson's disease. A complete neurologic examination should be performed on patients suspected of having disequilibrium, and should include careful testing of cerebellar functioning and gait and Romberg's test. Since the patient generally will not volunteer the information that her or his dizziness and falling is related to gait, one must observe the patient while walking, standing, and turning; perform Romberg's test; and observe tandem walking.[29] The condition may be multifactorial. A patient should be asked about medications, especially antidepressants and anticholinergics, that may produce dizziness[30] and about medication withdrawal.[31] It is important to inquire about falls and about dizziness while driving. Conditions that should be considered include cerebrovascular disease, cervical spinal problems, physical deconditioning, medication side effects, medication withdrawal, and vertigo. Chronic dizziness or disequilibrium often significantly impairs social and physical functioning in the elderly.[32,33] The treatment may be directed toward the most remediable problems.[34]

## REFERENCES

 1. Drachman D, Hart C: An approach to the dizzy patient. *Neurology* 1972; 22:323–334.
 2. Kroenke K, Lucas C, Rosenberg M, et al: Causes of persistent dizziness: a prospective study of 100 patients in ambulatory care. *Ann Intern Med* 1992; 117:898–904.
 3. Nedzelski J, Barber H, McIlmoyl L: Diagnosis in a dizziness unit. *J Otolaryngol* 1986; 15:101–104.
 4. Herr R, Zun L, Mathews J: A directed approach to the dizzy patient. *Ann Emerg Med* 1989; 18:664–672.
 5. Branch WT: Vertigo. In: Branch WT (ed): *Office Practice of Medicine,* 3d ed. Philadelphia, W. B. Saunders, 1994:715–729.
 6. Bass E, Hamilton M, Rothman W: Dizziness, vertigo, motion sickness, near syncope, syn-

cope and disequilibrium. In: Barker L, Burton J, Zieve P (eds.): *Principles of Ambulatory Medicine,* 3d ed. Baltimore, Williams & Wilkins, 1991:1114.

7. McGee S: Dizzy patient. Diagnosis and treatment. *West J Med* 1995; 162:37–42.

8. Dunniway H, Welling D: Intracranial tumors mimicking benign paroxysmal positional vertigo. *Otolaryngol Head Neck Surg* 1998; 118:429–436.

9. Wolfson R, Silberstein H, Marlowe F, Keels E: Vertigo. *Clin Symp* 1981; 33:1–32.

10. Hughes C, Proctor L: Benign paroxysmal positional vertigo. *Laryngoscope* 1997; 107:607–613.

11. Froehling D, Silverstein M, Mohr D, Beatty C: Does this dizzy patient have a serious form of vertigo? *JAMA* 1994; 271:385–388.

12. Katsarkas A, Kirkham T: Paroxysmal positional vertigo—a study of 255 cases. *J Otolaryngol* 1978; 7:320–330.

13. Kroenke K, Lucas C, Rosenberg M, et al: One-year outcome for patients with a chief complaint of dizziness. *J Gen Intern Med* 1994; 9:684–689.

14. Smouha E: Time course of recovery after Epley maneuvers for benign paroxysmal positional vertigo. *Laryngoscope* 1997; 1072:187.

15. Brandt T, Daroff R: Physical therapy for benign paroxysmal positional vertigo. *Arch Otolaryngol* 1980; 106:484–485.

16. Itaya T, Yamamoto E: Comparison of effectiveness of maneuvers and medication in the treatment of benign paroxysmal positional vertigo. *ORL J Otorhinolaryngol Relat Spec* 1997; 59:155–158.

17. Fujino A, Tokumasu K: Vestibular training for acute unilateral vestibular disturbances: its efficacy in comparison with antivertigo drug. *Acta Otolaryngol Suppl* 1996; 524:21–26.

18. Kentala E: Characteristics of six otologic diseases involving vertigo. *Am J Otol* 1996; 17:883–992.

19. Ishiyama A, Ishiyama G: Histopathology of idiopathic chronic recurrent vertigo. *Laryngoscope* 1997; 107:146.

20. Corsten M, Marsan J, Schramm D, Robichaud J: Treatment of intractable Meniere's disease with intratympanic gentamicin: review of the University of Ottawa experience. *J Otolaryngol* 1997; 26:361–364.

21. McFeely W, Singleton G, Rodriguez F, Antonelli P: Intratympanic gentamicin treatment for Meniere's disease. *Otolaryngol Head Neck Surg* 1998; 118:589–596.

22. Fisher C: Vertigo in cerebrovascular disease. *Arch Otolaryngol* 1967; 85:529–534.

23. Kim G, Heo J: Vertigo of cerebrovascular origin proven by CT scan or MRI: pitfalls in clinical differentiation from vertigo of aural origin. *Yonsei Med J* 1996; 37:47–51.

24. Becker K, Purcell L, Hackey W: Vertebrobasilar thrombosis: diagnosis, management, and the use of intra-arterial thrombolytics. *Crit Care Med* 1996; 24:1729–1742.

25. Harner S, Laws EJ: Clinical findings in patients with acoustic neuroma. *Mayo Clin Proc* 1983; 58:721–728.

26. Parker S, Weiss A: Some electronystagmographic manifestations of central nervous system disease. *Ann Otol Rhinol Laryngol* 1976; 85:127–130.

27. Rosenhall U, Johansson G, Orndahl G: Otoneurologic and audiologic findings in fibromyalgia. *Scand J Rehabil Med* 1996; 28:225–232.

28. Wood K, Drew B, Scheinman M: Frequency of disabling symptoms in supraventricular tachycardia. *Am J Cardiol* 1997; 79:145–149.

29. Fitzgerald D: Head trauma: hearing loss and dizziness. *J Trauma* 1996; 40:488–496.

30. McKiernan J, Lowe F: Side effects of terazosin in the treatment of symptomatic benign prostatic hyperplasia. *South Med J* 1997; 90:509–513.

31. Coupland M, Bell C, Potokar J: Serotonin reuptake inhibitor withdrawal. *J Clin Psychopharmacol* 1996; 16:356–362.
32. Fielder H, Denholm S, Lyons R, Fielder C: Measurement of health status in patients with vertigo. *Clin Otolaryngol* 1996; 21:124–126.
33. Grimby A, Rosehall U: Health-related quality of life and dizziness in old age. *Gerontology* 1995; 41:286–298.
34. Sloane P: Evaluation and management of dizziness in the older patient. *Clin Geriatric Med* 1996; 12:785–801.

DAVID B. DE LURGIO /
APRIL BARBOUR

# CHAPTER

# PALPITATIONS AND TACHYCARDIA

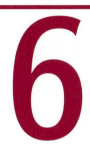

Palpitations may be defined as a disagreeable sensation of the heartbeat. Surveys of both medical and cardiology practices have found palpitations to be among the 10 most commonly reported symptoms, with up to 16 percent of patients in outpatient medical practices presenting with this complaint.[1,2] The most common descriptors offered are a sensation of "skipped beats" or "extra beats," a "fluttering" or "flip-flop," or of the heart briefly stopping. Many patients will describe pounding sensations and occasionally rapid, slow, or irregular heart rates. Some will have associated symptoms of anxiety, chest pain, syncope, or presyncope. The causes of palpitations range from the benign to potentially lethal. Initial evaluation includes a thorough history, physical examination, and 12-lead ECG and may require lab work, diagnostic tests, referral, or hospital admission. Ultimately, a diagnosis may be expected in more than 80 percent of patients.[3] Management by the primary care physician should identify individuals at risk for cardiac morbidity and result in a timely, safe, and cost-effective evaluation.

## ETIOLOGY

The list of causes of palpitations is quite extensive (Table 6-1). Useful differential diagnostic categories include cardiac, psychiatric, medical, drug-related, and unknown etiologies. These categories are guidelines to help understand the underlying pathophysiology responsible for palpitations. Often a patient will fall into more than one category. Usually, however, a primary cause can be determined. Evaluation of the patient with these general categories in mind is helpful in clarifying whether or not a patient requires further evaluation and/or treatment.

Cardiac etiologies of palpitations are identified most frequently and are the main focus of this chapter. Palpitations due to cardiac causes may be further subclassified as due to ectopic beats, supraventricular or ventricular tachyarrhythmias, episodic bradyarrhythmias, or valvular diseases.

**TABLE 6-1.   Etiologies of Palpitations**

Cardiac
  Premature atrial beats*
  Premature ventricular beats*
  Atrial fibrillation*
  Atrial flutter*
  Supraventricular tachycardia
  Sick sinus syndrome
  Ventricular tachycardia
  Valvular heart disease
  Artificial pacemaker malfunction
  Increased cardiac awareness

Psychiatric
  Panic disorder*
  Anxiety*
  Depression*
  Somatization
  Bereavement

Medical Illness
  Anemia
  Thyrotoxicosis
  High-output syndromes

Drugs
  Caffeine
  Nicotine
  Cocaine
  Amphetamines
  Beta agonists

Unknown

* Common in outpatient medical practices.

Ectopic atrial or ventricular complexes [premature atrial contractions (PACs) or premature ventricular contractions (PVCs), respectively] are perhaps the most frequent cause of palpitations encountered in medical practices; PACs and PVCs are ubiquitous and, in the absence of significant structural heart disease, innocuous. Most patients are unaware of ectopic beats, but, when perceptible, they may be disturbing or even disabling in some patients. Patients may note palpitations while resting in bed, especially in the left lateral decubitus position. The alteration in chest wall stimulation due to the premature beat and postcompensatory pause accentuation of contractility is the likely cause. With increased external stimuli and greater baseline heart rate during active hours, simple ectopic beats may be both less frequent and less noticed.

Tachycardias may also present as palpitations. Both supraventricular and ventricular tachycardias are discussed in detail in Chaps. 36 and 37. The complaint of a rapid, pounding heart rate naturally suggests tachycardia. The differential diagnosis must include sinus tachycardia, reentrant supraventricular tachycardias such as atrioventricular nodal reentrant tachycardia, orthodromic reciprocating tachycardia, automatic and reentrant atrial tachycardias, atrial fibrillation or flutter, and ventricular tachycardia.

Cardiac valvular disease may present as palpitations. Mitral valve prolapse has frequently been associated with the complaint of palpitations. It has been assumed that symptoms in these patients were due to an excess of cardiac arrhythmias. Indeed, many patients with mitral valve prolapse also have PACs and PVCs. Recent studies, however, have found that some patients with mitral valve prolapse may complain of palpitations during which no rhythm disturbances are present. This has led some investigators to conclude that palpitations associated with mitral valve prolapse are often functional in nature.[4] Mitral stenosis has been associated with palpitations, most likely as a result of an increased frequency of atrial fibrillation. Aortic regurgitation may produce palpitations as a result of the markedly increased stroke volume and increased cardiac activity. Aortic stenosis is not generally associated with palpitations unless the patient has related cardiac arrhythmias.

Psychiatric diagnoses and emotional instability are frequent causes of palpitations and must not be overlooked. In a recent prospective cohort study, the etiology of palpitations was panic attack, anxiety disorder, or somatization in 31 percent of 190 consecutive patients.[3] It has long been recognized that patients with panic disorders exhibit increased "cardiac awareness." Increased cardiac awareness refers to an enhanced sensation of the heartbeat, even though there may be no abnormality of rate or rhythm.[5] Patients with anxiety, panic, or depression tend to catastrophize this awareness, assuming that they suffer from a serious cardiac condition.[6] Isolated emotional events such as fear, anxiety, or bereavement may also cause palpitations and lead to an office visit. However, catastrophizing is not as prominent in these patients.

Important medical causes of palpitations must also be considered in the initial evaluation. Thyrotoxicosis may produce palpitations by several mechanisms, including increased forcefulness of the heartbeat, sinus tachycardia, and an increased frequency of ectopic beats, supraventricular tachycardia, and atrial fibrillation. Significant anemia may result in sinus tachycardia, forceful heartbeats (high-output state), and an increased likelihood of cardiac arrhythmias. Reactive hypoglycemia, orthostatic hypotension, and autonomic dysfunction may cause sudden sinus tachycardia that is perceived as palpitations. Rare medical conditions such as mastocytosis, carcinoid syndrome, and pheochromocytoma often have palpitations as part of the symptom complex.

Use of drugs (prescribed, illicit, and over-the-counter) is a frequent cause of palpitations. Cocaine and amphetamines cause sinus tachycardia and ectopy and have been linked to serious and occasionally lethal arrhythmias. Beta agonists, caffeine, and nicotine frequently produce ectopy and exacerbate supraventricular arrhythmias. Alcohol has been associated with atrial fibrillation (holiday heart). Drug or alcohol withdrawal must also be considered as a potential cause of palpitations in the appropriate setting.

## EVALUATION

At presentation in the primary care physician's office, patients usually are not having palpitations. The inital history, physical examination, laboratory work, and ECG, however, may establish the diagnosis in up to 40 percent of patients.[3] The nature, frequency, and duration of the palpitations and associated symptoms must be carefully assessed. Often symptoms characteristic of isolated ectopy may be elicited. These may include a characteristic description of a brief flip-flopping sensation or of the heart's briefly stopping, followed by a forceful beat. Question the patient carefully about time of day, association with exercise, emotional triggers, or association with caffeine or medications. If the patient complains of rapid or forceful beating, it may be helpful to have the patient tap out the rhythm. Alternatively, the physician may tap out various rhythms on the examination table or on the patient's chest. Attention to rate and regularity may help distinguish atrial fibrillation from ectopy or causes of rapid regular heart action. It is remarkable how often a patient can recognize the characteristics of ectopic beats or atrial fibrillation. Careful questioning about the onset of the palpitations is also useful. A sudden versus gradual onset or termination may help distinguish among reentrant and automatic mechanisms of arrhythmia and sinus tachycardia (Table 6-2).

Activity at onset or possible initiating factors should be explored. Onset during physical exertion or associated symptoms such as angina, diaphoresis, syncope, or presyncope may be evidence of underlying heart disease and should prompt a more urgent evaluation. Syncope from a cardiac cause is of far greater prognostic significance than isolated palpitations. A history of heart disease or a cardiac arrhythmia must not be discounted and greatly increases the probability of a cardiac cause of palpitations. In one large study, a history of heart disease predicted a cardiac cause of palpitations in nearly 50 percent of patients.[3] In this study, the mode of presentation was also very important. Nearly 50 percent of patients presenting to an emergency room with palpitations were found to have a cardiac cause versus only 20 percent of those presenting to an ambulatory medical clinic.

The history must also consider possible psychiatric etiologies of palpitations, such as depression, anxiety, somatization, or panic disorder. While most medical practitioners feel compelled to rule out medical or cardiac causes of palpitations first, a strong argument for early evaluation for psychiatric diagnoses can be made. The prospective study by Weber and Kapoor[3] identified a psychiatric cause of palpitations in 31 percent of that cohort. Another retrospective study found a history of psychiatric disease in 41 percent of patients presenting to an outpatient clinic with the complaint of palpitations.[7] These findings argue for an up-front consideration of these frequent causes of palpitations. A history that addresses this issue is essential. Useful tools that can be self-administered in the office setting include the General Health Questionnaire and a screening test for somatization.[8,9]

Physical examination of the patient with a history of palpitations must identify signs of underlying heart disease or medical causes of palpitations. Careful recording of the vital signs may supply the first clues to a diagnosis. The presenting heart rate may reveal unexpected tachycardia or bradycardia. The rhythm may be irregular or reveal the telltale signs of ectopic beats. The blood pressure reading may re-

**TABLE 6-2.   Physical Findings and Important History in Patients with Palpitations and Arrhythmias**

| Arrhythmia | Physical Findings | History |
|---|---|---|
| Sinus tachycardia | Regular rhythm, rate 100–170 beats per minute | Gradual onset, anxiety, drug use, medical illness |
| PACs, PVCs | Premature beat followed by compensatory or noncompensatory pause. Premature beat may have a diminished or absent pulse | Brief sensation of skipped beat or pause with postpause accentuation |
| Atrial flutter | Usually regular pulse at 150 beats per minute (2:1 conduction) Variable block may occur | Sudden onset, often coexistent lung or heart disease or hypertension (HTN) |
| Atrial fibrillation | Irregularly irregular rhythm, variable rate. May notice pulse dropout at periphery due to variability of diastolic filling | Sudden onset, often coexistent lung or heart disease, HTN, diabetes. Irregularity usually noted |
| Complete heart block | Jugular venous cannon a waves with variable amplitude, variable intensity of first heart sound | Fatigue, dyspnea on exertion, syncope or presyncope. Patient may sense cannon a waves as neck pounding |
| Supraventricular reentrant tachycardias | Rapid, regular rhythm, rate 160–220 beats per minute. May note prominent jugular venous pulsations due to contraction of atria against closed atrio ventricular valve | Sudden onset. Often a long history of recurrent symptoms. In some, neck pounding may be a clue to AV nodal reentry |
| Ventricular tachycardia | Rapid, regular rhythm. Often cannon a waves, variable first heart sound due to AV dissociation | Sudden onset; usually a history of coronary artery disease |

veal systemic hypertension, hypotension, or a wide pulse pressure. A febrile illness responsible for sinus tachycardia may occasionally be detected. Physical findings indicating a possible underlying medical cause of palpitations, such as perspiration, anxiety, exophthalmos, thyromegaly, or signs of anemia, should be sought. Findings suggestive of underlying atherosclerosis, such as xanthomata or arcus senilis, or signs of underlying genetic syndromes associated with heart disease (Marfan syndrome, Holt-Oram syndrome) should not be overlooked. Physical evidence of heart disease, such as elevated jugular venous pressure or an abnormal jugular venous waveform, delayed carotid upstroke, or carotid bruits, should be assessed. Cardiac enlargement on palpation may be the first sign of a cardiomyopathic process, and an $S_4$ or $S_3$ heart sound may support this diagnosis. Careful auscultation for a systolic click with or without a heart murmur may point to mitral valve prolapse. Other heart murmurs may indicate significant underlying heart disease such as mitral stenosis, aortic stenosis, or aortic regurgitation.

Occasionally, a patient will be experiencing palpitations at the time of evaluation. Physical findings during palpitations may suggest a diagnosis. Premature beats with a compensatory pause and postpause accentuation narrow the differential diagnosis to PACs or PVCs. An irregularly irregular rhythm strongly suggests atrial fibrillation. A tachycardia in the range of 100 to 170 beats per minute that transiently slows with vagal maneuvers such as carotid sinus massage is consistent with sinus tachycardia. A tachycardia at a rate of 150 beats per minute that abruptly blocks down with vagal maneuvers and quickly returns to 150 beats per minute is probably atrial flutter. Tachycardias that terminate with vagal maneuvers are typically supraventricular tachycardias, such as atrioventricular nodal reentrant or orthodromic reciprocating tachycardia. The jugular venous waveform may also provide important clues. Irregular cannon a waves during a slow rhythm indicate complete heart block. Irregular cannon a waves or cannon a waves occurring at a fixed ratio to the tachycardia rate suggests ventricular tachycardia. Table 6-2 lists characteristic physical findings and history in patients with ongoing arrhythmias and palpitations.

The baseline 12-lead ECG is helpful in ruling out significant organic heart disease and when normal is reassuring. Evidence of a prior myocardial infarction, chamber enlargement, conduction abnormalities or the presence of ectopy, QT prolongation, or a delta wave may support a working diagnosis. Electrocardiographic diagnosis of specific arrhythmias is discussed in Chap. 37. Laboratory work such as thyroid function studies, hematocrit, and electrolytes may be appropriate to rule out medical causes where indicated.

For patients with palpitations associated with significant symptoms suggestive of hemodynamic compromise, such as syncope or presyncope, or with significant heart disease, cardiology referral and possible electrophysiologic evaluation may be indicated. Patients with no cardiac disease in whom simple ectopy is strongly suspected may require no further evaluation. For the majority of patients, however, ambulatory electrocardiographic monitoring is a useful and safe method of evaluation for cardiac causes of palpitations. Traditionally, 24-h Holter monitoring has been used to assess cardiac rhythm and the occurrence of cardiac arrhythmias throughout the period of monitoring. The usefulness of this tool depends on the presence of cardiac events during a relatively short period of monitoring. Further complicating analysis is the occurrence of asymptomatic arrhythmias and the reporting of palpitations during periods of sinus rhythm. We have found event recorders to be more effective tools in this respect. For approximately the same cost as a 24-h Holter, patients may be provided for 30 days with a small device that is capable of saving and transmitting surface electrograms during palpitations. Devices that are pressed against the chest and activated during palpitations provide a real-time electrogram for a specified duration. We favor loop recorders in which two surface leads are left in place at all times. When the recorder is triggered by the patient, the loop is interrupted, storing an electrogram beginning a specified time *before* the patient triggered the device and continuing for a specified time. This event is stored in memory and can be transmitted over the telephone at the patient's convenience. The benefits of this type of ambulatory monitoring are the far greater duration of surveillance; less cumbersome equipment, allowing the patient to pursue normal activities; collection of electrograms directly related to symptomatic episodes; possible analysis of onset and termination of multiple episodes; and rapid

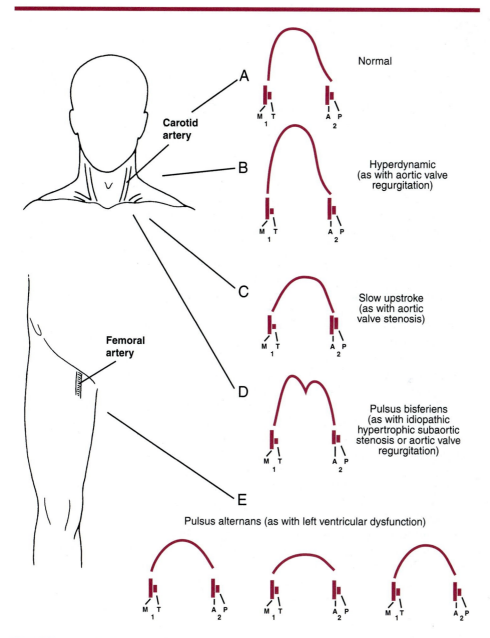

Figure 7-1   Arterial pulse contour.

# EXAMINATION OF THE NECK VEINS

## Mind-Set

The mind-set is to prove by observation that the external jugular veins are not abnormally distended and that no abnormal a wave, abnormal v wave, or abnormal x or y descents is apparent in the pulsations produced by the internal jugular veins.

## Technique of Examination

The patient should be examined initially in the supine position. Normally, the *external jugular veins* may be observed to be distended when the patient is in that position. The trunk of the patient should be elevated gradually until the distended external veins collapse. This normally occurs when the trunk of the patient is elevated less than 30° from the horizontal plane of the bed or examining table. Heart failure, some other cause of hypervolemia, or obstruction of the superior vena cava should be considered when distention of the external jugular veins persists when the trunk of the patient is elevated more than 30°.

The *internal jugular venous pulsations* are examined as follows: The internal jugular veins are located beneath the sternocleidomastoid muscles. Accordingly, the observer does not see the veins; only the movements can be seen. The patient should be examined initially in the supine position. The chin of the patient should be in the midline; turning the head to see the neck veins may obliterate the pulsations of the internal jugular veins because the action tightens the sternocleidomastoid muscle. It is useful to place a pillow under the head when the patient is supine in order to relax the sternocleidomastoid muscles. The line of the examiner's vision must be at right angles to the movement the examiner is trying to see. Small pulsations of the internal jugular veins may be seen normally when the patient is supine. The movements may become a little more apparent as the trunk of the subject is elevated a few degrees. The pulsations, if seen, disappear when the trunk of the patient is elevated 30° from the horizontal plane of the bed or examining table.

The neck vein pulsations should be observed while the observer listens to the heart because the first and second heart sounds become the reference points for the identification of the specific waves that compose the internal jugular venous pulse.

The examiner should diagram the heart sounds and the contour of the venous pulse on the patient's medical record.

## Normal and Abnormal Jugular Venous Pulsations

The *normal internal jugular* venous pulse is shown in Fig. 7-2A. The a wave is produced when the right atrium propels its contents of blood into the right ventricle during the last phase of right ventricular diastole. An a wave is not produced when there is atrial fibrillation (see Fig. 7-2B). When the a wave is easily seen, and its dis-

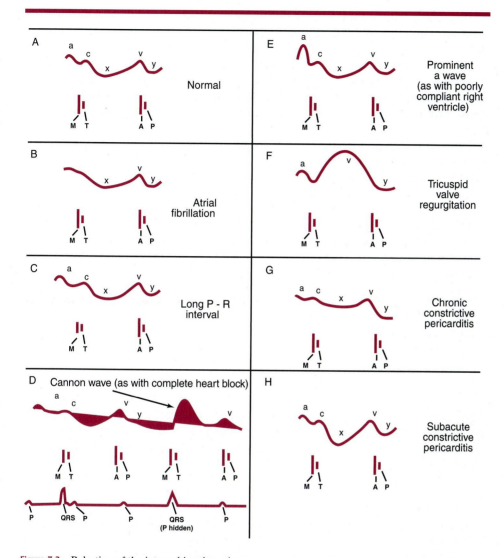

Figure 7-2  Pulsation of the internal jugular veins.

tance from the first heart sound seems to be longer than usual, the P-R interval may be longer than normal (see Fig. 7-2C). The a wave becomes very prominent when the right atrium contracts against a closed tricuspid valve, as it does when there is complete heart block or when there is ventricular tachycardia. These large a waves are called cannon waves (see Fig. 7-2D).

The a wave becomes prominent when there is tricuspid valve stenosis or when there is poor compliance of the right ventricle, as occurs with right ventricular hypertrophy (see Fig. 7-2E).

The c wave is due to the upward displacement of the tricuspid valve during early right ventricular systole. It is difficult to see and has no diagnostic value (see Fig. 7-2*A*).

The x descent occurs as blood flows into a relaxed right atrium during right atrial diastole and right ventricular systole (see Fig. 7-2*A*). The x descent decreases when there is atrial fibrillation (see Fig. 7-2*B*). A prominent x descent may be seen in patients with subacute constrictive pericarditis and pericardial effusion (see Fig. 7-2*H*).

The v wave normally occurs when the right atrium becomes filled with blood just before the tricuspid valve opens at the end of right ventricular systole (see Fig. 7-2*A*). A large v wave occurring during ventricular systole is usually due to tricuspid valve regurgitation (see Fig. 7-2*F*). It is an excellent sign of tricuspid valve regurgitation because a murmur may not be present.

The y descent occurs when the blood flows from the full right atrium into the right ventricle during early ventricular diastole (see Fig. 7-2*A*). The y descent is slowed when there is tricuspid valve stenosis and is more rapid when there is chronic constrictive pericarditis (see Fig. 7-2*G*).

# IDENTIFICATION OF PULSATION LOCATED ON THE FRONT OF THE CHEST

## Mind-Set

The mind-set should be to look for and exclude abnormal pulsations of the aorta, pulmonary artery, right ventricle, and left ventricle; atrial and ventricular gallop movements; and ectopic pulsations due to myocardial infarction or dilated cardiomyopathy.

## Technique of Examination

The movements made by the heart may be visible and palpable. In fact, some movements are more easily seen, and other movements are more easily felt. The patient should be lying supine, and the line of the examiner's vision must be at right angles to the direction of the movement that is being examined.

The first and second heart sounds should be used as reference points. The examiner should diagram the precordial movements in the patient's medical record.

## Normal and Abnormal Movements of the Anterior Portion of the Chest

Six areas of the precordium should be inspected and palpated (see Fig. 7-3*A*). No movement is normally seen or felt in area 1. A small systolic pulsation may be felt in area 2 in excited children. It is due to pulsation of the pulmonary artery. No movement is seen or felt in this area in normal adults. The pulsation of the normal right

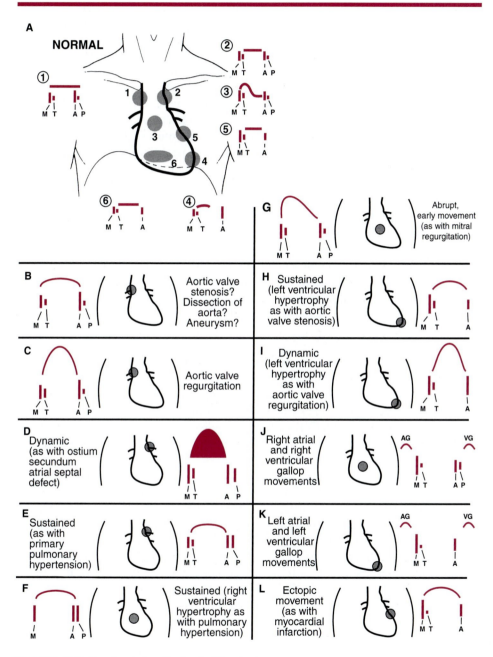

Figure 7-3   Pulsations located on the front of the chest.

ventricle may be felt in area 3. The movement of the normal left ventricle can be felt at the cardiac apex, which is located in the fourth or fifth intercostal space just to the right of the left midclavicular line (area 4). This area is smaller than a quarter, and the pulsation lasts about one-third of systole. Normally no pulsation is felt in area 5, and no pulsation is detected beneath the ensiform cartilage (area 6). The normal pulsations produced by the heart are shown in Fig. 7-3A.

An abnormal systolic movement may be detected in area 1 (see Fig. 7-3B). It may be caused by *dilatation of the aorta* in patients with aortic valve stenosis. In such a case, the movement is of low amplitude but sustained during systole. A similar pulsation may be felt in patients with a dilated aortic root due to an atherosclerotic aneurysm of the aorta and in patients with Marfan syndrome. Dissection of the aorta may produce a sustained prominent systolic movement in the same area; the sternoclavicular joint may move in systole in such cases.

A *dynamic pulsation* may be detected in area 1 in patients with aortic regurgitation (see Fig. 7-3C).

The pulsation of an *enlarged pulmonary artery* may be felt in systole in area 2. The movement in systole is dynamic when there is an increase in pulmonary blood flow, as there is in patients with an ostium secundum atrial septal defect (see Fig. 7-3D). A more sustained pulsation of the pulmonary artery may be felt when there is post-stenotic dilatation of the pulmonary artery due to pulmonary valve stenosis. An abnormal and sustained systolic pulsation may be detected when there is pulmonary artery hypertension from any cause (see Fig. 7-3E).

*Right ventricular hypertrophy* from any cause may produce a sustained systolic movement of area 3 (see Fig. 7-3F). This is almost always due to an increase in right ventricular systolic pressure, as occurs with pulmonary valve stenosis or pulmonary arterial hypertension from any cause. An exception is cor pulmonale due to obstructive lung disease, in which the abnormal pulsation of the right ventricle may be felt by the ends of the fingers when the fingers are placed beneath the ensiform cartilage in area 5.

Severe mitral valve regurgitation may produce a *brisk abnormal systolic movement* of area 3 (see Fig. 7-3G). This occurs because the left atrium is located in the center of the chest just anterior to the vertebral column. A rapidly expanding left atrium due to severe mitral regurgitation kicks the remainder of the heart anteriorly, producing an abnormal pulsation in area 3.

Left ventricular hypertrophy can be identified by studying area 4. The signs of left ventricular enlargement are as follows: The apex impulse may be located to the left of the midclavicular line in the fifth intercostal space, the apex impulse may be larger than a quarter, and the movement during systole may last longer than one-third of systole. The movement produced by left ventricular hypertrophy due to systolic pressure overload, such as that caused by valvular aortic stenosis, may be sustained and less dynamic (see Fig. 7-3H) than the movement produced by left ventricular hypertrophy due to diastolic overload of the left ventricle, as occurs with aortic valve regurgitation (see Fig. 7-3I).

*Right atrial and right ventricular gallop movements* may be detected in area 3 (see Fig. 7-3J). Detection of right atrial gallop movements suggests that there is poor compliance of the right ventricle. Identification of right ventricular gallop movements suggests that there is right ventricular dysfunction.

*Left atrial and left ventricular gallop movements* may be detected in area 4. These movements may be palpated when the gallop sounds are not heard because the very low frequency vibrations are barely within the range of audibility. The presence of an atrial gallop movement suggests that there is poor left ventricular compliance. The presence of a ventricular gallop movement suggests that there is left ventricular dysfunction (see Fig. 7-3K).

Area 5 is an ectopic area. An abnormal systolic movement can be felt in that area in some patients with *myocardial infarction* and in occasional patients with dilated cardiomyopathy (see Fig. 7-3L).

Area 6 is palpated when there is evidence of pulmonary emphysema. *Right ventricular hypertrophy* may be detected in such patients by pressing the ends of the fingers cephalad under the ensiform cartilage. The systolic movement of the large right ventricle strikes the ends of the fingers while the systolic movement of the aorta strikes the palmar surface of the fingers.

# AUSCULTATION OF THE HEART AND ELSEWHERE

On the one hand, auscultation of the heart is a simple act, but on the other hand, it is quite complex. No one has a problem hearing something, but hearing all that should be heard, deducing the physiologic phenomenon that causes the noises, and then deducing what the altered anatomy may be requires considerable skill and thought. Accordingly, not everyone who uses a stethoscope garners the same information. This problem has led to the overuse of expensive high technology, with the result that students do not master the skill of auscultation and the cost of medical care increases.

The stethoscope should have a bell and a diaphragm. To "play" the instrument, the examiner uses the bell to listen for low-pitched sounds and murmurs. This includes listening for atrial and ventricular gallop sounds and low-pitched rumbling diastolic murmurs at the cardiac apex. The bell should be applied lightly to the skin. The examiner should use the diaphragm to listen for high-pitched sounds and murmurs. This includes listening to aortic valve, mitral valve, tricuspid valve, and pulmonary valve closure sounds; ejection clicks; ejection sounds; an opening snap; systolic murmurs; and the murmurs of aortic valve regurgitation and pulmonary valve regurgitation. The diaphragm should be applied to the skin with firm pressure. The tubing should be as short as possible, but the comfort of the examiner must be maintained.

The usual auscultatory areas are shown in Fig. 7-4. They are the second right intercostal space near the sternum (area 1 in Fig. 7-4), the second left intercostal space near the sternum (area 2 in Fig. 7-4), the left sternal border (area 3 in Fig. 7-4), the midsternal area (area 4 in Fig. 7-4), the right sternal border (area 5 in Fig. 7-4), the cardiac apex (area 6 in Fig. 7-4), the lower sternal area (area 7 in Fig. 7-4), the neck, to the left of the cardiac apex, the back, and over the spine, sacrum, and head.

Figure 7-4   Where to place the end of the stethoscope.

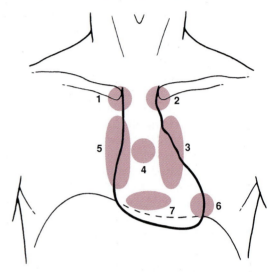

The position of the patient is important. The heart should be listened to when the patient is supine, when the patient is sitting and leaning forward, when the patient is in the left lateral recumbent position after exercise, when the patient is standing and squatting, and during inspiration and expiration.

## HEART SOUNDS

### Mind-Set

The mind-set should be to assume that the heart sounds are abnormal; the examiner's role is to exclude the presence of abnormal sounds. In other words, the examiner should assume that the mitral valve closure sound is abnormally loud; the pulmonary valve closure sound is abnormally faint or loud; the aortic valve closure sound is abnormally faint or loud; the second sound is widely split; the second sound is paradoxically split; there is fixed splitting of the second sound; there are left and right atrial gallop sounds and left and right ventricular gallop sounds; there is an ejection click; there is an ejection sound; there is an opening snap of the mitral valve; there is a pericardial friction sound. The act of excluding the presence of abnormalities implies that the examiner knows what to listen for, listens for it, and determines whether it is present or not. The old admonition is correct: One finds what one looks for.

### Technique of Examination

It is useful to listen initially in the second right intercostal space near the sternum because in this area (area 1 in Fig. 7-4) the normal second sound is always louder than the normal first sound. This permits the definite identification of systole and diastole. The examiner should then listen in sequence to the other areas shown in Fig. 7-4.

Finally, the examiner should be able to diagram the heart sounds and murmurs of a patient. The diagram should be placed in the patient's medical record.

**NORMAL HEART SOUNDS.**   Heart sounds are produced by a short series of vibrations. Murmurs are produced by a long series of vibrations. The first sound is produced by mitral valve closure; it is followed almost imperceptibly by tricuspid valve closure. The second sound is produced by aortic valve closure; it is followed by pulmonary valve closure. The comparative intensity of the two components of the two heart sounds varies according to the area where the examiner listens (see Fig. 7-5).

Normal children and adolescents may have a third heart sound in diastole at the apex. The sound coincides with the normal rapid inflow of blood into the left ventricle from the left atrium.

**ABNORMAL HEART SOUNDS.**   *Intensity of the First Heart Sound.*   The initial judgment about the intensity of the first heart sound is made by listening in the second right intercostal space adjacent to the sternum. As stated earlier, the second

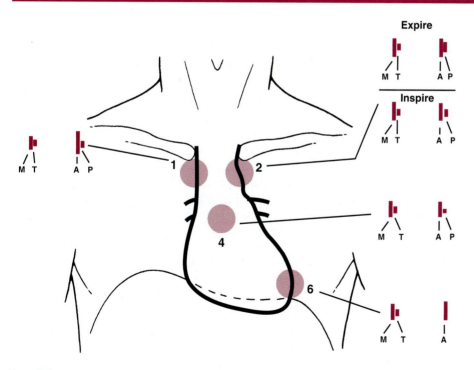

Figure 7-5   Normal heart sounds.

sound is normally louder than the first sound in this space; this is because the loud aortic valve closure sound contributes so much to the intensity of the second heart sound in this area (see Fig. 7-5). When the first heart sound, which is predominantly produced by mitral valve closure, is louder than the second heart sound in the second intercostal space near the sternum, the examiner must conclude that either the first heart sound is abnormally loud or the second heart sound is abnormally faint (see Fig. 7-6A). The usual cause of a faint second sound that is identified in the area being discussed is aortic valve stenosis. If the murmur of aortic valve stenosis is not heard, the examiner can conclude that the first heart sound is louder than the second heart sound because the mitral valve closure sound is abnormally loud. The most common cause of a louder than normal mitral valve closure sound heard in the second right intercostal space near the sternum is mitral valve stenosis.

The intensity of the first heart sound should also be judged while listening to the cardiac apex (area 6 in Fig. 7-5). The intensity of the first heart sound is determined by three variables.

1.   The most important factor that determines the intensity of the first heart sound is the interval of time between atrial contraction and ventricular contraction. When the interval of time is long, the first heart sound is faint (see Fig. 7-6B). When it is short, the first heart sound is loud (see Fig. 7-6C). The loudness of the first heart sound correlates with the duration of the P-R interval in the electrocardiogram; when the P-R interval is 0.20 to 0.24 s, the first sound is faint, and when the P-R interval is 0.14 to 0.16 s, the first heart sound is loud. Anyone trying to learn the skill of auscultation should correlate the intensity of the first heart sound with the P-R interval in the electrocardiogram.

2.   The structural characteristics of the mitral valve determine the flexibility of the leaflets. When the leaflets are destroyed by disease or cannot coapt properly because of dilatation of the mitral valve annulus, the first sound may be faint (see Fig. 7-6D). When the leaflets are thick, stiff, and fibrosed, as occurs in mitral stenosis, the first heart sound is often louder than average (see later discussion). Should the mitral valve leaflets become heavily calcified, they become immobile; when this occurs, the first heart sound may not be louder than average.

3.   The first heart sound may be louder than usual when the force of left ventricular contraction is greater than average, as it is with thyrotoxicosis or excitement. This factor, however, is not as important in determining the loudness of the first heart sound as the two factors mentioned previously.

***Abnormal Intensity of the Aortic Valve Closure Sound.***    The aortic valve closure sound may be louder than average in patients with systemic hypertension (see Fig. 7-6E). This abnormality is detected when listening to the heart in the second right intercostal space adjacent to the sternum. At times the aortic valve closure sound in such patients is said to have a tambour quality to it.

The aortic valve closure sound may become fainter than average when there is aortic valve stenosis (see Fig. 7-6F). This abnormality is detected while listening in the second right intercostal space next to the sternum. The aortic valve closure sound may not be heard at all when there is severe aortic valve stenosis. The inten-

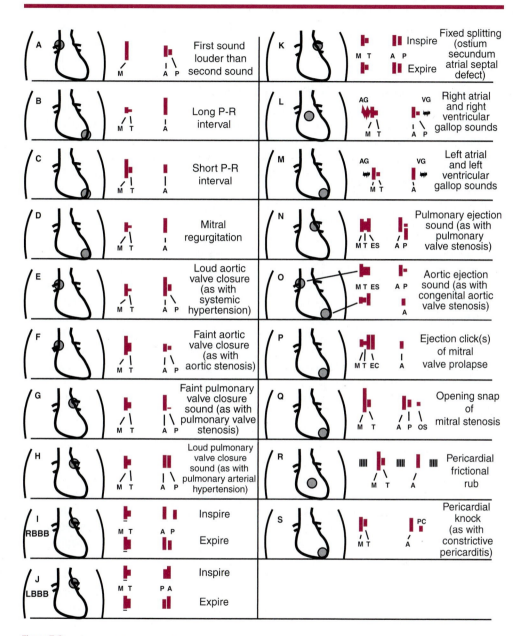

Figure 7-6   Abnormal heart sounds.

sity of the entire second heart sound may be diminished markedly when there is severe aortic valve stenosis, when there is paradoxical splitting of the second heart sound, and when the tail end of the systolic aortic murmur overrides the pulmonary valve closure sound.

***Abnormal Intensity of the Pulmonary Valve Closure Sound.***  The examiner should listen for the pulmonary valve closure sound in the second left intercostal space adjacent to the sternum. The pulmonary valve closure sound is abnormally faint when there is pulmonary valve stenosis (see Fig. 7-6G) and abnormally loud when there is pulmonary artery hypertension due to any of the many causes (see Fig. 7-6H). The latter is suspected when the pulmonary valve closure sound is easily identified, when it is equal to or louder than the aortic valve closure sound, or when it is heard at the cardiac apex (normally the pulmonary closure sound is not heard at the apex or, if it is, is very faint).

***Abnormal Splitting of the Second Heart Sound.***  Abnormal splitting of the second heart sound is identified while the examiner listens in the second left intercostal space near the sternum. Normally the two components of the second heart sound almost coincide during the time the patient expires and separate a little when the patient inspires (see Fig. 7-5). During inspiration, there is an increase in the blood rushing into the right ventricle. This prolongs right ventricular systole a fraction of a second. This, in turn, delays the closure of the pulmonary valve. This physiologic response should be sought each time the examiner listens to the heart.

Abnormal splitting of the components of the second heart sound occurs in the following three conditions:

1.  Wide splitting of the second heart sound occurs with right bundle branch block (see Fig. 7-6I). The components of the second heart sound are noted to be separated more than normal during the time the patient expires, and the split becomes even wider during the time the patient inspires. This occurs because there is a delay in the electrical activation and mechanical contraction of the right ventricle when there is right bundle branch block. This finding should be correlated with the finding of right bundle branch block in the electrocardiogram, and vice versa.
2.  Paradoxical splitting of the second heart sound occurs when there is left bundle branch block (see Fig. 7-6J) or severe aortic valve stenosis. The electrical excitation of the left ventricle and subsequent contraction are delayed when there is left bundle branch block. Accordingly, the closure of the aortic valve is delayed. This delay causes the aortic valve closure sound to occur after the pulmonary valve closure sound. So, when the patient inspires, the second sound becomes almost single, and when the patient expires, the second sound is split. This is, of course, opposite to normal. The examiner can become proficient by correlating the observation he or she makes by auscultation with the electrocardiogram.

3.  Wide fixed splitting of the second heart sound is almost diagnostic of ostium secundum atrial septal defect. The second heart sound is widely split on expiration and remains widely split on inspiration (see Fig. 7-5K). This occurs because the larger than normal amount of blood entering the right ventricle and traversing the pulmonary valve is the same during inspiration and expiration. Let us assume that the amount of blood entering the right atrium is 6 L. During inspiration, 4 L enters the right atrium via the superior vena cava and 2 L enters the right atrium through the shunt. During expiration, the reverse occurs, and so the amount of blood entering the right ventricle remains the same as during inspiration.

*Atrial Gallop Sound.*   A right atrial gallop sound may be heard to the left near the midportion of the sternum (see Fig. 7-6L). The sound is low-pitched and increases in intensity during inspiration. It is due to a poorly compliant (stiff) right ventricle such as occurs when there is right ventricular hypertrophy from any cause.

A left atrial gallop sound may be heard at the cardiac apex (see Fig. 7-6M). The sound is low-pitched and does not increase in intensity during inspiration. It is due to a poorly compliant left ventricle such as occurs with left ventricular hypertrophy from any cause.

*Ventricular Gallop Sound.*   A right ventricular gallop sound may be heard to the left of the midportion of the sternum (see Fig. 7-6L). The sound is low-pitched and increases in intensity during inspiration. It is a sign of right ventricular dysfunction due to one of many causes.

A left ventricular gallop sound may be heard at the cardiac apex (see Fig. 7-6M). The sound is low-pitched and does not increase in intensity during inspiration. With few exceptions, it is a sign of left ventricular dysfunction due to one of many causes. However, such a sound occurs normally in children, adolescents, and young adults, and may occur in patients with mild mitral valve regurgitation.

*Ejection Sound.*   This term should not be confused with the term *ejection click*. A pulmonary valve ejection sound is high-pitched and follows the first heart sound. It is heard best in the second left intercostal space near the sternum (see Fig. 7-6N). It may be present in patients with congenital pulmonary valve stenosis. In such a case, it is due to buckling of the dome-shaped pulmonary valve in early systole. It may also occur in patients with an ostium secundum atrial septal defect because the large systolic ejection of the right ventricle may produce an abrupt movement of the pulmonary artery.

An aortic ejection sound may be heard in patients with a congenital bicuspid aortic valve (see Fig. 7-6O). The sound is high-pitched in intensity and is heard best at the cardiac apex. It is due to buckling of the aortic valve. Such a sound may also be heard in the second right intercostal space near the sternum in patients with aortic valve regurgitation. It is due to a rapid movement of the aorta as a result of a rapid ventricular systolic ejection.

***Ejection Click.***    An ejection click is a high-pitched sound heard in early or mid-systole at the cardiac apex (see Fig. 7-6P). It may or may not be followed by the high-pitched systolic murmur of mitral regurgitation. The examiner should listen to the patient while the patient is standing. In this position, the ejection click becomes louder and moves toward the first heart sound. An ejection click, with or without a systolic murmur, occurs with mitral valve prolapse. Mitral valve prolapse is commonly due to myxomatous degeneration of the mitral valve leaflets and chordae tendineae.

***Opening Snap of the Mitral Valve.***    An opening snap of the mitral valve and a loud first heart sound are almost aways due to mitral valve stenosis which is secondary to rheumatic fever. These findings, which are heard at the cardiac apex, are widely distributed over the entire anterior surface of the chest. The opening snap is a high-pitched sound heard best at the apex (see Fig. 7-6Q). It is produced when the mitral valve buckles as the blood flows from the left atrium into the left ventricle during ventricle diastole. It occurs just after the second heart sound but earlier than the low-pitched sound of a left ventricular gallop. When the interval between the aortic valve closure sound and the opening snap is brief, this is a signal that the mitral stenosis is severe. When the interval between the aortic valve closure sound and the opening snap is relatively long, this is a signal that the mitral stenosis is mild.

A tumor "plop" due to a left atrial myxoma simulates an opening snap of the mitral valve.

***Pericardial Friction Rub.***    A series of high-pitched vibrations may be produced by pericarditis. A rub sounds like rubbing the finger briskly across sandpaper. The abnormal sounds are made when the heart moves during atrial systole, ventricular systole, and ventricular diastole (see Fig. 7-6R).

***Pericardial Knock.***    A pericardial knock occurs after the second heart sound. It is heard at the cardiac apex and is usually higher-pitched than a ventricular gallop sound (see Fig. 7-6S). It occurs in some patients with long-standing constrictive pericarditis.

# MURMURS

A short series of vibrations produces a sound and a long series of vibrations produces a murmur.

## Mind-Set

The mind-set of the examiner is that the patient has murmurs caused by aortic valve stenosis, aortic valve regurgitation, subaortic stenosis, pulmonary valve stenosis, pulmonary valve regurgitation, mitral stenosis, mitral valve regurgitation, tricuspid stenosis, tricuspid valve regurgitation, coarctation of the aorta, an interventricular septal defect, a patent ductus arteriosus, and a peripheral arteriovenous fistula. The examiner's job is to listen for all of these abnormal murmurs and be able to exclude their presence.

## Technique

The usual anatomic areas that should be auscultated are shown in Fig. 7-4.

The intensity (loudness) of murmurs is classified as follows by Freeman and Levine:[5]

Grade 1   The murmur is not heard immediately.
Grade 2   The murmur is heard immediately but is only slightly louder than a grade 1 murmur.
Grade 3   The murmur is moderately loud.
Grade 4   The murmur is louder than a grade 3 murmur but is not heard when a part of the rim of the stethoscope is applied to the chest wall.
Grade 5   The murmur is heard when a part of the rim of the stethoscope is applied to the chest wall.
Grade 6   The murmur is heard when the stethoscope is not applied to the chest wall.

## Observations Made by Listening in the Second Right Intercostal Space Adjacent to the Sternum

**AORTIC VALVE SCLEROSIS.**   The high-pitched systolic murmur of aortic valve sclerosis is diamond-shaped. The peak intensity is in midsystole or earlier. The second heart sound is normal (see Fig. 7-7*A*). It is caused by a stiffer than normal aortic valve. With the passage of time, the valve may become stenotic.

**AORTIC VALVE STENOSIS.**   The characteristics of the murmur of aortic valve stenosis depend upon the severity of the stenosis. *Mild aortic valve stenosis* produces a high-pitched, diamond-shaped murmur; the aortic valve closure sound may be slightly diminished in intensity. It may be about equal in intensity to the first heart sound, which is produced, for the most part, by mitral valve closure (see Fig. 7-7*B*). *Moderately severe aortic valve stenosis* produces a diamond-shaped murmur. The murmur may be a little more coarse than when there is mild aortic valve stenosis. The intensity of the murmur may peak at the end of the middle third of systole, and the aortic valve closure sound may be fainter than normal (see Fig. 7-7*C)*. As the severity of stenosis increases, the murmur may sound like "clearing the throat." *Severe aortic valve stenosis* produces a harsh systolic murmur; the intensity of the murmur peaks late in systole (see Fig. 7-7*D*). The aortic valve closure sound is delayed, and paradoxical splitting of the second sound may be present (not shown in illustration). The aortic valve closure sound may be faint or not heard at all. The tail end of the murmur may override and mask the pulmonary valve closure sound. The murmur may radiate to the right side of the neck and right shoulder.

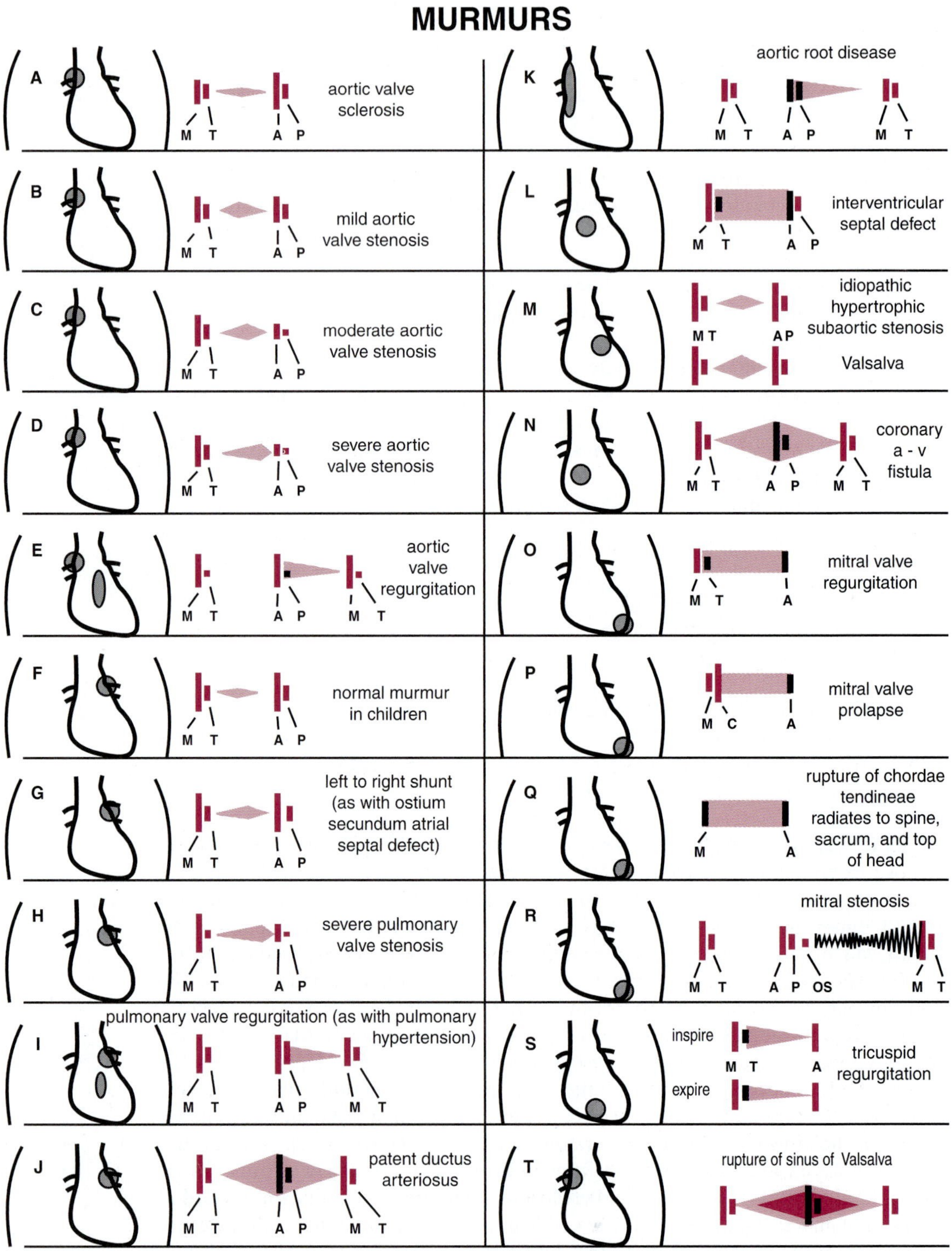

# MURMURS

**A** — aortic valve sclerosis
M T A P

**B** — mild aortic valve stenosis
M T A P

**C** — moderate aortic valve stenosis
M T A P

**D** — severe aortic valve stenosis
M T A P

**E** — aortic valve regurgitation
M T A P M T

**F** — normal murmur in children
M T A P

**G** — left to right shunt (as with ostium secundum atrial septal defect)
M T A P

**H** — severe pulmonary valve stenosis
M T A P

**I** — pulmonary valve regurgitation (as with pulmonary hypertension)
M T A P M T

**J** — patent ductus arteriosus
M T A P M T

**K** — aortic root disease
M T A P M T

**L** — interventricular septal defect
M T A P

**M** — idiopathic hypertrophic subaortic stenosis
M T A P
Valsalva
M T A P

**N** — coronary a - v fistula
M T A P M T

**O** — mitral valve regurgitation
M T A

**P** — mitral valve prolapse
M C A

**Q** — rupture of chordae tendineae radiates to spine, sacrum, and top of head
M A

**R** — mitral stenosis
M T A P OS M T

**S** — tricuspid regurgitation
inspire
M T A
expire

**T** — rupture of sinus of Valsalva

Figure 7-7   Murmurs.

A loud systolic murmur may be heard in patients with severe aortic valve regurgitation; it is due to the large systolic ejection of blood from the left ventricle.

Aortic valve stenosis may be congenital (bicuspid aortic valve) or may be caused by rheumatic heart disease or by calcific aortic valve disease of the elderly, which is believed by some to be atherosclerotic in origin.

**AORTIC VALVE REGURGITATION.**   The murmur of aortic valve regurgitation occurs in diastole. It is high-pitched and is heard best with the diaphragm of the stethoscope. The murmur begins with aortic valve closure and becomes less loud as diastole progresses; the murmur is said to be decrescendic. The murmur may be heard while listening in the second right intercostal space near the sternum but is more often heard along the left sternal border (see Fig. 7-7E). The examiner must listen at the left sternal border area of the patient when the patient is sitting, leaning forward, and when all the air has been exhaled from the lungs. The murmur of aortic regurgitation may also be heard at the cardiac apex.

When the murmur of aortic regurgitation is louder along the right sternal border than it is along the left sternal border, this is a clue that the patient may have aortic root disease (see later discussion).

Aortic valve regurgitation may be heard in patients with aortic valve disease due to rheumatic fever, systemic hypertension, myxomatous degeneration of the aortic valve, congenital bicuspid aortic valve, congenital heart disease with an interventricular septal defect and poorly supported aortic valve, acute dissection of the aorta, lupus erythematosus, osteogenesis imperfecta, rheumatoid arthritis, ankylosing spondylitis, trauma to the aortic valve, infective endocarditis, or syphilis.

## Observations Made by Listening to the Second Left Intercostal Space Adjacent to the Sternum

**NORMAL MURMUR.**   A systolic murmur may be heard in subjects with a normal heart who have a hyperdynamic circulation due to anemia, fever, or thyrotoxicosis or who are excited (especially children). If the examiner can distinguish this murmur by its setting and features from murmurs caused by valvular and other abnormalities, additional testing to characterize the murmur may be unnecessary. A normal murmur is usually grade 1 or 2 in intensity, and the first and second heart sounds are normal (Fig. 7-7F). Characteristically, a normal murmur peaks early in systole, less often in midsystole, as the hyperdynamic ventricular contraction produces an early peak to the murmur. The murmur should not be holosystolic or radiate to the axilla, but it may radiate minimally into the carotids. The carotid arterial upstroke is normal. The murmur is characteristically faint, with no accompanying thrill. Pregnancy in particular is often accompanied by a normal murmur. Experienced examiners can judge the extent to which the loudness and contour of the murmur are compatible with the patient's hyperdynamic state in pregnancy and other hyperdynamic disorders. The transient nature of some of these murmurs may be helpful to the examiner in distinguishing them from abnormal murmurs. The presence and intensity of a normal murmur should generally parallel the degree of hyperdynamic circulation. As the cause of the hyperdynamic circulation resolves, the murmur may diminish in intensity and eventually become inaudible.

**LEFT-TO-RIGHT SHUNTS WITH INCREASED PULMONARY BLOOD FLOW.**    A systolic murmur may be heard in the second left intercostal space near the sternum in patients with a left-to-right shunt at the atrial or ventricular level (see Fig. 7-7G). The murmur is due to the increase in blood flow across the pulmonary valve. The murmur is usually about grade 1 or 2 in intensity. Fixed splitting of the second heart sound during inspiration and expiration signals the presence of an ostium secundum atrial septal defect, and the murmur of an interventricular septal defect is almost diagnostic.

**PULMONARY VALVE STENOSIS.**    The murmur of pulmonary valve stenosis is diamond-shaped. It is located in the second left intercostal space near the sternum. It is usually heard best with the diaphragm of the stethoscope. The later the peak intensity occurs in systole, the more severe the stenosis is likely to be. The pulmonary valve closure sound may be fainter than normal (see Fig. 7-7H). When the stenosis is severe, the tail end of the murmur may override and mask the aortic valve closure sound, and the second sound may not be heard.

Pulmonary valve stenosis may be due to congenital heart disease or acquired carcinoid heart disease.

**PULMONARY VALVE REGURGITATION.**    The murmur of pulmonary valve regurgitation is usually high-pitched. It is heard best in the second left intercostal space near the sternum and along the left sternal border, where it may be confused with the murmur of aortic valve regurgitation. It is usually a sign of elevated pressure in the pulmonary artery. Accordingly, the pulmonary valve closure sound is commonly increased in intensity (see Fig. 7-7I). Pulmonary hypertension may be caused by Eisenmenger physiology, mitral stenosis, repeated pulmonary emboli, or primary pulmonary hypertension. Pulmonary valve regurgitation may also occur in patients with ostium secundum atrial septal defect in which there is dilatation of the pulmonary valve annulus and an increase in pulmonary blood flow, with or without pulmonary arterial hypertension.

Congenital pulmonary valve regurgitation is rare. When it is present, the diastolic decrescendic murmur is lower-pitched than it is when the murmur is caused by pulmonary artery hypertension.

**PATENT DUCTUS ARTERIOSUS.**    The murmur of patent ductus arteriosus is said to be continuous. It is almost always heard with maximum intensity in the second intercostal space next to the sternum (see Fig. 7-7J). The descriptive label suggests that the murmur lasts throughout systole and diastole. It is more accurate to view the murmur as being high-pitched, building in intensity during systole, masking the second heart sound, and decreasing in intensity during diastole. The systolic murmur "continues" through the second heart sound but may not continue through all of systole and diastole.

## Observations Made by Listening at the Left Sternal Border

The systolic murmur of aortic valve stenosis may be heard along the left upper sternal border (see the previous discussion of aortic valve stenosis). The murmur of aortic valve regurgitation may be heard best along the left sternal border (see Fig. 7-7E). In fact, it may be heard only in that location (see previous discussion).

## Observations Made by Listening at the Right Sternal Border

Whenever the high-pitched, diastolic murmur of aortic valve regurgitation is heard with maximum intensity along the right sternal border (area 5 in Fig. 7-4) as compared to its intensity along the left sternal border (area 3 in Fig. 7-4), it is wise to consider that it is caused by aortic root disease (see Fig. 7-7K). Aortic root disease may be due to dissection of the aorta or dilatation of the aorta in patients with Marfan syndrome.

## Observations Made at the Midsternal Area

The murmur of interventricular septal defect may be heard best in this location (area 4 in Fig. 7-4). The murmur lasts throughout systole (holosystolic) and is usually grade 3 to 4 in intensity (see Fig. 7-7L). This is usually a congenital defect but may be caused by rupture of the septum in patients with myocardial infarction and can be caused by trauma.

## Observations Made Halfway between the Second Right Intercostal Space near the Sternum and the Apex (Midpoint in Area 4 Shown in Fig. 7-4)

**IDIOPATHIC HYPERTROPHIC SUBAORTIC STENOSIS.**   The murmur of idiopathic hypertrophic subaortic stenosis is commonly heard best to the left of the midsternal area (see Fig. 7-7M). The second heart sound is commonly intact, aortic regurgitation is rarely evident, and the murmur decreases in intensity when the systolic blood pressure is increased with handgrip exercise. The murmur is increased in intensity when the patient does the Valsalva maneuver.

**MAMMARY SOUFFLE.**   A systolic bruit may be heard over the mammary artery in pregnant women. This is a normal finding caused by the increase in blood flow in the dilated mammary artery.

**CORONARY ARTERIOVENOUS FISTULA.**   Whenever a continuous murmur is heard in this area, it is more likely to be caused by a congenital coronary arteriovenous fistula (see Fig. 7-7*N*) than it is to be caused by a patent ductus arteriosus or rupture of the sinus of Valsalva.

## Observations Made at the Cardiac Apex

**MITRAL VALVE REGURGITATION.**   The systolic murmur of mitral valve regurgitation is high-pitched and is heard best with the diaphragm of the stethoscope. It may last throughout systole, be heard only during the last two-thirds of systole, or decrease in intensity during late systole. The louder the murmur, the more it tends to be heard laterally and over the base of the left lung.

*Rheumatic Mitral Valve Regurgitation.*   Rheumatic mitral valve regurgitation is now uncommon in the United States. The murmur may last throughout systole (see Fig. 7-7*O*). If this is an isolated finding, additional noncardiac information is needed in order to diagnose a rheumatic etiology.

*Mitral Valve Prolapse.*   This common condition may be mild, moderate, or severe (see Fig. 7-7*P*). The high-pitched murmur is ushered into systole by an ejection click or clicks. The murmur may be grade 1 to grade 4. The click becomes louder and moves toward the first heart sound when the patient stands. The condition is due to myxomatous degeneration of the mitral valve and chordae tendineae. It is usually benign but may produce arrhythmias or heart failure. One of the chordae tendineae may rupture, or the abnormal valve may be the site of bacterial endocarditis.

*Dilatation of the Left Ventricle.*   Mitral valve regurgitation may develop whenever the left ventricle becomes dilated. The anatomic distortion produced by left ventricular dilatation separates the papillary muscles so that they do not contribute normally to the closure of the mitral valve during ventricular systole. In addition to this, the mitral valve annulus dilates. This results in a systolic murmur due to mitral valve regurgitation.

*Rupture of the Chordae Tendineae.*   Acute rupture of the chordae tendineae of the mitral valve may produce acute pulmonary edema, hypotension, a loud left atrial gallop sound, and a loud, diagnostic systolic murmur at the cardiac apex (see Fig. 7-7*Q*). When the heart size is normal before the chordal rupture, it is likely to be normal immediately after the rupture. The heart rhythm is commonly normal unless it was abnormal before the rupture. The loud systolic murmur is located at the cardiac apex. The murmur usually radiates to the left. It may be heard over the vertebrae, over the cervical spine, over the sacrum, and at times on top of the head. This unusual radiation of the murmur is virtually diagnostic of rupture of the chordae tendineae.

Rupture of the chordae tendineae may be due to myxomatous degeneration of the mitral valve chordae, endocarditis, or trauma.

***Papillary Muscle Dysfunction and Rupture.***   Myocardial infarction may produce dyskinesis of the left ventricular myocardium located at the base of a papillary muscle. In addition, the papillary muscle itself may be ischemic. This produces poor contractility of the papillary muscle and leads to mitral valve incompetence. This causes a systolic murmur at the cardiac apex.

Papillary muscle rupture is usually due to myocardial infarction but may be caused by trauma. This may cause a systolic murmur due to mitral regurgitation. This murmur is usually heard at the cardiac apex, whereas the systolic murmur of a ruptured interventricular septum is heard near the midportion of the sternum. The murmur caused by papillary muscle rupture may not be very loud when there is systemic hypotension as a result of the myocardial infarction.

***Ostium Primum Atrial Septal Defect.***   A cleft mitral valve is commonly part of the congenital defect known as ostium primum atrial septal defect. This abnormality may produce a loud holosystolic murmur at the apex.

***Diastolic Rumble of Mitral Valve Blockade.***   The low-pitched diastolic rumble of mitral valve blockade is heard best with the bell of the stethoscope. The bell must be applied to the skin with light pressure. It is mandatory to listen to the cardiac apex when the patient is placed in the left lateral recumbent position after exercise.

*Mitral valve stenosis* may develop years after an episode of rheumatic fever. The loud first heart sound and opening snap are distributed all over the chest (see earlier discussions). The diastolic rumble, however, is localized to the cardiac apex (see Fig. 7-7R).

A *left atrial myxoma* is attached to a stalk that is anchored to the atrial septum. The tethered tumor can swing into and out of the mitral valve opening. A tumor "plop" emulates the opening snap of the mitral valve. The diastolic rumble may be louder when the patient sits. The tumor may beat against the valve leaflets until they are damaged, producing mitral valve regurgitation. This is known as the "wrecking ball" effect.

*Aortic valve regurgitation* may produce a low-pitched diastolic rumble at the apex. This murmur is known as an *Austin Flint murmur.* It is caused by partial closure of the mitral valve leaflets by the regurgitant stream of blood that occurs with aortic valve regurgitation. The other features of mitral stenosis are not present.

*Mitral regurgitation* of moderate degree can produce a diastolic rumble at the apex. It is due to the larger than normal volume of blood that must transverse the mitral valve during left ventricular diastole.

An *interatrial septal defect* may produce a tricuspid valve diastolic rumble which may be misinterpreted as emanating from the mitral valve. Patients with a *patent ductus arteriosus* or *interventricular septal defect* may have a diastolic rumble at the apex because the left-to-right shunts lead to a great increase in the amount of blood that must transverse the mitral valve during left ventricular diastole.

Many of the *prosthetic mitral valves* produce a diastolic rumble at the apex; there is often a small left atrial–left ventricular diastolic pressure gradient in these patients.

## Observations Made by Listening at the Lower End of the Sternum

**TRICUSPID REGURGITATION.**   Tricuspid regurgitation may produce a systolic murmur which is heard best at the lower end of the sternum (see Fig. 7-7S). The murmur increases in intensity during inspiration. The identification of a large, abnormal v wave in the deep jugular venous pulse due to tricuspid valve regurgitation occurs more often than the murmur.

Tricuspid regurgitation is usually due to dilatation of the right ventricle, which can be caused by severe left ventricular disease and heart failure, pulmonary disease, pulmonary hypertension from one of many causes, atrial septal defect, or carcinoid heart disease. The examiner should always consider the possibility of infective endocarditis as the cause of a new murmur due to tricuspid regurgitation in a febrile patient.

**TRICUSPID VALVE RUMBLE.**   Years ago tricuspid valve stenosis occurred occasionally as a result of rheumatic fever. Such patients usually had evidence of mitral and aortic valve disease. Today, when a low-pitched diastolic rumble is heard at the end of the sternum, the examiner should consider the possibility of carcinoid heart disease or that the rumbling, diastolic murmur is caused by a larger than normal blood flow across the tricuspid valve, as occurs with ostium secundum atrial septal defect. Fixed splitting of the second sound should clinch the latter diagnosis in such a patient.

## Observations Made at Nonconventional Locations

**RUPTURE OF A SINUS OF VALSALVA.**   This murmur develops suddenly and may be accompanied by acute dyspnea (see Fig. 7-7T). The new murmur is a continuous murmur. It is located in the second and third right intercostal spaces near the sternum. The continuous murmur caused by a patent ductus arteriosus is not heard with maximum intensity in that area.

**PERIPHERAL ARTERIOVENOUS FISTULA.**   The examiner should listen over every visible scar for a continuous murmur, regardless of the size of the scar. The examiner should listen over the sites where catheters or needles have been inserted previously as part of a diagnostic procedure. For example, if the femoral artery was used for cardiac catheterization, coronary arteriography, or coronary angioplasty, the astute examiner will listen over the puncture site even when no scar is seen.

**AUSCULTATION OF THE NECK, OVER THE RIBS, AND OVER THE KIDNEYS.** *Venous Hum.* A continuous murmur may be heard in the neck of normal young children. It is called a venous hum. It is caused by rapid blood flow in the veins of the neck of a normal child. It sounds like the roar of a large seashell. It is not heard when the child is recumbent but is heard when the child is sitting. The murmur becomes louder during inspiration, can be eliminated by appropriate pressure on the neck veins, and becomes higher-pitched when the head is turned and the neck is "stretched." A venous hum may be heard in adults with thyrotoxicosis or anemia and in pregnant women.

*Systolic Bruit in the Carotid Artery.* A systolic bruit may be heard in the left or right carotid artery. Such a finding usually signifies the presence of an atherosclerotic lesion in the carotid artery. It may, on rare occasions, be caused by fibromuscular hyperplasia. It is not always easy to separate a right carotid bruit from the murmur of aortic valve stenosis that radiates into the neck. Whenever there is a skip area below the bruit and the murmur of aortic valve stenosis is heard in the second right intercostal space, it suggests that both conditions are present.

*Coarctation of the Aorta.* This easily diagnosed condition may be recognized initially when bruits are heard over the tortuous intercostal arteries located in the back or when the murmur due to the coarctated segment of the aorta is heard over the midportion of the spine.

*Renal Artery Disease.* A systolic bruit may be heard over the kidneys when there is renal artery disease, such as atherosclerosis or fibromuscular hyperplasia. This examination should be performed in every patient with systemic hypertension.

---

### REFERENCES

1. Hurst JW: *Cardiovascular Diagnosis: The Initial Examination.* St. Louis, Mosby-Year Book, 1993:125–190.
2. Joint National Committee on Detection, Evaluation, and Treatment of High Blood Pressure: The Fifth Report of the Joint National Committee on Detection, Evaluation, and Treatment of High Blood Pressure (JNC V). *Arch Intern Med* 1993; 153:154–183.
3. Frank MJ, Casanegra T, Levinson GE: Evaluation of aortic insufficiency. *Circulation* 1963; 28:723.
4. Allen EV: Thromboangiitis obliterans; Methods of diagnosis of chronic arterial lesions distal to wrist with illustrative cases. *Am J Med Sci* 1929; 178:237–244.
5. Freeman AR, Levine SA: Clinical significance of systolic murmur: Study of 1,000 consecutive "non-cardiac" cases. *Ann Intern Med* 1933; 6:1371–1385.

THOMAS S. JOHNSTON

# EDEMA, ANASARCA, AND ASCITES

The edematous states are very common in clinical practice. In this chapter the pathophysiology, etiologies, differential diagnosis, and treatment of edematous states will be discussed.

## DEFINITIONS

Edema occurs when fluid accumulates in the interstitial tissues. Examination of the edematous patient reveals swelling of the extremities. Swelling with persistent indentation of the skin after pressure is applied is recognized as pitting edema. When the excess interstitial fluid is viscous, as occurs in lymphedema, for example, the skin is nonpitting, and no indentation is left after pressure is applied. Edema usually accumulates in dependent areas of the body. Therefore, edema is found in the lower extremities in ambulatory patients and in the sacral areas in bedridden patients. The interstitial volume must expand by several liters before edema is clinically apparent. Therefore, a weight gain of several pounds precedes edema formation. Anasarca is the term for generalized edema.

Ascites is the accumulation of fluid in the peritoneal space. Patients experience increasing abdominal girth and distention. On examination there is abdominal swelling, shifting dullness to abdominal percussion, and a demonstrable fluid wave on percussion of the abdomen.

## PATHOPHYSIOLOGY

Increased interstitial volume occurs when the net flux of fluid out of the capillary exceeds the capacity of the lymphatic system to carry the excess protein and water away from the interstitial space.[1] Starling's law governs the flux of fluid and protein out of the capillary; it is expressed as

$$\text{Net filtration} = K[(P_c - P_i) - (\pi_c - \pi_i)]$$

where $K$ is the filtration coefficient across the capillary membrane, $P_c$ is the hydrostatic pressure inside the capillary, $P_i$ is the hydrostatic pressure in the interstitium,

$\pi_c$ is the oncotic pressure of the plasma in the capillary, and $\pi_i$ is the oncotic pressure of the fluid in the interstitial space. Thus, increases in the capillary hydrostatic pressure, interstitial oncotic pressure, or capillary permeability favor edema formation. Furthermore, reduction in the plasma oncotic pressure also promotes edema.

When fluid moves from the vascular to the extravascular space, there is a fall in the plasma volume. Subsequently, in an attempt to maintain intravascular volume, the kidneys retain sodium and water. Some of this fluid remains in the blood vessels; however, a large amount crosses into the interstitial tissues, resulting in edema.[2]

In cases where the primary abnormality is inappropriate renal sodium retention, both the vascular and the interstitial volumes are expanded. This occurs mostly in primary renal diseases, but also as a result of hepatic failure and as a side effect of certain drugs.[2]

# ETIOLOGY OF EDEMATOUS STATES

There are numerous causes of edema. Table 8-1 lists the most common etiologies.

Congestive heart failure (CHF) is a syndrome characterized by the heart's inability at normal filling pressures to pump enough blood to meet the metabolic requirements of the body. The syndrome leads to symptoms of congestion (dyspnea, orthopnea, edema) and low cardiac output (fatigue, malaise). Low cardiac output leads to a decrease in effective circulating volume. Neurohormonal activation occurs in an attempt to maintain normal organ perfusion. The renin-angiotensin-aldosterone system and the sympathetic nervous system are activated. Vasopressin and endothelins are released. Despite simultaneous activation of counterbalancing vasodilatory and natriuretic substances, such as atrial natriuretic peptide, there is an increase in systemic vascular resistance as well as renal sodium and water retention. Increased blood volume results in an increased venous capillary hydrostatic pressure, thus promoting edema formation.[3]

Primary renal abnormalities prevent the excretion of sodium and water and lead to edema by increasing the plasma volume and increasing the venous capillary hydrostatic pressure. Most acute and chronic kidney diseases impair renal handling of sodium and water. Many medicines, including minoxidil, calcium channel blockers, $\beta$-adrenergic blockers, hydralazine, clonidine, methyldopa, nonsteroidal anti-inflammatory drugs, steroids, and estrogens, also lead to primary renal sodium retention. [2]

Nephrotic syndrome is caused by a variety of disorders and is characterized by an increased permeability of the glomerular capillary wall to protein. The clinical syndrome consists of hypoalbuminemia, edema, hyperlipidemia, lipiduria, and hypercoagulability. Hypoalbuminemia and the resultant reduction in plasma oncotic pressure favor the movement of fluid out of the vascular space into the interstitium. As with heart failure, this leads to a decreased effective circulating volume, neurohormonal activation, renal sodium and water retention, and edema. In addition, there may be primary sodium retention due to the underlying kidney disease, promoting

**TABLE 8-1.   Etiology of Edematous States**

***Increased capillary hydrostatic pressure***
  Increased blood volume due to renal $Na^+$ retention
    Heart failure
    Primary renal $Na^+$ retention
      Renal failure
      Drugs: minoxidil, calcium channel blockers, $\beta$-adrenergic blockers,
        hydralazine, clonidine, methyldopa, nonsteroidal anti-inflammatory drugs,
        steroids, estrogen
      ? Hepatic cirrhosis
      ? Idiopathic edema
    Pregnancy and premenstrual edema
  Venous obstruction
    Hepatic cirrhosis or hepatic venous obstruction
    Acute pulmonary edema
    Local venous obstruction

***Decreased plasma oncotic pressure***
  Protein loss
      Nephrotic syndrome
      Protein-losing enteropathy
  Reduced albumin synthesis
      Liver disease
      Malnutrition

***Increased capillary permeability***
  Burns
  Trauma
  Inflammation
  Allergic reactions
  Adult respiratory distress syndrome

***Increased interstitial oncotic pressure***
  Lymphatic obstruction
  Increased capillary permeability
  Hypothyroidism

*Source:* Rose BD: Clinical Physiology of Acid-Base and Electrolyte Disorders, 2d ed. New York, McGraw-Hill, 1984: 314, with permission.

further edema formation. The serum albumin is usually less than 2.5 g/dL, and more than 3.5 g of protein is lost in the urine during a 24-h period.[3]

The pathogenesis of ascites and edema formation in cirrhosis of the liver is complex. Irreversible chronic injury of the hepatic parenchyma leads to fibrosis, distortion of the hepatic vasculature, and nodular regeneration of the remaining liver parenchyma. The disrupted intrahepatic architecture leads to portal hypertension and an increase in splanchnic capillary bed pressure. This leads to hyperfiltration and extravasation of fluid from the capillary bed. Fibrotic changes in the liver parenchyma also impair lymphatic drainage. Increased production of vascular nitric oxide causes peripheral vasodilation.[4] The peripheral dilation leads to a relative underfilling of the circulation and a hyperdynamic circulatory state. This leads to neurohormonal activation, as occurs in heart failure, leading to renal sodium and water retention. There is less hepatic synthesis of proteins, leading to a reduction in serum albumin concentration. The resulting lower serum oncotic pressure also favors edema formation.  Because the failing liver is unable to metabolize aldosterone, circulating levels of this hormone are high, leading to more sodium retention.

Ascitic fluid can also accumulate in the peritoneal cavity when infection or peritoneal carcinomatosis produces inflammatory exudates faster than they can be resorbed.

During a normal pregnancy, the body's total water and sodium increases. Some 80 percent of pregnant women will experience edema during pregnancy, and this is considered normal.[5]

Idiopathic edema usually occurs in young, menstruating women in the absence of other medical illnesses that might cause edema. The etiology is unclear. Patients typically gain several pounds during the course of the day. Edema is generalized on the legs, hands, breasts, and abdomen. When the patient lies down, the edema is mobilized, and nocturia results in the overnight loss of the excess fluid. [2]

## DIFFERENTIAL DIAGNOSIS

A careful history and physical examination help determine the etiology of edema and ascites. The first step is to determine the distribution of the edema. Localized edema is usually due to obstruction of venous and/or lymphatic drainage. Generalized edema due to cardiac illness can be distinguished from edema from other causes by estimation of the central venous pressure through examination of the jugular veins. The serum albumin concentration and the degree of proteinuria aid in the diagnosis of nephrotic syndrome.

### Pulmonary Edema

Pulmonary edema is usually secondary to cardiac disease. The patient usually complains of shortness of breath, paroxysmal nocturnal dyspnea, and orthopnea. There are rales on auscultation of the lung. The cardiac examination usually reveals abnormal heart sounds, including gallops and murmurs. Chest x-ray confirms pulmonary edema. Pulmonary edema may also be noncardiac, as is the case with the adult respiratory distress syndrome. Primary renal sodium retention can also lead to pulmonary edema. Echocardiography and pulmonary artery catheterization can be helpful in distinguishing cardiac from noncardiac pulmonary edema. Interestingly, pulmonary edema does not occur as a result of hepatic cirrhosis or nephrotic syndrome because the fluid movement out of the intravascular space prevents the increase in venous return needed to increase left-sided filling pressures. Also, hypoalbuminemia does not lead to pulmonary edema because the pulmonary capillary is relatively permeable to albumin, and thus the pulmonary circulation does not depend on the oncotic pressure to hold fluid in the vascular space.[2]

## Bilateral Lower-Extremity Edema

Patients with CHF frequently have bilateral lower-extremity edema that is gradual in onset. There often is a past history of cardiac problems, such as coronary disease or hypertension. Symptoms of dyspnea on exertion, orthopnea, paroxysmal nocturnal dyspnea, and fatigue are often present. Physical examination reveals jugular venous distention and/or hepatojugular reflux. Most patients have abnormal heart sounds, including murmurs and gallops. Rales are heard at the bases of the lungs when pulmonary edema is present. Chest x-ray findings include cardiomegaly, engorgement of the pulmonary veins, cephalization of flow of the pulmonary vessels, and pulmonary edema. Echocardiography is often helpful in determining left and right ventricular function, valvular function, and the status of the pericardium.

Constrictive pericarditis may cause ascites and edema. Patients complain of weakness, fatigue, and shortness of breath. The neck veins are distended. There may not be the ordinary fall in venous pressure with inspiration (Kussmaul's sign), although this is difficult to recognize on physical examination. A pericardial knock, occuring shortly after $S_2$, is sometimes present on cardiac auscultation. Hepatic and splenic enlargement are common. Usually there is more ascites than peripheral edema. Electrocardiography shows diminished QRS voltage. Pericardial calcification is often seen on chest x-ray. Echocardiography, computed tomography (CT) of the chest, and cardiac magnetic resonance imaging (MRI) may show pericardial thickening.

In constrictive pericarditis, the hepatic enlargement and dysfunction associated with ascites may lead to the mistaken diagnosis of hepatic cirrhosis. Jugular venous distention distinguishes the diagnosis of constrictive pericarditis, however.

Cirrhotic patients may develop both ascites and bilateral lower-extremity edema. A history of chronic liver disease establishes the diagnosis. In hepatic cirrhosis, the jugular venous pulse is usually not elevated. In some patients, however, the etiology of the cirrhosis is cardiac, and the jugular veins may be distended. In cirrhosis there are usually other signs, including jaundice, parotid and lacrimal gland enlargement, clubbing of the fingers, palpable liver nodules, splenomegaly, distended abdominal wall veins, spider angiomata, palmar erythema, and testicular atrophy.

Patients with nephrotic syndrome have periorbital and bilateral lower-extremity edema. Occasionally ascites is present. The jugular veins are flat because there is relative hypovolemia as a result of the hypoalbuminemia. Patients have a serum albumin less than 2.5 g/dL and lose at least 3.5 g of protein in their urine in a 24-h period. The triglyceride level is usually elevated.

Patients with primary renal sodium retention are volume expanded and may have both pulmonary and peripheral edema. The neck veins are distended. Usually laboratory evaluation indicates severe renal failure. Cardiac examination is usually normal unless there is coexistent cardiac disease. Chest x-ray may show pulmonary edema. There is usually a normal cardiac silhouette. Echocardiography can assist in excluding cardiac causes of the edema.

Lymphedema and chronic venous stasis may involve one or more extremities. These entities are discussed below in the section on unilateral lower-extremity swelling.

## Unilateral Leg Swelling

Unilateral leg swelling is a very common clinical problem. The acuity of the edema is important in differentiating the cause. The physical examination of the lower extremity should focus on the size of the extremity, the presence of joint effusions, the circulation of the extremity, tenderness, and skin changes.

Causes of acute-onset (<72 h) unilateral leg swelling include acute deep venous thrombosis, popliteal (Baker's) cyst, rupture of the radial head of the gastrocnemius muscle, bacterial cellulitis, and erythema nodosum.[6]

Acute deep venous thrombosis is a common problem. Usually there are predisposing factors, such as recent trauma, immobilization, underlying malignancy, or hypercoagulable state. An acute onset of unilateral leg swelling and pain is typical. The edema is pitting, and the skin is frequently red and warm. The calf may be tender with a palpable venous cord. Homans' sign, calf discomfort when the foot is dorsiflexed, is unreliable in the diagnosis of deep venous thrombosis. Noninvasive venous duplex ultrasonography can detect areas of noncompressibility along the course of the affected veins (diagnostic of deep venous thrombosis). Venography, the gold standard, may be necessary to confirm the diagnosis. Acute deep venous thrombosis is an important consideration because of the risk of pulmonary embolism, a life-threatening complication.

A popliteal (Baker's) cyst may also cause unilateral leg swelling. Popliteal cysts are connected to the gastrocnemius membranous bursa in the calf, and synovial fluid can dissect from the knee bursa into the calf, inducing an inflammatory reaction. Typically patients have an underlying inflammatory joint disease, such as rheumatoid arthritis. The presentation consists of calf pain, unilateral leg edema, and the presence of a knee joint effusion. Ultrasonography and MRI can detect the abnormality and exclude acute deep venous thrombosis.

With rupture of the head of the gastrocnemius, there is severe calf pain at the time of the trauma, followed by calf swelling. In the case of bacterial cellulitis, there is spreading warmth, redness, and swelling in the involved extremity, along with fever and chills. Regional lymph nodes are enlarged and tender. Erythema nodosum is an inflammatory process that often results in unilateral swelling and red skin nodules. Constitutional symptoms such as fever, malaise, myalgias, and arthralgias are characteristic.

Etiologies of unilateral leg swelling of late onset (>72 h) are chronic venous insufficiency, lymphedema, reflex sympathetic dystrophy, congenital venous malformations, and malignancy.

Chronic venous insufficiency is a prevalent disease, affecting over 1.6 million Americans, and may cause either unilateral or bilateral edema. The most common causes are varicose veins, postthrombophlebitic syndrome, and congenital venous malformations. Venous valvular incompetence leads to increases in venous capillary pressure and ensuing accumulation of fluid, protein, and red blood cells in the interstitial space. Consequently, edema and a golden brown discoloration of the skin occur. Protein deposition in the skin leads to an inflammatory response that results in fibrosis and ulceration of the overlying skin. A common complaint is a deep dull ache in the affected extremity while standing that is relieved by elevation of the legs. Deep venous thrombosis must be considered.

Lymphedema is caused by malformation or obstruction of the lymphatic channels. The lymphatics drain proteinaceous fluid from the interstitium and return it to the systemic circulation. Obstruction of the lymphatics leads to painless edema. With time, the limb develops a woody texture and the edema is no longer pitting. Lymphedema may be congenital but more often is acquired as a consequence of cancer, trauma, surgery, radiation, or inflammation. A careful history and physical examination may identify the cause. Often supplemental testing with ultrasound, CT scanning, or MRI is required to make the diagnosis.

Reflex sympathetic dystrophy is characterized by burning pain, hyperesthesia, hyperhydrosis, trophic changes of the skin, and swelling of the affected extremity. Trauma, infection, and vascular insufficiency are etiologies of the syndrome. Central causes include brain tumors, cerebral infarctions, and spinal cord injuries. Paralysis can also reduce lymphatic and venous drainage of the affected side.

Bone and soft tissue tumors may also cause unilateral lower-extremity edema. Examination and x-rays usually clarify this diagnosis.

## Upper-Extremity Swelling

Upper-extremity swelling is an uncommon problem. Superior vena cava syndrome, lymphedema, and thoracic outlet syndrome are the most frequent etiologies. Obstruction or compression of the superior vena cava, usually by tumor, results in the superior vena cava syndrome. There is associated cyanosis and edema of the face, neck, and arms. The neck veins are dilated, and collateral veins on the anterior chest wall are seen. Compression of the subclavian artery and vein in the thoracic outlet results in edema and ischemia of the arm. Pain in the neck, shoulder, and arm is characteristic of the thoracic outlet syndrome. MRI or venography aids in the diagnosis.[7]

## Ascites

Chronic liver disease is the etiology of ascites in 80 percent of cases. Cardiac causes of ascites are associated with jugular venous distention and other cardiac findings. Nephrosis and malignancy are often easily recognized.

A paracentesis is indicated in all new cases of ascites. At a minimum, a complete blood count with differential, albumin level, and bacterial cultures should be obtained. In addition, cytology, an amylase level, Gram stain, and cultures and smear for acid-fast bacilli may also be helpful. The white blood cell count in the ascitic fluid is elevated in the case of bacterial peritonitis. Pancreatic ascites is associated with a high ascitic amylase level.

The serum-ascites albumin gradient can be used to distinguish the different etiologies of ascites. This gradient correlates directly with the portal pressure. The serum-ascites albumin gradient is calculated by subtracting the ascitic fluid albumin concentration from the serum albumin concentration at the time of the paracentesis. High-gradient ascites, indicating portal hypertension, is defined as a difference of 1.1 g/dL or more. Causes of high-gradient ascites include hepatic cirrhosis, heart failure, hepatic failure, Budd-Chiari syndrome, portal vein thrombosis, venoocclusive disease, extensive liver metastases, myxedema, and the fatty liver associated with pregnancy. For high-gradient ascites, a history and physical examination are usually sufficient to assess patients. When a patient with known liver disease develops high-gradient ascites, no additional evaluation is needed other than an ascitic fluid white blood count to exclude bacterial peritonitis. Causes of low-gradient (<1.1 g/dL) ascites are peritoneal carcinomatosis, tuberculosis, pancreatic ascites, bowel infarction or obstruction, nephrotic syndrome, infection, biliary ascites, postoperative lymphatic leakage, and serositis secondary to collagen vascular disease.[8]

## TREATMENT

Pulmonary edema is the only form of edema that necessitates urgent treatment. In other types of edema, the treatment can be more cautious, thus avoiding potential complications. The first step is treatment of the underlying disease process. After reversible causes of the edematous state have been eliminated, the next step is decreasing sodium in the diet. Avoidance of drugs that might promote edema, including nonsteroidal anti-inflammatory drugs, is important.

In cases of mild edema, a thiazide or low doses of a loop diuretic such as furosemide are usually sufficient to treat the swelling. In more severe cases, increasing dosages of loop diuretics are necessary. Potassium supplementation is often required. The addition of the potassium-sparing diuretic spironolactone also prevents hypokalemia.

Daily weighing at home is paramount in the care of the edematous patient. Weight gains can be treated with supplemental diuretics before clinically apparent edema occurs, preventing unnecessary emergency room visits and hospitalizations.

Risks of diuretic treatment include intravascular volume depletion resulting in orthostasis, weakness, fatigue, and azotemia. Teaching the patient how to recognize these symptoms at home before they become serious is important. Measurement of orthostatic blood pressures in the office and closely following serum electrolytes and renal function also is helpful.

With chronic venous insufficiency and lymphedema, patients should be advised to avoid prolonged standing. Frequent leg elevation is helpful. Graduated compression stockings should be worn during the day.

## REFERENCES

1.  Morrison RT: Edema and principles of diuretic use. *Med Clin North Am* 1997; 81:689–704.
2.  Rose BD: *Clinical Physiology of Acid-Base and Electrolyte Disorders,* 2d ed. New York, McGraw-Hill, 1984.
3.  Braunwald E: Edema. In: Fauci AS, Braunwald E, Isselbacher KJ, et al (eds): *Harrison's Principles of Internal Medicine,* 14th ed. New York, McGraw-Hill, 1998:210–214.
4.  Martin P, Schrier RW: Pathogenesis of water and sodium retention in cirrhosis. *Kidney Int* 1997; 51:S43–S49.
5.  Davison JM: Edema in pregnancy. *Kidney Int* 1997; 51:S90–S96.
6.  Merli GJ, Spandorfer J: The outpatient with unilateral leg swelling. *Med Clin North Am* 1995; 79:435–447.
7.  Powell AA, Armstrong MA: Peripheral edema. *Am Fam Physician* 1997; 55:1721–1726.
8.  Lipsky MS, Sternbach MR: Evaluation and initial management of patients with ascites. *Am Fam Physician* 1996; 54:1327–1333.

WILLIAM Z. H'DOUBLER /
ELLIOT L. CHAIKOF

CHAPTER

# THE COOL EXTREMITY

9

Initial evaluation of the cool extremity must assess the degree of ischemia and thus the acuity of need for referral. Patients can present with severe acute ischemia (usually secondary to an embolic event), acute ischemia (usually from thrombosis of a diseased vessel), or severe chronic ischemia. The etiologies, therapy, and prognosis vary with each presentation. This chapter will focus on identifying the acutely ischemic limb and evaluating severe chronic ischemia.

## ACUTE PERIPHERAL ARTERIAL OCCLUSION

Acute ischemia of the extremity requires prompt recognition and treatment. Delays in therapy can lead to severe functional deficits or limb loss. Acute arterial occlusion most commonly occurs secondary to embolus (usually cardiogenic) or thrombosis of diseased extremity vessels (Table 9-1).[1] Generally, patients with embolic phenomena have more severe ischemia and require emergency referral to a vascular surgeon. If they do not have previously formed collateral circulation, muscle necrosis can occur in less than 6 h from the onset of ischemia. Patients with acute thrombosis generally tolerate ischemia better, as they have developed collateral circulation. Regardless of the etiology, the history and physical examination determine the severity of the ischemia and thus the urgency of need for referral.

### Clinical Manifestations

The classic presentation of acute arterial ischemia is pain, pulselessness, pallor, paresthesia, paralysis, and poikilothermy (the six Ps). The main presenting complaint usually is severe, unrelenting pain in the affected limb. The pain is made worse with movement. Some 20 percent of patients will present with paresthesias manifested as tingling or "pins and needles" sensation in the foot.[2]

The differential diagnosis is limited. Phlegmasia cerulea dolens can progress to

**TABLE 9-1.**   Causes of Acute Arterial Ischemia

| |
|---|
| Arterial embolization (usually cardiac) |
| Thrombosis of atherosclerotic artery |
| Acute occlusion of a vascular graft |
| Atheroembolization |
| Arterial trauma |
| Thrombosis of popliteal or femoral aneurysm |
| Aortic dissection |

phlegmasia cerulea albans when the swelling occludes the arterial inflow. This can usually be distinguished from the more massive swelling characteristic of venous thrombosis. Low-flow states can lead to a cool extremity with decreased peripheral pulses. However, this entity would usually be encountered in the intensive care unit setting.

Pain is the most common manifestation of an acute arterial occlusion. The pain is often so abrupt in onset that the patient can relate the moment the symptoms occurred. The pain is constant in nature and is exacerbated by movement. As the ischemia progresses, sensory deficits may mask the pain and confuse the physician. Paresthesias are secondary to ischemia of peripheral nerves. Over time, the paresthesias will progress to loss of light touch sensation in the extremity. Later, more ominous symptoms of ischemia include loss of pressure and pain sensation and motor dysfunction. The examiner should elicit additional history about cardiac diseases and arrhythmia as well as any history of previous embolic events or prior anticoagulant use. A history of claudication, symptoms of rest pain, or other symptoms of chronic vascular disease make the diagnosis more likely to be an acute or chronic occlusion of a diseased vessel.

The physical examination proceeds in an orderly fashion, beginning with inspection and proceeding with palpation, feeling for pulses, and neurologic examination, specifically motor and sensory examination. Initially, the skin of the ischemic limb is white and cadaveric. Over time, the initial vasospasm eases and areas of local stasis develop, which leads to mottling of the skin. Capillary filling is absent or markedly delayed. Later signs of ischemia are skin blistering and necrosis. On palpation of the affected limb, one finds an ominously cool or cold extremity. The limb will be cool one joint below the site of occlusion. Thus iliac occlusion leads to a cool and mottled thigh, superficial femoral artery occlusion leads to the calf's being cool to touch, and popliteal or trifurcation occlusion leads to a cold foot. Absent pulses form the cornerstone of diagnosis. Pulses should be palpated with the examiner's dominant hand in a relaxed position to minimize the chance of the examiner's mistakenly feeling his or her own pulse. The contralateral extremity must also be examined. Signs of chronic ischemia in the uninvolved limb in conjunction with a history of claudication make the etiology more likely to be thrombosis of a diseased artery. As stated before, patients with thrombosis of a diseased vessel typically have less severe symptoms because of previously developed collateral circulation. Neurologic examination is critical in establishing the degree of ischemia and as a prognostic marker. Loss of light touch sensation is the earliest neurologic sign of ischemia. Typically the first area of anesthesia will be between the second and third toes of the ischemic extremity. Decreased motor function occurs after more prolonged ischemia and portends a more grim prognosis. Complete foot paralysis almost always requires amputation. Prolonged ischemia leads to muscle rigor, which always requires amputation.[3-5]

The hand-held Doppler should be used to examine the involved and uninvolved extremities. In the leg, the femoral, popliteal, dorsalis pedis, and posterior tibial vessels should be examined. When using the Doppler, it is important to distinguish venous from arterial signals. Venous sounds can exist with absent arterial signals.[6] Venous signals are more continuous but will often sound pulsatile. A helpful adjunct to distinguish venous from arterial Doppler signals is calf compression. Squeezing the calf while listening at the foot with the Doppler will augment the venous signal initially, and continued compression will eliminate the signal. Arterial flow will be heard despite manipulation of the calf.

If an arterial signal can be auscultated in the foot, then an ankle brachial index can be calculated. This is done by recording the highest systolic blood pressure from either arm and the highest pressure obtained from the dorsalis pedis or posterior tibial artery using a Doppler and blood pressure cuff. The brachial systolic pressure is divided by the ankle pressure.

Table 9-2 shows the clinical correlates with given ankle brachial indices. These values serve only to roughly quantitate extremity blood flow. This test is less helpful in the profoundly ischemic limb secondary to embolus, as frequently no arterial signal will be audible in the foot. Physical examination, especially the neurologic examination, is the best guide to the severity of the ischemia.

## Treatment and Complications

Initial therapy for patients with acute arterial occlusion begins with intravenous anticoagulation (heparin sodium 100 units per kilogram bolus). The heparin functions to prevent thrombosis in the microvasculature distal to the occlusion. It does not

**TABLE 9-2.   Lower-Extremity Ankle Brachial Indices and Corresponding Symptoms**

| | |
|---|---|
| Asymptomatic | ≥1.0 |
| Mild claudication | >0.8 |
| Moderate to severe claudication | 0.4–0.8 |
| Ischemic rest pain | <0.4 |
| Tissue loss | <0.5 |
| Limb-threatening ischemia | <0.15 |

lyse or open the occlusion. The patient with a cool extremity secondary to acute is-chemia should be immediately referred to a vascular surgeon for prompt manage-ment to optimize the outcome. After the diagnosis is made, patients with embolic disease and no prior peripheral vascular disease usually proceed quickly to the op-erating room for open embolectomy using catheters to extract the embolus and as-sociated thrombus. Arterial trauma is managed by direct repair of the injured seg-ment. Management of acute or chronic thrombosis varies depending on the severity of the ischemia. Therapy can involve endovascular techniques using catheter-directed thrombolytic therapy, operative thromboembolectomy, or operative by-pass. These patients usually undergo diagnostic arteriogram first because the less se-vere nature of the ischemia in this setting allows time for preoperative studies. It is better to study these patients first because they often have complex vascular disease, and an arterial road map greatly facilitates the conduct of the operation.[7] Compli-cations of acute arterial ischemia depend on the underlying pathology and the length of time from onset of the occlusion until restoration of flow. Patients may de-velop compartment syndrome, especially if the ischemic period is greater than 4 h. Sequelae of this include motor and sensory dysfunction, reperfusion injury (myo-globinuria, acute renal failure), and limb loss.

## Summary

The history and physical examination allow the physician seeing a patient with a cool extremity to establish a diagnosis and determine the acuity of need for treatment. The etiology of the ischemia can also usually be surmised. Because of the short time between the onset of symptoms and irreversible tissue loss, the clinician should quickly refer these patients to a vascular surgeon for expeditious treatment.

# SEVERE CHRONIC ARTERIAL INSUFFICIENCY

Chronic ischemia represents a spectrum of disease from asymptomatic to rest pain. Patients presenting with a cool extremity secondary to chronic ischemia usually have severe complex peripheral vascular disease and will frequently present with short-distance claudication, rest pain, ulceration, or gangrene of the affected limb.

## Clinical Manifestations

The history should focus on the time course of symptoms. The patient often relates a gradual onset and insidious progression of symptoms. The patient will often self-limit activity to avoid claudication and thus has an increasingly sedentary lifestyle until symptoms of pain at rest develop as a result of arterial insufficiency. Rest pain usually occurs at night with the patient supine. It is described as aching and burning in the forefoot. The pain is often relieved by hanging the foot in a dependent position. Other symptoms may include numbness or burning along ischemic nerves, disuse atrophy, cold sensitivity, or ulceration. Patients should be questioned about any past history of vascular disease or vascular surgical procedures. It is important that risk factors for vascular disease be defined. Cessation of smoking even in the setting of severe chronic ischemia can slow disease progression. Cigarette smoking stimulates atherogenesis and affects platelet function, lipid metabolism, and endothelial function. Acutely, smoking causes vasoconstriction and raises levels of carbon monoxide in the blood.[6,8] Other risk factors include diabetes mellitus, hypertension, and hyperlipidemia.

The physical examination should be unhurried and proceed in an orderly fashion. The limb should be inspected with the contralateral limb exposed to allow for comparison. The examiner looks for signs of infection, ulceration (especially between the toes), and old surgical scars. The chronic severely ischemic limb will be cool to the touch and show signs of inadequate nutrition, such as absent hair; thin, shiny skin; or thickened, hypertrophic nails.[9] Vascular disease is frequently symmetric; thus, the other limb should be inspected. The examiner checks pulses by first determining the patient's heart rate. This makes it easier to distinguish the examiner's pulse from the patient's pulse. Capillary refill is usually delayed in patients with chronic ischemia. Buerger's test can help assess the severity of ischemia. It is performed by elevating the limb, which leads to pallor of the extremity and often causes rest pain. The leg is then placed in a dependent position. Rubor develops in the foot and leg after it is dependent for several minutes. The neurologic examination should focus on motor and sensory function. The chronically ischemic extremity with evidence of anesthesia or motor weakness represents a threatened limb. These findings warrant prompt referral to a vascular surgeon.

As mentioned previously, the hand-held Doppler is an essential tool in evaluating the cool extremity without palpable pulses. An ankle brachial index should be calculated. Patients with calcified distal vessels (diabetics and patients with end-stage renal disease) will have artificially elevated ankle brachial indices. This test is of limited use in this group of patients.[10,11] In such patients, the noninvasive vascular laboratory can provide pulse volume recording studies which measure the volume changes (i.e., arterial inflow) in the limb and are not affected by arterial wall compliance. Absent or barely audible Doppler signals imply severe ischemia and impending tissue loss. This finding should lead to expeditious referral. Arteriography is not without risk and should be obtained only if surgical intervention is planned. Thus, an arteriogram to evaluate peripheral arterial occlusive disease is preferentially ordered by the consulting vascular surgeon.

## Treatment and Complications

Treatment of the severely ischemic limb usually requires surgical intervention. Arterial disease severe enough to cause a cool extremity is usually not adequately addressed with endovascular techniques alone. Patients with mild rest pain and no tissue loss can sometimes be managed nonoperatively, especially if they cease smoking. In this situation, the patient should be followed in conjunction with or by a vascular surgeon. The natural history of severe chronic ischemia is not clear. It is known that patients with rest pain and tissue loss usually require amputation if revascularization is not performed. Obviously, the most severe complication of chronic ischemia is major limb loss, often above or below the knee.

## Summary

The history and physical examination are essential in stratifying the patient with symptomatic chronic peripheral vascular disease. Use of the Doppler and noninvasive vascular laboratory studies provide additional information to localize the level of hemodynamically significant lesions. Patients with abnormal motor or sensory examination or absent or barely audible Doppler signals will benefit from early referral to a vascular surgeon. Intervention using either an endovascular or a classical operative approach will probably be required.

### REFERENCES

1. Dean RH, Yao JST, Brewster DC (eds): *Current Diagnosis and Treatment in Vascular Surgery*. Norwalk, Appleton and Lange, 1995.
2. Blaisdell FW, Steele M, Allen RE: Management of acute lower extremity ischemia due to embolism and thrombosis. *Surgery* 1978; 84:822.
3. Walker PM: Ischemia/reperfusion injury in skeletal muscle. *Ann Vasc Surg* 1991; 5:399–402.
4. Abbott WM, Maloney RD, McCabe CC, et al: Arterial embolism: A 44-year perspective. *Am J Surg* 1982; 143:460–464.
5. Connett MC, Murray DH Jr, Wenneker WW: Peripheral arterial emboli. *Am J Surg* 1984; 148:14.
6. Moore WS (ed): *Vascular Surgery: A Comprehensive Review*, 4th ed. Philadelphia, W. B. Saunders, 1993.
7. Rutherford RB: *Vascular Surgery*, 4th ed. Philadelphia, W. B. Saunders, 1995.
8. Rivers SP, Veith FJ, Ascer E, Gupta SK: Successful conservative therapy of severe limb-threatening ischemia: The value of nonsympathectomy. *Surgery* 1986; 99:759–767.
9. Goodreau JJ, Creasy JK, Flanigan DP, et al: Rational approach to the differentiation of vascular and neurogenic claudication. *Surgery* 1978; 84:749–757.
10. Ernst CB, Stanley JC (eds): *Current Therapy in Vascular Surgery*, 3d ed. St. Louis, Mosby-Year Book, 1995.
11. Veith FJ, Hobson RW, Williams RA, Wilson SE (eds): *Vascular Surgery*, 2d ed. New York, McGraw-Hill, 1987.

VICTOR J. WEISS / JOSEPH ANSLEY

# THE ASSESSMENT OF INTERMITTENT CLAUDICATION

As our patient population ages, the incidence of peripheral arterial disease continues to rise. A recent U.S. census estimates the number of individuals with peripheral arterial disease as 8.4 million, with half of those additionally diagnosed with intermittent claudication.[1] Intermittent claudication (derived from the Latin *claudicare,* meaning "to limp") refers to the symptoms produced by the limitation of blood flow to the lower extremities during a time of increased metabolic demand.

Although the differential diagnosis of leg pain is extensive, the diagnosis of intermittent claudication can be made with confidence based upon a focused history and physical examination. Furthermore, the location of the arterial lesion(s) can be determined without the need for elaborate vascular testing.

## PATHOPHYSIOLOGY

Repeated bouts of leg claudication can be viewed as a type of ischemia/reperfusion phenomenon, which is believed to potentially inflict oxidative free-radical injury.[1] This has led many to recommend walking to the point at which claudication begins and then resting, rather than attempting to "walk through" the pain.

Recent studies have provided new insight into the pathophysiology of intermittent claudication. Skeletal muscle calf biopsy in claudicants has revealed muscular denervation, which leads in part to the associated leg weakness.[2] Measurement of peak oxygen uptake demonstrates that these patients have a nearly 50 percent reduction in peak exercise capacity compared with healthy age-matched controls, placing them at a severity level similar to New York Heart Association class III heart failure patients.

# HISTORY

Studies have demonstrated that more than half of the patients with intermittent claudication never complain about this to their physicians, presumably believing that leg pain with ambulation is a natural consequence of aging.[1] Therefore, the symptoms of intermittent claudication should be actively sought, particularly in older patients with risk factors for peripheral vascular disease. These include the current or past use of tobacco, a history of diabetes, and a history of coronary or cerebrovascular occlusive disease.

The diagnosis of intermittent claudication is reliably made on the basis of historical assessment because the symptoms are quite characteristic. The onset of leg discomfort is a fairly reliable indicator of claudication. When asked about difficulty in walking, the patient with claudication typically describes symptoms that do *not* begin during the first few steps, but classically commence only after a certain distance has been traversed. The patient will also acknowledge that the discomfort abates after a minute or two of rest. Similarly characteristic is the finding that walking at a faster pace or up an incline (resulting in an increased metabolic demand) will accelerate the onset of these symptoms. The leg is typically asymptomatic at rest, unless a more severe degree of ischemia is present.

The nature of the discomfort described by the patient with intermittent claudication may vary. Calf claudication, the most common form of intermittent claudication, is typically characterized as a dull, cramping pain. Others may describe their symptoms as burning, as a sharp pain, or even simply as numbness. This sensation may or may not radiate up or down the leg. Thigh or buttock claudication tends to be more frequently described as a heaviness or tiredness. While both legs may be affected by claudication, one leg is typically more symptomatic. Many older patients will describe nocturnal muscle cramps of the lower extremities. This must be differentiated from vascular claudication, as it is not related to arterial occlusive disease. Many patients may also express concern over the feet often being cold. This correlates poorly with documented vascular disease.

The discomfort associated with intermittent claudication should be reliably relieved with rest. Pain that is unrelieved by a period of a few minutes of rest or discomfort that eases immediately with the cessation of activity would suggest a neurologic or musculoskeletal etiology for the symptoms. Patients with more severe ischemia and those who continue to ambulate during the pain of claudication may develop an ischemic myositis, which may lead to several days to weeks of painful ambulation and also to tenderness on examination, which is an unusual finding with claudication.

It is helpful to have the patient quantify the distance at which claudication is first noted, or at which he or she must stop walking because of the pain. While many authors quantify claudication in terms of city blocks (one block equals 300 feet), most patients living in rural areas are unable to use this system. Particular local landmarks, such as the number of houses on the patient's street or the number of shops in the mall, may be a more useful guide. A note about this distance should be kept in the patient's records, so that a benchmark may be determined, and improvement or progression of symptoms may be detected.

The location of claudication pain is a useful guide to the site of arterial obstruction, as the muscle groups affected are typically one joint distal to the impairment in blood flow. For example, the patient with calf claudication will most often have significant disease affecting the superficial femoral artery/popliteal artery segment. Likewise, patients with buttock claudication will be found to have aortoiliac disease. Foot claudication is unusual, but may accompany isolated tibial occlusions, as seen with Buerger's disease.

## PHYSICAL EXAMINATION

Physical findings will vary depending upon the degree of chronic ischemia. The limbs of the patient with intermittent claudication may appear normal upon inspection. With worsening ischemia, one may note hair loss, thinning of the skin, and thickening of the toenails. As the degree of ischemia progresses, one may find pallor with elevation and dependent rubor (Buerger's sign). Tissue ulceration or necrosis typically denotes limb-threatening ischemia.

Palpation of the limb in question may reveal a transition in skin temperatures, from a warmer upper leg to a cooler lower leg. Alternatively, no change in temperature may be noted. Pulse examination of the lower extremity begins with the common femoral artery, found at the midpoint between the pubic tubercle and the anterior superior iliac spine, just below the inguinal ligament. The popliteal artery is then located behind the knee with the knee in a slightly flexed position. The fingers of both hands are hooked into the popliteal fossa, with the thumbs pressing gently on an area from the superior edge of the patella to the tibial tubercle. The artery can be found slightly lateral to the midline and may be felt by compressing it against the femur or the tibia. The dorsalis pedis artery may be identified between the ankle and the distal third of the foot between the first two metatarsals. The posterior tibial artery is found posterior to the medial malleolus. The peroneal artery is located superior and anterior to the lateral malleolus. This artery is not palpable in this location, but should routinely be examined during Doppler assessment. If the pedal pulses are palpable, it is inaccurate to assume that the more proximal pulses will be intact. Frequently, patients with chronic superficial femoral arterial occlusion and well-formed geniculate collaterals may have diminished but palpable pedal pulses. Exercise to the point of claudication in these patients will cause the pedal pulses to disappear. Pulses are frequently graded on a four-point scale. Zero indicates nonpalpable pulses; 1+, a barely palpable pulse; 2+, a slightly diminished pulse; 3+, a normal pulse; and 4+, a hyperdynamic or aneurysmal pulsation.

Determination of vessel patency and measurement of ankle pressures with the hand-held Doppler is an integral aspect of the vascular examination. Any vessel without a palpable pulse should be assessed with the hand-held Doppler and a notation made as to the presence or absence of flow. Experience is necessary for the qualitative assessment of the Doppler signal, as it varies from its normal triphasic nature. A full description of Doppler flow characteristics is beyond the scope of this chapter, however. One must also be careful to distinguish the pulsatile arterial signal from the continuous "blowing" venous signal. Respiratory variation of the venous signal may also assist in distinguishing venous from arterial signals.

The most objective assessment of peripheral arterial disease can be made in the office by using the hand-held Doppler to measure ankle pressures. This simply refers to the pressure at which blood flow can be detected. A blood pressure cuff is inflated at a level above the ankle, and the Doppler probe is positioned over the dorsalis pedis or posterior tibial artery. As the cuff is slowly deflated, the pressure at which flow is first detected is noted. Similarly, the brachial artery systolic pressure is measured, and the ankle/brachial index (ABI) is calculated. Normally, the ankle systolic pressure exceeds the brachial pressure by 10 to 20 mmHg; therefore a normal ABI is 1.1 or greater. Abnormal ABIs are defined as less than 0.9 at rest and a 20 percent decrease after exercise. A resting ABI of less than 0.9 is believed to be associated with a 50 percent or greater vessel stenosis. Patients with claudication will typically have ABIs of 0.8 or less, and the ABI will drop further if taken following exercise (e.g., toe lifts). Ischemic rest pain typically does not occur until the ABI reaches 0.4 or less. Diabetic patients frequently have calcified vessels that are not compressible by cuff inflation. These patients typically have falsely elevated ankle/brachial indices and are more accurately assessed by measuring toe pressures in a more specialized noninvasive vascular laboratory. Patients with lower-extremity arterial occlusive disease may also have undiagnosed upper-extremity arterial lesions. Brachial pressures should therefore be measured in both arms, with the higher reading used for each ankle/brachial index.

The ankle/brachial index may be used in several different ways. At the initial patient encounter, the ABI may be useful in confirming the diagnosis of arterial insufficiency and may also determine the severity of the disease in an objective manner. Serial ABI readings can be used to follow the progression of the disease over extended periods of time. A sudden fall in ABI suggests progression of arteriosclerotic stenosis to occlusion, or the loss of collateral flow. The index should increase following arterial intervention, although improvements in claudication distance resulting from a walking program may fail to produce an elevation in the index.

## NATURAL HISTORY

The most feared consequence of peripheral vascular disease is worsening ischemia leading to amputation. Nearly all studies on the natural history of intermittent claudication using large patient samples have demonstrated that progression to amputation is an unusual event, occurring in about 12 percent of patients followed over a 10-year period.[3,4] A shortcoming of some of these earlier studies was that the diagnosis of claudication was based on symptoms alone, without any objective evaluation. More recent studies have painted a less optimistic picture. While the amputation rate has remained low, a third of patients will predictably have symptomatic or objective disease progression, with half of these patients requiring limb salvage procedures.[4] Most have found that continued tobacco use and diabetes mellitus correlate well with progression of the disease. The most important predictor of outcome has consistently been the severity of the disease, determined objectively by either noninvasive testing or arteriogram, at the initial patient encounter. Encouragingly, 50 to 80 percent of patients will have stability or improvement in symptoms.[4]

When discussing the meaning of intermittent claudication, it is helpful to inform patients that the risk of amputation is quite low. This is a frequent concern of the patient that often goes unmentioned. One must also inform the patient who uses tobacco that the ultimate fate of the extremity in question can in large part be influenced by whether the individual can overcome her or his tobacco addiction.

## CONCLUSION

The diagnosis of intermittent claudication can be reliably made based on history and physical assessment. Vascular surgeons have typically taken a conservative approach to the management of these patients, although the emergence of endovascular technology has led some to adopt a more aggressive treatment plan. The management of such patients is discussed in Chap. 35. Whatever treatment plan is adopted, it is crucial that these patients be followed for life. The exact interval of follow-up will be dictated by the severity of the disease. Follow-up is aimed at encouraging the patient to refrain from tobacco use and detecting progression of the disease so that intervention may occur prior to the development of tissue loss.

### REFERENCES

1. Hirsch AT, Hiatt WR (eds): An office-based approach to the diagnosis and treatment of peripheral arterial disease. *Am J Med* 1999; part IV:3–5.
2. Regensteiner JG, Wolfel EE, Brass EP, et al: Chronic changes in skeletal muscle histology and function in peripheral arterial disease. *Circulation* 1993; 87:413–421.
3. Imparato AM, Kim GE, Davidson F, et al: Intermittent claudication: its natural course. *Surgery* 1975; 78:795–799.
4. Nehler MR, Taylor LM, Moneta GL, Porter JM: Natural history, nonoperative treatment, and functional assessment in chronic lower extremity ischemia. In: Moore WS (ed): *Vascular Surgery: A Comprehensive Review.* Philadelphia, WB Saunders, 1998:251–264.

HALIT M. ISIKLAR /
WILLIAM T. BRANCH, JR./
ALAN B. LUMSDEN

# UNILATERAL LEG SWELLING AND POSTPHLEBITIC SYNDROME

A swollen limb is a common clinical presenting feature and may have a variety of causes. Basically, limb swelling results from excessive accumulation of interstitial fluid and may be a consequence of either too much production or impaired resorption. In defining a cause, however, one first has to determine whether there is unilateral or bilateral swelling. Typically, in most instances, bilateral swelling has a systemic cause (Table 11-1). Unilateral swelling usually has a local cause, which could be either venous (Table 11-2) or lymphatic (Table 11-3) in nature.

## ASSESSMENT

### Patient History

In evaluating a patient with a swollen limb, a careful history is taken and an initial examination is performed. A very important factor in the examination is the patient's age. Progressive unilateral enlargement of the limb in a child may be the result of hypertrophy arising from an arteriovenous fistula or lymphedema. Acute limb swelling in a hospitalized patient is most likely to represent deep venous thrombosis (DVT).

Pain, redness, and erythema may represent cellulitis or an acute DVT. A history of remote DVT is suggestive of postphlebitic syndrome. Progressive nonpitting edema involving the toes and dorsum of the foot, with episodes of cellulitis, is typical of lymphedema.

**TABLE 11-1.   Systemic Causes of Bilateral Swelling**

Congestive cardiac failure

Hypoproteinemia—nephrotic syndrome

Protein-losing enteropathy

Malnutrition

Cirrhosis

Hormone/drug therapy (calcium antagonists)

Myxedema

**TABLE 11-2.   Venous Causes of Unilateral Swelling**

| Causes | Results |
| --- | --- |
| Endoluminal obstruction | DVT |
| | Surgical ligation |
| Extrinsic compression | Arterial aneurysms |
| | Tumors |
| | Retroperitoneal fibrosis |
| Venous hypertension | Valvular dysfunction |
| | Arteriovenous fistula |

DVT, deep venous thrombosis.

**TABLE 11-3.   Lymphatic Causes of Unilateral Swelling**

| Causes | Results |
| --- | --- |
| Primary lymphedema | Congenital lymphedema |
| | Lymphedema praecox |
| | Lymphedema tarda |
| Secondary lymphedema | Radiation |
| | Surgical excision |
| | Infection: filariasis |
| | Limb inactivity |

## Bilateral Swelling

In an adult, bilateral swelling is most likely to be caused by systemic factors, as shown in Table 11-1. However, bilateral swelling can also be caused by intraabdominal problems leading to compression or occlusion of the central veins (Table 11-4). Extensive retroperitoneal malignancy permeating the lymphatic system can also cause bilateral swelling. Examination of the abdomen, with appropriate imaging techniques, is an important part of the evaluation process in patients with bilateral, yet otherwise unexplained, leg swelling.

## Unilateral Swelling

When unilateral swelling is encountered, a search for the cause focuses on the limb and pelvis, up to the confluence of the iliac veins with the inferior vena cava. Compression of the superficial femoral vein results in swelling from the knee down. Compression of the iliac vein in the pelvis results in unilateral swelling of the entire limb, while popliteal venous obstruction causes calf and ankle swelling. Simple physical examination can therefore direct the examiner to the level of the likely obstruction.

## Chronic Venous Hypertension

Chronic venous hypertension results from two principal processes:

- Valve dysfunction: primary (congenital; no known cause)
- Venous obstruction: secondary (postthrombotic, usually deep venous thrombosis)

There are two parallel venous systems within the leg: the deep venous system (the popliteal, peroneal, anterior tibial, and posterior tibial veins) and the superficial veins (the long and short saphenous system and the posterior arch vein). Obstruction or valve dysfunction in the deep system results in elevated deep venous pressure (Fig. 11-1). This is transmitted via perforating veins, which communicate

**TABLE 11-4.   Nonsystemic Causes of Bilateral Leg Swelling**

| | |
|---|---|
| IVC obstructions | Thrombosis |
| | Compression |
| Pelvic mass | Bilateral venous compression |
| Elevated intraabdominal pressure | Tumor |
| | Ascites |

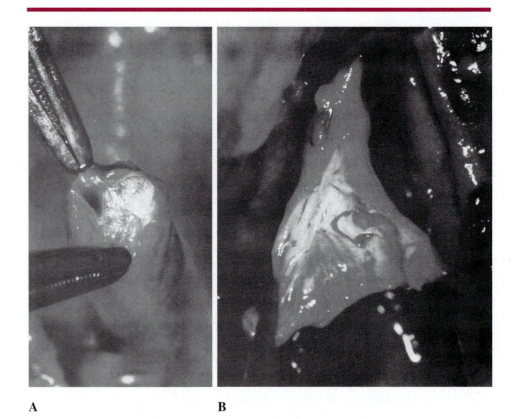

A                                    B

Figure 11-1   Typical appearance of a recanalized vein following DVT. This results in partial venous obstruction and valve dysfunction.

with the posterior arch vein above the medial malleolus (Fig. 11-2). Valves within the perforating veins normally direct flow from the superficial to the deep system; when these fail, high pressure is transmitted to the posterior arch vein above the medial malleolus. This is the typical location for cutaneous changes associated with chronic venous hypertension.

In a second scenario, once thought to be uncommon but now recognized as perhaps the most common cause of chronic venous hypertension, valve incompetence is limited to the superficial veins. This results in varicose vein development and in a small percentage of cases leads to skin changes above the medial malleolus, where the pressure is highest.

Regardless of the cause, venous hypertension is thought to create increased capillary pressure that leads to edema, fibrosis, hypoxia, and ultimately skin breakdown. It has also been hypothesized that stagnant capillary blood causes white blood cell trapping and activation, which adds to the inflammation.

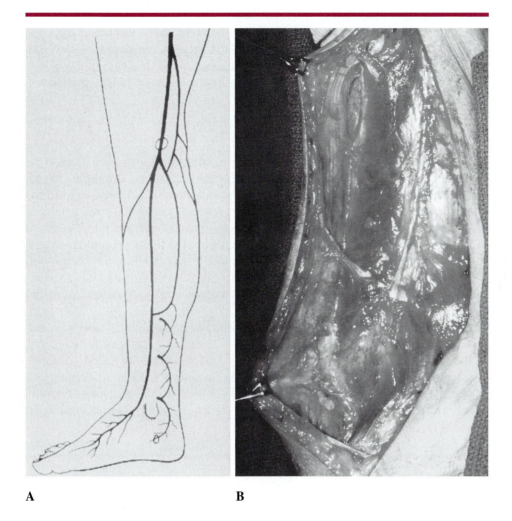

**A**                          **B**

Figure 11-2   Perforating veins communicate between the posterior tibial vein and the posterior arcuate vein.

The prevalence of venous ulceration due to chronic venous insufficiency has been estimated to be approximately 0.1 to 0.3 percent. In addition, for each patient with frank ulceration, there are up to 30 patients with lipodermatosclerosis. The management of ulceration associated with chronic venous insufficiency remains difficult and frustrating, and failure rates are high. Cutaneous venous hypertension occurs as a consequence of primary valvular incompetence (in up to 60 percent of patients), deep venous obstruction, or a combination of both in a series of cutaneous manifestations that, in their most severe forms, result in skin breakdown over the medial malleolus.[1,2]

Although superficial stripping, deep venous valve repair, and valve transfer all have their advocates, the mainstay of therapy has remained mechanical compression. External elastic stockings, worn by compliant patients, contribute to ulcer healing in 85 percent of cases. However, compliance is difficult to obtain in the elderly and infirm because of their difficulty in applying the stockings, and compliance is also poor in hot climates.

## Skin Changes

The mechanism of development of sequelae in chronic venous hypertension remains unclear.[3] Skin capillaries elongate and become tortuous, and these changes are associated with thickening of the capillary walls as well as increased filtration from the elevated pressure,[4] which further reduces resorption and results in edema. There is diapedesis of red blood cells into the interstitium, causing a breakdown which results in hemosiderin deposition and the development of typical brownish skin pigmentation. Fibrin is also deposited, resulting in a dense pericapillary cuff. The cuff represents a barrier to diffusion of oxygen and other nutrients. Some investigators suggest that skin oxygen tension is reduced, but this has been refuted.[5]

Margination, migration, and degranulation of white blood cells has also been suggested as contributing to the deleterious effects of venous hypertension.

The clinical manifestations include ankle and calf edema; brown skin pigmentation in the gaiter area, particularly above the medial malleolus; thickening and lichenification of the skin and subcutaneous tissue (lipodermatosclerosis); and ultimately recurrent ulceration. Pain is a significant feature only when ulceration develops (Fig. 11-3).

# TESTING

## Noninvasive Duplex Ultrasound

Duplex ultrasound scanning is a cheap and noninvasive technique for evaluating the swollen limb. As well as providing information on venous occlusion and extrinsic compression from a mass, it detects venous hypertension from an arteriovenous fistula and permits evaluation of valve function. Duplex ultrasound in some cases can provide imaging of the iliac veins up to the level of the inferior vena cava. Iliac veins may be obscured by bowel gas. Lack of respiratory variation in flow and venous distention suggests intraabdominal compression or occlusion.

## Ascending Venography

Ascending venography may still be necessary when imaging of the intraabdominal veins is required. This examination is best performed by direct femoral venous puncture and catheterization of the iliac vein. While ascending venography from the

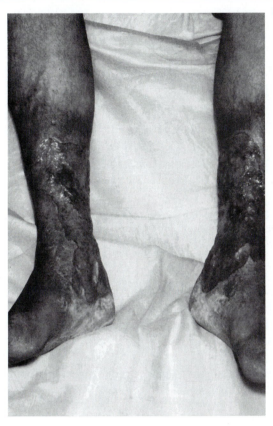

Figure 11-3 Skin changes typically develop above the medial malleolus.

foot is rarely required, descending femoral venography is used to demonstrate reflux down the leg through incompetent valves (Fig. 11-4).

# TREATMENT

## Chronic Venous Hypertension

**COMPRESSION THERAPY.** For most patients, external compression is adequate therapy and can be achieved in a number of ways. The most common approach is the use of elastic stockings. For patients with a history of DVT or skin changes, graduated compression stockings providing an ankle pressure of 30 to 40 mmHg are employed. We usually use below-knee stockings with a lighter pressure of 20 to 30 mmHg for patients with varicose veins because they are easier to put on and the compliance rate is improved. Patients with larger legs, however, may need made-to-measure stockings.

Circ-aid compression is a recently introduced form of nonelastic compression.

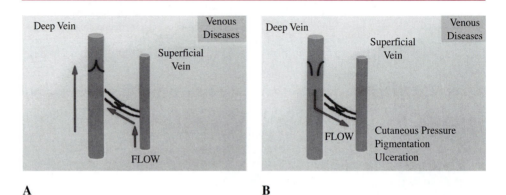

**A**                                                    **B**

Figure 11-4   *A.* Normally blood flows from the superficial to the deep venous system via perforating veins which contain unidirectional valves. *B.* Incompetence of the valves in the perforating veins results in reflux of high-pressure blood into the superficial veins.

This therapy consists of a series of Velcro straps, which when placed around the leg form an inelastic stocking that can be tightened as edema decreases. This is particularly useful when frequent dressing changes are necessary, since the straps are more durable than elastic stockings. Inelastic compression can also be provided by Unna boots or Profore dressing.

All of these techniques depend on the compressive device reducing cutaneous venous hypertension and thereby ameliorating its effect on the skin.

## Surgical Therapy

Surgery has always played a role in the management of these patients.[6-9] Linton proposed that those patients with perforator incompetence could be treated by directly dividing the offending perforators.[10] Unfortunately, in order to achieve this goal, a long incision through the medial skin from the knee to the medial malleolus was necessary. Perforators could then be identified below the fascia and divided. In concept, the procedure was sound. On average, 85 percent of patients remained ulcer-free in the long term. However, wound-related complications such as infection, flap necrosis, and delayed healing occurred in 17 percent of patients and caused the procedure to fall into disfavor. Although several modifications of the Linton procedure have been developed to minimize wound morbidity, such as the posterior stocking seam incision and parallel oblique incisions, it was not until the development of minimally invasive procedures, which permitted small, remote incisions, that the procedure began to be reevaluated.[11, 12]

Hauer, in Germany, used a mechanical system for endoscopic subfascial surgery and, to date, has the most experience.[13] O'Donnell, in the United States, employed saline infusion (because of concerns regarding $CO_2$ embolization) in the subfascial space to create an adequate optical space.[14] More recently, Gloviczki, in the United

States, employed $CO_2$ insufflation.[15] Renewed enthusiasm resulted from the increasing technical ease associated with $CO_2$ insufflation, and this was the technique used for most of the cases in our research.

The patients most appropriately treated with subfascial endoscopic perforator surgery (SEPS) include those with active ulcers, recurrent ulcers, or healed ulcers that were present for $> 4$ months. The underlying pathophysiologic process can be best defined using color flow duplex scanning. This procedure will document the presence of deep venous obstruction and superficial and deep venous reflux and also localize perforating veins and determine their competency.[16,17] Perforator vein incompetence can be demonstrated in 15 percent of patients without lipodermatosclerosis. In this operation, a scope is inserted into the leg through a 1-cm incision in the upper calf, and perforating veins are divided under the ulcer. This procedure has low morbidity and induces rapid ulcer healing (Fig. 11-5).

Patients with stigmata of chronic venous hypertension in whom reflux through the saphenofemoral junction is identified as the sole underlying process can be cured with saphenofemoral disconnection and stripping of the saphenous vein. Ulcer excision and skin grafting is also frequently employed, but this does nothing to

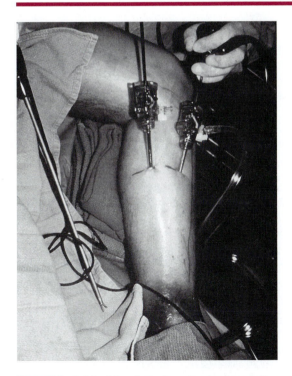

Figure 11-5   Subfascial endoscopic perforator interruption can be achieved through an endoscopic technique in which the incision can be placed high in the calf, remote from areas of lipodermatosclerosis.

**TABLE 11-5.   Treatment of Venous Stasis Ulcers**

Initial care

    Wash ulcer daily

    Cover with duoderm wafer

    Apply 30–40-mmHg compression stockings

    Keep legs elevated when nonambulatory

    Antibiotics if surrounding cellulitis

Investigations

    Duplex scan: define pathophysiology

Supplementary therapy

    Strip GSV if refluxing and no other pathology

    SEPS if deep venous reflux/occlusive disease

    SEPS if perforator incompetence

GSV, great saphenous vein; SEPS, subfascial endoscopic perforator surgery.

address the underlying pathophysiologic process, and continued compression is necessary (Table 11-5).

## REFERENCES

1. Shami SK, Shields DA, Scurr JH, Smith PDC: Leg ulceration in venous disease. *Postgrad Med J* 1992; 68:779–785.
2. Browse NL: Venous ulceration. *Br Med J* 1983; 286:1920–1922.
3. Anning ST: *Leg Ulcers: Their Causes and Treatment.* London, J & A Churchill, 1954.
4. Fagrell B: Microcirculatory disturbances—The final cause for venous ulceration. *Vasa* 1982; 11:101–103.
5. Coleridge Smith PD, Thomas P, Scurr JH, Dormandy JA: Causes of venous ulceration: A new hypothesis. *Br Med J* 1988; 296:1726–1727.
6. Kistner RL, Eklof B, Masuda EM: Deep venous valve reconstruction. *Cardiovasc Surg* 1995; 3:129–140.
7. Cikrit DF, Nichols WK, Silver D: Surgical management of refractory venous ulceration. *J Vasc Surg* 1988; 2:5–12.
8. Lumsden AB, Eaves FF III: Subcutaneous, video-assisted saphenous vein harvest. *Perspect Vasc Surg* 1994; 7:43–55.
9. Lumsden AB, Eaves FF, Jordan WD, Ofenloch JC: Subcutaneous, video-assisted saphenous vein harvest: A report of the first 30 cases. *Cardiovasc Surg* (in press).
10. Linton RR: The communicating veins of the lower leg and the operative technique for their ligation. *Ann Surg* 1938; 107:582–583.

11. Healy RJ, Healy EH, Wong R, Schaberg FJ: Surgical management of the chronic venous ulcer: The Rob procedure. *Am J Surg* 1979; 137:556–559.
12. De Palma RG: Surgical therapy for venous stasis. *Surgery* 1974; 76:910.
13. Hauer G, Barkun J, Wisser I, Deiler S: Endoscopic subfascial discussion of the perforating veins. *Surg Endosc* 1988; 2:5–12.
14. O'Donnell TF: Surgical treatment of incompetent communicating veins. In: Bergen JJ, Kistner RL (eds): *Atlas of Venous Surgery.* Philadelphia, W.B. Saunders, 1992: 111–124.
15. Gloviczki P, Cambria RA, Rhee YR, et al.: Surgical technique and preliminary results with endoscopic subfascial division of perforating veins. *J Vasc Surg* 1996; 23:517–523.
16. Sanjeev S, Scurr JH, Smith PDC: Medial calf perforators in venous disease: The significance of outward flow. *J Vasc Surg* 1992; 16:40–46.
17. Gloviczki P, Bergan JJ, Menawat SS, et al: Safety, feasibility and early efficacy of subfascial endoscopic perforator surgery (SEPS): A preliminary report from the North American Registry. *J Vasc Surg* (in press).

STEPHEN KONIGSBERG /
WILLIAM T. BRANCH, JR./
ALAN B. LUMSDEN

# VARICOSE VEINS

## LOWER-EXTREMITY VENOUS SYSTEM

The medical community has frequently underestimated varicose veins, often perceiving this pathologic condition as merely a cosmetic concern. In addition to the unpleasant appearance of varicose veins and the resulting distress experienced by those afflicted, they frequently result in pain and occasionally result in ulcer formation.

The venous system of the leg is composed of three networks: the superficial veins, the deep veins, and the perforating or communicating veins. These systems do not act independently and when one becomes dysfunctional, the entire complex is affected. When the superficial valvular system or any part thereof, particularly at the saphenofemoral junction, becomes incompetent, the superficial veins are placed under high pressure. They then dilate and become permanently enlarged to accommodate the extra blood volume. This appearance is known as varicose. Furthermore, blood refluxing down the superficial system can result in volume overload of the deep venous system, rendering those valves incompetent. The World Health Organization defines varicose veins as a "saccular dilatation of the veins which are often tortuous."[1]

The normal flow of blood through the lower-extremity venous system is dependent on two major factors. One of these is the pumping action of the calf, referred to as the calf pump. The other is the intact venous valves which prevent blood from refluxing back down the leg, creating superficial venous hypertension. Dysfunction of the valves results in varicose veins. Primary varicose veins result from congenital or acquired valvular incompetency somewhere in the superficial or perforating veins. In the otherwise healthy adult, varicosities occurring in the medial aspect of the thigh and calf are the result of valvular incompetence in the distribution of the great saphenous vein, including the saphenofemoral junction. Varicosities in the posterior and lateral calf are the result of valvular incompetence in the distribution of the lesser saphenous vein. In 60 to 70 percent of typical saphenous varicosities, the saphenofemoral junction will be found to be incompetent.[1a] Secondary varicose veins usually result from a direct valve injury from deep venous thrombosis.

Varices can be subdivided clinically into two groups comprising the five types of genuine varicose veins:

1. Large varicose veins
   a. Trunk varicosities
   b. Branch varicosities
   c. Incompetent perforators
2. Small varicose veins
   a. Reticular varicosities
   b. Telangiectasias (spider veins)[2]

This chapter will focus on large varicose veins, which have the potential for more debilitating symptoms than do small varicose veins.

## Presenting Symptoms

The typical patient seen in the office is a female in her twenties to fifties who complains of a history of lower-extremity varicose veins. They have been unsightly for many years but recently are becoming increasingly more painful. These women are often embarrassed to complain about the cosmetic aspect of the problem but should be encouraged to understand that their concern is perfectly reasonable.

The presence and degree of symptoms often do not equate with the severity of varicose veins observed. Presenting symptoms include throbbing or burning pain, itching, cramping, aching, heaviness, or tiredness. These symptoms are usually exacerbated by standing and relieved by lying down, elevating the legs, or walking, particularly in conjunction with the wearing of compression stockings. Symptoms may also be more severe during premenstrual periods and be relieved with weight loss. In a small percentage of patients who present with venous stasis ulcers, the cause can be traced to the existence of an incompetent superficial venous system with a completely competent deep venous system.

## Epidemiology

Varicose veins appear in a significant portion of the adult population, occuring more than twice as frequently in women as in men. Studies show that varicose veins are present in 8 percent of women between the ages of 20 and 29, 41 percent of women in their fifties, and 72 percent of women in their seventies. In men, however, 1 percent of the population demonstrate varicose veins in their thirties, 24 percent in their forties, and 43 percent in their seventies.[3–5]

## Differential Diagnosis

Symptoms from varicose veins typically are dull aches that worsen toward the end of the day and are exacerbated by standing rather than by exercise. History alone usually helps distinguish the patient with arterial insufficiency who complains of calf pain after ambulating. A simple examination of the pulses also helps distinguish venous from arterial disease. If pedal pulses are absent, further investigation is necessary to determine if arterial disease is the source of the symptoms. Another cause of leg symptoms is chronic venous hypertension secondary to deep venous thrombosis. If this is the case, the patient may be dependent on the superficial veins as a significant part of the overall venous system. A history of rapidly progressive lower-extremity or pelvic varicose veins, particularly with associated leg swelling, could also be the result of a pelvic tumor or an arteriovenous fistula, and a complete abdominal examination may be in order. The differential diagnosis may also include orthopedic or rheumatologic problems, which may need to be ruled out if suspected.

# ASSESSMENT

## History

The patient's background may be very important in determining the seriousness of his or her condition. The most aggressive symptoms occur in those patients who have a strong family history of varicose veins and whose varicosities began in their early twenties. A complete workup of such patients' lower-extremity venous system is indicated. Those patients who have a history of chronic significant superficial venous hypertension are at risk of developing disease of the perforator system, which in turn can lead to venous ulceration.

If the onset of varicose veins has been recent and rapid, particularly with a recent history of surgery, long travel, or immobilization, then a previously undiagnosed deep venous thrombosis needs to be considered.

## Physical Examination

An initial short physical examination can yield a significant degree of information about the status of a patient's complaints.

1. With the patient in the supine position, palpate the patient's femoral, dorsalis pedis, and posterior tibial pulses. If they are absent or severely diminished, then further assessment should be undertaken, using either ankle-brachial pressure indices or formal testing with pulse volume recording in a noninvasive lab.

2. With the patient in the standing position, observe and palpate the distribution of bulging varicosities in the thighs and calves.

3. Note any isolated bulges in the thigh or calf, which are indicative of incompetent perforators.

4. Look for dense spider veins around the ankle consistent with superficial venous hypertension. Dark pigmentation, induration, or ulcer formation in the lower leg may represent chronic deep venous hypertension.

5. Inspect the proximal thigh and buttocks. These areas may develop varicosities involving the pudendal or other pelvic vessels secondary to a pregnancy.

6. Inspect the pelvic and abdominal region for dilated veins, which may be the result of an earlier episode of iliofemoral venous thrombosis.

## Office Tests

**PERCUSSION (SCHWARTZ) TEST.**   This is a highly efficacious and simple test that can be performed in the examining room in a couple of minutes. With the patient in the standing position, the fingers or palm of the left hand is placed over the patient's inner thigh. The fingers of the right hand are then used to tap over the varicose vein below. If a pulse wave is felt over the distribution of the great saphenous vein, then the system between the two hands is probably incompetent because the pulse is being transmitted through a standing column of blood uninterrupted by competent valves. If you can trace the transmitted pulse all the way to the groin, the saphenofemoral junction is probably incompetent. Similarly, an incompetent lesser saphenous system can be detected by placing the left hand over the posterior calf just below the knee and tapping the varicose veins below.

**COUGH TEST.**   This is used to test for incompetency of the saphenofemoral system. With the patient in a standing position, the examiner's hand is placed over the saphenofemoral junction in the groin, and the patient is asked to cough. An incompetent saphenofemoral valve will produce a pulse wave transmitted from the vena cava. The accuracy of this test increases with the use of a Doppler probe instead of palpation. It is, however, a crude test, and negative results do not always prove valvular competency.

**BRODIE-TRENDELENBURG TEST.**   This valuable clinical test assesses the competency of not only the superficial system but also the perforator system. With the patient in the supine position, the leg is elevated and drained of venous blood so that any varicosities become flat. Compression is then applied to the upper thigh. A tourniquet or blood pressure cuff may be used, but the circumferential pressure may also occlude the deep veins. A more reliable method is to simply use direct pressure with the fingertips over the great saphenous vein. The patient is then instructed to stand, and the leg is observed for 30 s. There are three possible results:

1. *Positive.* The varicose veins remain flat below the point of compression until the finger pressure is released. When the fingers are removed, the veins quickly dis-

tend. This indicates reflux through the saphenofemoral junction and great saphenous vein.

2. *Double positive.* The varicose veins distend when the patient stands with the finger pressure firmly in place. Release of pressure causes further distention. This implies reflux both through the perforators and the saphenofemoral junction/great saphenous vein.

3. *Negative.* There is distention of the varicosities when the patient stands, and no additional distention is observed when finger pressure is released. This result indicates reflux through the perforating system only.

**BRACEY VARIATION.**    If one suspects that incompetent perforators are involved, their location can be determined through a useful test designed by Bracey in 1958.[6] With the patient in the standing position, a ring-shaped tourniquet designed to fit the calf is rolled over the foot and onto the lower calf. An occluding flat tourniquet is then placed just above the ankle to prevent filling of veins from upward flow. The ring is then rolled up the calf, emptying the varicose veins below it. As it passes over an incompetent perforator, the flattened varicosities will suddenly distend, indicating that the refluxing perforator is directly below the ring.

## Noninvasive Venous Testing

A variety of noninvasive procedures have been developed over the years for the evaluation of venous insufficiency. The most practical of these tests, in both ease of execution and the amount of useful data acquired, involve the deployment of the continuous-wave Doppler and the duplex scanner.

**DOPPLER ULTRASOUND.**    The use of the continuous-wave Doppler in the office setting is another practical and easy method of examining the patient for incompetency in the great saphenous venous distribution. With the patient in the standing position, the Doppler probe is placed over the great saphenous vein. The other hand is placed around the thigh below the probe, with the fingers over the great saphenous vein. The thigh is then squeezed several times, with pressure directed over the inner thigh, while the examiner listens for antegrade flow to finetune the placement of the probe. Squeezing and holding the thigh should produce a normal venous flow sound. Upon quick release of the hand, a competent vein will produce a very short signal, while an incompetent vein will produce a long refluxing sound as the blood returns down the leg in a retrograde direction. The level of valvular incompetency can then be traced up the thigh. At the saphenofemoral junction, however, it may be impossible to distinguish between valvular insufficiency of the saphenofemoral junction and of the deep venous system.

**DUPLEX SCANNING.**    Duplex scanning of the deep and superficial veins, in the hands of a trained technologist, is the most accurate method of examining the venous system. This imaging tool is capable of visualizing the entire venous system of the leg in real time, focusing on individual veins, identifying areas of incompetency, and quantifying the degree of reflux. When contemplating vein stripping, it is necessary to demonstrate incompetency of the saphenofemoral junction. More importantly, duplex scanning can rule out deep venous thrombosis, which may be a contraindication to vein stripping.

**AIR PLETHYSMOGRAPHY.**   This a noninvasive functional test which potentially provides a great deal of useful information regarding the movement of blood in an incompetent venous system.

**ASCENDING VENOGRAPHY.**   This test has largely been replaced by duplex scanning. Although it does provide an accurate picture of the deep veins, it is unnecessarily invasive.

**DESCENDING VENOGRAPHY.**   This test is also much less frequently used as a result of the increased popularity of duplex scanning. Descending venography is used specifically to evaluate reflux.

# TREATMENT

Conservative versus interventional treatment of varicose veins depends on several factors, which include the severity of the varicosities, the degree of discomfort they cause, the patient's perception of the cosmetic effects, and the severity of any other medical problems. Although venous stasis dermatitis and ulcer formation are usually caused by deep venous thrombosis, they can also be the result of pure, severe, and untreated superficial venous hypertension.

If conservative treatment is chosen, the use of prescription compression stockings is recommended. Worn when ambulating, they will significantly reduce venous hypertension while adding a degree of comfort. Persistent long-term use will help prevent the progression of the condition, as well as any possible complications.

## Sclerotherapy

Sclerotherapy of truncal varicose veins is a method of treatment that has been available for many years. It is often used to eliminate varicosities in patients who desire an alternative to surgery. The primary mechanism of action is the injection of a sclerosing agent that damages the endothelial lining of the vein wall, which in turn causes inflammation, spasm, and ultimately collapse of the vein.

There are many sclerosing agents available today, but the most widely used, in varying concentrations, is sodium tetradecyl sulfate (STS). The procedure can be done in the office setting. Butterfly needles with attached syringes containing 1% STS are inserted in the veins to be treated. The entire apparatus is taped to the leg. The patient's leg is then placed in a sling, and the table is tilted in the Trendelenburg position. From the very distally inserted butterfly and progressing cephalad, the sclerosing solution is slowly injected into the varicosities. After removal of the butterflies, beveled foam rubber strips are taped over the injected varicosities, and an elastic stocking rolled over the leg to provide continuous and constant compression for the next 48 h.

Although this is an effective method of treatment, the downside is that many of the sclerosed varicose veins will eventually recanalize and return. This regeneraton may take anywhere from months to years.

## Vein Stripping

The classic form of vein stripping involves tearing out segments of varicose veins through fairly large incisions; upon extraction, the veins are bunched and wrapped around an oversized acorn-shaped stripper head. This leaves behind large raw tracts which accumulate blood, resulting in pain, a long convalescent time, and sometimes cosmetically unacceptable scarring.[7] Fortunately, the present-day form of this process has been dramatically improved, and a minimally invasive technique is now utilized. When uncomplicated localized calf varicose veins need to be addressed, stab avulsion phlebectomy is used. This involves removing long segments of vein through 1/2-cm superficial incisions at several locations along the course of the varicosities.

When an incompetent great saphenous vein and saphenofemoral junction have been demonstrated, it becomes necessary to remove them to eliminate the pathway for venous hypertension. Saphenofemoral junction disconnection and inversion axial stripping remove the great saphenous vein in a relatively atraumatic manner. A 4-cm incision is made in the crease of the groin, and the saphenofemoral junction is ligated above the deep femoral vein. A pin stripper with a head smaller than the diameter of the vein is then passed through the length of the great saphenous vein, and the end is brought through a 1-cm incision made above the knee. With the end of the great saphenous vein tied to the end of the stripper, the vein is turned inside out and pulled through the small incision above the knee. This technique, termed inversion stripping, does a minimal degree of trauma to the vein bed, produces little bleeding, and allows the patient to ambulate at home within several hours with only mild pain. By the following day, the patient should be able to ambulate normally.

## SUMMARY

The approach to the patient with varicose veins should be one of both compassion for the disfiguring aspect of the disease and concern for the associated symptoms and potential for future complications. Modern methods of treatment offer patients real alternatives and effective modes of treatment. Patients may need to be reassured that their condition is neither life- nor limb-threatening, in addition to receiving advice on treatment options. If definitive treatment is sought, then referral to a vascular surgeon or dermatologist is indicated.

## REFERENCES

1. Prevovsky I: Disease of the veins, internal communication, MHO-PA 10964, World Health Organization.
1a. Goren G: *Office Phlebology: A Practitioner's Guide.* Encino, CA, Nerog-Hill Desktop Publishing, 1995:15.
2. Schultz-Ehrenburg U: Pretreatment testing of patients with varicose veins and telangiectatic blemishes. In: Bergan JJ, Goldman MP (eds): *Varicose Veins and Telangiectasias.* St. Louis, Quality Medical Publishing, 1993:85–99.
3. Coon WW, Willis PW III, Keller JB: Venous thromboembolism and other venous disease in the Tecumseh community health study. *Circulation* 1973; 48:839–846.
4. Lake M, Pratt GH, Wright IS: Arteriosclerosis and varicose veins: Occupational activities and other factors. *JAMA* 1942; 119:696.
5. Tianco EAV, Buendia-Teodosio G, Alberto NL: Survey of skin lesions in the Filipino elderly. *Int J Dermatol* 1992; 31:196.
6. Bracey DW: Simple device for location of perforating veins. *Br Med J* 1958; 2:101–106.
7. Goren G: Minimally invasive surgery for primary varicose veins. *Ann Vasc Surg* 1995; 9:401–414.

JAMES G. DROUGAS /
ELLIOT L. CHAIKOF

# ULCERS OF THE LOWER EXTREMITY

## OVERVIEW

Lower extremity ulcers are a common problem in the United States. They can be of venous, arterial, or neuropathic origin; however, their etiology is often multifactorial (Table 13-1). The majority of these lesions can be diagnosed in the office with minimal ancillary tests. Venous and neuropathic ulcers are generally best treated with nonsurgical therapy that can be performed on an outpatient basis. However, arterial ulcers usually require more invasive evaluation and treatment.

## VENOUS ULCERS

Venous ulcers are the sequelae of a condition termed *chronic venous insufficiency (CVI)*. This condition has a broad spectrum of symptoms; patients may be asymptomatic or may develop edema, hyperpigmentation, pain, and subsequently chronic ulceration. There are many terms in the literature that are applied to CVI. When the condition is preceded by a deep venous thrombosis (DVT), *postphlebitic* or *postthrombotic syndrome* is often used to describe it. However, there are two important mechanisms that produce venous insufficiency; valvular incompetence and venous obstruction. Often these two processes coexist and contribute to CVI.

### Incidence/Presentation

Venous ulcers have been recognized since antiquity. Yet their anatomic etiology was not elucidated until the twentieth century. Following DVT, recanalization of the vein occurs, with destruction of the valves. Numerous studies have shown that between 30 and 87 percent of patients with venous ulcer had a history suggestive of prior DVT. Estimates suggest that between 10 to 35 percent of the U.S. adult population

**TABLE 13-1.   Causes of Leg Ulcers**

Venous ulcer

Arterial insufficiency

Lymphatic obstruction

Neuropathic
  Diabetes, alcoholism, hemiplegia, polyneuritis, leprosy, tabes dorsalis

Traumatic
  Injury, burn, radiation, sclerotherapy

Vasculitic
  Systemic lupus erythematosus, polyarteritis nodosa, scleroderma,
    rheumatoid arthritis, allergic vasculitis

Infective
  Tropical ulcer (anaerobic infections, *Borrelia vincentii,* etc.)
  Syphilitic (ulcerated gummas)
  Tuberculous
  Fungal (blastomycosis, sporotrichosis, actinomycosis)
  Others (amebiasis, chancroid, yaws, kala-azar, tularemia, granuloma
    inguinale, leishmaniasis)

Neoplastic
  Squamous cell carcinoma
  Basal cell carcinoma
  Melanoma
  Lymphoma (mycosis fungoides)

Pyoderma gangrenosum
  Associated with inflammatory bowel disease

*Source:* Adapted from Veith FJ, Hobson RW, Williams RA, Wilson SE (eds): *Vascular Surgery: Principles and Practice,* 2d ed. New York, McGraw-Hill, 1994.

have some form of venous disorder, and among the most common chronic diseases, venous diseases rank seventh. Some 5 percent of the U.S. population has stasis changes of the skin, and as many as 500,000 Americans have venous ulcers.[1]

The typical presentation of CVI is a patient with an edematous leg with skin thickening and dermatitis involving the medial aspect of lower third of the leg. This area often has chronic inflammation and hyperpigmentation. As previously mentioned, there will often be a history of previous DVT. Other predisposing factors are previous major trauma, surgery, or less commonly, arteriovenous malformation. In the absence of these risk factors, primary valvular incompetence must be considered. Patients often complain of vague aches and night cramps in the leg. Relief of the symptoms with recumbency and elevation is common. If the patient has cellulitis or ulceration, local symptoms may be more severe and constitutional symptoms may be present. Less commonly patients may describe a throbbing pain with ambulation; this has been termed *venous claudication*. This pain is more severe in the thigh and is due to major venous obstruction.[2] One must be certain to rule out arterial insufficiency in these rare cases.

The swelling of the lower leg is described as a brawny or woody edema. It is caused by high venous pressure. This venous hypertension is transmitted to the capillary level, resulting in capillary rupture and diapedesis of erythrocytes into the interstitium. These red blood cells deposit hemosiderin, causing the typical brownish-purple hyperpigmentation of skin indicative of venous stasis. This pigmentation along with poor skin nutrition (venous eczema) causes severe pruritus. These skin changes are the earliest sign of CVI and often occur within 2 years of DVT. Ulceration generally does not occur until 2 to 5 years later, although this is extremely variable.[3]

The stasis or venous ulcers occur in the lower third of the leg and are usually superior and posterior to the medial malleolus of the ankle. This area is most commonly affected because the superficial and subcutaneous venous pressure is highest due to the proximity of incompetent perforator veins. They are typically oval and frequently multiple. There are often scars indicative of previously healed ulcers. The base of the ulcer is flat and covered with necrotic debris or infected slough (Fig. 13-1). The tissue beneath is also stiff and thickened. If infected, a surrounding rim of erythema is present. In long-standing chronic ulcers, squamous cell carcinoma can develop (Marjolin's ulcer). This is readily diagnosed by a punch biopsy of any suspicious areas.

Venous ulcers can occur in a corresponding area on the lateral side of the ankle, although this is much less common. In very severe cases, they can encircle the entire ankle. They do not occur on the foot; which distinguishes them from arterial and neuropathic ulcers.

Varicose veins may accompany other clinical features of CVI but are usually not causative. An exception to this is the patient with large primary varicose veins of the

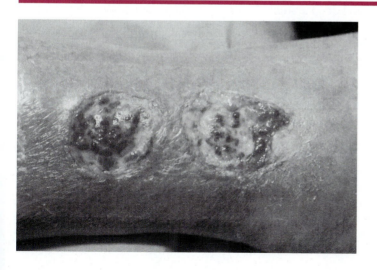

Figure 13-1 Characteristic venous ulcer of the lower extremity, usually located proximal to the medial malleolus.

greater or lesser systems that have been untreated for many years.[4] These can lead to perforator incompetence and subsequent CVI. Yet the misconception that varicose veins lead to venous ulcers persists.

## Assessment

Patients are first examined in the erect position. They are asked to stand for several minutes to allow filling of the leg veins. Any clinical features suggestive of CVI are noted, as well as sites of varicose veins. Saphenofemoral incompetence is initially judged by the presence of a transmitted cough pulsation in the greater saphenous vein. It is confirmed by Doppler examination. The saphenous vein is auscultated in the medial thigh. If it cannot be directly visualized, it is found by first identifying the arterial signal of the superficial femoral artery in the middle medial thigh. The greater saphenous vein is located several centimeters anterior to the artery. The venous Doppler signal is evaluated with compression of the thigh. A competent saphenofemoral junction will reveal antegrade flow in the saphenous vein without any retrograde flow. Valvular incompetence is demonstrated by significant retrograde flow with release of compression or Valsalva maneuver. Saphenopopliteal incompetence is assessed in a similar manner. Perforator incompetence is demonstrated by tourniquet occlusion of the superficial system with retrograde filling of perforators with gravity.

Duplex scanning has now become the initial imaging test for CVI. It can demonstrate reflux as well as obstruction. Valvular competence is assessed by flow direction, valve thickness, and valve coaptation. Abnormal retrograde flow greater than 10 mL/s is associated with a high incidence of venous ulceration.[5] Several studies have shown that up to 66 percent of venous ulcer patients have multisystem incompetence of the superficial, deep, and perforator systems.

Venography was the primary investigational modality prior to duplex scanning. Ascending venography is performed by cannulating a dorsal foot vein and placing a tourniquet above the ankle to preferentially fill the deep system. This provides good visualization of the deep system and of incompetent perforators. Venography is not indicated for uncomplicated CVI, but it may be helpful in severe cases or in patients being evaluated for operation. Venography can help identify presence of thrombus, areas of proximal obstruction, presence of incompetent perforators, and valvular deformity.

Venograhic assessment of the function of the deep valves requires descending venography through the femoral vein; this is performed in the semiupright position. Contrast is slowly injected, and reflux down the leg is observed with and without the Valsalva maneuver.

Ambulatory venous pressure is assessed by cannulating a vein on the dorsum of the foot. Pressure measurements are performed via a pressure transducer. This gives an accurate assessment of the deep venous pressure. Measurements are taken first during resting upright position, then during ankle plantarflexion standing on tiptoe, and finally during recovery. Venous pressure falls during exercise and gradually returns to the resting value when exercise stops. Normal resting pressure is 90 to

100 mmHg; pressure should fall to 20 to 30 mmHg with exercise and then gradually return to normal. In pathologic states, the pressure drop is markedly diminished and the subsequent rate of refilling is rapid. One study showed that if the ambulatory venous pressure can be brought below 45 mmHg, the risk of ulceration is zero, whereas if the pressure stays above 60 mmHg, the risk is greater than 50 percent.[6]

The examination of the leg must include an adequate assessment of the arterial system to rule out chronic arterial insufficiency. Table 13-1 reveals the differential diagnosis of leg ulcers.

## Management

**LOCAL WOUND CARE.**   Initial treatment is directed toward local measures of wound care. If cellulitis is present, systemic antibiotics are required. Often bacterial colonization of a chronic wound can be significant without overt signs of infection. This may inhibit wound healing. Antibiotics may be used empirically or, preferably, after a punch biopsy demonstrates greater than $10^6$ colony counts per gram of tissue. Concomitantly the patient is instructed to rest with the leg elevated, and a compression dressing is applied. Abscesses are drained if present. Occlusive compression dressings (e.g., Unna's boot or Primapore) have been the mainstay of treatment. These allow the patient to remain ambulant and are generally changed weekly. Exudate is absorbed by the dressing. Infected ulcers require more vigilant observation. There are various hydrocolloid and hydroactive dressings that may enhance healing when applied in conjunction with compression. Tissue-engineered skin equivalents (e.g., Apligraf) when applied topically have been shown to enhance the rate of healing for those ulcers present for more than 6 months. Refractory ulcers or long-standing ulcers should be biopsied to rule out squamous cell carcinoma.

If the ulcer heals with dressings, the patient must be vigilant with respect to prophylaxis. Graded compression stockings should be worn when erect. They should provide 30 to 50 mmHg compression at the ankle. Below-knee stockings are usually adequate and produce increased patient compliance compared to that for the above-knee style. These stockings require replacement at least every 6 months because of loss of elasticity.

Venous eczema also must be treated. Skin emollients are used liberally to prevent cracking, which can lead to infection or ulcer. Severe itching often responds to a short course of corticosteroid cream. The avoidance of trauma to the skin cannot be overemphasized.

**SURGICAL TREATMENT.**

*Ulcer Excision and Grafting.*   Before undertaking an operation, gross infection or cellulitis must first be controlled. Some chronic ulcers have very thick underlying tissue which requires excision and skin grafting. Wide excision of the ulcer base and surrounding abnormal tissue combined with skin grafting has been shown to have a 77 percent success rate at 5 years.[7] If there is exposed bone or tendon, a myocutaneous flap may need to be employed.

***Operations for Incompetent Perforators.***   There are numerous different approaches to dividing incompetent perforating vessels. The classic operation was described by Linton and entailed subfascial ligation of the perforating vein. This is performed through a longitudinal incision along the medial aspect of the leg. A major problem with this operation is healing of the operative incision; as it often traverses abnormal tissue planes. This complication is avoided by performing endoscopic subfascial ligation. This is a relatively new technique that employs a few small incisions in the proximal leg through normal tissue. Under endoscopic visualization, the incompetent perforators are divided.

These operations are palliative in that they do not improve deep venous function. However, in conjunction with long-term use of compression stockings, 80 to 95 percent of patients are free of recurrent ulcers at 2 to 5 years.

***Operations for Venous Obstruction.***   Patients with iliofemoral obstruction contributing to venous hypertension may benefit from either bypass or percutaneous transluminal angioplasty (PTA). An isolated iliac stenosis may be amenable to PTA and stenting. A more commonly encountered scenario is iliofemoral occlusion. In these settings, the contralateral greater saphenous vein can be used as a crossover graft to decompress the affected leg. Patency rates of as high as 75 percent have been reported with these bypasses.[8] A patent bypass generally relieves venous claudication but may not be sufficient to heal ulceration; however, subsequent ligation of perforators may further improve the situation.

A segmental femoral vein occlusion can be treated with a saphenopopliteal bypass. This requires an adequate caliber greater saphenous vein with competent valves. This vein is anastamosed to the popliteal vein below the level of the occlusion. Patency rates similar to those for the saphenofemoral crossover bypass have been reported.

***Venous Valve Surgery.***   Operative repair of damaged valves (valvuloplasty) has been advocated by some. Over 80 percent of the patients experience relief of their symptoms; however, recurrent ulceration is seen in 37 percent of patients over several years.[9] Incompetent deep vein valves can also be treated with vein segment transposition. A portion of valve-containing vein from the axillary or brachial vein is transposed to the popliteal vein to replace an incompetent system. Results with transposition are mixed with respect to ulcer healing.

## ARTERIAL ULCERS

Arterial ulcers are the result of inadequate blood flow being delivered to the tissues to meet the minimal metabolic requirements. They can be secondary either to occlusive disease within the arterial system or to arterial atheroemboli.

### Presentation

The clinical manifestations of chronic limb-threatening ischemia include ulceration, rest pain, and gangrene. Ischemic rest pain is typically described as a burning, dysesthetic pain involving primarily the forefoot over the location of the metatarsal heads and the toes. The pain is often aggravated by elevation of the foot and relieved by dependency, presumably because of the increase in arterial pressure with gravity. Classically, the term *ischemic ulcer* is used to indicate spontaneous development of a gangrenous toe as a result of distal arterial insufficiency, while a *nonhealing ulcer* is a traumatic wound of any part of the leg that is unable to heal due to inadequate blood supply (Fig. 13-2). Patients with occlusive disease generally do not have pedal pulses and may or may not have a popliteal pulse on exam. The chronically ischemic foot often demonstrates trophic changes, with hair loss; thin, shiny skin; and thickened nails. The foot may blanch with elevation and then develop rubor with dependency.

An ulcerated toe secondary to an atheroembolic process may appear similar to an ischemic ulcer on physical examination, but the history and physical examination will delineate these two processes. With an atheroembolic process, the onset of toe pain is sudden, and the patient first notices a purple digit, which may then progress to ulceration and gangrene (Fig. 13-3). This patient will have pulses throughout the entire length of the leg; the arterial system must be in continuity to deliver an embolus to the toe. One generally does not see trophic changes in the leg. Involvement of one leg suggests a source distal to the aortic bifurcation, while bilateral foot involvement suggests a more proximal source.

## Assessment

Initial assessment always begins with a thorough history and physical examination. Palpation of extremity pulses and measurement of blood pressure in all four extremities are extremely helpful. This allows calculation of the ankle-brachial index (ABI). A normal ABI is greater than 1.0, while an ABI less than 0.3 is indicative of

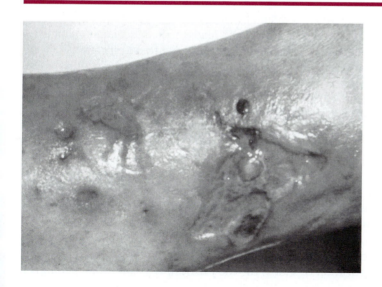

Figure 13-2  A nonhealing ulcer caused by significant peripheral vascular disease.

Figure 13-3   A purple and gangrenous toe often follows a distal atheroembolism.

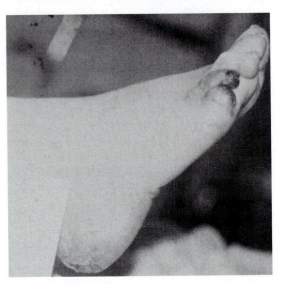

chronic ischemia that generally will not permit spontaneous healing of an ulcer.[10] Patients with calcified vessels, such as diabetics, often have a falsely elevated ABI. Assessment of segmental Doppler analog waveforms and toe pressures will provide both qualitative and quantitative assessment of the level and degree of the occlusive disease. A toe pressure greater than 30 mmHg is associated with a very high rate of healing following toe amputation. These tests can locate the level and extent of the occlusive disease in 90 percent of patients.[10] Peripheral vascular disease is a marker for generalized atherosclerosis, and evaluation for both coronary and extracranial carotid artery disease should be considered.

If the patient is considered a candidate for surgical intervention, the next step is arteriography. The arteriogram provides a road map for the vascular surgeon. PTA plays a very limited role in the management of ulcers due to chronic arterial insufficiency, since there is often segmental disease and PTA of the infrageniculate vessels has very poor patency rates.

The workup of patients with embolic disease also begins with arteriography. Concern regarding a proximal source of emboli warrants transesophageal echocardiography. This can assess the heart, ascending aorta, and proximal descending aorta.

## Management

Patients with occlusive disease who are acceptable surgical risks are then offered surgical treatment. Elderly patients who are nonambulatory may be best served by below-knee amputation in certain circumstances. Otherwise, revascularization, preferably with autologous vein graft, is the treatment of choice. Simple amputation of a gangrenous toe often results in nonhealing of the amputation site unless it is preceded by revascularization or unless the toe pressure is greater than 30 mmHg.

Often a combination of surgical bypass and PTA helps to diminish the degree of surgery required. An example is PTA and stenting of an iliac stenosis combined with an infrainguinal bypass.

Lifestyle modification plays a major role in the perioperative management of these patients. Smoking cessation is paramount. Some 90 percent of patients undergoing lower extremity amputation are smokers. Smoking cessation has been shown to improve walking distance in patients with chronic arterial insufficiency and to improve graft survival in those undergoing bypass. One study showed that 85 percent of patients with severe rest pain who stopped smoking avoided subsequent amputation.[11]

Pharmacologic treatment of arterial ulcers remains investigational. While pentoxifylline may play a role in the management of patients with claudication, it has no role in the treatment of patients with arterial ulcers. Use of growth factors and prostaglandins are currently being investigated in patients with severe rest pain and arterial ulcers in the United States. All patients with atherosclerosis should be on daily aspirin therapy unless this is contraindicated by allergy or intolerable side effects.

## Complications

Perioperative mortality ranges from 2 to 5 percent and is primarily related to coronary artery disease. Thus, thorough preoperative cardiac risk stratification is essential. Early complications include bleeding, infection, and graft thrombosis; these are seen in less than 5 percent of cases. Leg edema is a common problem but generally resolves within 6 weeks of operation. The major late complication is graft thrombosis. The 5-year patencies of above-knee, below-knee, and tibial vein grafts are 75, 70, and 67 percent, respectively.[12] With routine surveillance using duplex examination, the secondary patency rates of these grafts can be improved.

# NEUROPATHIC ULCERS

In the United States, neuropathic foot ulcers occur most commonly in diabetic patients, but they may also be seen in patients with any form of peripheral neuropathy (e.g., alcoholic, uremic, toxic, etc.). Management is generally the same regardless of etiology. The natural history of diabetic neuropathic foot ulcers has been most widely studied. Roughly 70 percent of long-term diabetics have some structural pathology of the foot, and 16 percent of these patients have a history of previous ulcer or amputation. It is estimated that 20 percent of diabetic hospital admissions are for foot problems.[13]

The etiology of neuropathic ulcers seems to be twofold; loss of pain and proprioception, and structural changes in the foot. The structural changes develop as a result of involvement of the motor nerves. The intrinsic muscles of the foot atrophy, causing an imbalance between the toe flexors and extensors which results in protrusion of the metatarsal heads. The result is increased force on the plantar aspect

**Figure 13-4** Malperforans ulcer on the insensate plantar aspect of the foot is most commonly seen in the diabetic patient with peripheral neuropathy.

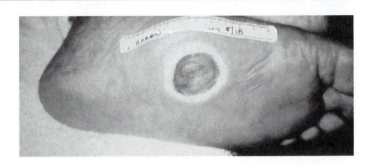

of the metatarsal heads. The sensory loss initiates a cycle of repetitive micro- or macrotrauma to the foot, often resulting in ulceration (Fig. 13-4).

## Assessment

Thorough assessment of the degree and proximal extent of the neuropathy is important. Often only the forefoot has sensory loss, while the hindfoot and lower leg have relatively normal sensation. Often ulceration is multifactorial, and arterial insufficiency must be ruled out; noninvasive testing is performed as previously described. A common scenario is the patient who presents with a plantar ulcer and palpable pedal pulses. The foot is often warm and dry, suggesting autosympathectomy. Roentgenograms of the foot are helpful in determining whether osteomyelitis is present. This can be followed by bone scans in equivocal cases. The ulcer should be probed to help determine its course and depth of invasion.

## Management

**LOCAL WOUND CARE.**   Subcutaneous sinuses should be unroofed. Conservative debridement of heaped-up calluses and necrotic tissue is indicated. If no cellulitis or osteomyelitis is present, antibiotics are not indicated. Ulcers confined to the skin and subcutaneous tissue often respond well to conservative measures of non-weight-bearing and local wound care. Unfortunately, patient compliance is often poor, requiring initial hospitalization.

**LOCAL RESECTION.**   For refractory ulcers over a metatarsal head, resection of the metatarsal head has a high success rate for healing. This is performed through a dorsal incision to avoid the weight-bearing surface. Along with removing the bony prominence, the often chronically infected metatarsal head is also removed.

**AMPUTATION.**   For patients with multiple plantar ulcers of the forefoot, consideration should be given to transmetatarsal amputation. This accomplishes two objectives. First, it removes all the ulcers and necrotic tissue in a single procedure. Second, it places the insensate skin on the non-weight-bearing surface of the foot. When performed in an adequately perfused foot, these amputations heal very well.

Following successful treatment of these ulcers, an aggressive protocol of foot care is mandatory. This entails orthotic shoes or inserts to increase the weight-bearing surface of the foot. Daily washing of feet with warm (not hot) water and mild soap is recommended. Soaking is to be avoided as it causes maceration. The feet should be dried and then lubricated with a lanolin-based preparation. This prevents cracking and encourages the patient to inspect his or her feet daily. The patient needs to be reminded that any injury to the feet may have major consequences and should be reported to a physician.

## SUMMARY

The treatment of patients with ulcers of the lower extremities begins with a thorough history and physical examination. Some 90 percent of all leg ulcers are due to venous disease, and their location and characteristics are usually sufficient to make the diagnosis. Arterial and neuropathic ulcers may be concomitant, requiring a multifaceted approach to treatment. Arterial ulcers invariably will require some form of surgical treatment, whereas the cornerstone of treatment for purely neuropathic ulcers begins with non-weight-bearing and local measures. Yet should these measures fail, surgery will often provide adequate palliation.

### REFERENCES

1.  Holewski JJ, Moss KM, Stess RM: Prevalence of foot pathology and lower extremity complications in a diabetic outpatient clinic. *J Rehab Res Dev* 1989; 26:35.
2.  Veith FJ, Hobson RW, Williams RA, Wilson SE (eds): *Vascular Surgery: Principles and Practice*, 2nd ed. New York, McGraw-Hill, 1994.
3.  Halliday P: Development of the postthrombotic syndrome: Its management at different stages. *World J Surg* 1990; 4:703.
4.  Henry ME, Fegan WG, Pegum JM: Five-year survey of the treatment of varicose ulcers. *Br Med J* 1971; 2:493.
5.  Vasdekis S: Doppler ultrasound in chronic venous insufficiency. In: Salmasi AM, Nicolaides AN (eds): *Cardiovascular Applications of Doppler Ultrasound.* London, Churchill Livingstone, 1989: 323–332.
6.  Nicolaides AN, Zukowski A, Lewis R: Venous pressure measurements in venous problems. In: Bergan JJ, Yao JST (eds): *Surgery of the Veins.* Orlando, FL, Grune & Stratton, 1985.
7.  Ackerman LV: *Surgical Pathology*, 6th ed. St. Louis, Mosby, 1981.
8.  Halliday JP, Harris JP, May J: Femoro-femoral crossover grafts (Palma operation): A long-term follow-up study. In: Bergan JJ, Yao JST (eds): *Surgery of the Veins.* Orlando, FL, Grune & Stratton, 1985.
9.  Raju S, Fredericks R: Valve reconstruction procedures for nonobstructive venous insufficiency: Rationale, techniques and results in 107 procedures with two- to eight-year follow-up. *J Vasc Surg* 1988; 7:301.

10. Rutherford RB (ed): *Vascular Surgery*, 4th ed. Philadelphia, WB Saunders, 1995.
11. Veith FJ: Femoral-popliteal-tibial occlusive disease. In: Veith FA (ed): *Vascular Surgery: A Comprehensive Review*, 4th ed. Philadelphia, WB Saunders, 1993: 463–469.
12. Whittemore AD: Infrainguinal bypass. In: Rutherford RB (ed): *Vascular Surgery*, 4th ed. Philadelphia, WB Saunders, 1995: 809.
13. Holewski JJ, Moss KM, Stess RM: Prevalence of foot pathology and lower extremity complications in a diabetic outpatient clinic. *J Rehab Res Dev* 1989; 26:35–44.

BYRON WILLIAMS

# CHAPTER
# 14

# CARDIAC TAMPONADE

The recognition of diseases of the pericardium has increased dramatically over the last quarter of a century, in large part because of improved detection by ultrasound. There are many processes that result in pericarditis and ultimately pericardial effusions. Currently, the most common etiologies recognized are postcardiac surgery, malignancy, radiation-induced, end-stage renal failure, viral, and connective tissue disorders. A more complete list of the causes of pericardial effusions can be found in Table 14-1. Cardiac tamponade occurs when there is compression of the heart by fluid under pressure within the pericardial sac, resulting in impaired diastolic filling of the ventricles.[1–4] The pericardium is made up of the visceral pericardium and the parietal pericardium, which create a potential space that is referred to as the pericardial sac. Normally there is approximately 50 mL or less of clear fluid in the pericardial sac. In the nonpathologic state, pericardial fluid serves as a lubricant between the two layers of pericardium.[4,5] The pericardium performs the function of preventing acute cardiac dilatation in volume overload states and also has a role in the distribution of hydrostatic forces throughout the various cardiac chambers.

As pericardial fluid accumulates, intrapericardial pressure increases, resulting in impaired diastolic filling of the ventricles. Impaired filling of the ventricles leads to elevated central venous pressure and ultimately decreased cardiac output. Patients can present with very large pericardial effusions—in fact, sometimes as much as 2 L of fluid—with minimal findings or symptoms of cardiac tamponade. Other patients, however, usually with trauma and acute hemorrhage into the pericardial space, can rapidly develop cardiac tamponade and hemodynamic collapse with less than 200 mL of pericardial fluid.[6] Normally, intrapericardial pressure is equal to atmospheric pressure and varies slightly with respiration.[1,3,5] Tamponade physiology can be variable in terms of its hemodynamic severity. Recognition of this variability and its translation to clinical findings in patients with pericardial effusions are very important. With only a slight increase in intrapericardial pressure to levels of 5 to 6 mmHg, the compression on the heart is minimal, since intracardiac diastolic pressures are usually greater than 5 to 6 mmHg. In situations of extreme volume depletion such as might be seen with gastrointestinal blood loss, vomiting, or profound diuresis, however, even small increases in intrapericardial pressure can result in

**TABLE 14-1.   Common Etiologies of Pericardial Effusion**

- Idiopathic

- Infectious—viral, bacterial, tuberculosis, fungal

- S/P cardiac surgery

- S/P myocardial infarction

- Malignancy

- Radiation induced

- Uremia

- Connective tissue disorders—scleroderma, lupus, rheumatoid arthritis, mixed connective disease, rheumatic fever, vasculitides

- Trauma

- Aortic dissection

- Drug induced—hydralazine, procainamide, penicillin, anticoagulant therapy, phenylbutazone, dilantin

- Miscellaneous—sarcoidosis, chylopericardium, amyloidosis, catheter perforation of heart or great vessels

tamponade physiology. In order to maintain a normal cardiac output and arterial blood pressure, compensatory mechanisms may be seen in mild to moderate tamponade. These mechanisms are tachycardia and arteriolar and venous constriction. Ultimately, compensatory mechanisms are overcome, and, in general, severe examples of cardiac tamponade are seen with intrapericardial pressures >15 mmHg.[3,4] This is often associated with moderate to large pericardial effusions involving volumes of at least 500 to 1000 mL of pericardial fluid. The pericardium has the capacity to stretch if the accumulation of this fluid is relatively slow and the state of the pericardium is otherwise normal. Development of asymptomatic large pericardial effusions may be seen with hypothyroidism or nephrotic syndrome. Thus, large pericardial effusions of 2000 mL or greater may develop with no or very few symptoms or signs of cardiac tamponade. With more rapid accumulation of fluid, however, the pericardium may not have the ability to stretch and accommodate the sudden increase in fluid. This situation might be seen clinically with catheter perforation of the ventricle or atrium. Untimely events like this have been reported with central venous catheter insertion and with invasive cardiology procedures.[6–10] Even small amounts of fluid, especially blood, can result in marked elevation of intrapericardial pressure with tamponade physiology.

The actual definition of cardiac tamponade and its translation to a meaningful clinical syndrome are somewhat controversial.[1–4] Physicians tend to have their own definition of what constitutes cardiac tamponade; thus there can be some confusion and debate regarding when tamponade physiology is really present in any one individual patient. Many clinicians reserve the term for situations in which there is true hemodynamic compromise and near circulatory collapse. In such a situation, the patient is hypotensive with signs of low cardiac output and poor organ perfusion, a syndrome very similar to shock.[11] This, of course, is an example of severe tamponade and is a true medical emergency that requires immediate life-saving relief of the pericardial fluid to restore more normal hemodynamics. It is better to use a broader definition and include patients with any evidence of hemodynamic derangement caused by increased pericardial fluid under pressure. In its mildest form, cardiac tamponade may present with only slight elevation of central venous pressure. More moderate forms of cardiac tamponade not only have elevated venous pressure but also show a decrease in cardiac output and usually blood pressure as well. In the most advanced form, the patient will be in a shocklike state, with elevated venous pressure, hypotension, decreased cardiac output, and tachycardia. The patient in shock is more easily recognizable as a patient with cardiac tamponade. When possible, it is best to recognize and manage cardiac tamponade at an earlier stage to avoid such a life-threatening situation.[4]

## SYMPTOMS OF CARDIAC TAMPONADE

Although very large pericardial effusions may accumulate without any symptoms, almost all patients with cardiac tamponade will be symptomatic.[4] The most prominent symptom is dyspnea. A vague anterior chest discomfort or classic pericarditis or pleuritic chest discomfort may also be present. Often abdominal visceral congestion can be the predominant symptomatology. When this is the case, the diagnosis is often delayed as the physician searches for other causes of abdominal discomfort. Other symptoms such as cough, hoarseness, and difficulty in swallowing may also confuse the issue. The symptoms of cardiac tamponade are frequently so nonspecific by themselves that the diagnosis is not suggested unless pericarditic symptoms are a prominent feature or other diagnostic modalities such as electrocardiogram, chest x-ray, or echocardiogram provide important clues.

## PHYSICAL SIGNS OF CARDIAC TAMPONADE

The classic triad described by Beck—hypotension, elevated systemic venous pressure, and a small, quiet heart—is not the usual clinical presentation.[12] This situation usually implies acute cardiac compression from intrapericardial bleeding and is most often seen with trauma, cardiac rupture, or aortic rupture. Many medical conditions lead to slower fluid accumulation with more subtle clinical findings, however.[13,14] Most patients do appear to be in some degree of distress or discomfort at the time of presentation if tamponade physiology is present. The arterial blood pressure is usually normal or only mildly decreased from baseline, but pulsus paradoxus is almost always present—in some series as high as 98 percent.[15] There is almost always some degree of sinus tachycardia, and, in contrast to Beck's triad, the heart sounds are usually not absent or muffled but more commonly can be heard. If a pericardial friction rub is heard, it certainly can be helpful in leading one to the right diagnosis, but this by itself does not indicate or exclude cardiac tamponade. The presence of a pericardial friction rub does confirm the presence of pericarditis. There is usually no third heart sound or pericardial knock, which is most commonly seen in constrictive pericarditis.[16] Since a left pleural effusion is commonly also present, as well as direct compression of the adjacent lung by the increasing cardiac size, a dullness to percussion over the left lower thorax can be found and is referred to as Ewart's sign.[17] Distended neck veins are almost always seen in cardiac tamponade but can be difficult to recognize. Patients with massive volume overload, such as that seen with chronic congestive heart failure (CHF), are more likely to have very prominent bulging external jugular veins that are very easy to recognize.[18] In cardiac tamponade the increase in blood volume is actually much less than that seen with CHF. Usually, there is associated venoconstriction as well. Thus, the external jugular veins may not be as prominent, and the clinician must search for elevated internal jugular veins. Kussmaul's sign, or a paradoxical increase in jugular venous pressure with inspiration, is commonly thought to be present in cardiac tamponade but is really a sign of constrictive pericarditis or right heart failure. It is rarely seen in uncomplicated cases of cardiac tamponade but can be seen if the patient has the so-called effusive constrictive physiology, which will be discussed somewhat later.[19]

Inspection of the neck veins is of extreme importance in making the diagnosis of cardiac tamponade. In fact, in the field of cardiac diseases, proper examination of the neck veins is one of the most important acts of the entire physical examination. It is often poorly understood, however, and frequently is not done well or even attempted.[18] The clinician performing the examination should identify both the external and internal jugular veins. The external vein should be assessed for distention, and the venous pulsation should be observed from the internal jugular veins. When the patient is fully reclining, the external jugular veins are normally distended, but they should disappear as the patient becomes more upright, at somewhere around 30° of truncal elevation.[18] Central venous pressure can be said to be abnormally elevated if the external jugular veins are distended when the patient's trunk is elevated more than 30° above the supine position.[18] In the majority of cases, this abnormality implies volume overload, with CHF being the most likely clinical diagnosis, but other causes of increased right heart pressures such as cardiac tamponade should be considered.

Jugular venous pulsations are observed by inspecting the internal jugular veins. When the patient is fully supine, the internal jugular vein is normally overdistended, and the pulsations cannot be easily seen. When the patient's trunk is elevated until maximum pulsations can be noted, which usually occurs somewhere between 20 and 30° of truncal elevation above the supine position, proper inspection of the pulsations can be made. If internal jugular venous pulsations are easily seen at more than 30° of truncal elevation, then central venous pressure is elevated. Confusing internal jugular venous pulsations with carotid artery pulsations is a common mistake. Very light compression with the clinician's finger will obliterate internal jugular venous pulsations but not carotid arterial pulsations to help in differentiating this. Typically in normal sinus rhythm there is an undulating and rhythmic motion to venous pulsations, as opposed to a singular large arterial pulsation from the carotid artery. In both constrictive pericarditis and cardiac tamponade, the internal jugular venous pulsations are very prominent and the a, c, and v waves become equally more prominent and confluent. The typical feature in constrictive pericarditis is a prominent Y descent, and this is usually not seen with tamponade physiology. In patients presenting with neck vein distention, the differential diagnosis should include CHF, cardiac tamponade, volume overload conditions not due to CHF, and superior vena cava syndrome. In addition, conditions associated with a noncompliant right ventricle should be considered, such as right ventricular hypertrophy secondary to pulmonary hypertension from any cause, right ventricular infarction, pulmonary emboli, or a cardiomyopathy, such as amyloidosis, affecting the right ventricle. Other conditions considered should be constrictive pericarditis, primary tricuspid valve disease, and pulmonic stenosis.

If there is one diagnostic physical finding for cardiac tamponade, it would be pulsus paradoxus.[1,15,20] Most patients with cardiac tamponade will have a paradoxical pulse. Recognition can be difficult in some patients without direct intraarterial pressure recordings. Pulsus paradoxus can also be present in other conditions, such as chronic obstructive pulmonary disease, asthma, right ventricular infarction, and some cases of constrictive pericarditis, especially in the setting of effusive constrictive physiology. Arrhythmias resulting in hypotension with a very narrow pulse pressure and severe left ventricular failure may also obscure the detection of pulsus paradoxus.[15,20] Difficulty in identifying a paradoxical pulse is more often due to the lack of experience of the examiner, as well as the inherent inexactness of the sphygmomanometric method of determination. As a general rule, it is considered normal to have less than 10 mmHg difference in systolic pressure between inspiration and expiration. When this difference exceeds 10 mmHg, pulsus paradoxus is said to be present.[20] In cases of severe cardiac tamponade, pulsus paradoxus usually exceeds 20 mmHg. (See Table 14-2 for reasons for the absence of a paradoxical pulse in patients with cardiac compression from tamponade.)

In summary, cardiac tamponade is likely to be present if elevated internal jugular venous pressure is observed in combination with a paradoxical pulse in the setting of a known pericardial effusion.

## TABLE 14-2.    Reasons for Absent Paradoxical Pulse

1. Localized right atrial compression

2. Severe left ventricular dysfunction with markedly elevated left ventricular end-diastolic pressure

3. Positive-pressure ventilation

4. Pulmonary arterial obstruction

5. Severe bi-ventricular hypertrophy

6. Atrial septal defect

7. Severe aortic regurgitation

# DIAGNOSTIC STUDIES IN CARDIAC TAMPONADE

After appropriate history and physical examination have been performed, if the patient has symptoms compatible with cardiac tamponade as well as physical findings of elevated central venous pressure and pulsus paradoxus, then diagnostic studies should be obtained to help confirm the diagnosis.[14]

The electrocardiogram is frequently performed in this setting, but it has only one finding that is highly suggestive of cardiac tamponade. That finding is electrical alternans (see the first example in Fig. 14-1).[21] Most of the time, the electrocardiogram is nonspecific, but there may be findings suggestive of pericardial disease. Some of those findings that might suggest pericardial effusion or pericarditis are (1) a low voltage, which can be seen in very large pericardial effusions; (2) electrocardiographic changes compatible with acute pericarditis, which characteristically are an abnormal ST-segment vector with ST elevation pointing toward the apex, often associated with P-R-segment depression in the limb leads; and (3) nonspecific ST-T abnormalities, which are often the evolutionary changes of acute pericarditis. Sinus tachycardia is usually present in patients with moderate to severe tamponade physiology, but this is a very nonspecific finding, since obviously many other conditions result in sinus tachycardia.[21,22]

The chest x-ray film is never diagnostic of cardiac tamponade, but it may be helpful in suggesting that a pericardial effusion is present.[14,23] There are some features of the chest x-ray film that should suggest pericardial effusion: an enlarged cardiac silhouette and an association with a left pleural effusion but no right pleural effusion or pericardial fat-pad displacement. The clinician must remember that the heart size can appear normal if acute intrapericardial bleeding has resulted in tamponade with less than 500 mL of fluid accumulation. Another point to remember is that in the chest x-ray film, a large pericardial effusion is often hard to distinguish from generalized cardiac enlargement but tends to have more of a "water-bottle" appearance than is seen in patients with four-chamber enlargement.

Newer imaging techniques have added much to the diagnosis of pericardial effusion. Computed tomographic (CT) scans and magnetic resonance imaging (MRI) are helpful in identifying the presence of a pericardial effusion and have been demonstrated to be very sensitive for the diagnosis.[24–28] In general, however, they do not determine when cardiac tamponade physiology is present. These radiologic studies are more useful in trying to determine whether constrictive pericarditis is present. In many cases of constriction, the pericardium is very thickened and usually measures greater than 3 mm in width by CT scan or MRI.[25,26] It has been reported that a CT scan is more sensitive in detecting pericardial calcification, which may imply constriction, than routine radiographs.[24,25] CT scanning and MRI can be useful in the differential diagnosis of other conditions that may either cause or mimic cardiac tamponade. One of those conditions that deserves consideration is acute aortic dissection with or without tamponade. Ultrafast CT is very effective in helping with the diagnosis of pulmonary embolism and can be useful in trying to determine whether one is dealing with restrictive cardiomyopathy or constrictive pericardial disease. In addition, malignant pericardial effusions, especially those related to lung or breast cancer, can sometimes be confirmed or strongly suspected when the primary tumor is seen with one of these imaging techniques in association with a pericardial effusion.

The most useful of the modern imaging techniques, however, is ultrasonography. Echocardiography remains the most reliable and readily accessible diagnostic tool.[3,14,17,19] This technique is widely available and easily transported to the patient's bedside in either the hospital or the emergency ward. It is quite helpful in facilitating a rapid diagnosis of a pericardial effusion. There continues to be some debate among experts as to whether the final arbiter for the diagnosis of cardiac tamponade is echocardiography, right heart catheterization, or physical examination.[2] The truth is that when one or any combination of these data sets is obtained, an experienced clinician can usually be very certain when cardiac tamponade physiology is present. None of these techniques in its own right is absolutely the final answer.

Many of the echocardiographic signs are listed in Table 14-3, but each may be misleading in its own right and must be combined with symptoms, physical findings, and other diagnostic tests that are available.[30–32] Some examples of abnormal echocardiographic findings are shown in Fig. 14-2.

Echocardiography has defined its role in the ability to diagnose the presence of pericardial effusion quite accurately, but it also is becoming increasingly utilized in helping to guide therapy.[29,33] Echocardiography can be used to guide pericardial drainage by the percutaneous technique and to demonstrate immediate improvement after drainage of the fluid has been successful.

In some cases, right heart catheterization, as well as intraarterial pressure monitoring, is needed to confirm the presence of tamponade physiology when other measures have failed to convince the clinician that tamponade physiology is definitely present. More typically, right heart catheterization is needed to confirm the presence of constrictive physiology prior to considering surgical intervention or after successful pericardiocentesis has been performed, yet the patient still has evidence of increased venous pressure.[19]

**TABLE 14-3.   Echocardiographic Features Commonly Found in Cardiac Tamponade**

1. Large pericardial effusion with swinging heart motion

2. Right ventricular diastolic collapse

3. Right atrial diastolic collapse

4. Abnormalities of tricuspid valve and mitral valve inflow. Velocity is determined by Doppler
   a. Inspiratory increase in tricuspid valve velocities
   b. Inspiratory decrease in mitral valve flow by greater than 15 percent

5. Inspiratory changes in right and left ventricular size, with increase in right ventricular size and decrease in left ventricular size

6. Plethora of the inferior vena cava
   a. Loss of respiratory variation of inferior vena cava
   b. Diameter of the inferior vena cava exceeds two times normal or more

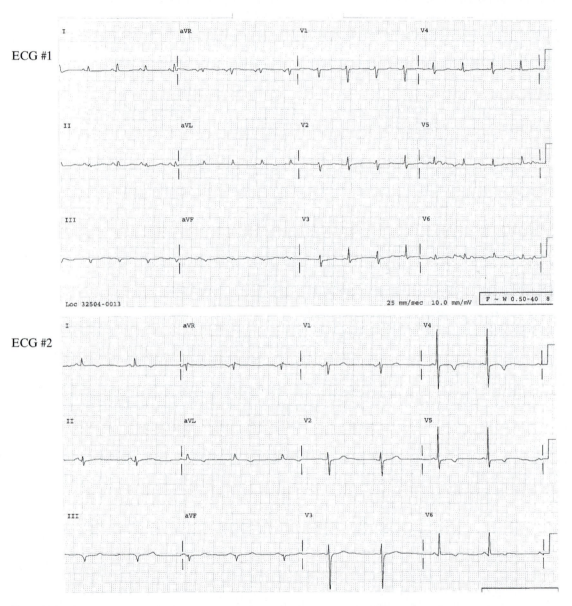

Figure 14-1   ECGs in patient with large pericardial effusion and tamponade. The first demonstrates electrical alternans (see lead $V_1$) and generalized low voltage. The second is approximately one week later, after pericardial effusion was drained. Notice the increased voltage and nonspecific T-wave changes.

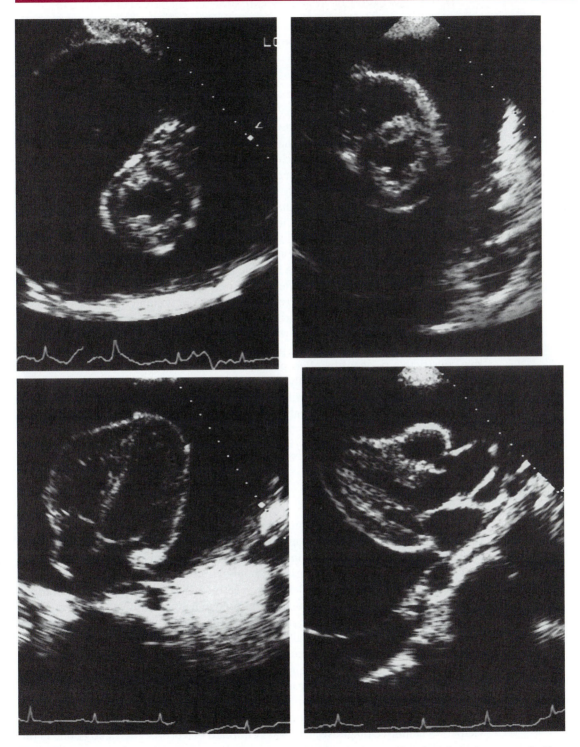

**Figure 14-2** Echocardiograms demonstrating a large pericardial effusion in a young female patient who presented with cardiac tamponade. The etiology was sytemic lupus erythematosus.

## SPECIAL SYNDROMES IN CARDIAC TAMPONADE

There are several unusual situations or syndromes in which cardiac tamponade may be present but may have atypical features, and these deserve further mention. Localized cardiac tamponade is considered to be present when the fluid is loculated and compressing only one or two chambers.[30,34] Often the chamber involved is the right atrium or right ventricle, but it can be any chamber of the heart. Localized tamponade typically occurs in the early stages after open-heart surgery.[27] At that point in time, it can be a rather difficult diagnosis to make because transthoracic echocardiograms are often technically difficult, with limited acoustical windows available. Usually transesophageal echocardiograms are used in this setting to confirm the diagnosis.[14,22,30,34] In patients with severe left ventricular hypertrophy, which most often is seen in our institution in the chronic dialysis patient, tamponade may affect only the right heart and a paradoxical pulse may be absent or barely detectable. In this situation, the picture is often confused with one of volume overload. Proper diagnosis is quite important, since further intravascular volume depletion will worsen the situation. Thus, recognition of the possibility of cardiac tamponade is essential in order to move forward with the proper treatment. Finally, the syndrome of effusive constrictive pericarditis often presents initially as tamponade, but constrictive physiology can be recognized only if hemodynamic monitoring is done during and after pericardiocentesis.[19] This situation seems to be increasing in frequency and is typically seen in etiologies of viral pericarditis, tuberculosis, radiation-induced, and post–open heart surgery.[19]

## TREATMENT OF CARDIAC TAMPONADE

In reality, there is only one treatment for cardiac tamponade, and that is drainage of the fluid to relieve the increased intrapericardial pressure. Conservative treatments with volume expansion and administration of pressors can be successful for a short period of time but should be considered only as a temporary measure as preparations are being made for more definitive treatment. There are just two indications for pericardiocentesis or pericardial drainage; one is for definitive therapy, and the other is for diagnosis. Primarily, pericardial drainage is for therapeutic relief of tamponade physiology, but occasionally pericardial drainage is indicated for diagnostic purposes. The so-called diagnostic tap in patients without elevated central venous pressure is rarely indicated, but on occasion there can be persistent concern regarding either a bacterial infection or a malignant effusion that may require pericardial drainage to make a definitive diagnosis. As a general rule, however, pericardial drainage and laboratory evaluation of the pericardial fluid have a relatively low yield for a definitive diagnosis. This was confirmed in a prospective study done in the early 1980s that showed a diagnostic yield of less than 10 percent in patients not clinically suspected of tamponade physiology.[35] Exceptions to this rule, however, are malignant effusions due to solid tumor involvement (often from lung or breast cancer) of the pericardial sac or the presence of a bacterial infection. The former etiology may have a positive cytology result approaching 85 percent from pericardiocentesis.[36–38] Tuberculous pericardial effusions are notoriously low yield with regard to a positive acid-fast bacilli culture and may require an open pericardial biopsy for definitive results.[39]

There are several methods of pericardial drainage that have become popular.[33,39–44] The longest experience is with percutaneous needle aspiration, and this is still the usual method of choice for most medical patients with cardiac tamponade. When the approach referred to as a pericardial window is applied to a patient with a pericardial effusion, there are three different procedures: (1) a subxiphoid surgical approach to pericardiostomy[39,40]; (2) a thoracoscopic approach, which is video-assisted and allows some localized pericardial resection; thoracoscopy can be done from either a subxiphoid approach or an anterolateral approach[42]; and (3) a percutaneous balloon pericardiostomy done with balloon dilatation over a needle-guided pericardiocentesis; this has been successfully used to create a pericardial window and has achieved modest popularity in recent times.[44]

One should also mention that medial sternotomy is the most effective surgical approach in dealing with pericardial disease but is reserved primarily for patients who are persistently symptomatic with constrictive physiology after the pericardial fluid has been removed. It is preferred in most patients with cardiac tamponade early after open-heart surgery.[34,39,40]

All of these approaches to pericardial drainage have a place in selected patients' situations. The surgical approaches are generally reserved for recurrent effusions after previous needle aspiration or when pericardial tissue is desired for diagnostic purposes. Occasionally, a surgical approach is needed for localized effusions that do not lend themselves to safe performance of the percutaneous needle aspiration technique. Also, surgical approaches are preferred in the early post–open heart patient with cardiac tamponade. Pericardial sclerosis for recurrent effusions is rarely used anymore, but it still has selective use in patients when surgery is not feasible or the patient's life expectancy is so limited that surgery is impractical.[41]

## SUMMARY

Pericardial effusions result from many different causes. Although often a benign observation made by echocardiography, pericardial effusion can result in hemodynamic embarrassment to the patient. In the worst-case scenario, cardiac tamponade is the syndrome that results from compression of the heart by pericardial fluid under pressure within the pericardial sac. There is no one physical finding, symptom, or diagnostic test that confirms for the physician that tamponade physiology is present. Careful inspection of the neck veins for elevated central venous pressure and of the blood pressure for a paradoxical pulse in the right clinical setting will usually bring the diagnosis into question, however. Confirmation by other diagnostic modalities, usually echocardiography, will then lead the clinician to the proper treatment. Most often that treatment is pericardial drainage. Advances in knowledge and experience with cardiac tamponade coupled with improved methods for safe and effective diagnosis and therapy have made this entity less of a clinical dilemma for both the patient and the clinician.

## REFERENCES

1. Starling EH: Some points in the pathology of heart disease. *Lancet* 1897; 1:652–655.
2. Fowler NO: Cardiac tamponade—a clinical or an echocardiographic diagnosis? *Circulation* 1993; 87:1738–1741.
3. Saah PK: Cardiac tamponade: pathophysiology, diagnosis and management. *Cardiol Clin* 1991; 9:665–674.
4. Hancock EW: Cardiac tamponade. *Heart Dis Stroke* May/June 1994; 3:155–159.
5. Fowler ND: Pericardial disease. In: *Atlas of Heart Disease,* vol. 2. Philadelphia, Current Medicine, 1995:13.1–13.16.
6. Friedrich SP, Berman AD, Baim DS, et al: Myocardial perforation in the cardiac catheterization laboratory. *Cathet Cardiovasc Diagn* 1994; 32:99–107.
7. Chabanier A, Davy F, Brutus P, et al: Iatrogenic cardiac tamponade after central venous catheterization. *Cardiol Clin* 1988; 11:91–99.
8. Aldridge HE, Jay AWL: Central venous catheters and heart perforation. *Can Med Assoc J* 1986; 135:1082–1084.
9. Greenspan AM, Spielman SR: Risks and complications of clinical cardiac electrophysiologic studies: a prospective analysis of 1,000 consecutive patients. *J Am Coll Cardiol* 1987; 9:1261–1268.
10. Bredlan CE, Roubin GS, Leinngruber PP, et al: In-hospital morbidity and mortality in patients undergoing elective coronary angioplasty. *Circulation* 1985; 72:1044–1052.
11. Rodgers KG: Cardiovascular shock. *Emerg Med Clin North Am* 1995; 13:793–810.
12. Beck CS: Two cardiac compression triads. *JAMA* 1935; 104:714–716.
13. Guberman BA, Fowler NO, Engel PJ, et al: Cardiac tamponade in medical patients. *Circulation* 1981; 64:633–640.
14. Chong HH, Plotnick GD: Pericardial effusion and tamponade evaluation, imaging modalities and management. *Compr Ther* 1995; 21:378–385.
15. Fowler NO: Pulsus paradoxus. *Heart Dis Stroke* 1994; 3:68–69.
16. Tyberg TI, Goodyer AVN, Langou RA: Genesis of pericardial knock in constrictive pericarditis. *Am J Cardiol* 1980; 46:570–575.
17. Fowler NO: Ewart's sign. In: Hurst JW (ed): *The Heart,* 3d ed. New York, McGraw-Hill, 1974; 1391.
18. Hurst JW: *Cardiovascular Diagnosis—The Initial Examination.* St. Louis, Mosby-Year Book, 1993:133–139.
19. Hancock EW: Subacute effusive constrictive pericarditis. *Circulation* 1971; 43:183–192.
20. Shabetai R: Pulsus paradoxus. In: *The Pericardium.* New York, Grune and Stratton, 1981; 279–324.
21. Spodick DH: Electrocardiographic changes in acute pericarditis. In: Fowler NO (ed): *The Pericardium in Health and Disease.* Mount Kisco, NY, Futura, 1985; 79–98.
22. Hurst JW: Ventricular electrocardiography. In: *Pericardial Disease.* New York, Gower Medical Publishing, 1991; 10.1–10.7.
23. Eisenberg MJ, Dunn MM, Kanth N, et al: Diagnostic value of CXR for pericardial effusion. *Circulation* 1974; 50:239–247.

24. Maish N: Pericardial diseases with a focus on etiology, pathogenesis, pathophysiology, new diagnostic imaging methods and treatment. *Curr Opin Cardiol* 1994; 9:379–388.

25. Tomoda H, Hoshiai M, Furuya H, et al: Evaluation of pericardial effusion with computed tomography. *Am Heart J* 1980; 99:701–706.

26. Mulvagh SL, Rokey R, Vick GW, et al: Usefulness of nuclear magnetic resonance imaging for evaluation of pericardial effusion and comparison with two dimensional echocardiography. *Am J Cardiol* 1989; 64:1002–1009.

27. Fuke FE, Tancredi RG, Shub C, et al: Detection of intra-pericardial hematoma after open heart surgery: the roles of echocardiography and computed tomography. *J Am Coll Cardiol* 1985; 5:1496–1499.

28. Schectem U, Tscholokoff D, Higgins CB: MRI at the abnormal pericardium. *Am J Radiol* 1986; 147:245–252.

29. Feigenbaum H, Waldhaussen JA, Hyde LP: Ultrasound diagnosis of the pericardial effusion. *JAMA* 1965; 191:107–111.

30. Troianos CA, Porembka DT: Assessment of left ventricular function and hemodynamics with transesophaegeal echocardiography. *Crit Care Clin* 1996; 12:253–272.

31. Armstrong WF, Schilt BF, Helper DJ, et al: Diastolic collapse of the right ventricle with tamponade: an echocardiographic study. *Circulation* 1982; 69:1491–1496.

32. Appleton CP, Hatle LK, Popp RL: Cardiac tamponade and pericardial effusion: respiratory variation in valvular flow velocities studied by Doppler echocardiography. *J Am Coll Cardiol* 1988; 11:1020–1030.

33. Callahan JA, Seward JB, Nishimura RA, et al: Two-dimensional echocardiography guided pericardiocentesis: experience in 117 consecutive patients. *Am J Cardiol* 1985; 55:476–479.

34. Ball JB, Morrison WL: Experience with cardiac tamponade following open heart surgery. *Heart Vessels* 1996; 11:39–43.

35. Permariyer Miralda G, Sagrista-Salueda J, Solar-Soler J: Primary acute pericardial disease: a prospective series of 231 consecutive patients. *Am J Cardiol* 1985; 56:623–630.

36. Zipf RE, Johnston WW: The role of cytology in the evaluation of pericardial effusions. *Chest* 1972; 62:593–596.

37. Edonte Y, Malberger E, Kutin A, et al: Symptomatic pericardial effusion in lung cancer patients: the role of fluid cytology. *J Surg Oncol* 1990; 45:121–123.

38. Meyers DG, Bouska DJ: Diagnostic usefulness of pericardial fluid cytology. *Chest* 1989; 95:1142–1143.

39. Tuna IC, Davidson GK: Surgical management of pericardial diseases. In: Shabeti R (ed): *Diseases of the Pericardium: Cardiology Clinics.* Philadelphia, W. B. Saunders, 1990; 683–696.

40. Moores DW, Dzuiban SW: Pericardial drainage procedures. *Chest Surg Clin North Am* 1995; 5:359–373.

41. Vaitkus PI, Herrman HC, LeWinter MM: Treatment of malignant pericardial effusion. *JAMA* 1994; 272:54–64.

42. Mack MJ, Aronoff RJ, Acuff TE, et al: Present role of thoracoscopy in the diagnosis and treatment of disease in the chest. *Am Thorac Surg* 1992; 54:403–409.

43. Mills SA, Julian S, Holliday RH, et al: Subxyphoid pericardial window for pericardial effusive disease. *J Cardiovasc Surg* 1989; 30:768–773.

44. Ziskind AA, Pearce AC, Lemmonn O, et al: Percutaneous balloon pericardiotomy for the treatment of cardiac tamponade and the large pericardial effusions. *J Am Coll Cardiol* 1993; 2:1–5.

OWEN B. SAMUELS / BARNEY J. STERN

# ISCHEMIC STROKE AND TRANSIENT ISCHEMIC ATTACKS

Most ischemic strokes are the outcome of long-standing atherosclerosis of the extracranial or intracranial arteries or the result of emboli from the heart. While major advances in diminishing the devastating effects of acute stroke are taking place, risk factor management and prevention remain the most effective strategies for reducing death and disability from stroke. This chapter will focus on stroke risk factors, stroke warning signs, mechanisms of infarction, and treatment strategies.

## TRANSIENT ISCHEMIC ATTACKS AND OTHER TRANSIENT NEUROLOGIC PHENOMENA

Transient ischemic attacks (TIAs) are warning signs of impending stroke and have been estimated to occur in 50 to 75 percent of patients with carotid artery territory stroke. The risk of suffering a stroke following a TIA is approximately 7 percent per year or 25 to 40 percent within 5 years after the first TIA, with the greatest risk occurring in the first month after TIA.

TIAs typically cause a sudden loss of neurologic function as a result of impaired blood flow to the brain. If symptoms last less than 24 h, by definition, the event is called a TIA. However, most TIAs resolve within 20 min, and 90 percent do so within 4 h. If symptoms persist for longer than 24 h, by arbitrary definition, the patient has suffered a stroke. Regardless of the duration of the TIA, both TIAs and strokes share a common pathomechanism, focal cerebral ischemia, and thus represent points on a continuum based on the persistence of symptoms and the intensity and duration of the ischemic insult.

Not all transient neurologic symptoms are ischemic in nature, and alternative causes such as seizures, mass lesions, migrainous phenomena, metabolic disturbances, or psychiatric illness should be considered when evaluating the patient. The history is the most important aspect in distinguishing ischemia from other causes of transient focal neurologic phenomena and must be obtained from the patient or other observers, since it is unlikely that the physician will be able to make a direct assessment. Long-standing symptoms without progression to permanent neurologic sequelae typically suggest a benign process. Alternatively, recent events occurring more frequently and with greater intensity warrant an expeditious evaluation. The presence of vascular and cardioembolic risk factors should always be sought.

The temporal onset, progression, and duration of the transient neurologic event are important clues to its etiology. For example, fortification spectra are common in migraine but rare in amaurosis fugax (transient monocular blindness) from carotid artery disease. Focal motor or sensory symptoms such as brief tingling or rhythmic shaking (positive symptoms) more often occur as a result of partial seizures, whereas cerebral ischemia causes loss of sensation and weakness (negative symptoms) or clumsiness. Migrainous phenomena tend to produce positive symptoms, causing a tingling that spreads or "marches" across a limb, whereas ischemia more typically affects an entire region simultaneously. Although headache is generally considered the hallmark of migraine, embolic stroke, large artery occlusion, arterial dissection, or ruptured cerebral aneurysm all can present with headache at onset. Unilaterality of the headache, a pulsatile quality, worsening with exertion, phonophobia, photophobia, and moderate nausea suggest migraine.

## MECHANISMS OF BRAIN ISCHEMIA

Pathogenesis of brain ischemia can be divided into three basic mechanisms: (1) cerebral embolism (cardioembolic, artery-to-artery), (2) arterial occlusive disease (extracranial large artery, intracranial large or medium artery resulting in distal hypoperfusion), and (3) small artery occlusive disease (lacunar). At times it is difficult to define a specific mechanism; some patients have multiple potential causes, and in others there is no obvious reason for the stroke.[1]

## CEREBRAL EMBOLISM

### Clinical Features

The classic clinical presentation of brain embolism is the abrupt onset of focal neurologic impairment, with maximal deficit at onset, occurring while the patient is awake, and often during periods of activity; only 5 percent of patients have a progressive or stuttering course. Headache occurs in approximately 20 percent of patients. The middle cerebral artery (MCA) is the artery most commonly involved. Emboli tend to lodge in distal arterial sites (M-1 or M-2 divisions), resulting in cortical deficits. Certain syndromes are particularly suggestive of embolism, such as isolated receptive aphasia (Wernicke's aphasia); middle cerebral artery branch occlusion, "top of the basilar syndrome," or isolated hemianopia (visual loss); and posterior cerebral artery occlusion. Multiple ischemic cortical infarcts in different vascular territories, in the absence of previous stereotypic TIAs, support a cardioembolic mechanism.

Cardiogenic embolism accounts for up to 20 percent of all ischemic strokes. This proportion is probably higher in younger patients. Approximately 80 percent of cardiogenic emboli affect the carotid circulation and 20 percent travel to the vertebrobasilar circulation, commensurate with the proportional cerebral blood flow in these two vascular territories. Angiographic evidence of an intraluminal filling defect that disappears on subsequent angiograms is suggestive of cardioembolism.

The likelihood of identifying a potential cardioembolic source depends on how extensively patients are evaluated and what lesions are accepted as potentially cardioembolic in nature. The diagnostic role of transesophageal echocardiography is evolving and has recently identified potential cardiogenic sources, including spontaneous contrast or "smoke" representing erythrocyte microaggregates in the left atrium, small septal defects (patent foramen ovale), and intraatrial septal aneurysms.

Numerous potential cardioembolic sources have been identified. These can be categorized into higher-risk and lower- or uncertain-risk sources of cardioembolism. High-risk sources include atrial fibrillation, mitral stenosis, mechanical heart valves, left ventricular thrombus, atrial myxoma, dilated cardiomyopathy, and infective or marantic endocarditis. Lower- or uncertain-risk cardioembolic sources are mitral valve prolapse with myxomatous changes, mitral annular calcification, patent foramen ovale, atrial septal aneurysm, calcified aortic stenosis, left ventricular wall motion abnormalities, and aortic arch atheromatous plaques.

## Nonvalvular Atrial Fibrillation

Nonvalvular atrial fibrillation (NVAF), a major source of cardioembolism, accounts for 50 percent of all cardioembolic strokes and is an independent risk factor for stroke. While the overall rate of ischemic stroke among patients with NVAF is 5 percent per year, the risk of cardioembolism is not uniform, and subgroups of patients with atrial fibrillation (AF) with higher or lower risks exist. Patients with "lone" AF and those younger than age 65 without previous stroke, TIA, or vascular risk factors have an annual stroke risk of <2 percent. High-risk patients include those with a history of prior TIA or stroke, diabetes, hypertension, or recent congestive heart failure (CHF). The risk of cardioembolism in these patients ranges from 7 to 18 percent per year and increases with age. Identification of high-risk patients is important when considering the risks and benefits of antithrombotic therapy.

Not all ischemic strokes or TIAs occuring in patients with AF are due to cardioembolism; therefore, other sources or mechanisms of stroke should be investigated. Nearly 30 percent of AF-associated strokes are due to other cardiac sources of embolism, arterial occlusive disease, or aortic arch atheroma. Of these patients, about 12 percent (typically elderly patients) have moderate to severe extracranial carotid stenosis.

Most cardiogenic emboli occuring after acute myocardial infarction (AMI) develop within the first 2 weeks from left ventricular thrombi. Left ventricular thrombi develop in 40 percent of anterior wall MIs, with subsequent cardioembolism occurring in 6 percent of patients. The risk of late cardioembolism falls sharply in the months following MI despite the persistence of left ventricular thrombus. The incidence of left ventricular aneurysm after MI is about 7 to 10 percent; however, the risk of clinically evident embolism is uncertain and is estimated in retrospective studies to be 4 to 6 percent per year.

Prosthetic heart valves account for approximately 10 percent of all cardioembolic strokes, with a thrombus forming either on the prosthesis or in the left atrium. Anticoagulated patients with mechanical valves have an embolic rate of 4 percent per year in the mitral position and 2 percent per year in the aortic position. Patients with bioprosthetic mitral and aortic valves who are treated with aspirin have a lower embolic rate of 1 to 3 percent per year.

Patent foramen ovale and small atrial septal defects (ASD) are more prevalent in young patients with stroke of "unknown cause." Although a paradoxical mechanism is hypothesized, venous thrombosis is rarely found.

# LARGE ARTERY DISEASE

## Aortic Arch Embolism

Atherosclerotic disease of the aortic arch is a potential source of brain embolism. Transesophageal echocardiography (TEE) allows the detection of aortic arch plaques that, when ≥4 mm in thickness and located proximal to the left subclavian artery, are associated with a ninefold increase in the risk of ischemic stroke. A mobile plaque component indicates an even higher risk of stroke.

## Anterior Circulation Ischemia

Atherosclerosis is the predominant disease process affecting the extracranial internal carotid artery (ICA) at its origin. High-grade stenosis may cause hemodynamic insufficiency in the distal regions of the ipsilateral hemisphere, so-called border-zone or watershed ischemia, or may serve as a source of artery-to-artery emboli obstructing the distal intracranial circulation. Less common causes of carotid occlusive and embolic disease include carotid dissection, fibromuscular dysplasia, and local radiation therapy.

**CAROTID BRUITS.**    The presence of a carotid bruit on neck auscultation should raise concern over occlusive disease of ICA origin. The quality of the bruit may vary and is not particularly predictive of the underlying degree of stenosis, although a diastolic component often suggests high-grade stenosis. Bruits tend to occur with moderate to severe stenosis and often disappear as the stenosis becomes near occlusive. Other cervical sounds can mimic ICA bruits, such as radiated cardiac murmurs, external carotid artery stenosis, nonstenosing lesions of the ICA (loops and kinks), and venous sounds.

The source of a cervical bruit should be investigated with noninvasive testing in asymptomatic and symptomatic patients. However, the absence of a bruit should not be construed as a reason to defer evaluation. Bruits are relatively poor predictors of carotid occlusive disease, with a sensitivity of 63 percent and specificity of 61 percent for detecting 70 to 99 percent stenosis in symptomatic patients. Importantly, carotid bruits are absent in over one-third of patients with high-grade stenosis (70 to 99 percent).

**CAROTID TERRITORY ISCHEMIA.**   TIAs are the principal warning symptoms of extracranial ICA occlusive disease. Transient monocular blindness (TMB) is common in patients with ≥70 percent ICA stenosis. Symptoms are typically brief, lasting less than 20 min, and characterized by painless monocular visual loss, described as a descending shade or window curtain. Many patients experience partial visual loss confined to a sector of the visual field. The pathomechanism of TMB in patients with vascular disease is a fibrin-platelet-cholesterol embolus from an atheromatous carotid plaque that travels to the ophthalmic artery, temporarily occluding the retinal circulation. Occasionally, cholesterol crystals, referred to as Hollenhorst plaques, can be visualized as bright spots on fundoscopy. Other potential causes of TMB are emboli derived from the heart or aortic arch, ocular migraine, temporal arteritis, antiphospholipid antibody syndrome, connective tissue disorders, blood dyscrasias, and vasospasm.

The most common features of hemispheral TIAs are contralateral motor and sensory loss (usually involving the face, arm, and leg) with language impairment (dominant hemisphere) or neglect syndromes (nondominant hemisphere). An unusual form of transient hemispheric ischemia has been referred to as "shaking limb" TIAs, characterized by limb trembling, shaking, twisting, or drawing up in a nonrhythmic, irregular manner. When "shaking limb" TIAs occur as the initial manifestation of carotid occlusive disease, differentiation of this disease from focal motor seizures can be difficult. A history of more typical carotid distribution TIAs in association with high-grade ICA stenosis suggests a vascular mechanism.

The clinical spectrum and severity of cerebral ischemia associated with carotid disease often depends on the mechanism, whether it be hemodynamic or embolic. If hemodynamic insufficiency results from near-occlusive ICA stenosis with insufficient collateral circulation, the brain tissue at particularly high risk for infarction is the "border zone," which occurs at the margins of vascular territories supplied by the major intracranial arteries. In these areas, circulation may be adequate under normal circumstances but becomes insufficient with systemic hypotension or severe arterial stenosis. Border-zone ischemia is categorized as anterior (territory between the anterior cerebral artery and the MCA) or posterior [territory between the MCA and the posterior cerebral artery (PCA)]. Neurologic symptoms suggestive of anterior watershed ischemia are contralateral arm and hand weakness, with relative sparing of the leg. Bilateral anterior watershed ischemia resulting in bilateral upper-extremity weakness with relative sparing of the legs is referred to as the "man in the barrel" syndrome. In the dominant hemisphere, transcortical motor aphasia (expressive aphasia with intact repetition) suggests anterior border-zone ischemia. Symptoms suggestive of posterior border-zone ischemia include hemianopia with a transcortical sensory aphasia (fluent aphasia with impaired comprehension, but with preserved ability to repeat), isolated word-finding difficulties (dominant hemisphere), and neglect syndromes (nondominant hemisphere). Anterior and posterior border-zone ischemia of either hemisphere may present with agitation and global confusion in the absence of focal neurologic deficits.

Bilateral severe ICA occlusive disease resulting in hemodynamic insufficiency can cause gait disturbances, dysequilibruim, dysarthria, and dysphagia. These features are more commonly seen in posterior circulation TIAs; when caused by carotid insufficiency, they are false localizing signs. Syncope may rarely result from severe bilateral ICA near-occlusive disease.

In contrast to border-zone ischemia, embolism from the extracranial ICA affects the MCA and its distal branches. Infarct location and symptoms will vary depending on the exact site of occlusion. If the MCA stem is occluded proximal to the lenticulostriate arteries, both the deep and superficial MCA territories are involved, resulting in contralateral hemiplegia and dense hemisensory loss, global aphasia (dominant hemisphere), neglect syndromes (nondominant hemisphere), and forced conjugate eye deviation toward the involved hemisphere. Although the sudden onset of severe hemispheric ischemia in the MCA distribution suggests an embolic occlusion, differentiating the source as cardiogenic versus arterial in origin is difficult on clinical grounds alone.

Atherosclerotic occlusive disease of the intracranial ICA and MCA is increasingly being identified as a mechanism for hemispheric ischemia. Recurrent, stereotypic TIAs in the absence of significant extracranial stenosis suggests intracranial occlusive disease. Mechanisms of ischemia are emboli (artery-to-artery) and hemodynamic compromise. Atherosclerosis of the carotid siphon commonly involves the cavernous portion distal to the origin of the ophthalmic artery, whereas MCA disease typically involves the main stem (M1 segment).

## Posterior Circulation Ischemia

Ischemia affecting the posterior circulation has mechanisms similar to those of anterior circulation ischemia. Emboli to the vertebrobasilar (VB) circulation tend to lodge in either the intracranial segment of the vertebral artery (VA), the apex of the basilar artery (BA), or the middle and distal segments of the PCA. Hemodynamic insufficiency occurs with BA or bilateral VA occlusive disease.

Posterior circulation ischemia causes slurred speech, weakness, numbness, and visual loss, all symptoms similar to those found with anterior circulation ischemia. Clinical features unique to the posterior circulation include vertigo, nystagmus (manifest as oscillopsia), diplopia, bilateral motor weakness or sensory loss, ataxia, and crossed findings of cranial nerve deficits and contralateral motor and sensory disturbances.

Discussions of posterior circulation ischemia symptoms often focus on vertigo as a primary feature, with vertigo being defined as a false sense of rotational motion. However, care must be taken to differentiate vertigo from dizziness without a sense of movement, which has little localizing value. Only a small proportion of patients with VB ischemia actually report being vertiginous; patients often use the term *dizzy,* which as an isolated symptom does not necessarily forecast cerebral ischemia.

Recurrent isolated dizziness lasting weeks to months is unlikely to be due to VB is-chemia. When vertigo is accompanied by other cardinal VB symptoms, such as diplopia, there is ample cause for concern. Less common features of VB ischemia in-clude a gritty sensation on the face, hiccups, sudden decreased hearing, a roaring sound in the ear, confusion, and amnesia. Rhythmic shaking movements of one or more limbs may rarely be seen in association with brainstem ischemia secondary to basilar artery occlusive disease. These movements may portend signs of acute de-cerebration associated with extensor posturing and may be mistaken for seizures.

Quadriplegia or alternating hemiparesis, a hallmark of VB disease, rarely presents as an isolated symptom and is usually accompanied by dysarthria or diplopia. When quadriplegia occurs in isolation, bilateral carotid disease is more likely. Syncope is rarely, if ever, caused by brainstem ischemia, and a cardiac etiology or hypotension should be pursued.

**SUBCLAVIAN ARTERY AND VERTEBRAL ARTERY ORIGIN DISEASE.** Atherosclerotic occlusive disease of the subclavian artery compromising perfusion of the VA can cause the syndrome of "subclavian steal." This occurs when there is severe stenosis or occlusion of the subclavian artery proximal to the origin of the VA causing low flow in the distal subclavian artery and a resultant "steal" effect from the contralateral VA. Symptoms may be vague, such as dizziness, numbness, blurred vision, or dysequilibrium. Many patients are asymptomatic and are identi-fied incidentally on angiography.

Atherosclerosis of the origin of the VA is an underrecognized cause of posterior circulation ischemia. This may be due to the difficulty of noninvasively imaging the aortic arch and the VA origins. If both VAs are of good caliber, progressive stenosis or occlusion of one VA origin is often asymptomatic, whereas if one vertebral artery is congenitally small or ends in the posterior inferior cerebellar artery (an anatomic variant), unilateral VA origin occlusive disease is often symptomatic and potentially life-threatening. Bilateral VA origin stenosis is also concerning, presenting with transient episodes of imbalance, blurred vision, diaphoresis, weakness, and rarely syncope. The attacks are often induced by an upright posture.

**INTRACRANIAL DISEASE OF THE VERTEBRAL AND BASILAR AR-TERIES.**   The intracranial segments of the VAs are common sites of atheroscle-rotic occlusive disease. Occlusion from a proximal embolic source such as the heart, the aortic arch, or the VA origin can occur. Abrupt occlusion of one of the intracra-nial vertebral arteries often causes the lateral medullary syndrome (Wallenberg's syndrome), leading to vertigo, lateropulsion toward the side of the lesion, ipsilateral limb ataxia, diplopia, Horner's syndrome, facial numbness, dysphagia, hiccups, and contralateral loss of temperature and pain sensation and temperature insensitivity of the arm and leg.

The proximal and middle portions of the BA are common sites of atherosclero-sis, whereas the distal portion is more frequently occluded by embolism. BA throm-bosis may have a stuttering progression of deficits over a period of hours to days, of-ten culminating in coma. Less commonly, patients may experience isolated pure motor hemiplegia (PMH) with dysarthria from atheromatous obstruction of the orifice of the paramedian penetrating arteries, branches of the BA. Ischemia from an embolus that lodges at the apex of the BA presents with a constellation of findings referred to as the "top of the basilar syndrome"; symptoms include sleepiness, impaired upgaze, visual loss, confusion, memory loss, and delirium.

# SMALL ARTERY OCCLUSIVE DISEASE (LACUNAR SYNDROMES)

Occlusive disease of the deep penetrating arteries of both the anterior and posterior circulation accounts for up to 20 percent of cerebral ischemia. "Lacunes" are the pathologic sequelae of small arterial occlusions, and lipohyalinosis of these small end arteries is the most common vascular pathologic finding at autopsy. Anterior circulation lacunar infarctions occur primarily in the territories of the lenticulostriate arteries, which are small branches of the proximal portions of the MCA and ACA supplying the internal capsule, caudate nucleus, and basal ganglia. Posterior circulation lacunar infarctions occur in the territories of the thalamoperforant branches of the PCA (which supply the midbrain and thalamus) and of the paramedian branches of the basilar artery (which supply the pons). These arteries are all end vessels without opportunity for collateral blood flow. Once they are occluded, infarction occurs.

Although several clinical features are considered typical of lacunar small artery disease, these presentations can be mimicked on occasion by both carotid and vertebrobasilar large artery occlusive disease, artery-to-artery embolism, and cardiogenic embolism. Clinical features such as pure motor hemiparesis or hemisensory loss are important diagnostic clues to the presence of lacunar disease. Lacunar infarctions tend to present in a stuttering tempo and worsen over a period of hours to days.

The most common lacunar syndromes include pure motor hemiparesis (internal capsule, pons), ataxic hemiparesis (internal capsule, pons), clumsy hand dysarthria (internal capsule, pons), and pure hemilateral sensory loss (thalamus). It is important to distinguish between capsular and brainstem localization, since PMH may reflect intrinsic BA occlusive disease, forecasting imminent basilar occlusion. Symptoms that favor a brainstem location of PMH include previous TIAs with dizziness, vertigo, alternating hemiplegia, or diplopia. These symptoms are referred to as a "herald hemiparesis."

# ARTERIAL DISSECTION

Dissection of the extracranial carotid or vertebral artery is relatively common, especially in younger individuals. Patients typically present with neck pain, facial pain, or headache, which can precede the development of ischemic symptoms by several days. Patients often do not have the usual stroke risk factors. Dissection may occur spontaneously, in the setting of trivial trauma, from whiplash injuries, from vigorous neck manipulation, or from iatrogenic trauma during central line placement. Patients with fibromuscular dysplasia are at the highest risk for spontaneous dissection. ICA redundancies, loops, and kinks are associated with spontaneous dissections. Less common conditions associated with dissection include Marfan's syndrome, pseudoxanthoma elasticum, and alpha$_1$-antitrypsin deficiency.

## HEMATOLOGIC CONDITIONS

The antiphospholipid antibody syndrome (APS) represents one of the most commonly identifiable causes of an acquired hypercoagulable state that produces cerebral ischemia. Stroke is the most common arterial thrombotic event associated with antiphospholipid antibodies and should be assayed for in young patients, especially women, with a history of recurrent thromboocclusive events. Clinical features include thrombotic events, both arterial and venous, marantic endocarditis, history of miscarriages, and migraine headaches associated with transient focal deficits. Ischemic strokes are generally in the territory of the MCA. Laboratory features of APS include a prolonged aPTT (activated partial thromboplastin time), false-positive VDRL test, thrombocytopenia, positive ANA, reduced complement $C_4$, and occasionally hemolytic anemia. The risk of recurrent stroke in patients with a prior event associated with APS is estimated to be 10 percent per year; patients with high titers of IgG anticardiolipin antibodies may be at greatest risk.

Deficiencies of proteins C and S and antithrombin III are most frequently associated with venous thrombosis, including cerebral vein and sagittal sinus thrombosis, but arterial thrombosis does occur. These deficiencies may be inherited, but can be acquired in protein-losing conditions such as nephrotic syndrome.

Activated protein C resistance [(APC-R) (factor V Leiden mutation)] is strongly linked to venous thrombosis and has been found in 20 to 60 percent of young patients with unexplained venous thrombosis. Although APC-R has been reported in several case series of ischemic stroke in the young, its significance is as yet unknown.

Stroke is the most common neurologic manifestation of sickle cell disease (SCD), which is the most frequent cause of stroke in children. As many as 17 percent of patients with SCD suffer a stroke, which is often hemorrhagic, by early adulthood. In addition to slugging and occlusion of small arteries, large vessel occlusive vasculopathy occurs in SCD.

## NEUROVASCULAR TESTING

Conventional cerebral angiography remains the gold standard for evaluating the extracranial and intracranial arteries. However, noninvasive techniques, such as duplex scanning, transcranial Doppler (TCD), and magnetic resonance angiography (MRA), have assumed a major role in stroke evaluation. Carotid duplex sonography has a sensitivity and specificity of over 80 to 90 percent for detecting stenosis at the ICA origin. Duplex scanning relies on velocity measurement, and therefore anatomic irregularities such as loops and kinks may result in false-positive tests for significant stenosis. MRA tends to overestimate moderate stenosis of ICA origin in the range of 50 to 70 percent. MRA and TCD are important screening methods for evaluating stenosis of the major intracranial arteries. In combination, MRA and TCD have a reported sensitivity of 80 to 90 percent for identifying intracranial stenosis.

# EVALUATION AND MANAGEMENT

## Approach to the Patient

TIAs should be considered the harbingers of a major stroke and require immediate evaluation[2] (see Fig. 15-1). From the initial encounter, the clinician should begin forming a hypothesis about the mechanism of ischemia, site of the vascular lesion, and localization of brain injury. A detailed history, with particular attention to the precise time of onset, the time course of neurologic symptoms, and relevant stroke risk factors, is essential. The medical and neurologic examinations should test clinical

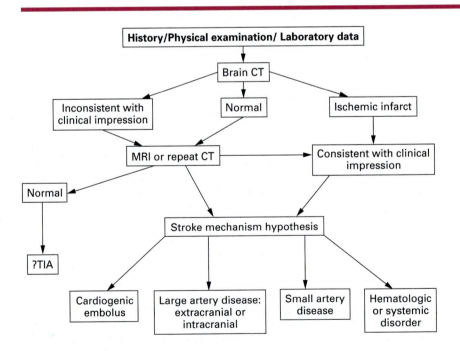

Figure 15-1    Ischemic stroke algorithm.

clues and hypotheses generated by the history, e.g., symptoms of transient hemispheric ischemia and TMB should direct a search for cervical bruits and retinal emboli. Posterior circulation TIAs should prompt a search for subclavian bruits, nystagmus, ataxia, or crossed sensorimotor deficits. When symptoms suggest embolism, murmurs of mitral stenosis and ECG abnormalities [AF, left ventricular hypertrophy (LVH)] are germane findings. Diagnostic tests such as MRA, duplex scanning, TCD, and echocardiogram should be prioritized in the order of clinical suspicion.

Since ischemia in younger patients is often due to etiologies other than atherosclerosis, arterial dissection, drug use, and hypercoagulable states should be considered. A recent history of neck pain, trauma, whiplash injuries, or neck manipulation should be elicited. A personal or family history of deep venous thrombosis, miscarriage, prior thromboembolic events, migraine headache, or concurrent use of oral contraceptives should be considered.

## Initial Emergent Evaluation and General Supportive Care

Patients with multiple TIAs within hours or days of presentation (so-called crescendo TIAs) or strokes should be admitted to the hospital for immediate evaluation.[3] Vital signs, including blood pressure, heart rate and rhythm, and oxygen saturation, should be closely monitored in patients with moderate to severe symptoms. Hematologic and chemistry profiles should be obtained in all patients. Serum glucose and, if clinically appropriate, a drug toxicology screen are indicated. Intravenous fluids should be limited to the replacement of losses in the acute setting unless hypovolemia is suspected. Isotonic saline without dextrose is preferred. Generally, hyperosmotic and dextrose-containing fluids should be avoided, since they can lead to an increase in regional lactate and worsen cerebral acidosis and edema. Blood pressure must be monitored closely. Though many stroke patients are hypertensive on acute presentation, the majority do not require treatment; their blood pressure will gradually drop over 24 h. Even in those with severe hypertension, blood pressure should be lowered cautiously because of the risk of cerebral hypoperfusion associated with neurologic deterioration. Agents that are easily titrated and have minimal effect on cerebral blood vessels (e.g., labetalol, enalapril) are preferred. Medications that may precipitously lower blood pressure, such as sublingual nifedipine, should be avoided. Treatment of blood pressure should be limited to patients with markedly sustained elevated blood pressures (mean arterial pressure >150 mmHg). Other general care measures include treatment of fever, swallowing evaluation and aspiration precautions, maintenance of nutrition, deep venous thrombosis and decubiti prophylaxis, management of bowel and bladder function, and early physical and occupational therapy.

## Neuroimaging

Once the patient is medically stable, early computed tomography (CT) imaging is important to differentiate a hemorrhage from an ischemic event and to exclude alternative causes of neurologic compromise. Conventional MRI is relatively insensitive for detecting early ischemia (<12 h) and therefore offers only a modest advantage over CT in the emergent setting. MRI diffusion and perfusion-weighted images, which promise early detection of focal ischemia, are under intensive clinical study, as are techniques to identify early parenchymal hemorrhages.

## Emergent Treatment of Acute Ischemia

Although, tradionally, an attempt is made to tailor stroke treatment to the pathophysiologic basis of an individual's stroke, the findings of the National Institute of Neurological Disorders and Stroke (NINDS) rt-PA Stroke Study Group pertain to all causes of ischemic stroke (specific stroke pathomechanistic-based treatment and management issues are discussed later in this chapter).[4] Tissue plasminogen activator (t-PA) administered within 3 h of symptom onset, 0.9 mg/kg (maximum dose 90 mg) infused over 1 h, is associated with a 30 percent greater likelihood of complete or near-complete recovery compared with placebo-treated patients.[4] This benefit was noted for all stroke subtypes, including cardioembolic, atherothrombotic, and lacunar strokes. The major complication of treatment is symptomatic intracranial hemorrhage (6.4 percent with t-PA versus 0.6 percent with placebo), although there was no significant difference in mortality at 3 months from treatment. Identifiable risk factors for symptomatic hemorrhage include elevated blood pressure, severe neurologic deficits on initial presentation, concurrent use of anticoagulants, and early CT changes suggesting edema or early infarction. Patient selection, t-PA dosing and administration, and patient monitoring, including close blood pressure management, must be done carefully in the setting of the emergency department or an intensive care unit to minimize treatment complications.

Intraarterial thrombolytic infusion into the occlusive thrombus of an intracranial vessel (e.g., MCA stem) via a superselective microcatheter has demonstrated clot lysis rates of 60 to 80 percent with clinical benefit in small case series. At present, intraarterial thrombolytic therapy is justified only in the setting of an investigational protocol. Other therapies under active investigation include neuroprotective agents targeting components of the ischemic cascade, various thrombolytic regimens, novel agents addressing platelet and white blood cell functions, and promoters of neuronal repair. These aggressive management strategies in concert with acute neurointensive monitoring promise to deliver significant improvements in the prognosis of the acute stroke patient.

## Anticoagulation in Acute Stroke

The use of intravenous anticoagulants such as heparin in the setting of acute ischemic stroke remains controversial.[5] On initial evaluation of stroke patients, it is not possible to determine if the neurologic deficit will resolve rapidly, remain fixed, or deteriorate. Progressing stroke, "stroke in evolution," occurs in a sizable number of patients. Because the specific pathogenesis of stroke in these patients is often difficult to elucidate in the emergent setting, some clinicians advocate intravenous heparin for patients with submaximal deficits. The rationale for early institution of heparin is twofold. Heparin may prevent recurrent embolism from a cardiac or proximal arterial source or prevent intraarterial thrombus propagation or reocclusion. Despite the absence of proven therapeutic efficacy, the use of intravenous heparin for acute ischemia should be considered in the following situations: (1) progressing stroke, (2) acute partial stroke with residual brain "at risk" in the compromised vascular territory, (3) crescendo TIAs or recent minor stroke, and (4) cardioembolic stroke. Complete blood count including platelets, coagulation profile (PT, aPTT), stool hemoccult, noncontrast CT, and prior bleeding history should be obtained before anticoagulation is instituted.

## Management of the Deteriorating Patient

Deteriorating patients should be evaluated to assess factors that might be contributing to the patient's decline. The blood pressure should not be so low as to impair cerebral perfusion or, at the opposite extreme, excessively high, promoting cerebral edema. Hydration should be adequate without the patient's being overhydrated, and proper oxygenation needs to be assured. The intensity of anticoagulation must be appropriate. The possibility of heparin-associated thrombosis should also be considered. A CT should be obtained to evaluate the possibility of intracranial hemorrhage or mass effect leading to brain shifts or increased intracranial pressure.

Aggressive but unproven therapeutic treatments include emergency carotid endarterectomy (CEA), hypervolemic hypertensive therapy with invasive monitoring of volume status, hyperventilation, hypothermia for treatment of elevated intracranial pressure, and decompressive hemicraniectomy. Surgical resection of an infarcted, edematous cerebellar hemisphere can be lifesaving.

## Cardiogenic Embolism

When a cardioembolic source is suspected, the rationale for the early institution of anticoagulant therapy is the possibility of recurrent emboli, estimated to be 1 percent per day or 20 percent over 2 weeks following the initial event. Anticoagulation may be postponed for 3 to 7 days in patients with severe neurologic deficits to diminish the risk of hemorrhagic conversion of large ischemic brain areas, leading to clinical deterioration.

Patients presenting with atrial fibrillation in the setting of an ischemic stroke have a high risk of recurrent stroke (12 percent per year). Institution of warfarin is recommended [international normalized ratio (INR) 2.5 to 3.0] while the patient is being treated with heparin. Since anticoagulation is recommended for all patients with AF-associated stroke who can safely receive it, the need for an echocardiogram is debatable. However, in patients with relative contraindications to anticoagulation, TFE evidence of a clear cardioembolic source ("smoke" or atrial thrombus) in high-risk patients may influence the risk-benefit decision. Management of these patients is often tempered by advanced age, disabling neurologic deficits, and comorbid medical conditions. Aspirin should be used when anticoagulants cannot be given safely; however, it provides only a modest relative risk reduction of 15 percent in high-risk patients.

Coexistent extracranial ICA occlusive disease in patients with AF-associated stroke should be investigated in those patients with anterior circulation stroke. These patients are potential candidates for carotid endarterectomy if ipsilateral ICA stenosis exceeds 70 percent.

Warfarin (INR 2 to 3) is effective (risk reduction 68 percent) and relatively safe for primary and secondary prevention of stroke in high-risk AF-patients (prior stroke or TIA, hypertension, dilated cardiomyopathy, diabetes, recent MI, or mitral stenosis) 75 years of age or younger; in older patients, a lower INR (~2.0) is recommended to minimize the risk of hemorrhage. Aspirin (75 to 325 mg) is active in preventing stroke in AF-patients who are not warfarin candidates, but is substantially less effective (risk reduction 20 percent). Patients <60 years with "lone" AF may not benefit from warfarin therapy given their low annual risk of stroke. Empiric use of aspirin, although not of proven benefit, is a reasonable approach in these patients. The key to effective and safe selection of antithrombotic prophylaxis in AF-patients is stroke risk stratification.[6,7]

Patients with mechanical prosthetic heart valves require higher levels of anticoagulation (INR 3 to 4). Early anticoagulation is recommended in patients undergoing surgery for bioprosthetic valves, given the high risk of embolism in the first 3 months; subsequent long-term aspirin (325 mg) is then recommended.

In the setting of an acute transmural MI, anticoagulation with heparin reduces the risk of early stroke. Long-term anticoagulation (3 to 6 months) is recommended in patients with a left ventricular thrombus or a large hypokinetic segment.

The definitive management of patients with a patent foramen ovale (PFO) or atrial septal aneurysm (ASA) is controversial. For patients with a PFO/ASA and otherwise unexplained TIA or stroke without evidence for a venous embolic source, antiplatelet therapy is reasonable. Surgical correction is not of proven efficacy. Treatment for patients with PFO/ASA with recurrent TIAs or strokes on antiplatelet therapy must be decided on an individual basis; anticoagulation and surgical repair are alternative options.

# ARTERIAL OCCLUSIVE DISEASE

## Symptomatic Extracranial Carotid Artery Disease

Carotid endarterectomy reduces the risk of recurrent stroke from 26 to 9 percent over 2 years in patients with a TIA or minor stroke ipsilateral to a 70 to 99 percent stenosis of the ICA (perioperative complication rate <6 percent).[8] The potential benefit of CEA in patients with moderate stenosis (30 to 69 percent) has not yet been established; antiplatelet therapy may be appropriate for the majority of these patients. Surgery for patients with <30 percent ICA origin stenosis is of no proven benefit. In patients undergoing surgery, excluding those with major deficits, early CEA (days to weeks after stroke) is recommended because of the high risk of early recurrent stroke. Careful postoperative blood pressure control is important to minimize reperfusion injury, which can result in seizures, hemorrhage, and brain edema. Optimal medical management of symptomatic high-grade stenosis in surgically high-risk patients has not yet been defined. Warfarin may be used in these patients if symptoms recur on antiplatelet agents. Carotid angioplasty and stenting is technically feasible if surgery is deemed too high risk; however, its safety and long-term efficacy is yet to be demonstrated in a large randomized clinical trial. Patients with total occlusion of the extracranial ICA do not warrant surgery; short-term warfarin (3 months) may be used to prevent distal stump emboli, followed by long-term antiplatelet treatment.

The benefit of carotid endarterectomy for patients with asymptomatic ICA origin disease remains somewhat controversial. The Asymptomatic Carotid Atherosclerosis Study (ACAS) demonstrated an annual absolute reduction of 1 percent per year in the risk of ipsilateral stroke with CEA (perioperative risk <3 percent) versus medical therapy. The benefit of surgery was not appreciated until the third of 5 years of follow-up. Asymptomatic patients at greatest risk may include those with >80 percent stenosis with multiple vascular risk factors; these patients may particularly benefit from surgery.

The medical management of carotid occlusive disease consists of vigilant attention to vascular risk factors and antithrombotic therapy. Antiplatelet agents, such as aspirin (75 to 1300 mg) or ticlopidine, are recommended for both medical and post-CEA management.[9,10]

## Posterior Circulation

Antithrombotic strategies for occlusive disease are similar for both the anterior and posterior cerebral circulations. Symptomatic patients with VA origin stenosis often respond to antiplatelet therapy. If ischemic events persist, warfarin treatment can be instituted, but the benefit of long-term anticoagulation has not been proven. VA origin angioplasty is an emerging technique in patients who respond poorly to medical therapy. Anticoagulation is often recommended in patients with acute VA thrombosis to prevent propagation of the clot or distal embolism; warfarin can be used for several months, followed by antiplatelet therapy. Patients who suffer hemispheric cerebellar infarction are at risk for hydrocephalus and brain herniation. If the patient is deteriorating, urgent surgical decompression is required.

## Intracranial Disease

Therapeutic guidelines for patients with stenosis or occlusion of a major intracranial artery have not been established.[11] Warfarin (INR 2 to 3) may be more effective than aspirin in preventing recurrent stroke in patients with intracranial stenosis.

Bypass extracranial-intracranial (EC-IC) surgery for patients with intracranial ICA or MCA stenosis is ineffective for preventing stroke. Bypass surgery in the posterior circulation is rarely used for the treatment of intracranial VA or BA occlusive disease. Transluminal angioplasty of the intracranial ICA, MCA, vertebral, and basilar arteries in patients refractory to maximal antithrombotic therapy is another therapeutic option.

Patients with basilar artery thrombosis require urgent evaluation and intensive monitoring. Anticoagulation with heparin is recommended, particularly if there are fluctuating neurologic findings. Because of the poor prognosis of basilar occlusion, there is recent interest in thrombolysis and angioplasty. These high-risk procedures should be limited to experienced neurointerventional centers.

Lacunar disease is presently treated by most physicians with long-term antiplatelet therapy, either aspirin or ticlopidine.[12] Given that lacunar disease can coexist with other stroke-prone lesions, patients should be evaluated for other potential causes of stroke to define treatment options.

## Arterial Dissection

The majority of patients with ICA and VA dissections do well regardless of their treatment. Nevertheless, empiric anticoagulation for 3 to 6 months to reduce the likelihood of distal embolization and arterial occlusion, followed by antiplatelet treatment, is recommended.

# RISK FACTORS FOR ISCHEMIC STROKE

Although stroke can be caused by a number of different pathologic processes (large artery extracranial atherosclerosis, intracranial atherosclerosis, lacunar disease, and cardiac embolism), predisposing risk factors for each stroke subtype are often similar. Increased age, hypertension, cigarette smoking, diabetes, and hypercholesterolemia are common risk factors for strokes of all types.[13] There is compelling evidence for aggressive treatment of hypertension, given the direct relationship between the incidence of stroke and increasing blood pressure.[14] Even patients with borderline isolated systolic hypertension have an increased incidence of stroke or transient ischemia attack. Acute myocardial infarction, CHF, atrial fibrillation, and left ventricular hypertrophy are well-established stroke risk factors. Recently, increased levels of total homocysteine have been related to the prevalence of extracranial common carotid artery stenosis. Early studies of high-dose formulations of oral contraceptives (>50 $\mu$g estrogen) demonstrated an increased risk of stroke, especially in hypertensive cigarette smokers. More recent studies of lower-dose estrogen-containing oral contraceptives (<50 $\mu$g estrogen) have reported a considerably lower risk of stroke, which supports the current recommended practice of prescribing the lowest doses of estrogen and progestin and restricting the use of oral contraceptives in women who smoke cigarettes or who have other stroke risk factors.

# NEUROREHABILITATION

The extent of brain injury generally determines the need for and effectiveness of rehabilitation. Approximately 70 percent of stroke patients may benefit from outpatient or intensive inpatient rehabilitation, with improvement most likely to occur within the first 3 months after stroke. When neurologic recovery does not occur or is incomplete, rehabilitation programs are directed at improving function and performance in daily activities. Depression, a frequent complication of stroke affecting up to 50 percent of patients, requires prompt recognition and treatment. Aggressive treatment of depression can improve outcome and enhance overall quality of life. Central nervous system depressants such as benzodiazepines should be avoided. Current evidence supports stroke rehabilitation as being efficacious and cost-effective.

## REFERENCES

1. Bamford J, Sandercock P, Dennis M: Classification and natural history of clinically identifiable subtypes of cerebral infarction. *Lancet* 1991; 337:1521–1526.
2. Feinberg WM, Sandercock P, Dennis M: Guidelines for the management of transient ischemic attacks. From the ad hoc committee on guidelines for the management of transient ischemic attacks of the Stroke Council of the American Heart Association. *Stroke* 1994; 25:1320–1335.
3. Adams HP, Brott TG, Crowell RM, et al: Guidelines for the management of patients with acute ischemic stroke: a statement for healthcare professionals from a special writing group of the Stroke Council, American Heart Association. *Circulation* 1994; 90:1588–1601.
4. The National Institute of Neurological Disorders and Stroke rt-PA Stroke Study Group: Tissue plasminogen activator for acute ischemic stroke. *N Engl J Med* 1995; 333:1581–1587.
5. Counsell C, Sandercock P: The efficacy and safety of anticoagulant therapy in patients with acute presumed ischemic stroke: a systematic review of the randomized trials comparing anticoagulants with control. *The Cochrane Database of Systematic Reviews,* 1997.
6. Atrial Fibrillation Investigators: Risk factors for stroke and efficacy of antithrombotic therapy in atrial fibrillation: analysis of pooled data from five randomized clinical trials. *Arch Intern Med* 1994; 154:1949–1957.
7. Hart RG, Boop B, Anderson DC: Oral anticoagulants and intracranial hemorrhage: facts and hypothesis. *Stroke* 1995; 26:1471–1477.
8. North American Symptomatic Carotid Endarterectomy Trial Collaborators: Beneficial effect of carotid endarterectomy in symptomatic patients with high-grade carotid stenosis. *N Engl J Med* 1991; 325:445–453.
9. Barnett HJM, Eliaszim M, Meldrum HE: Drugs and surgery in the prevention of ischemic stroke. *N Engl J Med* 1995; 4:238–248.
10. Moore WS, Barnett HJ: Guidelines for carotid endarterectomy: a multidisciplinary consensus statement from the ad hoc committee, American Heart Association. *Stroke* 1995; 26:188–201.

11. Selwa LS, Chimowitz MI: Atherosclerotic intracranial large artery occlusive disease. *Neurologist* 1995; 1:53–64.
12. Antiplatelet Trialist's Collaboration: Collaborative review of randomized trials of antiplatelet therap:. I. Prevention of death, myocardial infarction, and stroke by prolonged antiplatelet therapy in various categories of patients. *Br Med J* 1994; 308:81–106.
13. Wolf PA, Lewis A: Conner memorial lecture. Contributions of epidemiology to the prevention of stroke. *Circulation* 1993; 88:2471–2478.
14. SHEP Cooperative Research Group: Prevention of stroke by antihypertensive drug treatment in older persons with isolated systolic hypertension. Final results of the Systolic Hypertension in the Elderly (SHEP). *JAMA* 1991; 265:3255–3264.

TAREK ABDELAZIM SALAM /
ATEF A. SALAM

# ABDOMINAL AORTIC ANEURYSMS

While there is some controversy as to what constitutes an aortic aneurysm, there is general agreement that a 50 percent increase in the size of the aorta—compared to its diameter proximal to the dilatation—should be considered an aortic aneurysm.

The contemporary incidence of abdominal aortic aneurysm ranges between 30 to 60 per 1000 persons. As aging of the population and improvement of the screening and diagnostic tools increase, this incidence seems to be rising in both the United States and other Western countries.[1,2] The average age of patients presenting for evaluation of aortic aneurysm is between 60 and 70 years, with men being more commonly affected than women by a ratio of 4:1.[3,4] There is also a definite familial tendency for abdominal aortic aneurysms, with the estimated frequency of family history for aortic aneurysm ranging from 11 to 30 percent.[4,5] The incidence is also higher among patients with other atherosclerotic lesions, being about 5 percent in patients with coronary artery disease and 10 percent in patients with peripheral vascular disease. Aneurysms are about eight times more frequent among cigarette smokers than nonsmokers. Hypertension is another commonly associated factor, noted in about 40 percent of patients with aortic aneurysms.[6]

## ETIOLOGY AND PATHOLOGY

The most common type of abdominal aortic aneurysm, accounting for over 90 percent of infrarenal aortic aneurysms, results from nonspecific aortic degenerative disease. The term *nonspecific,* which has been suggested by the Society for Vascular Surgery and the International Society for Cardiovascular Surgery Committee on Standards in Reporting of Vascular Disease as the etiologic relationship of atherosclerosis to aneurysm disease, has been questioned in recent years. Most patients with aneurysms have no associated peripheral vascular disease. It has been estimated that less than 25 percent of aortic aneurysms are associated with significant occlusive disease.[3,7] The development of fusiform aneurysms in animal models of atherosclerosis is also very rare.

While the exact mechanism of formation of aortic aneurysms remains unclear, several studies have shown decreased quantitites of both elastin and collagen bundles in the wall of the aneurysm.[8] This results in replacement of the elastic media by a much thinner layer of collagen, rendering the resulting thin aortic wall more prone to progressive dilatation. Several mechanisms have been suggested to explain this process, including excessive activity of collagenase and/or elastase or reduction of their naturally occurring inhibitors in the aortic wall.[7]

Once an aneurysm develops, regardless of the mechanism of its formation, its enlargement becomes governed by Laplace's law (tension = pressure × radius). This law states that the wall tension is proportionate to the radius for a given transmural pressure and explains why large aneurysms are more prone to disruption and why hypertension is an important risk factor for aneurysm rupture.

Most abdominal aortic aneurysms are infrarenal in location. The reason for this remains speculative, although both hemodynamic and structural factors have been suggested.[9] About 5 percent are juxtarenal, with no normal aorta between the upper end of the aneurysm and the renal artery, and only 2 to 5 percent are suprarenal, with involvement of one or more of the visceral arteries.

Other much less common causes for abdominal aortic aneurysm include congenital lesions, connective tissue disorders, Marfan's syndrome, Ehlers-Danlos syndrome, cystic medial necrosis, Behçet's disease, and other inflammatory, traumatic, and infectious etiologies.

## CLINICAL PRESENTATIONS

About three-quarters of abdominal aortic aneurysms are asymptomatic at the time of presentation. They are usually discovered either during a routine physical examination or during radiological evaluation for an unrelated abdominal complaint. Occasionally an aortic aneurysm is first discovered during laparotomy performed for some other unrelated abdominal condition.

Abdominal aortic aneurysms become symptomatic when they expand rapidly or rupture. Virtually any type of abdominal, flank, or back pain can be noted in this situation. Because of the very high mortality associated with aneurysm rupture, all symptomatic aneurysms—with or without hemodynamic instability—should be considered to be leaking aneurysms and handled as such until proven otherwise; errors or delays in making the diagnosis can result in catastrophic rupture. Rupture most commonly occurs into the posterolateral aspect of the retroperitoneum or, less frequently, into the free peritoneal cavity. The incidence of free rupture into the peritoneal cavity is probably higher than that reported in most series, as most of these patients die of hypovolemic shock before reaching the hospital. Aneurysms rarely rupture into the inferior vena cava or left renal vein, causing an aortocaval or aortorenal fistula, or into the duodenum, causing an aortoenteric fistula. Large aneurysms can also cause symptoms by eroding the spine, resulting in severe back pain in the absence of rupture. Aneurysm thrombosis or distal embolization is rather uncommon with abdominal aortic aneurysms.

# DIAGNOSIS

Plain x-ray films of the abdomen may show a fine rim of calcification outlining the aortic wall. However, this is noted in less than two-thirds of cases. A negative film cannot be relied upon to exclude the diagnosis of abdominal aortic aneurysm.

B-mode ultrasonography can reliably confirm the presence of an aneurysm and can accurately determine its size. When compared to operative measurements, ultrasonic measurements are accurate to within ±3 mm.[10] Ultrasonography is the modality of choice for initial evaluation of pulsating abdominal masses, screening of patients for abdominal aortic aneurysms, and follow-up surveillance of aneurysms to determine the increase in size. This is due to its wide availability, noninvasive nature, and relatively low cost. Unfortunately, ultrasonography has not been as useful for imaging the thoracic or suprarenal aorta because of the overlying air-filled lungs. Similarly, morbid obesity and bowel distention can reduce confidence in the ultrasound images. In such instances, a computed tomography (CT) or magnetic resonance imaging (MRI) scan may be preferable.

Computed tomography imaging provides more precise definition of the size and longitudinal extent of the aneurysm, and, unlike ultrasonography, it is not affected by bowel gas or obesity. It provides accurate measurements of the aorta in the abdomen and in the chest; and it can often identify the celiac, superior mesenteric, renal, and iliac arteries. Thinner slices are usually helpful for this purpose. Computed tomography also helps to identify major venous anomalies and ectopic or horseshoe kidneys. Contrast enhanced CT scans are very reliable for assessing the retroperitoneum for the purpose of excluding aneurysm rupture; it is claimed that as little as 10 mL of blood may be detected in this situation. They are also very useful in identifying retroperitoneal fibrosis associated with inflammatory aortic aneurysms.

A CT scan requires more time and is more expensive than ultrasound. Furthermore, it entails exposure to ionizing radiation and contrast injection, and its images can be degraded by patient motion and the presence of metallic surgical clips. New software is now available that allows CT data to be displayed as three-dimensional reconstruction similar to those provided by MRI. The advantage of this spiral CT scan over the conventional study in clinical practice is yet to be demonstrated.

Magnetic resonance imaging is the most recent imaging modality for evaluation of aortic aneurysms.[11] A complete picture of the aorta can be created that is much more detailed than that available with ultrasonography or CT scan. Magnetic resonance imaging can clearly distinguish arteries and veins from surrounding structures. It is superior to CT and ultrasound in demonstrating involvement of branch vessels, especially the renal arteries. It can provide three-dimensional projections that can clearly identify the aneurysm neck and the origin of the renal arteries. Periaortic structures and anomalies such as retroaortic vena cava can also be easily seen on MRI. Another advantage of MRI over CT scan is the lack of ionizing radiation and the need for toxic contrast agents.

Several problems, however, are associated with the use of MRI technology. Because of its very high cost, MRI is not as widely available as ultrasound or CT, and interpretation of the image requires considerable experience and skill. The presence of metallic surgical slips, cardiac pacemakers, or monitoring equipment makes performance of MRI impossible. Extreme obesity may preclude imaging because the patient's girth may extend beyond the magnetic field. Finally, some patients cannot tolerate the confinement and the noise of the MRI scanner.

## Aortography

Because of the wide availability and accuracy of the aforementioned modalities, aortography is not required for diagnosing the presence of abdominal aortic aneurysm. Furthermore, aortography cannot be relied upon to determine the diameter of the aneurysm because of the mural thrombus, which reduces the aneurysm lumen size. However, aortography provides valuable information in the preoperative evaluation of patients with aneurysms. It allows identification of iliac artery involvement and of suprarenal extension. Most importantly, it provides precise assessment of associated occlusive disease of the peripheral, renal, and mesenteric arteries. Because knowledge of these factors can contribute to better planning of the operative approach, routine angiography has been adopted by some surgeons.

Nevertheless, aortography is an invasive procedure and is associated with definite risks, including the risk of contrast nephropathy; distal embolization from the laminated thrombus during manipulation of the angiography catheter; and certainly the catheter entry-site complications such as hematomas, pseudoaneurysms, and arteriovenous fistulas. Digital subtraction techniques have decreased, but not eliminated, these complications. Because of the associated risks, it is probably more prudent to perform angiography on a selective basis. The usual indications for obtaining the study include (1) evidence of peripheral vascular occlusive disease, such as claudication or diminished distal pulses; (2) severe hypertension or suspicion of renovascular disease; (3) suspected mesenteric vascular disease; (4) suprarenal or thoracoabdominal aneurysm on CT scan; and (5) the presence of femoral aneurysm.

## Preoperative Decision Making

Because the operative mortality for ruptured aortic aneurysm is approximately 50 percent in most series and has not shown significant improvement over the years,[12] there is general agreement that aortic aneurysms should be repaired electively before rupture occurs.

When considering repair of an asymptomatic abdominal aortic aneurysm, the main issue to be resolved is whether the risk of rupture exceeds the risk of elective operation.

## Risk of Aneurysm Rupture

The size of the aneurysm must be considered. In general terms, the risk of rupture correlates directly with size. The average rate of aneurysm enlargement is 0.4 to

0.5 cm per year. As mentioned earlier in this text, the rate of expansion is higher for larger aneurysms (Laplace's law). The calculated 5-year rupture rate for aneurysms less than 5 cm in diameter is about 20 percent; for a 5 to 6 cm aneurysm, it is about 35 percent; and if the aneurysm exceeds 7 cm, the rupture rate is 95 percent at 5 years.[13] Consequently, the current recommendation is to repair aortic aneurysms measuring 5 cm or more in diameter. The operation is also recommended for aneurysms 4 to 5 cm in diameter in good-risk patients who are relatively young and have a life expectancy of 10 or more years. Aneurysms measuring 4 cm or less in diameter can safely be observed every 6 months using follow-up ultrasound scans. When progressive enlargement is documented, or if the aneurysm becomes symptomatic at any time, surgical reconstruction should be considered.[14]

Another factor is aneurysm configuration. Saccular aneurysms are considered by some to be an indication for repair regardless of the size, because of their high propensity for rupture and their unpredictable rate of expansion compared to that of fusiform aneurysms.

## Risk of Surgical Repair

There has been a steady improvement in the results of elective repair of abdominal aortic aneurysms; the current operative mortality for most centers ranges between 1 and 5 percent. The mortality rate is influenced by two groups of factors:

(1) *Comorbid conditions:* Of these, cardiac disease is the most important. Manifestations of significant heart disease include previous myocardial infarction, unstable angina, congestive heart failure (CHF), left ventricular ejection fraction less than 30 percent, and ventricular arrhythmias.

Pulmonary disease manifested by $P_{O_2} < 60$ mmHg or $P_{CO_2} > 50$ mmHg on room air or forced expiratory volume at 1 s ($FEV_1$) <1 L, also constitutes a high risk factor.

Renal disease manifested by serum creatinine >3 mg/dL or 24-h creatine clearance <30 mg/min is another bad prognostic factor for postoperative renal failure and mortality.

Other comorbid factors include liver disease and morbid obesity. It is to be noted that age per se should not be considered a contraindication. Reports on aneurysm repair in octogenarians have shown acceptable morbidity and mortality rates.[15] Thus, when otherwise indicated, aneurysm repair should not be withheld on the basis of age alone.

(2) *Technical factors related to the aneurysm:* Several technical issues can complicate the operative procedure and can increase the mortality rate accordingly. These include the hostile abdomen with multiple previous laparotomies, previous radiation, the presence of colostomies or ileostomies, etc. Operative repair can be further complicated by venous anomalies such as double inferior vena cava and retrocaval left renal vein, and by renal anomalies such as horseshoe kidneys and ectopic kidneys. Inflammatory aortic aneurysms with marked retroperitoneal fibrosis, suprarenal or juxtarenal aneurysms, and the need for adjunctive revascularization

of the visceral or renal arteries are all technical issues that can significantly affect the operative mortality.

In summary, elective aneurysm repair should be considered for asymptomatic patients with abdominal aortic aneurysms 5 cm or larger in diameter who have an acceptable operative risk. Smaller aneurysms should also be considered for elective repair in good-risk patients, especially if they are hypertensive or live in remote areas where facilities for aneurysm repair are not readily available. Aneurysms smaller than 5 cm in diameter should otherwise be followed by serial imaging, and repair should be recommended if enlargement in size is documented on serial scans. All symptomatic aneurysms, on the other hand, should be considered for urgent repair.

## TECHNIQUE OF OPERATIVE REPAIR

As with other major vascular procedures, patients undergoing abdominal aortic aneurysm repair require placement of arterial and venous cannulas, a central venous line, and a urinary bladder catheter. Patients with compromised cardiac function may require the insertion of a flow-directed balloon-tipped pulmonary artery catheter (Swan-Ganz catheter). The use of a cell-saver autotransfusion device is now routine in most major centers, minimizing the need for transfusion of banked blood.[16] Broad-spectrum antibiotic coverage is required, as a synthetic vascular prosthesis is implanted.

Aortic exposure is usually done via a midline or transverse abdominal incision. The left retroperitoneal exposure (with or without extension into the chest) is favored by some, but is usually reserved for patients with hostile abdomen, juxtarenal or suprarenal aneurysm, morbid obesity, or some renal anomalies.[17] This incision provides good access to the suprarenal aorta and is claimed to have less postoperative complications and a shorter period of postoperative ileus. Access to the right iliac artery, as well as exposure of the right renal artery, through this incision is usually limited. Following systemic heparin administration, vascular clamps are applied at the neck of the aneurysm and distally at the common iliac arteries. The aneurysm sac is then opened, the intima and the laminated thrombus are removed, and back bleeding from the lumbar arteries is controlled by suture ligation. An appropriately sized vascular graft is employed, with the choice of the graft material usually being the surgeon's preference, since there is no proven superiority of one graft type over another. A tube graft should be used whenever feasible, but a bifurcated graft is inserted if iliac aneurysmal or occlusive disease is present. All anastomoses are constructed using running polypropylene sutures. After ensuring adequate perfusion of the lower extremities and the left colon, the graft is isolated from the overlying bowel by careful closure of the aneurysm sac over the graft. This is followed by standard closure of the abdominal incision.

# COMPLICATIONS OF AORTIC ANEURYSM REPAIR

As mentioned earlier in this discussion, in recent years the mortality rate following abdominal aortic aneurysm repair has declined to under 5 percent in most centers. The most frequent cause of death is myocardial infarction (MI). This underscores the importance of good cardiac evaluation with appropriate intervention as needed before embarking on aneurysm repair.

## Declamping Hypotension

*Declamping hypotension* can occur at the time of restoring perfusion to the extremities; it is avoided by very gradual release of the distal clamp while the blood pressure is carefully monitored. For bifurcated grafts, flow is restored to one extremity at a time. Rapid infusion of intravenous fluids at the time of reperfusion may also be necessary to maintain adequate blood pressure.

## Microembolization

*Microembolization* to the digital arteries of the feet (commonly known as "trash feet"), or less frequently macroembolization to the major arteries of the lower extremities, can occur from the laminated thrombus or the underlying atheroma. This should be avoided by appropriate flushing prior to restoring perfusion and by restoring blood flow to the hypogastric arteries before the external iliac arteries are unclamped.

## Left Colon Ischemia

Adequate perfusion of the left colon should always be confirmed at the conclusion of the procedure. Suture ligation of the inferior mesenteric artery should be done from within the aneurysm sac to avoid disturbing any collateral blood supply to the colon. If the inferior mesenteric artery is excessively large, or if the circulation to the left colon or sigmoid is impaired at the end of the operation, reimplantation into the aortic prosthesis should be done. This is accomplished by implanting a patch of native aortic wall around the orifice of the inferior mesenteric artery (Carrel patch) into the aortic graft. Maintaining adequate perfusion to at least one internal iliac artery is another essential precaution to avoid left colon ischemia.

## Paraplegia

This catastrophic complication is a well-recognized problem after thoracoabdominal aortic aneurysm repair. The incidence ranges between 5 and 15 percent and is higher with more proximal extension of the aneurysm. Paraplegia is rarely seen after surgical repair of infrarenal aortic aneurysm; the estimated incidence is 1 in 400.[18] The precise mechanism of spinal cord injury is still unclear, and, unfortunately, this complication is unpredictable. It has been suggested that perioperative cerebrospinal fluid drainage following thoracoabdominal aneurysm repair may reduce the incidence of this complication.

## Renal Failure

The incidence of renal failure after abdominal aortic aneurysm repair has declined significantly in recent years. Possible mechanisms of renal failure include hypotension, atheroembolism to the renal arteries during manipulation of the perirenal aorta, suprarenal clamping, and occasionally aggravation of preexisting renal dysfunction by preoperative contrast studies. Adequate hydration and administration of mannitol during cross-clamping of the aorta are important measures for preventing renal dysfunction.

## Special Problems with Aortic Aneurysm Repair

**RUPTURED AORTIC ANEURYSM.**   The critical step in this situation is rapid proximal control of the aorta, which can usually be expeditiously obtained by compression of the aorta at the diaphragmatic hiatus, and by rapid exposure and clamping of the aorta through the lesser omentum. The suprarenal clamp is replaced by an infrarenal clamp as soon as feasible. Systemic heparin is best avoided for patients with ruptured aortic aneurysms. Once the proximal anastomosis is completed, balloon catheters should be used to extract any clots that might have formed distally  as a result of the combined effect of aortic clamping and hypotension.

**INFLAMMATORY AORTIC ANEURYSM.**   This type of aneurysm is associated with dense inflammatory fibrotic reaction in the retroperitoneum that incorporates adjacent structures, especially the duodenum (90 percent) and the inferior vena cava, left renal vein, and ureters. The reported incidence of inflammatory aortic aneurysm is between 3 and 10 percent.[19]

Clinically the triad of abdominal pain, tenderness, and elevated erythrocyte sedimentation rate and white blood count in a patient with abdominal aortic aneurysm is highly suggestive of inflammatory aneurysm. Excessive thickening of the aneurysm wall and obliteration of planes in the tissues around it can be readily seen on CT scan. At the time of surgery, the aneurysm is usually encased in dense, shiny, white fibrotic reaction in the retroperitoneum surrounding the aortic aneurysm. The surgical approach should be modified instantly to avoid duodenal injury.

**JUXTARENAL/SUPRARENAL EXTENSION.**   For juxtarenal aortic aneurysm, proximal aortic clamping is temporarily obtained at the supraceliac level while the proximal anastomosis to the juxtarenal cuff is constructed. Upon completion of this anastomosis, the graft is occluded just distal to the suture line and the proximal clamp is removed, restoring blood flow to the renal and visceral arteries.

## Note on Endovascular Repair of Abdominal Aortic Aneurysm

Thanks to advances in vascular imaging, catheter delivery systems, and arterial stenting techniques, endovascular aortic aneurysm repair has become feasible in recent years. A graft can be introduced through the femoral artery and anchored by endovascular stents to a nondilated arterial segment at both ends of the aneurysm. Graft attachment must be secure, accurate, and hemostatic, both proximally and distally. The avoidance of an abdominal operation and general anesthesia are the main advantages of this technique. The appeal of endovascular grafting in high-risk patients is obvious.[20]

While the early results of this technique have been encouraging, long-term follow-up data comparing it to standard operative repair are not yet available. At the present time, endovascular aortic grafting should still be considered a technique in evolution, and its utilization should be limited to academic institutions until its long-term safety and efficacy have been firmly established.

## REFERENCES

1. Melton L, Bickerstaff L, Hollier LH: Changing incidence of abdominal aortic aneurysms: A population-based study. *Am J Epidemiol* 1984; 120:379–386.
2. Castleden W, Mercer J: Abdominal aortic aneurysms in Western Australia: Descriptive epidemiology and patterns of rupture. *Br J Surg* 1985; 72:109–112.
3. Tilson MD, Stansel HC: Differences in results for aneurysm vs. occlusive disease after bifurcation grafts. *Arch Surg* 1980; 115:1173–1175.
4. Taylor LM, Porter JM: Basic data related to clinical decision making in abdominal aortic aneurysms. *Ann Vasc Surg* 1980; 1:502–504.
5. Thurmond AS, Semler JH: Abdominal aortic aneurysm. Incidence in a population at risk. *J Cardiovasc Surg* 1986; 27:457–460.
6. Spittel JA: Hypertension and arterial aneurysms. *J Am Coll Cardiol* 1983; 1:533–540.
7. Dobrin PB: Pathophysiology and pathogenesis of aortic aneurysms Current concepts. *Surg Clin North Am* 1989; 69:687–703.
8. Dobrin PB, Baker WH, Gley WC: Elastolytic and collagenolytic studies of arteries: Implications for the mechanical properties of aneurysms. *Arch Surg* 1984; 119:405–409.
9. Powell J, Greenhalgh RM: Cellular, enzymatic, and genetic factors in the pathogenesis of abdominal aortic aneurysms. *J Vasc Surg* 1989; 9:297–303.
10. Gomes MN, Choyke PL: Preoperative evaluation of abdominal aortic aneurysms: Ultrasound or computed tomography? *J Cardiovasc Surg* 1987; 28:159–165.
11. Lee JKT, Ling D, Heiken JP: Magnetic resonance imaging of abdominal aneurysms. *AJR* 1984; 143:1197.
12. Hardman TA, Fisher CM, Patel MB, et al: Ruptured abdominal aortic aneurysm: Who should be offered surgery? *J Vasc Surg* 1996; 23:123–129.

13. Limet R, Sakalihassan N, Albert A: Determination of the expansion rate and incidence of rupture of abdominal aortic aneurysms. *J Vasc Surg* 1991; 14:540–548.

14. Katz DA, Littenberg B, Cronenwett JL: Management of small abdominal aortic aneurysms: Early surgery vs watchful waiting. *JAMA* 1992; 268:2678–2686.

15. O'Hara PJ, Hertzer NR, Krajewski LP, et al:: Ten-year experience with abdominal aortic aneurysm repair in octogenarians: Early results and late outcome. *J Vasc Surg* 1995; 21:830–838.

16. Kelly-Patterson C, Ammar AD, Kelley H: Should the cell- saver autotransfusion device be used routinely in all infrarenal abdominal aortic bypass operations? *J Vasc Surg* 1993; 18:261–265.

17. Shepard AD, Tollefson DFJ, Reddy DJ, et al: Left flank retroperitoneal exposure: A technical aid to complex aortic reconstruction. *J Vasc Surg* 1991; 14:283–291.

18. Szilagi DE: A second look at the etiology of spinal cord damage in surgery of the abdominal aorta. *J Vasc Surg* 1993; 17:1111–1113.

19. Pennel RC, Hollier LH, Lie JT: Inflammatory abdominal aortic aneurysms: A 30-year review. *J Vasc Surg* 1985; 2:859–869.

20. Parodi JC, Palmaz JC, Barone HD: Transfemoral intraluminal graft implantation for abdominal aortic aneurysms. *Ann Vasc Surg* 1991; 5:491–499.

# Part

# 2

# PREVENTION OF CARDIOVASCULAR DISEASES

WILLIAM T. BRANCH, JR./
ROBERT C. SCHLANT

# ROUTINE SCREENING

Preventive care is much of the work of a primary care physician. Many preventive measures focus on cardiovascular disease. The primary care physician engages in cardiovascular prevention in the context of an overall preventive care package, tailored for each patient by age, sex, and other known risk factors.[1,2] This chapter will review current recommendations for preventive care.

Primary care physicians should also be aware of the national quality standards set by the Health Plan Employer Data and Information Set (HEDIS), which have been developed by the National Committee for Quality Assurance.[3] These measures are in voluntary use by the Health Care Financing Administration (HCFA) and many excellent managed care companies. Quality indicators developed for HEDIS III, the most recent version, continue to focus on preventive measures. Indicators for adult patients include cholesterol screening, mammography, and Pap smears. These indicators are considered to be minimal quality standards and are used by Medicare, Medicaid, and private companies to monitor quality and by employers to help make purchasing decisions. The American Heart Association has published excellent guidelines for the primary prevention of cardiovascular diseases.[4]

The history, including an initial database on every patient, and physical examination remain central to preventive care. The history, database, and physical examination identify many patients at above-average risk who require targeted preventive measures. Among the special factors to be identified are those that place patients at risk of suicide (recent divorce, unemployment, depression, alcohol or other drug abuse, medical illness, living alone, recent bereavement), those that involve health habits (smoking, alcohol abuse, drug abuse, obesity, unhealthy diet, lack of exercise), those that place patients at risk of disease (multiple sexual partners, sexual partner with multiple contacts, living in a high-prevalence area for infection, high-risk sexual habits), those involving the care of others (prevention of falls of elderly adults in the home, car seats for infants), and those involving abuse (sexual abuse in childhood, physical abuse by a partner).

There are also special parts of the physical examination for persons with higher than average risk. These include the complete skin examination and search for malignant melanomas in individuals with occupational or recreational sun exposure or a family history of malignant melanoma. One should seek thyroid nodules in persons with a history of upper body irradiation; perform complete oral cavity examination in those with tobacco and/or excessive alcohol exposure; perform annual clinical breast examinations in young women with a family history of premenopausal breast cancer in a first-degree relative; perform testicular examination in young males with testicular atrophy, cryptorchidism, or orchiopexy; auscultate for carotid bruits in middle-aged individuals with hypertension, smoking, diabetes, or other risk factors for atherosclerotic disease; and carefully palpate the peripheral arteries in those with risk factors for peripheral vascular disease.

It should be pointed out that although a complete history; database including social, family, and occupational history and review of systems; and physical examination are not specifically recommended by all expert bodies, these standard parts of the medical examination have not been studied in detail. Because of their importance in establishing an overall plan for the patient, it is presumed that every patient should have a complete history and physical examination at some point. Expert bodies recommend periodic updating of the database and examination every 3 to 5 years in young persons, 2 to 3 years in middle-aged persons, and 1 to 2 years in older individuals.[1,2] Because each part of the evaluation, performed incrementally, takes little time once the patient is in the doctor's office, it is likely that some standard measures, such as the rectal examination, which might not be cost-effective to perform alone, are reasonable to perform as part of an overall examination.

## CARDIOVASCULAR SCREENING

Several preventive measures are particularly important in prevention of cardiovascular diseases. Treatment of hypertension, smoking cessation, and lipid disorders are discussed in detail in other chapters. Diabetic patients are especially in need of aggressive management of blood pressure and lipids to prevent vascular and other complications. In women of child-bearing age, establishing immunity or administering rubella vaccine is essential for prevention of congenital heart disease.[4a] Sexually active, inner-city teenaged girls and institutionalized females represent populations in whom testing for immunity to rubella is often overlooked, but they are at risk of pregnancy.[4b]

## BREAST CANCER SCREENING

Annual or every-2-year screening for women ages 50 to 70 is now well accepted. A paucity of data in women over the age of 70 years limits official recommendations, but most experts believe that continuing to screen with mammography into the seventies is reasonable. Controversy has focused on women ages 40 to 49. Although much has been written regarding this controversy, it can be summarized by saying that a meta-analysis of randomized trials suggests that after 10 to 12 years of follow-up, women ages 40 to 49 benefit from annual mammography by an approximately 7 to 16 percent decrease in breast cancer mortality.[5,6] Those who debate this issue have reached different conclusions regarding the amount of benefit based on removing or not removing some of the trials from analysis.[7] Reanalysis may focus on the age at which a woman's breast cancer was actually detected in the trials, as results to date have reported benefit based on age of enrollment.[8] Hence, the conclusion that young women benefit could still be altered by additional analysis or additional data. Another caveat is the relatively high number of cases of ductal carcinoma in situ detected by screening: approximately 25 percent of all cases detected. There is no consensus on treatment for ductal carcinoma in situ: Some experts recommend removal by breast-conserving surgery followed by watchful waiting and aggressive screening to detect an invasive cancer, whereas others recommend mastectomy.[8a] Those who urge caution in adopting screening guidelines in women 40 to 49 years of age argue that a program designed to detect ductal carcinoma in situ is not warranted based on current understanding. Despite all of the controversy, there does appear to be benefit from performing mammography routinely every 1 to 2 years in women aged 40 to 49 years, and such is the current recommendation of the National Cancer Institute.[8b]

Mammography and/or other screening measures should be performed annually in young women at increased risk of breast cancer. These include those with a personal history of breast cancer; a mother, sister, daughter, or two other close relatives with breast cancer; BRCA 1 or BRCA 2 positivity; 75 percent of breast tissue too dense for interpretation by mammography; first child at age 30 years or older; and/or two breast biopsies previously performed for benign disease.

## COLON CANCER SCREENING

Three large randomized trials have demonstrated that screening for colon cancer with the stool hemoccult test reduces mortality from that disease. A Scandinavian and a British trial showed ~20 percent reduced mortality with few false-positive hemoccults and a reasonably small number of colonoscopies performed in the study population.[9,10] A large American trial revealed a 33 percent reduction in mortality but used rehydration to enhance the sensitivity but lower the specificity of stool hemoccults, leading to many more colonoscopies being performed.[11] Expert bodies currently do not recommend rehydration.[2] Most recommend annual screening with three stool hemoccults of all persons at average risk over the age of 50 years.[12] More aggressive screening is indicated for individuals with familial polyposis syndromes, ulcerative pancolitis of more than 10 years' duration, or a strong family history of colon cancer. No randomized trial has been published on sigmoidoscopy, but this procedure appears to be complementary to the stool hemoccult. Large cohort studies and a well-designed case control study suggest benefit in the range of 40 percent reduced mortality from colorectal cancer within reach of the sigmoidoscope.[13] Based on decision analysis, many experts recommend that sigmoidoscopy be performed every 5 to 10 years in persons of average risk over the age of 50 years.

## LUNG CANCER SCREENING

Although it is possible to identify a population at high risk of developing lung cancer (heavy smokers), trials to date have not documented a significant benefit from aggressive screening programs.[2] Programs including periodic chest films and sputum cytologies have had little or no effect on outcome from lung cancer once one accounts for lead-time bias. Screening asymptomatic persons for lung cancer by chest roentgenography is not recommended.

## PROSTATE CANCER SCREENING

The prostate-specific antigen (PSA) test offers high sensitivity for the early detection of prostate cancer. Studies suggest that the PSA detects 50 to 80 percent of clinically important asymptomatic prostate cancers, whereas the digital rectal examination of the prostate detects 20 to 30 percent in primary care practices.[2] Several variations of the PSA test have been studied to see if they enhance sensitivity or specificity. Attempting to correct the PSA level for size of the prostate has not increased the accuracy of the test because of difficulty in accurately and reproducibly defining the size of the prostate gland.[14] Measuring free versus bound PSA (with bound being more characteristic of prostate cancer) adds specificity and may be useful in the decision to rule out biopsy of patients whose PSA is borderline elevated.[15–17] An increase of more than 0.7 unit in PSA per year on patient follow-up may help in the decision to rebiopsy someone with a suspiciously elevated PSA whose initial biopsies were negative.[18,19] The major controversy lies in whether or not to recommend wide-scale screening with PSA of all males. No large randomized trial has been underway for sufficient time to determine if patient outcomes are benefited or harmed by this strategy. Treatment with radical prostatectomy or radiotherapy can produce complications, including impotence and incontinence, and carries a small risk of death. Decision analysis suggests that younger men with moderately or poorly differentiated tumors may benefit from treatment.[19a] Patients with well-differentiated tumors and those over the age of 75 years appear to do as well with watchful waiting as they do with treatment, so they probably will not benefit from screening. However, the majority of prostate cancers in younger individuals are moderately differentiated. Because of the smaller incidence of false-positive results and greater likelihood of benefit, PSA screening, if done, might best be targeted to patients in their fifties.[20] Several expert bodies have not recommended wide-scale screening with PSA.[2] A reasonable strategy would be to discuss the pros and cons of screening with individual patients and to make a mutually informed decision based on patient preferences.[2,21]

# CERVICAL CANCER SCREENING

There is now overwhelming evidence from large numbers of patients enrolled in studies that the Pap smear for detection of cervical dysplasia and/or carcinoma in situ (cervical intraepithelial neoplasia) and effective local treatment of this disorder prevents development of invasive cervical cancer and thereby prevents mortality from this disease.[2] Effective screening programs conducted for 10 years or more may diminish mortality rates by more than 80 percent. The long latency period of cervical intraepithelial neoplasia before the development of invasive cancer suggests that screening less often than annually could be effective. Decision analysis suggests that screening should begin at the age of onset of sexual activity or age 18 in women, that it be performed at least every 2 or 3 years, and that it not be discontinued unless there are three well-documented normal Pap smears within the past decade in women 65 years of age or older. Because invasive cancer develops most commonly in older women, even though cervical intraepithelial neoplasia is generally a disease of young women, physicians are encouraged to obtain Pap smears in older women if there is any doubt about the adequacy of previous screening. The strong correlation of sexual activity with cervical intraepithelial neoplasia, whose etiology is thought to be human papillomavirus acquired sexually, suggests that women known never to have had sexual activity need not be screened. For Pap smear screening to be effective, the examiner must be competent to obtain smears from both within the cervical os by brush or Q-Tip and from the cervix itself by scraping.[22] The squamocolumnar juncture must be sampled. The laboratory interpreting the smear must be properly certified.

Table 17-1 summarizes recommendations for screening of healthy adults.[1,2] Additional case-focused screening should be performed in individuals identified as being at higher than average risk for disease as outlined above.[1,2] Physicians engaging in primary care must be competent in delivering preventive care. Detailed familiarity with the recommendations for screening, competence in performing the screening procedures, and a well-organized office that is capable of monitoring and following results are essential. Nowadays, the physician is often responsible not only for individual patients seen in his or her office but also for a population of patients who may be assigned to receive their care from the practice. Patient education is increasingly important. Patients must be informed of the need to receive preventive care routinely and must have access to care so that it can be delivered. Patients with cardiovascular disorders are likely to see the physician but may be in danger of having their care too focused on the cardiac problem. The physician's judgment is needed to determine how aggressive a screening program should be in someone with underlying cardiac disease. In general, preventive medicine remains important in these individuals, whose cardiac problems may be adequately treated. This provides them with a good prognosis for expected life span and the opportunity to benefit from early detection and effective treatment of noncardiac disease.

**TABLE 17-1.    Minimum Preventive Measures for Nonpregnant, Healthy Adults**

| Routine Examination | Age of Patients | | |
| --- | --- | --- | --- |
| | 19–39 years | 40–64 years | 65 years and over |
| History | Dietary intake<br>Physical activity<br>Tobacco, alcohol, or drug use<br>Sexual practices<br>Depressive symptoms | Dietary intake<br>Physical activity<br>Tobacco, alcohol, or drug use<br>Sexual practices<br>Depressive symptoms | Functional status<br>Dietary intake<br>Physical activity<br>Tobacco, alcohol, or drug use<br>Symptoms of transient ischemic attack<br>Depressive symptoms<br>Abnormal bereavement<br>Changes in cognitive function<br>Medications that increase risk of falls |
| Physical examination | Height and weight, waist-to-hip ratio<br>Blood pressure, at least every 2 years<br>Clinical breast examination for women<br>Tooth decay or gingivitis<br>Signs of physical abuse | Height and weight<br>Blood pressure<br>Clinical breast examination (annually for women)<br>Signs of phyical abuse<br>Malignant skin lesions<br>Tooth decay, gingivitis, loose teeth | Height and weight<br>Blood pressure<br>Vision and hearing<br>Clinical breast examination (annually for women)<br>Signs of physical abuse or neglect<br>Malignant skin lesions<br>Peripheral arterial disease<br>Tooth decay, gingivitis, loose teeth |
| Laboratory/ diagnostic procedures | Cholesterol and HDL-cholesterol every 5 years<br>Papanicolaou smear (every 1–3 years) | Cholesterol and HDL-cholesterol<br>Papanicolaou smear (every 1–3 years)<br>Mammogram (annually for women ages 50–70; every 1 to 2 years in women aged 40–49)<br>Fecal occult blood testing (annually over age 50)<br>Flexible sigmoidoscopy (every 5–10 years, beginning at age 50) | Thyroid function test (for women)<br>Papanicolaou smear (unless three previously normal)<br>Mammogram (until age 75–80)<br>Fecal occult blood testing (annually)<br>Flexible sigmoidoscopy (every 5–10 years) |
| Counseling | Diet and exercise: fat, cholesterol, fiber, iron (for women), calcium (for women), caloric balance, selection of exercise program | Diet and exercise: fat, cholesterol, complex carbohydrates, fiber, calcium (for women), caloric balance, selection of exercise program | Diet and exercise: fat, cholesterol, complex carbohydrates, fiber, calcium (for women), caloric balance, selection of exercise program |

**TABLE 17-1.   Minimum Preventive Measures for Nonpregnant, Healthy Adults** *(continued)*

| Routine Examination | Age of Patients | | |
|---|---|---|---|
| | 19–39 years | 40–64 years | 65 years and over |
| | Substance use: tobacco cessation; alcohol and other drugs: limiting alcohol consumption during driving or other dangerous activities, Counseling for abuse Sexual practices: sexually transmitted diseases, partner selection, condoms, anal intercourse, unintended pregnancy, and contraceptive use Injury prevention: safety belts, use of safety helmets, smoke detectors, no smoking near bedding or upholstery Violent behavior (for men), firearms (for men) Dental health: regular tooth brushing, flossing, dental visits | Hormone replacement therapy (peri- and postmenopausal women) Substance use: tobacco cessation; alcohol and other drugs: limiting alcohol consumption during driving or other dangerous activities Counseling for abuse Sexual practices: sexually transmitted diseases, partner selection, condoms, anal intercourse, unintended pregnancy, and contraceptive options Injury prevention: safety belts, use of safety helmets, smoke detectors, no smoking near bedding upholstery or Dental health: regular tooth brushing, flossing, dental visits | Postmenopausal hormone replacement Substance use: tobacco cessation; alcohol and other drugs: limiting alcohol consumption especially if prone to falls or if taking psychoactive pre-scription medications Counseling for abuse Injury prevention: prevention of falls, use of safety belts, smoke detectors, no smoking near bedding or upholstery, safe hot water temperature, use of safety helmets Dental health: regular dental visits, tooth brushing, flossing Other primary preventive measures: glaucoma testing by eye specialist |
| Immunizations | Tetanus-diphtheria booster (every 10 years) Measles-mumps (persons born after 1956 not known to be immune to measles) Rubella (women without documented immunity) Hepatitis B (all persons at risk) | Tetanus-diphtheria booster (every 10 years) | Tetanus-diphtheria booster (every 10 years) Influenza vaccine (annually) Pneumococcal vaccine |

*Source:* Adapted and modified with permission from Branch W T Jr, Lawrence RS: Periodic health assessment of asymptomatic adults. In: Branch WT Jr (ed): *Office Practice of Medicine,* 3d ed. Philadelphia, W. B. Saunders Co., 1994:908; U.S. Preventive Services Task Force: *Guide to Clinical Preventive Services,* 2d ed. Baltimore, Williams & Wilkins, 1996; and American Heart Association Guide to primary prevention of cardiovascular diseases. *Circulation* 1997; 95:2329–2331.

## REFERENCES

1. Sox HC Jr: Current concepts: Preventive health services in adults. *N Engl J Med* 1994: 330:1589–1595.
2. U.S. Preventive Services Task Force: *Guide to Clinical Preventive Services,* 2d ed. Baltimore, Williams and Wilkins, 1996.
3. National Committee for Quality Assurance: *Health Plan Employer Data and Information Set.* Washington, DC, National Committee for Quality Assurance, 1993.
4. Grundy SM, Balady GJ, Criqui MH, et al: Guide to primary prevention of cardiovascular diseases. A statement for health care professionals from the Task Force on Risk Reduction. *Circulation* 1997; 95:2329–2331.
4a. Watson JC, Hadler SC, Dykewicz CA, et al: Measles, mumps, and rubella—vaccine use and strategies for elimination of measles, rubella, and congenital rubella syndrome and control of mumps: Recommendations of the Advisory Committee on Immunization Practices (ACIP). *MMWR* 1998; 47:1–57.
4b. Olsen ME, Olsen NM, Breuel K, et al: Rubella serology in mentally retarded adults. *South Med J* 1998; 91:842–846.
5. Mettlin C, Murphy GP: Breast cancer screening in premenopausal women: Current recommendations and opportunities for research. *Ann Intern Med* 1995; 27:461–465.
6. Kerlikowske K, Grady D, Rubin SM, et al: Efficacy of screening mammography: A meta-analysis. *JAMA* 1995; 273:149–154.
7. Fletcher SW, Black W, Harris R, et al: Report of the International Workshop on Screening for Breast Cancer. *J Natl Cancer Inst* 1993; 85:1644–1656.
8. Margolese R: Screening mammography in young women: A different perspective. *Lancet* 1996; 347:881–882.
8a. Steering Committee on Clinical Practice Guidelines for the Care and Treatment of Breast Cancer—Canadian Association of Radiation Oncologists. *CMAJ* 1998; 10:527–534.
8b. Final mammography recommendation? *JAMA* 1997; 227:1181.
9. Kronborg O, Fenger C, Olsen J, et al: Randomized study of screening for colorectal cancer with faecal occult blood test. *Lancet* 1996; 348:1467–1471.
10. Hardcastle JD, Chamberlain JO, Robinson MH, et al: Randomized controlled trial of faecal occult blood screening for colorectal cancer. *Lancet* 1996; 348:1472–1477.
11. Mandel JS, Bond JH, Church TR, et al: Reducing mortality from colorectal cancer by screening for fecal occult blood. *N Engl J Med* 1993; 328:1365–1371.
12. Lieberman D, Sleisenger MH: Is it time to recommend screening for colorectal cancer? *Lancet* 1996; 348:1463–1464.
13. Selby JB, Friedman GD, Quesenberry CP, et al: A case-control study of screening sigmoidoscopy and mortality from colorectal cancer. *N Engl J Med* 1992; 326:653–657.
14. Raviv G, Zlotta RA, Janssen TH, et al: Do prostate specific antigen and prostate specific antigen density enhance the detection of prostate carcinoma after initial diagnosis of prostatic intraepithelial neoplasia without concurrent carcinoma? *Cancer* 1996; 77:2103–2108.
15. Elgamal AA, Cornillie FJ, Van Poppell HP, et al: Free to total prostate specific antigen ratio as a single test for detection of significant stage T1c prostate cancer. *J Urol* 1996; 156:1042–1049.
16. Murphy GP, Barren RJ, Erickson SJ, et al: Evaluation and comparison of two new prostate carcinoma markers. Free prostate specific antigen and prostate specific membrane antigen. *Cancer* 1996; 78:809–818.

17. Demura T, Shinorhara N, Tanaka M, et al: The proportion of free to total prostate specific antigen: A method for detecting prostate carcinoma. *Cancer* 1996; 77:1137–1143.

18. Keetch DW, McMurtry JM, Smith DS, et al: Prostate specific antigen density vs. prostate specific antigen slope as predictors of prostate cancer in men with initially negative prostate biopsies. *J Urol* 1996; 156:428–431.

19. Urstelling JE: Age specific references ranges for serum PSA. *N Engl J Med* 1996; 335:345–346.

19a. Fleming C, Wasson JH, Albertsen PC: A decision analysis of alternative treatment strategies for clinically localized prostate cancer. *JAMA* 1993; 269:2650–2658.

20. Partin AW, Criley SR, Subong ENP, et al: Standard vs. age specific prostate specific antigen references ranges among men with clinically localized prostate cancer: A pathologic co-analysis. *J Urol* 1996; 155:1336–1339.

21. Wolf A, Nassar JF, Wolf AM, Schorling JB: The impact of informed consent on patient interest in prostate specific antigen screening. *Arch Intern Med* 1996; 156:1333–1336.

22. Henderson IC, Branch WT Jr, Sheets EE: Case finding for cancer. In: Branch WT Jr (ed): *Office Practice of Medicine,* 3d ed. Philadelphia, W. B. Saunders Co., 1994:914–926.

W. VIRGIL BROWN /
TERRY A. JACOBSON

# CHAPTER

# THE MANAGEMENT OF LIPOPROTEIN DISORDERS

# 18

The blood plasma lipoproteins perform the vital functions of transporting large amounts of energy from organ to organ and also maintaining appropriate redistribution of cholesterol and fat-soluble vitamins among the tissues. This system, however, is full of potential pitfalls that are generated by both common human genetic variations and environmental influences. These often result in elevated low-density lipoprotein cholesterol (LDL-C), elevated triglycerides, and reduced plasma concentrations of high-density lipoprotein cholesterol (HDL-C). Our recently developing understanding of the various plasma lipoproteins and their metabolism has been associated with an equally rapid elucidation of the pathogenesis of arteriosclerosis.[1] A powerful series of clinical trials using both diet and lipoprotein-modifying drugs has demonstrated that reducing elevated levels of LDL-C can be considered both effective prevention of arteriosclerosis[2–4] and treatment of the disease after it is clinically manifest.[5–9] This evidence has stimulated an effort to identify persons with blood lipoprotein concentrations that confer risk and to provide them with appropriate guidance in achieving more healthful blood lipid levels.

In the United States, more than 50 medical, governmental, and public health organizations have collaborated to organize the National Cholesterol Education Program (NCEP).[10] This has led to the development of a series of recommendations that would change the personal diet and exercise habits for much of our population. It has also provided physicians with specific guidance in identifying persons with lipoprotein disorders, in setting of goals for individuals, and in choosing the therapeutic options that might best achieve those goals. This endeavor, which has been very successful, began in 1987 and has continued, with revision in 1993.[10] These guidelines are becoming widely accepted as defining the "standard of care" for patients all over North America and in other parts of the world. Widespread adherence to these guidelines could lead to a marked reduction in the incidence of myocardial infarction (MI), coronary death, stroke, congestive heart failure (CHF), revascularization procedures, and hospitalization for unstable angina pectoris. Cardiovascular disease is such an overwhelming front runner among all serious diseases

201

in the United States that changes in these clinical events could also have a marked effect on expenditures for medical care and would produce a sizable decline in total death rates in America.[11,12]

This chapter utilizes the 1993 report of the Adult Treatment Panel to the NCEP as a guide to the identification and classification of persons who would benefit from the management of their lipoprotein-related risk by a primary care physician. It is important to recognize that many risk factors accelerate development of arteriosclerotic lesions; risk management must consider all of those that occur frequently in our population. The accumulation of several risk factors in a given individual may alter the treatment modalities that are recommended for a given modifiable risk factor, such as LDL-C. Successful reduction of LDL-C in one person may require achieving a plasma concentration much lower than that recommended for another person with less total risk. Applying treatment of moderate cost in a population at low total risk may lead to a high cost for any measurable benefit, since many individuals may need to be treated for years for every event prevented. Treating high-risk patients with coronary artery disease (CAD) using an effective LDL-C-reducing regimen has been shown to actually produce an overall cost savings, however.[12] Therefore, having a systematic approach to patients that identifies and sets goals in conjunction with total risk assessment will lead to the most efficient use of resources.

# INITIAL IDENTIFICATION OF LIPOPROTEIN-RELATED CARDIOVASCULAR RISK

Initial assessment of risk in a primary care practice should include the measurement of total plasma cholesterol and HDL-C. Taken in conjunction with age, gender, blood pressure, weight, and height and also with assessment of a history of diabetes or cigarette smoking and a family history of cardiovascular disease, these values provide for the basic planning of risk factor modification. All adult patients should receive such an assessment at least once every 5 years. Children should receive a similar assessment if there is a family history of early coronary heart disease (CHD) or if there is known hypercholesterolemia in first-degree relatives. This initial evaluation does not require fasting and can be done anytime, without concern about a recent meal.

All adults should be screened for

1. *Elevated* total cholesterol
2. *Reduced* HDL cholesterol

In certain individuals, the LDL-C should be assessed. That is done by measuring the blood plasma triglyceride concentration, total cholesterol, and HDL-C and then calculating the LDL-C. These measurements should be made after approximately 12 h of fasting, since triglycerides may be increased significantly by a single fat-containing meal. It is possible to obtain a direct measure of LDL-C in many laboratories, but this is not necessarily more accurate. Furthermore, there is information in the triglyceride measurement that will be useful clinically, and it is wise to confirm any HDL-C measurement, since such measurements tend to be subject to considerable laboratory error. This fasting plasma lipoprotein assessment should be made in all patients who have (1) arteriosclerotic vascular disease, (2) high total plasma cholesterol levels (>240 mg/dL), or (3) low HDL-C (<35 mg/dL). In those with no clinical evidence of vascular disease, the presence of other risk factors should guide further lipoprotein measurements. The NCEP guidelines also call for these fasting lipoprotein measurements to be completed in anyone with two major risk factors and total plasma cholesterol >200 mg/dL. The diagnosis of type 2 diabetes mellitus implies a high risk of vascular disease and is frequently associated with other major risk factors, such as high blood pressure, low HDL, and elevated triglycerides. The American Diabetes Association has therefore recommended that these patients should also have a lipoprotein analysis on fasting blood plasma. The possibility of significant hypertriglyceridemia should also be considered when on examination (1) the plasma is lipemic, (2) lipemia retinalis or eruptive xanthomata are present, (3) the spleen or liver is enlarged, (4) pancreatitis is present, or (5) unexplained abdominal pain is present.

Fasting blood should be obtained to measure

1. Triglycerides
2. HDL cholesterol
3. LDL cholesterol

when the clinical findings include

1. Clinically evident arteriosclerosis
2. Diabetes mellitus
3. HDL-C <35 mg/dL
4. Blood cholesterol >240 mg/dL
5. Blood cholesterol >200 mg/dL and two risk factors
6. Symptoms or signs suggesting hypertriglyceridemia

Certain cardiovascular risk factors are so dominant in population-based studies that they maintain strong associations with clinically significant vascular events even after adjusting for relationships with other characteristics of the individual. These are referred to as independent risk factors and should be given careful consideration in determining the assessment strategy and the setting of goals for treatment. The presence of two or more of these should cause the person to be considered to be in a "high-risk" state, and the target for LDL-C should be adjusted accordingly.

Major independent risk factors for cardiovascular disease are

1. Age over 45 if a man
2. Postmenopausal if a woman
3. High blood pressure, even if treated

4.  Cigarette smoking (>10 per day)
5.  Diabetes mellitus
6.  Family history of early vascular disease in close relatives (men <55 or women <65 years of age)
7.  HDL-C <35 mg/dL

There are also other characteristics of the plasma lipoproteins that have statistical associations with vascular disease and may play some role in the pathogenesis of vascular disease. Perhaps most studied and debated is the problem of elevated plasma triglycerides. Plasma triglycerides under 150 mg/dL seems to be desirable. This is associated with desirable or higher HDL-C and with LDL-C of normal level and composition. When the circulating triglycerides are higher, the HDL-C is often (but not always) lower. Many community studies have classified triglyceride concentrations as elevated when they are above 200 mg/dL and have noted a rising incidence of vascular disease in those persons with concentrations above this level— usually up to approximately 400 mg/dL. It is interesting that in the Framingham Heart Study, above 400 mg/dL the risk does not appear to rise further.[13] In this 200- to 400-mg/dL range, one finds the cholesterol-rich lipoproteins LDL and HDL to be modified: They are smaller and relatively cholesterol depleted. This reduced cholesterol content belies the relative number of particles, and some have theorized that these small, dense LDL particles play a key role in the pathogenesis of arteriosclerotic vascular disease.[14] There seems little doubt that the patients with this cluster of changes, which includes elevated fasting very-low-density lipoproteins (VLDL) and triglycerides, reduced and smaller HDL, and smaller cholesterol-depleted LDL, are at risk from deranged lipoprotein metabolism. Which of these is the operative factor remains unclear, however. Until defining studies are completed, control of the triglycerides while lowering LDL should be the focus. Quantitating additional lipoprotein risk factors provides little further guidance in treatments that have been documented by clinical trials.

The measurement of Lp(a) lipoprotein may prove to be an exception to this advice.[15] Lp(a) represents an LDL molecule that is covalently linked through a disulfide bridge with apo B-100, the major structural protein of LDL. The plasma concentration of Lp(a) ranges from 1 to over 300 mg/dL in different persons. The mean concentration in Caucasian and oriental populations is approximately 10 mg/dL, with the upper limit of normal at 30 mg/dL. In those of African descent, the mean value approaches 30 mg/dL. The concentration in any given individual is determined primarily by genetic influences, presumably controlling the rate of synthesis of the "a" protein. Members of some families with very high levels (well above 30 mg/dL) often have vascular disease early in life, particularly when these levels are associated with elevated LDL-C. An association with disease incidence has been found in several but not all community-based epidemiologic studies. To date, there are no studies that have proven benefit from using drugs that lower Lp(a), although those with elevated Lp(a) seem to be particularly benefited by reduction in elevated LDL-C. In those subjects with a strong family history of vascular disease and with early onset, measuring Lp(a) may provide an explanation and guide treatment.

## OTHER RISK FACTORS

A large number of other clinical findings have been associated with an increased incidence of ischemic events due to coronary, cerebrovascular, and peripheral vascular disease. These include obesity (particularly increased intraabdominal fat), glucose intolerance, elevated clotting factors [fibrinogen, factor VIIa, plasminogen activator inhibitor 1 (PAI-1)], platelet aggregability, increased number of circulating white blood cells, and increased plasma homocysteine and ferritin. Dietary factors are also related, including increased intake of saturated fat and cholesterol or reduced intake of unsaturated fats, certain vitamins (vitamin E, vitamin C), and fish. In managing most persons at risk of vascular disease, there is little practical value in quantitating any of these factors, with the exception of obesity. Increased body fat (particularly intraabdominal fat) amplifies elevated blood pressure, insulin resistance, and several lipoprotein abnormalities.[16,17] Diets high in calories as well as cholesterol and saturated fat should be assessed in qualitative terms and altered appropriately. The benefits of these actions are well documented.

Although homocysteine levels are now well correlated with increasing risk over a range of values commonly seen in practice,[18] evidence of benefit in the prevention of vascular disease as a result of direct treatment with vitamin combinations (folate, $B_6$, and $B_{12}$) has not been obtained. Although this measurement may provide a clue to the reason for strongly inherited coronary disease, the measurement is expensive and problematic. The blood should be drawn in preservative and cooled, and plasma should be removed from the cells immediately and properly analyzed. Furthermore, the folate occurring in the food supply is now being supplemented by folate added to flour and meal. It may prove far more cost-effective to simply advise those at risk to take a daily multivitamin with 400 $\mu$g of folate.

## FAMILY SCREENING

Genetics play a crucial role in determining lipoprotein concentrations. In a few patients, this can be traced to a specific molecular defect; however, in many individuals with elevated blood cholesterol or triglycerides, no genetic abnormality has been defined, although a clear familial pattern of inheritance can be demonstrated. In most, the inheritance is not definable, and it appears that the cause is polygenic, i.e., several minor genetic factors from both parents have clustered in the individual to produce the abnormal lipoprotein levels. Some of these genetic variations may result in vulnerability to environmental influences such as diets high in saturated fat and cholesterol. The absorption of dietary cholesterol in different individuals may range from 10 to 90 percent of that consumed, presumably as a result of such genetic determinants. Learned behavior patterns (diet, cigarette smoking, etc.) can also cause clustering of cardiovascular disease in a family.

There are three common lipoprotein abnormalities that are inherited as dominant traits.[19–21] These may be the result of many different molecular variations at the level of the gene, leading to a final common pathway of physiologic response. When first-degree relatives (parents, siblings, and children) are screened by appropriate testing, one-half are expected to have these disorders.

**1.**   *Familial hypercholesterolemia.* This rather general designation has come to be reserved for a clinical syndrome characterized by a marked elevation of LDL-C (usually >190 mg/dL). This disorder is fully expressed from early childhood and leads to vascular disease 10 to 15 years earlier than in persons with similar risk factors and average LDL-C. The underlying defect is usually due to reduced or dysfunctional LDL receptors on the surface of cells.[21] Since both genes coding for these receptors are required in order to develop a fully functional clearance system for LDL, a single abnormal gene leads to reduced removal of LDL from the plasma. LDL concentrations range from approximately 190 to 350 mg/dL in persons heterozygous for this disorder. Homozygous or mixed heterozygous patients with two dysfunctional genes may have LDL-C of 400 to 1000 mg/dL. The latter may develop coronary disease in the first decade of life. Both heterozygous and homozygous patients have a high frequency of tendon xanthomata, xanthelasma, and corneal arcus. Patients with the most severe forms of these disorders should usually also consult a lipid specialist.

**2.**   *Familial combined hyperlipidemia.* Patients with this syndrome are characterized by elevation of both VLDL and LDL. As a result, both plasma cholesterol and triglycerides are elevated. There is considerable variability in the lipoprotein levels over time, however, and at some point either of these lipoproteins may predominate as deviating the most from normal. On screening of family members, half of the first-degree relatives are expected to be affected but this may be expressed as elevation in either or both lipoprotein concentrations. HDL-C may be reduced, particularly if the triglycerides are elevated above 300 mg/dL. The basic physiology appears to be overproduction of VLDL by the liver, which leads to increased LDL as the VLDL particles are metabolized by the lipase enzymes. Full expression is usually seen after age 30. Affected children have lipid levels at or above the upper end of the expected concentrations for their age and sex. Diabetes accentuates the VLDL elevation. The specific molecular mechanism for patients with this syndrome is not yet defined. An association with arteriosclerosis is evident in many studies. Xanthomata and other clinical findings such as corneal arcus are not frequently observed. This familial disorder is frequently observed, with prevalence of over 1 percent reported in population studies. It is responsive to weight change and diet. Treatment designed to lower triglycerides often leaves the LDL-C elevated, so that combined therapeutic regimens are required.

**3.**   *Familial hypertriglyceridemia.* Plasma triglyceride elevations with near-normal LDL cholesterol, occuring with an autosomal dominant pattern of inheritance, are seen in 1/2 to 1 percent of the population in the United States. These individuals may have moderately elevated VLDL (triglyceride concentrations of 200 to 400 mg/dL), or they may manifest markedly elevated VLDL and chylomicrons in fasting blood plasma, with total triglycerides exceeding 5000 mg/dL. LDL concentrations may be quite low compared to the normal range, and HDL-C is usually reduced. Since the VLDL contains one part cholesterol by weight for each five parts of triglyceride, very high VLDL will also cause the total cholesterol to be above normal. There is a moderately strong association with vascular disease, but this is primarily predicted by the reduced HDL-C. Treatment of the lipoprotein abnormality with weight loss or drugs that lower triglycerides usually produces a satisfactory lipoprotein profile, including a desirable LDL-C concentration. The HDL-C may not return to a significantly higher range, however.

# SECONDARY HYPERLIPOPROTEINEMIAS

Selective laboratory tests should be combined with the medical history and physical examination to rule out other diseases and drugs that can markedly accentuate both elevated LDL-C and hypertriglyceridemia. These conditions are most commonly proteinuria (nephrotic syndrome), hypothyroidism, diabetes mellitus, and obstructive liver disease. Thiazide diuretics, progestogens, isotretinoin, protease inhibitors, cyclosporine, and anabolic steroids are among the potential causes of elevated VLDL and LDL-C. Estrogens taken orally may markedly accentuate elevated triglycerides, although commonly reducing LDL-C and raising HDL-C in those with normal lipids. Transdermal or vaginal administration of estrogenic compounds is less prone to cause this problem. Alcohol intake of more than two drinks per day may also raise triglycerides, particularly in those with some forms of genetic hypertriglyceridemia. In those with normal VLDL concentrations, HDL-C may be increased from 5 to 15 percent by moderate alcohol intake. This effect may partially explain the population studies suggesting a reduced incidence of CAD in persons who regularly consume small amounts of alcohol. No randomized clinical trials have been completed to establish that this is a protective factor independent of other economic and behavioral characteristics, however. Alcohol is not sufficiently documented to be safe or effective in preventing vascular disease and should not be prescribed for this purpose.

# TREATMENT GOALS

## Goals for LDL-C Reduction

Establishing an optimal LDL-C (see Table 18-1) should be the first consideration in managing lipoprotein disorders when the major goal is the prevention of myocardial infarction, stroke, and vascular death. In general terms, the higher the overall risk for future events, the lower should be the LDL-C. Those patients with proven cardiovascular disease are at very high risk and should maintain an LDL-C below 100 mg/dL. Those middle-aged patients with diabetes mellitus are at similar risk, and accordingly, the same goal, LDL-C <100 mg/dL, is appropriate. In those without significant evidence of arteriosclerosis, the presence of two or more risk factors (see above) places the patient in a high-risk category, and the goal in these persons is recommended to be <130 mg/dL by the NCEP. The LDL-C in low-risk individu-

**TABLE 18-1.   Threshold Cholesterol Levels According to Risk Factors**

| Category | Threshold for Initiating Dietary Therapy, mg/dL | | Threshold for Initiating Drug Therapy, mg/dL | | Goal for LDL Cholesterol, mg/dL |
| --- | --- | --- | --- | --- | --- |
| | Total Cholesterol | LDL Cholesterol | Total Cholesterol | LDL Cholesterol | |
| 0 or 1 risk factor | 240 | 160 | 275 | 190 | <160 |
| ≥2 risk factors | 200 | 130 | 240 | 160 | <130 |
| Cardiovascular disease | 160 | 100 | 200 | 130 | <100 |

als with one or fewer risk factors in middle life should be <160 mg/dL. There are, however, healthy young persons whose *only* risk factor is an elevated LDL-C and who can anticipate 20 or more years of life free of any clinical vascular event. These persons might be safely left with LDL-C in the 190 to 220 mg/dL range for a few years without drug therapy while the importance of diet, exercise, and other life style changes that reduce risk is emphasized to them.

| *Patient Risk Status* | *LDL-C Goals:* |
| --- | --- |
| Arteriosclerosis present | <100 mg/dL |
| Diabetes mellitus present | <100 mg/dL |
| No known arteriosclerosis | <130 mg/dL |
| Two or more major risk factors | |
| Men over 35 and women over 50 | <160 mg/dL |
| One or no major risk factors | |
| Premenopausal women and | <190 mg/dL |
|   men less than 35 years with | |
|   no other risk factors | |

When LDL-C is found to be above these goals, all patients should have careful evaluation of their diet and exercise patterns and be given the appropriate counseling to achieve meaningful changes. In general, drug therapy might be considered in those who remain above these targeted values after monitoring at approximately 8-week intervals. LDL-C concentrations 30 mg/dL above the goal should result in the introduction of the appropriate drug unless there are definite contraindications to such treatment. Once drugs are introduced, the LDL-C should be titrated to the goals above.

## Goals for Triglyceride Reduction

Triglycerides should be considered as elevated in adults when they are over 200 mg/dL. Over 400 mg/dL, they should be considered very high, and over 1000 mg/dL, they should be considered dangerously elevated. Any associated cardiovascular risk appears to reach full expression at levels around 400 mg/dL and is associated with the commonly found low HDL-C concentrations in these hypertriglyceridemic patients. Triglyceride elevations are frequently associated with increased LDL-C (as in familial combined hyperlipidemia), insulin resistance, high blood pressure, and central obesity. The specific molecular causes of increased arteriosclerosis in patients with this constellation of findings remain controversial.[21,22] Treatment of the hypertriglyceridemia frequently improves several of these disorders, however. Whenever possible, the goal should be to reduce fasting plasma triglycerides to 200 mg/dL or less.

Persons with triglycerides in excess of 1000 mg/dL are vulnerable to sudden further elevations into the 3000 to 10,000 mg/dL range, where fasting chylomicrons dominate the plasma lipoprotein spectrum. The massive buildup of these particles is associated with organ dysfunction, such as acute hemorrhagic pancreatitis, nausea, vomiting, diarrhea, peripheral neuropathy, central nervous dysfunction, dyspnea, and worsening of congestive heart failure (CHF). Although the specific etiology of this so-called hyperchylomicronemic syndrome is not fully understood, it probably involves the plugging of capillaries by clumps of chylomicrons, with regional ischemia and dysfunction in vulnerable organs.[23] The minimal goal in such patients is to maintain triglycerides at less than 1000 mg/dL and below 200 mg/dL if possible.

## DIETARY MODIFICATION

A two-tiered approach to dietary modification is advocated by the NCEP.[10] For patients without a history of myocardial infarction (MI) or other evidence of CAD, the Step I diet is recommended (Table 18-2). The Step II diet is a more stringent regi-

TABLE 18-2.   Nutrient Intake Guidelines for the Step I and Step II Diets in the Management of Hypercholesterolemia

| Nutrient | Recommended Intake (% of Total Calories) | |
| --- | --- | --- |
| | Step I Diet | Step II Diet |
| Total fat | <30 | <30 |
| Saturated fatty acids | <10 | <7 |
| Polyunsaturated fatty acids | <10 | <10 |
| Monounsaturated fatty acids | <15 | <15 |
| Cholesterol | <300 mg/day | <200 mg/day |
| Carbohydrates | >55 | >55 |
| Protein | ~15 | ~15 |

men that calls for 7 percent of total calories as saturated fatty acids and only 200 mg/day of cholesterol; it is advisable for patients who have experienced an MI or who have failed a Step I diet.[24–26] In collaboration with a registered dietitian, it is possible to achieve even more restrictive diets that are palatable and well balanced in protein, vitamins, and minerals and that reduce LDL-C more effectively.

In practice, it is possible to go well beyond the current dietary guidelines with benefit to the patient. Habitual diets in several societies contain 4 to 7 percent saturated fats and less than 100 mg/day of cholesterol. These can maintain caloric contributions of 15 percent from protein, 25 to 30 percent from total fat, and 55 to 60 percent from carbohydrate by following a few simple rules. These include (1) selecting most foods from vegetable, fruit, and grain sources; (2) restricting meat to a single portion of approximately 4 oz (1/4 lb) per day; and (3) eliminating egg yolks, dairy fats, heavily hydrogenated fats, and coconut oils. The diet is then vegetarian except for one meal per day, and all added fats are naturally occurring vegetable oils that are high in unsaturated fats and very low in saturated fats (e.g., safflower, sunflower, canola, and olive oils). All meats should be selected to be lean, have the fat trimmed, and be cooked so that the fat can drain in the process. Substituting fish for two of the meat entrees each week is advisable, since this level of fish consumption has been found to be associated with less vascular disease in several population studies. These simple rules can be taught by a physician and other office staff, but the important finer points and the answers to many questions are best provided by a trained nutritionist.

Acceptance and long-term adherence is essential if dietary therapy is to work. The recording and careful consideration of food habits and preferences can allow a highly competent dietitian to offer an eating plan that fits the patient's tastes and remains within the guidelines. Adherence to the diet requires both the patient and other members of the family to understand the principles and establish daily habits, and family members must also provide ongoing support and reinforcement at home. It is therefore most important to provide dietary instruction to the spouse and other influential members of the household. It requires at least 8 weeks to demonstrate successful dietary effect on LDL-C in an outpatient setting.[26] Further counseling after this point may correct misconceptions and induce further important changes. The physician should inquire about dietary adherence at every visit. This reinforces the commitment of the patient because it demonstrates the important place this issue occupies in the overall therapeutic regimen. True dietary change seldom fails to achieve some degree of improvement in lipid profiles. At a minimum, reduction in the dose of a cholesterol-lowering drug is a common benefit. In general, one should recommend avoiding fad diets that have very poor supporting data documenting long-term safety and benefit. These include diets that restrict protein or fat to 10 percent or less of calories and certainly those that recommend very high meat and fat intakes. Short-term weight loss with such diets is no help in achieving long-term cardiovascular health. If the patient does not achieve LDL-C reduction and HDL-C elevation for at least 5 years, the full initial benefits are not achieved. The same is certainly true with weight loss. Lifelong benefits require lifelong risk factor control.

Control of elevated triglycerides is best done with a similar dietary recommendation while emphasizing reduction in body weight to a desirable range. Setting standards too strictly can be detrimental in some cases, however. A moderate reduction of 5 or 10 lb can have dramatic effects on triglyceride levels in many patients. Once improvement has been achieved, sustained calorie restriction and a regular exercise program are the keys to long-term success.[27]

# DRUG THERAPY

## HMG-CoA Reductase Inhibitors (Statins)

After a test of diet and lifestyle change has been conducted, drug therapy may be needed to reach the desired range for LDL-C or triglyceride concentrations. A predrug trial period of only 8 weeks might be appropriate for patients who have known vascular disease. For young persons with no other risk factors, several years of working on lifestyle issues may be safe and more cost-effective even though LDL-C remains above the desirable range. When drugs are indicated, several classes are available; these provide a choice of mechanisms, one or more of which will be most effective when matched with the underlying lipid disorder and the specific lipoprotein goals. A recent review gives guidance on choosing specific drugs (see Table 18-3).[21]

Never before has the utility of lipid-lowering agents in reducing coronary morbidity and mortality been more clearly evident. In the past 5 years, several landmark clinical trials have demonstrated that treatment with 3-hydroxy-3-methylglutaryl coenzyme A (HMG-CoA) reductase inhibitors (statins) confers substantial cardioprotective benefits, sharply reducing coronary morbidity and mortality in patients with or without a prior history of MI.[3–9]

**MECHANISM OF ACTION.**   Statins, a competitive substrate for the enzyme HMG-CoA reductase, the rate-limiting step in hepatic cholesterol biosynthesis (the conversion of HMG to mevalonate), decrease the formation of cholesterol, which in turn leads to upregulation of LDL receptors and enhanced clearance of LDL cholesterol from serum.[28] Statins may also attenuate hepatic output of VLDL.[29]

**DOSAGE/ADMINISTRATION.**   Because cholesterol biosynthesis peaks in the evening, statins are generally administered before bedtime or with the evening meal. Although the absorption of most statins is relatively independent of food intake, lovastatin absorption is enhanced in the presence of food, while pravastatin absorption is decreased by food. The typical dosages presented in Table 18-3 may need to be diminished in the setting of hepatic disease (e.g., primary biliary cirrhosis) or renal insufficiency, or in the elderly.

**EFFECTS ON LIPIDS.**   At typical dosages, statins decrease LDL cholesterol by about 25 to 60 percent. In the settings of both primary[3,4] and secondary[5–9] coronary

**TABLE 18-3.   Lipid-Lowering Agents**

| Category | Mechanism of Action | Dosage | Effects on Lipoproteins |
|---|---|---|---|
| HMG-CoA reductase inhibitors (statins) | ↑LDL receptors<br>↓Cholesterol biosynthesis | (mg/day)<br>Atorvastatin, 10–80<br>Cerivastatin 0.2–0.4<br>Fluvastatin, 20–80<br>Lovastatin, 20–80<br>Pravastatin, 10–40<br>Simvastatin, 10–40 | ↓LDL-C, 24–60%<br>↑HDL-C, 6–12% |
| Niacin | ↓VLDL/LDL synthesis through ↑free fatty acid mobilization | 50–100 mg tid/titrate to 1.0–2.5 g tid<br><br>Niaspan (extended-release niacin) 1000–2000 mg qhs (titrated in 375–500-mg increments) | ↓LDL-C, 15–25%<br>↓VLDL-C, 25–35%<br>↓TG, 25–70%<br>↑HDL, 15–30% |
| Bile acid–binding resins (sequestrants) | ↑Incorporation of cholesterol into bile acids<br>↑LDL receptors | Cholestyramine, 8–12 g bid or tid<br>Colestipol, 10–15 g bid or tid | ↓LDL-C, 20–30%<br>↑HDL-C, TG |
| Fibric acid derivatives | ↑LPL activity/↑TG hydrolysis<br>↓VLDL synthesis<br>↑LDL catabolism | Gemfibrozil, 600 mg bid<br>Clofibrate, 2 g/day<br>Fenofibrate, 67 mg tid | ↓TG, 25–40%<br>↑HDL-C<br>↓LDL-C |

LDL-C = low-density lipoprotein cholesterol; HDL-C = high-density lipoprotein cholesterol; ULN = upper limit of normal; CY = cytochrome; VLDL = very-low-density lipoprotein; TG = triglycerides; NIDDM = non-insulin-dependent diabetes mellitus; bid = twice a day; tid = three times a day.

*Source:* Ginsberg HN, Goldberg IJ: Disorders of lipoprotein metabolism. In: Fauci AS, Braunwald E, Isselbacher KJ, et al (eds): *Harrison's Principles of Internal Medicine,* 14th ed. New York, McGraw-Hill, 1998:2138–2149.

prevention, treatment with pravastatin, lovastatin, or simvastatin has resulted in approximately 25 to 35 percent declines in coronary event rates, cardiovascular mortality, the need for revascularization, and all-cause mortality. A reduction in stroke risk using the statins has also been demonstrated in secondary prevention trials.

| Adverse Effects | Contraindications | May Interact With | Safe to Combine With |
|---|---|---|---|
| ↑Liver enzymes (2–3 × ULN) Muscle pain Abdominal pain, nausea, diarrhea | Myositis + renal failure, severe hepatic disease Treatment with strong inhibitors of CY P-450-3A4 enzyme, except for pravastatin, fluvastatin, and cerivastatin | Gemfibrozil, cyclosporine, warfarin, ketoconazole, and many others | Bile acid–binding resins |
| Cutaneous (e.g., flushing, pruritus, dry skin), nausea, abnormal hepatic function/hepatitis diarrhea, peptic ulcer disease, acid reflux, supraventricular arrhythmias ↑Uric acid ↓Glucose disposal (hyperglycemia) | NIDDM, gout, peptic ulcer disease, liver disease | Ganglionic-blocking agents | Bile acid–binding resins, statins, gemfibrozil |
| Constipation, nausea, gastric discomfort | Obstruction of biliary tract or gastric outlet, hypertriglyceridemia | Absorption of digitalis, thiazide diuretics, phenylbutazone, phenobarbital, thyroid hormones, certain antibiotics | Niacin, statins, gemfibrozil |
| Abnormal liver function, myositis, nausea ↑Bile lithogenicity | Hepatic/biliary disease (↓dose in renal insufficiency) | Anticoagulant activity of warfarin | Bile acid–binding resins |

Further, the Cholesterol and Recurrent Events (CARE) trial[6] and the Long-Term Intervention with Pravastatin in Ischaemic Disease (LIPID) Trial[7] demonstrated that statins are effective in preventing a second coronary event even when baseline LDL cholesterol concentrations are not markedly elevated.

Other favorable effects induced by statins at typical dosages include a 20 to 40 percent decrease in total cholesterol, a 10 to 35 percent decline in triglycerides, and a 6 to 12 percent rise in HDL cholesterol. After the initial reduction achieved with the starting dose, doubling the dosage of a statin results in a decline in LDL cholesterol of only 6 percent. Compared with other HMG-CoA reductase inhibitors, simvastatin and atorvastatin *(at half the dose)* offer the greatest LDL-C reduction. At very high doses, they reduce LDL cholesterol in the range of 47 to 60 percent. Many patients do not need such marked change to achieve the desirable range, however, and several of the drugs in this class are satisfactory. The thousands of patients treated with pravastatin[3,6,7] and lovastatin in controlled clinical trials offer a very large data set against which to judge both safety and efficacy in risk reduction.

Although the statins are not first-line therapy for hypertriglyceridemia, they may be effective as an adjunct in treating hypertriglyceridemia[22] (e.g., both LDL and VLDL elevations), decreasing this parameter by a maximum of 35 to 40 percent.[30,31] In addition to polygenic (type IIa/IIb) hypercholesterolemia, statins may be effective in treating familial combined hyperlipidemia (often in combination with another agent) as well as dyslipidemias associated with non-insulin-dependent diabetes mellitus. The statins may also favorably influence putative CAD risk factors, improving endothelial vasomotor tone as well as suppressing cholesterol esterification in macrophage cultures.[32,33]

**SIDE-EFFECTS PROFILE.**   Statins are exceedingly well tolerated. Because HMG-CoA reductase inhibitors can induce isolated [i.e., 1.5 times the upper limits of normal (1.5 x ULN)], asymptomatic rises in liver enzymes [i.e., alanine aminotransferase (ALT) and aspartate aminotransferase (AST)], liver function tests should be conducted at 6 and 12 weeks after therapy is instituted and at 6-month intervals thereafter during long-term treatment.[31] Recently, the FDA has eased the number of liver function tests required after 12 weeks for some of the statins, so long as no dosage changes are made or other drugs introduced that have the potential of slowing metabolism and excretion of the statin. Aminotransferase elevations are typically transient, or levels may be restored to normal upon dosage adjustment. HMG-CoA reductase inhibitors should be discontinued if ALT or AST values rise to more than 3 x ULN, an event that occurs in 2 to 3 percent of patients over 5 years compared to a rate of 1 to 2 percent in placebo-treated patients for the same period.[31] Hepatotoxicity may be more likely in recipients of high statin doses but occurs in less than 1 percent of such patients.[31,34]

Muscle discomfort is an important symptom because it may herald severe myopathy (e.g., rhabdomyolysis with renal failure secondary to myoglobinuria) when the symptoms are associated with profound creatine phosphokinase elevations on the order of 10 x ULN. This finding should cause immediate discontinuation of statin therapy. Although myopathy was observed in only 0.2 percent of patients in a large, long-term clinical trial of lovastatin,[34] its frequency may reach 5 percent when statins are administered in combination regimens with the fibric acid derivative gemfibrozil, and may also be elevated when administered concomitantly with cyclosporine (e.g., in heart transplant patients), itraconazole, fluconazole, or the macrolide antibiotics erythromycin and clarithromycin,[35,36] especially in elderly patients with renal insufficiency.[37]

Other side effects of statins experienced by relatively small proportions of patients include gastrointestinal (GI) discomfort, sleep disturbances, rash, peripheral neuropathy, and headache. For hypercholesterolemic patients who experience sleep disturbances during statin treatment, the use of statins (e.g., pravastatin or fluvastatin) that do not penetrate the central nervous system[31] may be a more logical choice. In addition, these two statins (pravastatin and fluvastatin) are not metabolized by the hepatic cytochrome-P450 3A4 enzyme system,[31] potentially diminishing the prospect of certain drug-drug interactions with other agents metabolized by this system (see Table 18-3). Finally, statins are teratogenic and should not be administered to pregnant women or those of childbearing potential who are not using reliable contraception.

## Niacin (Nicotinic Acid)

**MECHANISM OF ACTION.** Although its mode of action is not completely understood, niacin probably improves lipid profiles by inhibiting hepatic output of apo B-100-containing lipoproteins (Table 18-3). This results in diminished VLDL synthesis and, possibly, reduced conversion of VLDL to LDL. There is also evidence of enhanced clearance of VLDL through as yet undisclosed mechanisms.[38] Niacin tends to reduce lipolysis in adipose tissue through transient suppression of hormone-sensitive lipoprotein lipase activity. This is probably not a major factor in its prolonged effect, however.

**DOSAGE/ADMINISTRATION.** Of the lipid-lowering agents discussed in this review, niacin was the first available—it has been in continuous use for nearly 40 years.[31] Its use has been limited by the frequent adverse effects, including unpleasant cutaneous vasodilation (with or without pruritus). This "flushing" may be readily managed by administering low-dose (325 mg) aspirin within an hour before niacin dosing and instituting therapy at relatively low entry doses (e.g., 100 mg qid) and titrating upward by doubling the dosage after 3 to 7 days to 1 g tid or more (Table 18-3). In addition, the development of an FDA-approved extended-release niacin (Niaspan) has been associated with significantly less flushing and better long-term compliance.

Like statins, delayed-release niacin is often administered in the evening because it appears to be more efficacious at that time. This may be related to the observation that there is increased hepatic synthesis of both cholesterol and triglycerides during the nocturnal hours.[40] Thus, HMG-CoA reductase inhibitors and niacin (1.5 to 2 g/day) can be combined conveniently in the setting of elevated LDL and low HDL cholesterol, eliciting synergistic benefits on the lipoprotein profile without producing additive adverse events,[41–43] although the risk of myositis (<1 percent) must be considered. In patients with familial combined hyperlipidemia, which affects 10 to 15 percent of patients with CAD before the age of 60 (<2 percent of the general population),[19] niacin (3 to 4 g/day) can also be combined with bile acid–binding resins.

**EFFECTS ON LIPIDS.** Niacin is arguably the most versatile lipid-lowering agent, substantially improving virtually every lipoprotein fraction. Typical favorable effects achieved by niacin include declines of 15 to 25 percent in total and LDL cholesterol, 25 to 35 percent in triglycerides in those with moderate hypertriglyceridemia, and 35 to 70 percent in triglycerides in those with markedly elevated triglycerides (>500 mg/dL). It is the most effective of all drugs in raising HDL cholesterol, with changes on the order of 15 to 25 percent commonly observed (Table 18-3). In addition, niacin may reduce levels of two putative CAD risk factors: Lp(a) (by 30 percent)[44] and fibrinogen. Niacin may also be capable of transforming small, dense LDL particles into more cholesterol-rich forms as triglycerides are reduced.

**SIDE-EFFECTS PROFILE.**    Flushing may be a matter of particular concern to certain patients, such as perimenopausal women experiencing hot flashes. Troublesome truncal and facial flushing can engender covert noncompliance among patients, compromising the efficacy of niacin.

Niacin can also have undesirable metabolic effects, elevating serum uric acid levels and perturbing normal glucose disposal, with attendant glucose intolerance. Because of these effects, type II diabetes is a relative contraindication, and gout definitely contraindicates niacin use. Hepatotoxicity, including fulminant hepatitis, has been observed principally after administration of high-dose timed-release, rather than crystalline (plain), formulations.[38,45] Interestingly, the Niaspan formulation has not been reported to cause severe liver damage. Modest fluctuations in ALT and AST values are often observed but may be secondary to lipid lowering per se. Other side effects include rash, GI disturbances (e.g., indigestion, nausea, diarrhea), supraventricular arrhythmias, conjunctivitis, and nasal congestion. The frequency of GI complaints may also be higher in patients treated with some timed-release niacin preparations than in those treated with immediate-release formulations.[45] There are many small suppliers of niacin, and the adverse event rate appears to vary with the source. Finding a product that is documented gives added safety and freedom from some of the annoying and occasionally quite serious adverse events noted above.

## Bile Acid–Binding Resins (Sequestrants)

**MECHANISM OF ACTION.**    By disrupting enterohepatic circulation of bile acids, resins increase the conversion of cholesterol into bile salts, thereby reducing the hepatic cholesterol content, with a resulting upregulation of LDL receptor expression.

**DOSAGE/ADMINISTRATION.**    The bile acid sequestrants colestipol and cholestyramine are formulated as powders to be mixed in water or juice and taken with meals. Typical dosages range from 4 to 8 g bid to 12 g tid for cholestyramine, and from 5 to 10 g bid to 15 g tid for colestipol (Table 18-3).

**EFFECTS ON LIPIDS.**    Dose-dependent decreases of about 20 to 30 percent in LDL cholesterol are effected by resins.[2,46,47] The sequestrants modestly increase HDL cholesterol. In addition to enhancing cholesterol clearance, these agents may also induce a compensatory increase in VLDL output, potentially elevating serum triglycerides. This effect is minimal in normal persons but can be quite exaggerated in some patients with hypertriglyceridemia. Sequestrants may be used to reduce LDL-C after triglycerides are controlled by other therapy.

Although in use for approximately three decades, bile acid–binding resins have largely been consigned to adjunctive roles in combination regimens with fibrates, niacin, or HMG-CoA reductase inhibitors. These often provide for additive reduction in LDL-C, since their mechanism of action is different from that of any other drug. They are particularly helpful in combination with statins when attempting to diminish very high LDL-C, as in some patients with familial hypercholesterolemia. The inhibition of cholesterol biosynthesis simultaneously with an increase in hepatic cholesterol loss through the bile acid pathway amplifies the induction of LDL receptors. Bile acid sequestrants also tend to increase HDL cholesterol when added to HMG-CoA reductase inhibitor regimens.

**SIDE-EFFECTS PROFILE.**   Because resins act within the GI tract and are thus not considered systemic agents, their safety profiles are relatively favorable, and the sequestrants may thus be appropriate for young men, premenopausal women, and even children with hypercholesterolemia. On the other hand, many patients find the powders unpalatable and may also complain of GI discomfort (e.g., constipation, bloating, gas, nausea). Some of these adverse effects can be relieved by the simultaneous use of vegetable fiber supplements (e.g., psyllium). Mixing the vegetable fibers with the resin also gives a more natural "mouth feel" and improves the palatability of the preparation. Resins can also bind to and reduce the absorption of a variety of other drugs, including digoxin, warfarin, and thiazide diuretics. All drugs should be taken at least 1 h before or more than 4 h after the resins. Finally, high doses of bile acid–binding resins can also cause more serious complications in small children, including obstructions of the biliary tract or gastric outlet and hyperchloremic acidosis.[47]

## Fibric Acid Derivatives (Fibrates)

This group of drugs has been tested in long-term clinical trials involving hundreds of patients and has proven most effective in patients with high triglycerides, low HDL-C, and desirable or moderately elevated LDL-C.[48,49]

**MECHANISM OF ACTION.**   When fibrates are administered to humans, a series of changes in lipoprotein metabolism occurs. The major effect is a reduction in triglycerides, both VLDL and (if elevated) chylomicrons. This is due primarily to an increase in clearance of these lipoproteins from the plasma. Although fibrates increase lipoprotein lipase,[50] the major effect may be due to their changing the apolipoprotein composition of these triglyceride-rich lipoproteins by reducing the content of apo C-III.[51,52] This protein acts as a surface stabilizing agent but also slows both lipase action[53] and remnant clearance by the liver.[52] Fibrates inhibit apo C-III synthesis in the liver. They also decrease hepatic synthesis of VLDL triglycerides by enhancing free fatty acid oxidation in the liver. LDL and HDL usually become larger and more cholesterol-rich.[54] In patients with normal triglycerides, fibrates can provide significant reduction of LDL-C,[55] perhaps through their ability to increase hepatic output of cholesterol in bile.

**DOSAGE/ADMINISTRATION.** Gemfibrozil is administered at a dosage of 600 mg bid and clofibrate at 1 g bid (Table 18-3). Fenofibrate tablets are administered 67 mg tid. The usual dose is 201 mg/day.

**EFFECTS ON LIPIDS.** Fibrates reduce serum triglyceride levels by approximately 25 to 40 percent. The percent reduction usually increases in proportion to the baseline triglyceride concentration, with maximum effects seen in those over 1000 mg/dL. An accompanying rise in HDL-C is also greatest in those with severe hypertriglyceridemia, ranging from 4 to 20 percent. The very low LDL-C seen in such patients usually increases as well but rarely rises above 130 mg/dL unless the underlying disorder is combined familial hyperlipidemia. Much of the LDL-C increase is due to the greater cholesterol content found in each LDL particle; the number of particles may not change. In persons with triglyceride levels less than 200 mg/dL, LDL-C usually falls 15 to 25 percent.[56]

Fibrates are indicated principally for patients with pronounced hypertriglyceridemia (>1000 mg/dL) and low HDL cholesterol, as well as in combination regimens with niacin in the setting of elevated triglycerides and LDL cholesterol.

**SIDE-EFFECTS PROFILE.** The most common adverse event with fibrate therapy is abdominal pain, probably attributable to direct gastric or intestinal irritation. It was the only symptom that was increased significantly in the Helsinki Heart Study,[48] and although annoying, it was without further complications. Fibrates, by increasing the relative excretion of cholesterol, can induce lithogenic bile and over a long period induce cholelithiasis. Abnormal ALT and AST profiles are observed in less than 5 percent of patients and have always been reversible. Rarely, myositis, myopathy, or rhabdomyolysis has been reported, particularly when fibrates are administered together with lovastatin or other drugs that inhibit cytochrome P-450-dependent metabolism of these drugs. This is particularly of concern in patients with renal insufficiency.[35] Both clofibrate and gemfibrozil are potentially teratogenic. Caution should be exercised when treating pregnant women, particularly in the first trimester. These drugs have been used, however, in severe hypertriglyceridemia seen in the latter stages of pregnancy in some patients with genetic hyperlipidemia. The dosage of certain fibrates may need to be adjusted according to prothrombin times when administered concomitantly with warfarin.

## CONCLUSIONS

Although it exacts a heavy toll in terms of coronary mortality, morbidity, and costly revascularization procedures, CAD is an eminently preventable condition. In concert with reduction of other CAD risk factors and limitation of dietary saturated fat and cholesterol, a series of effective drugs can be used to lower LDL-C and raise HDL-C with documented benefit to patients. After appropriate goals for LDL-C and triglycerides are set, the statins, niacin, bile acid–binding resins, and fibric acid derivatives constitute a potent clinical armamentarium in primary and secondary prevention of CAD.

## REFERENCES

1. Levine GN, Kearney JF Jr, Vita JA: Cholesterol reduction in cardiovascular disease: clinical benefits and possible mechanisms. *N Engl J Med* 1995; 332:512–521.
2. Lipid Research Clinics Coronary Primary Prevention Trial results: I. Reduction in incidence of coronary heart disease. *JAMA* 1984; 251:351–364.
3. Shepherd J, Cobbe SM, Ford I, et al, for the West of Scotland Coronary Prevention Study Group: Prevention of coronary heart disease with pravastatin in men with hypercholesterolemia. *N Engl J Med* 1995; 333:1301–1307.
4. Downs JR, Clearfield M, Weis S, et al: Primary prevention of acute coronary events with lovastatin in men and women with average cholesterol levels: results of AFCAPS/TEXCAPS. *JAMA* 1998; 279(20):1615–1622.
5. Scandinavian Simvastatin Survival Study Group: Randomized trial of cholesterol lowering in 4444 patients with coronary heart disease: the Scandinavian Simvastatin Survival Study. *Lancet* 1994; 344:1383–1389.
6. Sacks FM, Pfeffer MA, Moyle LA, et al, for the Cholesterol and Recurrent Events Trial Investigators: The effect of pravastatin on coronary events after myocardial infarction in patients with average cholesterol levels. *N Engl J Med* 1996; 335:1001–1009.
7. The Long-Term Intervention with Pravastatin in Ischaemic Disease (LIPID) Study Group: Prevention of cardiovascular events and death with pravastatin in patients with coronary heart disease and a broad range of initial cholesterol levels. *N Engl J Med* 1998; 339:1349–1357.
8. The Post Coronary Artery Bypass Graft Trial Investigators: The effect of aggressive lowering of low-density lipoprotein cholesterol levels and low-dose anticoagulation on obstructive changes in saphenous-vein coronary-artery bypass grafts. *N Engl J Med* 1997; 336:153–162.
9. Pitt B, Waters D, Brown WV, et al, for the Atorvastatin versus Revascularization Treatment Investigators: Aggressive lipid-lowering therapy compared with angioplasty in stable coronary artery disease. *N Engl J Med* 1999; 341:70–76.
10. Expert Panel: Summary of the second report of the National Cholesterol Education Program (NCEP) Expert Panel on Detection, Evaluation, and Treatment of High Blood Cholesterol in Adults (Adult Treatment Panel II). *JAMA* 1993; 269:3015–3023.
11. Hebert PR, Gaziano JM, Chan KS, Hennekens CH: Cholesterol lowering with statin drugs, risk of stroke and total mortality. An overview of randomized trials. *JAMA* 1997; 278:313–321.
12. Pearson TA, Swan HJ: Lipid lowering: the case for identifying and treating the high-risk patient. *Cardiol Clin* 1996; 14:117–130.
13. Castelli WP: Cholesterol and lipids in the risk of coronary artery disease: the Framingham Heart Study. *Can J Cardiol* 1998; 4(suppl A):5A–10A.
14. Austin MA, King MC, Vranizan KM, Krauss RM: Atherogenic lipoprotein phenotype, a proposed genetic marker for coronary heart disease risk. *Circulation* 1990; 82:495–506.
15. Uterman G: Lipoprotein(a). In: Scriver CR, Beaudet AL, Sly WS, Valle D (eds): *The*

*Metabolic and Molecular Bases of Inherited Disease.* New York, McGraw-Hill, 1995:1887–1912.

16. Bjorntorp P: Body fat distribution, insulin resistance and metabolic diseases. *Nutrition* 1997; 13:795–803.

17. Wickelgren I: Do "apples" fare better than "pears"? *Science* 1998; 280:1365.

18. Welch GN, Loscalzo J: Homocysteine and atherothrombosis. *N Engl J Med* 1995; 332:1491–1498.

19. Goldstein JL, Schrott HG, Hazzard WR, et al: Hyperlipidemia in coronary heart disease: II. Genetic analysis of lipid levels in 176 families and delineation of a new inherited disorder, combined hyperlipidemia. *J Clin Invest* 1973; 52:1544–1568.

20. Havel RJ, Rapaport E: Management of primary hyperlipidemia. *N Engl J Med* 1995; 332:1491–1498.

21. Ginsberg HN, Goldberg IJ: Disorders of lipoprotein metabolism. In: Fauci AS, Braunwald E, Isselbacher KJ, et al. (eds): *Harrison's Principles of Internal Medicine,* 14th ed: Vol 2. New York, McGraw-Hill, 1998:2138–2149.

22. Ginsberg HN: Is hypertriglyceridemia a risk factor for atherosclerotic cardiovascular disease? A simple question with a complicated answer. *Ann Intern Med* 1997; 126:912–914.

23. Brunzell JD, Bierman EL: Chylomicronemia syndrome: interaction of genetic and acquired hypertriglyceridemia. *Med Clin North Am* 1982; 66:455–468.

24. Denke MA: Cholesterol-lowering diets: a review of the evidence. *Arch Intern Med* 1995; 155:17–26.

25. Retzlaff BM, Walden CP, McNeney WB, et al: Nutritional intake of women and men on the NCEP Step I and Step II diets. *J Am Coll Nutr* 1997; 16:52–61.

26. Knopp RH, Walden CE, Retzlaff BM, et al: Long-term cholesterol-lowering effects of 4 fat-restricted diets in hypercholesterolemic and combined hyperlipidemic men: the Dietary Alternatives Study. *JAMA* 1997; 278:1509–1515.

27. Denke MA, Sempos CT, Grundy SM: Excess body weight: an underrecognized contributor to high blood cholesterol levels in white American men. *Arch Intern Med* 1993; 153:1093–1103.

28. Bilheimer DW, Grundy SM, Brown MS, Goldsterin JL: Mevinolin and colestipol stimulate receptor-mediated clearance of low-density lipoprotein from plasma in familial hypercholesterolemia heterozygotes. *Proc Natl Acad Sci U S A* 1983; 80:4124–4128.

29. Arad Y, Ramakrishnan R, Ginsberg HN: Effects of lovastatin therapy on very-low-density lipoprotein triglyceride metabolism in subjects with combined hyperlipidemia: evidence for reduced assembly and secretion of triglyceride-rich lipoproteins. *Metabolism* 1992; 421:487–493.

30. Bakker-Arkema RG, Davidson MH, Goldstein RJ, et al: Efficacy and safety of a new HMG-CoA reductase inhibitor, atorvastatin, in patients with hypertriglyceridemia. *JAMA* 1996; 275:128–133.

31. *Physicians' Desk Reference,* 53d ed. Montvale, NJ: Medical Economics, 1999.

32. Vaughan CJ, Murphy MB, Buckley BM: Statins do more than just lower cholesterol. *Lancet* 1996; 348:1079–1082.

33. Cignarella A, Brenhausen B, von Eckardstein A, et al: Differential effects of lovastatin on the trafficking of endogenous and lipoprotein-derived cholesterol in human monocyte-derived macrophages. *Arterioscler Thromb Vasc Biol* 1998; 18:1322–1329.

34. Bradford RH, Shear CL, Chremos AN, et al: Expanded Clinical Evaluation of Lovastatin (EXCEL) study results: I. Efficacy in modifying lipoproteins and adverse event profile in 8245 patients with moderate hypercholesterolemia. *Arch Intern Med* 1991; 151:43–49.

35. Smit JWA, Jansen GH, de Bruin TWA, Erkelens DW: Treatment of combined hyper-lipidemia with fluvastatin and gemfibrozil, alone or in combination, does not induce muscle damage. *Am J Cardiol* 1995; 76:126A–128A.

36. Illingworth DR, Tobert JA: A review of clinical trials comparing HMG-CoA reductase inhibitors. *Clin Ther* 1994; 16:366–385.

37. Pierce LR, Wysowski DK, Gross TP: Myopathy and rhabdomyolysis associated with lovastatin-gemfibrozil therapy. *JAMA* 1990; 264:71–75.

38. Knopp RH, Ginsberg J, Albers JJ, et al: Contrasting effects of unmodified time-release forms of niacin on lipoproteins in hyperlipidemic subjects: clues to mechanism of action of niacin. *Metabolism* 1985; 34:642–650.

39. Altschul R, Hoffer A, Stephen JD: Influence of nicotinic acid on serum cholesterol in man. *Arch Biochem Biophys* 1955; 54:558–559.

40. Schlierf G, Dorow E: Diurnal patterns of triglyceride, free fatty acids, blood sugar, and insulin during carbohydrate-induction in man and their modification by nocturnal sup-pression of lipolysis. *J Clin Invest* 1973; 52:732–740.

41. Davignon J, Roederer G, Montigny M, et al: Comparative efficacy and safety of pravastatin, nicotinic acid and the two combined in patients with hypercholesterolemia. *Am J Cardiol* 1994; 73:339–345.

42. Stein EA, Davidson MH, Dujovne CA, et al: The efficacy and tolerability of low dose simvastatin and niacin, alone and in combination, in patients with combined hyperlipid-emia: a prospective trial. *J Cardiovasc Pharmacol Therapeut* 1996; 1:107–116.

43. Jacobson TA, Chin M, Fromell G, et al: Fluvastatin, with and without niacin, for hyper-cholesterolemia. *Am J Cardiol* 1994; 74:149–154.

44. Knopp RH, Alagona P, Davidson M, et al: Equivalent efficacy of a time-release form of niacin (Niaspan) given once a night vs. plain niacin in the management of hyperlipid-emia. *Metabolism* 1998; 47:1097–1104.

45. McKenney JM, Proctor JD, Harris S, Chinchili VM: A comparison of the efficacy and toxic effects of sustained vs immediate-release niacin in hypercholesterolemic patients. *JAMA* 1994; 271:672–677.

46. Pravastatin Multicenter Study Group II: Combined efficacy and safety of pravastatin and cholestyramine alone and combined in patients with hypercholesterolemia. *Arch Intern Med* 1993; 153:1321–1329.

47. Packard CJ, Shepherd J: The hepatobiliary axis and lipoprotein metabolism: effects of bile acid sequestrants and ileal bypass surgery. *J Lipid Res* 1982; 23:1081–1098.

48. Frick MH, Elo O, Haapa K, et al: Helsinki Heart Study; primary prevention trial with gemfibrozil in middle-aged men with dyslipidemia: safety in treatment, changes in risk factors and incidence of coronary heart disease. *N Engl J Med* 1987; 317:1237–1245.

49. Rubins HB, Robins SJ, Collins D, and the Veterans Affairs HDL Intervention Trial (VA-HIT) Study Group: Gemfibrozil for the secondary prevention of coronary heart disease in men with low levels of high-density lipoprotein cholesterol. *N Engl J Med* 1999; 341:410–418.

50. Boberg J, Boberg M, Gross R, et al: The effect of treatment with clofibrate on hepatic triglyceride and lipoprotein lipase activities of post-heparin plasma in male patients with hyperlipoproteinemia. *Atherosclerosis* 1977; 27:499–503.

51. Auwerx J, Schoonjans K, Fruchart J-C, Staels B: Transcriptional control of triglyc-eride metabolism: fibrates and fatty acids change the expression of the LPL and apo CIII genes by activating the nuclear receptor PPAR. *Atherosclerosis* 1996; 124(suppl): S29–S37.

52. Staels B, Dallongeville J, Auwerx J, et al: Mechanisms of action of fibrates on lipid and lipoprotein metabolism. *Circulation* 1998; 98:2088–2093.

53. Brown WV, Baginsky ML: Inhibition of lipoprotein lipase by an apoprotein of human very low density lipoprotein. *Biochem Biophys Res Com* 1972; 375–381.

54. De Graaf J, Hendricks JC, Demacker PN, Stalenhoef AE: Identification of multiple dense LDL subfractions with enhanced susceptibility to in vitro oxidation among hypertriglyceridemic subjects: normalization after clofibrate treatment. *Arterioscler Thromb Vasc Biol* 1993; 13:712–719.

55. Brown WV, Dujovne CA, Farquhar WJ, et al: Effects of fenofibrate on plasma lipids: double-blind, multicenter study in patients with type IIA or IIb hyperlipidemia. *Arteriosclerosis* 1986; 6:670–678.

SUNIL KRIPALANI / TERRY A. JACOBSON

# TOBACCO ABUSE— CARDIOVASCULAR EFFECTS AND STRATEGIES FOR CESSATION

## EPIDEMIOLOGY AND COSTS

By recent estimates, 23.2 percent of Americans smoke.[1] What is of even more concern is that tobacco use is responsible for more than 400,000 deaths annually in the United States alone, and exposure to secondhand smoke may contribute to another 50,000 deaths. More than 170,000 of these deaths are from cardiovascular causes. Altogether, cigarettes are a factor in more than 20 percent of all deaths in the United States, or approximately 1000 deaths per day, making tobacco use the leading preventable cause of death in our society. Not surprisingly, smokers have nearly double the overall mortality of nonsmokers.[2] Smoking also costs the U.S. economy nearly $100 billion annually. This figure includes not only the direct expenses of smoking-related medical care but the indirect costs, such as lost wages and productivity.[3]

## EFFECTS ON THE CARDIOVASCULAR SYSTEM

Compared to nonsmokers, smokers have two to six times the risk of suffering a myocardial infarction, one and one-half times the risk of stroke, and two to three times the risk of death from ruptured aortic aneurysm.[2] Environmental tobacco smoke is also associated with an increased risk for premature cardiovascular disease and death.[4,5]

Of the more than 4000 adverse chemicals found in cigarettes, carbon monoxide and nicotine are probably the most important in terms of their effects on the cardiovascular system. Nicotine, an adrenergic agonist which elevates catecholamine levels, increases myocardial demand by raising both heart rate and blood pressure. At the same time, carbon monoxide interferes with the oxygen-carrying capacity of hemoglobin, reducing oxygen delivery to the myocardium. Furthermore, smoking even one cigarette increases coronary vascular resistance and decreases blood flow, even in the absence of atherosclerosis. In some individuals, this effect is so pronounced as to cause sudden arterial vasoconstriction and angina.[6]

Smoking accelerates atherogenesis through a number of mechanisms. It causes injury and inflammation to the arterial endothelium in a dose-dependent fashion, an effect which is at least partially mediated by free-radical formation. It also has an adverse effect on the lipid profile, increasing total cholesterol and decreasing high-density lipoprotein (HDL) levels. While low-density lipoprotein (LDL) levels do not change significantly, smoking oxidizes the LDL molecule and makes it more susceptible to oxidation from other sources. Oxidized LDL is thought to be one of the major initiators of the atherosclerotic process. Levels of platelet-derived growth factor increase with smoking, and this, in turn, promotes smooth muscle growth and atherogenesis. By increasing platelet reactivity and fibrinogen levels, smoking also creates a thrombogenic state.[6]

According to the 1990 Surgeon General's report on tobacco, the effects of smoking on the cardiovascular system start to reverse with cessation. This beneficial effect occurs more rapidly than the reduction in pulmonary disease and cancer. Within 1 year of quitting, smokers reduce their risk of premature coronary heart disease by one-half. After 10 to 15 years, overall mortality is reduced nearly to the levels of nonsmokers.[7] The benefits of smoking cessation also extend to older individuals, those with documented coronary heart disease, and even those who have undergone revascularization procedures.[6]

## SMOKING CESSATION

### Opportunities for Intervention

Given the high prevalence of smoking in the United States and the tremendous impact it has on morbidity and mortality, physicians must address tobacco use as an active medical problem. The first step is to diagnose patients who are current or former smokers. Physicians should chart tobacco use as a fifth vital sign and consider adding stickers to identify the charts of smokers.[8]

Each year, at least 70 percent of smokers have an office visit with a physician, creating a number of opportunities for intervention. Physician advice, even if limited to a few minutes, is effective in motivating cessation. Physicians are also a valuable source of patient education, particularly since many Americans are not fully aware of the health risks of tobacco. When patients present with illnesses that are clearly exacerbated or caused by smoking, a "teachable moment" arises, along with a potential motivator to quit. Similarly, when patients are hospitalized (frequently for smoking-related illnesses) and often must remain smoke-free for several days, physicians should encourage long-term cessation and initiate pharmacologic therapy if appropriate. Other common opportunities for counseling include routine adult physicals and adolescent athletic physicals, as well as visits when a child exposed to secondhand smoke presents with respiratory symptoms.

The office environment can be a useful adjunct to physicians' efforts. A smoke-free office with a designated stop smoking coordinator is the first step. Antismoking posters, educational materials in the waiting room, and reading material that is free of cigarette advertising all send a message to patients as well.

## Behavioral Interventions

Although physician advice to quit smoking is clearly beneficial, only half of smokers are urged by their physicians to quit.[9] There are a number of barriers to physician intervention. The limited time available (the average outpatient encounter lasts only 12 min) often does not permit in-depth counseling. Furthermore, in spite of abundant evidence concerning the cost-effectiveness of smoking cessation, many health insurance plans do not provide reimbursement.[10] Other physician barriers include a lack of skills, a lack of resources, and the perception that cessation efforts are not rewarding or worthwhile because rates of success are low.[11] However, if physicians attained only a 5 percent success rate in their cessation efforts, an additional 2 million smokers would quit each year.[12]

The U.S. Agency for Health Care Policy and Research (AHCPR) recently developed clinical guidelines for primary care physicians (Table 19-1).[13,14] The panel recommends taking advantage of every opportunity to identify and counsel smokers,

**TABLE 19-1.   Actions and Strategies for the Primary Care Physician—The Four A's**

*Step 1. Ask*—Systematically identify all tobacco users at every visit
- Take smoking status as a fifth vital sign

*Step 2. Advise*—Strongly urge all smokers to quit
- Use a clear, strong, and personalized approach
- Encourage clinic staff to reinforce the cessation message
- Identify smokers willing to make a quit attempt at this time

*Step 3. Assist*—Aid the patient in quitting
- Set a quit date and help the patient prepare for quitting
- Encourage nicotine replacement therapy
- Give advice on how to make the attempt more successful
- Provide educational materials

*Step 4. Arrange*—Schedule follow-up contact
- Contact the patient soon after the quit date to congratulate success and encourage against relapse
- Use relapses as a learning tool for the next quit attempt, not as a sign of failure

*Source:* Adapted from The Agency for Health Care Policy and Research Smoking Cessation Clinical Practice Guideline. *JAMA* 1996; 275:1270–1280, with permission.

tailoring the message to the individual patient. To begin with, it is sometimes beneficial to ask patients if they understand the consequences of continued smoking. Physicians can then provide information about the health risks of tobacco use, the benefits of quitting, and the nature and time course of withdrawal. They should also help patients recognize personal factors which may make relapse more likely, such as being around other smokers, using alcohol, taking even a single puff after the quit date, and not coping well with stressors. While the most effective behavioral interventions are intense, consisting of several sessions lasting 20 to 30 min over 2 weeks, shorter messages are also helpful in promoting cessation.

Many patients will have tried to quit smoking unsuccessfully or will not be ready to set a quit date at the time of the encounter. These patients may be uninformed about the benefits of quitting, concerned about withdrawal symptoms, or frustrated by previous failure. Physicians should still make an effort to discuss reasons for quitting and ways to overcome individual barriers in order to motivate future attempts. Successful clinical interventions often incorporate the four R's: relevance, risks, rewards, and repetition (Table 19-2).[13]

Another useful approach for guiding physician counseling is the stages of change counseling model, which assesses a patient's readiness to initiate behavioral change. Three key questions are used to assess a smoker's readiness to quit:

1. Do you intend to quit smoking in the next 6 months?
2. Do you intend to quit smoking in the next month?
3. Have you tried to quit smoking in the past year?

Patients who are not ready to quit in the next 6 months, who account for 30 percent of smokers, are in the *precontemplation* stage. For these individuals, physicians should provide advice regarding the health consequences of smoking and personal reasons for cessation, with a goal of helping them think seriously about quitting. Peo-

**TABLE 19-2.   Components of Clinical Interventions which Enhance Motivation to Quit Smoking—The Four R's**

*Relevance.* Tailor motivational information to a patient's individual concerns and disease status, such as frequent respiratory infections, children at home, or experiences during prior cessation attempts

*Risks.* Ask the patient to identify the negative consequences of smoking and highlight those that are most relevant to him or her

*Rewards.* Ask the patient to list the benefits of quitting smoking and highlight those that are most relevant to him or her

*Repetition.* Repeat the motivational intervention at every patient encounter

*Source:* Adapted from The Agency for Health Care Policy and Research Smoking Cessation Clinical Practice Guidelines. *JAMA* 1996; 275:1270–1280, with permission.

ple in the *contemplation* stage (about 60 percent) intend to quit in the next 6 months but not in the next month; they frequently need to build confidence in their ability to quit. Physicians should assist these patients by providing them with reasons to quit and informing them about self-help methods and specific strategies for overcoming their personal barriers to cessation. Follow-up to discuss plans for quitting is also important. In the *preparation* stage, smokers are taking some steps toward quitting, such as significantly reducing their daily number of cigarettes, and are often prepared to take action. Individuals in the *action* stage represent 10 percent of all smokers. They have tried to quit in the past year and plan to quit in the next month. The best approach here is for the physician to set a quit date with the patient, in addition to all of the above interventions. Follow-up during a quit attempt provides an opportunity to discuss particular difficulties with the attempt and may help prevent relapse. The final stage, which begins 6 months after the successful quit attempt, is *maintenance* or relapse prevention. During this time, counseling should be supportive and should reinforce the reasons for quitting, as well as emphasizing any early benefits that have been achieved, such as a reduction in respiratory symptoms or improved taste for food. Physician interventions which are matched to the smoker's stage of change are more effective in reaching the eventual goal of cessation.[15]

Allied health providers (i.e., health educators, nurse practitioners, and physician assistants) can bolster physicians' efforts, since they frequently possess additional skills in behavioral counseling. In fact, the team leader for a smoking cessation program is often not a physician. Nurse-managed interventions have been shown to be effective in a variety of settings, including smoking cessation.[16] The programs usually include algorithms for monitoring patients' progress, frequently through telephone follow-up. Patient satisfaction has been high, and cost savings are evident even over a short period of time. An additional advantage of such programs is that the allied health provider can initiate contact with hospitalized patients and follow up through the outpatient program, lending continuity to the smoking cessation effort.

## Pharmacologic Therapy

Nicotine replacement therapy (NRT) is a valuable adjunct to cessation efforts and should be offered to every patient who is trying to quit. Multiple clinical trials of NRT have demonstrated double the quit rate, compared to placebo. Even better results are obtained when NRT is combined with behavioral therapy. Most experts recommend using the patch rather than nicotine gum because of greater compliance and ease of use.[13] Treatment for 8 weeks or less is sufficient with the patch, but nicotine gum is often used for 12 weeks or longer. Physicians should caution patients not to smoke while using the patch or gum. There is little research on the use of these products in light smokers (i.e., less than half a pack per day), and a lower starting dose should be considered in such patients. (See Tables 19-3 and 19-4 for prescribing information.) The nicotine nasal spray and nicotine inhaler are additional options, but they are available by prescription only. The spray is dosed one to two times per hour for 3 months; it is the most rapid method of nicotine delivery. The inhaler,

TABLE 19-3.   Prescribing Information for Nicotine Patch

| Brand | Duration of Step, weeks | Dose, mg/h |
|---|---|---|
| Nicoderm and Habitrol | 4 | 21/24 |
| | 2 | 14/24 |
| | 2 | 7/24 |
| Prostep | 4 | 22/24 |
| | 4 | 11/24 |
| Nicotrol | 4 | 15/16 |
| | 2 | 10/16 |
| | 2 | 5/16 |

*Source:* The Agency for Health Care Policy and Research Smoking Cessation Clinical Practice Guideline. *JAMA* 1996; 275:1270–1280.

a plastic rod with a nicotine plug, bears some resemblance to cigarettes. It delivers its medication locally to the buccal mucosa, with pharmacokinetics similar to that of nicotine gum.[17]

Potential side effects of the patch are a local, self-limited skin reaction in up to 50 percent of patients; this can usually be helped by rotating the patch location daily or by topical application of 5% hydrocortisone or 0.5% triamcinolone cream. Nicotine gum commonly causes mouth soreness, dyspepsia, hiccups, and jaw ache. Most patients using the nasal spray experience irritation in the nose and throat, accompanied by rhinorrhea and watery eyes. The nicotine inhaler may cause a mild cough.

There is little definitive data regarding the safety of NRT in patients with *stable* coronary disease or arrhythmias. A large observational study with over 5000 patients and three smaller experimental trials did not show any increased risk of acute coronary events in patients receiving NRT. One explanation is that nicotine levels are no higher with NRT than with cigarette smoking. Furthermore, the deleterious

TABLE 19-4.   Prescribing Information for Nicotine Gum

- Chew until a peppery taste emerges, then place between cheek and gums for better absorption
- Intermittently chew and hold for about 30 min
- For better absorption, avoid eating and drinking anything except water for 15 min before and during chewing
- Chewing gum on a fixed schedule of at least 1 piece every 1 to 2 h may be better than prn use, as many patients do not use enough gum to get the maximum benefit

*Source:* Adapted from The Agency for Health Care Policy and Research Smoking Cessation Clinical Practice Guideline. *JAMA* 1996; 275:1270–1280, with permission.

effects of smoking seem to be mediated largely by a hemodynamic milieu (i.e., hypercoagulability, increased myocardial demand, and carbon monoxide–mediated hypoxemia), which is not found in patients receiving NRT. For these reasons, NRT is considered safe in patients with stable cardiovascular disease, since the risks are greatly outweighed by the potential benefits of smoking cessation.[18] There is less information regarding the safety of NRT in individuals with *unstable* coronary disease. While NRT is not considered to be an independent risk factor for cardiovascular events, it should be used cautiously in this group of patients (i.e., those with myocardial infarction in the past 4 weeks, severe or worsening angina, or serious arrhythmias).[13,18] Pregnant or lactating women should first be encouraged to try quitting without pharmacologic therapy, but nicotine replacement may be used if necessary.[13,19]

The use of bupropion to aid cessation efforts was recently approved by the FDA and has also been found to double the quit rate. The slow-release form, given in a dose of 150 to 300 mg/day over 7 to 12 weeks, may be appropriate for smokers who do not wish to try, or who have failed with NRT.[20] To achieve adequate blood levels, the medication should be started 1 week prior to the quit date. Physicians should be cautious in prescribing bupropion (Wellbutrin) to patients with a seizure disorder, since earlier studies using a higher dose suggested an increased risk of seizures.[17]

## Relapse

Relapse is most common within the first 6 months, particularly in the first 2 to 4 weeks. Rates are higher in patients with a high level of nicotine dependence, psychiatric comorbidity, low levels of motivation to quit, low self-efficacy or self-confidence, environmental risks (i.e., other smokers at home or in the workplace), and high stress level. Postpartum females and younger individuals are also vulnerable to relapse.[13]

Ideally, relapse prevention strategies should be used with every smoker who quits. Follow-up in the office within 1 to 2 weeks is best, but telephone calls and letters are alternative methods of delivering formal congratulations and encouragement. Although physicians are the best individuals to perform the follow-up telephone contact, programs which use allied health providers or nursing staff have been successful as well. A second follow-up appointment in 1 to 2 months provides an opportunity for physicians to review with their patients the health benefits of quitting, progress of withdrawal symptoms, stressors threatening the success of the effort, and ways to deal with those factors. Difficulties such as weight gain, depression, prolonged withdrawal symptoms, or lack of support may require additional intervention. Weight gain usually totals less than 10 lb and is more common in females, African Americans, heavy smokers, and smokers under age 55. Patients must be clearly counseled that the benefits of smoking cessation greatly outweigh the risks associated with weight gain. Although there are no proven strategies for preventing weight gain in ex-smokers, nicotine replacement (particularly the gum) can delay postcessation weight gain.[12,13]

**TABLE 19-5.**   Resources for Primary Care Physicians and Patients

| Organization | Phone Number | E-mail | Web Site |
|---|---|---|---|
| American Academy of Family Physicians | 816-333-9700 | fp@aafp.org | www.aafp.org |
| American Cancer Society | 1-800-ACS-2345 | (via Web site) | www.cancer.org |
| American Lung Association | 1-800-LUNG-USA | (via Web site) | www.lungusa.com |
| Centers for Disease Control and Prevention | 404-639-3311 | (via Web site) | www.cdc.gov |
| Doctors Ought to Care | 713-528-1487 | | www.bcm.tmc.edu/doc |
| DOC Washington chapter | 206-326-2894 | washdoc@wln.com | www.kickbutt.org |
| National Cancer Institute | 1-800-4-CANCER | (via Web site) | www.nci.nih.gov |

# RESOURCES FOR THE PRIMARY CARE PHYSICIAN

Some patients may benefit from referral to tobacco cessation specialists, who generally have more structured resources than the average primary care physician, allowing them to utilize a multidisciplinary approach to smoking cessation, with close follow-up of patients. In addition, a number of national organizations offer helpful materials for both patients and physicians (Table 19-5). Additional materials are available from the American Academy of Family Physicians, American Cancer Society, Doctors Ought to Care (DOC), National Cancer Institute, American Lung Association, Centers for Disease Control and Prevention, and numerous other organizations.

## REFERENCES

1. Centers for Disease Control and Prevention: State-specific prevalence among adults of current cigarette smoking and smokeless tobacco use and per capita tax-paid sales of cigarettes—United States, 1997. *MMWR* 1998; 47:922–926.
2. Frank E: Benefits of stopping smoking. *West J Med* 1993; 159:83–87.
3. Herdman R, Hewitt M, Laschober M: Smoking-related deaths and financial costs: Office of Technology Assessment estimates for 1990. Congress of the United States, Office of Technology Assessment, 1993.
4. Taylor AE, Johnson DC, Kazemi H: Environmental tobacco smoke and cardiovascular disease: a position paper from the Council on Cardiopulmonary and Critical Care, American Heart Association. *Circulation* 1992; 86:699–702.
5. Glantz SA, Parmley WW: Passive smoking and heart disease: mechanisms and risk. *JAMA* 1995; 273:1047–1053.

6. Rigotti NA, Pasternak RC: Cigarette smoking and coronary heart disease: risks and management. *Cardiol Clin* 1996; 14:51–68.
7. U.S. Department of Health and Human Services: The health benefits of smoking cessation: a report of the Surgeon General. Atlanta, GA, U.S. Department of Health and Human Services, Public Health Service, Centers for Disease Control and Prevention, Center for Chronic Disease Prevention and Health Promotion, Office on Smoking and Health, 1990. DHHS publication CDC 90–8416.
8. Robinson MD, Laurent SL, Little JM Jr: Including smoking status as a new vital sign: it works! *J Fam Pract* 1995; 40:556–561.
9. Centers for Disease Control and Prevention: Physician and other health-care professional counseling of smokers to quit—United States, 1991. *MMWR* 1993; 42:854–857.
10. Cromwell J, Bartosch WJ, Fiore MC, et al: Cost-effectiveness of the clinical practice recommendations in the AHCPR guideline for smoking cessation. Agency for Health Care Policy and Research. *JAMA* 1997; 278:1759–1766.
11. Coultas DB: The physician's role in smoking cessation. *Clin Chest Med* 1991; 12:755–768.
12. Glynn TJ, Manley MW: How to help your patients stop smoking: a National Cancer Institute manual for physicians. Bethesda, MD, U.S. Department of Health and Human Services, Public Health Service, National Institutes of Health, National Cancer Institute, 1990. NIH publication 90-3064.
13. The Agency for Health Care Policy and Research Smoking Cessation Clinical Practice Guideline. *JAMA* 1996; 275:1270–1280.
14. Fiore MC, Wetter DW, Bailey WC, et al: Smoking cessation. Clinical Practice Guideline No 18. Rockville, MD, U.S. Department of Health and Human Services, Public Health Service, Agency for Health Care Policy and Research, 1996. AHCPR Publication No. 96-0692.
15. Prochaska JO, Goldstein MG: Process of smoking cessation: implications for clinicians. *Clin Chest Med* 1991; 12:727–735.
16. Taylor CB, Houston-Miller N, Killen JD: Smoking cessation after acute myocardial infarction: effects of a nurse managed intervention. *Ann Intern Med* 1990; 113:118–123.
17. Hughes JR, Goldstein MG, Hurt RD, Shiffman S: Recent advances in the pharmacotherapy of smoking. *JAMA* 1999; 281:72–76.
18. Benowitz NL, Gourlay SG: Cardiovascular toxicity of nicotine: implications for nicotine replacement therapy. *J Am Coll Cardiol* 1997; 29:1422–1431.
19. Benowitz NL: Nicotine replacement therapy during pregnancy. *JAMA* 1991; 266:3174–3177.
20. Hurt RD, Sachs DPL, Glover ED, et al: A comparison of sustained-release bupropion and placebo for smoking cessation. *N Engl J Med* 1997; 337:1195–1202.

GERALD FLETCHER

CHAPTER

# 20

# EXERCISE PROGRAMS AND POSTMYOCARDIAL INFARCTION REHABILITATION THERAPY

Exercise has become an important component of management in most subjects with cardiovascular disease. Exercise activities may take place in group supervised programs or in medically directed home programs with appropriate health professional guidance and follow-up.

Substantial data exist supporting the benefits of physical activity in both the primary and secondary prevention of cardiovascular disease. These data are well documented in existing position statements of the American Heart Association,[1,2] the current Surgeon General's report,[3] and population studies.[4–8] The following discussion will delineate basic fundamentals for the implementation of physical activity programs in both primary and secondary prevention of cardiovascular disease.

## PRIMARY PREVENTION

Physical activity in primary cardiovascular prevention should begin in early school years and continue throughout life. Schools must specifically designate physical education programs to provide and teach aerobic activities for children at early ages. Programs should include recreational sports such as running, dancing, or swimming and also selected types of resistance exercises using free weights and/or certain machines. In addition, there should be support for an active lifestyle for children at home.

In the "patient visit" setting, physicians and their staff should discuss physical activity and specify exercise prescriptions for patients and their families, especially children. In certain instances, suggestions should be made with regard to configuration of work sites in order to implement physical activity recommendations.

Intensity, duration, and frequency, as well as mode and progression, should be considered in all types of physical activity programs. As children and adolescents become adults and are no longer engaged in the athletic endeavors found in elementary school, high school, and college, primary prevention must involve a plan for appropriate physical activity throughout one's lifetime. Ideally, this activity should be done for at least 30 to 60 min four to six times weekly[1] or 30 min on most days of the week.[3] The frequency, duration, and intensity of the activity, along with mode and progression, should be individualized, taking in consideration the subject's convenience and satisfaction. Subjects may employ individual end points of exercise intensity such as breathlessness and/or a fatigue level considered *somewhat hard* to *hard* based on the Borg perceived exertion scale.[9] Heart rates that are designated by standardized charts may be helpful in determining heart rate end points that can be measured immediately after exercise.[10] Exercises should include aerobic activities such as bicycling (stationary or routine), walking-jogging protocols, swimming, and other active recreational-leisure sports. Proper shoes and clothing should be worn, with clothing appropriately adjusted for extremes of heat, cold, and humidity.

Resistance exercises using free weights or standard machines should be done two to three times weekly. These should include 8 to 10 different exercise sets with 10 to 15 repetitions per set (arms, shoulders, chest, trunk, back, hips, legs), performed at a moderate intensity. If one uses free weights, 15 to 30 lb is adequate. Resistance exercises tend to supplement aerobic exercise in that some training effect is realized. However, development of muscle tone is more important, and strengthening of body musculature is important as adults age.[1]

The long-term effect of any physical activity program is affected by compliance. In today's mobile society, one must make plans for business trips and vacations. Such settings may not have convenient exercise facilities, and in such instances one must "improvise." For example, if one is a "walker-jogger," it is important to have walking or running shoes available and find a safe place to walk or run in order to maintain one's activity level. Most hotels or motels have some type of exercise facility with track or treadmill, exercise cycle, and weights. These can be utilized and one's routine adapted to them so that one can maintain an exercise program while traveling or otherwise away from a normal schedule.

Physical activity should be measured in terms of total time or kilocalories per week and may be scheduled in various ways, such as 10 to 15 min in the morning, a similar noontime period, and/or an afternoon-evening session. Many subjects may schedule longer and less frequent periods of exercise. As intensity decreases, frequency and duration should increase, and vice versa (Fig. 20-1). The "dosage," or total calorie expenditure per week, must be individualized for each subject.

When illnesses such as influenza syndromes or respiratory conditions occur, exercise should be decreased or discontinued for a period of time until the illness has resolved. If the period of time exceeds more than 2 to 3 weeks, the individual should resume activity at a lower level to compensate for the slight loss of training effect.

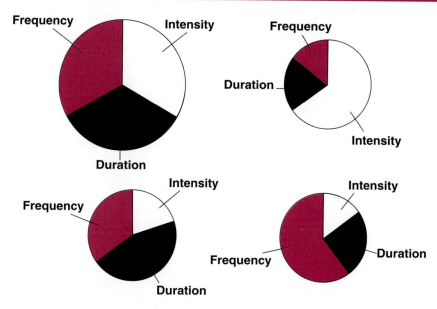

**FIGURE 20-1**   Graphic display of four different combinations of intensity, duration, and frequency of exercise that can be utilized in exercise prescriptions.

Various types of exercise testing that measure functional capacity are of interest but are not necessary in subjects for primary prevention. Many athletically inclined individuals desire to have oxygen consumption measurements done periodically to assess level of training, but this is not routinely recommended. However, exercise testing should be done in those who are considered at high risk for cardiovascular disease (for example, those with hypertension or abnormal blood lipids).

A lifestyle including physical activity from childhood throughout the adult years fosters health and longevity.[1] This improved state of health is enhanced by weight control, restricted saturated fat and cholesterol intake, abstention from cigarette smoking, and control of high blood pressure and glucose intolerance.

# SECONDARY PREVENTION[2]*

## Early Activity

The emphasis of exercise within the first 2 weeks after myocardial infarction or coronary bypass surgery should be to offset the effects of bed rest or former periods of inactivity. When the individual is stable, as measured by symptomatic standards, echocardiogram (ECG), and vital signs, he or she should begin to increase the

---

* (After established coronary artery disease, i.e., myocardial infarction, coronary bypass surgery, or angioplasty with or without stent.)

activity program. Although this activity is well tolerated and safe, certain precautions are recommended, such as awareness of chest discomfort, faintness, and dyspnea.

Walking is the recommended mode of activity unless the individual can attend supervised classes in which other activities can be provided. Table 20-1 details the types of activities utilized in supervised classes. Walking should at first be limited and continue slowly, with a gradual increase until 5 to 10 min of continuous movement has been achieved. Active but nonresistance range of motion exercises of the upper extremities are also well tolerated early as long as they do not stress or impair healing of the sternal incision after coronary bypass surgery.

Initial activities should be supervised, with symptoms, rating of perceived exertion, heart rate, and blood pressure recorded. When safety and tolerance have been documented, the activity can be performed without supervision.

## Late Activity[2]

A symptom-limited exercise test is often performed after the individual is stable (as early as 2 to 6 weeks after the coronary event). Such testing is desirable in all subjects in secondary prevention prior to their beginning a physical activity program. If more studies, such as echocardiography or angiography, are not indicated, a regular conditioning program can be initiated, with a careful prescription of activity based on results of the exercise test.

For conditioning purposes, large-muscle group activities should be performed for at least 20 min (preceded by warm-up and followed by cooldown) at least three to four times weekly. Initially, supervised group sessions are often recommended to enhance the exercise educational process, ensure that the participant is tolerating the program, confirm that progress is occurring, and provide medical supervision in

**TABLE 20-1.**   Types of Physical Activities Utilized in Supervised Classes of Cardiac Rehabilitation

Warm-up and cooldown (stretching, walking)

Aerobic—dynamic
    Walking, treadmill, stationary bicycle (leg, arm/leg)
    Rower
    Stairclimber
    Water aerobics

Resistance
    Arm ergometry
    Free weights
    "Machine" activities

Team
    Volleyball (court and pool)
    Ping-Pong

high-risk situations.[2] Home programs without supervision can be utilized by low-risk individuals who are motivated and who understand the basic principles of exercise training.

## General Principles of Exercise Prescription in Secondary Prevention

**PRESCRIPTION IN THE ABSENCE OF ISCHEMIA OR SIGNIFICANT AR-RHYTHMIAS (LOW RISK).[2]**   Exercise intensity should approximate 50 to 80 percent of maximal oxygen consumption ($V_{O2max}$), as determined by an exercise test. If a test is not done initially, a target of 20 beats per minute above resting heart rate is adequate until testing is performed.

The exercise training heart rate should be designated as 50 to 75 percent of heart rate reserve [(maximal heart rate − resting heart rate) × 50 to 75%] plus resting heart rate. Activities should be prescribed to provide the work intensity that achieves the training heart rate after 5 to 10 min at the same workload (steady state). This may be expressed as watts on an ergometer, speed on a treadmill, or metabolic equivalents (one metabolic equivalent equals 3.5 mL/kg/min of oxygen consumed). When an individual cannot assess exercise intensity, heart rate counting (manually or with a cardiotachometer) becomes especially useful. Heart rate counters are widely available and are generally accurate for low- to moderate-intensity exercise.

If an individual intends to walk on a level surface, the step rate needed to generate the desirable heart rate, found on a treadmill, can be prescribed. The step rate is the number of steps taken in 15 s while walking at the desired speed on the treadmill. Step rate can be easily counted, as it requires less skill than counting heart rate. If this approach is used, individuals should be cautioned to avoid hills. Walking in shopping malls or gymnasiums allows subjects to avoid inclement weather and utilize a flat surface. Exercise should ideally be supervised for the first few sessions to ensure that the instructions are understood and the activity is well tolerated.[2]

Individuals can also quite accurately judge the intensity of exercise through the rating of perceived exertion, which can be equated to desirable heart rate and to their activities during laboratory exercise. The original scale is a 15-grade category scale ranging from 6 to 20, with a verbal description at every odd number beginning at 7, or very, very light, and progressing to 19, or very, very hard.

The following rating of perceived exertion values should be followed: <12, perceived as fairly light (light intensity), 40 to 60 percent of maximal heart rate; 12 to 13, perceived as somewhat hard (moderate intensity), 60 to 75 percent of maximal heart rate; 14 to 16, perceived as hard (high intensity), 75 to 90 percent of maximal heart rate.

Activities can progress as tolerance is demonstrated. An appropriate initial intensity of training is 60 to 75 percent of maximal heart rate (moderate) or a rating of perceived exertion of 12 to 13. However, many individuals may need to begin at

40 to 60 percent of maximal heart rate (light). After safe activity levels have been established, duration is increased by a 5-min increment each week. Later, as a training effect develops and heart rate response to exercise decreases with conditioning, intensities can be increased with a frequency of 3 to 6 times weekly. At this point, limited resistance exercises can be added, as described previously. These have been proved both safe and effective in secondary prevention.[2]

## PRESCRIPTION FOR EXERCISE IN THE PRESENCE OF ISCHEMIA OR SIGNIFICANT ARRHYTHMIAS (MODERATELY HIGH RISK).[2]

An *exercise test* and *medical supervision*[2] *are essential* for this type of prescription. The manifestations of arrhythmias or ischemia that require such precautions can vary but usually include ventricular tachycardia (3 to 4 beats or less), any arrhythmia that is symptomatic or causes hemodynamic instability, anginal chest discomfort, ECG ST depression of 2 mm or more, or a fall in exercise systolic blood pressure of 20 mmHg or more from baseline.

Exercise testing is performed in the usual fashion, but the conditioning (training) work intensity is derived from the *heart rate associated with the abnormality*. If the exercise test continues to a high level of effort, the heart rate at 50 to 60 percent of heart rate maximum can be used if it falls at least 10 beats per minute below the abnormal level. Otherwise, the recommended peak training heart rate is 10 beats per minute *less than that associated with the abnormality*. It is desirable that these individuals have medically supervised cardiac rehabilitation and reevaluation, with the hope that they can be reclassified as a lower risk.[2] Exercise testing should be repeated at least yearly.

As the population ages and more elderly subjects survive coronary events, there will be increasing numbers who will need appropriate physical activity. Most of these subjects will benefit initially from supervised exercise for a brief period of time. This is primarily to introduce the subject to exercise (which he or she may not have done before) and to have the subject evaluated for possible complications of exercise, such as arrhythmias, evidence of heart failure, anginal chest pain, or abnormal ECG ST segments. Based on this, the subject can be categorized as low risk or moderate to high risk and appropriate cardiac rehabilitation precautions utilized.[2]

Most subjects in secondary prevention can soon be reclassified as low risk and have an exercise prescription that can be implemented at home or in a community program. In this setting, the previously mentioned primary prevention guidelines apply as well. The intensity may be much less and the frequency may be greater, with appropriate changes in duration. Exercise testing is recommended at least yearly, and the modification of other coronary risk factors should be aggressive.[11] This aggressive risk modification applies specifically to smoking cessation and blood pressure and blood lipid control, but also to the other factors designated in Table 20-2.

In summary, in designing physical activity program strategies for both primary and secondary prevention, physicians should consider the "dosing effect," or kilo-

TABLE 20-2.    Guidelines for Aggressive Risk Factor Modification

| Risk Intervention | Recommendation |
| --- | --- |
| Smoking | Goal: Complete cessation.<br>Strongly encourage patient and family to stop smoking.<br>Provide counseling, nicotine replacement, and formal cessation programs as appropriate. |
| Lipid management | Primary goal: LDL<100 mg/dL.<br>Secondary goal: HDL >35 mg/dL; TG <200 mg/dL.<br>Start AHA Step II diet in all patients: ≤30% fat, <7% saturated fat, <200 mg/day cholesterol.<br>Assess fasting lipid profile. (In postmyocardial infarction patients, lipid profile may take 4 to 6 weeks to stabilize.) Add drug therapy according to accepted guidelines. |
| Weight management | Start intensive diet and appropriate physical activity, as outlined above, in patients >120% of ideal weight for height.<br>Particularly emphasize need for weight loss in patients with hypertension, elevated triglycerides, or elevated glucose levels. |
| Antiplatelet agents | Start aspirin 81 to 325 mg/day if not contraindicated. |
| Blood pressure control | Goal: ≤140/90 mmHg.<br>Initiate lifestyle modification—weight control, physical activity, alcohol moderation, and moderate sodium restriction—in all patients with blood pressure >140 mmHg systolic or 90 mmHg diastolic.<br>Add blood pressure medication, individualized to other patient requirements and characteristics (i.e., age, race, need for drugs with specific benefits) if blood pressure is not less than 140 mmHg systolic or 90 mmHg diastolic in 3 months or if *initial* blood pressure is >160 mmHg systolic or 100 mmHg diastolic. |

LDL = low-density lipoproteins; HDL = high-density lipoproteins; TG = triglycerides; AHA = American Heart Association.

*Source:* Information used to construct table is from Smith SC Jr, Blair SN, Criqui MH, et al: Preventing heart attack and death in patients with coronary disease. *Circulation* 1995; 92:2–4.

calorie expenditure over a unit of time, usually a week (Fig. 20-2). The program should, if possible, entail 5 to 6 h weekly of various physical activities. The exercise routine must be individualized for each subject and should include both aerobic and resistance exercises. As noted previously, the benefits of exercise have been well established in population studies and studies of secondary prevention.[4–8] These benefits will be enhanced with good to excellent compliance with exercise and appropriate lifestyle modifications.

FIGURE 20-2   Graphic display of the fundamentals of kilocalo-
rie expenditure by altering intensity, duration, and frequency
of exercise. (Reproduced with permission from Miller TD,
Balady GJ, Fletcher GF: Exercise and its role in the prevention
and rehabilitation of cardiovascular disease. *Ann Behav Med*
1997; 19:225.)

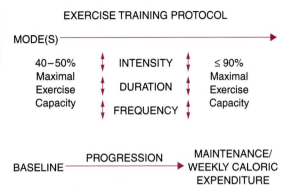

## REFERENCES

1. Fletcher GF, Balady G, Blair SN, et al: Statement on exercise. Benefits and recommendations for physical activity programs for all Americans. A statement for health professionals by the Committee on Exercise and Cardiac Rehabilitation of the Council on
   Clinical Cardiology, American Heart Association. *Circulation* 1996; 94:857–862.
2. Fletcher GF, Balady G, Froelicher VF, et al: Exercise standards. A statement for healthcare professionals from the American Heart Association Writing Group. *Circulation*
   1995; 91:580–615.
3. U.S. Department of Health and Human Services: *Physical Activity and Health: A Report
   of the Surgeon General.* Atlanta, GA: U.S. Department of Health and Human Services,
   Centers for Disease Control and Prevention, National Center for Chronic Disease Prevention and Health Promotion, The President's Council on Physical Fitness and Sports,
   1996.
4. Morris JN, Clayton DG, Everitt MG, et al: Exercise in leisure time: Coronary attack and
   death rates. *Br Heart J* 1990; 63:325–334.
5. Blair SN, Kohl HW III, Paffenbarger RS Jr, et al: Physical fitness and all-cause mortality. A prospective study of healthy men and women. *JAMA* 1989; 262:2395–2401.
6. Blair SN, Kohl HW III, Barlow CE, et al: Changes in physical fitness and all-cause mortality. A prospective study of healthy and unhealthy men. *JAMA* 1995; 273:1093–1098.
7. Lee IM, Hsieh CC, Paffenbarger RS Jr: Exercise intensity and longevity in men. The
   Harvard Alumni Health Study. *JAMA* 1995; 273:1179–1184.
8. O'Connor GT, Buring JE, Yusuf S, et al: An overview of randomized trials of rehabilitation with exercise after myocardial infarction. *Circulation* 1989; 80:234–244.
9. Borg GA: Psychophysical bases of perceived exertion. *Med Sci Sports Exerc* 1982;
   14:377–381.
10. Sheffield LT, Ratman D, Reeves TJ: Hemodynamic consequences of physical training af-
    ter myocardial infarction. *Circulation* 1968; 37:192–202.
11. Smith SC Jr, Blair SN, Criqui MH, et al: Preventing heart attack and death in patients
    with coronary disease. *Circulation* 1995; 92:2–4.

THOMAS M. GUEST /
W. ROBERT TAYLOR

# CORONARY ATHEROSCLEROSIS— EFFECTS OF ASPIRIN, OXIDATIVE STRESS, ALCOHOL, AND PSYCHOLOGICAL FACTORS

The development of atherosclerotic cardiovascular disease (ASCVD) is a multifactorial process. There is a vast literature that defines the major cardiovascular risk factors, such as hypertension, lipid disorders, tobacco use, and diabetes. This chapter explores the roles of oxidative stress, alcohol, and psychological factors in the development of coronary atherosclerosis. The role of aspirin in the primary and secondary prevention of coronary atherosclerosis also is examined. Continuing research on less well-described risk factors may help to elucidate primary mechanisms of atherogenesis.

## ASPIRIN AND CORONARY ARTERY DISEASE

### Coronary Artery Thrombosis

Platelets are circulating, membrane-bound fragments of megakaryocytes. They are known to be important in the pathogenesis of atherosclerosis, as well as in the pathophysiology of acute coronary events. Following endothelial injury, exposure of subendothelial collagen and microfibrils stimulates platelet adhesion and aggregation. Activation of the intrinsic and extrinsic pathways of coagulation leads to thrombin generation, fibrin deposition, and thrombus growth. Thrombus formation contributes to the development of ASCVD via release of a number of vascular mitogens. In the acute settings of unstable angina and myocardial infarction (MI), coronary artery thrombosis on a disrupted plaque results in a sudden and severe decrease in distal blood flow. Aspirin, as a platelet cyclooxygenase inhibitor, acts to reduce the initial adherence of platelets to the disrupted endothelium, as well as blunting platelet activation and the subsequent generation of thrombin. As understanding of the importance of thrombosis in coronary artery disease increased, a number of studies evaluating the utility of aspirin in acute coronary syndromes and in the primary and secondary prevention of ASCVD have been completed (see Table 21-1).

## Primary Prevention

Aspirin as a means of primary prevention of ASCVD was prospectively evaluated in the Physicians' Health Study.[1] In this study of more than 22,000 male physicians followed for an average of 5 years, aspirin prophylaxis decreased the risk of MI by 44 percent, although there was no overall cardiovascular mortality benefit. A slightly increased, but not statistically significant, risk of hemorrhagic stroke was seen among those subjects taking aspirin. Further analyses revealed that although the reduction in the risk of MI was present at all cholesterol levels, the beneficial effect was limited to those subjects 50 years of age and older. These data are in contrast with those from a much smaller study of British physicians, which did not show a benefit of aspirin prophylaxis (500 mg per day), although the number of events was low, resulting in wide confidence intervals.[2] Of concern in this study is the significant increase in the incidence of disabling stroke. To date, there are no randomized primary prevention trials that include significant numbers of women, although three prospective cohort studies with conflicting results have been published.[3–5]

The U.S. Preventive Services Task Force currently recommends low-dose aspirin on alternate days for men over age 50 for the primary prevention of MI. Official recommendations for aspirin use in women are likely to await completion of randomized trials; thus at this point individual guidance for women at high risk for ASCVD must be given on a case-by-case basis. The American Heart Association and American College of Cardiology have yet to issue practice guidelines for aspirin use in the primary prevention of ASCVD.

## Secondary Prevention

A number of medium-sized, prospective secondary prevention trials have studied the long-term use of aspirin following MI. Individually, these trials have not provided convincing data to suggest a benefit or lack of benefit of aspirin use, but a meta-analysis of the available studies that combines over 18,000 patients provides

**TABLE 21-1.   Selected Prospective and Randomized Studies of the Relationship between Aspirin and CAD**

| Study | Study Population | Findings |
|---|---|---|
| **Primary Prevention** | | |
| Hammond and Garfinkel[3] | >1,000,000 men and women | No CAD risk reduction in men or women |
| Manson, Stampfer, Colditz, et al[5] | 87,678 female nurses | 32% reduction in risk of first MI with use of one to six aspirin per week |
| Physicians' Health Study[*1] | 22,071 U.S. male physicians | 44% reduction in risk of first MI with use of aspirin every other day |
| Peto, Gray, Collins, et al[*2] | 5139 British male physicians | No CAD risk reduction |
| **Secondary Prevention** | | |
| Antiplatelet Trialists' Collaboration[6] | >18,000 men and women with prior MI (meta-analysis) | 31% reduction in risk of nonfatal MI, 13% decrease in vascular mortality |
| **Unstable Coronary Syndromes** | | |
| VA Cooperative Study[*8] | 1266 U.S. military veterans with unstable angina | 51% reduction in death or MI |
| Canadian Multicenter Trial[*9] | 555 Canadian patients with unstable angina | 56% reduction in nonfatal MI, 30% decrease in cardiac death |
| Theroux, Ouimet, McCains, et al[*10] | 479 patients with unstable angina | 25% reduction in MI |
| ISIS-2[*11] | 17,187 patients with suspected acute MI | 50% reduction in reinfarction, 23% decrease in vascular death |

CAD = coronary artery disease; MI = myocardial infarction; ISIS-2 = Second International Study of Infarct Survival.
[*] Denotes randomized study.

clinical guidance.[6] This study demonstrated that antiplatelet therapy (some of the included studies used dipyridamole or sulfinpyrazone in addition to aspirin) decreased the risk of nonfatal MI by 31 percent, strokes by 42 percent, and vascular mortality by 13 percent in patients with prior MI.

The American Heart Association and American College of Cardiology have recommended that all patients presenting with MI be given aspirin, 160 to 325 mg per day, with the initial dose given in the emergency room and daily administration continued indefinitely.[7] The data regarding long-term use of other antiplatelet agents post-MI are not yet convincing.

## Unstable Coronary Syndromes

The data regarding aspirin therapy in the face of unstable angina or acute myocardial infarction (AMI) provide the strongest indication for aspirin use in coronary artery disease. In the face of unstable angina, prompt aspirin therapy will decrease the incidence of in-hospital infarction from 12 to 3 percent.[8] The magnitude of the change is roughly equivalent to that seen with intravenous heparin therapy. In this situation, continuation of aspirin therapy as an outpatient will decrease the risk of MI and sudden cardiac death by 50 percent.[9,10] In the Second International Study of Infarct Survival (ISIS-2), aspirin therapy (160 mg per day) started within 24 h of hospital admission and continued for 1 month was shown to decrease the risk of vascular death at 5 weeks by 23 percent and the risk of reinfarction by 50 percent.[11]

The American Heart Association and American College of Cardiology jointly recommend the use of aspirin, 160 to 325 mg per day, for patients presenting with unstable angina or MI. The initial dose should be given in the emergency department and daily administration continued indefinitely.[7] It is important to note that patients requiring warfarin therapy for cardiovascular or neurologic disease still benefit from specific antiplatelet therapy. In this situation, the common practice is to continue warfarin therapy and treat with aspirin at 81 mg per day.

# ANTIOXIDANTS AND CORONARY ARTERY DISEASE

## The Oxidative-Modification Hypothesis of Atherosclerosis

There is a growing body of in vitro and in vivo data suggesting that free-radical formation can result in cellular damage. Oxygen free-radicals are produced by many oxidative reactions in the body and have been implicated in a number of chronic disease processes, including ASCVD. The oxidative-modification hypothesis of atherosclerosis postulates that modification of low-density lipoprotein (LDL) cholesterol by oxygen free-radicals, also termed lipid peroxidation, is a central feature in the development of ASCVD. Minimally modified LDL cholesterol is known to accumulate in the extracellular subendothelial space, where it participates in the recruitment of monocytes to the arterial wall. Once within the arterial wall, monocytes differentiate to macrophages and ultimately form lipid-laden foam cells as they internalize completely oxidized LDL particles. Oxidized LDL cholesterol and reactive oxygen species produced within the vessel wall also have direct cytotoxic effects on endothelial and vascular smooth muscle cells. The cellular injury enhances further infiltration of LDL cholesterol into the arterial wall, production of chemotactic factors, and numerous growth factors that promote cell proliferation and the secretion of extracellular matrix. In sum, alterations in vascular oxidative stress promote vascular alterations characteristic of ASCVD. In response to this growing body of data implicating oxidative stress in the development of ASCVD, investigators have begun to explore the clinical role of free-radical scavengers in the prevention of ASCVD.

## Micronutrient Antioxidants

**VITAMIN E.**   Vitamin E comprises a group of similar compounds that share the biologic activity of $\alpha$-tocopherol. These compounds are chain-breaking antioxidants, capable of scavenging oxygen radicals and terminating free-radical chain reactions. Although 80 to 90 percent of the body's vitamin E stores are within adipose tissue, most of the circulating fraction is in direct association with LDL particles. In Western diets, vegetable oils are the primary source of vitamin E, with olive, canola, safflower, and sunflower oils probably having the greatest antioxidant properties. Fruits and vegetables, cereals, peanut butter, eggs, and nuts represent other sources of vitamin E. The recommended daily allowance of vitamin E is 15 IU for men. The gastrointestinal absorption is 20 to 40 percent and can be enhanced by dietary fats. The rate of absorption decreases with supplementation.

**CAROTENOIDS.**   Carotenoids are a group of pigments found in plants and microorganisms, but not synthesized in eukaryotic cells. These pigments can directly scavenge free radicals. Most of the circulating carotenoids are in association with lipoproteins. A number of the carotenoids can be metabolized to retinol and function as vitamin A precursors. Interestingly, though, once they are converted to vitamin A, very little antioxidant activity remains. Fruits and vegetables are the primary source of carotenoids in Western diets. The gastrointestinal absorption is 10 to 30 percent; like that of vitamin E, it decreases with supplementation and is enhanced by dietary fats. Dietary fiber inhibits carotenoid absorption.

**VITAMIN C.**   Vitamin C, or ascorbic acid, is capable of scavenging superoxide and hydroxyl radicals and acts as a chain-breaking antioxidant in lipid peroxidations. A number of investigators also postulate that vitamin C has an indirect antioxidant effect via its ability to regenerate the active form of membrane-bound vitamin E after it has scavenged a free radical. This raises the possibility that vitamins E and C function synergistically in vivo. The main dietary source of vitamin C is fruits and vegetables, particularly citrus fruits, green vegetables, peppers, tomatoes, berries, and potatoes. Gastrointestinal absorption is 70 to 90 percent, but falls appreciably with supplementation. Osmotic diarrhea and gastrointestinal discomfort with supplementation are most commonly due to unabsorbed vitamin C and can be avoided by spacing smaller doses throughout the day.

## Clinical Studies

A number of epidemiologic studies have suggested a cardiovascular benefit from antioxidant supplementation. Early cross-sectional and case-control studies suggested that dietary micronutrient antioxidants were protective for angina pectoris, angiographically evident CAD, and cardiovascular mortality.[12–15] More recent prospective and randomized trials have attempted to confirm the relationship (see Table 21-2).

The prospective cohort studies include the Nurses' Health Study[16] and the Health Professionals' Follow-up Study (HPFS),[17] which demonstrate a 34 to 41 percent decline in the incidence of nonfatal MI and cardiovascular mortality in

**TABLE 21-2.   Selected Prospective and Randomized Studies of the Relationship between Antioxidants and CAD**

| Study | Study Population | Findings |
|---|---|---|
| **Vitamin E** | | |
| HPFS[17] | 39,910 U.S. male health professionals without known CAD | 36 to 37% reduction in the risk of developing CAD |
| Nurses' Health Study[16] | 87,245 U.S. female nurses without known CAD | 34 to 41% reduction in the risk of developing CAD |
| CHAOS[*19] | 2002 British men and women with angiographic CAD | 77% reduction in nonfatal MI, no overall benefit in cardiovascular mortality |
| ATBC[*20] | 1862 Finnish male smokers with previous myocardial infarction | 38% reduction in nonfatal MI, no overall benefit in cardiovascular mortality |
| **Carotenoids** | | |
| HPFS[17] | 39,910 U.S. male health professionals without known CAD | 40 to 70% decrease in risk of CAD for smokers only |
| Physicians' Health Study[*1] | 22,071 U.S. male physicians | No association with risk of CAD |
| ATBC[*20] | 1862 Finnish male smokers with previous MI | 58 to 75% increase in cardiovascular mortality |
| **Vitamin C** | | |
| HPFS[17] | 39,910 U.S. male health professionals without known CAD | No association with risk of CAD |
| NHANES[18] | 11,348 U.S. men and women | 25 to 42% reduction in cardiovascular mortality |

ATBC = Alpha-Tocopherol, Beta Carotene Cancer Prevention Study; CAD = coronary artery disease; CHAOS = Cambridge Heart Anti-oxidant Study; HPFS = Health Professionals' Follow-up Study; MI = myocardial infarction; NHANES = National Health and Nutritional Examination Survey.

[*] Denotes randomized study.

subjects taking supplemental vitamin E. The greatest benefit was seen in subjects taking 100 to 250 IU per day. Little additional benefit was seen at higher doses of vitamin E, and little benefit was seen in patients during the first 2 years of treatment. The HPFS also showed that carotene intake was associated with a lower risk of coronary disease among current and former smokers, but not among non-smokers. Prospective data regarding vitamin C intake and cardiovascular disease have yielded mixed findings and have not yet been evaluated in a randomized fashion.[17,18]

The Cambridge Heart Antioxidant Study (CHAOS) evaluated high-dose α-tocopherol (400 or 800 IU daily) in a randomized, double-blind, placebo-controlled study involving more than 2000 patients with angiographically proven CAD.[19] The primary endpoints were cardiovascular death and nonfatal MI. This study demonstrated a 77 percent reduction in nonfatal MI but no statistically significant change in cardiovascular mortality with the use of α-tocopherol supplements. Beneficial effects were seen after as little as 1 year of treatment. CHAOS was followed by the Alpha-Tocopherol, Beta Carotene Cancer Prevention Study (ATBC), which followed almost 2000 Finnish smokers with previous myocardial infarction; it also showed no benefit in fatal ischemic heart disease and a 38 percent reduction in nonfatal myocardial infarction with lower-dose α-tocopherol supplements (50 mg or ~75 IU daily).[20] This project also evaluated β-carotene supplementation (20 mg daily) and revealed a surprising excess of fatal ischemic heart disease in subjects receiving β-carotene alone or in combination with α-tocopherol. The lack of cardiovascular benefit with β-carotene supplementation has been seen in other studies as well.[21]

Selenium and flavonoids are other dietary antioxidants that have not been shown to have a strong relationship to the primary or secondary prevention of ASCVD in cohort or case-control studies. No randomized clinical trials to further evaluate these two micronutrients have been proposed thus far.

## Summary

There is a growing body of data linking antioxidants and a reduction in coronary artery disease events. Generally, the cross-sectional, case-control, and prospective cohort studies have described an inverse relationship between dietary antioxidants and ASCVD, whereas the randomized trials have thus far shown a probable benefit with vitamin E at higher doses (400 to 800 IU daily) but no benefit with β-carotene supplementation. Potential side effects of long-term vitamin E supplementation are unknown, and the potential for increased cardiovascular mortality with supplementation, as suggested in CHAOS and the ATBC study, is concerning. Thus the establishment of clinical practice guidelines awaits the completion of several large ongoing randomized trials, including the Women's Health Study, a continuation of the Physicians' Health Study, the Heart Outcome Prevention Evaluation Study, and the Heart Protection Study in the United Kingdom.

# PROOXIDANTS AND CORONARY ARTERY DISEASE

## Homocysteine

Elevated plasma homocysteine levels appear to be an independent risk factor for ASCVD.[22–24] The mechanism for this is uncertain, but may involve direct lipid peroxidation, arterial smooth muscle cell proliferation, and/or endothelial dysfunction. Homocysteine levels are elevated with nutritional deficiencies of folate and vitamins $B_6$ and $B_{12}$. In the United States, more than 90 percent of adults consume less than 400 mg of folic acid per day. An elevated homocysteine level can be effectively lowered with supplemental folic acid. Caution must be taken, though, as supplemental folic acid may mask the signs and symptoms of a vitamin $B_{12}$ deficiency. To date, no randomized clinical trials have evaluated the effect of folic acid on homocysteine and the development of ASCVD.

## Iron

Iron is known to possess prooxidant properties. In a prospective study involving nearly 2000 Finnish men, a positive association between total iron intake, serum ferritin levels, and risk of MI was described.[25] The observed increase in risk of MI, adjusted for plasma levels of cholesterol but not for other dietary factors, was 5 percent for a 1-mg increase in daily iron intake. In the Health Professionals' Follow-up Study, only intake of heme iron (mainly from red meat) was associated with an increased risk of MI and fatal coronary disease.[26] Additional data are needed to further define the association between iron and cardiovascular disease.

# ALCOHOL AND CORONARY ARTERY DISEASE

Over the past three decades, a considerable body of epidemiologic data has been developed to suggest that low to moderate consumption of alcohol is associated with a decreased incidence of coronary heart disease (CHD) and cardiovascular mortality. These studies have included both men and women, have been carried out in at least 20 countries, and include case-control, prospective cohort, autopsy, and arteriographic studies. The major case-control studies looking at the association of alcohol consumption and CHD have described risk reduction of 30 to 70 percent.[27]

The precise cardioprotective mechanisms are unknown, but probably involve an increase in high-density lipoprotein (HDL) cholesterol subfractions. Additionally, alcohol ingestion confers an antithrombotic effect via an increase in the prostacycline/thromboxane ratio, decreased platelet aggregability, enhanced release of plasminogen activator, and lowered fibrinogen. It has been suggested that red wine is more cardioprotective than other forms of alcohol; this may be due to its unique antioxidant properties, but the analysis is difficult, as red wine drinkers tend to have a better cardiovascular risk profile, are better educated, and smoke less.[27] Based on a large meta-analysis of 30 cohort studies, the cardioprotective effects of alcohol seem to follow an L-shaped saturation curve—thus the full preventive effect can be seen with consumption of as little as one-half drink per day.[28] The cardioprotective effects of alcohol are dependent on delivery in frequent small amounts and are not evident when periods of heavy drinking alternate with periods of abstinence.

Caution must be used in making recommendations to patients regarding the protective effects of alcohol consumption. Alcohol is a drug with an unusually high abuse potential, and excessive use is clearly a preventable cause of morbidity and mortality. Indeed, even within the cardiovascular system, excessive alcohol use is strongly associated with hypertension, arrhythmias, and dilated cardiomyopathy. Alcoholism is a major public health concern and is estimated to afflict 5 to 17 million people in the United States. Thus, in the absence of evidence that encouraging low to moderate alcohol use as a cardiopreventive measure does not increase abuse, discretion must be used in making recommendations to patients.

# PSYCHOLOGICAL FACTORS AND CORONARY ARTERY DISEASE

Epidemiologic research on the development of ASCVD has identified several important psychosocial risk factors. Both the Framingham Study and the Western Collaborative Group Study have described a twofold increase in the risk of coronary heart disease associated with type A personality patterns.[29,30] The type A personality is characterized as highly competitive, ambitious, and in constant struggle with the environment. Recently, the type D personality, in which there is a tendency to suppress emotional distress, has also been proposed as an independent predictor of cardiac mortality.[31]

The mechanisms by which personality may influence the development of ASCVD are not known. It is possible that an imbalance between sympathetic and parasympathetic tone results in acute or chronic increases in blood pressure. It has also been suggested that lipid disorders exist more frequently in persons who perceive themselves to be under stress.

Behavioral counseling with stress management has been advocated as a means of primary and secondary prevention of ASCVD. Although this type of counseling will decrease a patient's reaction to stressful situations, its effect on CAD has not yet been evaluated in a prospective fashion.

REFERENCES

1. Steering Committee of the Physicians' Health Study Group: Final report on the aspirin component of the ongoing Physicians' Health Study. *N Engl J Med* 1989; 321:129–135.

2. Peto R, Gray R, Collins R, et al: Randomised trial of prophylactic daily aspirin in British male doctors. *Br Med J* 1988; 296:313–316.

3. Hammond E, Garfinkel L: Aspirin and coronary heart disease. *Br Med J* 1975; 2:269–271.

4. Paganini-Hill A, Chaos A, Ross R, Henderson B: Aspirin use and chronic diseases. *Br Med J* 1989; 299:1247–1250.

5. Manson J, Stampfer M, Colditz G, et al: A prospective study of aspirin use and primary prevention of cardiovascular disease in women. *JAMA* 1991; 226:521–527.

6. Antiplatelet Trialists' Collaboration: Secondary prevention of vascular disease by prolonged antiplatelet treatment. *Br Med J* 1988; 296:320–331.

7. Ryan TJ, Anderson JL, Antman EM, et al: ACC/AHA guidelines for the management of patients with acute myocardial infarction: a report of the American College of Cardiology/American Heart Association Task Force on Practice Guidelines (Committee on Management of Acute Myocardial Infarction). *J Am Coll Cardiol* 1996; 28:1328–1428.

8. Lewis HD Jr, Davis JW, Archibald DG, et al: Protective effects of aspirin against acute myocardial infarction and death in men with unstable angina: results of a Veterans Administration Cooperative Study. *N Engl J Med* 1983; 309:396–403.

9. Cairns JA, Gent M, Singer J, et al: Aspirin, sulfapyrazine, or both in unstable angina: results of a Canadian Multicenter Trial. *N Engl J Med* 1985; 313:1369–1375.

10. Theroux P, Ouimet H, McCains J, et al: Aspirin, heparin, or both to treat acute unstable angina. *N Engl J Med* 1988; 319:1105–1111.

11. ISIS-2 (2nd International Study of Infarct Survival) Collaborative Group: Randomized trial of streptokinase, oral aspirin, both, or neither among 17,187 cases of suspected acute myocardial infarction: ISIS-2. *Lancet* 1988; 2:349–360.

12. Verlangieri AJ, Kapeghian JC, el-Dean S, Bush M: Fruit and vegetable consumption and cardiovascular disease mortality. *Med Hypotheses* 1985; 16:7–15.

13. Gey KF, Puska P: Plasma vitamins E and A inversely correlated to mortality from ischemic heart disease in cross-cultural epidemiology. *Ann NY Acad Sci* 1989; 570:268–282.

14. Riemersma RA, Wood DA, Macintyre CCH, et al: Risk of angina pectoris and plasma concentrations of vitamins A, C, and E, and carotene. *Lancet* 1991; 337:1–5.

15. Ramirez J, Flowers NC: Leukocyte ascorbic acid and its relationship to coronary heart disease in man. *Am J Nutr* 1980; 33:2079–2087.

16. Stampfer MJ, Hennekens CH, Manson JE, et al: Vitamin E consumption and the risk of coronary disease in women. *N Engl J Med* 1993; 328:1444–1449.

17. Rimm EB, Stampfer MJ, Ascherio A, et al: Vitamin E consumption and the risk of coronary disease in men. *N Engl J Med* 1993; 328:1450–1456.

18. Enstrom JE, Kanim LE, Klein MA: Vitamin C intake and mortality among a sample of the United States population. *Epidemiology* 1992; 3:194–202.

19. Stephens NG, Parsons A, Schofield PM, et al: Randomised controlled trial of vitamin E in patients with coronary disease: Cambridge Heart Antioxidant Study (CHAOS). *Lancet* 1996; 347:781–786.

20. Rapola JM, Virtamo J, Ripatti S, et al: Randomised trial of alpha-tocopherol and beta-carotene supplements on incidence of major coronary events in men with previous myocardial infarction: The Alpha-Tocopherol, Beta Carotene Cancer Prevention Study Group. *Lancet* 1997; 349:1715–1720.

21. Hennekens CH, Buring JE, Manson JE, et al: Lack of effect of long-term supplementation with beta carotene on the incidence of malignant neoplasms and cardiovascular disease. *N Engl J Med* 1996; 334:1145–1149.

22. Bousney CJ, Beresford SAA, Omenn GS, Motulsky AG: A quantitative assessment of plasma homocysteine as a risk factor for vascular disease. *JAMA* 1995; 274:1049–1057.
23. Graham IM, Daly LE, Refsum HM, et al: Plasma homocysteine as a risk factor for vascular disease: The European Concerted Action Project. *JAMA* 1997; 277:1775–1781.
24. Nygard O, Nordrehaug JE, Refsum H, et al: Plasma homocysteine levels and mortality in patients with coronary artery disease. *N Engl J Med* 1997; 337:230–236.
25. Salonen JT, Nyyssonen K, Korpela H, et al: High stored iron levels are associated with excess risk of myocardial infarction in Eastern Finnish men. *Circulation* 1992; 86:803–811.
26. Ascherio A, Willett WC, Rimm EB, et al: Atherosclerosis in coronary heart disease: dietary iron intake and risk of coronary disease among men. *Circulation* 1994; 89:969–974.
27. Kannel WB, Ellison RC: Alcohol and coronary heart disease: the evidence for a protective effect. *Clin Chim Acta* 1996; 246:59–76.
28. Maclure M: Demonstration of deductive meta-analysis: ethanol intake and risk of myocardial infarction. *Epidemiol Rev* 1993; 15:328–351.
29. Eaker ED, Abbott RD, Kannel WB: Frequency of uncomplicated angina pectoris in type A compared with type B persons. The Framingham Study. *Am J Cardiol* 1989; 63:1042–1045.
30. Rosenman RH, Friedman M, Straus R, et al: A predictive study of coronary heart disease. The Western Collaborative Group Study. *JAMA* 1964; 189:15–22.
31. Denollet J, Sys SU, Stroobant N, et al: Personality as an independent predictor of long-term mortality in patients with coronary heart disease. *Lancet* 1996; 347:417–421.

SALLY E. McNAGNY /
NANETTE K. WENGER

CHAPTER

# THE CONTROVERSY OF POSTMENOPAUSAL HORMONE REPLACEMENT THERAPY AND CARDIOVASCULAR RISK REDUCTION

**22**

## CORONARY HEART DISEASE AND WOMEN

Coronary heart disease (CHD) is the leading cause of death in postmenopausal women, accounting for over 250,000 deaths in U.S. women annually. Over the rest of her lifetime, the average 50-year-old U.S. woman has a 46 percent probability of developing CHD and a 31 percent probability of dying from CHD.[1] Of concern, once women develop CHD, their prognosis may be worse than that of men, as evidenced by higher mortality rates after myocardial infarction (MI), percutaneous transluminal coronary angioplasty (PTCA), and coronary artery bypass grafting (CABG).[2] Thus, an intervention that prevents or delays the development of CHD will have a powerful impact on women's health.

# HORMONE REPLACEMENT THERAPY: INTERPRETING STUDY RESULTS

In a review of the literature on hormone replacement therapy (HRT) and CHD, several key issues make combining studies into meta-analyses or generalizing from one study to another problematic. First, the HRT epidemiologic and animal model literature involves studies of both estrogen alone and estrogen plus a progestin. Second, different HRT studies use different estrogen preparations, different progestins, and different dosages of both. Third, study outcomes differ. For instance, CHD outcomes may include angina, MI, combined CHD events, and/or CHD mortality, and all may have different durations of follow-up. Fourth, relative risk estimates are adjusted differently, ranging from age adjustment alone to adjustment for multiple cardiac risk factors. Finally, and most crucial, results from all observational studies have inherent bias, since the women under investigation are free to make their own decisions about using HRT, and recommendations by their personal physicians may vary. This chapter highlights results from randomized clinical trials and summarizes significant biases inherent in observational studies.

# THE ASSOCIATION OF ESTROGEN AND PRIMARY PREVENTION OF CHD

## Epidemiologic Evidence

An early link between estrogen status and cardiovascular disease was the discovery that women who were estrogen-deficient secondary to bilateral oophorectomy had rates of coronary artery lesions almost comparable to those of men of the same age.[3] In contrast, women without oophorectomy had a delay in the onset of CHD of 10 years and of MI of 20 years, compared to men.[4] A recent study of over 12,115 postmenopausal women showed a 2 percent cardiovascular mortality risk decrease for every year's delay in the menopause.[5] These studies suggest that endogenous estrogen may offer cardioprotection.

There are no large randomized trials of HRT for the primary prevention of CHD. Since 1970, more than 30 observational studies have examined the relationship between estrogen and CHD risk reduction.[6] Follow-up ranges from 1 to 19 years, and primary outcomes include angina, MI, all cardiovascular events (CVD), and/or nonfatal MI plus CHD death. Estrogens include estradiol, conjugated equine estrogen, and unspecified estrogens. Five studies reported a significant decrease in CHD risk ranging from 30 to 70 percent, and five found no significant difference. Only the Framingham Heart Study reported a significant *increase* in CHD risk of 80 percent[6]; when the data were analyzed later excluding angina as an endpoint, the increased risk disappeared.[7]

Several comprehensive meta-analyses calculated a significant CHD risk reduction of 35 to 50 percent with estrogen replacement therapy.[6] The findings of observational studies are strong and are consistent with the hypothesis that HRT reduces the likelihood of developing CHD.

## Biological Plausibility

Multiple biological mechanisms by which estrogen may be cardioprotective have been reviewed.[8] The major categories include favorable effects on lipid metabolism, coagulation and fibrinolysis, and the hemodynamic/vascular system. Unopposed oral conjugated equine estrogen (CEE), 17-$\beta$-estradiol, esterified estrogen, estropipate, and ethinyl estradiol all lower low-density lipoprotein cholesterol (LDL-C) and increase high-density lipoprotein cholesterol (HDL-C) and triglycerides within the first year of treatment.[9–12] The long-term lipid effects of estrogen have been studied only with CEE.[13] After 3 years, women randomized to unopposed CEE had average changes from baseline of LDL-C, HDL-C, and triglyceride levels of $-14.5$ mg/dL, $+5.6$ mg/dL, and $+13.7$ mg/dL, respectively.[13] Thus, while all oral estrogens improve HDL-C and LDL-C and have the undesirable effect of raising triglyceride levels, these changes are modest with long-term treatment. Estrogen also decreases lipoprotein (a) and inhibits LDL oxidation, which is important because oxidized LDL inhibits nitric oxide.[8]

The favorable lipid effects of HRT explain only about 25 to 50 percent of the lower CHD risk in large prospective studies.[6] HRT may be cardioprotective by decreasing hemostatic factors, including fibrinogen, antithrombin III, and PAI-1, and by decreasing platelet aggregation.[8] Estrogen may provide benefit through receptor-dependent and receptor-independent hemodynamic and vascular effects. Estrogen receptors are present in the muscularis of arteries,[8] and evidence from both animal and human studies shows that estrogen (with and without micronized progesterone) improves blood flow in the coronary arteries.[8]

Estrogen may also decrease levels of endothelin, a potent vasoconstrictor.[14] Another possible mechanism by which estrogen may be cardioprotective is its favorable effect on homocysteine metabolism. In a small randomized trial, homocysteine levels were significantly lowered by 12.6 percent from baseline by estradiol and cyclical dydrogesterone.[15]

## The Addition of a Progestin

Addition of a progestin is necessary in order to offset the increased risk of endometrial cancer caused by unopposed estrogen in women without hysterectomy.[13] Progestins blunt some of estrogen's beneficial effects on lipoproteins, particularly HDL-C levels, in a direct relation to the dose and androgenicity of the progestin.[8,10,12,13] In the Postmenopausal Estrogen/Progestin Interventions (PEPI) Trial, HDL-C in women taking CEE without a progestin increased by an average of 5.6 mg/dL, compared to smaller increases of 4.1 mg/dL and 1.2 mg/dL when micronized progesterone or medroxyprogesterone acetate (MPA), respectively, was added.[13]

When norethindrone was added to estrogen, HDL-C did not significantly improve from baseline.[16] Addition of methyltestosterone significantly *decreased* HDL-C by 16 mg/dL.[12] Thus, to maximize estrogen's beneficial effects on HDL-C, the progestin of choice is micronized progesterone or MPA.

Despite attenuation of estrogen's beneficial effect on the lipid profile, animal[17,18] and large observational studies do not show an adverse effect of added progestins.[6] In the Nurses' Health Study, among 120,000 nurses followed since 1976, women who chose to use estrogen (predominantly Premarin) and progestin (predominantly MPA or Provera) were 60 percent less likely to develop CHD, compared to women not using HRT.[6] Another observational study also reported cardioprotection of 50 percent for the estrogen-progestin combination of estrogen and levonorgestrel, compared to women not using HRT.[6] Therefore, observational study results support the hypothesis that combination therapy of estrogen and progestin may be cardioprotective. Randomized trials are necessary to confirm and quantitate the benefit of estrogen for primary prevention of CHD.[6]

## The Postmenopausal Estrogen/Progestin Interventions Trial

Despite the use of HRT for more than 30 years, PEPI[13] (see Table 22-1) was the first large randomized placebo-controlled trial to examine the long-term impact of HRT on heart disease risk factors—lipids, fibrinogen, glucose, insulin, body weight, and blood pressure. Between 1989 and 1991, 875 healthy postmenopausal women aged 45 to 64 years were randomized to placebo; Premarin 0.625 mg daily; or Premarin combined with either MPA 2.5 mg daily, cyclic MPA 10 mg for 12 days/month, or cyclic micronized progesterone (MP) 200 mg for 12 days/month and followed for an average of 3 years. Women with serious chronic medical illnesses or prior history of breast or uterine cancer were excluded from the study.

The PEPI participants were predominantly Caucasian and middle class. The average age was 56.1 years, and more than 50 percent had completed college. Approximately 80 percent of hysterectomized women and 75 percent of women with a uterus reported taking more than 80 percent of their study pills at study completion. Table 22-1 presents the changes in lipoproteins, fibrinogen, and weight among the treatment groups. Oral estrogen alone or in combination with a progestin modestly decreased LDL-C and raised HDL-C and triglycerides. MP had the most favorable effect on HDL-C when compared to MPA. HRT lowered fibrinogen levels without detectable effects on postchallenge insulin or blood pressure. Women in the hormone groups did not gain more weight than women in the placebo group.

Women with a uterus assigned to unopposed estrogen had significantly more adenomatous or atypical endometrial hyperplasia, a precursor of endometrial cancer, compared to placebo (41 versus 2), and were also more likely to have a hysterectomy during the course of the study. Therefore, the high rate of endometrial hyperplasia with estrogen without a progestin restricts its use to women without a uterus.

**TABLE 22-1.  Results of the Postmenopausal Estrogen / Progestin Intervention (PEPI) Trial***

| | Treatment Group** | | | | | $p$ |
| | Placebo | CEE Only | CEE + MPA (cyc) | CEE + MPA (con) | CEE + MP (cyc) | Bonferroni |
| --- | --- | --- | --- | --- | --- | --- |
| Lipoproteins, mg/dL | | | | | | |
| HDL-C | −1.2 [−2.2, −1.2] | 5.6 [4.5, 6.7] | 1.6 [0.5, 2.7] | 1.2 [0.1, 2.2] | 4.1 [3.1, 5.1] | <.001 |
| LDL-C** | −4.1 [−6.5, −1.8] | −14.5 [−16.8, −12.1] | −17.7 [−20.1, 15.4] | −16.5 [−18.8, −14.2] | −14.8 [−17.0, −12.5] | <.001 |
| Triglycerides† | −3.2 [−7.2, 0.7] | 13.7 [9.3, 18.0] | 12.7 [8.5, 16.8] | 11.4 [7.0, 15.9] | 13.4 [9.1, 17.7] | <.001 |
| Fibrinogen, g/L**† | 0.10 [0.04, 0.16] | −0.2 [−0.08, 0.04] | 0.06 [0.00, 0.12] | 0.01 [−0.04, 0.07] | 0.01 [−0.04, 0.7] | <.001 |
| Weight, kg | 1.3 [0.8, 1.8] | 0.4 [0.3, 1.2] | 0.8 [0.4, 1.2] | 0.6 [0.2, 1.0] | 0.6 [0.2, 1.1] | .03 |

* Data expressed as unadjusted mean changes (i.e., average of all follow-up data minus average of all baseline data) and associated 95 percent confidence interval [brackets].

** Adjusted for baseline differences among randomized cohorts.

† Computed from log transformed data.

HDL-C and LDL-C = high- and low-density lipoprotein cholesterol, respectively; CEE = conjugated equine estrogen; MPA = medroxyprogesterone acetate; cyc = cyclic administration (days 1 through 12 of each month); con = administration daily for 1 month; MP = micronized progesterone.

*Source:* Data abstracted from The Writing Group for the PEPI Trial: Effects of estrogen or estrogen/progestin regimens on heart disease risk factors in postmenopausal women. The Postmenopausal Estrogen/Progestin Interventions (PEPI) Trial. *JAMA* 1995; 273:199–208.

# THE ASSOCIATION OF HRT AND SECONDARY PREVENTION OF CHD

## Epidemiologic Evidence

The first randomized trial to assess the effect of HRT on secondary prevention of CHD was conducted in men in the 1960s. Male survivors of Q-wave MI were randomized to placebo or conjugated equine estrogen 2.5 mg or 5 mg daily, among other lipid-lowering agents.[19] Both the hormone arms of the trial were stopped prematurely because of a significant *increase* in myocardial infarction and venous thromboembolic disease in the estrogen-treated men.

To evaluate the effect of self-selected HRT use in women with CAD, women with angiographically proven CAD were followed for 10 years.[20] Of the 644 women with mild to moderate disease, 10-year survival was 96 percent for estrogen users compared to 85 percent for nonusers ($p = .027$). Of the 1178 women with severe coronary stenosis (70 percent stenosis of one or more major coronary arteries), the 10-year survival was 97 percent in the estrogen users and 60 percent in the nonusers ($p = .007$). Only a small proportion of the women enrolled at baseline were followed for 10 years. These findings are consistent with the hypothesis that HRT is cardioprotective in women with established CHD. Encouraged by such results, investigators designed the Heart and Estrogen-Progestin Replacement Study (HERS), the first randomized placebo-controlled trial to assess the effect of HRT in the secondary prevention of CHD in postmenopausal women.

## The Heart and Estrogen/Progestin Replacement Study

HERS[21] is the first large randomized, double-blind, placebo-controlled trial to test the effect of HRT on new CHD events in postmenopausal women with established CHD. Between 1993 and 1994, 2763 postmenopausal women were randomized at 20 U.S. clinical centers, receiving either placebo or Premarin 0.625 mg plus MPA 2.5 mg daily.

Eligible women were postmenopausal, less than age 80, with an intact uterus, and with established CHD. Established CHD was defined as a documented MI, CABG, or PTCA or a cardiac catheterization demonstrating angiographic evidence of greater than 50 percent narrowing of a major coronary artery. Women with a CHD event within 6 months prior to randomization were excluded, as were women with severe heart failure. Other major exclusion criteria included a history of venous thromboembolic disease, breast or uterine cancer, a fasting triglyceride level greater than 300 mg/dL, or a fasting blood glucose level greater than 300 mg/dL. The primary outcome measure was the combined endpoint of nonfatal MI and CHD death.

The HERS participants were predominantly Caucasian (89 percent) and well educated, with an average age of 67 years. There were no significant differences between the hormone and the placebo group in any baseline characteristics. In the hormone group, 13 percent were current smokers, 19 percent were diabetic, the average LDL-C was 145 mg/dL, and the average HDL-C was 50 mg/dL. Use of daily medications included aspirin (78 percent), beta blockers (33 percent), and lipid-lowering agents (45 percent). At the end of the third year, 75 percent of women in the hormone group and 81 percent in the placebo group reported taking the study medication.

Results of HERS are presented in Table 22-2. After a mean of 4.1 years of followup, despite favorable changes in lipid levels, there was no significant difference between the hormone and control groups in the primary outcome (nonfatal MI + CHD death) or in multiple secondary cardiovascular outcomes. Of note, in the first year there was a significant 52 percent increase in CHD primary outcome events in the hormone versus the control group. There was a statistically significant time trend, with more CHD events in the hormone than in the placebo group in year 1 and fewer events in years 4 and 5. Because of the increased risk of CHD events in the first year, this HRT regimen is not recommended for secondary prevention of CHD. However, given the favorable pattern of CHD events after the first year of therapy, it may be appropriate for women with CHD who are already receiving HRT to continue therapy.

HERS did not address the use of unopposed estrogen, the use of HRT in women without preexisting CHD, or the use of other forms of estrogen or progestin. The majority of women were Caucasian, and therefore results may not be generalizable to other ethnic groups.

**TABLE 22-2.   Results of the Heart and Estrogen/Progestin Replacement Study (HERS)***

|  | Estrogen/Progestin ($n = 1380$) | Placebo ($n = 1383$) | RH [95% CI] | $p$ value |
|---|---|---|---|---|
| Primary CHD events** | 172 | 176 | 0.99 [0.80–1.22] | .91 |
| CHD death | 71 | 58 | 1.24 [0.87–1.75] | .23 |
| Nonfatal MI | 116 | 129 | 0.91 [0.71–1.17] | .46 |
| Primary CHD events[†] |  |  |  |  |
| Year 1 | 57 | 38 | 1.52 [1.01–2.29] | $p$ value for |
| Year 2 | 47 | 48 | 1.00 [0.67–1.49] | trend |
| Year 3 | 35 | 41 | 0.87 [0.55–1.37] | .009 |
| Years 4 and 5 | 33 | 49 | 0.67 [0.43–1.04] |  |

* Each row represents the number of women with the designated event; women with more than one type of event may appear in more than one row.

** Primary CHD events include coronary death and nonfatal MI. Among the 245 nonfatal MIs, there were 7 silent MIs found on annual electrocardiogram. There were 26 women with nonfatal MI who subsequently suffered CHD death.

[†]Primary CHD events include nonfatal myocardial infarction and CHD death.

RH = relative hazard; CI = confidence interval; CHD = coronary heart disease; MI = myocardial infarction.
*Source:* Results from Hulley S, Grady D, Bush T, et al: Randomized trial of estrogen plus progestin for secondary prevention of coronary heart disease in postmenopausal women. *JAMA* 1998; 280:605–613.

# RETHINKING THE POSSIBLE CARDIOPROTECTION OF HRT

## Bias in Observational Studies

The apparent cardioprotection reported in observational and case-control studies may not be caused by HRT, but may instead be a result of fundamental differences between women who choose to take HRT and those who do not.[6] For example, women who choose to use HRT, compared to women who do not, have better metabolic risk factors *before the menopause,* have healthier lifestyles, are more highly educated, and are more likely to be adherent with medication. These are all factors associated with overall disease risk reduction.[6]

As described in the editorial accompanying HERS, being a "good adherer" is significantly associated with cardiovascular risk reduction.[22] Subjects in the Coronary Drug Project who were adherent to placebo were 30 percent less likely to develop CHD than nonadherent subjects taking placebo. In the Beta-Blocker Heart Attack Trial, being a good adherer in the placebo group was also associated with a significant 60 percent reduction of CHD risk, compared to subjects who did not take their placebo pill regularly.[22] Thus, good adherence is powerfully associated with CHD risk reduction and is likely to be a marker for other healthy behaviors.

## Post-HERS: Reconsidering the Data

In 1991–1992, three meta-analyses concluded that postmenopausal estrogen decreases CHD risk by 35 to 40 percent.[6] In 1992, major medical organizations such as the American College of Physicians and the American College of Obstetricians and Gynecologists extrapolated these observational study results to encourage the use of HRT for cardiovascular risk reduction.[1,23] By 1996, conjugated equine estrogen (Premarin) was the most frequently dispensed medication in the United States.

A post-HERS review of the association of HRT and CHD concluded that until findings from randomized trials could confirm the benefit of HRT in prevention of CHD, HRT should not be routinely recommended solely for CHD prevention.[6] HERS did not address CHD risk reduction in women without preexisting heart disease. Both observational studies and biological mechanisms support the hypothesis that HRT may be effective in primary prevention of CHD. Despite such potentially promising results, treating women with HRT solely for the primary prevention of CHD is not recommended for the following reasons: (1) observational data may be incorrect secondary to inherent biases, and (2) HRT has established risks and side effects. If physicians choose to prescribe HRT solely for the primary prevention of CHD, it is recommended that they document that the patient understands that this is a *potential* benefit of HRT and that the patient has been informed of both established and potential risks.

## The Established and Potential Risks of HRT

In a randomized trial, HRT significantly increased the risk of venous thromboembolic events (VTE) threefold.[21] In healthy women, the absolute number of *extra* cases of deep vein thrombosis attributed to HRT appears to be only about 1 in 5000 users per year and that of pulmonary embolus only 1 in 20,000 users per year[24]; therefore, the absolute increase in risk is small. However, in an older population of women with established CHD, HRT use was associated with 1 extra case of VTE per 62 women during 4 years.[21] Therefore, although the absolute impact of HRT on VTE risk is extremely small in healthy women, the excess incidence of VTE in older women with CHD is several orders of magnitude greater.

Symptomatic gallbladder disease is also significantly increased, by approximately 40 percent, in older women with CHD using HRT (these studies involve only oral CEE and MPA), of whom 89 percent required gallbladder surgery.[21] The 40 percent increase in risk translates to 1 extra case per 62 women during a 4-year period.[21] Although surgery was required for 90 percent of women with cholecystitis, none of the gallbladder events were fatal.[21]

More than 50 epidemiologic studies have explored the relationship between HRT and breast cancer.[25] Despite continued uncertainty, three meta-analyses and several consensus panels agree that there is no evidence to suggest an increase in breast cancer risk when HRT is used for less than 5 years.[25] In contrast, there may be an increased risk of breast cancer of approximately 30 percent in women who use HRT for more than 5 years.[25]

During 3 years of follow-up in PEPI, there was no increased risk of endometrial hyperplasia or cancer with estrogen-progestin combination therapy compared to placebo.[13] However, there is some evidence that HRT may increase the risk of endometrial cancer, despite appropriate doses of progestin, when women use HRT for more than 5 years.[26]

Other potential risks of HRT include increases in benign breast disease[27] and a possible decrease in sensitivity and specificity of screening mammography in women using HRT.[28]

## The Established and Potential Benefits of HRT

HRT is highly effective in treating estrogen-deficient hot flashes and atrophic vaginal changes. HRT also prevents and treats osteoporosis, although improvement in bone mineral density from HRT is not maintained after cessation of treatment.[29] Benefits of HRT that have not yet been confirmed in randomized trials include a possible reduction in risk of Alzheimer's disease and of colorectal cancer.[30,31]

Confirmation of the suggested risks and benefits of HRT await results from large randomized trials such as the Women's Health Initiative (WHI) Hormone Trial, a randomized, placebo-controlled trial designed to assess the risks and benefits of HRT in over 27,000 women.[32] Results are not expected until after the completion of the trial in 2005. A comparable trial is currently underway in the United Kingdom.

## SUMMARY

Despite favorable observational data and plausible biological mechanisms, it is unknown whether HRT reduces the risk of developing CHD. There are established risks and side effects of HRT, as well as noncoronary benefits. Therefore, until findings from randomized trials establish cardioprotection, HRT should not be prescribed *solely* for the primary prevention of CHD.

In postmenopausal women with established CHD, results from a large randomized trial of secondary prevention of CHD (HERS) indicate that this combination of estrogen and progestin does not reduce the rate of MI and CHD death. Of concern, women in the hormone group had a significant 52 percent increase in MI and CHD death during the first year of treatment, compared to women in the placebo group. Therefore, this hormone regimen should not be prescribed for the secondary prevention of CHD.

## REFERENCES

1. Grady D, Rubin SM, Petitti DB, et al: Hormone therapy to prevent disease and prolong life in postmenopausal women. *Ann Intern Med* 1992; 117:1016–1037.
2. Marrugat J, Sala J, Masia R, et al: Mortality differences between men and women following first myocardial infarction. *JAMA* 1998; 280:1405–1409.
3. Wuerst JH, Dry TJ, Edwards JE: The degree of coronary atherosclerosis in bilaterally oophorectomized women. *Circulation* 1953; 7:801–809.
4. Kannel WB: Metabolic risk factors for coronary heart disease in women: perspective from the Framingham Study. *Am Heart J* 1987; 114:413–419.
5. van der Schouw YT, van der Graff Y, Steyerberg EW, et al: Age at menopause as a risk factor for cardiovascular mortality. *Lancet* 1996; 347:714–718.
6. Barrett-Connor E, Grady D: Hormone replacement therapy, heart disease, and other considerations. *Annu Rev Public Health* 1998; 19:55–72.
7. Eaker E, Castelli W: Coronary heart disease and its risk factors among women in the Framingham Study. In: Eaker E, Packard B, Wenger N, et al (eds): *Coronary Heart Disease in Women.* New York, Haymarket Doyma, 1987:122–132.
8. Chae CU, Ridker PM, Manson JE: Postmenopausal hormone replacement therapy and cardiovascular disease. *Thromb Haemost* 1997; 78:770–780.
9. Genant H, Lucas J, Weiss S, et al: Low-dose esterified estrogen therapy: effects on bone, plasma estradiol concentration, endometrium, and lipid levels. Estratab/Osteoporosis Study Group. *Arch Intern Med* 1997; 157:2609–2615.
10. Miller VT, Muesing RA, LaRosa JC, et al: Quantitative and qualitative changes in lipids, lipoproteins, apolipoprotein A-I, and sex hormone-binding globulin due to two doses of conjugated equine estrogen with and without a progestin. *Obstet Gynecol* 1994; 83:173–179.

11. Speroff L, Rowan J, Symons J, et al: The comparative effect on bone density, endometrium, and lipids of continuous hormones as replacement therapy (CHART Study). A randomized controlled trial. *JAMA* 1996; 276:1397–1403.

12. Watts NB, Notelovitz M, Timmons MC, et al: Comparison of oral estrogens and estrogens plus androgen on bone mineral density, menopausal symptoms, and lipid-lipoprotein profiles in surgical menopause. *Obstet Gynecol* 1995; 85:529–537.

13. The Writing Group for the PEPI Trial: Effects of estrogen or estrogen/progestin regimens on heart disease risk factors in postmenopausal women. The Postmenopausal Estrogen/Progestin Interventions (PEPI) Trial. *JAMA* 1995; 273:199–208.

14. Polderman KH, Stehouwer CDA, van Kamp GJ, et al: Influence of sex hormones on plasma endothelin levels. *Ann Intern Med* 1993; 118:429–432.

15. Mijatovic V, Kenemans P, Jakobs C, et al: A randomized controlled study of the effects of 17-beta-estradiol-dydrogesterone on plasma homocysteine in postmenopausal women. *Obstet Gynecol* 1998; 91:432–436.

16. Taitel H, Kafrissen M: Norethindrone—a review of therapeutic applications. *Int J Fertil* 1995; 40:207–223.

17. Adams MR, Kaplan JR, Manuck SB, et al: Inhibition of coronary artery atherosclerosis by 17-beta estradiol in ovariectomized monkeys. Lack of an effect of added progesterone. *Arteriosclerosis* 1990; 10:1051–1057.

18. Clarkson T, Shively C, Morgan T, et al: Oral contraceptives and coronary artery atherosclerosis of cynomolgus monkeys. *Obstet Gynecol* 1990; 75:217–222.

19. Coronary Drug Project Research Group: The Coronary Drug Project: findings leading to discontinuation of the 2.5-mg/day estrogen group. *JAMA* 1973; 226:652–657.

20. Sullivan J, Zwaag R, Hughes J, et al: Estrogen replacement and coronary artery disease. *Arch Intern Med* 1990; 150:2557–2562.

21. Hulley S, Grady D, Bush T, et al: Randomized trial of estrogen plus progestin for secondary prevention of coronary heart disease in postmenopausal women. *JAMA* 1998; 280:605–613.

22. Petitti D: Hormone replacement therapy and heart disease prevention. *JAMA* 1998; 280:650–652.

23. American College of Obstetricians and Gynecologists: Hormone replacement therapy. *Technical Bulletin*, vol. 166. Washington, DC, American College of Obstetricians and Gynecologists, 1992.

24. Grady D, Hulley S, Furberg C: Venous thromboembolic events associated with hormone replacement therapy. *JAMA* 1997; 278:477.

25. Collaborative Group on Hormonal Factors in Breast Cancer: Breast cancer and hormone replacement therapy: collaborative reanalysis of data from 51 epidemiological studies of 52,705 women with breast cancer and 108,411 without breast cancer. *Lancet* 1997; 350:1047–1053.

26. Beresford S, Weiss N, Voigt L, McKnight B: Risk of endometrial cancer in relation to use of oestrogen combined with cyclic progestogen therapy in postmenopausal women. *Lancet* 1997; 349:458–461.

27. Berkowitz GS, Kelsey JL, Holford TR, et al: Estrogen replacement therapy and fibrocystic breast disease in postmenopausal women. *Am J Epidemiol* 1985; 121:238–245.

28. Laya MB, Larson EB, Taplin SH, White E: Effect of estrogen replacement therapy on the specificity and sensitivity of screening mammography. *J Natl Cancer Inst* 1996; 88:643–649.

29. National Osteoporosis Foundation: *Physician's Guide to Prevention and Treatment of Osteoporosis.* Washington DC, National Osteoporosis Foundation, 1998.

30. Yaffe K, Grady D, Pressman A, Cummings S: Serum estrogen levels, cognitive performance, and risk of cognitive decline in older community women. *J Am Geriatr Soc* 1998; 46:816–822.
31. Grodstein F, Martinez E, Platz E, et al: Postmenopausal hormone use and risk for colorectal cancer and adenoma. *Ann Intern Med* 1998; 128:705–712.
32. The Women's Health Initiative Group: Design of the Women's Health Initiative clinical trial and observational study. *Controlled Clin Trials* 1998; 19:61–109.

MARIO DI GIROLAMO /
JACQUELINE FINE

**CHAPTER**

# OBESITY

# 23

Obesity has become a prevalent disorder in the developed countries and is fast becoming a significant problem in the developing countries. In the United States, one out of three adults is obese, and among Hispanics and African Americans, the number is one out of two.[1,2] A variety of conditions influence the development of obesity: Genetic expression, environmental factors, inactivity, behavior, underlying illness, and socioeconomic status all play a role.[3,4] For this reason, obesity has been called a multifactorial disorder, although an imbalance between calories ingested and calories utilized is usually present, particularly in the early stages of obesity development.

The importance of obesity in clinical medicine resides in the link between obesity and several severe health risk factors.[5] Obesity predisposes to or aggravates hypertension, hyperlipidemia, carbohydrate intolerance and diabetes, atherosclerotic heart disease, restrictive lung disease, gout, cholelithiasis, infertility, degenerative arthritis, and some types of cancer.[6–9] Insurance companies have recognized for many decades the association of obesity with increased morbidity and mortality.[10]

## WHO IS OBESE?

A practicing physician has no difficulty in recognizing obesity in one of his or her patients. Increased fat accumulation in the subcutaneous region, around the neck, buttocks, thighs, and abdomen, is often clearly evident at physical examination.

It is harder, however, to quantitate the degree of obesity. Obesity can be defined as an *excessive accumulation of body fat.* But, since it is difficult to determine the amount and location of body fat, body weight has been used as a surrogate parameter.

There are two general ways to list normative values: (1) relative body weight and (2) body mass index.

### Relative Body Weight

Although imprecise, relative body weight gives the physician or nurse a practical and simple tool for assessing the patient's overall nutritional status. A normal body weight for the patient's height and gender can be determined from tables provided by Metropolitan Life Insurance Company.[10] Alternatively, the Hamwi formula can be used:[11]

- For a female, 100 lb are allotted for 5 ft of height, plus 5 lb for each additional inch.
- For a male, 106 lb are allotted for 5 ft, plus 6 lb for each additional inch. Once the normal, "desirable" weight has been defined for a given subject (100 percent), the relative weight (i.e., the percent above or below the desirable or ideal body weight) can be calculated. The normal relative body weight range is 90 to 109 percent of ideal body weight. Below 90 percent, individuals are considered *underweight*.

Individuals with relative body weight in excess of 110 percent are considered *overweight*. Of these, those classified as *preobese* have relative body weight of 110 to 119 percent; those who are *obese Class I*, 120 to 149 percent; those who are *obese Class II*, 150 to 199 percent; and those who are *obese Class III*, over 200 percent of ideal body weight.

## Body Mass Index

The body mass index (BMI) is a relatively new and convenient measure of body mass (and indirectly of body fat) that is independent of gender. The BMI can be calculated as weight in kilograms divided by height in meters squared ($BMI = kg/m^2$).[12]

A recent task force has defined the normal BMI range to be between 18.5 and 24.9.[13] A BMI below 18.5 is seen in *underweight* subjects. A BMI over 25 indicates *overweight*. The *preobese* have a BMI of 25 to 29.9; the *obese Class I*, a BMI of 30 to 34.9; the *obese Class II*, a BMI of 35 to 39.9; and the *obese Class III*, a BMI of over 40 (see Table 23-1).

It has to be recognized that some individuals are overweight (i.e., BMI > 25) but do not have excessive body fat, as their lean body mass is enhanced (football players, weight lifters, etc.). Conversely, some inactive individuals may have a body weight within the ideal range or a normal BMI, but their bodies may contain excessive body fat as a result of diminished lean body mass. A body fat in excess of 22 percent of body weight in males and of 32 percent in females is considered abnormal. Although knowledge of body fat content is not strictly necessary for medical practice, it is often a useful parameter to follow, particularly in sedentary individuals who initiate an activity program.

Underwater weighing, bioelectrical impedance, or dual energy x-ray absorptiometry offer the best estimates of absolute or relative body fat mass.[14–16] Circumferences (waist, hip, and thigh) and skinfold thickness in four to six affected sites can also be used to estimate regional fat distribution.[17,18] The reader may need to consult more specialized literature for more information on these techniques.

**TABLE 23-1.** Overweight and Obesity Classification

|  | BMI (kg/m$^2$) |
|---|---|
| Underweight | < 18.5 |
| Normal range | 18.5–24.9 |
| Overweight | 25.0–29.9 |
| Obesity |  |
|    Class I | 30.0–34.9 |
|    Class II | 35.0–39.9 |
|    Class III | >40 |

*Source:* Adapted from Expert Panel on the Identification, Evaluation, and Treatment of Overweight in Adults: Clinical guidelines on the identification, evaluation, and treatment of overweight and obesity in adults: Executive summary. *Am J Clin Nutr* 1998; 68:899–917 (public domain).

# WHAT ARE THE RISKS OF OBESITY?

Excess accumulation of body fat is associated with many adverse health consequences (see Table 23-2). Furthermore, increases in mortality rates relative to increases in body weight are more precipitous for persons younger than 50 than for the more geriatric population and are related directly to the severity and duration of obesity.[5]

**TABLE 23-2.** Health Risks of Obesity

1. Hypertension, hyperlipidemia
2. Insulin resistance, carbohydrate intolerance, and diabetes
3. Elevated uric acid and gout
4. Cholelithiasis
5. Cardiovascular disease and strokes
6. Venous insufficiency and thrombophlebitis
7. Restrictive lung disease and pulmonary insufficiency
8. Infertility
9. Degenerative arthritis of weight-bearing joints
10. Certain types of cancer
11. Increased mortality

Primary and secondary risks of obesity probably derive from the interaction among genetics, diet, exercise habits, and other factors such as smoking that increase morbidity. Each increment in body fat carries with it an increased risk for disease. For example, many studies have shown that individuals who are 15 to 20 percent overweight have up to an eightfold increase in risk for hypertension.[5] Other studies have shown that every 10 percent increase in relative body weight is associated with a 12-mg/dL increase in plasma cholesterol.[19] The same connection between increment in BMI and increased risk for disease has been observed for non-insulin-dependent diabetes mellitus (NIDDM);[5,20] gallbladder disease;[21] respiratory disease, such as sleep apnea;[22] and some forms of cancer (colorectal and prostate cancers in men; endometrial, gallbladder, cervical, ovarian, and breast cancers in women).[5]

In addition to its role as an independent risk factor for coronary heart disease, obesity also can augment other risk factors that lead to coronary heart disease morbidity (see Table 23-3).[5] The *direct* relation between obesity and death is less clear, as the number of studies that show a negative association are almost as numerous as the number that demonstrate a positive association. This may be due to several factors, including the fact that, in some studies, the body weights of lean individuals may have been the result of a disease process rather than a more healthy lifestyle.[23,24] In addition, because obesity exerts some of its effects through amplification of other risk factors, as described above, its direct role in mortality is more difficult to discern.[5] More controlled studies of cohorts of nonsmokers, however, reveal a significant trend toward increasing mortality rate with increased body mass index.[25]

**TABLE 23-3.   Degree of Health Risk as Related to Regional Fat Deposition and to Waist Circumference**

**A. Regional Fat Deposition**

| Region | Abdominal visceral | Abdominal subcutaneous | Gluteal-femoral subcutaneous |
|---|---|---|---|
| Risk | High | Moderate | Low |

**B. Waist Circumference**

| | Waist Circumference | |
|---|---|---|
| | **Men** | **Women** |
| Low risk | < 102 cm<br>< 40 in. | < 88 cm<br>< 35 in. |
| High risk | > 102 cm<br>> 40 in. | > 88 cm<br>> 35 in. |

*Source:* Adapted from Expert Panel on the Identification, Evaluation, and Treatment of Overweight in Adults: Clinical guidelines on the identification, evaluation, and treatment of overweight and obesity in adults: Executive summary. *Am J Clin Nutr* 1998; 68:899–917 (public domain).

# WHAT ARE THE EFFECTS OF REGIONAL FAT DISTRIBUTION ON THE RISKS OF OBESITY?

Body fat is not a unitary organ. Anatomically discrete adipose depots have region-specific responses to changes in age, nutritional status, and systemic hormonal milieu that lead to preferential accumulation of excess lipid by some depots.[26] The selective accretion of upper-body fat, and abdominal fat in particular, occurs with aging in both sexes. There are, however, gender-based differences in the temporal onset of this process. Men show continuous increases in the ratio of upper- to lower-body fat with age.[27] In contrast, females tend to maintain a stable total fat mass, but show a *redistribution* of body fat with advancing age, with increases in upper-body fat and reductions in lower-body fat.[27] In addition, increases in the visceral fat mass by males are almost three times those of premenopausal women.[28] Menopause markedly accelerates the accumulation of intraabdominal visceral fat and abolishes the gender differences just described.[28]

In humans of both genders, the accumulation of visceral rather than subcutaneous fat has been associated with many of the metabolic abnormalities and secondary health consequences of obesity discussed above (see Table 23-3).[5] In fact, there are many data that suggest that the abdominal localization of body fat is almost *more* important than the total amount of body fat in the prediction and development of NIDDM, cardiovascular disease, hyperinsulinemia, elevated serum triglyceride levels, and stroke.[5,29,30] There also are indications that obese children store a higher percentage of their fat internally and that this may be a harbinger of the visceral adipose tissue deposition found in obese adults with metabolic difficulties, such as the increase in insulin resistance that precedes NIDDM.[31]

# ENDOCRINE AND METABOLIC ABNORMALITIES ASSOCIATED WITH OBESITY

Adipose tissue is a unique organ in the body. It has the greatest capacity to store calories, because of a small water content (usually less than 10 percent its weight) and a large storage of neutral fat, triglycerides (1 g = 9 cal). Adipose tissue is present all over the body, but approximately 50 percent of it is present in the subcutaneous region. Its main cellular components are adipocytes, specialized cells containing a large lipid droplet with a rim of cytoplasm where most of the metabolic activity is carried out.

In normal lean individuals, adipose tissue performs important metabolic and non-metabolic functions. Some of these functions become altered with the development of obesity. A lean male individual usually has 12 to 18 percent of body weight as fat and has 80,000 to 120,000 cal stored in adipose tissue. A lean female usually has 18 to 28 percent of body weight as fat and about 90,000 to 140,000 cal stored in adipose tissue. In moderately and severely obese individuals, body fat can reach 35 to 50 percent of body weight, and calories stored in adipose tissue can reach 250,000 to 500,000.

Nonmetabolic functions of adipose tissue include insulation from heat loss and provision of a movable subcutaneous cushion to protect the skeleton, vessels, and skin from trauma-related damage.[32]

A major metabolic function of adipose tissue is related to its participation in daily metabolic exchanges. During fasting, adipocytes break down stored triglycerides and mobilize glycerol and fatty acids into the circulation; following a meal, adipose tissue liberates lipoprotein lipase, an enzyme which helps to remove circulating triglyceride-rich lipoproteins. Adipose tissue takes up glucose and free fatty acids, and synthesizes and stores triglycerides. Fat cells are exquisitely sensitive to the effect of insulin in promoting glucose utilization and in suppressing lipolysis; they also respond to a variety of lipolytic hormones, catecholamines, parathyroid hormone, glucocorticoids, etc., which stimulate triglyceride breakdown and lipid mobilization.[32]

A lesser-known metabolic function of adipose tissue involves the capacity of fat cells to convert glucose to lactate and then release lactate into the circulation. Lactate is a major precursor of gluconeogenesis and glycogen synthesis in the liver.[32]

Other functions of adipose tissue include conversion of androgens to estrogens by aromatase enzymes, and synthesis and release of many cytokines, in particular leptin, a newly identified hormone with multiple sites of action, which provides information to the hypothalamus concerning the amount of energy stored in peripheral adipose tissues.[32] Excessive accumulation of adipose tissue in the body, as seen in moderate or severe obesity, leads to several endocrine and metabolic abnormalities.[33]

With obesity, insulin resistance develops in muscle and in adipose tissue. The precise origin of the insulin resistance is unknown, but it may be linked to excessive production of free fatty acids and lactate.[32] These substrates could be used preferentially to glucose and thus lead to carbohydrate intolerance. Insulin resistance is accompanied by insulin overproduction by the pancreas and circulating hyperinsulinemia. Excessive production of insulin by the pancreas has been linked to "pancreatic exhaustion."[32] When the pancreas fails to keep up with the insulin needed to overcome insulin resistance, frank hyperglycemia of diabetes (NIDDM) ensues.

Hyperlipidemia is frequently observed in obesity, usually linked to excessive very-low-density lipoprotein production; it probably results, in part, from excessive arrival of free fatty acids to the liver.

Additionally, obesity is associated with menstrual irregularities, probably because of imbalance between gonadal hormone production and storage in adipose tissue.

At times, patients with obesity are referred to an endocrinologist because of suspicion of Cushing's syndrome (hypertension, moon facies, buffalo hump, occasional striae). In obesity, glucocorticoid production by the adrenal gland and urinary excretion are moderately increased, but plasma cortisol levels are usually normal. In equivocal cases, suppression of plasma cortisol in the morning (below 5 μg/dL) following ingestion of 1 mg dexamethasone at midnight rules out adrenal hyperfunction. With obesity, circulating levels of growth hormone are decreased.[33]

## OBESITY MANAGEMENT

A thorough history and physical examination is necessary at a first office visit and should include the following:

1. Possible underlying endocrine and nonendocrine etiologies of the obesity problem should be assessed. Endocrine dysfunctions such as hypothyroidism, Cushing's syndrome, hyperinsulinemia of insulinoma, polycystic ovarian syndrome, and hypogonadism need to be ruled in or out; if any of these is ruled in, correction of the underlying endocrine abnormality is often helpful in the management of obesity. Other less frequent abnormalities include hypothalamic-pituitary disorders and rare genetic syndromes associated with obesity.
2. Behavioral and psychological factors should be identified. Clarifications of personal factors or family and environmental issues that may have influenced the development of obesity are often very important. Some of these issues may need to be resolved prior to, or in parallel with, management of obesity by diet, exercise, and behavior modification.
3. Assessment of nutritional factors, such as size and frequency of meals, diet composition, ingestion of alcohol, and social eating opportunities, must be done, together with gathering of information on type, frequency, and pattern of physical activity. A diet and weight history, including maximum weight and attempts to lose weight by various methods, may be very useful.
4. Physical examination should include height and weight, waist and hip circumferences, and, in some instances, measurement of skinfold thickness to identify regional body fat distribution (upper-body segment or lower-body segment obesity). Presence, location, and color of striae (abdomen, thighs, etc.) or presence of buffalo hump should be noted.

### Diet

Even though all kinds of diet have been extolled in the scientific and lay press, most experts on obesity recommend a diet balanced among protein (10 to 15 percent of calories), fat (20 to 30 percent of calories), and nonrefined carbohydrates (45 to 55 percent of calories), with strong emphasis on ingestion of fruits and vegetables. Three meals a day, with an occasional snack at bedtime, for a caloric deficit of 500 to 700 cal from estimated caloric maintenance (based on patient's age, gender, weight, and degree of physical activity), should lead to weight loss of approximately 0.5 to 1 lb per week, 2 to 4 lb per month. Patients should be encouraged to weigh themselves in the morning, on a bathroom scale, at least once a week, wearing minimal clothing. Initially, patients should visit the doctor's office at least monthly to monitor compliance with the regimen planned, to continue the dietitian's education efforts, and to receive feedback and encouragement. The success of the dietary effort is linked to clear understanding of proximate and ultimate goals of reasonable body weight, continuing education on dietary principles and practice, motivation of the patient, and support by family and environment. Occasionally, in subjects with life-threatening conditions, when more rapid weight loss is recommended, more drastic caloric restriction (i.e., 1000 to 1200 cal below maintenance) under stricter medical supervision may be needed.

## Exercise

A plan for a progressive effort to reach a new level of acceptable and enjoyable *daily* physical activity is probably as important as the dietary plan in achieving weight loss and changes in body composition (decreased fat mass and increased lean body mass).

The physician should explore the patient's preference and the ability to initiate a new level of exercise. Simple and enjoyable exercise has more chance of being accepted than complex forms of exercise utilizing specialized equipment. For example, walking (initially slow, later brisk walking), water aerobics, team sports, tennis, or gardening can provide a daily energy expenditure of 300 to 400 cal. A weekly caloric expenditure of 1800 to 2500 cal through added physical activity is considered an ideal adjuvant to the diet in promoting weight loss and facilitating body weight maintenance after weight loss.

Exercise has been shown to have multiple beneficial effects on the organism: It reduces insulin level and improves lipid levels and carbohydrate tolerance; it helps in reducing blood pressure, and it provides the patients, particularly the elderly patients, with increased muscle strength, renewed vigor, and elevation of mood.

## Behavior Modification

Simple rules of behavior modification in addition to diet and exercise have contributed to successful weight loss.[34]

Shopping for food after dinner (rather than on an empty stomach) leads to the purchase of less food and avoidance of less healthy products. Eating slowly, at times laying the fork on the table between mouthfuls, increases the time to complete the meal and allows satiety to set in before large amounts of food are ingested. Keeping a food diary that can be checked by a dietitian helps a patient to define the amount and content of food ingested. Other, more specialized recommendations are often offered to the motivated patient in individual or group sessions. In well-run studies, the beneficial effects of this adjuvant approach have been described.[34]

## Drugs

The pharmacologic approach to the management of obesity has been emphasized in recent years, and several new drugs have reached the market. Unfortunately, each drug has several, at times serious, side effects.[35] Recently, the FDA has removed two widely used drugs because of serious heart valve complications. Furthermore, the availability of some of these drugs and their overprescription by physicians and others have led to improper use by a large number of patients who desire rapid cosmetic results without paying due attention to diet, exercise, and behavior modification.

Some of the new drugs can provide an additional stimulus and, thus, contribute to weight loss when used properly under a doctor's supervision. Presently, phentermine is available for certain patients, and another drug (Orlistat) has received FDA approval. Analysis of the better studies presented in the last decade, however, indicates that the addition of a drug usually increases the weight loss promoted by diet and exercise by only 7 to 10 lb a year. This beneficial effect must be weighed against possible harmful side effects.

Obesity drugs have different underlying mechanisms of action. Some produce a degree of anorexia by promoting the release, or blocking the reuptake, of neurotransmitters such as dopamine, norepinephrine, and serotonin.[34] Others reduce nutrient utilization by interfering with the normal digestion and absorption of nutrients. Some reduce fat synthesis and accumulation, whereas others accelerate fat mobilization and heat production (thermogenesis).

Even though a particular drug may help certain patients to get through difficult times or temporary relapse, the physician should monitor the patient carefully for possible side effects of the drugs. In addition, until better drugs become available, the physician should insist that the patient use these drugs *temporarily*, and only as an adjunct to diet, exercise, and some form of behavior modification.

## Surgery

In severe obesity, when other treatments have failed, and when complications such as diabetes, thromboembolism, or cardiovascular disease may be life-threatening, surgical approaches have been successful in achieving a rapid and substantial weight loss[36] with improvement or resolution of some obesity-related health risks.

The reader is directed to specialized literature[37] for more comprehensive information on and assessment of the various forms of gastric stapling or bypass, including the newest laparoscopic approach.

With regard to another surgical approach, suction lipectomy, this intervention is almost always ineffective in the reduction of excessive adipose mass in obesity. Animal studies have shown clear evidence of regeneration of adipose tissue in the same site or in vicarious sites.[38] Lipectomy can be of some use, however, in the removal of small, localized accumulations of adipose tissue (e.g., lipomas), with some valid cosmetic results.

## Comprehensive Approach

A motivated patient who is eager to learn and apply information on quality and quantity of the diet can be successfully helped to lose body weight and maintain it at the newly acquired level by a caring physician and a team that includes a nutritionist, a nurse, and possibly a behavior expert. A well-balanced diet, with a reduction from maintenance calories of 500 to 700 cal per day, reduction in fat content of the diet to less than 30 percent of calories, and generous intake of vegetables and fruit, is the main feature of a correct dietary approach. Daily exercise of 30 to 40 min and simple measures of behavior modification can contribute to the expected reduction in body weight and to improved body composition.

## OBESITY PREVENTION

Obesity, as measured by changes in body weight, often is insidious in onset, with gains of 8 to 10 lb per year. Once a stage of obesity is reached and maintained for many years, it becomes harder to lose weight, i.e., "obesity defends itself." This statement is supported by many studies that indicate several mechanisms that contribute to weight regain after weight loss. Persistence of elevated lipoprotein lipase enzyme and smaller fat cells with enhanced insulin sensitivity lead to lipid (triglyceride) reaccumulation by the fat cells. A reduced metabolic rate, in part linked to some loss of lean body mass, makes it harder for patients to maintain their body weight at the acquired level with a reduced caloric intake.[39]

For all these reasons, educational efforts directed toward an understanding of "desirable" body weight in adults and in children can alert the physician and the patient when an early, modest weight gain occurs. This is the time for intervention with diet and exercise to prevent further weight gain and to promote judicious loss of the excess fat. In children and adolescents, dietary restriction needs to be monitored so that growth is not negatively affected.

In a broader sense, a healthy lifestyle, with a balanced diet rich in fruit and vegetables and a plan of steady exercise 4 to 7 days a week, for a caloric expenditure of 1800 to 2500 cal a week, is usually sufficient to promote a healthy body weight and body composition and to prevent the development of obesity.

## WHEN TO REFER A PATIENT FOR OBESITY MANAGEMENT

Many internists and family practice physicians see patients daily who have various degrees of obesity. Often the patient is receptive, in the early stages of obesity development, to recommendations concerning "desirable" body weight, proper diet, and a plan for enhanced physical activity. This can be achieved in the doctor's office with a proper interaction between the patient, the doctor, and a nurse who can take a diet history and provide simple dietary and exercise instructions.

Occasionally, patients with more severe obesity (Class I or higher), whose attempts to lose weight by individual efforts or through commercial enterprises have failed, may need to be referred to physicians, or groups headed by physicians, who have specialized knowledge and provide a team approach to the treatment of moderate or severe obesity.

Usually these teams include a nutritionist and a psychologist consultant in addition to the physician and nurse. Office equipment, or referral opportunities, for measuring body weight, anthropometric indices, and body composition may be necessary to fully evaluate the severity of the problem and institute a plan of action involving frequent visits, dietary instruction, and enhanced physical activity. In this setting, it may be easier to prescribe an obesity drug for a limited time and monitor carefully both the beneficial effects and possible deleterious side effects.

In extreme cases of obesity—BMI over 40, or BMI over 35 with severe and life-threatening complications—it may be at times advisable to refer the patient to a specialized surgical facility where bariatric surgery can be considered and offered to the patient.[36,37]

## CONCLUSIONS

The prevalence of obesity has reached alarming levels in the United States and in many other developed countries. The nature of the obesity problem, and of the many and severe associated complications, is such that it may be necessary to develop new and more effective ways to identify patients with established or developing obesity, and to manage them in the same fashion that chronic conditions such as diabetes or hypertension are managed. This may require government intervention, creative new approaches, and improved third-party payments for a problem that can be managed and even prevented, so that the obesity-related health risk hazards can be reduced or prevented.

### REFERENCES

1. Wickelgren I: Obesity: How big a problem? *Science* 1998; 280:1364–1366.
2. Popkin BM, Doak CM: The obesity epidemic is a worldwide phenomenon. *Nutr Rev* 1998; 56:106–114.
3. Bray GA: Obesity: Historical development of scientific and cultural ideas. *Int J Obes* 1990; 14:909–926.
4. Bouchard C: Genetics and the metabolic syndrome. *Int J Obes* 1995; 19 (suppl. 1): S52–S59.
5. Pi-Sunyer FX: Health hazards of obesity. *Ann Intern Med* 1993; 119:655–660.
6. Klatsky A, Armstrong M: Cardiovascular risk factors among Asian Americans living in northern California. *Am J Public Health* 1991; 81:1423–1428.
7. Alexander JK: The heart and obesity. In: Alexander RW, Schlant RC, Fuster VA (eds): *Hurst's The Heart*, 9th ed. New York, McGraw-Hill, 1998:2407–2412.
8. Matsuzawa YS, Tokunaga FK, Seichiro T: Classification of obesity with respect to morbidity. *Proc Soc Exp Biol Med* 1992; 200:197–201.
9. Welty T, Lee E, Yeh J, et al: Cardiovascular disease risk factors among American Indians: The Strong Heart Study. *Am J Epidemiol* 1995; 142:269–287.
10. Metropolitan Life Insurance Company: New weight standards for men and women. In: *Statistical Bulletin Metropolitan Life Insurance Company*, 1983; 64:2–9.

11. Hamwi GJ: Therapy: Changing dietary concepts. In: Danowski, TS (ed): *Diabetes Mellitus: Diagnosis and Treatment*. New York, American Diabetes Association, 1964:73–78.

12. Quetelet LAJ: *Antropometrics pour mesure des differentes facultés de l'homme*. Brussels, Belgium, C. Muguardt, 1981:479.

13. International Obesity Task Force: Obesity: Preventing and managing the global epidemic. Geneva, World Health Organization, 1988.

14. Siri WE: Body composition from fluid spaces and density: Analysis of methods. In: Brozack J, Henschel A (eds): *Techniques for Measuring Body Composition*. Washington, DC, National Academy of Sciences, 1969:223–244.

15. Schoeller DA: Update: NIH consensus conference. Bioelectrical impedance analysis for the measurement of human body composition: Where do we stand and what is the next step? *Nutrition* 1996; 12:760–762.

16. Laskey A: Duel-energy x-ray absorptiometry and body composition. *Nutrition* 1996; 12:45–51.

17. Forbes GB, Brown MR, Griffiths HJ: Arm muscle plus bone area: Anthropometry and CAT scan compared. *Am J Clin Nutr* 1988; 47:929–931.

18. Goodman-Gruen D, Barret-Connor E: Sex differences in measures of body fat and body distribution in the elderly. *Am J Epidemiol* 1996; 143:898–906.

19. Kannel WB, Gordon T: Physiological and medical concomitants of obesity: The Framingham Study. In: Bray G (ed): *Obesity in America*. Bethesda, MD, U.S. Department of Health, Education, and Welfare, Public Health, Health Service, National Institutes of Health, 1979:123–163.

20. Knowler WC, Narayan KMV, Hanson RL, et al: Perspectives in diabetes. Preventing non-insulin-dependent diabetes. *Diabetes* 1995; 44:483–488.

21. Rimm AAL, Werner H, Yserloo BV, Bernstein RA: Relationship of obesity and disease in 73,532 weight-conscious women. *Public Health Rep* 1975; 90:44–54.

22. Remmers JE, deGroot WJ, Sauerland EK, Anch AM: Pathogenesis of upper airway occlusion during sleep. *J Appl Physiol* 1978; 44:931–938.

23. Andres R, Muller DC, Sorkin JD: Long-term effects of change in body weight on all-cause mortality. A review. *Ann Intern Med* 1993; 119:737–743.

24. Cornoni-Huntley JC, Harris TB, Everett DF, et al: An overview of body weight of older persons, including the impact on mortality. The National Health and Nutrition Examination Survey I—Epidemiologic Follow-up Study. *J Clin Epidemiol* 1991; 44:743–753.

25. Gordon T, Doyle JT: Weight and mortality in men: The Albany Study. *Int J Epidemiol* 1988; 17:77–81.

26. Bjorntorp P: The regulation of adipose tissue distribution in humans. *Int J Obes Relat Metab Disord* 1996; 20:291–302.

27. Horber FF, Gruber B, Thomi F, et al: Effect of sex and age on bone mass, body composition and fuel metabolism in humans. *Nutrition* 1997; 13:524–534.

28. Kotani K, Tokunaga K, Fujioka S, et al: Sexual dimorphism of age-related changes in whole-body fat distribution in the obese. *Int J Obes* 1994; 18:207–212.

29. Anderson KM, Kannel WB: Obesity and disease. In: Bjorntorp P, Brodoff BN (eds): *Obesity*. Philadephia, J.B. Lippincott Co., 1992:465–473.

30. Gautier JF, Mourier A, de Kerviler E, et al: Evaluation of abdominal fat distribution in noninsulin-dependent diabetes mellitus: Relationship to insulin resistance. *J Clin Endocrinol Metab* 1998; 83:1306–1311.

31. Fox K, Peters D, Armstrong N, et al: Abdominal fat deposition in 11-year-old children. *Int J Obes* 1993; 17:11–16.

32. Di Girolamo M, Newby FD, Lovejoy J: Lactate production in adipose tissue: A regulated function with extra-adipose implications. *FASEB J* 1992; 6:2405–2412.

33. Di Girolamo M: Cellular, metabolic, and clinical consequences of adipose mass enlargement in obesity. *Nutrition* 1991; 7:287–289.

34. Expert Panel on the Identification, Evaluation, and Treatment of Overweight in Adults: Clinical guidelines on the identification, evaluation, and treatment of overweight and obesity in adults: Executive summary. *Am J Clin Nutr.* 1998; 68:899–917.

35. Wolthers T, Grofte T, Norrelund H, et al: Differential effects of growth hormone and prednisolone on energy metabolism and leptin levels in humans. *Metabolism* 1998; 47:83–88.

36. Yale CE: Surgery for morbid obesity. Selecting the patient and procedure. *Postgrad Med* 1988; 83:173–175.

37. Watson DI, Game PA: Hand-assisted laparoscopic vertical banded gastroplasty. Initial report. *Surg Endosc* 1997; 11:1218–1220.

38. Mauer MM, Bartness TJ: Body fat regulation after partial lipectomy in Siberian hamsters is photoperiod dependent and fat pad specific. *Am J Physiol* 1994; 266:R870–R878.

39. Leibel R, Hirsch J: Diminished energy requirements in reduced-obese patients. *Metabolism* 1984; 33:164–170.

STEPHEN D. CLEMENTS /
LARRY RAY

# ANTIBIOTIC PROPHYLAXIS FOR THE PREVENTION OF BACTERIAL ENDOCARDITIS

Endocarditis and endarteritis are dreaded complications of cardiovascular disease and are associated with a high mortality and morbidity despite modern treatment regimens; therefore, prevention is very important.

Over the years, our understanding of the pathogenesis of endocarditis has come a long way. In the presence of structural heart disease, bacteremia can result in colonization and invasion of valvular endocardial surfaces, followed by the clinical syndrome of bacterial endocarditis.

Dental procedures, including dental cleaning, scaling, and some surgical procedures (those not involving a sterile surgical field) and instrumentations, result in transient bacteremia lasting up to 15 or 20 min. These procedures place individuals with valve disease at risk of developing endocarditis. Prophylactic measures are directed at the bacteremia associated with these procedures and offer some hope for prevention.

Not all individuals with endocarditis have had preceding procedures that can be identified as a source of bacteremia. Also, observations suggest that only certain bacteria are prone to cause endocarditis. From this information, an approach to prevention has been developed. These recommendations are made with the knowledge that there are no carefully controlled studies that offer conclusive proof that current regimens are fully effective.

Fortunately, the incidence of endocarditis is low even in the presence of bacteremia; and the risk is higher with valve disease and some cardiac conditions than with other conditions. Antibiotics are not without risk and are not inexpensive, so they must be carefully considered.

Given this background knowledge, recommendations for endocarditis prophylaxis have been developed by a group appointed by the American Heart Association; these recommendations were most recently revised and published in 1997.[1]

Certain cardiac conditions can be categorized as high risk and moderate risk according to the potential outcome if endocarditis occurs (Table 24-1).

Mitral valve prolapse deserves special attention. Mitral valve prolapse without regurgitation does not require prophylaxis; however, when regurgitation is present, prophylaxis is required. Controversy exists concerning patients with isolated nonejection clicks, since some of these individuals have intermittent mitral regurgitation. Similar controversy exists concerning those with thickened anterior mitral valve leaflets. These must be considered on an individual basis.

Significant bacteremia following certain procedures can potentially result in endocarditis. Dental procedures are high on the list (Table 24-2), and the bacteremia

## TABLE 24-1.   Cardiac Conditions Associated with Endocarditis

### Endocarditis Prophylaxis Recommended

High-risk category
   Prosthetic cardiac valves, including bioprosthetic and homograft valves
   Previous bacterial endocarditis
   Complex cyanotic congenital heart disease (e.g., single ventricle states,
      transposition of the great arteries, tetralogy of Fallot)
   Surgically constructed systemic pulmonary shunts or conduits

Moderate-risk category
   Most other congenital cardiac malformations (other than above and below)
   Acquired valvular dysfunction (e.g., rheumatic heart disease)
   Hypertrophic cardiomyopathy
   Mitral valve prolapse with valvular regurgitation and/or thickened leaflets[*]

### Endocarditis Prophylaxis Not Recommended

Negligible-risk category (no greater risk than the general population)
   Isolated secundum atrial septal defect
   Surgical repair of atrial septal defect, ventricular septal defect, or patent ductus
      arteriosus (without residua beyond 6 months)
   Previous coronary artery bypass graft surgery
   Mitral valve prolapse without valvular regurgitation[*]
   Physiologic, functional, or innocent heart murmurs[*]
   Previous Kawasaki disease without valvular dysfunction
   Previous rheumatic fever without valvular dysfunction
   Cardiac pacemakers (intravascular and epicardial) and implanted defibrillators

* See text for further details.

*Source:* From Dajani AS, Taubert KA, Wilson W, et al: Prevention of bacterial endocarditis: Recommendations by the American Heart Association. *JAMA* 1997; 277:1794–1801, with permission. Copyright 1997, American Medical Association.

**TABLE 24-2.  Dental Procedures and Endocarditis Prophylaxis**

| Endocarditis Prophylaxis Recommended* |
|---|
| Dental extractions |
| Periodontal procedures including surgery, scaling and root planing, probing, and recall maintenance |
| Dental implant placement and reimplantation of avulsed teeth |
| Endodontic (root canal) instrumentation or surgery only beyond the apex |
| Subgingival placement of antibiotic fibers or strips |
| Initial placement of orthodontic bands but not brackets |
| Intraligamentary local anesthetic injections |
| Prophylactic cleaning of teeth or implants where bleeding is anticipated |
| **Endocarditis Prophylaxis Not Recommended** |
| Restorative dentistry[†] (operative and prosthodontic) with or without retraction cord[‡] |
| Local anesthetic injections (nonintraligamentary) |
| Intracanal endodontic treatment; postplacement and buildup |
| Placement of rubber dams |
| Postoperative suture removal |
| Placement of removable prosthodontic or orthodontic appliances |
| Taking of oral impressions |
| Fluoride treatments |
| Taking of oral radiographs |
| Orthodontic appliance adjustment |
| Shedding of primary teeth |

[*] Prophylaxis is recommended for patients with high- and moderate-risk cardiac conditions.

[†] This includes restoration of decayed teeth (filling cavities) and replacement of missing teeth.

[‡] Clinical judgment may indicate antibiotic use in selected circumstances that may create significant bleeding.

*Source:* From Dajani AS, Taubert KA, Wilson W, et al: Prevention of bacterial endocarditis: Recommendations by the American Heart Association. *JAMA* 1997; 277:1794–1801, with permission. Copyright 1997, American Medical Association.

that follows these procedures is related in part to the state of oral hygiene. Excellent oral hygiene is the best prophylaxis for limiting bacteremia.

If unexpected bleeding occurs during a procedure that is not ordinarily treated prophylactically, antibiotics can be given effectively within 2 h. After 4 h, antibiotics probably have no benefit.

When several procedures are needed, they should be grouped as much as possible in order to avoid development of a resistant organism population. Intervals of 9 to 14 days between procedures have been recommended.[1]

Bacteremia associated with respiratory tract procedures depends on the procedure (Table 24-3). Bronchoscopy using a flexible bronchoscope, with or without biopsy, produces only a low incidence of bacteremia; however, use of a rigid bronchoscope may result in more disruption of the mucosa and, therefore, more bacteremia. Endocarditis prophylaxis is indicated for procedures with the rigid bronchoscope but not the flexible one.

Routine endoscopic procedures including transesophageal echocardiography are associated with a low incidence of bacteremia, and prophylaxis is optional for high-risk individuals, such as those with prosthetic valves. This includes procedures with biopsy or polypectomy.

Other procedures associated with a high incidence of bacteremia and thus warranting prophylactic antibiotics include dilation of esophageal strictures, sclerosis of esophageal valves, and especially biliary tract procedures and surgery.

The genitourinary tract is not a common source of endocarditis but is second to the oral cavity as an entry area. Bacteremia after genitourinary manipulation is more common in the presence of urinary tract infections. Care should be taken to avoid this situation by identifying the offending organism, eradicating the infection with the appropriate antimicrobial, and then proceeding. Prophylaxis should be guided by culture information, with the most likely organisms being enterococcus or *Klebsiella*.

Uncomplicated vaginal delivery is associated with a low incidence of bacteremia, and endocarditis following this procedure is uncommon. Prophylaxis is, therefore, not recommended. Cervical biopsy and intrauterine device insertion do not require prophylaxis, but removal of an intrauterine device probably does.

Individuals taking antibiotics for the prevention of rheumatic fever are not protected from bacteremia—penicillin-resistant *Streptococcus viridans* or other organisms require the use of clindamycin or azithromycin or clarithromycin. If possible, a delay of 9 to 14 days is desirable in order for usual mouth flora to return.

Infected tissues should be approached with the most likely organism in mind (Tables 24-4 and 24-5). Antistaphylococcal penicillins, first-generation cephalosporins for routine non-oral cavity organisms, and clindamycin or even vancomycin for more virulent organisms, including methicillin-resistant *Staphylococcus aureus,* should be used. Urinary tract infections may require aminoglycosides or third-generation cephalosporins.

Cardiac surgery requires special consideration, since the consequences are very serious. Dental health should be optimized before surgery is performed, even if this

## TABLE 24-3. Other Procedures and Endocarditis Prophylaxis

### Endocarditis Prophylaxis Recommended

Respiratory tract
  Tonsillectomy and/or adenoidectomy
  Surgical operations that involve respiratory mucosa
  Bronchoscopy with a rigid bronchoscope

Gastrointestinal tract*
  Sclerotherapy for esophageal varices
  Esophageal stricture dilation
  Endoscopic retrograde cholangiography with biliary obstruction
  Biliary tract surgery
  Surgical operations that involve intestinal mucosa

Genitourinary tract
  Prostatic surgery
  Cystoscopy
  Urethral dilation

### Endocarditis Prophylaxis Not Recommended

Respiratory tract
  Endotracheal intubation
  Bronchoscopy with a flexible bronchoscope, with or without biopsy†
  Tympanostomy tube insertion

Gastrointestinal tract
  Transesophageal echocardiography†
  Endoscopy with or without gastrointestinal biopsy†

Genitourinary tract
  Vaginal hysterectomy†
  Vaginal delivery†
  Cesarean section
  In uninfected tissue:
    Urethral catheterization
    Uterine dilatation and curettage
    Therapeutic abortion
    Sterilization procedures
    Insertion or removal of intrauterine devices

Other
  Cardiac catheterization, including balloon angioplasty
  Implanted cardiac pacemakers, implanted defibrillators, and coronary stents
  Incision or biopsy of surgically scrubbed skin
  Circumcision

* Prophylaxis is recommended for high-risk patients; optional for medium-risk patients.

† Prophylaxis is optional for high-risk patients.

*Source:* From Dajani AS, Taubert KA, Wilson W, et al: Prevention of bacterial endocarditis: Recommendations by the American Heart Association. *JAMA* 1997; 277:1794–1801, with permission. Copyright 1997, American Medical Association.

**TABLE 24-4.   Prophylactic Regimens for Dental, Oral, Respiratory Tract, or Esophageal Procedures**

| Situation | Agent | Regimen* |
|---|---|---|
| Standard general prophylaxis | Amoxicillin | Adults: 2.0 g; children: 50 mg/kg orally 1 h before procedure |
| Unable to take oral medications | Ampicillin | Adults: 2.0 g intramuscularly (IM) or intravenously (IV); children: 50 mg/kg IM or IV within 30 min before procedure |
| Allergic to penicillin | Clindamycin *or* | Adults: 600 mg; children: 20 mg/kg orally 1 h before procedure |
|  | Cephalexin[†] or cefadroxil[†] *or* | Adults: 2.0 g; children: 50 mg/kg orally 1 h before procedure |
|  | Azithromycin or clarithromycin | Adults: 500 mg; children: 15 mg/kg orally 1 h before procedure |
| Allergic to penicillin and unable to take oral medications | Clindamycin *or* | Adults: 600 mg; children: 20 mg/kg IV within 30 min before procedure |
|  | Cefazolin[†] | Adults: 1.0 g; children: 25 mg/kg IM or IV within 30 min before procedure |

* Total children's dose should not exceed adult dose.

† Cephalosporins should not be used in individuals with immediate-type hypersensitivity reaction (urticaria angioedema, or anaphylaxis) to penicillins.

*Source:* From Dajani AS, Taubert KA, Wilson W, et al: Prevention of bacterial endocarditis: Recommendations by the American Heart Association. *JAMA* 1997; 277:1794–1801, with permission. Copyright 1997, American Medical Association.

means that a delay in the surgery is necessary. Responsible organisms are most commonly *S. aureus*, coagulase-negative or diphtheroids. Staphylococcus and fungal infections are not as common. First-generation cephalosporins are most often used; however, if other organisms are anticipated, then antibiotics should be tailored for them, such as vancomycin for methicillin-resistant *S. aureus*. Antibiotics should be started immediately before the procedure and continued for no more than 24 h.

Some cardiac procedures, such as valve replacement, result in perpetual increased risk of endocarditis. With others, such as closure of a ventricular septal defect or patent ductus arteriosus, the risk of endocarditis falls to the level of the general population 6 months after the procedure. Vascular grafts that are not coronary probably warrant prophylaxis for 6 months. Coronary bypass procedures require antibiotic prophylaxis for the procedure itself but not thereafter. Post-heart transplant patients with immunosuppression probably do require prophylaxis.

Although endocarditis prophylaxis regimens have not been proven to prevent all

**TABLE 24-5.   Prophylactic Regimens for Genitourinary Gastrointestinal (Excluding Esophageal) Procedures**

| Situation | Agents* | Regimen† |
|---|---|---|
| High-risk patients | Ampicillin plus gentamicin | Adults: ampicillin 2.0 g intramuscularly (IM) or intravenously (IV) plus gentamicin 1.5 mg/kg (not to exceed 120 mg) within 30 min of starting the procedure; 6 h later, ampicillin 1 g IM/IV or amoxicillin 1 g orally |
| | | Children: ampicillin 50 mg/kg IM or IV (not to exceed 2.0 g) plus gentamicin 1.5 mg/kg within 30 min of starting the procedure; 6 h later, ampicillin 25 mg/kg IM/IV or amoxicillin 25 mg/kg orally |
| High-risk patients allergic to ampicillin/amoxicillin | Vancomycin plus gentamicin | Adults: vancomycin 1.0 g IV over 1–2 h plus gentamicin 1.5 mg/kg IV/IM (not to exceed 120 mg); complete injection/infusion within 30 min of starting the procedure |
| | | Children: vancomycin 20 mg/kg IV over 1–2 h plus gentamicin 1.5 mg/kg IV/IM; complete injection/infusion within 30 min of starting the procedure |
| Moderate-risk patients | Amoxicillin or ampicillin | Adults: amoxicillin 2.0 g orally 1 h before procedure, or ampicillin 2.0 g IM/IV within 30 min of starting the procedure |
| | | Children: amoxicillin 50 mg/kg orally 1 h before procedure, or ampicillin 50 mg/kg IM/IV within 30 min of starting the procedure |
| Moderate-risk patients allergic to ampicillin/amoxicillin | Vancomycin | Adults: vancomycin 1.0 g IV over 1–2 h; complete infusion within 30 min of starting the procedure |
| | | Children: vancomycin 20 mg/kg IV over 1–2 h; complete infusion within 30 min of starting the procedure |

* Total children's dose should not exceed adult dose.

† No second dose of vancomycin or gentamicin is recommended.

*Source:* From Dajani AS, Taubert KA, Wilson W, et al: Prevention of bacterial endocarditis: Recommendations by the American Heart Association. *JAMA* 1997; 277:1794–1801, with permission. Copyright 1997, American Medical Association.

cases of endocarditis, they are the best that can be put forth at this point in time. They represent the best effort of the ad hoc group appointed by the American Heart Association and should be carefully applied to current clinical situations.

---

## REFERENCES

1.  Dajani AS, Taubert KA, Wilson W, et al: Prevention of bacterial endocarditis: Recommendations by the American Heart Association. *JAMA* 1997; 277:1794–1801.

# MANAGEMENT OF CARDIOVASCULAR DISEASES

J. JEFFREY MARSHALL

# OUTPATIENT TREATMENT OF STABLE ANGINA PECTORIS

Ischemic heart disease is a heterogeneous array of clinical entities linked by the common etiology of coronary atherosclerosis. These clinical syndromes vary from the asymptomatic phases of coronary plaque growth that occur in the second and third decades of life, to the abrupt clinical manifestation of sudden cardiac death in previously asymptomatic patients, to stable angina pectoris, and finally to end-stage patients with congestive heart failure (CHF) from multiple myocardial infarctions (MIs). Each of these cardiovascular diagnoses obviously falls within the spectrum of ischemic heart disease. The treatments for these diverse disease states or diagnoses, however, are as far as the east is from the west. Thus, when approaching the outpatient management of ischemic heart disease, one must identify a more singular diagnosis in your patient. This chapter will focus on the clinical entity of stable angina, one type of ischemic heart disease.

## PREVALENCE AND ECONOMIC IMPACT

The exact prevalence of stable angina pectoris in the United States is not known with certainty. In an adult primary care practice, however, it is certainly one of the most common diagnoses requiring aggressive, frequent, chronic medical therapy. Several facts and estimates support the idea that the diagnosis of chronic stable angina pectoris is a frequent clinical problem in the outpatient setting. Coronary artery disease remains the number one cause of death in the United States[1] and is responsible for more than 20 percent of all deaths in America. The death rates as compared to those from the second most common killer in America, cancer, are shown in Table 25-1. In approximately one-half of all patients with coronary artery disease (CAD), the initial diagnostic feature is stable angina pectoris. The American Heart Association (AHA) has estimated that 6.2 million Americans have chest pain.[2] The American

TABLE 25-1.   Death Rates per 100,000 Population (Not Adjusted for Age)

| Patient Group | Diseases of the Heart | Cancer |
|---|---|---|
| Caucasian males | 297.9 | 228.1 |
| African American males | 244.2 | 209.1 |
| Caucasian females | 297.4 | 202.4 |
| African American females | 231.1 | 159.1 |

*Source:* Adapted from National Center for Health Statistics: Report of final mortality statistics, 1995. *Monthly Vital Statistics Report,* vol 45, no. 11. Hyattsville, MD, Public Health Service, 1997.

College of Cardiology (ACC) and American Heart Association guidelines on chronic stable angina[3] estimate that up to 16.5 million Americans may have chest pain syndromes consistent with stable angina pectoris. This estimate may even be less than the actual prevalence, as it does not include patients who choose not to seek medical attention. The conversion from stable angina pectoris to one of the acute (unstable) coronary syndromes results in more than 6 million encounters in emergency rooms in the United States.[1] Of these patients visiting the emergency room, more than 1.1 million will have an acute myocardial infarction (AMI).

The economic impact of stable angina pectoris is staggering. Diagnosis-related group data from Medicare patients show that approximately $7.5 billion is spent on direct care of patients with chronic stable angina. If one conservatively assumes that the cost for the remainder of the patients with the same diagnosis (those not covered by Medicare) is about the same, then the direct costs for patients with stable angina pectoris probably exceed $15 billion annually!

## DEFINITION

Stable angina pectoris is said to be present when the angina has persisted unchanged in frequency, duration, and precipitating causes for 60 days.

A comprehensive understanding of the pathophysiology, diagnosis, risk stratification, appropriate testing, and efficient treatment and follow-up of patients with stable angina pectoris is essential for primary care physicians, especially in the outpatient practice setting.

## PATHOPHYSIOLOGY

The pathophysiology of stable angina pectoris is quite different from that of the acute coronary syndromes of (1) sudden cardiac death, (2) unstable angina pectoris, and (3) AMI. In the acute coronary syndromes, coronary thrombosis is the major pathophysiologic event, resulting in a decrease in blood supply (Fig. 25-1*B*). In stable angina pectoris, however, coronary thrombosis is not a major contributor to the development of symptoms. Anginal symptoms in stable angina pectoris usually result from an imbalance between myocardial oxygen demand and the available myocardial oxygen supply (Fig. 25-1C). The lack of adequate coronary blood flow can occur, in a binary model, from either decreased supply or increased demand (Fig. 25-1). In the decreased supply scenario (Fig. 25-1B), an episode of angina at a relatively low cardiac workload may be caused by reduced blood flow through narrowed, atherosclerotic coronary arteries supplying a specific zone of myocardium (i.e., deficiency in supply). Alternatively, in the increased demand scenario (Fig. 25-1C), the reduced amount of coronary blood flow occurs secondary to increased demand for myocardial oxygen delivery. In this instance, blood and oxygen delivery are adequate at rest, but during exercise, the myocardial need for oxygen is higher

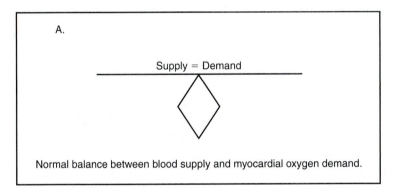

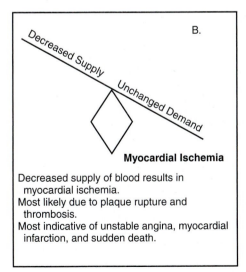

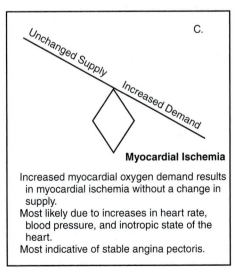

Figure 25-1.  Pathophysiology of ischemic syndromes.

than the diseased coronary arteries can supply because of increased heart rate, blood pressure, and inotropic state of the myocardium. In reality, this is not simply a binary system of increased demand or reduced supply, but rather a dynamic system with interacting supply and demand issues that result in an imbalance between the supply and demand and results in angina.

The initial pathophysiologic process that leads to stable angina pectoris is coronary atherosclerosis. Although a full discussion of the pathogenesis of atheroslcerosis is beyond the scope of this chapter, an understanding of the atherosclerotic process is required for an appropriate diagnosis and treatment of stable angina pectoris.

Atherosclerosis of coronary blood vessels occurs because of an either inherited or acquired dysfunction of the blood vessel wall. In order to appreciate the ways in which dysfunction of the blood vessel wall leads to symptoms in stable angina pectoris, one must first understand the normal coronary artery function. In the normal coronary artery, the intima (composed of endothelial cells and the internal elastic lamina) is a smooth, mirror-like surface that acts as the interface between the vessel wall and the circulating blood elements. The intima of a coronary artery serves as a permeability barrier, provides the antithrombotic surface that is exposed to the circulating blood, and is the metabolic factory of the blood vessel wall. The media of a coronary artery is composed of vascular smooth muscle and connective tissue. The main function of the media is to control the minute-to-minute diameter of the artery in response to vasoactive substances secreted by the intima, excreted by the formed blood elements, or derived from exogenous medications. The balance between vasoconstriction and vasodilation is an important determinant of the total amount of blood flow delivered to the distal myocardium. The adventitial layer of a coronary artery is composed mainly of connective tissue elements that serve to hold the blood vessel in place on the surface of the beating heart muscle. Additionally, the adventitia contains the vaso vasorum, the microscopic blood supply of the coronary artery.

The first stage of atherosclerosis involves endothelial injury. Several cardiac risk factors are known to injure the endothelium. Diabetes mellitus, hypertension, cigarette smoking, and hypercholesterolemia are all known to damage the protective attributes of the vascular endothelium in the intima. These risk factors promote oxidative stress in the blood vessel wall and promote an inflammatory response. This inflammatory response promotes the expression of certain receptors on the surface of the vascular endothelium that allow white blood cells (WBCs) and circulating monocytes to invade the vessel wall. In addition, the protective endothelial barrier now becomes more permeable to cholesterol, particularly the low-density lipoprotein (LDL) particle.

The next step of the atherosclerotic process involves a complex interaction between the WBCs, monocytes, LDL, and the constitutive cells within the blood vessel wall (i.e., vascular smooth muscle cells and connective tissue cells). The WBCs and monocytes, now within the blood vessel wall, attack and oxidize the LDL. This oxidized LDL further promotes the inflammatory process within the vascular wall and leads to the growth of smooth muscle cells and their migration from the media to the intima. This leads to the growth of the atherosclerotic plaque, or blockage, within the intima of the coronary artery. Pools or deposits of cholesterol then begin to coalesce into "lipid lakes" within the plaque. These lipid lakes are one of the key anatomic features of a complex plaque. These complex plaques then grow by a cycle of plaque rupture, thrombosis, and fibrosis. When plaques occupy more than 70 percent of the cross-sectional area of the lumen of the coronary artery, they may become flow-limiting and cause effort-induced angina in patients with stable angina.

## DIAGNOSIS

As stated earlier, and restated here for emphasis, stable angina pectoris is defined as chest discomfort having the characteristics described below that is unchanged for 60 days.

The diagnosis of angina remains a clinical diagnosis that is made from the history and physical examination. Angina is defined as a *discomfort in the chest* or adjacent areas (neck, jaw, shoulder, humerus, or epigastrium) that is due to myocardial ischemia. The discomfort is often described as a "heaviness," a "pressure-like sensation," a "vice-like feeling," or a "constricting" or "crushing" sensation. Some patients describe the sensation of angina as "something swelling up inside" the chest. Sharp, stabbing, or fleeting chest pain is not indicative of angina pectoris. Not all patients, however, manifest myocardial ischemia as chest pain or discomfort. Indeed, some patients, especially diabetics, have no symptoms at all. This is termed *silent ischemia.* The reason that some patients have silent ischemia is not clear. It may be because of autonomic denervation. Still other patients experience anginal equivalents (nonanginal symptoms of myocardial ischemia). Common anginal equivalents include exertional dyspnea, fatigue, and faintness. In both patients with silent ischemic and patients with anginal equivalents, it has been well demonstrated that ischemia electrocardiographic changes are present in the absence of chest pain or during the anginal equivalent, respectively.

The *site* of the discomfort is usually retrosternal, and radiation of the discomfort to the ulnar surface of either arm, the neck, the jaw, or the throat commonly occurs. It is uncommon for the discomfort to radiate above the mandible or inferior to the epigastrium.

The appropriate *duration* of chest discomfort is suggestive of the diagnosis of anginal chest pain. Anginal discomfort in patients with stable angina is usually precipitated by exertion and lasts 5 to 10 min after physical activity is stopped. The response of anginal chest discomfort to medications and cessation of exercise is also helpful in making the diagnosis of angina pectoris. When exertion is ceased, anginal chest discomfort usually takes 5 to 10 min to abate. The response to sublingual nitroglycerine can also be used as a diagnostic tool. In patients with true anginal chest pain, the administration of nitroglycerine results in chest pain relief within 30 s to 5 min. Thus, chest discomfort that lasts for days or that is relieved immediately with nitroglycerine is unlikely to be angina pectoris. Chest discomfort thought to be due to myocardial ischemia that lasts 30 min or more or chest pain that occurs at rest suggests MI and should be treated aggressively in the hospital, not in the outpatient setting.

Anginal chest pain should be classified in every patient. One important distinction should be made before classifying all comers. That is, "Does this patient have stable or unstable angina?" Angina that is designated as stable must not have changed in 60 days. Unstable angina is angina at rest, severe new-onset angina, and increasing frequency of angina (or angina that is precipitated by a lower exercise threshold or is longer in duration). Unstable angina should be managed in the inpatient setting. Stable angina is most commonly classified by the Canadian Cardiovascular Society Classification System (see Table 25-2), which uses common daily activities as a guideline to stratify patients with angina pectoris.

Most patients with stable angina pectoris have fixed-threshold angina. Fixed-threshold angina is defined as angina that occurs with a constant amount of physical exertion. Thus, patients will complain of anginal chest discomfort each time they walk to the mailbox or after climbing one flight of stairs. Patients often complain that activities involving motions or an exercise requiring the use of their hands and arms above their heads most predictably precipitates angina at a fixed threshold. Hurrying also tends to precipitate angina at a predictable workload. Fixed-threshold angina is due to an increase in myocardial oxygen demand. As the patient exercises to the threshold of precipitating angina, the heart rate, blood pressure, and inotropic state of the heart increase. These increases result in increased myocardial oxygen demand (see Fig. 25-1C). The diseased coronary arteries cannot meet the de-

**TABLE 25-2.   Canadian Cardiovascular Society Classification of Anginal Symptoms**

*Class I*

Ordinary physical activity does not cause angina, such as walking or climbing stairs. Angina occurs with strenuous activity or with rapid or prolonged exertion at work or recreation.

*Class II*

Slight limitation of ordinary activity. Angina occurs on walking or climbing stairs rapidly, walking uphill, walking or stair climbing after meals, or in cold, or in wind, or under emotional stress, or only during the few hours after awakening. Angina occurs on walking more than two blocks on the level and climbing more than one flight of ordinary stairs at a normal pace and in normal condition.

*Class III*

Marked limitations of ordinary physical activity. Angina occurs on walking one to two blocks on the level and climbing one flight of stairs in normal conditions and at a normal pace.

*Class IV*

Inability to carry on any physical activity without discomfort; anginal symptoms may be present at rest.

*Source:* Campeau L: Grading of angina pectoris. *Circulation* 1976; 54:522, with permission of the publisher and author.

mand for oxygen, however, because of fixed atherosclerotic plaques that impede blood flow. Therefore, the heart muscle becomes ischemic. The myocardial ischemia leads to the sensation of anginal chest pain and signals the patient to stop the activity at a relatively fixed threshold of exertion.

Not all patients with stable angina demonstrate the clinical pattern of fixed-threshold angina. Some patients demonstrate variable-threshold angina. Variable-threshold angina is defined as angina precipitated at variable amounts of physical activity. Thus, these patients will state that they have "good days" and "bad days." On good days, they can engage in much more physical activity without any episodes of angina. On bad days, very little physical exertion results in angina pectoris. Patients with variable-threshold angina will often complain of chest discomfort following meals, chest pain precipitated by cold weather, and even chest pain at rest. Vasoconstriction at sites of coronary artery blockages (plaques) or even at "normal" sites causes variable-threshold angina. The ensuing vasoconstriction leads to a decrease in myocardial oxygen supply (see Fig. 25-1B) and results in ischemia. The myocardial ischemia causes anginal chest pain, and this occurs at varying levels of physical exertion because it is due to changes in supply, not changes in demand.

Most patients fall into either the fixed-threshold or the variable-threshold angina category. A minority of patients, however, fall in between these two classifications of anginal patterns. These patients, who have some features of fixed-threshold angina and some features of variable-threshold angina, are said to have mixed angina. The presumed pathophysiology in this group of patients is that they have fixed coronary blockages (plaques) that account for the fixed-threshold, increased-demand-mediated angina and they have an element of vasoconstriction that accounts for the variable-threshold component of angina. These diagnostic classifications of the different types of anginal patterns are helpful in selecting treatments.

The presence or absence of cardiac *risk factors* is important in helping the clinician evaluate the likelihood that the chest pain experienced by the patient is angina. Smoking more than half a pack of cigarettes per day within the last 5 years increases the probability of coronary artery disease. If the patient is diabetic (fasting blood glucose >140 mg/dL on two occasions) or hyperlipidemic (total cholesterol >250 mg/dL), then the likelihood of coronary disease and angina is significantly increased. Of these three risk factors, diabetes mellitus is the most powerful predictor in a model of predicting coronary disease risks from the history and physical examination.[4] Surprisingly, family history of coronary disease and hypertension, although very important risk factors for developing coronary disease and angina, were not statistically significant as independent predictors for the presence of coronary disease and angina from the history and physical examination alone.

## Other Causes of Chest Discomfort

Not all chest pain is anginal, and the differential diagnosis of chest pain can be quite challenging. Many patients believe that any chest pain on the left side of the chest or the left arm must be originating from the heart and may seek medical attention. Several other clinical diagnoses can cause chest discomfort, however.

*Esophageal disorders* are frequent causes of chest pain. The chest pain from esophageal disorders can mimic the pain from myocardial ischemia (i.e., angina). Reflux of the acidic gastric contents into the lower esophagus can cause retrosternal discomfort. This discomfort is more often described as a burning or "heartburn" sensation and may be associated with reflux of acidic-tasting fluid into the oropharynx. Esophageal spasm may also cause chest discomfort. This type of pain may be constant in nature and may be relieved by sublingual nitroglycerine. Esophageal discomfort often occurs in relation to the intake of food or may awaken patients at night. These precipitating factors may make it more difficult to distinguish esophageal pain from angina. Unlike angina, esophageal pain may respond to antacids, milk, or food, and occasionally may be ameliorated by the consumption of warm liquids.

*Biliary colic* may also produce symptoms similar to angina. The pain results from increased biliary pressure secondary to obstruction of the cystic duct. The location of biliary colic pain may be epigastric, retrosternal, or in either the right or left upper quadrant of the abdomen. Unlike angina, the pain usually lasts for 2 to 4 h and is generally constant.

*Musculoskeletal disorders* can also masquerade as angina pectoris. Costochondritis may cause severe chest pain and discomfort. The pain is usually precordial, at or near the costochondral junctions. The pain may be sharp, aching, or dull in nature. Palpation of the inflamed costochondral junctions causes pain and is useful in diagnosing this syndrome. This is a common disorder, and the presence of tender costochondral junctions does not exclude the concomitant presence of angina pectoris. Cervical and thoracic nerve root pain can mimic anginal chest pain. This discomfort is often precordial, scapular, or in the shoulder or neck. Unlike in angina, there is often a hyperalgesic area of the skin that can be noted by running a finger down the back of the patient.

There are several *cardiopulmonary disorders* that can cause symptoms similar to angina pectoris. Pulmonary embolism is a cause of chest pain, but this is usually pleuritic in nature. A pulmonary embolus is usually associated with dyspnea, and this can be confused with the shortness of breath experienced by patients with prolonged bouts of angina with resultant left ventricular dysfunction and pulmonary congestion. Unlike in angina, the pleuritic nature of the pain and the presence of a pleural rub tend to point toward pulmonary emboli as an etiology of this symptom/sign complex.

*Aortic dissection* is another cardiovascular cause of chest pain. The discomfort of an aortic dissection is usually retrosternal and radiates through to the back. It is often described as a tearing or ripping pain, and patients may call it the "worst pain they've ever had." A past history of hypertension is common, and the physical examination often reveals a pulse and blood pressure deficit between the right and left arms.

*Pericarditis* is also a cause of chest pain. The pain, at times, can be difficult to distinguish from anginal chest pain. It tends to occur in younger patients, and the pain is often pleuritic and exacerbated by positional changes. The pain of pericarditis is often alleviated by sitting up and leaning forward, but is worse with inspiration and lying supine. The physical examination may disclose a pericardial friction rub that is suggestive of pericardial inflammation; although a friction rub can occur with an AMI, it does not occur with angina.

The *general physical examination* is aimed at detecting signs of *cardiac risk factors*. The examination of the head and neck may reveal xanthomas or xanthelasma, indicative of hyperlipidemia. Corneal arcus in young men may also be indicative of elevated lipids. The presence of an earlobe crease in patients less than 50 years of age, except in Native Americans and Asian Americans, has been correlated with a higher incidence of CAD and cardiovascular mortality. The presence of bruits over the carotid and femoral arteries is indicative of peripheral arterial occlusive disease and is suggestive of the presence of CAD. A careful examination of the peripheral pulses may also identify patients with peripheral arterial occlusive disease, a finding that increases the likelihood of finding coronary artery disease.

The cardiac examination in patients with a history of chest pain is often entirely normal if it is performed at a time when the patient is not actively having chest pain. A cardiac examination made while the patient is having pain, however, may demonstrate several helpful findings. The presence of a new third or fourth heart sound, a paradoxically split $S_2$, a new murmur of mitral regurgitation, or new rales with chest pain is highly suggestive of angina and significant CAD.

## DIAGNOSTIC TESTING AND RISK STRATIFICATION

Even though a highly suggestive history and physical examination has a high predictive value in the diagnosis of ischemic heart disease and angina, many times the history and physical examination are not conclusive and suggest an intermediate risk of the patient's having CAD and stable angina. In this group of patients, noninvasive testing is necessary to confirm the possible diagnosis of CAD and angina. Several testing modalities are available and are discussed below.

A *resting electrocardiogram* (ECG) is an important diagnostic tool and should be obtained in every patient being evaluated for a history of chest pain. Unfortunately, the resting (non-chest pain) ECG is normal in approximately one-half of patients who do indeed have coronary artery disease and stable angina pectoris, and so a normal ECG does not exclude the presence of severe disease. The finding of left bundle branch block in a patient with a good history for angina increases the likelihood of multivessel CAD and carries a poor prognosis. On the other hand, incomplete right bundle branch block has no increased predictive value of cardiovascular events in the patient with presumed angina. An ECG obtained during an episode of chest pain is a very powerful diagnostic tool if it is positive for ischemia. A finding of ≥1 mm of flat or downsloping ST depression, dynamic symmetrically inverted T waves, or transient ST elevation is diagnostic of CAD and angina. The converse finding, however, is not helpful in eliminating angina as a diagnosis; that is, a normal ECG done during an episode of chest discomfort does not rule out the presence of ischemic heart disease and angina.

A *chest x-ray film* is recommended in the evaluation of a patient with presumed coronary artery disease and stable angina. Although it is normal in over 50 percent of patients, it can be useful in diagnosis if certain findings are discovered. The presence of coronary artery calcifications would be diagnostic of coronary artery disease and would support the diagnosis of angina in a patient with a history of chest pain. The x-ray film of the chest may show signs of cardiac enlargement in some patients who have had a prior MI and pulmonary venous congestion consistent with left ventricular dysfunction and heart failure. However, the x-ray film of the chest is usually normal in patients with angina pectoris.

*Laboratory blood work* is useful in the evaluation of a patient with a history of chest pain. In the most recent guidelines from the AHA and ACC, a fasting glucose, a fasting lipid profile [total cholesterol, high-density lipoprotein (HDL) cholesterol, calculated LDL cholesterol, and triglycerides], and a hemoglobin are the recommended studies. Other studies should be obtained as suggested by the clinical history. For example, one should check thyroid-stimulating hormone (TSH) in an elderly patient with signs and symptoms of hyperthyroidism and new onset of anginal-quality chest discomfort. Importantly, in this example, it is obvious that a TSH is not indicated in the evaluation of every patient who presents with chest pain.

*Exercise electrocardiography,* or exercise stress testing or exercise tolerance testing (all three are synonymous), has long been the cornerstone of noninvasive testing for patients with a history of chest pain and possible angina. Stress testing is performed to answer several clinical questions. The most common question is, "Does my patient have CAD, and is his/her chest pain history really angina?" In other words, the exercise test is done for diagnostic reasons. A second question is, "What is the long-term prognosis of my patient with established or possible CAD and chest pain?" That is, the reason for requesting the test is to risk-stratify a patient with possible angina. A third question is, "What is the exercise capacity of my patient with chest pain or dyspnea?" This third reason to request an exercise test is to measure, as objectively as possible, the patient's response to and tolerance for exercise—that is, to make a functional exercise assessment. In this chapter, the first two indications for stress testing will be highlighted.

When referring a patient whose chest pain is not diagnostic of angina but in whom angina is possible for exercise stress testing, several practical issues need to be addressed before scheduling the examination. The first is to determine which of the three questions needs to be answered. Next, there are contraindications to stress testing that should be carefully considered before performing an exercise test. Absolute contraindications include patients with unstable angina pectoris, MI, left main CAD, severe or symptomatic aortic stenosis, symptomatic heart failure, cardiac arrhythmias causing symptoms of hemodynamic compromise, acute pulmonary embolus or infarction, and acute aortic dissection. Relative contraindications include moderate aortic stenosis, electrolyte disturbances, systolic hypertension >200 mmHg, diastolic hypertension >110 mmHg, tachy- or bradyarrhythmias, idiopathic hypertrophic subaortic stenosis (IHSS), high-degree atrioventricular block, and inability to exercise safely. Finally, there are some conditions in which a standard exercise ECG stress test is not indicated because they impair the interpretation of the ST segment of the ECG that is needed for the correct diagnosis. These include complete left bundle branch block, left ventricular hypertrophy with repolarization abnormalities, electronically paced rhythm, Wolff-Parkinson-White syndrome, and patients on digoxin.

The next important consideration before performing a stress test on a patient to confirm the suspected diagnosis of CAD and stable angina is the probability that a positive test will actually "prove" that the patient has the disease. The probability that a positive test will confirm that the patient has CAD is actually a science unto itself and is, in part, quite dependent on the pretest likelihood that a specific patient has CAD. In brief, consider three patients being evaluated for the diagnosis of CAD and angina. The first is a 55-year-old man with a typical history for angina pectoris. This man has a 93 percent chance of having CAD before any tests are performed. *Thus, an ECG stress test is unlikely to add much to the probability that this man has coronary disease and that his chest pain is truly angina.* A positive test might increase the probability from 93 to 95 percent, not much help in the management of this man. Thus, performing an ECG exercise test on this man will not greatly help in establishing a diagnosis because he is already at high probability for having the disease. This man might be exercised in order to determine his prognosis and severity of disease or to establish his exercise tolerance, however. *In reality, this patient might be best diagnosed and risk-stratified by coronary angiography (cardiac catheterization).* Next, consider a 40-year-old man with an atypical history for angina (e.g., sharp chest pain that is not predictably precipitated by exercise). In this example, the pretest likelihood of this specific patient's having CAD, and his chest pain's being angina, is approximately 50 percent. A positive ECG exercise test for ischemia will increase the probability that this man has the disease from 50 up to around 90 percent, depending on how positive the test is. *So for this patient with an intermediate pretest risk, an exercise ECG test is an excellent test for diagnosis and risk stratification.* Finally, consider a 30-year-old female patient with atypical chest pain for angina. This patient has a pretest probability of coronary disease in the 2 percent range. Even if she were exercised on a regular ECG treadmill test and had a positive test, the probability that she truly has coronary disease and angina is only around 25 to 30 percent. *Therefore, performing a routine ECG stress test on this woman would not help in confirming the diagnosis of CAD and angina because she has such a low pretest probability of having CAD.* In the best treatment circumstances, this patient would need no diagnostic test but simply reassurance that her chest pain was not anginal. If the patient needed further documentation that she did not have CAD (e.g., if she were an airline pilot), then a diagnostic test with a higher sensitivity and specificity, like a thallium stress test, could rule out CAD.

From these examples, it becomes obvious that for patients at the extremes of pretest probabilities, both high and low, there is little diagnostic benefit from routine ECG exercise testing. These high- and low-pretest-probability patients need diagnostic tests that are more sensitive and specific. It is those patients with an intermediate pretest likelihood of having disease that can be best diagnosed and stratified with routine ECG stress testing. For a full treatise on the pre- and posttest probabilities of exercise testing, the reader is referred to the joint ACC/AHA guidelines for stress testing.[5]

Diagnostic ECG stress testing also yields valuable information regarding the severity of CAD and the attendant prognosis associated with certain test results. The findings indicative of three-vessel or left main coronary artery disease (i.e., coronary anatomy that identifies a high-risk patient with angina) are (1) exercise-induced hypotension, (2) ST-segment change >2 mm, (3) persistent ST depression >5 min in duration, (4) an early positive stress test, within the first stage of a standard Bruce protocol, and (5) high-grade ventricular ectopy with exercise. These are patients that have a poor prognosis for life-threatening complications from their CAD and angina.

The addition of *thallium* or *sestamibi imaging* to an ECG exercise test is a common practice in the noninvasive testing of patients with presumed or confirmed coronary artery disease and chronic stable angina. This test utilizes a radioactive tracer, thallium or sestamibi, that is administered intravenously when the patient is at peak exercise. Two separate imaging scans are then performed, one just after maximal exercise and one at rest. The two images are then compared to determine what areas of myocardium are either (1) viable and nonischemic (well perfused at rest and during stress), (2) viable but ischemic (well perfused at rest and underperfused during stress), or (3) nonviable scar (not perfused at rest or during stress). This technique markedly improves the sensitivity and specificity of routine ECG stress testing from the 50 to 60 percent range to the 85 to 90 percent range. Indications for this test include stress testing in those patients listed above who are not suited for routine ECG stress testing because of electrocardiographic contraindications (i.e., left bundle branch block, Wolff-Parkinson-White syndrome, patients on digoxin, left ventricular hypertrophy with strain, electronic pacing). Another indication for thallium or sestamibi stress testing is high and low pretest probabilities for coronary disease and angina. Because of improved sensitivity and specificity, negative tests are less likely to be falsely negative and more likely to truly indicate no significant coronary disease, and positive tests are more likely to be truly indicative of significant coronary disease and "real" angina. Finally, this test is often used because it allows the clinician to get an estimate of the amount of myocardium at risk and can localize which zone(s) of myocardium (anterior, inferior, septal, or posterior-lateral) is ischemic or scar.

Several other imaging techniques coupled with exercise or pharmacologic stress have been developed and validated. Many of these are in use in hospitals and clinics and are available for primary care physicians to utilize for the evaluation of their patients with chest pain. These include but are not limited to combinations of thallium, sestamibi, positron emission tomography (PET) scanning, magnetic resonance imaging (MRI), or echocardiographic imaging techniques and dobutamine, adenosine, or persantine pharmacologic stress modalities. Thus in some localities, persantine or adenosine PET scans may be available, whereas in other geographic areas, persantine thallium, dobutamine echo, or adenosine sestamibi tests are utilized. The sensitivities and specificities of the various tests are nearly comparable except for PET scanning and MRI, which may be significantly more sensitive and specific. Thus, the decision on which test to order should be based on the local expertise in a specific testing modality, the relative local sensitivities and specificities, and the cost of the examination.

One newer imaging modality that may be used to help in the work-up of patients without a previous diagnosis of coronary artery disease and angina is the *electron-beam computed tomography (EBCT) scan.* This technique, unlike the others listed above (which utilize perfusion markers and imaging to diagnose coronary atherosclerosis), capitalizes on the presence of coronary calcifications in the coronary arteries as a marker for coronary atherosclerosis. This novel idea is based on the pathophysiologic fact that the atherosclerotic process up-regulates the expression of a gene coding for a protein called osteopontin. Osteopontin is the same protein that causes cartilage to ossify (calcify) into bone. This occurs normally within the marrow space of bones but is distinctly abnormal in coronary arteries unless atherosclerosis is present. This test takes a fraction of the time that one of the other imaging/perfusion modalities would take and makes an image of the heart and its coronary blood vessels in situ. The EBCT scanner can make an image of the heart fast enough to "freeze" the motion of the heart, and it produces tomographic slices of the heart and its arterial blood supply. This allows visualization of the coronary arteries so that a calcium score (based on the quantity of calcium deposits seen within the coronary blood vessels) can be calculated. These calcium scores have now been correlated with the presence of disease by angiography, and the extent of calcification has been correlated with severity of disease. Prognostic studies linking high calcium scores to patients with a poor prognosis have also been performed.[6] The current indications for this test are somewhat "under construction," but it can be used instead of an exercise test. Thus, patients with intermediate pretest risks for coronary disease and chronic stable angina can be diagnosed and risk-stratified with this procedure. In addition, this test is ideal for the "worried well," who may have a family history of coronary disease but no symptoms. The test is easy to perform and provides a picture of the patient's heart that can easily be used as a motivational tool for lifestyle change and risk modification. There is even recent evidence that serial changes in EBCT calcium scores can be positively affected by therapeutic interventions.

The final diagnostic test for patients with a history of chest pain suggestive of angina and possible coronary artery disease is *coronary angiography,* commonly referred to as cardiac catheterization. This is certainly the most invasive testing modality, but it is also the gold standard for diagnosing occlusive coronary artery disease. The risks of major complications (MI, stroke, and death) vary extensively with the patient's age and gender, the experience of the operator, and the state and severity of the patient's disease; however, a global major risk estimate is approximately 1 in 1000. This is significantly higher than the major risks from exercise testing, which run between 1 in 2500 and 1 in 10,000. The indications for this procedure in the work-up of patients with stable angina include (1) patients with disabling stable angina (Canadian Cardiovascular Society classes III and IV) that cannot be managed with medications, (2) patients with high-risk positive noninvasive tests regardless of anginal severity, (3) patients with angina who have survived sudden cardiac death or serious ventricular arrhythmias, (4) patients with angina and symptoms of CHF, (5) patients with a high likelihood of severe CAD (left main and three-vessel CAD). The decision to proceed with coronary angiography should be made in consultation with a cardiovascular disease specialist with a high level of experience with cardiac catheterization and coronary interventions (percutaneous transluminal coronary angiography, stent placement, etc.) because data confirm that complication rates are lower when the procedure is performed by high-volume angiographers.

Coronary angiography and contrast ventriculography (an angiographic picture of the contracting left ventricle) are the most powerful predictors of long-term outcome, despite the fact that coronary angiography has its own cadre of limitations. The Coronary Artery Surgery Study (CASS) is a particularly robust and mature database that demonstrates the importance of left ventricular systolic function and the severity of CAD (left main, three-vessel, two-vessel, or single-vessel disease or no CAD) as powerful prognostic indicators in patients with angina.[7] The most important predictor of long-term survival in patients with angina is the ejection fraction as obtained by contrast ventriculography. Patients with ejection fractions in the 50 to 100 percent range have a 12-year survival rate of 54 percent, whereas those patients with an ejection fraction <35 percent have a 12-year survival rate of only 21 percent. Likewise with severity of CAD: Patients with normal coronary arteries have a 91 percent 12-year survival rate compared to 74 percent for those with single-vessel disease, 59 percent for two-vessel disease, and 40 percent for three-vessel disease.

# TREATMENT

Patients with stable angina as the manifestation of their ischemic heart disease are well suited for outpatient therapy because stable angina is a chronic disease with no known cure for which there are several effective forms of therapy. Aggressive treatment plans with proven therapies can therefore be beneficial to our patients and gratifying for the organized healthcare providers. For most patients, this disease is in large part a disease of lifestyle. Several of the cardiac risk factors are controllable through lifestyle changes and compliance with dietary and medical therapies including smoking cessation, alteration of sedentary lifestyle, elimination of obesity, diabetic blood sugar control, compliance with antihypertensive medications, and adherence to a low-fat, low-cholesterol diet.

## Patient Education

As with all diseases partially attributable to lifestyle, patient education must be a major thrust of therapy. There are several excellent approaches to the educational directives given to patients with ischemic heart disease.[8] These directives, however, all have eight common thrusts: (1) access the patient's baseline understanding of the disease process; (2) evoke the patient's desire for information, utilizing whatever the patient's agenda may be; (3) use evidence-based medicine and epidemiology to demonstrate the effectiveness of "proven" therapies; (4) utilize ancillary personnel to extend the teaching times and interactions; (5) distribute professional resources when available (see http://www.americanheart.org); (6) develop a written plan with the patient, including medication charts; (7) involve family members and significant others to help motivate the patient; and (8) remind, repeat, and reinforce! Other specific information that the patient must be taught includes the appropriate time to seek emergency care (chest pain >30 min in duration that does not respond to sublingual nitroglycerine), the importance of prompt aspirin use, having an action plan that includes activating 911, knowing which local hospitals have 24-h emergency cardiac care, and the need for cardiopulmonary resuscitation training for family members. Unfortunately, patient and family education is the most difficult, time-consuming, and poorly reimbursed aspect of the care of patients with stable angina and ischemic heart disease, despite evidence that aggressive programs may improve outcomes.[9] Nevertheless, when well organized, professionally presented, and persistently pursued, patient education can have a large impact on the well-being of our patients, their perception of their health status and quality of life, and their adherence to medical therapy.

## Exercise Prescription

There are several theoretic benefits from an organized exercise therapy/cardiac rehabilitation program for patients with stable angina. Regular exercise is likely to help patients achieve their ideal body weight and reduce obesity. This can positively affect blood pressure control in hypertensive patients, positively affect blood sugar control in diabetics, increase HDL levels, promote a less atherogenic blood lipid profile, and improve exercise capacity and patient well-being. The recommended minimal amount of exercise is brisk walking three to five times a week for 30 to 60 min continuously per session. Unfortunately, the data for objective improvement from exercise training in patients with stable angina is quite limited. The best data for exercise training are in patients with previous MI, and these data are not readily transferable to the group of patients with stable angina. Despite the lack of clear scientific evidence for outcome benefits, the recommendations stand for encouragement of walking 30 to 60 min three to five times per week.

## Control of Risk Factors

Reduction in cardiac risk factors is one of the mainstays of therapy for patients with stable angina pectoris. The risk factor reductions for which there is definite evidence of reduction in the incidence of coronary disease events in patients with stable angina are smoking cessation, reduction in LDL cholesterol, control of hypertension and reduction in left ventricular hypertrophy, tight control of diabetes mellitus, and reduction in thrombogenic factors with aspirin therapy.

Cigarette smoking impairs the secretion of endothelial-derived nitric oxide in human coronary arteries and promotes systemic endothelial cell damage and vasoconstriction.[10] These deleterious effects help initiate and promote coronary atherosclerosis and lead to a 50 percent increase in cardiovascular mortality in patients who smoke. There is an established dose-response relationship between cigarette smoking and cardiovascular disease events in men and women.[11,12] Patients who continue to smoke following an AMI have a 22 to 47 percent increased risk of death. Although no randomized clinical trials of smoking cessation in patients with stable angina have been performed, several studies of primary prevention of cardiovascular disease events have been completed and demonstrated a 7 to 47 percent reduction in events in patients who stopped smoking. Unfortunately, only about a third of patients will stop smoking at the time of a cardiac event. This number can be nearly doubled by enrolling patients in a nurse-managed smoking cessation program.[13] Nicotine patches and antidepressant-type medications may be helpful in the motivated patient. No medication alone can break the addiction to cigarettes, however. A carefully implemented and supportive smoking cessation class must be an integral part of a comprehensive program. Extensive smoking cessation guidelines can be obtained from the U.S. Department of Health and Human Services.[14] This publication proposes a five-part plan for assisting patients to discontinue cigarette smoking: (1) ask about smoking at every visit, (2) advise and strongly urge smokers to quit, (3) identify smokers who are willing to attempt to quit, (4) assist those who are motivated to quit, and (5) arrange follow-up contact for the smoker trying to quit.

There is little doubt that increased LDL cholesterol promotes cardiovascular disease event rates and results in increased cardiovascular death rates. Even the early bile-acid sequestrant trials showed a consistent trend of reduced cardiovascular event rates with modest reductions in total cholesterol (6 to 15 percent reductions). Direct evidence regarding the correlation between LDL cholesterol reduction and decreased mortality rates and major coronary event rates was first reported from the Scandinavian Simvastatin Survival Study trial of simvastatin versus placebo in patients with known CAD and high total cholesterol levels (around 270 mg/dL, mean). The relative reduction in mortality was approximately 30 percent, and the comparable reduction in major coronary event rates was 35 percent.[15] Similar effects were seen in patients with recent MIs and average total cholesterol levels of 209 mg/dL in the Cholesterol and Recurrent Events trial.[16] Patients were randomized to receive pravastatin or placebo, and there was a 24 percent reduction in the risk of nonfatal MI and coronary death in the group receiving statin therapy. These data compel the clinician to aggressively treat elevated LDL cholesterol in patients with stable angina pectoris. The current National Cholesterol Education Program adult treatment panel II guidelines[17] suggest treating LDL cholesterol levels if they are >100 mg/dL and the patient has known CAD. Treatment should be initiated with a diet first and then statin therapy to reduce the LDL level to <100 mg/dL. For elevated triglycerides, niacin and fibrates are recommended for triglycerides between 200 and 400 and >400 mg/dL, respectively.

## Control of Hypertension

Hypertension is another risk factor that deserves aggressive treatment. Hypertension causes direct endothelial and vascular injury via mechanical forces and inflammatory mediators [via the angiotensin-converting enzyme (ACE) pathway] and through its effects on myocardial oxygen demand. As blood pressure increases, myocardial wall stress is increased, as is aortic impedance, resulting in a greater myocardial oxygen demand. The Veterans Administration cooperative studies were the first to unequivocally demonstrate the benefits of hypertension control for reducing cardiovascular disease risk.[18,19] Blood pressure control in the elderly is especially important, as treatment in this patient population may result in nearly twice the mortality reduction seen in younger patient cohorts.[20] The new guidelines for blood pressure goals are to reduce systolic blood pressure to <130 mmHg and to reduce diastolic blood pressure to <85 mmHg. Lifestyle changes including routine exercise, achievement of ideal body weight, monitoring of sodium intake, and moderation in alcohol intake are the first steps in treatment. Individualization of antihypertensive medications is based on age, race, and the need for drugs with specific benefits for individual patients. For example, in patients with stable angina and hypertension who have had a previous MI and left ventricular hypertrophy, a beta blocker would be one drug of choice. In a diabetic with reduced left ventricular function, an ACE inhibitor would be preferable. A younger patient with normal left ventricular function, hypertension, no prior MI, and no diabetes might be best treated with a long-acting calcium channel blocker. The use of short-acting, first-generation, dihydropyridine calcium blocking agents (e.g., nifedipine, nisoldipine, etc.) is not recommended.

## Drug Treatment

The pharmacologic treatment of patients with stable angina has a robust armamentarium, and the choice from among the several drug classes available should be highly individualized. A mnemonic for the initial treatment of patients with stable angina has been suggested[3]:

A = Aspirin and Antianginal therapy
B = Beta blocker and Blood pressure
C = Cigarette smoking and Cholesterol
D = Diet and Diabetes
E = Education and Exercise

Some medications are obviously indicated in all patients without specific allergies to them because of their low side effect to therapeutic benefit ratio and their low cost. The prototypical medication for the prevention of MI in patients with stable angina is aspirin. Aspirin has been demonstrated to reduce adverse cardiac events by 33 percent in patients with stable angina.[21,22] Even though it does not reduce anginal episodes, it is indicated as a preventive measure in all patients who are not aspirin-allergic. The recommended dose is 81 to 325 mg daily. If patients have a true aspirin allergy, then ticlopidine or clopidogrel is a reasonable alternative. These drugs act by inhibiting platelet aggregation via an ADP-dependent mechanism. Clopidogrel has been studied in a randomized trial (Clopidogrel versus Aspirin in Patients at Risk of Ischaemic Events,[23] comparing aspirin with clopidogrel in patients with prior MI, prior stroke, or a history of peripheral vascular disease. Clopidogrel was slightly more effective than aspirin in reducing the combined risk of MI, stroke, and vascular death. Current recommendations suggest its use as an aspirin alternative. It is noteworthy that it costs much more than aspirin. The other drug that should be prescribed for all patients with stable angina pectoris is sublingual nitroglycerine or a nitroglycerine spray for breakthrough episodes of angina. Patients should be instructed carefully on how to take their nitroglycerine and counseled to seek urgent medical attention if three sublingual nitroglycerine tablets do not ameliorate an episode of angina within 30 min.

Antianginal and anti-ischemic therapy is important in symptom control, and some classes of drugs within this schema have been shown to reduce cardiovascular mortality in patients with prior myocardial infarctions and chronic stable angina. Beta-blocking agents are among the preferred medications in a tailored pharmacopoeia for individual patients. The data on suppression of anginal episodes are quite good. Beta blockers mechanistically reduce myocardial oxygen demand by reducing heart rate, reducing the inotropic state of the myocardium, and causing blood pressure reduction. Indeed, beta blockers are probably the best available oral agents for reducing myocardial oxygen demand. Additionally, numerous beta blockers that do not have intrinsic sympathomimetic activity have been shown to reduce cardiovascular morbidity and mortality in large randomized clinical trials. Thus, if a patient with stable angina does not have a contraindication to beta blockade (high-degree atrioventricular block, unstable CHF, sick sinus syndrome, severe bronchospasm, or severe depression), a beta blocker is one of the drugs of choice.

Calcium channel blocking agents have effectiveness similar to that of beta blockers at reducing anginal episodes in patients with stable angina. Calcium channel blockers work by reducing the inotropic state of the heart, decreasing heart rate (in the nondihydropyridine calcium blocking agents), and vasodilating epicardial coronary arteries as well as peripheral and coronary microvascular arterial beds. These actions result in both increased coronary blood supply and reduced myocardial oxygen demand. Therefore, calcium channel blockers are useful in fixed- and variable-threshold angina, and also mixed angina. Furthermore, calcium channel blockers are one of the drugs of choice in the rare patient with pure coronary artery spasm as the etiology of stable angina pectoris. In general, this class of drugs is extremely well tolerated and is without the central nervous system side effects that accompany the beta blockers. Short-acting dihydropyridine should be used with great care in patients with heart failure because of their negative inotropic effect, which may increase the likelihood of a mortality. Also, heart rate–modulating calcium channel blockers may be contraindicated in patients with bradycardia. The second-generation, long-acting, vasoselective dihydropyr-idines (amlodipine and felodipine) have been used in patients with severe left ventricular dysfunction without adverse effects on cardiovascular morbidity or mortality.

Organic nitrates are the third type of antianginal medication. Organic nitrates have been utilized in the treatment of angina for over 150 years, but their mecha-nism of action has been elucidated only in the past 10 years. All clinically utilized nitrates (nitroglycerine, sodium nitroprusside, nitroglycerine ointment, and nitro-glycerine patches) are considered nitrovasodilators and are essentially nitric oxide donors. These drugs also have effects on platelets, inhibiting platelet aggregation, and reduce preload via capacitance vein dilation. This reduction in preload may indirectly affect myocardial oxygen demand, but most of the actions of the or-ganic nitrates serve to increase myocardial oxygen supply. Organic nitrates have been shown to increase treadmill walking time in patients with stable angina but have not been shown to alter cardiovascular mortality. Nitrates should be used with caution in combination with other drugs that lower blood pressure. One of the most important aspects of the appropriate use of long-acting nitrates (patches, oral mono- and dinitrates) is the avoidance of tolerance. The most effective method to avoid tolerance is a 12-h nitrate-free period during every 24-h time period.

In patients with stable angina, combination therapy with aspirin, beta blockers, ni-trates, calcium channel blockers, ACE inhibitors, hypolipidemic agents, other anti-hypertensive agents, and drugs for the treatment of other concomitant conditions is often necessary. With such a broad and effective pharmacopoeia, clinicians can of-ten maintain a patient in a stable pattern of angina if the patient can remain com-pliant with multiple drugs and drug schedules. Follow-up of patients with stable angina pectoris is recommended at intervals of every 4 to 6 months for the first year and then every 4 to 12 months thereafter. The treatment goal for patients with sta-ble angina is to convert their angina to Canadian Cardiovascular Society Classifica-tion class I. Any acceleration to class II should alert the clinician to escalate the medical therapy by adding other drugs or by boosting the dosages of currently pre-scribed drugs. When patients "break through" their antianginal regimes, however, there are other modes of therapy to restabilize them, specifically revascularization therapies.

## Revascularization Procedures

When patients cannot be stabilized on medical therapy alone, it is appropriate for the primary care provider to refer the patient quickly to a cardiovascular disease specialist for consideration of percutaneous transluminal angioplasty, coronary artery bypass surgery (CABS), or, on the horizon, therapeutic angiogenesis for pa-tients whose anatomy is not conducive to traditional revascularization. For a dis-cussion of the relative merits of each of these treatment options, the reader is re-ferred to the ACC/AHA/ACP-ASIM Guidelines for the Management of Patients with Chronic Stable Angina.[3]

## SUMMARY

In summary, stable angina pectoris occurs as a result of atherosclerotic coronary vascular disease and can be diagnosed primarily through a thorough history and physical examination. It is a common diagnosis in the United States and may account for a significant proportion of adult outpatient medical care by primary care physicians. Diagnostic testing to confirm the diagnosis of stable angina is needed in those patients who have an intermediate pretest risk of having the disease. Tailoring these tests to individual patients is important so that the appropriate diagnostic, prognostic, and risk-stratification information can be gathered efficiently. The severity of angina as graded on the Canadian Cardiovascular Society scale is an important element in risk stratification. The concept of coronary blood supply and myocardial oxygen demand is important in treating patients with fixed-threshold, variable-threshold, and mixed angina. A large number of medical therapies are available for patients with chronic stable angina, and maintaining CCS class I is an achievable goal for most patients. When patients become unstable on medical therapy, referral to a cardiovascular disease specialist can provide further therapies for these patients.

### REFERENCES

1. American Heart Association: *Biostatistical Fact Sheet.* Dallas, American Heart Association, 1997:1–29.
2. American Heart Association: *1999 Heart and Stroke Statistical Update.* Dallas, American Heart Association, 1999.
3. Ritchie JL, Gibbons RJ, Cheitlin MD, et al: ACC/AHA/ACP-ASIM guidelines for the management of patients with chronic stable angina. *J Am Coll Card* 1999; 33:2092–2197.
4. Diamond GA, Forrester JS: Analysis of probability as an aid in the clinical diagnosis of coronary-artery disease. *N Engl J Med* 1997; 300:1350–1358.
5. Gibbons RJ, Balady GJ, Beasley JW: ACC/AHA guidelines for exercise testing: executive summary. A report of the American College of Cardiology/American Heart Association Task Force on Practice Guidelines (Committee on Exercise Testing). *Circulation* 1997; 96:345–354.
6. Rumberger JA, Simons DB, Fitzpatrick LA, et al: Coronary artery calcium area by electron-beam computed tomography and coronary atherosclerotic plaque area: a histopathologic correlative study. *Circulation* 1995; 92:2157–2162.
7. Emond M, Mock MB, Davis KB: Long-term survival of medically treated patients in the Coronary Artery Surgery Study (CASS) Registry. *Circulation* 1995; 90:2645–2657.
8. Kinsbury K: Taking AIM: How to teach primary and secondary prevention effectively. *Can J Cardiol* 1998; 14(suppl A):22A–26A.
9. The Multiple Risk Factor Intervention Trial (MRFIT). A national study of primary prevention of coronary heart disease. *JAMA* 1976; 235:825–827.
10. Winniford MD, Jansen DE, Reynolds GA: Cigarette smoking-induced coronary vasoconstriction in atherosclerotic coronary artery disease and prevention by calcium antagonists and nitroglycerin. *Am J Cardiol* 1987; 59:203–207.

11. Doll R, Peto R: Mortality in relation to smoking: 20 years' observations on male British doctors. *Br Med J* 1976; 2:1525–1536.

12. Willett WC, Green A, Stampfer MJ: Relative and absolute excess risks of coronary heart disease among women who smoke cigarettes. *N Engl J Med* 1990; 322:213–217.

13. Taylor CB, Houston-Miller N, Killen JD: Smoking cessation after acute myocardial infarction: effects of a nurse-managed intervention. *Ann Intern Med* 1990; 113:118–123.

14. Fiore MC, Bailey WC, Cohen JJ: Smoking cessation. *Clinical Practice Guideline No. 18.* AHCPR Publication no. 96-0692. Rockville, MD, Agency for Health Care Policy and Research, Public Health Service, U.S. Department of Health and Human Services, 1996.

15. Randomised trial of cholesterol lowering in 4,444 patients with coronary heart disease: the Scandinavian Simvastatin Survival Study (4S). *Lancet* 1994; 344:1383–1389.

16. Sacks FM, Pfeffer MA, Moye LA: The effect of pravastatin on coronary events after myocardial infarction in patients with average cholesterol levels. Cholesterol and Recurrent Events Trial investigators. *N Engl J Med* 1996; 335:1001–1009.

17. Summary of the second report of the National Cholesterol Education Program (NCEP) Expert Panel on Detection, Evaluation, and Treatment of High Blood Cholesterol in Adults (Adult Treatment Panel II). *JAMA* 1993; 269:3015–3023.

18. Effects of treatment on morbidity in hypertension: results in patients with diastolic blood pressures averaging 115 through 129 mmHg. *JAMA* 1967; 202:1028–1034.

19. Effects of treatment on morbidity in hypertension: II. Results in patients with diastolic blood pressure averaging 90 through 114 mmHg. *JAMA* 1970; 213:1143–1152.

20. Cutler JA, Psaty BM, McMahon S, Furberg CD: Public health issues in hypertension control: what has been learned from clinical trials. In: Laragh JH, Brenner BM (eds): *Hypertension: Pathophysiology, Diagnosis, and Management.* New York, Raven Press, 1995:253–270.

21. Ridker PM, Manson JE, Gaziano JM, et al: Low-dose aspirin therapy for chronic stable angina. A randomized, placebo-controlled clinical trial. *Ann Intern Med* 1991; 114:835–839.

22. Antiplatelet Trialists Collaboration: Collaborative overview of randomised trials of antiplatelet therapy: I. Prevention of death, myocardial infarction and stroke by prolonged antiplatelet therapy in various categories of patients. *Br Med J* 1995; 308:81–106.

23. CAPRIE Steering Committee: A randomised, blinded, trial of clopidogrel versus aspirin in patients at risk of ischaemic events (CAPRIE). *Lancet* 1996; 348:1329–1339.

R. WAYNE ALEXANDER /
DAVID L. ROBERTS

# CHAPTER
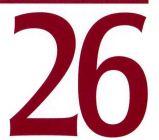

# ACUTE MYOCARDIAL INFARCTION AND UNSTABLE ANGINA

---

## ACUTE MYOCARDIAL INFARCTION

### Background and General Principles

The demonstration in the late 1970s of the role of thrombus formation in the pathogenesis of acute myocardial infarction (AMI) quickly led to the systematic testing of thrombolytic strategies to abort the event. Major multicenter clinical trials on the treatment of AMI demonstrated the efficacy of streptokinase and recombinant tissue plasminogen activator in reducing mortality.[1,2] Thus, large, adequately powered, randomized studies in this area have helped set a new standard for and approach to the goal of treating AMI. The availability of data from clinical trials has permitted the development of practice guidelines for the treatment of AMI.[3]

The progress that has been made in treatment of AMI has resulted in substantial improvement in outcomes. The increased use of standard coronary care unit (CCU) procedures—including electrocardiographic and hemodynamic monitoring, defibrillation, beta blockers, and, more recently, thrombolytics, coronary interventions, and aspirin—has decreased the mortality, under the best of circumstances, to 5 percent or less.

Increased understanding of the pathophysiologic mechanisms of AMI has in turn led to greatly expanded understanding of the spectrum of ischemic heart disease, which ranges from stable angina to unstable angina to non-Q-wave MI to, at the extreme, MI with ST-segment elevation resulting from total coronary occlusion. The common underlying event is breakdown of the integrity of the arterial intima related to atherosclerotic coronary artery disease, with resulting thrombus formation. Disruption in the integrity of the intima represents the transition from stable atherosclerotic disease to the acute coronary ischemic syndromes, with their attendant risk of AMI and sudden death. The clinical manifestations are dependent upon the extent to which the thrombus occludes the coronary artery and the duration of the occlusion. Unstable angina and non-Q-wave MI usually cannot be distinguished on clinical grounds alone and account for the majority of CCU admissions in which a diagnosis of acute coronary artery disease syndromes has been established.

## Clinical Aspects

**PREDISPOSING CHARACTERISTICS AND CIRCUMSTANCES.**   The risk factors for the development of coronary artery disease are dyslipidemia, family history, relative age, male gender, cigarette smoking, diabetes mellitus, and hypertension. Careful consideration of the probability of the presence of coronary artery disease is centrally important in the initial assessment and evaluation of testing results of any patient with chest pain. AMI or unstable angina occurs as a result of the disruption of a plaque at a site of a high density of inflammatory cells. Thus, the acute coronary syndromes result from the acute exacerbation of a chronic inflammatory response.

**PRECIPITATING EVENTS.**   An association has been noted between AMI and antecedent mild respiratory syndromes. A more specific relationship between AMI and an infectious agent has been posited in the case of *Chlamydia pneumoniae*.[4]

AMI has been associated with emotional or environmental stresses that activate the sympathetic nervous system and with increases in catecholamines. These factors can lead to plaque rupture in an area weakened by inflammation. High catecholamine levels can increase thrombus formation by activating platelets.

Any stressful event can precipitate AMI in a patient with "active," susceptible coronary atherosclerotic lesions. Anesthesia and surgery are well known to enhance the risk of MI, and cardiac events are the leading cause of perioperative morbidity.

**SYMPTOMS.**   *Prodromal symptoms* antedating AMI are common and occur in at least 60 percent of patients.[5] Most of these symptoms are anginal or angina-like, especially when assessed retrospectively in the context of the character of the pain of the acute infarct. New-onset angina or a worsening of preexisting anginal symptoms is a hallmark of unstable angina and frequently represents an ominous antecedent of AMI. Considering the general feeling of malaise and fatigue that many patients have prior to AMI, it is obviously relatively unusual for the event to be totally unheralded.

The *classic symptoms* of AMI involve chest discomfort that is commonly retrosternal or precordial in *location* and is described as pressure, aching, burning, crushing, squeezing, heavy, swelling, or bursting in *quality*. The location of chest pain is usually of little help in differentiating ischemia/infarction from other causes, but severe chest pain (as opposed to vague discomfort) and the presence of *associated symptoms* (dyspnea, nausea, diaphoresis, and vomiting) are more commonly associated with MI. The discomfort often *radiates* over the anterior chest and frequently into the left arm or both arms (particularly the medial aspect) and/or into the neck or jaw. In unusual instances, the pain may be in the back, particularly between the scapulae. There may be skip areas with retrosternal pain, associated with jaw, ante-cubital fossa, or wrist pain, or there may be no pain in between the two sites. More-over, the pain may appear only in the referral area. The *duration* of the pain is pro-longed, lasting by definition longer than 15 min. While the intensity of the pain is usually steady following an initial crescendo, there is occasionally some waxing and waning. Sudden relief of pain may accompany reperfusion. Marked apprehension is common. Occasionally, presenting symptoms include syncope, acute confusion, agi-tation, stroke, or palpitations.

Approximately 23 percent of MIs go unrecognized because of the absence of symptoms or the lack of recognition of the significance of symptoms. The common symptoms in this latter instance are nonclassic or atypical pain, dyspnea, nausea, vomiting, and/or epigastric pain. A MI may also masquerade as the development or worsening of congestive heart failure (CHF), the appearance of an arrhythmia, an overwhelming sense of apprehension, profound weakness, acute indigestion, peri-carditis, embolic stroke, or peripheral embolus. Presentation with painless MI is more common in the elderly than in the nonelderly, and this subgroup has an in-creased frequency of CHF as the initial presenting symptom.

## PHYSICAL FINDINGS.

*General Examination.*    The patient with unstable angina may have a normal presentation, except for the history, unless he or she is having pain at the time of the examination. The patient with AMI is frequently sitting up because of a sense of suf-focation or shortness of breath.[5] Most patients have some sense of impending doom, which is reflected in their facial expression. They may have a grayish appear-ance, or one of panic or exhaustion. Diaphoresis is frequent. In severe cases, patients may be quite anxious, with an ashen or pale face beaded with perspiration.

It is important to rapidly ascertain the vital signs and the nature, character, and rhythm of the arterial pulse; to observe the jugular venous pulse; to check the pe-ripheral pulses; to palpate the precordium; and to auscultate the chest and pre-cordium. Examination of the extremities should include subjective assessment of the temperature and color of the feet. The presence of very cool feet, especially with acrocyanosis in the setting of tachycardia, suggests low cardiac output.

The heart rate and rhythm in AMI are very important indicators of cardiac func-tion. A normal rate usually indicates absence of significant hemodynamic compro-mise. In patients with inferior MI, heart rates in the fifties and sixties are very com-mon, especially during the first few hours. The bradycardia may be associated with secondary hypotension resulting from vagal stimulation. *Persistent sinus tachycardia beyond the initial 12 to 24 h is predictive of a high mortality rate.* The pulse may be low in volume, reflecting decreased stroke volume. The blood pressure is usually normal, but it may be increased secondary to anxiety or decreased from cardiac fail-ure. All peripheral pulses should be examined to exclude current occlusion and to provide a baseline in case of future embolic events. The carotid pulse is most useful in assessing systolic upstroke time and stroke volume, which are decreased with a low-output state. The rhythm of the pulse is very important because of the fre-quency of ectopic atrial and, in particular, ventricular beats in AMI.

The respiratory rate is usually within the normal range. However, patients who are extremely anxious often exhibit hyperventilation, and those with pulmonary edema and cardiac failure also may exhibit shallow inspirations.

Examination of the jugular venous pulse is important with AMI, especially in patients with an inferior infarction, because insights can be gained into possible involvement of the right ventricle. It may be manifest by elevated jugular venous pressure or by a prominent a wave because of the decreased compliance of the right ventricle (RV). Kussmaul's sign, or an increase in the venous pressure on inspiration, may also be seen in right ventricular infarction because of decreased RV compliance.

***Examination of the Lungs.***   Basilar rales are frequently detected in AMI. Cardiac failure diagnosed on the basis of mild signs of pulmonary congestion occurs transiently in 30 to 40 percent of otherwise uncomplicated patients. Patients with just unstable angina usually have a normal pulmonary examination.

***Cardiac Examination.***   Between episodes of pain, patients with unstable angina usually have a normal cardiac examination or, minimally, one that is unchanged from baseline. During active episodes of pain and ischemia, results of examination of the heart may not be dissimilar from those in AMI. In AMI, palpation of the precordium may reveal evidence of regional wall motion abnormalities and should be performed with the patient initially lying supine; this often is adequate to ascertain whether there is a localized normal apical impulse or a dyskinetic impulse. In the left lateral decubitus position, one may palpate a diffuse rather than a localized apical impulse, akinesis, or a paradoxical bulging during late systole; and in some patients, a palpable atrial contraction corresponding to an audible $S_4$ gallop may be present.

The first and second heart sounds are often soft because of decreased contractility. The second heart sound is usually normally split with inspiration; however, with extensive damage, it may be single. Paradoxical splitting may reflect severe left ventricular dysfunction. A fourth heart sound is often audible. A third heart sound is heard in probably only about 15 to 20 percent of patients. A pericardial friction rub is heard in only about 10 percent of patients, usually 48 to 72 h after onset. The crescendo-decrescendo, midsystolic murmur of papillary muscle dysfunction is relatively common early and reflects ischemia of the papillary muscle or the myocardial attachment rather than irreversible injury. This murmur usually disappears after the first 12 to 24 h if it is soft, but if it is moderate to loud in intensity, it may persist much longer. Mitral regurgitation is most commonly due to ischemia of the posteromedial papillary muscle.

## Diagnosis of Acute Myocardial Infarction and Unstable Angina

**DIFFERENTIAL DIAGNOSIS.**   Myocardial infarction has typically been diagnosed on the basis of the triad of chest pain, electrocardiographic (ECG) changes, and elevated plasma enzyme activity. Unstable angina is a diagnosis of exclusion, with symptoms and frequently (as discussed below) ECG changes consistent with ischemia but with the absence of enzyme changes. Although AMI may occur without chest pain (20 to 25 percent of cases), chest pain is usually responsible for the patient's presentation. The differential diagnosis of prolonged chest pain is presented in Table 26-1. It is often impossible to distinguish ischemia or infarction from other causes of chest pain on the basis of history alone. Most patients at risk for MI will be admitted for evaluation unless definite noncardiac causes of chest pain— such as chest wall pain, hyperventilation, pleurisy, gastrointestinal pain, and so on— that are not imminently dangerous can be identified. Only about 20 percent of patients admitted with chest pain have AMI.

**ELECTROCARDIOGRAPHIC DIAGNOSIS.** The ECG is very sensitive for detecting ischemia and infarction but is frequently not powerful enough to differentiate ischemia (unstable angina) from necrosis. Serial ECGs during AMI will show some evolutionary changes in the majority of patients. An ECG obtained during cardiac ischemic pain frequently exhibits changes in repolarization. The absence of ECG changes during pain provides evidence but not proof that the pain is not ischemic in nature. The early ECG changes of T-wave inversion or ST-segment depression may reflect ischemia or infarction. ST-segment elevation is more specific for AMI and reflects the epicardial injury–associated total occlusion of an epicardial coronary artery. The hallmark of AMI is the development of abnormal Q-waves,

### TABLE 26-1. Differential Diagnosis of Prolonged Chest Pain

AMI/acute coronary syndromes

Aortic dissection

Pericarditis

Atypical angina pain associated with hypertrophic cardiomyopathy

Esophageal, other upper gastrointestinal, or biliary tract disease

Pulmonary disease
   Pleurisy: infectious, malignant, or immune disease–related
   Embolus with or without infarction
   Pneumothorax

Hyperventilation syndrome

Chest wall
   Skeletal
   Neuropathic

Psychogenic

*Source:* Adapted from Alexander RW, Pratt CM, Roberts R: Diagnosis and management of patients with acute myocardial infarction. In: Alexander RW, Schlant RC, Fuster V, et al (eds): *Hurst's The Heart,* 9th ed. New York, McGraw-Hill, 1998.

which appear, on the average, 8 to 12 h after the onset of symptoms but may not develop for 24 to 48 h. Abnormal Q-waves usually reflect tissue death and the development of an electrical dead zone but are not useful in initial diagnostic management and triage except to indicate presence of prior MI. The diagnostic serial ECG changes consist of ST-segment elevation with the development of T-wave inversion and the evolution of abnormal Q-waves. The appearance of abnormal Q-waves is very specific to AMI; however, these waves are present in less than 50 percent of patients with documented AMI. Most of the other patients who have AMI will have ECG changes restricted to T-wave inversion or ST-segment depression or no change at all and represent the group with non-Q-wave infarction.

The misnomers *transmural* and *nontransmural infarction* have been replaced by the terms *Q-wave infarction* and *non-Q-wave infarction,* respectively.[6] The evolution of a non-Q-wave infarction is characterized by the appearance of reversible ST-T-wave changes with ST-segment depression that usually return to normal over a few days but are occasionally permanent. The ST-segment (usually depression) and T-wave changes in unstable angina are usually transient and last for the duration of the pain. There are major differences in the pathogenesis, clinical manifestations, treatment, and prognosis of Q-wave and non-Q-wave MI. The initiating events are identical, namely, thrombus superimposed upon vasoconstriction. In non-Q-wave infarction, early spontaneous reperfusion occurs, limiting the extent of necrosis. In contrast, in Q-wave infarction, the coronary occlusion is sustained for a period that is at least long enough to result in extensive necrosis.

The ECG criteria for the diagnosis of AMI are the presence, in the setting of chest pain, of any one of the following: (1) new, or presumably new, Q waves (at least 30 ms wide and 0.20 mV deep) in at least two leads from any of the following: (a) leads II, III, or $aV_F$; (b) leads $V_1$ through $V_6$; or (c) leads I and $aV_L$; (2) new or presumably new ST-T-segment elevation or depression (>0.10 mV measured 0.02 s after the J point in two contiguous leads of the above-mentioned lead combinations); or (3) a new, complete left bundle branch block in the appropriate clinical setting.

The ECG diagnosis of RV infarction offers special challenges. RV infarction occurs in the presence of inferior left ventricular infarction; the resulting ST-segment elevation in the conventional precordial leads overlying the RV ($V_2$ and $V_3$) is usually overwhelmed by the ST-segment elevation in the opposing left ventricular myocardium on the inferior surface. ST-segment elevation must be sought in the right chest leads, $V_1$, and $V_3R$ to $V_6R$; when found, this provides reasonably strong evidence for the presence of RV infarction.

In view of a lack of sensitivity and specificity of the chest pain history or of the ECG, confirmation of the diagnosis of AMI is based on elevated plasma levels of cardiac-specific isoenzymes.[5]

**DIAGNOSTIC MARKERS IN PLASMA.**   Myocardial necrosis is associated with the release of a variety of proteins that have been evaluated as diagnostic markers for AMI.[7] The use of creatine kinase (CK) and MB-CK has become routine; these are highly sensitive, specific, and cost-effective for diagnosing MI. The cardiac troponin I radioimmunoassay is very specific for myocardial injury. It is also very sensitive. The assay for plasma cardiac troponin T is also very specific but may be less sensitive.

***Temporal Profiles of Plasma MB-CK, Myoglobin, Troponin I, and Troponin T.***
Plasma MB-CK activity following MI is significantly elevated, and reliable diagnostic sensitivity (>90 percent) is reached within 12 to 16 h of the onset of symptoms. Maximal levels are reached between 14 and 36 h, and levels return to normal after 48 to 72 h. Reliable diagnostic sensitivity (≥90 percent) with plasma troponins I and T is reached by 12 to 16 h, and maximal activity is reached by 24 to 36 h. Plasma myoglobin is increased within 2 h of the onset of symptoms and remains increased for at least 7 to 12 h.

***Early Diagnosis (6 to 10 h of Onset): MB-CK Subforms and Myoglobin.***
Early, rapid diagnosis is required in order to triage patients with chest pain so as to reduce costs and to select appropriate therapy because of the difficulty in distinguishing cardiac ischemia from infarction based on clinical criteria and because of the frequent absence of diagnostic ECG changes. The only two plausible candidates as early (<6 h) diagnostic markers are MB-CK subforms and myoglobin.

When MB-CK is released into plasma after myocardial injury, the parent form (MB-2) is converted into MB-1 by proteolytic activity, and the subforms can be rapidly separated and detected by electrophoresis.[8] The total assay can be performed in less than 1/2 h. Normally, MB-1 and MB-2 are in equilibrium with a ratio of 1 to 1. When infarction occurs, MB-2 initially is released into the circulation in minute amounts, so that total MB-CK remains within the normal range, but the ratio of MB-2 to MB-1 changes markedly and provides the basis for an early diagnosis of MI.

MB-CK subforms afford a sensitivity and specificity of about 90 percent for the diagnosis of AMI within 6 h of the onset of symptoms. Myoglobin has a sensitivity of 83 percent. Thus, *if a patient has a negative MB-CK subform test at 6 h after the onset of symptoms, one can reliably conclude that the patient does not have infarction.* The total MB-CK (activity or mass assay) and troponins T and I afford a sensitivity of only 65 percent within the first 6 h. For the same time intervals, myoglobin had a sensitivity of 83 percent. Total MB-CK and troponins I and T have high sensitivity and specificity for the diagnosis of MI from 10 to 14 h from the onset of symptoms. The enzymatic criteria for diagnosis of acute MI are summarized in Table 26-2.

***Diagnosis of Acute Myocardial Infarction 48 h or More from the Onset of Symptoms.***   In patients admitted 48 to 72 h after the onset of symptoms, particularly when associated with minimal myocardial damage, the preferred diagnostic marker has become troponin I or T. Both remain elevated for 10 to 14 days.

## NONINVASIVE IMAGING IN ACUTE MYOCARDIAL INFARCTION.
***Chest Roentgenogram.***   The chest roentgenogram (x-ray) is important and may help to exclude causes of chest pain such as pneumothorax, pulmonary infarction

**TABLE 26-2.   Enzymatic Criteria for Diagnosis of Myocardial Infarction**

| |
|---|
| Serial increase, then decrease of plasma MB-CK or subform ratio, with a change >25% between any two values |
| MB-CK >10–13 U/L or >5% total CK activity |
| Increase in MB-CK activity >50% between any two samples, separated by at least 4 h |
| If only a single sample available, MB-CK elevation >twofold |
| Beyond 72 h, an elevation of troponin T or I |

*Source:* From Alexander RW, Pratt CM, Roberts R: Diagnosis and management of patients with acute myocardial infarction. In: Alexander RW, Schlant RC, Fuster V, et al (eds): *Hurst's The Heart,* 9th ed. New York, McGraw-Hill, 1998.

with effusion, aortic dissection, skeletal fractures, and so on. In the patient with AMI, the chest film can be useful in establishing the presence of pulmonary edema, in assessing heart size to assist in determining whether or not cardiomegaly is present, and in deciding whether heart failure or myocardial or valvular disease is acute or chronic.

***Echocardiography.*** Two-dimensional and Doppler echocardiography are very useful tools in the assessment of the patient with AMI, especially in the patient with a nondiagnostic ECG.[5] The presence of a regional wall motion abnormality provides strong supportive evidence of acute coronary ischemia and is generally present in Q-wave MI. Wall motion abnormalities are less common but still frequently present in non-Q-wave infarction. Echocardiography also provides an assessment of ventricular function; it is useful in predicting the prognosis and in diagnosing RV infarction. It can also provide information concerning alternative diagnoses such as aortic dissection and, coupled with Doppler, can provide information on such complications as ruptured chordae tendineae with mitral regurgitation and ventricular septal defect. It is useful in detecting ventricular thrombus and pericardial fluid.

**MEASUREMENT OF MYOCARDIAL INFARCT SIZE.** The major determinant of both acute and long-term prognosis following MI is the extent of myocardial damage.

***Electrocardiographic Estimates of Infarct Size.*** The ECG has long been used to obtain a semiquantitative assessment of the extent of MI. In general, it has been found, for example, that patients with anterior infarcts who develop Q waves in leads $V_1$ to $V_6$ usually have extensive damage and an unfavorable prognosis. In general, there is a direct relationship between the number of leads showing ST-segment elevation and mortality.

*Infarct Size Assessment by Imaging.*    For practical reasons, echocardiography is the most commonly used imaging modality in the acute evaluation.

## Prehospital Care

Modern in-hospital care of the patient with an acute coronary ischemic syndrome has resulted in a substantial reduction in mortality. Some 40 to 65 percent of deaths from AMI, however, occur within an hour of the onset of symptoms and prior to arrival at a hospital. Most of these deaths are attributable to ventricular fibrillation. Substantial further reductions in acute mortality rates are likely to require marked improvements in prehospital care and in patient responsiveness to symptoms. The goals for community Emergency Response Services (EMS)[5] include the availability of 911 telephone access and of personnel trained in defibrillation and, potentially, in initiation of out-of-hospital thrombolysis.

The major contribution that the physician can make to minimizing delay between the time that patients first appreciate subjective manifestations of AMI and the time they present at the Emergency Department (ED) is in educating patients beforehand as to the proper responses to ischemic coronary symptoms. The guiding principles are *recognition* and *response.* Thus, the patient should be taught to recognize and appreciate chest pain as potentially representing coronary ischemia and, if sustained, threatened AMI. Patients should be warned specifically of the dangers of rationalizing the pain as having a noncardiac origin or of trying extensive "diagnostic trials" of home remedies. They should be instructed in the standard protocol for using nitroglycerin. That is, at the onset of pain, the patient should immediately use nitroglycerin in a form that is absorbed rapidly from the oral mucosa. If the pain is not relieved within 5 min, the dosing should be repeated. If the discomfort persists for another 5 min, a third dose should be administered. If at this point no relief is obtained, the patient should proceed immediately to the nearest emergency department (ED). The potential risk of fatal arrhythmia in the early course of AMI should be explained. *Educating patients about this protocol is one of the most important functions of the physician caring for patients with coronary artery disease (CAD).*

## Evaluation and Management of the Chest Pain Patient in the Emergency Department

**BACKGROUND.**    The goals of the ED with respect to chest pain patients are as follows: to rapidly identify those patients with AMI with both typical and atypical presentations, so that appropriate therapy can be initiated; to recognize those patients with acute coronary syndromes (unstable angina) but without MI who are thus at high risk; and to assess accurately those patients at low risk who are candidates for noninvasive evaluation and early discharge. The earlier reperfusion therapy is initiated in the subset of patients with diagnostic ST-segment elevation, the more favorable the clinical results.[9]

An important objective, obviously, should be a triage system that minimizes the number of patients at high risk (AMI or unstable angina) who are inadvertently discharged from the ED while also minimizing the admission to high-intensity CCUs of low-risk patients without AMI.

Misdiagnosis of AMI is commonly associated with misinterpretation of the ECG. A major contributing problem to the difficulty of diagnosing AMI is that even experienced clinicians appear to be able to achieve sensitivity and specificity of only about 80 percent in the diagnosis of AMI on clinical grounds alone. The problem extends also to diagnosing unstable angina in the absence of infarction. These patients with coronary instability are also at high intermediate-term risk. *The clinical focus in the ED should not be simply to "rule out" AMI but, taking a proactive approach, to "rule in" either acute infarction or unstable angina in an expeditious manner.* If these urgent conditions can be excluded or ascertained to be of low probability, the next level of concern is determining the presence of other acute cardiovascular or cardiopulmonary conditions, such as aortic dissection, pulmonary embolus, pericarditis, and so on.

**INITIAL APPROACH, DETECTION, AND ASSESSMENT OF RISK.**   A major goal in dealing with chest pain patients is establishment of a routine approach that leads to a rapid (10-min) preliminary evaluation, acquisition of a 12-lead ECG, and establishment of intravenous access, continuous electrocardiographic monitoring, and supplemental oxygen (Fig. 26-1). The initial assessment is guided by the differential diagnosis of chest pain, with the goal of establishing whether or not myocardial ischemia is a likely or possible diagnosis. Blood is drawn for baseline cardiac marker levels; if coronary ischemia is suspected and there are no contraindications, the patient is given aspirin of 160 to 325 mg to chew and swallow. Also, the patient with suspected coronary ischemia is given sublingual nitroglycerin unless the systolic blood pressure is less than 90 mmHg. This should be avoided with severe bradycardia or tachycardia. The history of chest pain alone usually dictates entry into the system for evaluation. In general, the only chest pain patients not systematically evaluated for myocardial ischemia would be those in whom a clear noncardiac cause, such as chest wall tenderness, can be demonstrated unequivocally to be the etiology of the presenting symptoms. Continuous ECG monitoring is essential because of the propensity of any patient with an acute coronary ischemic syndrome to develop sudden and potentially lethal ventricular arrhythmias. Intravenous access is essential for therapeutic interventions under such circumstances as well as for more general purposes. Additionally, paroxysmal changes in the ST-segment may be recognizable on the monitor. The causes of chest pain that are not the result of acute pathologic changes compromising the structural integrity of the large coronary arteries are listed in Table 26-3.

*As a general rule, one should begin the evaluation of the chest pain patient with the assumption that one is dealing with myocardial ischemia until proven otherwise.* The three most serious and urgent alternative diagnoses that need to be considered specifically during the initial evaluation are *aortic dissection, acute pulmonary embolus,* and *acute pneumothorax. Acute pericarditis* and *myopericarditis* need to be considered as well.

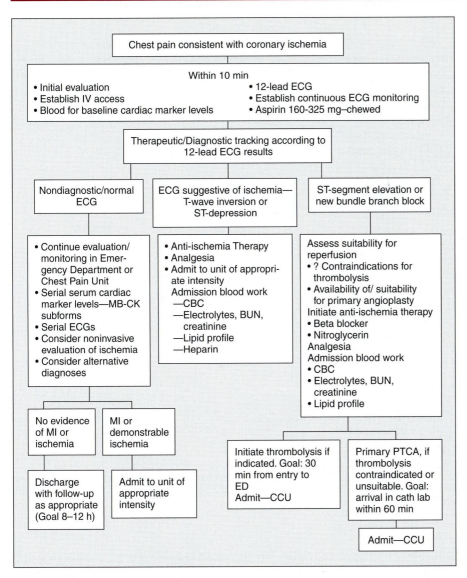

**Figure 26-1** Algorithm for the initial assessment and evaluation of the patient with acute chest pain in the emergency department. The emergency department should be organized to facilitate the rapid triage of chest pain patients so that the initial evaluation, obtaining a 12-lead ECG, and establishing intravenous access and continuous monitoring are accomplished within 10 min. The path in the decision tree is determined by the results of the 12-lead ECG. The presence of ST-segment elevation diagnostic of AMI or of presumptively new BBB suggestive of this diagnosis should lead to the immediate consideration of the suitability of the patient for reperfusion therapy, which, if indicated, should be initiated within 30 min of the patient's arrival. The primary PTCA option is applicable only in those settings in which it is immediately available and can be performed by highly qualified interventional cardiologists. In general, patients should not be transferred for angioplasty if thrombolysis is an option. Thrombolysis is not indicated in patients with only ST-segment depression. [From Alexander RW, Pratt CM, Roberts R: Diagnosis and management of patients with acute myocardial infarction. In: Alexander RW, Schlent RC, Fuster VC, et al (eds): *Hurst's The Heart,* 9th ed. New York, McGraw-Hill, 1998.]

**TABLE 26-3.   Causes of Chest Pain Other than Acute Coronary Artery Syndromes**

Cardiovascular
   Aortic dissection
   Aortic stenosis
   Pericarditis
   Mitral valve prolapse
   Microvascular angina
      Hypertrophic cardiomyopathy
      Syndrome X
   Pulmonary embolus
   Arrhythmia/palpitations

Noncardiovascular
   Pleurisy
   Pneumonia
   Pneumothorax
   Costochondritis
   Gastrointestinal
      Esophageal spasm/reflux
      Acid peptic disease
      Cholecystitis
      Gastritis

Psychiatric
   Panic attack
   Cardiac neurosis
   Depression

Malingering

*Source:* From Alexander RW, Pratt CM, Roberts R: Diagnosis and management of patients with acute myocardial infarction. In: Alexander RW, Schlant RC, Fuster V, et al (eds): *Hurst's The Heart,* 9th ed. New York, McGraw-Hill, 1998.

Aortic dissection must be considered and ruled in or out during the initial evaluation, since specific intervention can decrease its high mortality. Furthermore, administration of thrombolytic agents in the presence of aortic dissection is associated with high mortality. Suspicion of dissection should be heightened in hypertensive patients or in those with marfanoid habitus.

Pulmonary embolus can be life-threatening and should be suspected in anyone with a sudden onset of shortness of breath and chest pressure or pain, especially if there is a history of being sedentary or immobilized and/or a history of deep venous thrombosis.

Acute pericarditis may mimic AMI in that the pain can be substernal and persistent. Frequently, however, there will be a positional component as well as characteristics of pleurisy, with accentuation by deep breathing. Furthermore, the diffuse ST-segment elevation may lead to a misdiagnosis of MI. The key differentiating features in pericarditis include PR depression, the diffuse nature of ST-segment elevation in most leads, and the absence of reciprocal changes.

Esophageal disorders are very common in patients presenting with chest pain in whom cardiac ischemia is ruled out. Because of the high frequency of gastrointestinal disease in chest pain patients, "GI cocktails" or antacids have been used as a diagnostic tool to guide triage and disposition. Only 25 percent of patients with esophageal pain, however, have been reported to obtain pain relief with antacids.[10] Furthermore, coincidental, spontaneous relief of ischemic chest pain at the time of administration of the GI cocktail could be misleading. Similarly, administration of nitroglycerin as a diagnostic strategy for ischemic disease could be misleading because it can relieve esophageal spasm. Moreover, pain relief after nitroglycerin does not predict unstable angina or AMI. The use of these "response-to-treatment" strategies as major decision points in the evaluation of chest pain has been discouraged.

***Detection.***    The results of the 12-lead ECG guide the next level of decision making for the patient with chest pain thought to be compatible with myocardial ischemia (Fig. 26-1). The ECG interpretation is assigned to one of three categories: (1) ST-segment elevation in two or more leads or a presumptively new left bundle branch block, implicating acute coronary occlusion, usually thrombotic; (2) ST-segment depression and/or T-wave inversion, implying subtotal occlusion and nontransmural ischemia; and (3) normal or nondiagnostic. The group with ST-segment elevation or a left bundle branch block is particularly important to define, as it is this group that has been shown to benefit from thrombolytic therapy. There is no indication as yet of the benefit of thrombolytic therapy or primary angioplasty in those patients without ST-segment elevation or bundle branch block.

The measurement of serum markers of myocardial damage plays a major role in diagnosis, as discussed. Measurement of MB-CK is the benchmark laboratory test, and the specificity and sensitivity of samples taken 2 h apart during serial sampling have been reported to be 91 and 94 percent, respectively.

Two-dimensional echocardiography can be useful as an adjunctive modality. It may be especially useful in detecting wall motion abnormalities in the presence of conduction abnormalities on the ECG.

***Risk Stratification.***    Stratifying risk in the patient with acute myocardial infarction or unstable angina is an essential part of the management strategy during all phases of care.

Predictors of an increased risk include the following: ECG evidence of ST-segment elevation or Q waves in two or more leads that are not known to have been present previously; ST-segment depression or T-wave inversions consistent with myocardial ischemia and not known to be present previously; pain worse than prior angina or the same as that experienced with prior MI; systolic blood pressure of less than 100 mmHg; or rales bilaterally.[5]

Blood levels of cardiac markers are prognostically important. In particular, the levels of troponins (I and T) at presentation appear to be strong predictors of risk in patients with acute ischemic syndromes.[11,12]

***Initial Management.***    As discussed, one frequently does not have a definitive diagnosis of AMI in the chest pain patient in the emergency department. Nevertheless, the initial general treatment of the acute coronary syndromes including unstable angina is the same.

*Routine General Measures.*

**1.**   *Oxygen administration.* Hypoxemia is not uncommon in patients with AMI, even with an uncomplicated course. Nasal oxygen should be administered to all AMI patients with pulmonary congestion and $SaO_2$ of less than 90 percent. $O_2$ should be administered to all uncomplicated AMI patients for the first 2 to 3 h. There appears to be little justification for extending use of oxygen administration beyond 2 to 3 h in uncomplicated MI with an $SaO_2$ of greater than 90 percent or in the case of unstable angina. Oxygen administration should be continued in patients with pulmonary congestion and desaturation.

**2.**   *Analgesia.* The alleviation of pain and anxiety remains an essential element in the care of the patient with AMI. The pain and accompanying anxiety contribute to excessive activity of the autonomic nervous system and to restlessness. These factors, in turn, increase the metabolic demands of the myocardium.

The approach to pain consists of relieving ischemia and attacking the pain directly. Anti-ischemic therapy consists of reperfusion, beta blockers (if appropriate), nitrates, and oxygen administration. Morphine is the drug of choice in most instances, since it is well tolerated and offers analgesia without significant cardiac depression. It also relieves anxiety and the feeling of doom that is commonly described. Morphine sulfate can be given intravenously at doses of 2 to 4 mg every 15 min until adequate relief has been obtained, which in some patients may require 25 to 30 mg. If the patient's anxiety is not controlled by the administration of narcotics, mild sedation with a benzodiazepine is appropriate. Diazepam in doses of 5 mg orally every 8 to 12 h or alprazolam in doses of 0.25 mg every 8 h are most often used. In patients with unstable angina without frequent episodes of prolonged pain, analgesia is obviously less imperative.

**3.**   *Nitroglycerin.* This should be administered for the first 24 to 48 h to AMI patients with CHF, large anterior MI, persistent recurrent angina, or persistent pulmonary congestion. Nitroglycerin in an oral or topical form should be considered beyond 48 h in patients with large or complicated AMI.

Nitroglycerin has become very widely used in the treatment of AMI. It is an anti-ischemic agent not only by virtue of its actions to decrease preload and afterload, and thus to decrease oxygen demand but also because of its vasodilator actions on epicardial coronary arteries and on coronary collaterals. The early administration of nitroglycerin limits the extent of myocardial damage and favorably affects survival.

*Complications and limitations.* The most serious complication of nitroglycerin is hypotension. Thus, nitroglycerin should be avoided in patients with a systolic pressure of less than 90 mmHg or in the case of severe bradycardia. Caution should be exercised in the case of inferior wall infarction because of the possibility of right ventricular involvement. Nitroglycerin should be used only with extreme caution, if at all, in right ventricular infarction, because the right ventricle in this circumstance becomes extremely dependent upon preload, which can be diminished by the veno-dilating properties of the drug.[13]

*Dosage of nitroglycerin.* Long-acting nitrates should generally not be used as initial therapy in AMI. Intravenous nitroglycerin is preferable. Dose titration can be assessed by frequent determinations of blood pressure and heart rate. Invasive monitoring is not essential but is probably prudent if high doses are required or if there is hemodynamic instability or uncertainty about the adequacy of ventricular preload.

Treatment should be initiated with a bolus injection of 12.5 to 25 $\mu$g and should be followed by infusion by pump of 10 to 20 $\mu$g/min with increases of 5 to 10 $\mu$g every 5 to 10 min while assessing hemodynamic and clinical responses. Control of symptoms is a major end point; in the case of high left ventricular filling pressure, the objective is a decrease of 10 to 30 percent in pulmonary artery wedge pressure. Limitations of nitroglycerin dosing are as follows: (1) a decrease in mean arterial pressure of 10 percent in normotensive patients; or (2) a decrease of 30 percent in hypertensive patients but not below a systolic pressure of 90 mmHg; or (3) an increase in heart rate of 10 beats per minute, not to exceed 110 beats per minute.

Doses of nitroglycerin of greater than 200 $\mu$g/min are associated with an increased risk of hypotension. Requirements this high may indicate tolerance, and alternative drugs such as angiotensin-converting enzyme (ACE) inhibitors or nitroprusside should be considered. If tolerance is the issue, responsiveness should return after a 12- to 18-h period off nitroglycerin.

**4.** *Aspirin.* The antiplatelet agent aspirin reduces the incidence of vascular events in patients with AMI at 1 month, and the patient suspected of having a coronary ischemic syndrome and without contraindication should receive, early in the course, 160 to 325 mg of non-enteric-coated aspirin, which is chewed. If CAD is confirmed, aspirin treatment should be continued indefinitely.

**MANAGEMENT AFTER TRIAGE INTO ECG SUBGROUPS.** The initial ECG, as a first approximation, permits assignment of patients with chest pain into subgroups distinguishable by therapeutic responsiveness and risk, as discussed previously. It must be kept in mind that these initial categorizations do not necessarily define ultimate outcome. Thus, patients with no ST-segment elevation at presentation may, in fact, have unstable angina and ultimately have no infarction or may progress to have either a Q-wave or a non-Q-wave infarction. Similarly, those presenting with ST-segment elevation may have a non-Q-wave infarction, although the majority of these will develop Q waves. This potential for variable outcomes provides the underlying rationale for close monitoring and continuous reassessment of clinical course, risk, and therapeutic strategies during the period of observation and for monitoring both in the ED and subsequently in other hospital units.

***Approach to the Patient with ST-Segment Elevation.*** The approach to the patient with chest pain and ST-segment elevation is guided heavily by the evidence that members of this subgroup have a high frequency of epicardial coronary artery occlusion by a thrombus and that, in them, thrombolytic therapy has shown clinical benefit. Evaluation and management of the patient with ischemic chest pain and ST-segment elevation is focused on the rapid assessment of suitability for and delivery of reperfusion therapy (Fig. 26-2).[3]

Initial evaluation and management have been discussed. The appropriate next steps are to administer a beta-adrenergic blocker if not contraindicated and to ini-

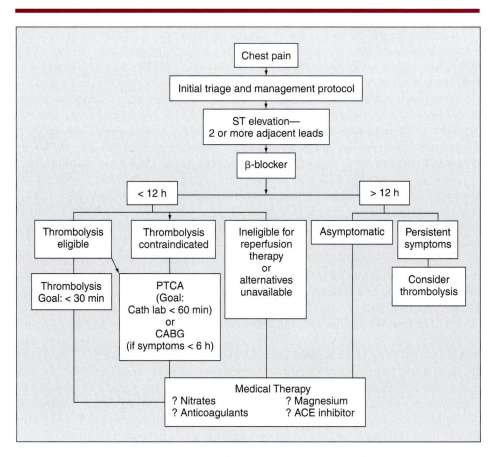

**Figure 26-2**   Evaluation of patients with ST-segment elevation. Algorithm for initial decision making in regard to reperfusion therapy in patients with suspected AMI and ST-segment elevation. Whether or not to administer thrombolytics or to perform primary PTCA is determined by the time from onset of symptom. For patients in whom more than 12 h have elapsed since the onset of symptoms, reperfusion should be considered only if there are persistent or recurrent symptoms associated with ST-segment elevation. For patients with ST-segment elevation and duration of symptoms between 7 and 12 h, the decision to proceed with a reperfusion strategy requires careful clinical judgment in weighing the risk/benefit issues, as discussed in the text. (Reproduced with permission. Ryan TJ, Anderson JL, Antman EM, et al: ACC/AHA Guidelines for the Management of Patients with Acute Myocardial Infarction. *J Am Coll Cardiol* 1996; 28:1328–1428. Copyright ©1996 American College of Cardiology and American Heart Association, Inc.)

tiate evaluation for reperfusion therapy. The 12-h point defines the time frame in which the risk/benefit ratio is clearly favorable for administering thrombolytic therapy—although, obviously, the earlier the better.

*Beta-Adrenergic Receptor Blockers.*   Beta-adrenergic receptor blockers interfere with the positive inotropic and chronotropic effects of catecholamines and therefore reduce myocardial oxygen consumption.

*The available data strongly support the use of beta blockers early in the course of acute Q-wave MI in the absence of contraindications, irrespective of concomitant thrombolytic therapy.*[3] Patients with continuing or recurrent ischemic pain or with tachyarrhythmias, such as atrial fibrillation with rapid ventricular response, should also be considered for beta-blocker therapy. The evidence for beta-blocker therapy in non-Q-wave AMI is less compelling. Patients with moderate or severe congestive heart failure or other contraindications should not receive beta blockers. While metoprolol and atenolol are the only beta blockers approved by the FDA for use in the United States for AMI, *therapeutic efficacy is a class effect of beta blockers lacking intrinsic sympathomimetic activity.*

The relative contraindications to beta-blocker therapy are as follows:[3] (1) heart rate less than 60 beats per minute; (2) systolic blood pressure less than 100 mmHg; (3) moderate or severe left ventricular failure; (4) signs of peripheral hypoperfusion; (5) PR interval greater than 240 ms; (6) second- or third-degree atrioventricular (AV) block; (7) severe chronic pulmonary disease; (8) history of asthma; (9) severe peripheral vascular disease; and (10) diabetes mellitus requiring insulin. Since these contraindications are relative and not absolute, the clinician has the option of assessing the effects of beta blockade with the short-acting, intravenous beta blocker esmolol, which has an onset of action within 5 to 10 min and a half-life of about 30 min.

*Thrombolysis.*

**1.** *Indications for thrombolytic therapy.* Reperfusion therapy should be given immediate consideration in all patients presenting with AMI. The primary indication for attempts at reperfusion, given an appropriate history, is the findings on the ECG, as discussed above. Patients with ST-segment elevation (>0.1 mV) in two or more contiguous leads or a bundle branch block (BBB) masking ST-segment changes occurring within 12 h of onset of symptoms are candidates for thrombolytic therapy.[9] *Patients with ongoing symptoms should be repeatedly evaluated by 12-lead ECGs as frequently as every 10 to 15 min in order to identify ST-segment elevation as soon as possible.* Conversely, ST-segment elevation in the absence of suggestive symptoms should suggest such possibilities as early repolarization, pericarditis, and previous infarction with aneurysm formation. Elderly patients should not be excluded from thrombolytic therapy primarily because of their age or because of the increased risk of bleeding.

Large, placebo-controlled clinical trials have consistently demonstrated reduced mortality in patients receiving thrombolytic therapy within 6 h of the onset of an

AMI. Because of the suggestion of benefit between 6 and 12 h, it has been recommended that the time limit for therapy be up to 12 h from the onset of symptoms. The benefit of thrombolytics given between 6 and 12 h postevent is greater in patients classified as high-risk, such as those with severe heart failure and large infarctions. Thrombolysis can be considered in the case of ongoing pain and marked ST-segment elevation at times between 12 and 24 h from onset, although there is only a trend for benefit under these circumstances in clinical trials. Patients with ST-segment depression, T-wave inversion, or no ECG changes have not been shown to benefit from thrombolytic therapy.

The potential for therapeutic benefit of thrombolysis in the setting of high risk of MI when the blood pressure is markedly elevated (>180 mmHg systolic and/or >110 mmHg diastolic) has to be carefully weighed against the increased risk of intracranial hemorrhage under these circumstances. Lowering the blood pressure pharmacologically before administering thrombolytics has been recommended but is of unproven benefit. If available, coronary artery bypass grafting or primary percutaneous transluminal coronary angioplasty (PTCA) should be considered.[3]

**2.** *Contraindications to thrombolytic therapy.* The absolute and relative contraindications to thrombolytic therapy are summarized in Table 26-4.

**3.** *Choice of thrombolytic agent.* Four thrombolytic agents have been approved in the United States for routine use: streptokinase (SK), recombinant tissue plasminogen activator (rt-PA), anistreplase (APSAC), and reteplase (r-PA).[5] Each has been shown to limit infarct size, preserve ventricular function, and improve survival rates.

**4.** *Dose and administration of thrombolytic agents.* Streptokinase is given in a dose of 1.5 million units intravenously over 30 to 60 min. Since antibodies develop and may persist for several years, a subsequent need for thrombolytic therapy, as for early or late reocclusion, would require the use of rt-PA or r-PA. APSAC is identical to SK as a thrombolytic agent but can be given as a rapid infusion of 30 units over 5 to 10 min. The FDA-approved dose of rt-PA is an initial bolus of 15 mg, followed by an infusion of 50 mg or 0.75 mg/kg of body weight over the next 30 min and an infusion of 35 mg or 0.50 mg/kg of body weight over the subsequent 60 min, for a total of up to 100 mg given over 90 min. Reteplase is given as an initial bolus of 15 megaunits (MU), followed by a second bolus of 15 MU in 30 min. Thrombolytic therapy is rapidly evolving, and both the specific agent and various combinations as well as the specific doses and regimens of administration are changing rapidly.

*Overall Strategy for Reperfusion of Patients with Acute Myocardial Infarction.* The criteria for initiating thrombolytic therapy are as follows (Table 26-5):

1. Patients presenting with chest pain suggestive of myocardial ischemia who have ST-segment elevation greater than 1 mm in two contiguous limb leads or greater than 2 mm in two contiguous precordial leads or new left bundle branch block and who are within 6 h of the onset of symptoms should receive thrombolytic therapy if there are no contraindications. In patients presenting between 6 and 12 h, the bias should be toward thrombolytic therapy the higher the risk of the

**TABLE 26-4.   Absolute and Relative Contraindications to Thrombolytic Therapy**

| Absolute Contraindications | Relative Contraindications |
| --- | --- |
| Active internal bleeding | History of nonhemorrhagic cerebrovascular accident in distant past with complete recovery |
| Intracranial neoplasm or recent head trauma | Recent trauma or surgery >2 weeks previously |
| Prolonged, traumatic CPR | Active peptic ulcer disease |
| Suspected aortic dissection | Hemorrhagic retinopathy |
| Pregnancy | History of severe hypertension with diastolic blood pressure >100 |
| History of hemorrhagic cerebrovascular accident or recent nonhemorrhagic cerebrovascular accident | Bleeding diathesis or concurrent use of anticoagulants |
| Recorded blood pressure >200/120 | Previous treatment with SK or APSAC if being considered (does not apply to rt-PA) |
| Trauma or surgery that is a potential bleeding source within previous 2 weeks | |
| Allergy to SK or APSAC if being considered | |

Key: CPR = cardiopulmonary resuscitation; SK = streptokinase; APSAC = anistreplase; rt-PA = recombinant tissue plasminogen activator.

*Source:* From Alexander RW, Pratt CM, Roberts R: Diagnosis and management of patients with acute myocardial infarction. In: Alexander RW, Schlant RC, Fuster V, et al (eds): *Hurst's The Heart,* 9th ed. New York, McGraw-Hill, 1998.

AMI. Patients presenting after 12 h are not routinely considered for thrombolytic therapy.

2. Contraindications for thrombolytic therapy are absolute or relative, as discussed earlier (Table 26-4).

3. In patients receiving rt-PA or r-PA, it is recommended that heparin be given as a bolus infusion of 5000 units, followed by a continuous infusion of 1000 units/h, adjusted to keep the partial thromboplastin time (PTT) at one and one-half to two times the normal control for 24 to 48 h. Heparin should be given in patients who have received SK or APSAC who are at high risk for systemic embolization. Aspirin (160 to 325 mg) should be administered as soon as possible and continued indefinitely. Beta blockers, nitrates, and occasionally calcium blockers may be given as indicated with or without thrombolytic therapy.

**TABLE 26-5.   Criteria for Initiating Thrombolytic Therapy**

Chest pain consistent with angina

ECG changes
   ST increased >1 mm, >2 contiguous limb leads
   ST increased >2 mm, >2 contiguous precordial leads
   New left bundle branch block

Absence of contraindications

*Source:* From Alexander RW, Pratt CM, Roberts R: Diagnosis and management of patients with acute myocardial infarction. In: Alexander RW, Schlant RC, Fuster V, et al (eds): *Hurst's The Heart,* 9th ed. New York, McGraw-Hill, 1998.

4. Patients allergic to SK or APSAC who require thrombolytic therapy should receive rt-PA or r-PA. Patients who have received SK or APSAC and who again require thrombolytic therapy should receive rt-PA or r-PA.
5. Patients presenting with ST-segment depression and chest pain are not candidates for thrombolytic therapy and need to be triaged, as indicated in Fig. 26-1.
6. PTCA, as a primary procedure, is an alternative to thrombolytic therapy only if performed in a timely fashion by individuals skilled in the procedure and supported by experienced personnel in high-volume centers. PTCA is indicated in patients with a contraindication to thrombolytic therapy or those in cardiogenic shock.
7. Elective angioplasty should be reserved for patients who develop ischemia or reinfarction or in whom thrombolytic therapy appears ineffective. In patients in whom angioplasty cannot be performed and who develop recurrent ischemia with possible infarction, the possibility of readministering a thrombolytic agent should be considered.

*Heparin as Conjunctive or Adjunctive Therapy.*   After thrombolytic therapy is given, it is recommended that heparin not be started immediately but that an activated partial thromboplastin time (aPTT) be drawn at 4 h and that heparin be started when the aPTT returns to less than twice control (about 70 s). Lysis of a thrombus by any thrombolytic agent induces a highly thrombogenic surface. Furthermore, lysis with either rt-PA or SK is associated with marked elevation of plasma levels of thrombin. The use of heparin during the initial 24 to 48 h is critical to prevent rethrombosis and reocclusion.

Heparin is not necessary in order to achieve reperfusion but is essential in the first 24 h to maintain patency rates with rt-PA. While heparin may be beneficial when SK is being used, subcutaneous administration of heparin appears adequate in this circumstance. At present, heparin is recommended in a bolus of 5000 units intravenously followed by an infusion of 1000 to 1200 units/h to keep the PTT at one and one-half to two times normal. It is recommended that the PTT not be measured until 4 h after initiating heparin therapy, because it has not yet reached a steady state.

If the PTT has increased more than twofold over the normal level, the same dose of heparin should be continued; if the PTT exhibits less than a twofold increase, the infusion rate of heparin should be increased. Initiation of heparin is recommended either during or following completion of thrombolytic therapy, and in the uncomplicated patient it should be maintained for 24 to 48 h.

The use of heparin has also been recommended conjunctively in patients with AMI who are not being treated with the drug for other reasons, i.e., postthrombolysis or post-primary PTCA. Currently, guidelines recommend heparin 7500 units twice daily subcutaneously as prophylaxis against deep venous thrombosis. Given the enhanced risk of stroke after acute myocardial infarction in patients with atrial arrhythmias, those with large and especially anterior and apical infarction, and those with a history of previous stroke, guidelines have incorporated this recommendation for broader prophylaxis against systemic embolization.[3] In high-risk patients, the intravenous route is probably preferable. Heparin therapy should be continued for 48 h, and a judgment about continuation should be made at that point based on individual patient characteristics.

As more studies become available, and once therapeutic regimens are tested and standardized, the use of low-molecular-weight heparins may replace many of the recommendations above.

***Early Coronary Angiography in Patients with ST-Segment Elevation not Undergoing Primary PTCA.***   Routine immediate or delayed angioplasty is not recommended as a standard mode of therapy following thrombolysis. At present, the most widely accepted recommendation is to perform cardiac catheterization for possible angioplasty or bypass surgery in patients who develop angina or manifest evidence of myocardial ischemia during submaximal exercise testing or who develop hemodynamic or ischemic instability.[3] Thus, if intervening with PTCA generally offers no demonstrable benefit after thrombolysis, there is little apparent reason to perform early coronary angiography routinely.

Patients with cardiogenic shock have a very high (>70 percent) mortality with or without thrombolysis, and some rather small series have provided evidence that outcomes are improved with an aggressive reperfusion strategy. Successful PTCA in conventionally treated patients who had cardiogenic shock reduced mortality from greater than 80 to about 30 percent. Thus, an aggressive interventional strategy including PTCA seems reasonable, based on available data, in appropriate patients with cardiogenic shock who have failed thrombolysis therapy.

***Emergency or Urgent Coronary Artery Bypass Surgery.***   In the presence of cardiogenic shock, coronary artery bypass grafting in patients in whom other strategies either have failed or have not been indicated has been associated with mortality rates from about 10 to 40 percent.[14] These results are generally better than those associated with PTCA. Thus, AMI patients with multivessel CAD or cardiogenic shock who have had unsuccessful thrombolysis and/or PTCA and are within 4 to 6 h of the onset of symptoms should be considered for emergency coronary artery bypass grafting.[3]

### Arrhythmias Early in the Course of Acute Myocardial Infarction.

*Bradycardia.*   Bradyarrhythmias are relatively common (30 to 40 percent) early in the course of AMI, especially in inferior infarction or after reperfusion of the right coronary artery. Atropine, because of its anticholinergic effects, can be very useful in this situation, since it enhances the discharge rate of the sinus node and facilitates AV conduction, as well as reversing the peripheral effects of excessive cholinergic activity, such as vasodilation with associated hypotension. Parasympathomimetic effects, with bradycardia, hypotension, and nausea and vomiting, are also produced by morphine and can be reversed by atropine.

*Sinus Bradycardia, Atrioventricular Block, or Ventricular Asystole.*   Atropine is indicated for the treatment of type I Wenckebach second-degree AV block (progressive prolongation of the PR interval before a dropped QRS complex), especially when it is complicating inferior MI, and is useful at times in third-degree AV block at the AV node in restoring AV conduction or for increasing the junctional response rate.[3] Treatment of sinus bradycardia or first- or type I second-degree AV block is generally not indicated in the absence of hemodynamic compromise,[3] and atropine should seldom be used in the treatment of type II AV block (location of the block below the AV node). *Symptomatic bradycardia that is unresponsive to atropine should be treated with pacing.* Atropine should be administered intravenously at a dosage of 0.5 to 1.0 mg and titrated carefully as necessary to achieve an adequate heart rate (50 to 60 beats per minute), with doses as needed every 3 to 5 min, up to a total maximum dose of 2.5 mg, which gives complete vagal blockade.[3]

*Heart Block.*   Heart block (complete or third-degree) develops in about 10 percent of patients with AMI and is associated with an increased mortality during hospitalization, but does not predict long-term mortality in those who survive to be discharged. Intraventricular conduction delay or bundle branch block is also associated with increased in-hospital mortality. The increase in mortality associated with heart block reflects the extent of myocardial damage. Thus, heart block in the setting of anterior MI reflects extensive infarction and concomitant destruction of the conduction system and is associated with relatively high mortality. In contrast, heart block with inferior MI may reflect primarily ischemia of the AV node rather than extensive tissue damage and is associated with a more favorable prognosis. Because of the overwhelming effect of the extent of myocardial damage on prognosis, pacing has not been shown to lessen mortality associated with AV block or bundle branch block. In AMI, the risk of developing heart block is augmented by the presence of any evidence of conduction system abnormality, including first-degree AV block, Mobitz type I or II AV block, left anterior or posterior hemiblock, or a left or right bundle branch block.[3]

*Temporary Pacing Early in the Course of Acute Myocardial Infarction.*   Recent guidelines place increased emphasis on transcutaneous pacing in view of the availability of new systems that provide standby status for pacing in AMI in patients who do not require immediate pacing and are at intermediate risk for developing heart block.[3] These systems use a single pair of multifunctional electrodes, permitting ECG monitoring, transcutaneous pacing, and defibrillation. Transcutaneous pacing does not entail the risk and complications of transvenous pacing and, because invasive procedures may be avoided or delayed, is well suited for use in the patient who has undergone thrombolysis. Percutaneous pacing is painful; if prolonged pacing is required, the patient should be switched to transvenous systems.

The following conditions are indications for placement of patches or activation (demand) of transcutaneous pacing:[3] (1) sinus bradycardia (rate less than 50 beats per minute) with symptoms of hypotension unresponsive to drug therapy; (2) Mobitz type II (absence of a QRS complex after a normal P wave without antecedent progressive prolongation of the PR interval) second-degree AV block; (3) third-degree heart block; (4) bilateral bundle branch block (alternating left and right bundle branch block or right bundle branch block with alternating left anterior and posterior fascicular block); (5) newly acquired or age-indeterminant left bundle branch block, or right bundle branch block and anterior or posterior fascicular block; (6) right or left bundle branch block and first-degree AV block.

As noted, transcutaneous pacing is intended to be temporary; if prolonged pacing is required, transvenous pacing should be instituted (discussed subsequently). In addition, patients with a high probability of requiring pacing should have it instituted early on.[3]

*Ventricular Ectopy, Tachycardia, and Fibrillation.*   Ventricular rhythm abnormalities are common during the early phases of AMI, with an incidence of ventricular fibrillation (VF) within the first 4 h, so-called primary VF, of 3 to 5 percent, which declines rapidly thereafter. Primary VF is associated with increased in-hospital mortality, but not with increased long-term mortality for patients who survive and are discharged.

Post-AMI ventricular tachycardia (VT) occurs in about 15 percent of patients and is also most commonly manifested during the relatively early period. VT is classified according to its electrocardiographic morphology (monomorphic or polymorphic) and by its duration and consequences: sustained (lasting more than 30 s and/or causing hemodynamic compromise earlier, which requires intervention) and nonsustained (not resulting in hemodynamic compromise and lasting less than 30 s).[3] Short runs (5 beats or less) of nonsustained VT are very common in the early post-MI period and do not require specific treatment.

Accelerated idioventricular rhythm normally occurs frequently during the first hours of AMI[3] and occurs after thrombolysis as a reperfusion arrhythmia. In neither case is it a premonitory rhythm for VT/VF. *Accelerated idioventricular rhythm should ordinarily be observed and not treated specifically.*[3]

Formerly, it was common practice to treat patients prophylactically with lidocaine in order to prevent VT/VF. Currently, *routine use of prophylactic lidocaine in AMI in the presence or absence of thrombolysis is not recommended.* Two prophylactic approaches to the prevention of VT/VF are recommended, however.[3] Routine administration of beta blockers, as described previously, has been shown to reduce the incidence of VT/VF. Also, since evidence suggests that hypokalemia is a risk factor for VT/VF, it is recommended that serum potassium levels be kept above 4.0 mEq/L by supplementation, as necessary.

*Treatment of Ventricular Tachycardia/Fibrillation.* Electrical cardioversion of VT that is hemodynamically compromising should be performed immediately. Rapid polymorphic VT should be considered the equivalent of VF and cardioverted with an unsynchronized shock of 200 J; monomorphic VT at a rate of greater than 150 beats per minute can be treated initially with a synchronized discharge of 100 J.[3] Urgent cardioversion for VT with rates of under 150 beats per minute is usually not needed. VT that is tolerated hemodynamically can be approached initially with trials of lidocaine, procainamide, or amiodarone.

Ventricular fibrillation should initially be treated with an unsynchronized shock of 200 J, then incrementally at 200 to 300 J, and finally at 360 J as needed. The advanced cardiac life support (ACLS) protocol recommends the following hierarchical approach, as needed, to adjunctive therapy of resistant VF: (1) epinephrine (1 mg IV); (2) lidocaine (1.5 mg/kg IV); (3) bretylium (5 to 10 mg/kg IV). Intravenous amiodarone (150 mg IV bolus) may also be used.[3] In the case of resistant or recurrent VT/VF, electrolyte imbalances should be sought and corrected, and ongoing ischemia should be suspected. Beta-adrenergic blockers should be used in recurrent VT or primary VF to decrease sympathetic input to the heart and to decrease ischemia.[3] If ongoing ischemia is involved, intraaortic balloon pumping or emergency revascularization should be considered.

### Approach to the Patient with Ischemic-Type Chest Pain and without ST-Segment Elevation.

As discussed, the initial criterion for differentiating patients with symptoms compatible with AMI for therapeutic purposes is the presence or absence of ST-segment elevation; this is a distinction of importance because in the absence of ST-segment elevation, there is no therapeutic benefit of thrombolysis. AMI in which Q waves do not develop is categorized as *non-Q-wave MI (NQWMI)*, and most patients (90 percent) present with ST-segment depression.

NQWMI is precipitated by plaque disruption.[15] Total coronary occlusion demonstrated angiographically is much less common than in Q-wave MI. Because of the residual noninfarcted myocardium at risk distal to a disrupted plaque, moreover, patients with NQWMI have a high propensity for recurrent ischemia, infarction, and death and present an opportunity for secondary prevention. Two important conclusions can be derived from the available data: (1) Thrombolysis cannot be recommended in AMI patients without ST-segment elevation, and (2) in the NQWMI group, based on the admission ECG, there is a graded, decremental spectrum of risk ranging from ST-segment depression to T-wave inversion to normal.

*Management of Non-Q-Wave Myocardial Infarction.* Initially, the NQWMI patient, who by definition does not have diagnostic ST-segment elevation, cannot be distinguished from the patient with unstable angina and no myocardial necrosis. Thus, patients are admitted to the coronary care unit, and *other than avoiding thrombolytic therapy,* the initial pharmacological approach is identical (Fig. 26-1).

Because NQWMI is associated with either transient or nonocclusive thrombus formation, therapy should include the use of heparin for at least 48 h. The potential usefulness of platelet GPIIb/IIIa inhibitors to diminish risk of thrombus formation is currently an area of active investigation. Serial ECGs and cardiac marker measurements should be performed, and in the case of recurrent pain with the development of ST-segment elevation, thrombolysis or primary PTCA should be performed. If the patient has recurrent, stuttering symptoms, angiography should be performed.

Non-dihydropyridine calcium entry blockers such as diltiazem and verapamil have been shown to reduce reinfarction rate in patients with NQWMI with preserved left ventricular function. Most clinicians would use diltiazem in NQWMI in the presence of atrial fibrillation with rapid ventricular response unresponsive to beta blockers and with preserved left ventricular function. Some would use diltiazem or verapamil as prophylaxis after 24 h and for 1 year in all patients with NQWMI and preserved left ventricular function. In a recent trial comparing PTCA with conventional therapy, there was a decrease in mortality associated with diltiazem in the arm comparing conventional medical management with and without diltiazem. Parenthetically, there were more deaths in the invasive than in the conservative arm.

It seems prudent to recommend aspirin (160 to 325 mg/day) in addition to heparin, as noted, for NQWMI and—in patients without evidence of CHF, pulmonary congestion, or left ventricular dysfunction—to add diltiazem to standard therapy after the first 24 h and to continue it for 1 year.[3] Generally beta blockers have shown no effect on the reinfarction rate in patients recovering from NQWMI. Beta blockers may be given to relieve pain or arrhythmia, as discussed previously for Q-wave MI.

## Management after Hospital Admission

**GENERAL APPROACH.**    The general issues involved in the management of the patient with suspected or manifest AMI in the intensive or moderate care unit are to provide for adequate monitoring for the detection of arrhythmia, ischemia, and hemodynamic instability; to provide the patient with a calm, supportive, and reassuring environment; to control the level of activity; to begin the education process for a lifetime of living with coronary heart disease; to control pain and inappropriate anxiety; and to treat adverse events promptly. It is assumed, as previously discussed, that oxygen therapy, beta-adrenergic blockers, aspirin, thrombolytics, heparin, and nitroglycerin have been begun or given, as appropriate, in the emergency department.

*Activity.*    Minimizing physical exertion is an important approach to minimizing sympathetic nervous system drive concomitantly with administering beta-adrenergic blockers to decrease myocardial oxygen demand and thus myocardial ischemia and necrosis. Controlling pain and excessive anxiety is also important in this regard. *Prolonged bed rest and a severe limitation of activities such as self-feeding are no longer recommended except in the case of continuing ischemic pain and/or hemodynamic instability.* Constipation should be avoided, and stool softeners should be routinely prescribed. A bedside commode is preferable to a bedpan in all but the most unstable patients.

***Analgesics and Anxiolytics.***   The importance of controlling chest pain and excessive anxiety and the use of morphine and diazepam have been discussed. Anxiolytics may be useful in treating symptoms of nicotine withdrawal in smokers. Intravenous haloperidol, or other such agents, can be useful and safe in treating intensive care unit (ICU) psychosis, particularly in the elderly.

***Education.***   Education of the AMI patient, both by the CCU staff and by the physician, with information about the management of symptoms and the prevention of their recurrence, gives a sense of empowerment that is associated with changes in behavior and decreases in anxiety. Because of the substantial risk of cardiac arrest in the 18 months after AMI, family members should be taught cardiopulmonary resuscitation (CPR).

**ADJUNCTIVE THERAPY DURING THE EARLY IN-HOSPITAL PERIOD.**
***Angiotensin-Converting Enzyme Inhibitors.***   ACE inhibitors reduce left ventricular dysfunction and dilatation and slow the progression to CHF in patients with left ventricular dysfunction after AMI.[16,17] Efficacy may be greatest in those at highest risk—i.e., patients with worst left ventricular function. Oral therapy with low doses should begin within the first 24 h after hemodynamic stabilization whether or not thrombolytic therapy has been administered. ACE inhibitors should not be given if systolic blood pressure is below 100 mmHg. If there is no evidence of left ventricular dysfunction at 4 to 6 weeks, therapy can be stopped. With significant left ventricular dysfunction (left ventricular ejection fraction <40 percent), therapy should probably be continued indefinitely.

**MANAGEMENT OF THE LOW-RISK PATIENT.**   The patient with AMI who has an uncomplicated initial course and is at low risk for development of complications is a candidate for transfer out of the CCU within 24 to 36 h. These patients, including those who have had thrombolysis, may be candidates for early discharge at 3 to 4 days. Excessive diagnostic testing in all post-AMI patients, especially those at low risk, should be discouraged.[3]

If AMI is effectively ruled out using serum markers in the low-risk patient (i.e., one with normal ECG and absence of the characteristics noted above, especially the absence of prolonged initial pain or the recurrence of pain), noninvasive testing can establish the safety of early discharge (3 to 12 h) from the ED or CCU for further evaluation as an outpatient. In general, such patients do not need to be admitted to the CCU unless noninvasive testing is positive for ischemic heart disease. Patients with ischemic-type chest discomfort and intermediate probabilities of AMI (i.e., duration of chest pain greater than 20 to 30 min and nondiagnostic ECG changes without significant ST-segment elevation or depression, T-wave inversion, or bundle branch block) and without known CAD should be admitted to an observation unit or to the CCU. They should be placed on a fast track to rule in AMI or unstable angina. If the clinical course is unrevealing and serum marker enzymes are negative, stress testing and further evaluation can be planned. Clinical decisions can usually be made within 12 h in this setting.

**MANAGEMENT OF THE HIGH-RISK PATIENT WITH ACUTE MYOCAR-DIAL INFARCTION.**   The high-risk AMI patient is defined by the presence of one or more of the following: recurrent chest pain; CHF and low cardiac output; arrhythmias, in particular recurrent or sustained ventricular tachycardia or fibrillation; mechanical cardiac complications of AMI such as ruptured papillary muscle or intraventricular septum; and/or inducible ischemia and extensive CAD. *In general, cardiology consultation should be sought in all high-risk patients.*

*Recurrent Chest Pain.*   The most common causes of recurrent chest pain after AMI are coronary ischemia and pericarditis.

*Recurrent Ischemia.*   Recurrence of chest pain in the AMI patient is a serious development and requires immediate diagnosis and treatment, especially if the pain represents recurrent ischemia. Postinfarction angina is chest pain occurring at rest or with limited activity during hospitalization 24 h or more after onset of the AMI. Three categories of patients are at high risk: (1) patients with NQWMI; (2) patients who have received thrombolysis; and (3) patients with multiple risk factors.

The approach to recurrent ischemia is similar to that for the original episode. Coronary arteriography generally should be performed; if a high-grade stenosis is found, PTCA should be performed (if the lesion is suitable) or, if there is associated ST-segment elevation, additional thrombolysis should be administered if mechanical reperfusion is not feasible or available. If multiple high-grade stenoses are found, coronary artery bypass grafting should be considered.

*Early Postinfarction Pericarditis.*   Early postinfarction pericarditis, as reflected by pain and a friction rub, occurs in about 10 percent of patients, usually between days 2 and 4. The treatment of choice is aspirin (160 to 325 mg daily), although higher doses (650 mg every 4 to 6 h) may be required;[3] however, other nonsteroidal anti-inflammatory drugs (NSAIDs) may be used. The use of anticoagulants is relatively contraindicated in AMI complicated by pericarditis.

*Heart Failure in Acute Myocardial Infarction.*
*Pathophysiology and Hemodynamics.*   Cardiac failure develops when left ventricular function is reduced to 30 percent or more of normal and usually occurs within minutes or hours of onset of a large infarction. Some compromise of cardiac function is associated with perhaps more than two-thirds of cases of AMI and is transient (24 to 72 h). The severity of the failure, its duration, and whether or not it is reversible are predominantly dependent on infarct size.

*Right Ventricular Infarction.*   Inferior MI associated with right ventricular infarction defines a high-risk subset with a mortality rate of 25 to 30 percent.[18] This group should be approached aggressively, with consideration of reperfusion therapy. Right ventricular involvement should always be considered and should be specifically sought out in inferior MI with clinical evidence of low cardiac output, because the therapeutic approaches in the presence of right ventricular involvement are quite different from those for predominantly left ventricular failure.

ST-segment elevation in lead $V_{4R}$, as noted, is the single most powerful predictor of right ventricular involvement in inferior infarction and identifies a patient subset with a markedly increased in-hospital mortality. All patients with inferior infarction should be screened by recording ECG lead $V_{4R}$. Echocardiography can also be useful as an adjunctive diagnostic approach.

*Treatment of Right Ventricular Ischemia/Infarction.*   The major objectives in treating right ventricular infarction are to maintain right ventricular preload, to provide inotropic support, to reduce afterload of the right ventricle, and to achieve early reperfusion. The recommendations are summarized in Table 26-6.

*Management of Congestive Heart Failure in Acute MI—General Issues.*
**1.**   *Hemodynamic Monitoring.* The balloon flotation (Swan-Ganz) catheter funda-

**TABLE 26-6.   Treatment Strategy for Right Ventricular Ischemia/Infarction**

Maintain right ventricular preload
    Volume loading (IV normal saline)
    Avoid use of nitrates and diuretics
    Maintain AV synchrony
        AV sequential pacing for symptomatic high-degree heart block unresponsive to
            atropine
    Prompt cardioversion for hemodynamically significant SVT

Inotropic support
    Dobutamine (if cardiac output fails to increase after volume loading)

Reduce right ventricular afterload secondary to left ventricular dysfunction
    Intraaortic balloon pump
    Arterial vasodilators (sodium nitroprusside, hydralazine)
    ACE inhibitors

Reperfusion
    Thrombolytic agents
    Primary PTCA
    CABG (in selected patients with multivessel disease)

Key: IV = intravenous; AV = atrioventricular; SVT = supraventricular tachycardia; ACE = angiotensin-converting enzyme; PTCA = percutaneous transluminal coronary angioplasty; CABG = coronary artery bypass graft.

Reproduced with permission. Ryan TJ, Anderson JL, Antman EM, et al: ACC/AHA Guidelines for the Management of Patients with Acute Myocardial Infarction. *J Am Coll Cardiol* 1996; 28:1328–1428. Copyright © 1996 American College of Cardiology and American Heart Association, Inc.

mentally permits one, in the setting of low cardiac output, to distinguish between in-adequate ventricular filling pressures and inadequate systolic function. The former is treated with volume expansion and the latter with inotropic support and, fre-quently, afterload reduction. The catheter, even when used correctly, is not totally benign. Indications for insertion generally are severe or progressive CHF or shock and suspected mechanical complications (ventricular septal defect, papillary muscle rupture, tamponade).[3]

Arterial monitoring in AMI is useful in all hypotensive patients, but especially in those in shock. Arterial monitoring is also recommended in patients receiving vaso-pressor agents. The radial artery is the preferred site, although the brachial and femoral arteries can be used.[3]

**2.** *Intraaortic Balloon Counterpulsation.* The intraaortic balloon pump reduces af-terload during ventricular systole and increases coronary perfusion during diastole. The decrease in afterload and increased coronary perfusion account for its efficacy in cardiogenic shock and ischemia. It is particularly useful as a stabilizing bridge to facilitate diagnostic angiography as well as revascularization and repair of mechan-ical complications of AMI.

**3.** *Diuretics and Positive Inotropic Agents.*

*Diuretics and cardiac failure in AMI.* Diuretics generally should not be the drugs used initially in the treatment of pulmonary congestion in AMI because in-travascular volume is initially normal (unless there was preexisting CHF). Their use early in the course should usually be guided by hemodynamic measurements from a Swan-Ganz catheter. Diuretic therapy may become appropriate later if salt and water retention occur and left ventricular filling pressures become excessively high.

*Inotropic agents in congestive heart failure.* Digoxin is not the drug of choice in acute heart failure in MI. The primary use of digoxin in AMI is to control heart rate in atrial fibrillation. Dobutamine has favorable pharmacologic properties for use in heart failure in MI. Dopamine has a tendency to in-crease heart rate more than dobutamine. With higher doses, it may increase peripheral resistance and increase filling pressures, thus offsetting some of the positive inotropic effects.

*Management of Uncomplicated Cardiac Failure after AMI.*   In patients with un-complicated AMI, there is no need to perform invasive monitoring if careful clini-cal observations are made.[3]

If cardiac failure is not complicated by mechanical factors—such as mitral valve rupture, ventricular septal rupture, pulmonary embolus, or tamponade—the failure in most patients is transient and of mild to moderate severity. If the cardiac output is normal, aggressive treatment is often not recommended. In patients with rales at the base of the lungs with only minimal increase in heart rate and no other signs of hypoxemia, conventional therapy with morphine, nasal oxygen, nitrates (intra-venous, oral, or transdermal), and bed rest is adequate. In patients with extensive pulmonary edema who are normotensive and exhibit hypoxia and dyspnea, the treatment of choice is nitroglycerin given intravenously at 0.1 $\mu$g/ kg of body weight per minute and increased in increments of 5 to 10 $\mu$g/min, stopping at a dose that does not decrease the systolic blood pressure below 100 mmHg. It is preferable that hemodynamics be monitored invasively (Swan-Ganz catheter) when one gives a vasodilator to reduce the ventricular filling pressure to 15 to 17 mmHg. An intravenous inotropic agent may be needed. The inotropic agents are generally dobutamine and dopamine, with dobutamine being the preferred agent. The infusion should be initiated at 2 to 5 $\mu$g/kg of body weight per minute, and should be increased such that adequate systemic pressure is maintained and the heart rate does not increase by more than 10 to 15 percent. The ventricular filling pressure should be decreased to a range of 14 to 18 mmHg while maintaining adequate cardiac output and blood pressure.

In patients with borderline blood pressure and evidence of peripheral hypoperfusion, therapy should be initiated with an inotropic agent and not a vasodilator. Low doses of dopamine (2 to 7 $\mu$g/kg of body weight per minute) are usually given and are associated with an increase in stroke volume, cardiac output, renal blood flow, and peripheral resistance to a modest degree. Higher doses of dopamine induce significant vasoconstriction and increase in left ventricular filling pressure. Diuretics should be used with caution. If high filling pressure (>18 to 20 mmHg) persists after achieving adequate output with positive inotropic agents and/or vasodilators, diuretics may be added.

*Complicated Heart Failure after MI.*   In fulminating heart failure, administration of high concentrations (60 to 100 percent) of oxygen via a face mask is essential, and endotracheal intubation may be needed. Invasive hemodynamic monitoring is particularly useful in these patients. The therapy for severe pulmonary edema should include intravenous morphine. If systolic blood pressure is adequate ($\geq$100 mmHg), nitroglycerin is administered intravenously. In severe pulmonary edema, nitroprusside may be essential to reduce afterload. If the systolic blood pressure is <100 mmHg, treatment should be initiated with a positive inotropic agent, with the subsequent addition of a vasodilator if adequate blood pressure is achieved.

**1.** *Hypotension and cardiogenic shock.* As a result of massive ischemia and necrosis, cardiogenic shock usually occurs within hours of the onset of infarction.[5] Reversible causes must be excluded. These include mitral valve rupture, ventricular septal rupture, right ventricular infarction, pulmonary embolus, and cardiac tamponade.

The approaches to pulmonary congestion include the use of morphine and the maintenance of adequate oxygenation together with endotracheal intubation and mechanical ventilation if necessary. Pulmonary artery and arterial catheters should be placed. Urinary output is monitored using an indwelling catheter. The cornerstones of therapy are inotropic and vasopressor agents. If the systemic arterial vasopressure is below 80 to 90 mmHg, a pressor agent such as dopamine should be infused as described. If high doses of dopamine are necessary to maintain adequate perfusion (and pressure of 90 to 100 mmHg), a change to norepinephrine infusion should be considered. On occasion, the severity of cardiac pump dysfunction will require the combined use of nitroprusside and dopamine. Stabilization in cardiogenic shock may be achieved by the intraaortic balloon. Aortic counterpulsation is usually reserved for patients with a potentially reversible condition or those in whom cardiac transplantation is being considered.

Restoration of coronary blood flow will probably be the most effective therapy in salvaging patients with cardiogenic shock. Mechanical revascularization appears to improve survival in cardiogenic shock complicating AMI.

**2.**   *Mechanical dysfunction contributing to cardiac failure. Papillary muscle rupture* is manifested by the sudden appearance of pulmonary edema, usually 2 to 7 days after the infarction. A mid- or holosystolic murmur with wide radiation is usually audible. The diagnosis can be established by Doppler echocardiographic studies.

Immediate recognition and treatment are essential. Intraaortic counterpulsation alone, or with vasodilator and inotropic therapy, is frequently required for temporary stabilization. The patient should undergo cardiac catheterization to define coronary anatomy, and surgery for mitral valve replacement or repair and coronary artery bypass grafting should be performed.

**3.**   *Papillary muscle dysfunction.* The sudden development of an apical systolic murmur after a MI is much more often secondary to papillary muscle dysfunction than to rupture. Papillary muscle dysfunction is frequently compatible with long-term survival.

Echocardiography coupled with Doppler flow studies will confirm the presence of mitral regurgitation, grade its severity, and permit assessment of left ventricular function. Ordinarily papillary muscle dysfunction will require no specific therapy; the unusual patient with severe regurgitation should be treated like one with papillary muscle rupture. In intermediate cases, afterload reduction with ACE inhibitors should be considered.

**4.**   *Ventricular septal rupture.* There is a higher prevalence of ventricular septal rupture in first infarctions, and the majority occur within the first week. Ventricular septal rupture is usually manifested by the appearance of a new harsh, holosystolic murmur along the left sternal border (often associated with a thrill) and sudden clinical deterioration with hypotension and pulmonary congestion. Often the event is heralded by a recurrence of chest pain. The diagnosis can be established by two-dimensional and Doppler echocardiographic studies. Results of these studies and/or the oxygen stepup on right heart catheterization would confirm the presence of septal rupture.

Medical therapy can be expected to be ineffective. Prompt but temporary stabilization can be achieved with intraaortic balloon counterpulsation alone or in conjunction with vasodilator and inotropic drug therapy. Cardiac catheterization should be performed in an expeditious manner. An aggressive approach of immediate operative repair of these patients results in a short-term survival rate of 42 to 75 percent.

### *Arrhythmias and Conduction Disturbances Complicating AMI.*

**1.**   *Ventricular ectopy, ventricular tachycardia, and ventricular fibrillation.* The management of ventricular tachycardia and fibrillation after the first 24 h of hospitalization for AMI is similar to that for the early phase.[5] The occurrence of symptomatic, sustained ventricular tachycardia or ventricular fibrillation in the later phases of the hospital course, however, suggests that a chronic arrhythmogenic focus may be developing in the damaged ventricle. These ventricular arrhythmias are classified as *secondary* and indicate an increased risk of subsequent sudden cardiac death.

**2.** *Sinus tachycardia or atrial premature beats.* Sinus tachycardia following AMI is common and is frequently an unfavorable prognostic sign. Patients with a large area of infarcted myocardium may have sinus tachycardia on the basis of left ventricular dysfunction, which causes reflex sympathetic nervous system activation. Frequent atrial premature complexes are relatively common in AMI, and no specific therapy is indicated.

**3.** *Paroxysmal supraventricular tachycardia.* Episodes of paroxysmal supraventricular tachycardia occur rather commonly in AMI and usually are transient. Rate control is essential, and the therapeutic approaches may include carotid sinus massage, adenosine, digoxin, verapamil, and diltiazem.

**4.** *Atrial flutter and atrial fibrillation.* Atrial flutter is relatively uncommon in AMI, whereas atrial fibrillation has an incidence of 10 to 15 percent. Atrial fibrillation is associated with an increased in-hospital mortality rate. A rapid ventricular response can worsen ischemia and infarction. Risk of systemic embolization is increased in AMI in the presence of atrial fibrillation. Thus, heparin therapy is indicated in patients not already receiving it. If the patient experiences new or worsening pain, ischemic ST changes, or hemodynamic instability during atrial fibrillation with a rapid ventricular response rate, immediate electrical cardioversion is indicated.

**5.** *Heart block.* First-degree block is seen frequently in AMI, especially in inferior MI. This is attributable to ischemia or enhanced vagal activity. Treatment is seldom required.

Second-degree AV block is also relatively common, especially Mobitz type I or Wenckebach block. It is associated with a narrow QRS complex and is frequently the result of AV node ischemia in inferior MI. It is usually transient, and its presence does not affect the prognosis. Mobitz type II block is uncommon but is associated with more serious complications and a worse prognosis. It usually occurs with anterior MI and reflects trifascicular block. It is characterized by a wide QRS complex and a nonvarying PR interval before a nonconducted atrial beat. Heart block may develop suddenly and is an ominous sign, with a mortality of about 80 percent. It is usually permanent.

Third-degree AV block, or complete heart block, occurs in about 5 percent of patients with AMI and is most commonly seen with inferior infarction, usually with the block at the AV node. There is some increase in in-hospital mortality rates in this setting, but complete heart block in inferior MI is not an independent predictor of poor long-term prognosis. In contrast, patients with anterior infarction who develop third-degree AV block have a high mortality rate of 80 percent.

**6.** *Indications for temporary transvenous pacing.* The indications for temporary pacemaker insertion in AMI that have been generally agreed on include asystole, complete heart block in the setting of anterior MI, new onset of right or left bundle branch block with persistent Mobitz type II second-degree AV block in the setting of anterior MI, or other symptomatic bradycardias unresponsive to atropine. Bundle branch block in the setting of AMI identifies a population at risk for both electrical and mechanical complications. Such patients must be monitored for evidence of transient high-degree heart block.

**7.** *Permanent pacing.* The use of permanent pacemakers is reviewed extensively in the American College of Cardiology/American Heart Association guidelines for pacemaker implantation[19] and is summarized in Chap. 34 of *Hurst's The Heart,* 9th ed.[20] The fact that temporary pacing may have been required in the course of AMI does not necessarily indicate the need for permanent pacing. Patients who have had permanent pacemakers inserted after AMI usually have a relatively unfavorable prognosis that is primarily related to the extensiveness of the underlying disease and myocardial damage.[3]

***Discharge from the Coronary Care Unit.***   The length of stay in the CCU should be based on the risk of developing ventricular tachycardia and ventricular fibrillation. The risk of developing primary ventricular fibrillation after AMI decreases exponentially, with the majority of arrhythmic deaths occurring within the first 24 h. A patient with an uncomplicated infarction can be transferred from the CCU on the third day, although some patients need more prolonged cardiac monitoring. Those patients who are prime candidates for late-hospital sudden death manifest, while in the CCU, one or more of the following: (1) the arrhythmias of pump failure (sinus tachycardia, atrial flutter, or atrial fibrillation), (2) the arrhythmias of electrical instability (ventricular tachycardia or ventricular fibrillation), (3) acute interventricular conduction disturbances, (4) evidence of circulatory failure (CHF, pulmonary edema, or significant hypotension), or (5) large anterior infarction. The effectiveness of prolonged monitoring of this select group of patients in an intermediate care unit following CCU discharge is evident in a doubling of the rate of successful resuscitations.

In an uncomplicated MI, the patient does not need to be confined to bed for longer than 24 h. Upon transfer from a CCU, the patient should be started on a progressive ambulation program. The speed with which the patient progresses from one stage to the next depends on the severity of the infarction, the presence or absence of complications, the patient's age, and the presence of comorbid conditions. The length of hospitalization following an AMI should likewise depend on these same factors. If the patient has not experienced complications during the first 4 days of hospitalization, he or she is very unlikely to do so at any later time. This patient could probably be discharged after 7 or fewer days in the hospital. The last 2 to 3 days of the hospitalization are generally necessary to resolve the questions pertaining to residual ventricular function, the presence or absence of ventricular ectopy, and the adequacy of the remainder of the coronary circulation. In addition, time is needed for instruction in risk-factor modification.

***Noninvasive Risk Stratification in Patients Surviving AMI.***   Survivors of AMI have a substantial risk of subsequent cardiovascular events. Noninvasive risk assessment provides useful information to individualize the extent of further work-up and therapy: (1) targeting specific long-term therapies, (2) identifying high-risk patients requiring aggressive diagnostic testing, (3) counseling the patient on prognosis, (4) developing an exercise program, and (5) planning modifications of lifestyle.

Three interrelated prognostic factors are the focus of predischarge assessment: (1) assessment of left ventricular function, (2) detection of residual myocardial ischemia (jeopardized myocardium), and (3) assessment of the risk of arrhythmic (sudden cardiac) death. High-risk patients can be identified clinically because of the presence of one or more of the following: decompensated CHF, angina associated with electrocardiographic changes, in-hospital cardiac arrest, spontaneous sustained ventricular tachycardia, or the development of a high-degree heart block. In the majority of patients who have a relatively benign hospital course, noninvasive testing can accurately identify a group at very low risk whose annual mortality is 1 to 3 percent. The practical consequence of identifying a low-risk group is that emphasis is focused on early discharge, lifestyle modification, and targeted prophylactic medical therapy rather than on expensive, invasive diagnostic testing.

Early coronary angiography and aggressive interventional therapy are indicated for patients with recurrent episodes of spontaneous or induced (with low-level exercise testing) angina or ischemia or with evidence of persistent pulmonary congestion, clinical left ventricular dysfunction, or cardiogenic shock.[3] There is general agreement that there is not adequate evidence to support routine coronary angiography for the initial assessment in asymptomatic patients; therefore, the guidelines dissuade its use as the primary tool for diagnostic evaluation.[3]

*Assessment of Left Ventricular Function and Left Ventricular Ejection Fraction.* Ventricular function is an important determinant of long-term survival after AMI regardless of reperfusion status and, in general, should be assessed by noninvasive or, if otherwise indicated, by angiographic techniques.

*Assessment of Myocardial Ischemia—Clinical Significance of Predischarge Submaximal Exercise Testing in Uncomplicated Patients.* Predischarge exercise testing consistently identifies a group at high risk for recurrent cardiac events (MI, unstable angina, etc.) or mortality in the first year after the AMI. Exercise testing also identifies a group at very low risk (1 to 3 percent mortality rate for the first year). A negative test should promote early discharge as well as discourage an aggressive diagnostic approach. Submaximal exercise testing in *uncomplicated* patients, including those who have had thrombolysis, before discharge has a class I indication.[3]

The presence of ischemia generally mandates cardiac catheterization to define the coronary anatomy and to consider revascularization. A recommended approach to post-AMI risk stratification is summarized in Fig. 26-3.[3]

*Assessment of the Risk of Arrhythmic (Sudden Cardiac) Death.* The identification of patients who are asymptomatic but at high risk for arrhythmic death after AMI has not been associated with the delineation of a successful treatment strategy. Although the presence of asymptomatic spontaneous ventricular arrhythmias as detected on ambulatory monitoring is predictive of increased arrhythmic (sudden) death, the positive predictive value is poor. The dearth of safe, effective antiar-

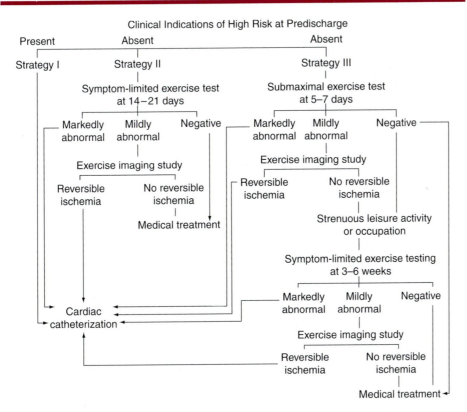

**Figure 26-3**   Strategies for exercise test evaluations soon after MI. If patients are at high risk for ischemic events based on clinical criteria, they should undergo invasive evaluation to determine if they are candidates for coronary revascularization procedures (strategy I). For patients initially deemed to be at low risk at time of discharge after MI, two strategies for performing exercise testing can be used. One is a symptom-limited test at 14 to 21 days (strategy II). If the patient is on digoxin or if the baseline ECG precludes accurate interpretation of ST-segment changes (e.g., baseline left BBB or left ventricular hypertrophy), then an initial exercise imaging study can be performed. Results of exercise testing should be stratified to determine need for additional invasive or exercise perfusion studies. A third strategy is to perform a submaximal exercise test at 5 to 7 days after MI or just before hospital discharge. The exercise test results could be stratified using the guidelines in strategy I. If exercise test studies are negative, a second symptom-limited exercise test could be repeated at 3 to 6 weeks for patients undergoing vigorous activity during leisure or at work. (Reproduced with permission. Ryan TJ, Anderson JL, Antman EM, et al: ACC/AHA Guidelines for the Management of Patients with Acute Myocardial Infarction. *J Am Coll Cardiol* 1996; 28:1328–1428. Copyright ©1996 American College of Cardiology and American Heart Association, Inc.)

rhythmic drugs has limited the usefulness of routinely evaluating the asymptomatic post-AMI patient in this regard.

*Assessing Arrhythmic Death: Conclusions.*   None of the noninvasive (ambulatory monitoring) or invasive (electrophysiologic testing) techniques is generally agreed upon to be beneficial, useful, and effective in assessment of arrhythmic death.[3] No clinical trial has demonstrated that the use of any one or a combination of these modalities of testing identifies a high-risk population in whom intervention can result in clinical benefit.

***Coronary Angiography and Percutaneous Transluminal Coronary Angioplasty.*** The selection of patients for cardiac catheterization and coronary angiographic studies prior to hospital discharge should be based on identification of those at risk for ischemic events and on whether or not the information provided by cardiac catheterization and coronary angiography will change patient management. In general, studies that have compared acute or early cardiac catheterization to a more conservative approach of performing cardiac catheterization and coronary angiographic studies only for patients with spontaneous recurrent angina or exercise-induced ischemia have demonstrated no benefit to the strategy of routine catheterization.[3,21] Patients who have a complicated clinical course characterized by refractory cardiac failure, unstable angina, an episode of sustained ventricular tachycardia, or cardiac arrest should be studied.

The recommended algorithm for selecting asymptomatic, uncomplicated post-AMI patients for cardiac catheterization is presented in Fig. 26-3. Decision making focuses on the presence or absence of myocardial ischemia. When patients have received thrombolytic therapy, it seems reasonable that those who have evidence of residual ischemia are still at increased risk of future ischemic events and should undergo coronary angiography. Consideration of PTCA following coronary angiographic studies should be based on established clinical and anatomic guidelines.[3] Coronary artery bypass surgery (CABS) should be considered in those groups in whom it has been shown to be of proven benefit: patients with triple-vessel disease, patients with ischemia, and those with significant left ventricular dysfunction.

## Secondary Prevention and Cardiac Rehabilitation

**RISK-FACTOR REDUCTION.**   There is now abundant evidence that risk-factor reduction will reduce coronary events in susceptible patients. Thus, since those who have had AMI are among those at highest risk for recurrence, management strategies to mitigate this risk are very important.

***Smoking.***   Smoking cessation is an essential goal after AMI, since the recurrence and death rates after AMI are doubled by the continuation of smoking, and since the risk associated with smoking declines rapidly, within 3 years, to that of the nonsmoking cohort survivors. The role of the physician in motivating the patient to quit smoking is extremely important, and the likelihood of success appears to be directly related to the extent of his or her involvement.

***Dyslipidemia.***   Recent large secondary prevention trials have provided compelling evidence that after AMI, therapy with HmG-CoA reductase inhibitors to lower serum cholesterol levels that were initially either elevated, as in the Scandinavian Simvastatin Survival Study (4S),[22] or within "average" range, as in the Cholesterol and Recurrent Events trial (CARE),[23] was effective in reducing both cardiovascular and total mortality as well as cardiovascular events. The guidelines of the expert panel of the National Cholesterol Education Program provide target goals for patients with manifest coronary artery disease. These goals are LDL cholesterol <100 mg/dL (2.59 mmol/L); HDL cholesterol >35 mg/dL (0.91 mmol/L). *All AMI patients should have serum lipids evaluated and treated intensely in order to achieve target goals.* Treatment should start in the hospital with initiation of the AHA step II diet.

*Inactivity.*    A sedentary lifestyle is a risk factor for coronary artery disease. Meta-analysis of cardiac rehabilitation studies has shown a reduction in mortality in the exercise group as opposed to a control group. The greatest benefits of exercise are those observed with moderate, regular exercise as contrasted with no exercise.

Regular aerobic exercise should be prescribed for post-AMI patients in stable condition at an intensity, duration, and frequency as determined by formal testing and clinical judgment. Optimum benefit is achieved in a supervised program, although asymptomatic, stable patients can exercise without direct supervision. They should, however, receive regular monitoring by a physician.

## DRUG THERAPY.

*Beta-Adrenergic Blockers.*    The benefits of beta-blocker therapy given early in the course of AMI were discussed. Multiple clinical trials have also demonstrated the benefits of long-term treatment of post-AMI patients with beta blockers. Mortality has been shown to be reduced by about 25 to 35 percent. The beneficial effect is highest in high-risk patients with large (usually anterior) MI and compensated left ventricular dysfunction. The beneficial effects in low-risk patients are less clear, but the consensus is that these patients probably should be treated because of the relatively favorable side-effect profile.[3] Beta blockers with intrinsic sympathomimetic activity should not be used in this context.

*Aspirin.*    The role of aspirin during the early phases of AMI was discussed. Aspirin use over the long-term after AMI is also associated with a reduction in mortality. Aspirin at relatively low doses (81 to 325 mg/day) is recommended for all patients with AMI in the absence of contraindications.

*Anticoagulation.*    Anticoagulation can reduce mortality, recurrent MI, and stroke after AMI. The role of warfarin is limited to those at increased risk for developing mural thrombi. In addition, those post-AMI patients with demonstrable left ventricular thrombus and atrial fibrillation should be anticoagulated. The duration of anticoagulation should be limited to 3 months in the case of left ventricular thrombus.

*Angiotensin-Converting Enzyme Inhibitors.*    The ACE inhibitors and recommendations for their use early in the course of AMI were discussed. Recent studies have documented their efficacy in secondary prevention. Thus, ACE inhibitors are recommended for chronic use after AMI in those patients with significant left ventricular dysfunction (ejection fraction <35 to 40 percent), and their use should be considered in those with only mild to moderate left ventricular dysfunction (ejection fraction <45 percent).

**MODIFICATION OF LIFESTYLE AND CARDIAC REHABILITATION AFTER AMI.**   Because of the relatively high risk of recurrence and the need for lifelong modification of lifestyles and risk factors, most post-AMI patients should be enrolled in a cardiac rehabilitation program that emphasizes dietary modification, risk-factor reduction, and exercise. The low-risk patient does not require prolonged supervised exercise. All patients, however, can benefit from a structured environment to launch a lifetime of healthy living. Cardiac rehabilitation is discussed in detail in Chaps. 47[5] and 55[24] of *Hurst's The Heart,* 9th ed; risk factors and the prevention of coronary artery disease are discussed in Chap. 41[25] of the same edition.

# UNSTABLE ANGINA

As alluded to previously, in many instances unstable angina represents a transitional state of an atherosclerotic lesion from stable obstruction to disruption of structural integrity and nonocclusive mural thrombus formation.[26] This condition is reflected in a change in clinical state, with either the development of angina in someone who was previously asymptomatic or a worsening of an established pain pattern. The characteristics of the pain are as described earlier for AMI, except that the pain is usually not prolonged. Cases of unstable angina associated with change in structural integrity of an atherosclerotic plaque in the coronary artery are defined as primary unstable angina. A clinical syndrome resembling primary unstable angina can be precipitated when, in the presence of an obstructive lesion, myocardial oxygen demands become excessive or the capacity to deliver oxygen to the myocardium is markedly diminished. Primary unstable angina is associated with a markedly increased risk for the development of acute myocardial infarction and thus represents a condition to which a physician must respond promptly and purposefully.

## Definition

Unstable angina is manifested by a range of clinical symptoms intermediate between those of stable angina and those of AMI. An essential element is the presence of an evolving pattern of chest discomfort or pain that is new or that departs from the previous pattern of chest pain in the patient with angina. In the case of preexisting angina, instability may be reflected in a change of threshold for inducing angina, an increase in the duration of discomfort, a requirement for more nitroglycerin to relieve the pain, or the new development of rest angina. This scenario has been described variously as progressive angina or perhaps crescendo angina. De novo angina is the new development of symptoms consistent with angina pectoris.

It is extremely important to recognize that many patients who go on to develop AMI give, in retrospect, a history of a few antecedent episodes of chest discomfort that was new to their experience. Obviously, recognition of this symptom complex prior to the development of AMI is of the utmost clinical importance.

## Classification

As stated, unstable angina can be classified as primary or secondary.[27] The secondary form usually occurs in the presence of an obstructive coronary artery plaque but may occur in the presence of normal coronary arteries. The syndrome is caused by excessive myocardial oxygen demand and/or decreased capacity of oxygen delivery. The causes can be divided into extracoronary factors resulting in enhanced oxygen demand by increasing heart rate (anemia, fever, tachyarrhythmias, thyrotoxicosis), increase in inotropic state (high adenergic state, use of sympathomimetic drugs), increase in afterload (aortic stenosis, obstructive hypertrophic cardiomyopathy, severe hypertension), and interference with oxygen delivery (anemia, hypoxemia, polycythemia, high blood viscosity). Intrinsic coronary factors include hyperadenergic stimulation, cocaine or amphetamine intoxication, thrombotic CAD as in sickle cell anemia or polycythemia, coronary emboli, coronary vasculitis, and trauma.

**PRIMARY UNSTABLE ANGINA.**   Several classification schemes have been developed to allow patients with unstable angina to be placed in risk categories varying from high to low to guide clinical responses and decision making. One of the most frequently used is the Braunwald classification, which divides patients into three levels of severity in the context of the clinical circumstances.[27] These levels (in ascending order of severity) are: (I) new onset of severe or accelerated angina without rest pain; (II) a history of angina at rest within the past month, but not within the immediately preceding 48 h; and (III) angina at rest within the preceding 48 h. Primary unstable angina is further subdivided according to clinical circumstances. The most dangerous category is that occurring within 2 weeks post-AMI. Thus, a patient who has had episodes of pain within the past month but none within the past 48 h could potentially be evaluated in the office or over the next few days as an outpatient, whereas the patient who has had pain within the last 48 h would be hospitalized minimally with telemetry and probably on a CCU if this occurred in the setting of a recent AMI or if the patient is having recurrent, prolonged episodes. Short-term indicators of adverse prognosis are, incrementally, persisting instability with episodes of chest pain within the last 48 h to 1 week; crescendo angina with prolonged episodes of 20 min or greater and persisting ECG changes within the preceding 48 h; and refractory instability with persistent chest pains and ECG changes while on full medical therapy.

*Diagnosis and Clinical Presentation.*   Unstable angina is diagnosed based on the clinical presentation, which includes the changing symptom complex as previously described. Two key features are either new onset of pain consistent with coronary ischemia or a worsening of symptoms and especially a change in threshold. The key point clinically is for the physician to have a high index of suspicion. *In the appropriate clinical setting of the presence of known coronary disease or of multiple risk factors such as strong family history, diabetes, hyperlipidemia, and/or hypertension, together with postmenopausal state in females, a new or changing chest discomfort should be considered as potentially being cardiac in origin until proven otherwise.*

The clinical background can be very important. The high-risk status of a patient with unstable angina who has had a recent MI has been alluded to previously. Similarly, patients with unstable angina who have had previous coronary artery bypass surgery are a relatively high-risk subgroup because of the extensive nature of their disease.[5] Finally, recurrent angina in a patient with previous PTCA within the preceding 6 months may well represent restenosis, and in this setting the clinical prognosis is more favorable because the episode possibly represents restenosis of the previously dilated segment rather than activation of a new lesion. Pain occurring beyond 6 months is more likely to represent activation of another lesion and thus would have the same implications as in someone with established coronary artery disease.

*Electrocardiogram.*   ST-segment depression is the most common abnormality seen in unstable angina and non-Q-wave MI (about 30 percent of patients). T-wave inversions are reported in about 20 percent, and ST-segment elevation, indicating transient total occlusion, is seen in about 5 percent of patients. The absence of ECG changes does not exclude the presence of unstable angina. ECG changes are of greater diagnostic significance when they evolve and change with episodes of pain. In general, the more severe and more prolonged the ECG changes, the worse the prognosis.

*Cardiac Enzymes.*   As indicated previously, unstable angina becomes a diagnosis of exclusion of non-Q-wave MI by the absence of significant MB-CK enzyme elevations indicating myocardial necrosis. However, it has become apparent that the troponins are released with severe myocardial cell injury that is not necessarily fatal for the cell. Evidence is clear that unstable angina patients with elevations of troponin I or troponin T even in the presence of a normal MB-CK have a less favorable prognosis.[12]

**MANAGEMENT AND TREATMENT.**   Patients with active unstable angina should be hospitalized. High-risk and low-risk patients are characterized in Table 26-7. Low-risk patients (low probability of coronary artery disease, no chest pain within the past 48 h to 1 week, and without ECG changes) can be dealt with expeditiously in a chest pain unit or through prompt office evaluation with stress electrocardiography and, frequently, nuclear imaging. Those with inducible ischemia are defined as being at higher risk.

Management of the acute phase of the high-risk patient is identical to that previously described for the initial management of AMI except for the use of thrombolytic agents, which are not indicated in the absence of appropriate ST-segment el-

**TABLE 26-7.   Markers of Risk in Unstable Angina Associated with an Adverse Outcome***

|  | High Risk | Low Risk |
|---|---|---|
| Clinical presentation | Prolonged chest pain (>20 min)<br>Repetitive pain<br>Nocturnal pain<br>Hemodynamic instability | De novo angina<br>Effort angina<br>Little progression |
| Clinical background | Positive risk factors<br>Previous MI<br>Previous CABG | Low probability of CAD |
| ECG | ST-segment depression ≤1 mm<br>Deeply inverted T waves | ECG normal or minimal changes |
| Clinical evolution | Persistent instability on<br>treatment | No recurrence of pain |
| Blood markers | Elevated CK values<br>Elevated troponin T or I level<br>Inflammatory markers | Normal |
| Extent of CAD | Positive treadmill at low level<br>Significant perfusion defects | Negative treadmill or positive at high<br>level |

*Risk evaluation is performed at admission and updated as clinical status evolves.
CAD = coronary artery disease; MI = myocardial infarction; CABG = coronary artery bypass graft.
*Source:* From Theroux P, Waters D: Diagnosis and management of patients with unstable angina. In: Alexander RW, Schlant RC, Fuoster V, et al (eds): *Hurst's The Heart,* 9th ed. New York, McGraw-Hill, 1998.

evation. Aspirin is administered to all patients in the absence of contraindications. The dose should be between 160 and 325 mg and, initially, should be chewed. Heparin is also indicated in all patients with any one of the high-risk features. Anti-ischemic therapy, including intravenous nitroglycerin, is also recommended. Beta blockers are indicated for angina control. The dose should be adjusted to achieve a target heart rate of 50 to 60 beats per minute. Diltiazem or verapamil is a good alternative choice if beta blockers are contraindicated. Dihydropyridine calcium entry blockers as single therapy are not recommended. Three-drug therapy with beta blockers, nitroglycerin, and a calcium antagonist is recommended in patients with recurrent angina. Patients who do not stabilize on intense medical management and who show evidence of recurrent pain and ischemia should proceed to cardiac catheterization. Those who stabilize over 24 to 48 h are then risk-stratified. Their therapy is switched to a more chronic mode. Aspirin, beta blockers, and calcium channel blockers are continued generally. Heparin may be discontinued. While clinical practice varies, the best recent evidence suggests that patients who stabilize rapidly on therapy do not necessarily have to proceed to cardiac catheterization. They should be risk-stratified for inducible ischemia as reflected in exercise testing, frequently with nuclear imaging. The presence of inducible ischemia identi-

**TABLE 26-8.  Acute Management of Unstable Angina**

|  | High/Intermediate Risk | Low Risk |
|---|---|---|
| Treatment setting | Coronary care unit | Wards/home |
| Antithrombotic therapy | Aspirin and heparin | Aspirin |
| Anti-ischemic therapy | IV nitroglycerin + beta blocker and/or diltiazem or verapamil | Nitrates and beta blocker or diltiazem or verapamil |
| If persisting pain | Beta blockers + calcium antagonist<br>Consider intraaortic counterpulsation<br>Cardiac catheterization |  |

*Source:* From Theroux P, Waters D: Diagnosis and management of patients with unstable angina. In: Alexander RW, Schlant RC, Fuster V, et al (eds): *Hurst's The Heart,* 9th ed. New York, McGraw-Hill, 1998.

fies the patient as being in a high-risk category and should lead to cardiac catheterization.

Cardiac catheterization will identify culprit lesions and lead to a decision either for PTCA or for coronary artery bypass grafting. Recent evidence suggests that outcomes are improved in unstable angina and in PTCA performed in this setting with the use of new GIIb/IIIa platelet inhibitors.[29] It is likely that use of these drugs together with heparin and aspirin will become standard therapy in unstable angina. It should also be noted that low-molecular-weight heparin may be a suitable alternative to the use of standard heparin in the treatment of non-Q-wave MI and unstable angina.

The acute management of unstable angina is summarized in Table 26-8.

Chronic therapy for a patient recovering from unstable angina is the same as that previously discussed for the patient recovering from AMI and involves the use of aspirin, lipid-lowering drugs, and frequently beta blockers, and somewhat less frequently calcium entry blockers. These patients require long-term follow-up for their *atherosclerotic cardiovascular disease.*

## REFERENCES

1. GISSI (Gruppo Italiano per lo Studio della Streptochinasi nell'Infarto Miocardio): Effectiveness of intravenous thrombolytic treatment in acute myocardial infarction. *Lancet* 1986; 1:397–402.
2. GUSTO Investigators: An international randomized trial comparing four thrombolytic strategies for acute myocardial infarction. *N Engl J Med* 1993; 329:673–682.
3. Ryan TJ, Anderson JL, Antman EM, et al: ACC/AHA guidelines for the management of

patients with acute myocardial infarction: a report of the American College of Cardiology/American Heart Association Task Force on Practice Guidelines (Committee on Management of Acute Myocardial Infarction). *J Am Coll Cardiol* 1996; 28:1328–1428.

4. Miettinen H, Lehto S, Saikku P, et al: Association of *Chlamydia pneumoniae* and acute coronary heart disease events in non-insulin dependent diabetic and non-diabetic subjects in Finland. *Eur Heart J* 1996; 17:682–688.

5. Alexander RW, Pratt CM, Roberts R: Diagnosis and management of patients with acute myocardial infarction. In: Alexander RW, Schlant RC, Fuster V, et al (eds): *Hurst's The Heart,* 9th ed. New York, McGraw-Hill, 1998; chap 47.

6. Spodick DH: Q-wave infarction versus S-T infarction: nonspecificity of electrocardiographic criteria for differentiating transmural and nontransmural lesions. *Am J Cardiol* 1983; 51:913–915.

7. deWinter RJ, Koster RW, Sturk A, Sanders GT: Value of myoglobin, troponin T, and CK-MB mass in ruling out an acute myocardial infarction in the emergency room. *Circulation* 1995; 92:3401–3407.

8. Puleo PR, Meyer D, Wathen C, et al: Use of rapid assay of subforms of creatine kinase MB to diagnose or rule out acute myocardial infarction. *N Engl J Med* 1994; 331:561–566.

9. Fibrinolytic Therapy Trialists' (FTT) Collaborative Group: Indications for fibrinolytic therapy in suspected acute myocardial infarction: collaborative overview of early mortality and major morbidity results from all randomized trials of more than one-thousand patients. *Lancet* 1994; 343:311–322.

10. Levene DL: Chest pain: prophet of doom or nagging neurosis? *Acta Med Scand Suppl* 1981; 644:11–13.

11. GUSTO IIA Investigators, Ohman EM, Armstrong PW, Christenson RH, et al: Cardiac troponin T levels for risk stratification in acute myocardial ischemia. *N Engl J Med* 1996; 335:1333–1341.

12. Antman EM, Tanasijevic MJ, Thompson B, et al: Cardiac-specific troponin I levels to predict the risk of mortality in patients with acute coronary syndromes. *N Engl J Med* 1996; 335:1342–1349.

13. Kinch JW, Ryan TJ: Right ventricular infarction. *N Engl J Med* 1994; 330:1211–1217.

14. Hochman JS, Boland J, Sleeper LA, et al: Current spectrum of cardiogenic shock and effect of early revascularization on mortality: results of an International Registry. SHOCK Registry Investigators. *Circulation* 1995; 91:873–881.

15. Fuster V, Badimon L, Badimon JJ, Chesebro JH: The pathogenesis of coronary artery disease and the acute coronary syndromes (2). *N Engl J Med* 1992; 326:310–318.

16. Pfeffer MA, Braunwald E, Moye LA, et al: Effect of captopril on morbidity and mortality in patients with left ventricular dysfunction after myocardial infarction: results of the Survival and Ventricular Enlargement Trial. The SAVE Investigators. *N Engl J Med* 1992; 327:669–677.

17. SOLVD Investigators: Effect of enalapril on survival in patients with reduced left ventricular ejection fractions and congestive heart failure. *N Engl J Med* 1991; 325:293–302.

18. Zehender M, Kasper W, Kauder E, et al: Right ventricular infarction as an independent predictor of prognosis after acute inferior myocardial infarction. *N Engl J Med* 1993; 328:981–988.

19. Dreifus LS, Fisch C, Griffin JC, et al: Guidelines for implantation of cardiac pacemakers and antiarrhythmia devices: a report of the American College of Cardiology/American Heart Association Task Force on Assessment of Diagnostic and Therapeutic Cardiovascular Procedures (Committee on Pacemaker Implantation). *J Am Coll Cardiol* 1991; 18:1–13.

20. Mitrani RD, Myerburg RJ, Castellanos A: Cardiac pacemakers. In: Alexander RW, Schlant RC, Fuster V, et al (eds): *Hurst's The Heart,* 9th ed. New York, McGraw-Hill, 1998; chap 34.

21. TIMI Study Group: Comparison of invasive and conservative strategies after treatment with intravenous tissue plasminogen activator in acute myocardial infarction. Results of thrombolysis in myocardial infarction (TIMI) phase II trial. *N Engl J Med* 1989; 320:618–627.

22. Scandinavian Simvastatin Survival Study Group: Randomised trial of cholesterol lowering in 4444 patients with coronary heart disease: the Scandinavian Simvastatin Survival Study (4S). *Lancet* 1994; 344:1383–1389.

23. Sacks FM, Pfeffer MA, Moye LA, et al: The effect of pravastatin on coronary events after myocardial infarction in patients with average cholesterol levels. Cholesterol and Recurrent Events (CARE) Trial. *N Engl J Med* 1996; 335:1001–1009.

24. Wenger NK: Rehabilitation of the patient with coronary heart disease. In: Alexander RW, Schlant RC, Fuster V, et al (eds): *Hurst's The Heart,* 9th ed. New York, McGraw-Hill, 1998; chap 55.

25. Maron DJ, Ridker PM, Pearson TA: Risk factors and the prevention of coronary heart disease. In: Alexander RW, Schlant R, Fuster V, et al (eds): *Hurst's The Heart,* 9th ed. New York, McGraw-Hill, 1998; chap 41.

26. Theroux P, Waters D: Diagnosis and management of patients with unstable angina. In: Alexander RW, Schlant RC, Fuster V, et al (eds): *Hurst's The Heart,* 9th ed. New York, McGraw-Hill, 1998.

27. Braunwald E: Unstable angina: an etiologic approach to management [editorial]. *Circulation* 1998; 98:2219–2222.

28. Farkouh ME, Smars PA, Reeder GS, et al: A clinical trial of a chest-pain observation unit for patients with unstable angina. Chest Pain Evaluation in the Emergency Room (CHEER) Investigators. *N Engl J Med* 1998; 339:1882–1888.

29. PRISM-PLUS Study Investigators: Inhibition of the platelet glycoprotein IIb/IIIa receptor with tirofiban in unstable angina and non-Q-wave myocardial infarction. Platelet Receptor Inhibition in Ischemic Syndrome Management in Patients Limited by Unstable Signs and Symptoms (PRISM-PLUS) Study Investigators. *N Engl J Med* 1998; 338:1488–1497.

ANDREW L. SMITH /
CLYDE PARTIN

# HEART FAILURE

Heart failure management has changed dramatically over the past two decades. Current treatment strategies are directed not only toward the relief of symptoms and edema but also toward reducing mortality and hospitalizations. Additionally, medications may improve myocardial function long-term, a benefit not known to occur with prior strategies. Findings from large-scale clinical trials, particularly in patients with systolic dysfunction, have resulted in evidence-based practice guidelines for managing patients with heart failure.

It is recognized that the heart failure syndrome derives not only from the heart, but importantly from the complex response of the body to the failing heart. In fact, there has been a shift from treatments aimed primarily at increasing cardiac contractility to those that counteract the deleterious responses of the body. These maladaptive responses include activation of endogenous neurohormonal systems and the sympathetic nervous system. It is this complex interaction of myocardial disease with neural, endocrine, vascular, skeletal muscle, and renal alterations that ultimately determines a patient's symptoms and physical findings. Through the recognition of this complexity, one should no longer be surprised at the observations that most positive inotropic agents given chronically worsen heart failure and increase mortality and, conversely, that drugs such as beta-adrenergic blockers have beneficial effects in chronic heart failure.

Primary care physicians are often the sole providers of care for patients with the syndrome of heart failure. Primary care providers are faced with a wide spectrum of medical care delivery, from dealing with those at risk for heart failure to dealing with those in the terminal phases of pump failure. Prophylactic strategies are now aimed at preventing initial cardiac injury as well as delaying the progression to symptomatic disease in patients who have systolic dysfunction. At the other end of the spectrum, there are management strategies that can potentially take the patient with severe left ventricular dysfunction and severe symptoms to a normal or near-normal activity level with or without direct improvement in systolic function.

This chapter will review our current understanding of the epidemiology, pathophysiology, and management of patients with congestive heart failure (CHF).

## DEFINITION

Heart failure is a clinical syndrome in which a variety of symptoms, physical signs, or laboratory abnormalities are due to disordered cardiac function. Pathophysiologically, heart failure may be defined as the inability of the heart to pump enough blood at normal filling pressures to meet the metabolic demands for ordinary activity. Although clinicians commonly refer to heart failure as a "problem," it is more appropriate to consider heart failure as a physiologic manifestation of one of several cardiovascular disease processes. There are numerous cardiac disease states that may cause heart failure. Likewise, a variety of diseases and physiologic processes peripheral to the heart may contribute to this syndrome. The clinical manifestations of heart failure generally include dyspnea, fatigue, and fluid retention. In most patients, heart failure is not only a symptom complex but also a progressive disorder in which a natural decline in cardiac function and progression of symptoms occurs over time.

## EPIDEMIOLOGY AND COST

Efforts to describe the epidemiology of heart failure are flawed because clinical heart failure is a syndrome and not a specific illness. Naturally, it is simpler to define a specific problem, e.g., acute myocardial infarction (AMI), than to agree on criteria for a syndrome that has various clinical manifestations. Statistics related to heart failure vary depending on whether cohorts are identified from patients with prior hospitalizations, identified from patients in the outpatient setting, or selected based on laboratory data such as ejection fraction.

It is estimated that there are currently 4.8 million people in the United States with the syndrome of CHF and that there are more than 400,000 new cases per year.[1] Heart failure is the leading cause of hospitalization in patients over age 65. More than 6 percent of patients greater than age 65 and more than 10 percent of patients over age 75 have congestive heart failure.[2] Overall, mortality at 5 years remains high, approaching 50 percent in trials of patients with moderate symptoms at the time of enrollment. Approximately 300,000 patients die each year with heart failure, and about half of these deaths are sudden.[3–5]

In an era in which other major cardiovascular disorders are decreasing, the prevalence of heart failure is increasing. The major factor responsible for this is the aging population. Additionally, patients are now more likely to survive myocardial infarctions (MIs) and thus are developing symptomatic heart failure at a later time as a consequence of ventricular dysfunction. Over the last 40 years, there has been a significant shift in the etiology of heart failure from hypertension and rheumatic valvular heart disease to coronary heart disease and diabetes.[6,7]

Studies of outpatient care delivery have documented that management of heart failure has been a neglected problem.[7] A focus on outpatient heart failure management is now emerging, based upon the considerable economic costs of managing this chronic condition. Managed care organizations, state and federal governments, and hospitals are becoming increasingly aware of this economic burden. Heart failure accounts for 3 to 5 percent of total health care costs. Hospitalizations account for approximately half of these costs. Hospitals often are faced with financial shortages in providing care to patients with heart failure because of inadequate insurance reimbursement. Targeting improved outpatient care will reduce hospitalizations and have a favorable impact on costs.[8]

# ETIOLOGIES OF HEART FAILURE

The symptoms of fatigue and dyspnea and the physical findings of rales and edema may be indicative of the syndrome of heart failure. The astute clinician, however, will develop a mental checklist of potential cardiac and noncardiac conditions that may result in this clinical presentation. Dyspnea and fatigue are not specific to heart failure. Likewise, all that rattles and swells may not be indicative of heart disease. Noncardiac disorders that may mimic heart failure include lung disease, thyroid disorders, anemia, hypoalbuminemia, pulmonary embolism, and idiopathic edema. Heart failure, when present, may occur as a result of a variety of conditions.

Acute causes of myocardial failure include severe ischemia, MI, valvular rupture (endocarditis, myxomatous degeneration), myocarditis, and myocardial contusion. Pressure overload from hypertensive crisis or pulmonary embolism may result in acute left or right ventricular failure, respectively. Pericardial tamponade may result in acute heart failure.

"High-output" heart failure is the presence of congestion in the setting of a supranormal cardiac output. There is generally vasodilatation, with physical findings of a widened pulse pressure and warm extremities. Potential causes of high-output failure include hyperthyroidism, arteriovenous fistula (following trauma or as a complication of cardiovascular procedures or hemodialysis), beriberi, and Paget's disease. Severe anemia may result in high-output failure.

Right heart failure is most commonly due to left heart failure. Certain conditions are associated specifically with right-sided heart failure, however. Causes of pulmonary hypertension resulting in right heart failure include obstructive lung disease, congenital heart disease, primary pulmonary hypertension, pulmonary thromboembolic disease, and collagen vascular diseases. Right heart failure may also occur in the setting of normal pulmonary artery pressures as a result of right ventricular infarction, arrhythmogenic right ventricular dysplasia, or pulmonary or tricuspid valvular heart disease.

Chronic heart failure may result from abnormalities of the valves, pericardium, endocardium, great vessels, or myocardium. Cardiac failure may be due to systolic dysfunction, diastolic dysfunction, or both. It is estimated that a significant percentage of patients with heart failure have predominantly abnormalities that involve diastolic dysfunction.[9] Diastolic dysfunction is defined as impaired filling of one or both ventricles.

## Diastolic Heart Failure

Common causes of diastolic dysfunction are as follows:

- Systemic hypertension
- Coronary artery disease
- Hypertrophic cardiomyopathy
- Infiltrative cardiomyopathies (amyloid, hemochromatosis)
- Aortic stenosis
- Aging

In isolated diastolic dysfunction, there is a normal-sized ventricle with normal emptying (normal ejection fraction) but with elevated diastolic pressures. In severe forms, cardiac output may be compromised because of inadequate stroke volume resulting from diminished diastolic filling. The clinical manifestations of diastolic dysfunction, which include exertional dyspnea, pulmonary congestion, and peripheral edema, are indistinguishable from signs and symptoms of disorders of systolic dysfunction.

Myocardial abnormalities that cause diastolic dysfunction are often the result of myocardial hypertrophy or ischemia.[10] Pressure overload states such as systemic hypertension or aortic stenosis cause concentric hypertrophy, in which an increase in ventricular wall thickness but no increase in ventricular chamber diameter occurs. Volume overload may cause eccentric hypertrophy, in which the ventricle wall thickness and ventricular chamber diameter increase proportionately. Concentric hypertrophy is more closely associated with diastolic function abnormalities. The myocyte mass in concentric hypertrophy may lead to inadequate capillary density, resulting in ischemia or fibrosis. Diastolic dysfunction is associated with slowed myocardial relaxation and increased ventricular passive chamber stiffness due to hypertrophy and fibrosis.[11]

Diastolic myocardial relaxation is an active process involving actin-myocin cross-bridge dissociation. Impaired relaxation may occur as a result of intracellular calcium overload in the setting of tachycardia, myocardial ischemia, or increased afterload states.[10] Patients with diastolic dysfunction are prone to increasing symptoms with activities that increase heart rate and blood pressure.

Diastolic dysfunction is suspected in the patient with a history of exertional dyspnea or congestion and a normal heart size on chest x-ray. Echocardiography helps exclude systolic dysfunction and may provide evidence of hypertensive left ventricular hypertrophy, hypertrophic cardiomyopathy, or aortic stenosis. Restrictive cardiomyopathy or pericardial restriction may cause diastolic dysfunction with normal ventricular cavity size and thickness. Suggestive echocardiographic features include enlarged atria in the setting of normal ventricular dimensions.

Evaluation of cardiac hemodynamics with noninvasive techniques such as Doppler, echocardiography, or radionuclide ventriculography may provide clues to the presence of diastolic dysfunction. However, these techniques are dependent on preload conditions and lack sensitivity in establishing a diagnosis.[12] Patients with sudden episodes of dyspnea at rest or on exertion should be evaluated for coronary artery disease (CAD).

To date, large-scale clinical trials have not addressed the chronic medical management of patients with heart failure due to diastolic dysfunction. Of note, there are no true "lusitropic" agents that selectively improve diastole without having inotropic effects.[13] In general, medical management is directed at treating the etiology of the disorder, such as lowering blood pressure in systemic hypertension and preventing ischemia in CAD.

As is the case with heart failure from systolic dysfunction, diuretics are necessary for patients with diastolic heart failure who have edema. Patients with diastolic dysfunction are sensitive to changes in preload, and excessive diuresis may result in reduced cardiac output and hypotension. Direct-acting vasodilators may be poorly tolerated in this condition. The reduction in vascular resistance in diastolic dysfunction may not increase cardiac output and thus may cause hypotension.

Increasing diastolic filling time by slowing heart rate is of benefit in the treatment of symptomatic diastolic dysfunction. This may be accomplished with beta blockers and calcium channel blockers. There are no convincing data showing that these agents directly improve diastolic relaxation in patients with diastolic dysfunction. Activity-related hypertension appears to worsen symptoms and hemodynamics in patients with diastolic dysfunction. Pharmacologic therapies that reduce exercise-mediated hypertension may improve symptoms.[14]

Angiotensin-converting enzyme (ACE) inhibitors and angiotensin receptor blockers are being investigated in diastolic dysfunction. Myocardial tissue ACE activity is up-regulated in pressure-overload hypertrophy, and theoretically these agents may have beneficial direct myocardial effects in patients with diastolic dysfunction.[11] Digoxin is generally not indicated in the treatment of heart failure related to diastolic dysfunction.

## Systolic Heart Failure

Patients are generally considered as having heart failure from systolic dysfunction when the left ventricular ejection fraction is less than 40 to 45 percent. Common causes of systolic heart failure are as follows:

- Coronary artery disease
- Myocarditis
- Toxins (alcohol, anthracyclines)
- Infiltrative diseases
- Valvular/congenital disorders
- Chronic tachycardia
- Thyroid disorders
- Sleep apnea syndrome

In recent large-scale clinical trials involving systolic heart failure in the United States, coronary artery disease accounts for over 60 percent of patients. Approximately 40 percent of patients have coexistent systemic arterial hypertension.[2] Excessive alcohol use may result in systolic dysfunction, a problem that is potentially reversible with cessation of ethanol. Increasing use of the anthracycline chemotherapeutic agents in treating cancer has resulted in an increased number of patients with anthracycline-related systolic dysfunction.[15] The toxicity from the anthracyclines is dose-related, with the incidence increasing significantly when over 550 mg/m$^2$ of daunorubicin has been administered. The development of symptoms of heart failure in this setting may not occur until several decades later. Myocarditis, often related to viral illnesses, may be an underlying cause of dilated cardiomyopathy; however, documentation is usually absent.[16] There is growing evidence that dilated cardiomyopathy may be associated with a variety of genetic mutations.[17] Thyroid disorders, including hyperthyroidism and hypothyroidism, may be contributing causes of systolic dysfunction. Patients with chronic tachyarrhythmias may develop "tachycardia-mediated dilated cardiomyopathy," an entity that may be reversible with interventions that restore normal heart rate.[11,18]

## Pathophysiology of Chronic Heart Failure

Traditional medical teachings have focused on the concepts related to the pathophysiology of acute heart failure. In this scenario, acute damage to the heart results in decreased cardiac output and activation of compensatory mechanisms. These compensatory mechanisms include sympathetic activation, redistribution of cardiac output to the vital organs, enhanced renal salt retention, tachycardia, increased tissue oxygen extraction, and enhanced contractility due to Frank-Starling mechanisms. Acute hemodynamic abnormalities such as elevation of the left ventricular end-diastolic pressure and a decrease in cardiac output are clinically manifest as dyspnea, edema, and fatigue. Based on this understanding of pathophysiology, acute management strategies have been targeted to lower preload, lower afterload, and increase cardiac output.

Numerous observations over the past two decades have resulted in a separation in the understanding of the pathophysiology of acute heart failure and that of chronic heart failure.[19] Part of this knowledge has come from the results of large therapeutic trials, both favorable and unfavorable, involving patients with chronic heart failure. Many pharmacologic strategies that improve acute heart failure have been shown to have no impact on or to adversely affect the prognosis of patients with systolic dysfunction. There are many inotropic agents and arterial vasodilators that have theoretically appeared useful for heart failure management but that when clinically evaluated had adverse consequences when given chronically. For instance, milrinone, a phosphodiesterase inhibitor, improved short-term hemodynamics and exercise tolerance but increased mortality when given orally in a chronic heart failure trial.[20]

There are other examples of the lack of correlation between acute hemodynamic effects and chronic outcome. Drugs that do produce long-term improvement, such as ACE inhibitors, may have their maximum hemodynamic effects early, but may not maximally affect symptoms or exercise tolerance for several months.[21] Medications such as beta-adrenergic blockers may worsen hemodynamics early but be beneficial in the long term.

It is now recognized that the progression of chronic heart failure is linked closely to "inappropriate" activation of the sympathetic nervous system and to activation of neurohormones, including renin, angiotensin II, aldosterone, endothelin, and arginine vasopressin, as well as vasoconstrictor prostaglandins. Interestingly, these are the same hormones that are activated as a result of volume depletion. In essence, in chronic heart failure, the body is unable to recognize the difference between volume depletion and congestion. Activation of these neurohormonal mechanisms results in tachycardia, fluid retention, increased thirst, and vasoconstriction. Prolonged activation of the sympathetic nervous system and the neurohormonal axis is postulated to cause myocyte damage, in part independent of hemodynamic alterations resulting from this activation. Thus the chronic heart failure state results in a downward clinical spiral in which cardiac deterioration further activates the body to release substances that increase cardiac work and exacerbate congestion. Chronic pharmacologic strategies are now targeted at blocking these maladaptive responses.

One manifestation of the progression of systolic dysfunction following myocardial damage is an increase in left ventricular size and the formation of a more globular ventricular geometry. The left ventricle dilates, in part because of hypertrophy of myocytes, but also because of alterations of the cytoskeletal network. This process is referred to as ventricular remodeling.[22] Associated with this is diminished systolic performance (as measured by ejection fraction) and an increase in mitral regurgitation as a result of dilatation of the mitral annulus. The increase in mitral regurgitation results in elevated left atrial pressure and a decrease in forward cardiac output. Traditionally, much attention has been paid to the concept of Starling forces, where an increase in myocardial stretch results in increased contractility. This has resulted in the dogma of avoiding lowering the left ventricular end-diastolic pressure excessively. This dogma is based on studies with acute heart failure. In the setting of a chronically hypokinetic dilated ventricle, however, an attempt to decrease the diastolic left ventricular pressure to normal may actually reduce mitral regurgitation and improve cardiac output.[23] Therefore, maintaining a higher volume status in an attempt to keep the left ventricular diastolic pressure above normal and provide further stretch on myocytes may have the consequence of worsening mitral regurgitation and have adverse clinical consequences.

Abnormal vascular endothelial function has been documented in chronic heart failure.[24] This results in impaired vasodilatation and may affect exercise performance. Skeletal muscle changes due to neuroendocrine activation and physical deconditioning contribute to poor exercise tolerance in this condition.[25] Respiratory muscle abnormalities may also contribute to dyspnea.[26] Renal retention of sodium is a hallmark of the heart failure syndrome but varies among individuals with some patients experiencing more problems with edema than others.

The pathophysiology of chronic heart failure is complex. It is therefore not surprising that research demonstrates a poor correlation between symptoms and ejection fraction. There are many patients with very low ejection fractions (<15 percent) who are asymptomatic or minimally symptomatic on medical therapy. There are other patients who have minimal decreases in their ejection fraction but are quite debilitated. Differences in diastolic function abnormalities may contribute to these differences.[27]

In chronic heart failure, physical findings may be misleading in determining the degree of hemodynamic deterioration.[28,29] A patient with chronic heart failure may not develop pulmonary rales even in the setting of a very high pulmonary capillary wedge pressure. This is in part secondary to the marked increase in lymphatic drainage that occurs in the pulmonary lymphatics. Additionally, a patient on medical therapy may not develop lower-extremity edema until he or she is 7 to 10 lb volume overloaded. Many patients will redistribute their sodium retention to the liver and abdomen and not to the feet.

Patients with heart failure are at risk for sudden death. Ventricular dilatation, myocardial hypertrophy, and myocardial fibrosis, seen in patients with heart failure, are important factors contributing to the development of ventricular rhythm disturbances. Activation of the sympathetic nervous system and neuroendocrine systems may predispose an individual to sudden cardiac death from ventricular rhythm disturbances. In severe heart failure, sudden death is frequently the direct result of pump failure. Rhythm disturbances prior to "sudden" death may be bradycardic and may not necessarily be related to ventricular tachycardia or fibrillation.[30]

## CLINICAL ASSESSMENT

Early identification of patients with heart failure and those with asymptomatic left ventricular systolic dysfunction has become increasingly important. Clinical trials have demonstrated the benefits of early initiation of medical therapy in preventing hospitalizations, delaying the progression of heart failure symptoms, and reducing mortality. Additionally, there is the practical benefit of beginning management of a chronic illness prior to a preventable acute emergency room presentation.

The physician should have a heightened awarness for heart failure when examining a patient with a history of MI, hypertension, or diabetes, particularly if the patient has exertional fatigue or dyspnea. Markers of left ventricular systolic dysfunction include a displaced point of maximal impulse (PMI) on physical examination, third heart sound, murmur of mitral regurgitation, enlarged cardiac silhouette on chest x-ray, and poor R-wave progression or Q waves on the electrocardiogram. As discussed previously, with the gradual development of heart failure, patients often do not have pulmonary rales or peripheral edema on examination.

It is recommended that patients with new onset of dyspnea on exertion, orthopnea, or paroxysmal dyspnea undergo evaluation for heart failure unless the history and physical examination are indicative of another cause. According to published guidelines,[31] patients with symptoms that are highly suggestive of heart failure should undergo assessment of the left ventricular ejection fraction. This can be done by techniques such as echocardiography or radionuclide ventriculography. Patients with less specific symptoms, including fatigue or lower-extremity edema, require such testing only if there are physical or radiographic signs that suggest heart failure.

The primary care physician may be faced with the challenge of diagnosing heart failure in a previously healthy individual. Young patients presenting with dilated cardiomyopathy may be mistakenly diagnosed with "bronchitis" when the initial symptoms are dyspnea and cough. Abdominal symptoms including early satiety, abdominal bloating, or right upper quadrant discomfort may mimic a primary gastrointestinal illness. A careful physical examination may help sidestep these pitfalls. The absence of rales or edema on physical examination is an insensitive physical finding and may mislead the clinician away from the diagnosis of heart failure in the absence of a careful cardiac examination. Palpation for displacement of the PMI and listening for a third heart sound or murmurs of mitral regurgitation are likely to help identify these patients earlier. Recognition of jugular venous pressure elevation by neck vein examination may prevent an unnecessary delay in making the proper diagnosis.

Sound clinical practice involves not only identifying the patient with heart failure but also not overdiagnosing heart failure. There are numerous conditions that mimic heart failure, including lung disease, anemia, renal insufficiency, thyroid disorders, and nephrotic syndrome. Patients presenting with new-onset heart failure should be evaluated for these conditions. Specific tests for patients with signs or symptoms of heart failure are listed in Table 27-1.[31]

Once it is established that the patient has heart failure and concomitant diseases have been identified, the evaluation for the etiology of heart failure is performed. The framework for evaluating etiology is listed in Fig. 27-1. Ejection fraction should be assessed to differentiate etiologies associated primarily with diastolic dysfunction from those associated with systolic dysfunction. If there is systolic dysfunction, with a left ventricular ejection fraction less than 40 percent, attention should be focused on determining if the patient has underlying CAD.

Patients with angina pectoris and heart failure should be considered for coronary angiography unless the patient has a contraindication to a revascularization procedure.[32] With improvement in surgical techniques, coronary artery bypass surgery (CABG) can be performed successfully even in the setting of an ejection fraction below 20 percent. Patients with heart failure who have a high ischemic burden have a poor prognosis with medical therapy. Although randomized trials of CABG have generally excluded patients with heart failure or severe left ventricular dysfunction, there are center-specific reports that suggest that revascularization improves symptoms and survival in this group.[33] It is estimated that over 75 percent of heart failure patients with significant concomitant angina have surgically correctable disease.

Patients with no angina but a prior history of MI should be considered for a physiologic test such as stress nuclear testing or stress echocardiography. If the findings suggest ischemia, cardiac catheterization should be performed.[32] An alternative approach is to perform coronary arteriography to identify multivessel disease and plan further evaluation based upon the results.

There are few data to support a specific diagnostic approach for coronary disease in patients without angina and with no prior history of MI. It is reasonable to evaluate patients based upon their risk factors for coronary artery disease. Following clinical assessment, it may be appropriate not to pursue further testing for coronary disease, to use noninvasive tests to detect myocardial ischemia, or to perform coronary angiography. In patients with a high likelihood of CAD, more aggressive strategies such as cardiac catheterization should be considered.

**TABLE 27-1.  Recommended Tests for Patients with Signs or Symptoms of Heart Failure**

| Test Recommendation | Finding | Suspected Diagnosis |
| --- | --- | --- |
| Electrocardiogram | Acute ST-T-wave changes | Myocardial ischemia |
| | Atrial fibrillation, other tachyarrhythmia | Thyroid disease or heart failure due to rapid ventricular rate |
| | Bradyarrhythmias | Heart failure due to low heart rate |
| | Previous MI (e.g., Q waves) | Heart failure due to reduced left ventricular performance |
| | Low voltage | Pericardial effusion |
| | Left ventricular hypertrophy | Diastolic dysfunction |
| Complete blood count | Anemia | Heart failure due to or aggravated by decreased oxygen-carrying capacity |
| Urinalysis | Proteinuria | Nephrotic syndrome |
| | Red blood cells or cellular casts | Glomerulonephritis |
| Serum creatinine | Elevated | Volume overload due to renal failure |
| Serum albumin | Decreased | Increased extravascular volume due to hypoalbuminemia |
| $T_4$ and TSH (obtain only if atrial fibrillation, evidence of thyroid disease, or patient age $> 65$) | Abnormal $T_4$ or TSH | Heart failure due to or aggravated by hypo/hyperthyroidism |

MI = myocardial infarction; TSH = thyroid-stimulating hormone.
*Source:* Heart Failure Guideline Panel: *Heart Failure: Evaluation and Care of Patients with Left Ventricular Systolic Dysfunction.* Clinical Practice Guideline No. 11, AHCPR Publication 94-0612. Rockville, MD, U.S. Department of Health and Human Services, Agency for Health Care Policy and Research, 1994.

Patients with CAD may have left ventricular systolic dysfunction that is potentially reversible. "Hibernating" myocardium is myocardial dysfunction resulting from chronic ischemia without infarction. Several noninvasive tests are available to detect chronically ischemic or hibernating myocardium. Quantitative thallium scintigraphy using exercise and late redistribution or reinjection at rest is available at many medical centers. Of note, technetium 99m sestamibi is helpful in determin-

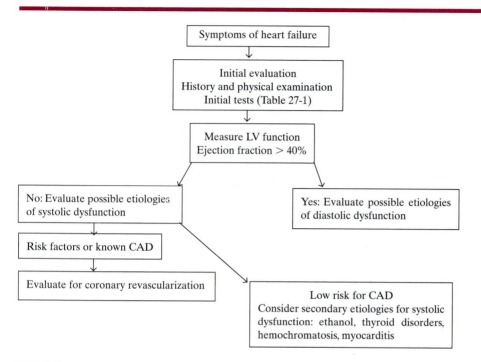

**Figure 27-1** Algorithm for evaluation of patients with heart failure. LV = left ventricular; CAD = coronary artery disease. (Adapted from Heart Failure Guideline Panel: *Heart Failure: Evaluation and Care of Patients with Left Ventricular Systolic Dysfunction.* Clinical Practice Guideline No. 11, AHCPR Publication 94-0612. Rockville, MD, U.S. Department of Health and Human Services, Agency for Health Care Policy and Research, 1994.)

ing ischemia but is of less value in differentiating between infarcted and hibernating muscle. Positron emission tomography is considered the best test for myocardial viability but is not widely available. Stress echocardiography with exercise or dobutamine is an alternative to nuclear testing.[32]

When coronary disease has been considered but excluded, the focus should then be centered on other etiologies for the dilated dysfunctional ventricle. Patients with nonischemic dilated left ventricular systolic dysfunction should not be designated as having "idiopathic dilated cardiomyopathy" until other etiologies have been considered. Reversible causes of systolic dysfunction, including ethanol abuse and thyroid disorders, should be excluded. Preferably, if no cause is apparent, the patient should be considered as having "dilated cardiomyopathy of uncertain etiology."

There are a variety of conditions that may cause systolic dysfunction (see "Systolic Heart Failure"). It is recognized that cardiac biopsy performed in patients with suspected myocarditis has a low yield. When strict histologic criteria for active myocarditis are applied, the yield is less than 15 percent in patients with systolic dysfunction and recent onset of heart failure symptoms. Of note, the Myocarditis

Treatment Trial[16] found no beneficial effect of immunosuppression with prednisone combined with either azathioprine or cyclosporine in patients with histologic evidence of myocarditis. Therefore, an aggressive approach with either cardiac biopsy or a panel of blood tests to support evidence of suspected myocarditis is rarely indicated.

Electrocardiography is a standard part of the evaluation of the heart failure patient. A normal electrocardiogram is rare in patients with symptomatic heart failure due to systolic dysfunction. Left bundle branch block and intraventricular conduction delays are common in patients with myocardial damage from either ischemic or nonischemic etiologies. Low QRS voltage may be present in pericardial and infiltrative disorders as well as in myocarditis or dilated cardiomyopathy. Conduction system disease, including heart block, may be a presenting finding in cardiac sarcoidosis or Lyme myocarditis.[34] The electrocardiogram is also useful in showing evidence of arrhythmias, previous MI, or left ventricular hypertrophy. Patients with very wide QRS complexes (greater than 140 ms) generally have significant myocardial disease and generally have a worse prognosis.[35]

Chest radiography may be the first objective indicator of undiagnosed cardiac disease. Cardiomegaly, indicated by an increased cardiothoracic ratio of greater than 0.50 on the posterior-anterior (PA) film, may be an indicator of increased diastolic volume. The chest x-ray may provide clues to the presence of congenital heart disease, valvular heart disease, or pericardial disease. Caution should be exercised in attempting to determine the hemodynamic status of a patient by chest x-ray. In the patient with chronic CHF, the chest x-ray is an insensitive test for predicting elevation of the pulmonary capillary wedge pressure.[28] Therefore, chest x-rays on office follow-up are an insensitive and expensive means of assessing volume status.

Echocardiography is helpful in differentiating systolic from diastolic dysfunction, in assessing ventricular chamber size, and in documenting valvular disease and congenital heart disease. Clinicians often focus on the measurement of the ejection fraction, but numerous other features recorded on the echocardiogram report may have important clinical significance. Attention should be paid to the left ventricular diastolic diameter. This, in addition to the ejection fraction, has prognostic value. Patients having left ventricular diastolic diameters greater than 7 cm have a less favorable outlook. Regional wall motion abnormalities on echocardiography may suggest CAD, particularly if the abnormal segments fit a vascular distribution. Hypertrophy, seen in hypertrophic cardiomyopathy and systemic arterial hypertension, is well assessed by echocardiography. Abnormal texture on two-dimensional echocardiography may be a clue to infiltrative diseases such as amyloid, but this finding is not specific. Doppler evaluation is useful in assessing the presence and severity of valvular regurgitation and in assessing hemodynamic gradients in hypertrophic cardiomyopathy with outflow obstruction. Additionally, evidence of pulmonary artery hypertension can be obtained by evaluation of the velocity of tricuspid regurgitation: Estimated right atrial pressure $+ 4 \times velocity^2 =$ estimated systolic pulmonary artery pressure.

# CLINICAL HISTORY IN THE PATIENT WITH ESTABLISHED HEART FAILURE

This section will focus on information that should be obtained in patients with established heart failure during the initial or follow-up visits. A detailed history will help direct the physician to an appropriate clinical assessment of the etiology and physiology of the patient's illness.

Common symptoms related to CHF are as follows:

- Dyspnea—at rest, at night, with activity, etc.
- Fatigue
- Cough
- Nausea/anorexia
- Abdominal pain or bloating
- Thirst
- Weight fluctuation
- Edema
- Palpitations/dizziness
- Chest discomfort
- Impotence

Review of symptoms with the patient is important; not only will it aid in medical diagnosis and management, but discussion of the basis for symptoms will help the patient recognize that many seemingly non-heart-related symptoms are in fact "heart failure" symptoms. Additionally, patients often confuse symptoms of worsening heart failure with side effects from their medications. For instance, patients with heart failure have excessive thirst (in part secondary to increased vasopressin levels). They may blame this thirst on taking diuretics, when it may actually be a manifestation of worsening heart failure. Likewise, nausea secondary to hepatic congestion is commonly interpreted by patients as a medication side effect.

Certain symptoms in the patient with heart failure may indicate the need to adjust medical therapy. Orthopnea, nocturnal cough, and paroxysmal nocturnal dyspnea (PND) are usually indicative of volume overload and the need for increased diuresis even in the absence of edema. Likewise, abdominal bloating, right upper quadrant abdominal discomfort, and early satiety may indicate hepatic congestion. These symptoms often abate after adequate diuresis.

Correlation of symptoms with changes in the patient's weight is useful. For instance, a patient may notice chest tightness with activity, but only on days when his or her weight has increased, thus indicating a primary problem with fluid retention. The types and duration of activities that cause symptoms should be reviewed and correlated with variables related to daily living. Sleep disturbances, common in patients with heart failure, should be reviewed in detail. Often these disturbances are secondary to fluid retention and improve with medical treatment, but in selected populations, sleep apnea may be the underlying etiology, and formal testing may be required to guide appropriate therapy.[36]

A careful dietary history is time-consuming but invaluable in managing patients with problems of fluid retention. The statement "I do not eat salt" indicates that a patient is unaware of the sodium that is in our diet. A description of the amounts and types of foods and fluids that a patient consumes each day should be elicited. Questioning about the intake of alcoholic beverages in the past as well as currently may help identify a contributing factor to heart failure. Patients are often surprised to learn that as little as two alcoholic beverages a day may have a significant depressor effect on myocardial function.

The medication history includes review of all medications and allergies. Ability to purchase medications should be reviewed. Patients should be questioned as to which medications they take for pain relief or cold symptoms. Aspirin and non-steroidal anti-inflammatory medications are known to interfere with ACE inhibitors and with diuretics.[37] Acetaminophen in high doses may potentiate the effects of warfarin. Ephedrine may cause vasoconstriction.

Patients with chronic heart failure are at increased risk for pulmonary infections and may be at high risk for complications from influenza. Vaccination status, including pneumococcal vaccine and influenza vaccine, should be reviewed.

One of the more important questions, often unasked, is, "Do you weigh yourself daily?" Noting an increase in weight of 3 to 4 lb in several days can provide the earliest possible recognition of fluid retention. This may be a sign of inadequate diuretics or excessive sodium intake.

The history at each follow-up visit should include a review of potential complications that occur in patients with heart failure. Sudden dizziness, palpitations, and syncope or near-syncope are clues to potentially fatal cardiac dysrhythmias. Patients with suspected rhythm disturbances require further evaluation. Transient focal weakness may suggest transient ischemic attacks from embolism from intracardiac thrombi. Postural hypotension from excessive diuresis may be indicated by orthostatic weakness or dizziness.

At each follow-up visit, changes in the patient's symptoms should be assessed. Symptoms of dyspnea at rest or with exertion, presence of PND or orthopnea, episodes of dizziness, or prolonged palpitations should be noted. The presence or absence of chest discomfort should be elicited. The level of activity should be reviewed and New York Heart Association[38] functional status established. Medication compliance, including a review of time intervals of various medications, should be reviewed. It is helpful for the patient to keep a written log of his or her daily weights. Dietary compliance should be noted in the medical record.

## PHYSICAL EXAMINATION

The physical findings in CHF have been well described and are familiar to the practicing physician. The differentiation between the physical findings of acute heart failure and those of chronic heart failure has received less attention, however. Physical signs of acute left heart failure resulting from AMI have been shown to corre-late well with measures of hemodynamics. The presence of a third heart sound and rales on pulmonary examination are generally indicative of a pulmonary capillary wedge pressure greater than 18 to 22 mmHg. In chronic CHF, the pulmonary ex-amination is less reliable. Less than 25 percent of chronic heart failure patients with pulmonary capillary wedge pressures greater than 22 mmHg will have rales on ex-amination.[28] Additionally, an $S_3$ gallop is absent in one-third of patients with pul-monary capillary wedge pressures greater than 18 mmHg. Examination for jugular venous distention at rest or by the hepatojugular reflux test is a relatively sensitive and specific finding in predicting elevation of left heart pressures in patients with chronic left ventricular dysfunction, however.[28] Proper evaluation of heart failure requires the ability to assess neck veins.

With the above limitations in mind, the following directed heart failure examina-tion should be performed during each encounter (see Table 27-2). Pulse, blood pres-sure, and weight should be obtained. On the initial visit and on follow-up visits in which patients complain of orthostasis, blood pressure should be taken in the supine, seated, and standing positions. A drop in systolic blood pressure of greater than 10 mmHg may be indicative of volume depletion or autonomic neuropathy or be related to vasodilator therapy (particularly if it occurs on initiation of therapy). The pulse should be assessed for rate, regularity, and quality. Pulsus alternans is a specific finding for ventricular failure. A weak or thready pulse may be indicative of a low cardiac output. Patients with acute heart failure should be assessed for pulsus paradoxus, seen in pericardial tamponade. Patients with atrial fibrillation should have the heart rate documented by cardiac auscultation. In the evaluation of the pa-tient with atrial fibrillation, it is useful to assess the heart rate at rest and after ac-tivity such as walking in the hallway. An inappropriately rapid rate response at low activity levels may lead to exertional fatigue and dyspnea. Therapies targeted at pre-venting exercise-related tachycardia may improve outcome.

Respiratory rate and pattern should be observed. The Cheyne-Stokes breathing pattern, in which there is hyperpnea followed by apnea, is seen in patients with ad-vanced hemodynamic derangement.

Estimation of the jugular venous pulse should be made at each encounter. This is accomplished by examining the patient at a 45° angle from the horizontal plane. The

**TABLE 27-2.   Heart Failure Evaluation at Each Visit**

- Pulse, blood pressure, weight
- Jugular venous pulse
- Cardiac palpation and auscultation
- Lung examination
- Liver examination
- Extremity examination

jugular venous pulsation should be less than 4 cm above the sternal angle. Alternatively, if the internal jugular venous pulsation is visible with the patient sitting upright, the jugular venous pressure is increased. The hepatojugular reflex (HJR) is elicited when gentle continuous compression on the abdomen results in the prolonged distention of the neck veins. When present, the HJR indicates volume overload.

Cardiac examination should be performed with the examiner on the patient's right side. Palpation of the point of maximal impulse inferiorly and to the left occurs with ventricular dilatation. The PMI is best appreciated with the patient rotated laterally to the left. A parasternal pulsation may indicate right ventricular volume or pressure overload. On auscultation, the intensity of the first heart sound is often diminished in heart failure. An increase in the pulmonic closure sound ($P_2$) occurs when there is pulmonary hypertension.

Auscultation for gallops is best done with the bell of the stethoscope, with the patient in the left lateral decubitus position. When sinus rhythm is present, a fourth heart sound is often present in patients with diastolic dysfunction related to left ventricular hypertrophy. A third heart sound may indicate elevated left ventricular end-diastolic pressure, as discussed previously. When tachycardia is present, the third and fourth heart sounds occur simultaneously, resulting in a "summation" gallop. Mitral regurgitation is common in patients with left ventricular dilatation. The murmur is holosystolic, heard best at the apex with radiation to the left lateral chest. Likewise, tricuspid regurgitation is common with right ventricular dilatation. This holosystolic murmur increases on inspiration. Regurgitant murmurs may disappear with measures that reduce ventricular volume or afterload. The third heart sound may disappear with improvement in the patient's hemodynamic status.

Pulmonary examination consists of chest percussion to seek evidence of dullness over the posterior thorax, suggestive of pleural effusion. This is more frequently present on the right. The patient should be assessed for rales. A pleural friction rub may be indicative of pulmonary embolism. Wheezing or "cardiac asthma" may occur with pulmonary edema.

The liver should be palpated for assessment of enlargement indicative of fluid congestion or tricuspid regurgitation. Findings suggestive of ascites may be present with long-standing right heart failure. Lower-extremity edema is generally indicative of an excess of 5 L of fluid volume. Thus peripheral edema is an insensitive finding for the presence of volume overload. When pedal edema is present, it generally indicates that decompensation has been present for several days. Peripheral cyanosis and cool extremities are findings that suggest a low cardiac output and peripheral vasoconstriction. In summary, physical findings can be useful in determining whether patients have fluid retention and congestion as well as in assessing whether there is adequate tissue perfusion.

# TREATING CHRONIC HEART FAILURE

The goals of heart failure treatment are to reduce morbidity and mortality and to maintain or improve quality of life. From a public health perspective, heart failure treatment should also involve effective strategies to prevent diseases that can result in cardiac dysfunction and symptomatic heart failure. CAD and hypertension are the most common etiologic factors in heart failure. Prevention and treatment of these factors can reduce the risk of developing heart failure. Cigarette smoking and lipid disorders are major contributors to coronary artery disease.

During the past 15 years, there has been remarkable improvement in the pharmacologic management of heart failure. However, nonpharmacologic strategies such as changes in daily living routines may be equally important. Numerous specialized heart failure treatment centers, including our own, have seen patients with "refractory heart failure" display marked improvement in symptoms and physical findings following dietary counseling and appropriate lifestyle alterations. Topics for patient and family education and counseling are listed in Table 27-3.

The primary care physician faces the challenge of both implementing effective medical therapy and giving proper educational instruction. This is particularly difficult with the time constraints of a modern office practice. The patient with congestive heart failure usually has two to four concomitant problems that may require specific attention. Therefore, the physician needs to develop an organized plan for approaching heart failure education and management. Written or video educational materials are available and helpful, but are not a substitute for direct discussion with patients and family members. This type of education is often best done by a patient educator such as a nurse or dietitian with reinforcement from the physician. Many hospitals have now developed heart failure clinics aimed at improving the education and management of heart failure patients. This approach is in some respects similar to the previous development of diabetes clinics at many hospitals. It is important for both the patient and the medical provider to recognize that in most cases the heart failure syndrome will not disappear but will be present for life. A time commitment on the "front end" to educate patients properly is likely to result in a decrease in complications, including hospitalizations, long term.[7,39,40]

When counseling patients about the signs and symptoms of heart failure, it is important to emphasize that symptom improvement is an expected result of compliance with the medical regimen. Emphasis should be placed on measuring body weight daily. Instructing the patient to call the office or to do self-adjustment of diuretics in the event of a 3- to 4-lb weight gain over a short period of time can prevent symptomatic deterioration.

It is important to discuss with the patient that "heart failure" is actually a poor term. It does not mean that the patient cannot engage in any activities or that his or her heart is about to stop. Discussing the heart's function as a pump and why symptoms develop when the pump has been damaged may help the patient understand his or her condition. It is useful to explain to the patient that deteriorating symptoms may be due to inappropriate responses by the body and not necessarily to a sudden deterioration in the heart. Telling a patient that the body cannot "tell the difference between dehydration and heart failure" may improve recognition of the need to limit salt and fluid intake.

**TABLE 27-3.   Topics for Education of Patients and Family**

General Counseling
  Explanation of heart failure and the reason for symptoms
  Cause or probable cause of heart failure
  Expected symptoms
  Symptoms of worsening heart failure
  What to do if symptoms worsen
  Self-monitoring with daily weights
  Explanation of treatment/care plan
  Clarification of patient's responsibilities
  Importance of cessation of tobacco use
  Role of family members or other caregivers in the treatment/care plan
  Availability and value of qualified local support group
  Importance of obtaining vaccinations against influenza and pneumococcal disease

Prognosis
  Life expectancy
  Advance directives
  Advice for family members in the event of sudden death

Activity Recommendations
  Recreation, leisure, and work activities
  Exercise
  Sex, sexual difficulties, and coping strategies

Dietary Recommendations
  Sodium restriction
  Avoidance of excessive fluid intake
  Fluid restriction (if required)
  Alcohol restriction

Medications
  Effects of medications on quality of life and survival
  Dosing
  Likely side effects and what to do if they occur
  Coping mechanisms for complicated medical regimens
  Availability of lower-cost medications or financial assistance

Importance of Compliance with the Treatment/Care Plan

*Source:* Adapted from Heart Failure Guideline Panel: *Heart Failure: Evaluation and Care of Patients with Left Ventricular Systolic Dysfunction.* Clinical Practice Guideline No. 11, AHCPR Publication 94-0612. Rockville, MD, U.S. Department of Health and Human Services, Agency for Health Care Policy and Research, 1994.

Traditionally, there has been an overemphasis on the need for rest in patients with diminished ejection fractions. Rest is indicated for patients during acute decompensation or during periods of diuretic resistance. Patients who have stabilized should be encouraged to engage in activities. Exercise helps to avoid deconditioning. Periods of at least 10 continuous minutes of uninterrupted walking daily are beneficial in improving the patient's activity level and overall sense of well-being. Isometric exercises should be discouraged, but upper-extremity tone may be maintained through the use of multiple repetitions with 3- to 5-lb arm weights. The patient should understand that physical activity will not improve the contractile function of the heart directly but that avoiding deconditioning allows the heart to function more efficiently.[41]

Recommendations regarding employment should take into account the fact that patients on medical therapy for CHF may not tolerate extremes of heat or cold. Patients may have periods of temporary instability, making jobs involving climbing perilous. Jobs involving heavy lifting may put a sudden strain on the heart, potentially initiating ventricular rhythm disturbances.

Dietary restrictions of sodium include limitation to 3 g of sodium daily in patients with milder forms of heart failure and 2 g/day in patients requiring loop diuretic therapy. Liquid intake should be reduced to less than 2 qt/day in patients with symptomatic heart failure who have episodes of fluid retention. Alcohol use should be discouraged. Many patients with coronary artery disease are aware of the potential benefits of alcohol consumption on lipid abnormalities. They need to recognize, however, that as little as two drinks daily of alcohol may worsen symptoms in the setting of systolic dysfunction.

The benefits and potential side effects of medications should be discussed. Evidence of efficacy (determined from the very large heart failure trials) should be shared with patients. Patients need to understand that their medical regime is aimed at not only improving symptoms but also preventing complications and prolonging life. Patients need to understand that they have a responsibility for improving their health. Instructions for patients with CHF are listed in Table 27-4.

**TABLE 27-4.   Instructions for the Patient with Heart Failure**

- Weigh yourself every morning: if weight of 3–4 lb is gained in 1–2 days, adjust diuretic or call physician.

- Limit sodium and fluids.

- Limit alcohol.

- Activity as tolerated (see discussion).

- Call physician's office if you experience chest pain, pressure, persistent cough, dizziness, nausea, increased shortness of breath, weight gain, swollen feet, or abdominal discomfort.

- Take medications as prescribed.

- Your next appointment is _____

- Medication changes today are _____

# PHARMACOLOGIC THERAPY FOR ASYMPTOMATIC LEFT VENTRICULAR SYSTOLIC DYSFUNCTION

Asymptomatic patients with moderate or severe left ventricular systolic dysfunction (left ventricular ejection fractions less than 35 to 40 percent) should be treated with an ACE inhibitor unless there is a specific contraindication.[42] Absolute contraindications to ACE inhibitor therapy include angioedema, hyperkalemia, symptomatic hypotension, and pregnancy. In the Survival and Ventricular Enlargement (SAVE) trial,[43] patients with recent MI and systolic dysfunction were randomized to placebo or captopril (target dose of 50 mg three times daily). At follow-up (average 42 months), there was a decrease in the development of heart failure by 22 percent and a decrease in all-cause mortality by 19 percent. In the Studies of Left Ventricular Dysfunction (SOLVD) Prevention trial,[44] patients with left ventricular ejection fractions less than 35 percent were randomized to enalapril (target dose 10 mg bid). At an average follow-up of 3 years, there was a 36 percent reduction in hospitalization for heart failure and a trend toward a decrease in mortality that did not reach statistical significance.

In addition to ACE inhibitor therapy, beta-blocker therapy may prevent the development of heart failure. Beta-blocker therapy following MI has the greatest mortality benefit in patients with reduced cardiac contractility. Therefore, a low ejection fraction post-MI in the absence of heart failure symptoms may be considered an indication and not a contraindication to beta blockade. Combined beta-blocker therapy and ACE inhibitor therapy has additive beneficial effects.[45]

Patients are generally screened for asymptomatic left ventricular systolic dysfunction by echocardiography or radionuclide gated imaging. Asymptomatic patients with evidence of cardiomegaly and those with physical findings such as murmurs of mitral regurgitation or ventricular gallops should be considered for screening. Patients generally should be screened for systolic dysfunction following MI. Such screening may be optional for certain patients who are at lower risk for systolic dysfunction. This includes post-acute MI patients with no previous history of MI, no Q waves on electrocardiogram, an uncomplicated clinical course, infarction isolated to inferior location, and only a modest increase in cardiac enzymes.[31]

# PHARMACOLOGIC THERAPY FOR SYMPTOMATIC HEART FAILURE

Treatment of patients with symptomatic heart failure with appropriate medications is based on the premise that drugs have acute effects that are generally related to changes in hemodynamics and chronic effects that are more complex and involve many mechanisms that alter myocardial and vascular functions. The results of clinical trials in symptomatic heart failure have allowed us to identify those medications that have beneficial chronic effects. As mentioned previously in this chapter, numerous medications with acute beneficial effects have "failed" when used chronically. Therefore, it is important not only to know the pharmacology of the various medicines but also to understand the implications of the results of the large clinical heart failure trials. Common drugs used in the treatment of heart failure will be reviewed.

## Diuretics

There have been no long-term studies assessing the effects of diuretics on morbidity and mortality in heart failure. The majority of patients with chronic heart failure will require a diuretic. Diuretics are necessary in patients with evidence of fluid retention. Appropriate use of diuretics is essential in achieving the maximum benefit of therapy with other agents, such as ACE inhibitors or beta blockers.

The loop diuretics are most frequently selected for patients with CHF. Loop diuretics are secreted in the proximal tubule and act from the luminal side of the loop of Henle. In situations where heart failure is advanced, or in other situations where there is a decrease in drug absorption or glomerular filtration rate, a higher dose of diuretic is required.[46] Thiazide diuretics may be used alone in patients with mild heart failure, but they generally lose their effectiveness when the creatinine clearance is less than 30 mL/min.

The use of diuretics can be divided into two phases. In the initial phase, the physician chooses a diuretic or combination of diuretics to relieve congestion and restore appropriate volume status. During this phase, the patient should notice an increase in urination within several hours of initiation of drug administration. The patient should notice weight loss the following day. If the patient does not respond to the initial oral dose, the dose should be increased until a diuretic response is achieved. Furosemide is generally the agent of choice because of its low cost. However, torsemide, which appears to be better absorbed and have an earlier peak effect than furosemide, may be the preferred loop diuretic when resistance to diuresis is encountered.[47] Intravenous diuretics in the clinic or inpatient setting may be necessary in some patients. An alternative approach is to use a thiazide diuretic or metolazone in combination with a loop diuretic. This approach should be used with caution, however, because of the potential for a very brisk diuresis with resultant life-threatening electrolyte or volume depletion.

The second phase of diuretic therapy is the maintenance phase. In this phase, a lower dose of the diuretic is necessary to maintain diuresis long-term in patients who have achieved appropriate volume status. Patients should not necessarily be prescribed a fixed dose of the diuretic; instead, they should be prescribed a daily dose and then instructed to adjust diuretic therapy based upon daily weights. For instance, a patient may be instructed to take 40 mg of furosemide daily, but if his or her weight increases by 2 to 3 lb in a day, to take an additional 40 mg in the evening. A change on the scale may be the first evidence of fluid retention. Patients who cannot be relied on to properly adjust the diuretic dose should notify the physician's office for instructions concerning diuretic dose adjustment when there is weight gain.

The risks of treatment with diuretics include electrolyte depletion, with the potential for cardiac rhythm disturbances; volume depletion, with resultant hypotension and azotemia; and neurohormonal activation, potentially resulting in worsening heart failure. Patients on diuretics require monitoring of potassium to avoid hypokalemia, which may precipitate ventricular ectopy. The majority of patients on loop diuretics with normal renal function will require potassium supplementation, unless they are on an aldosterone antagonist such as spironolactone.[21] Concomitant administration of magnesium should be considered in patients with hypokalemia requiring high-dose potassium supplementation in the setting of hypomagnesemia. Although hypomagnesemia may potentially aggravate ventricular arrhythmias, there is no long-term outcome data on magnesium supplementation in heart failure.

The aldosterone antagonist spironolactone generally has weak diuretic properties but may prevent electrolyte depletion through potassium-sparing effects. Spironolactone reduces mortality when added to standard heart failure therapy in patients with advanced symptoms of heart failure[21] (see "Aldosterone Antagonism" later in this chapter).

Although hypotension and azotemia may result from overdiuresis, inadequate diuresis is a very common mistake in the management of heart failure. It is not uncommon to see the blood urea nitrogen (BUN) concentration rise during the initiation or intensification phase of diuretic therapy; nevertheless, if there are physical signs of fluid retention, diuretic therapy should be continued. If there is evidence of hypoperfusion, including a narrow pulse pressure, hypotension, or cool extremities, adding short-term inpatient inotropic support should be considered.

## ACE Inhibitors

ACE inhibitors should be given to all patients with systolic dysfunction, regardless of symptoms. Recommended dosages of ACE inhibitors are shown in Table 27-5. In symptomatic patients, ACE inhibitors have been demonstrated to decrease mortality, improve symptoms, and reduce hospitalizations. The impact on mortality is related to decreasing the risk of progressive heart failure. There is no clear impact on

**TABLE 27-5.   Recommended Doses of ACE Inhibitors in Heart Failure**

| Drug | Initial Dose (mg) | Target Dose (mg) | Major Adverse Reactions |
|------|-------------------|------------------|-------------------------|
| Enalapril | 2.5 bid | 10 bid | Hypotension, hyperkalemia, renal insufficiency, cough, skin rash, angioedema, neutropenia |
| Captopril | 6.25–12.5 tid | 50 tid | Same |
| Lisinopril | 5 qd | 20 qd | Same |
| Quinapril | 5 bid | 20 bid | Same |

sudden death. ACE inhibition decreased mortality 16 percent in the SOLVD treatment trial with captopril (predominantly NYHA class II-III) and 27 percent in the CONSENSUS trial[48] with enalapril (predominantly NYHA class IV).

In the United States, studies suggest that ACE inhibitors are significantly underprescribed for CHF. In over 30 percent of patients who should be receiving these medicines, the drug is absent from the medical regimen. Additionally, these drugs are often prescribed in clinical practice at dosages that are much lower than those that have been used in the controlled clinical trials.[49] In controlled clinical trials of ACE inhibitors, the dosages have been titrated to a target dose and not to a specific therapeutic response such as improvement of symptoms. The Assessment of Treatment with Lisinopril and Survival Study (ATLAS) supports the use of target doses of ACE inhibitors. In this trial, more than 30 mg/day of lisinopril was shown to have an increased benefit compared to low doses (2.5 to 5 mg/day).[50]

Underprescribing of ACE inhibitors has occurred in part because of concerns about the risks of ACE inhibitor treatment. These risks include hypotension, worsening renal function, and hyperkalemia. In clinical trials, however, over 95 percent of patients tolerate ACE inhibitors long term. When hypotension or azotemia is encountered during therapy with ACE inhibitors, volume depletion should be excluded as a cause. For instance, the patient admitted to the hospital and given intravenous diuretics who experiences a drop in blood pressure after ACE inhibitor therapy may be volume depleted and not ACE inhibitor intolerant. Diuretics should be appropriately decreased. Approximately 5 to 15 percent of patients will develop a dry cough on an ACE inhibitor. This cough is related to an increase in bradykinin levels, which does not occur with the angiotensin-receptor blockers.

Patients with advanced heart failure are prone to the hypotensive effects of ACE inhibitors. However, ACE inhibition has the greatest relative benefit in those with the most advanced heart failure.[48] Therefore, efforts should be made to slowly titrate the doses of these medicines in patients with marginal hemodynamic status. This may be done over a period of weeks to months.

Patients with severe heart failure, particularly in combination with chronic hypotension, are at risk for renal deterioration when treated with ACE inhibitors. Patients with renal vascular disease, diabetes, and intrinsic renal disease are most at risk. The development of mild azotemia is not a contraindication to ACE inhibitor treatment.[21] Generally, ACE inhibitors should be continued unless there is a clear relationship between the medication and progressive renal deterioration.

During initiation of ACE inhibitor therapy, the patient should be checked for signs of excessive diuresis, including measurement of orthostatic blood pressures. Doses can generally be titrated up to maximum dose within 4 to 6 weeks. Patients may be advised not to expect maximum improvement in symptoms until up to 3 months after achieving maintenance therapy. Although low systolic blood pressure is not a contraindication to ACE inhibitor therapy, care should be taken in initiating therapy in patients with systolic blood pressure less than 100 mmHg. Systolic blood pressures in the 80 to 90 mmHg systolic range are acceptable as long as the patient is asymptomatic. One should consider referral of patients who do not tolerate ACE inhibitors because of symptomatic hypotension to a cardiology heart failure specialist. Such patients have difficult to manage heart failure and may benefit from specialized heart failure therapy.

The various ACE inhibitors have differences in pharmacologic activity, including differences in tissue selectivity and duration of action. There are minimal data comparing one ACE inhibitor to another. Review of clinical trials suggests that there are no major differences among the ACE inhibitors in their effects on symptoms and cardiovascular events. Current recommendations are to focus on achieving a target dose with a particular agent, with less concern about the specific agent used. Considerations such as patient compliance, insurance formulary, and medication expense are clinically more important than theoretical issues related to pharmacology. The emerging use of beta blockers has increased the clinical controversy about ACE inhibitor dosage. It may be more important to aim to treat patients with combinations of therapy rather than to push one particular agent to a maximum level at the expense of not prescribing the other medication.

## Digitalis

Cardiac glycosides exert their effect by inhibiting the sodium–potassium–adenosine triphosphatase pump. One result is an increase in cardiac contractility. The clinical benefits of digitalis may be secondary to its effects in other tissues, however. In chronic heart failure, the cardiac baroreceptors are desensitized. Digoxin resensitizes baroreceptors and thus reduces sympathetic outflow and subsequent sodium retention in the kidneys.[51] Digitalis may therefore act primarily by decreasing neurohormonal activation and not as a positive inotropic agent.

Digitalis is indicated in patients with heart failure and atrial fibrillation with uncontrolled heart rate. Digitalis is quite effective at lowering the resting heart rate in atrial fibrillation; however, exercise- or catecholamine-stimulated increases in heart rate often require the addition of other agents, including beta blockers.[52]

There has been controversy about the use of digitalis in patients with systolic heart failure and normal sinus rhythm. Several trials have demonstrated that digoxin improves symptoms and exercise tolerance in patients with mild to moderate heart failure and sinus rhythm.[21] Withdrawal of digoxin from stable patients has resulted in clinical deterioration in up to one-third of patients over a period of months.[53] There is only one placebo-controlled trial that has evaluated the effects of digoxin on mortality in patients with chronic heart failure. The Digitalis Investigation Group (DIG) trial evaluated patients with ischemic and nonischemic etiology of heart failure. Patients with mild to moderate heart failure were randomized to placebo or digoxin in addition to standard therapy with diuretics and ACE inhibitors. Overall, there was no effect on survival. There was a small decreased risk of death from heart failure and a small increased risk of death from arrhythmias. Hospitalizations for heart failure were reduced by 28 percent, although overall hospitalizations were reduced by only 6 percent.[54]

The usual dose of oral digoxin is 0.25 mg/day unless the patient is elderly or has renal insufficiency. No loading dose is necessary for treating chronic heart failure. There is little evidence to support the monitoring of digoxin levels to achieve maximum efficacy. Levels are helpful in assessing patients for toxicity or when poor patient compliance is suspected. Prescribing large doses of digoxin does not appear to be more effective than using small doses in the treatment of heart failure.[21]

Digoxin is generally not indicated as an acute treatment for heart failure with rapid loading, but should be viewed as chronic therapy. Digoxin may be initiated early in a patient's clinical symptomatic course or may be reserved for those patients who do not respond symptomatically to treatment with ACE inhibitors, diuretics, and possibly beta-blocker therapy. There are no data that support the use of digoxin in patients with asymptomatic left ventricular dysfunction.

## Beta-Adrenergic Receptor Blockers

Traditionally beta-adrenergic receptor blockers have been contraindicated in patients with CHF. These agents have acute negative inotropic effects and can worsen hemodynamics in the patient with decompensated heart failure. It is now recognized, however, that beta-adrenergic blockers, properly prescribed, are of major benefit in the treatment of chronic heart failure due to systolic dysfunction. Emerging clinical trials suggest that the relative benefits of beta-blocker therapy may actually exceed those seen with the ACE inhibitors.

The rationale for the use of beta blockers is derived from studies that indicate that chronic activation of the sympathetic nervous system is deleterious in heart failure. Sympathetic activation results in maladaptive responses, including cardiac hypertrophy, myocyte ischemia, apoptosis, peripheral vasoconstriction, and renal retention of sodium. These effects are mediated through $beta_1$-, $beta_2$-, and $alpha_1$-adrenergic receptors.[21] Beta blockers have been shown to reduce sympathetic activation and to have favorable effects in terms of reducing vasoconstrictors and restoring myocardial contractile properties.

The first suggestion that beta blockade was beneficial in heart failure was from a report of seven patients in 1975.[55] Since that time, there have been more than 10,000 patients studied in chronic heart failure trials evaluating beta blockade.[21] Most of these data have been reported in the past 3 years. These trials indicate that in patients with systolic dysfunction and New York Heart Association class II or III symptoms of heart failure, beta blockers have very beneficial effects when added to therapy with ACE inhibitors and diuretics.

Carvedilol, a combined nonselective beta and $alpha_1$ blocker, has been evaluated in four trials totaling over 1100 patients with predominantly NYHA class II or III symptoms of heart failure.[56] These trials were terminated prematurely when a 65 percent reduction in mortality was noted (3.2 versus 7.8 percent after approximately 1 year). This included a reduction in deaths due to progressive heart failure as well as a reduction in sudden deaths. There was a 27 percent reduction in need for hospitalization. The degree of mortality benefit has been questioned owing to the fact that mortality was not a prospectively designed clinical end point. Overall, clinical benefit was obvious, resulting in approval of carvedilol by the Food and Drug Administration for the indication of heart failure. Interestingly, the adverse event of worsening heart failure was less frequent with carvedilol compared to placebo.

Metoprolol, a beta$_1$-selective blocker, has been evaluated in several trials, the largest being the MERIT-HF trial.[21,57] In this trial, 3991 patients with ischemic or nonischemic cardiomyopathy were enrolled in a study evaluating extended-release metoprolol (100 to 200 mg/day). This study was terminated prematurely when a 35 percent reduction in mortality was noted with metoprolol therapy.[21]

The CIBIS II trial[58] evaluated 2647 patients randomized to the selected beta$_1$ blocker bisoprolol versus placebo. Treatment with bisoprolol resulted in a 34 percent reduction in mortality, a 32 percent reduction in heart failure hospitalizations, and a 20 percent reduction in hospitalization for any reason.

The results of these beta-blocker trials have led to recently published consensus recommendations by heart failure specialists[21] to include a beta blocker as part of the standard therapy for patients with stable NYHA class II or class III heart failure due to left ventricular systolic dysfunction. There are inadequate data to recommend use of beta blockers in NYHA class IV patients; these trials are currently being conducted.

Initiation of beta-blocker therapy for heart failure should be done with the recognition that acute benefit is unlikely and early clinical deterioration is possible. Therefore, appropriate patients for beta-blocker therapy are nonhospitalized patients with mild to moderate symptoms of heart failure (New York Heart Association class II or class III) due to systolic dysfunction (left ventricular ejection fraction to less than 35 to 40 percent) who are not edematous or receiving intravenous therapy for heart failure. Initial doses of beta blockers should be very low. The clinical trials typically used a starting dose that was less than one-eighth the eventual maintenance dose. Dose titration usually consists of doubling the dose every 2 to 4 weeks. Close outpatient monitoring is required during this period. Doses of diuretics or ACE inhibitors may require adjustment. In patients with very mild symptoms of heart failure, beta blockade has at most a modest impact on improving symptoms. The importance of beta-blocker therapy in this setting is the benefit from prevention of progression to more advanced symptoms and possibly improvement of cardiac function. Of all the classes of medications for heart failure, beta blockers are the most likely to improve the left ventricular ejection fraction. This result does not occur acutely but has generally been noted at 6 to 12 months following therapy. In patients with dilated cardiomyopathy, the average improvement in the left ventricular ejection fraction has been approximately 10 percent in clinical trials. Improvement of approximately 5 percent has been noted in studies of combined ischemic/nonischemic etiologies.[59] Chronic beta-blocker therapy provides stabilization of the pathophysiologic processes in the heart failure patient and does not result in the long-term exacerbation of CHF. Therefore, there are few data to suggest discontinuation of chronic beta-blocker therapy in the event of symptomatic deterioration, an expected consequence in the natural history of heart failure. In fact, abrupt discontinuation of beta-blocker therapy may result in clinical deterioration.

It is uncertain whether a particular beta blocker is preferable to another in heart failure management. Agents are different with regard to both beta-selectivity and alpha-receptor blockade. Experimental data indicate that in chronic heart failure, there is a decrease in myocardial beta$_1$-receptor density and a relative increase in beta$_2$ receptors. Alpha$_1$ receptors are present in the myocardium as well. Theoretically, because of the different myocardial and vascular effects of these agents, there may be differences in outcomes from nonselective and selective adrenergic blockade in heart failure. A trial comparing the nonselective agent carvedilol to the selective agent metoprolol is currently being conducted.

## Aldosterone Antagonism

Aldosterone may have adverse effects on myocardial and vascular structure and function in chronic heart failure. These effects appear to be in part independent of the consequences of angiotensin II. The Randomized Aldactone Evaluation Study (RALES) evaluated 1663 patients with severe heart failure (recent or current NYHA class IV) treated with spironolactone versus placebo. There was a 27 percent decrease in mortality and a 36 percent reduction in the combined risk of death or hospitalization for heart failure. Spironolactone reduces the need for potassium supplementation in patients on loop diuretics. Spironolactone therapy should be considered for patients with severe symptoms of heart failure.[21]

## Angiotensin Receptor Blockers

The angiotensin receptor blockers are currently under investigation in the therapy of chronic heart failure. These agents do not cause cough and are currently the therapy of choice for patients intolerant of ACE inhibitors because of cough. Whether these agents are a substitute for or preferred choice over ACE inhibitors in patients with heart failure is unresolved.[21]

## Other Vasodilator Therapy

Hydralazine and isosorbide dinitrate given in combination have been documented to improve ejection fraction and exercise tolerance and have a questionable impact on survival. Hospitalizations for heart failure were not decreased in the Vasodilator Heart Failure Trial (V-HeFT 1), however.[60] This combination may be considered for patients who are intolerant of ACE inhibitors as a result of hypotension or worsening renal function.[21]

Calcium channel blockers are generally not indicated for heart failure therapy and may be deleterious when given chronically to patients with systolic dysfunction. Amlodipine, a long-acting agent, may be the exception. This agent does not appear to adversely affect survival and is being investigated as a therapy for nonischemic dilated cardiomyopathy.[21]

## Antiarrhythmic Agents

Patients with severe left ventricular dysfunction are at risk for sudden cardiac death. Empiric antiarrhythmic therapy is generally not indicated. In the setting of left ventricular dysfunction, many antiarrhythmic drugs have proarrhythmic properties.

There is lack of convincing data that even amiodarone, the least proarrhythmic and most effective agent, prevents sudden death in heart failure. Patients with symptomatic ventricular rhythm disturbances, unexplained dizziness or syncope, or frequent episodes of nonsustained ventricular tachycardia should be referred to a cardiologist for further evaluation.

## Anticoagulation

Patients with atrial fibrillation and heart failure are at high risk for thromboembolic complications and should be anticoagulated unless there are specific contraindications. There is controversy regarding whether patients with sinus rhythm and severely depressed ventricular function should receive warfarin. No well-designed clinical trials have addressed this issue. Therefore, the decision about which patients should receive anticoagulation with warfarin is based on the individual patient's characteristics, as well as the biases of the prescribing physician.

## SUMMARY

Heart failure therapy is based on an understanding of the individual patient's disease state, fluid status, and clinical status. Major advances have been made in the treatment of systolic dysfunction. Implementation of recommended clinical practices should result in improving long-term outcomes, as well as providing symptomatic relief to patients with this syndrome.

### REFERENCES

1. American Heart Association: *1998 Heart and Stroke Statistical Update*. Dallas, TX, American Heart Association, 1997.
2. Massie BM, Shah NB: Evolving trends in the epidemiologic factors of heart failure: rationale for preventive strategies and comprehensive disease management. *Am Heart J* 1997; 133:703–712.
3. The SOLVD Investigators: Effect of enalapril on survival in patients with reduced left ventricular ejection fractions and congestive heart failure. *N Engl J Med* 1991; 325:303–310.
4. Francis GS: Congestive heart failure management: the impact of medication therapy on survival. *Am Heart J* 1998; 115:699–701.
5. Stevenson WG, Stevenson LW, Middlekauff HR, Saxon LA: Sudden death prevention in patients with advanced ventricular dysfunction. *Circulation* 1993: 88:2953–2961.
6. Kannel WB, Belanger AJ: Epidemiology of heart failure. *Am Heart J* 1991; 121:951–957.
7. Cardiology Roundtable: *Beyond Four Walls. Cost-Effective Management of Chronic Congestive Heart Failure*. Washington, DC, The Advisory Board Company, 1994.
8. O'Connell JB, Bristow MR: Economic impact of heart failure in the United States: time for a different approach. *J Heart Lung Transplant* 1994; 13:5107–5112.
9. Grossman W: Diastolic dysfunction in congestive heart failure. *N Engl J Med* 1991; 325:1557–1564.

10. Bonow RO, Udelson JE: Left ventricular diastolic dysfunction as a cause of congestive heart failure. *Ann Intern Med* 1992; 112:502–510.

11. Schlant RL, Sonnenblick EH, Katz AM: Pathophysiology of heart failure. In: Alexander RW, Schlant RC, Fuster V, et al (eds): *Hurst's The Heart,* 9th ed. New York, McGraw-Hill, 1998:682–726.

12. Nishamura RA, Tajik AJ: Evaluation of diastolic filling of left ventricle in health and disease: Doppler echocardiography is the clinician's Rosetta stone. *J Am Coll Cardiol* 1997; 30:8–18.

13. Nishamura RA, Schwartz RS, Holmes DR Jr, Tajik AJ: Failure of calcium channel blockers to improve ventricular relaxation in humans. *J Am Coll Cardiol* 1993; 21:180–188.

14. Warner JG Jr, Metzger DC, Kitzman DW, et al: Losartan improves exercise tolerance in patients with diastolic dysfunction and a hypertensive response to exercise. *J Am Coll Cardiol* 1999; 33:1567–1572.

15. Shan K, Lincoff AM, Young JB: Anthrocycline-induced cardiomyopathy. *Ann Intern Med* 1996; 125:47–58.

16. Mason JW, O'Connell JB, Herskowitz A, et al, and the Myocarditis Treatment Trial Investigators: A clinical trial of immunosuppressive therapy for myocarditis. *N Engl J Med* 1995; 323:269–275.

17. Ledan JM: The genetics of dilated cardiomyopathy—emerging clues to the puzzle. *N Engl J Med* 1997; 337:1080–1081.

18. Parker DL, Bardy GH, Wesley SJ, et al: Tachycardia-induced cardiomyopathy: a reversible form of left ventricular dysfunction. *Am J Cardiol* 1986; 57:563–570.

19. Packer M: The neurohormonal hypothesis: a theory to explain the mechanism of disease progression in heart failure. *J Am Coll Cardiol* 1992; 20:248–254.

20. Packer M, Carver JR, Rodeheffer RJ, et al, for the PROMISE Study Research Group: Effect of milrinone on mortality in severe chronic heart failure. *N Engl J Med* 1991; 325:1468–1475.

21. Packer M, Cohn JN: Consensus recommendations for the management of chronic heart failure. *Am J Cardiol* 1999; 83(2A):1A–79A.

22. Cohn JN: Structural basis for heart failure: ventricular remodeling and its pharmacologic inhibition. *Circulation* 1995; 91:2504–2507.

23. Stevenson LW: Tailored therapy for symptomatic heart failure. *Heart Failure* 1995; 11:87–107.

24. Katz S: Mechanisms and implications of endothelial dysfunction in congestive heart failure. *Curr Opin Cardiol* 1997; 18:259–264.

25. Wilson JR, Martin JL, Ferraro N: Impaired skeletal muscle nutritive flow during exercise in patients with congestive heart failure: role of cardiac pump dysfunction as determined by the effect of dobutamine. *Circulation* 1993; 87:470–475.

26. Mancini DM, Henson D, LaManca J, Levine S: Respiratory muscle function and dyspnea in patients with chronic congestive heart failure. *Circulation* 1992; 86:909–918.

27. Franciosa JA, Park M, Levine TB: Lack of correlation between exercise capacity and indexes of resting left ventricular performance in heart failure. *Am J Cardiol* 1981; 47:33–39.

28. Butman SM, Ewy GA, Standen JR, et al: Bedside cardiovascular examination in patients with severe chronic heart failure: implications of rest or inducible jugular venous distension. *J Am Coll Cardiol* 1993; 22:968–974.

29. Stevenson LW, Perloff JK: The limited reliability of physical signs for estimating hemodynamics in chronic heart failure. *JAMA* 1989; 26:884–888.

30. Luu M, Stevenson WG, Stevenson LW, et al: Diverse mechanisms of unexpected sudden death in advanced heart failure. *Circulation* 1989; 80:1673–1680.

31. Heart Failure Guideline Panel: *Heart Failure: Evaluation and Care of Patients with Left Ventricular Systolic Dysfunction*. Clinical Practice Guideline No. 11, AHCPR Publication 94-0612. Rockville MD, U.S. Department of Health and Human Services, Agency for Health Care Policy and Research, 1994.

32. ACC/AHA Task Force on Practice Guidelines: Guidelines for the evaluation and management of heart failure. *Circulation* 1995; 92:2764–2784.

33. Elefteriades JA, Tolis G Jr, Levi E, et al: Coronary artery bypass grafting in severe left ventricular dysfunction: excellent survival with improved ejection fraction and functional state. *J Am Coll Cardiol* 1993; 22:1411–1417.

34. Cox J, Krajden M: Cardiovascular manifestations of Lyme disease. *Am Heart J* 1991; 122:1449–1455.

35. Shamin W, Francis DP, Yousufuddin M, et al: Intraventricular conduction delay. A predictor of mortality in chronic heart failure? *Eur Heart J* 1998; 19:926A.

36. Javaheri S, Parker TJ, Liming JS, et al: Sleep apnea in 81 ambulatory male patients with stable heart failure. Types and their prevalences, consequences and presentations. *Circulation* 1998; 92:2154–2159.

37. Hall D, Zeitler H, Rudolph W: Counteraction of the vasodilator effects of enalapril by aspirin in severe heart failure. *J Am Coll Cardiol* 1992; 20:1549–1555.

38. New York Heart Association: *Nomenclature and Criteria for Diagnosing Diseases of the Heart and Great Vessels,* 9th ed. Boston, Little, Brown, 1994.

39. Rich MW, Beckham V, Wittenberg C, et al: A multidisciplinary intervention to prevent the readmission of elderly patients with congestive heart failure. *N Engl J Med* 1995; 333:1190–1195.

40. Stevenson WG, Stevenson LW, Middlekauff HR, et al: Improving survival for patients with advanced heart failure: a study of 737 consecutive patients. *J Am Coll Cardiol* 1995; 26:1417–1423.

41. Braith RW, Welsch MA: Exercise training. In: Mills RM, Young JB (eds): *Practical Approaches to the Treatment of Heart Failure*. Baltimore, Williams and Wilkins, 1998:125–196.

42. Packer M: Do angiotension-converting enzyme inhibitors prolong life in patients with heart failure treated in clinical practice? *J Am Coll Cardiol* 1996; 28:1323–1327.

43. Pfeffer MA, Braunwald E, Moy LA, et al, on behalf of the SAVE Investigators: Effect of captopril on mortality and morbidity in patients with left ventricular dysfunction after myocardial infarction: results of the Survival and Ventricular Enlargement Trial. *N Engl J Med* 1992; 327:669–677.

44. The SOLVD Investigators: Effect of enalapril on mortality and the development of heart failure in asymptomatic patients with reduced left ventricular ejection fractions. *N Engl J Med* 1992; 327:685–691.

45. Vantrimpont P, Rouleau JI, Wun CC, et al, for the SAVE Investigators: Additive beneficial effects of beta-blockers to angiotensin-converting enzyme inhibitors in the Survival and Ventricular Enlargement (SAVE) Study. *J Am Coll Cardiol* 1997; 29:229–236.

46. Cody RJ, Kubo SH, Pickworth KK: Diuretic treatment for the sodium retention of congestive heart failure. *Arch Intern Med* 1994; 154:1905–1914.

47. Vargo DL, Kramer WG, Black PK, et al: Bioavailability, pharmacokinetics, and pharmacodynamics of torsemide and furosemide in patients with congestive heart failure. *Clin Pharmacol Ther* 1995; 57:601–609.

48. The CONSENSUS Trial Study Group: Effects of enalapril on mortality in severe congestive heart failure: results of the Cooperative North Scandinavian Enalapril Survival Study (CONSENSUS). *N Engl J Med* 1987; 316:1429–1435.

49. Havranck EP, Abrams F, Stevens E, Parker K: Determinants of mortality in elderly patients with heart failure: the role of angiotension-converting enzymes inhibitors. *Arch Intern Med* 1998; 158:2024–2028.

50. Packer M, Poole-Wilson P, Armstrong P, et al: Comparative effects of low-dose versus high-dose lisinopril on survival and major events in chronic heart failure: the Assessment of Treatment with Lisinopril and Survival Study (Atlas). (Abstr.) *Eur Heart J* 1998; 19(suppl): 142.

51. Gheorghiade M, Ferguson D: Digoxin. A neurohormonal modulator in heart failure? *Circulation* 1991; 84:2181–2186.

52. David D, Segni ED, Klein HO, Kaplinsky E: Inefficacy of digitalis in the control of heart rate in patients with chronic atrial fibrillation: beneficial effect of an added beta adrenergic blocking agent. *Am J Cardiol* 1979; 44:1378–1382.

53. Packer M, Gheorghiade M, Young JB, et al, for the RADIANCE Study: Withdrawal of digoxin from patients with chronic heart failure treated with angiotensin-converting enzyme inhibitors. *N Engl J Med* 1993; 329:1–7.

54. The Digitalis Investigator Group: The effect of digoxin on mortality and morbidity in patients with heart failure. *N Engl J Med* 1997; 336:525–533.

55. Waagstein F, Hjalmarson A, Varnauskas E, et al: Effect of chronic beta-adrenergic blockade in congestive cardiomyopathy. *Br Heart J* 1975; 37:1022–1036.

56. Packer M, Bristow MR, Cohn JN, et al, for the U.S. Carvedilol Heart Failure Study Group: The effect of carvedilol on mortality in patients with chronic heart failure. *N Engl J Med* 1996; 334:1349–1355.

57. The International Steering Committee: Rationale, design, and organization of the Metoprolol CR/XL Randomized Intervention Trial in Heart Failure (MERIT-HF). *Am J Cardiol* 1997; 80(suppl 9B):54J–58J.

58. CIBIS II: Investigators and committees. The Cardiac Insufficiency Bisoprolol Study (CIBIS II): a randomized trial. *Lancet* 1999; 353:9–13.

59. Kukin ML, Kalman J, Charney RH, et al: Prospective, randomized comparison of effect of long-term treatment with metoprolol or carvedilol on symptoms, exercise, ejection fraction and oxidative stress in heart failure. *Circulation* 1999 99:2645–2651.

60. Cohn JH, Johnson G, Ziesche S, et al: Effect of vasodilator therapy on mortality in chronic congestive heart failure: results of the veterans Administration Cooperative Study. *N Engl J Med* 1996; 314:1547–1552.

# CARDIOMYOPATHY

JERRE F. LUTZ

## CARDIOMYOPATHY

### Definition

Cardiomyopathy is a disorder of heart muscle characterized by abnormal cardiac performance.

### Classification

The various forms of cardiomyopathy may be classified according to function, etiology, histology, genetics, and therapeutic response.[1] The only currently used classification developed by consensus is the World Health Organization (WHO) and International Society and Federation of Cardiology classification, devised in 1980 and revised in 1995,[2] in which the cardiomyopathies are classified according to pathophysiology unless etiologic or pathogenetic factors are known. Others favor the terms *primary* and *secondary cardiomyopathy* to identify cardiomyopathies on a clinical basis.[3]

This chapter will concentrate on those forms of cardiac dysfunction classified according to pathophysiology in which there is no known etiology.

## DILATED CARDIOMYOPATHY

### Definition

The term *dilated cardiomyopathy* is used to describe heart muscle disease in which the left ventricle exhibits increased systolic and diastolic volumes along with an ejection fraction less than 40 percent.[4]

## Etiology

Although there is a wide variety of systemic or cardiac processes that can produce dilated cardiomyopathy, most of these should be characterized as secondary cardiomyopathies. The term *idiopathic dilated cardiomyopathy* should be reserved for primary heart muscle disease without known cause. It is estimated that idiopathic dilated cardiomyopathy has a familial basis in about one-quarter of cases, with autosomal dominant, autosomal recessive, and X-linked transmission reported. No candidate genes have as yet been identified.[4]

## Pathology

On gross examination, the weight of the heart is increased and all four cardiac chambers are dilated. The walls of the left ventricle are not thickened due to massive dilatation. Myocardial scars are common despite normal epicardial vessels. Intracardiac thrombi and mural endocardial plaques secondary to organized thrombi are found in about half of cases.[4] Systemic and pulmonary emboli are more common in those patients in whom intracardiac emboli are found at autopsy.

Pathologic and physiologic differences between the most common forms of cardiomyopathy are found in Table 28-1.

On microscopic examination, myocytes are hypertrophied, with large, bizarre nuclei. Other cellular changes include mitochondrial abnormalities, T-tube dilatation, and increased intracellular lipids. Interstitial, parenchymal, and perivascular focal infiltrates are not specific and are not associated with adjacent myocyte necrosis. Fibrosis is not uncommon and is most frequently found in the subendocardium.[4]

**TABLE 28-1.   Physiologic Changes in Untreated Patients with Cardiomyopathy**

|  | Dilated Cardiomyopathy | Hypertrophic Cardiomyopathy | Restrictive Cardiomyopathy |
|---|---|---|---|
| End-diastolic volume | ⇑ | N or ⇓ | N |
| End-systolic volume | ⇑ | ⇓ | ⇓ |
| Ejection fraction | ⇓ | ⇑ | N |
| Hypertrophy | N or ⇓ | ⇑⇑⇑ | N or slight ⇑ with infiltrative |
| Filling pressure | ⇑ | ⇑ | ⇑ |
| Restriction to filling | Possible | ⇑ | ⇑⇑⇑ |

N = normal, ⇑ = increased, ⇓ = decreased. With treatment, abnormalities may correct toward normal. In end-stage hypertrophic and restrictive cardiomyopathy, ejection fraction may ⇓ and volumes may ⇑.

## Pathophysiology

Dilated cardiomyopathy is the most common form of primary myocardial disease referred to specialty centers. Regardless of the etiology, the primary insult leads to systolic dysfunction. Compensatory stabilizing mechanisms are invoked, including an increased heart rate, volume expansion (to utilize the Frank-Starling mechanism), and myocyte hypertrophy. These changes are mediated via the reninangiotensin system and the adrenergic nervous system. Although these mechanisms are designed to maintain perfusion pressure, compensatory overshoot results in an increased vascular resistance, which in turn decreases the systolic function of the left ventricle. Sodium retention, designed to improve left ventricular contractility utilizing the Frank-Starling mechanism, leads to pulmonary congestion.

## Clinical Manifestations

**SUBJECTIVE.**   Some patients are asymptomatic, and the process is discovered by way of an abnormal electrocardiogram (ECG) or chest roentgenogram.

Fatigue due to decreased cardiac output or exercise intolerance (dyspnea on exertion) may occur earlier in the process than paroxysmal nocturnal dyspnea, ascites, or peripheral edema.

Chest pain is common, and the character is often suggestive of angina pectoris. Pleuritic chest pain may occur as a result of pulmonary infarction.

Palpitations and syncope due to arrhythmias are common.

**OBJECTIVE.**   The systolic blood pressure is normal or low. The pulse pressure is often low as a result of the decreased stroke volume. Pulsus alternans is present only with advanced left ventricular failure.

The apical impulse is often enlarged and displaced. Gallop cadences may be both audible and palpable. The second heart sound may be paradoxically split in the setting of a left bundle branch block. With pulmonary hypertension, the second sound is split narrowly and the pulmonic component is increased in intensity.

A murmur compatible with atrioventricular valve regurgitation due to dilatation of the valvular apparatus (mitral or tricuspid regurgitation) or pulmonary hypertension (tricuspid regurgitation) is frequently audible.

Jugular venous distention is seen with right ventricular failure, whereas an enlarged a wave is compatible with diminished right ventricular compliance. A large R or c–v wave may be seen as a result of tricuspid regurgitation. Ascites, peripheral edema, and a pulsatile liver indicate advanced right heart failure.

**THE ELECTROCARDIOGRAM.**   Sinus tachycardia is frequent. Atrial and ventricular dysrhythmias are common, as are interventricular conduction delays, especially left bundle branch block. A left atrial abnormality suggests abnormal left ventricular compliance. Poor R-wave progression of the QRS complex in the precordial leads or frank Q waves (pseudoinfarction pattern) are frequently seen.

**THE CHEST ROENTGENOGRAM.**   The cardiac silhouette is moderately to severely enlarged. There is evidence of pulmonary hypertension. Pleural effusions are seen following advanced chronic pulmonary congestion.

**THE ECHOCARDIOGRAM.**   The left ventricular cavity is dilated and the ejection fraction is diminished. The atria are enlarged, with increased diastolic pressures. Abnormal mitral valve motion is seen, with abnormal compliance and increased pressures. Severe tricuspid or mitral regurgitation may be seen as a result of ventricular chamber dilatation and increased diastolic pressures.

**SPECIAL DIAGNOSTIC TESTS.**   Left ventricular dilatation and dysfunction may be quantitated on radionuclear ventriculography. Abnormal thallium-201 fixed defects are common in dilated cardiomyopathy even in the absence of coronary disease. Reversible defects are not as specific for coronary disease as one would hope but are as good as present methods allow for screening noninvasively for significant coronary artery obstructions.

An abnormal blood test for human immunodeficiency virus and abnormal serum levels of phosphate, calcium, thyroid hormones, and iron may all indicate the cause of secondary cardiomyopathy.

## Natural History

Dilated cardiomyopathy has a high prevalence and a high morbidity rate. The median survival is 1.7 years for men and 3.2 years for women.[5] Dilated cardiomyopathy is more common in males and African-Americans than in females and Caucasians. The prognosis is poorer in African-Americans.[3]

The single most powerful predictor of death is left ventricular ejection fraction.[6] Treatment that improves left ventricular function improves prognosis, whereas treatment that ultimately decreases left ventricular function, such as many positive inotropic agents, can be associated with a poorer prognosis.[7]

Marked limitation of cardiopulmonary exercise function, manifest as reduced maximal systemic oxygen utilization, reliably predicts future mortality and is an indication for consideration of cardiac transplantation.

## Differential Diagnosis

Idiopathic dilated myopathy should be reassigned to the alcohol-induced category if the patient has consumed more than 100 g of alcohol per day for a substantial time. Similarly, reassignment to the hypertensive group should occur if the patient has had documented blood pressures >160/100 mmHg for years.

Coronary artery bypass grafting (CABG) in patients with substantial stunned or hibernating myocardium and advanced left ventricular dysfunction can result in an 80 to 83 percent 3-year survival rate.[8] It is thus important to differentiate patients with irreparable disease due to dilated myopathy who have normal coronary arteries from those with ischemic chronic myopathy who cannot be improved with revascularization and those patients who would benefit.

Surgery is of greatest benefit to patients with significant left ventricular dysfunction who also have severe class III or IV angina, those in whom symptoms of angina exceed congestive symptoms, those with the more severe coronary obstructions, and those with significant left main occlusion.[9]

## Medical Therapy

Nonpharmacologic interventions include sodium and fluid restriction. Walking should be encouraged, but strenuous exercise, especially isometrics, is prohibited. Digitalis, diuretics, and either angiotensin-converting enzyme inhibitors or hydralazine/nitrate combinations should be instituted. Studies of Left Ventricular Dysfunction (SOLVD) showed that enalapril improved symptoms and survival rates in patients with class II or III congestive heart failure (CHF).[10] In the SOLVD prevention trial, there was no survival benefit in class I patients treated similarly, but there was a significant decrease in hospitalization and a delay in onset of clinical heart failure.[11]

Beta blockade should be added to the above regimen for persistent symptoms or tachycardia.[12] Carvedilol is a nonselective vasodilating beta-blocking agent with antioxidant properties. Improvement in symptoms has been shown in patients given carvedilol,[12] bisoprolol,[13,14] or metoprolol.[15] Improved survival has been seen with carvedilol[16] and bisoprolol.[14] Improved ejection fraction has been seen with carvedilol.[17] Beta blockade is currently recommended for NYHA class II and III patients. Ongoing clinical trials are evaluating the use of beta blockers in severe class IV patients, patients with heart failure after acute myocardial infarction (AMI), and asymptomatic patients with left ventricular dysfunction.

Calcium antagonists that suppress left ventricular function are contraindicated, whereas those calcium antagonists that vasodilate without myocardial suppression may be added to angiotensin-converting enzyme inhibitors in selected cases.

Coumadin is indicated in the setting of atrial fibrillation, a history of systemic or pulmonary emboli, and demonstration of intracardiac thrombus. Many cardiologists will start Coumadin for an ejection fraction of less than 30 percent in the absence of contraindications.

There are no data showing that prophylactic antiarrhythmic agents prolong life or prevent sudden death; therefore, treatment is confined to symptomatic arrhythmias.[18] Many agents either suppress ventricular function or are proarrhythmic in this setting. Amiodarone may be instituted even in the presence of severe left ventricular dysfunction. An implantable defibrillator may be recommended in patients with poor left ventricular function and frequent runs of nonsustained ventricular tachycardia. Electrophysiology studies are hazardous and of limited reliability in determining those patients with severe left ventricular dysfunction who are at risk for sudden death.[19]

Although intravenous infusion of positive inotropic agents may improve symptoms and hemodynamics on a short-term basis, either increased mortality or failure to reduce mortality has been associated with intermittent intravenous dobutamine infusion, oral amrinone, milrinone, enoximone, flosequinon, and high-dose vesnarinone.[20]

## Surgical Therapy

Patients with poor left ventricular function and severe mitral regurgitation are at high risk for valve replacement but may benefit from a mitral valve ring repair.

Dynamic cardiomyoplasty[21] and partial ventricular resection (Batista procedure[22]) have had variable results with high morbidity/mortality rates and thus have not become commonly utilized procedures.

# HYPERTROPHIC CARDIOMYOPATHY

## Definition

Hypertrophic cardiomyopathy is a primary form of cardiac muscle disease characterized by a thick left ventricle with a nondilated cavity in the absence of other cardiac disease capable of producing hypertrophy. The left ventricle is usually hyperdynamic. The term *hypertrophic subaortic stenosis* is not utilized, since most patients do not have a systolic gradient and the outflow tract is usually not stenotic. Suggested causes of the hypertrophy include (1) abnormal calcium kinetics, (2) abnormal sympathetic stimulation, (3) myocardial ischemia of intramyocardial vessels, (4) ischemic alteration of calcium metabolites, and (5) structural abnormalities leading to hypertrophy and muscle disarray.

## Etiology

Hypertrophic myopathy is a genetically transmitted mutation caused by one of multiple genes that encode protein on the cardiac sarcomere.[23] About half of cases involve autosomal dominant transmission; the remainder are of unknown etiology.[3]

## Pathology

Left ventricular hypertrophy is usually diffuse but can be isolated to the septum. The posterior segment of the free wall is least often involved. The left ventricular cavity is not dilated. Average wall thickness is 21 to 22 mm.[24] The atria are enlarged and the mitral valve leaflets elongated. Most hearts at autopsy show a plaque on the septum resulting from contact with the mitral valve. Left ventricular muscle thickness increases before age 18 and stabilizes thereafter. The decreased thickness seen in the elderly may be due to regression of muscle mass or to premature death of younger patients who are more severely affected.

Intramural coronary arteries have thick-ended arterial walls but decreased luminal cavity size.

Histologic examination shows (1) disarray of muscle cells, (2) replacement fibrosis, and (3) normal small intramyocardial cells.[24]

## Pathophysiology

A subaortic gradient may be seen in only a minority of patients with hypertrophic myopathy. Contributing factors include diminished left ventricular outflow tract dimensions, asymmetric septal hypertrophy, an anteriorly displaced mitral valve, increased size of the mitral valve leaflets, hyperdynamic left ventricular function (Venturi effect pulling the mitral valve through the outflow tract), and malposition of the papillary muscle insertion.

Diastolic dysfunction is seen in the majority of patients. Myofibrillar disarray and interstitial fibrosis may contribute to the increased stiffness and impaired relaxation of the myocardium.

Myocardial ischemia has been attributed to abnormal intramyocardial vessels, increased oxygen demand, and prolonged diastolic relaxation associated with increased wall tension.

Arrhythmias may relate to impaired transmission of normal electrophysiologic forces through the abnormal whorls of myocardial tissue.[4]

## Clinical Manifestations

**SUBJECTIVE.**   The majority of patients are asymptomatic or minimally symptomatic[3] Dyspnea is the most common symptom, followed by chest pain often suggestive of angina. Orthopnea and paroxysmal nocturnal dyspnea are uncommon symptoms.

In children, presyncope and near-syncope identify some patients at risk of sudden death. There is a higher sudden death mortality in younger patients than in older patients. Unfortunately, the first symptom of hypertrophic cardiomyopathy can be sudden death.

**OBJECTIVE.**   Since the majority of patients do not have outflow tract obstruction, the presence of an abnormal physical is not required for diagnosis. An $S_4$ gallop suggestive of abnormal compliance is common.

Abnormal findings in the setting of significant outflow tract obstruction include (1) abnormal jugular venous pulses with a prominent a wave due to abnormal ventricular compliance, (2) a bifid carotid with a dart and dome configuration, coinciding with (3) a harsh systolic murmur that increases with increased contractility (Isuprel or exercise) or decreased arterial pressure or left ventricular volume (Valsalva or antihypertensive agents). The murmur decreases with decreased contractility (beta blocker) or increased left ventricular volume (squatting or vasoconstrictor drugs). The second sound may be widely split with outflow tract obstruction.

**ELECTROCARDIOGRAM.**   The electrocardiogram is abnormal in the vast majority of patients. Common findings include left ventricular hypertrophy, ST–T-wave changes, a left atrial abnormality, and abnormal Q waves in the absence of coronary artery disease (pseudoinfarct pattern).

Arrhythmias are common, including premature ventricular contractions, ventricular tachycardia, and nonsustained ventricular tachycardia. Sustained monomorphic ventricular tachycardia is uncommon.

**CHEST ROENTGENOGRAM.**   If abnormal, the chest x-ray will include mild to moderate cardiomegaly and an enlarged left atrial shadow.

**ECHOCARDIOGRAPHY.**   The echocardiogram is most useful for initial diagnosis and screening of relatives. Abnormal features may include asymmetric septal hypertrophy, narrowed left ventricular outflow tract, or systolic anterior motion of the mitral valve. The left ventricular cavity is usually small or normal in size.

**SPECIAL TESTING.**   Electrophysiology does not convincingly add data that predict mortality and morbidity. Abnormal thallium scanning in the absence of coronary artery disease is not uncommon.

## Medical Therapy

Genetic evaluation of the patient and family may be warranted. Echocardiographic evaluation of family members and children until age 18 is suggested in order to closely observe them during the age of most rapid progression of this illness.

In asymptomatic patients, there are no data indicating that beta blockers or calcium antagonists influence left ventricular hypertrophy or prevent sudden death. Amiodarone or automatic implantable cardioverter defibrillators are utilized in high-risk patients in hope that sudden death can be prevented. Amiodarone is the only pharmacologic agent that prevents sudden death.[25, 26] Automatic implantable cardiac defibrillators, with or without amiodarone, are indicated for survivors of sudden death.

Symptoms of chest pain and dyspnea are often alleviated by beta blockers, calcium antagonists (especially verapamil), and disopyramide. Decreasing heart rate, decreasing oxygen consumption, and improving filling parameters seem to be the mechanism of symptom relief.

Antibiotics for subacute bacterial endocarditis prophylaxis are indicated.

Many patients experience episodes of atrial fibrillation over a lifetime. Beta blockers and calcium antagonists may slow the rate of the conduction, but amiodarone appears to be the best agent to prevent occurrences.

Sinus node dysfunction and atrioventricular block are indications for pacing in patients with hypertrophic myopathy.[19] Dual-chamber pacing with a short atrioventricular delay has been associated with brief periods of symptomatic and hemodynamic improvement, but there is no concomitant evidence of improved exercise tolerance.[27] In a study comparing dual-chamber pacing with standard therapy, peak oxygen consumption was not improved with pacing. Some patients improved symptomatically, some remained unchanged, and some deteriorated. Thus, routine dual-chamber pacing cannot be recommended.[28]

## Surgical Therapy

Surgical intervention is indicated for relief of incapacitating symptoms not responsive to medications and for normalization of an increased left ventricular end-diastolic pressure. Ventricular septal myotomy and myoectomy (Morrow procedure) is the procedure of choice, but mitral valve replacement has also been performed. The operative mortality of the Morrow septal myectomy is 1 to 2 percent.[29]

# RESTRICTIVE/INFILTRATIVE MYOPATHY

## Definition

Restrictive myopathy is a systemic or idiopathic disorder of the myocardium characterized by restrictive diastolic filling and thus simulating constrictive pericarditis. Systolic function is normal. There is no outflow tract obstruction or stenotic valvular disease. Infiltrative disease of the myocardium is a secondary disorder with similar physiology.

## Pathology

Restrictive myopathy is characterized by idiopathic fibrosis or minimal changes. Amyloid or infiltrative process due to the specific underlying disorder may be seen in secondary restrictive myopathies.

## Physiology

End-diastolic volumes are diminished, whereas end-systolic volumes and ejection fractions are normal. Filling pressures are high relative to the degree of filling. In diastole, filling occurs normally in the initial phase but rapidly reaches a maximum distention that cannot be exceeded.

## Clinical Manifestations

**SUBJECTIVE.**   Exercise intolerance is frequent, whereas chest pain is infrequent. Many patients present with advanced pulmonary congestion (dyspnea, orthopnea, and paroxysmal nocturnal dyspnea) and systemic congestion (edema and ascites).

**PHYSICAL EXAMINATION.**   Jugular venous pulsations are elevated, with prominent x and y descents. An inspiratory increase in venous pressure (Kussmaul's sign) may be seen. Pulse pressures may be decreased as a result of decreased stroke volumes, and tachycardia is frequent. Atrioventricular valve regurgitation (either tricuspid or mitral) may be evident. An $S_3$ gallop coinciding with abrupt cessation of diastolic filling may be audible. Ascites, hepatomegaly, and anasarca may be seen in advanced cases. Signs of primary amyloid (macroglossia) or secondary amyloid (lymphadenopathy, splenomegaly, hepatomegaly) due to diseases such as rheumatoid arthritis or tuberculosis may be seen when one of those diseases is the underlying disorder.

**ELECTROCARDIOGRAM.**   The electrocardiogram is usually abnormal. Left bundle branch block is common. Decreased QRS voltage is common in amyloid. Atrial fibrillation and atrioventricular block are frequently seen.

**CHEST ROENTGENOGRAM.**   The atria are enlarged, and there is evidence of pulmonary congestion with restrictive myopathy. The ventricles are not enlarged.

**ECHOCARDIOGRAPHY.**   The ventricles are usually normal in size, while the atria are enlarged. Tricuspid and mitral regurgitation are common. The ventricular walls may be thick as a result of infiltration. There is no pericardial thickening, but a pericardial effusion may be present with volume overload or pericardial involvement with amyloid. There is a restrictive filling pattern of the ventricles, with rapid filling in early diastole and virtually none in the last two-thirds of diastole.

**SPECIAL TESTING.**   Computed tomography or magnetic resonance imaging may be utilized to delineate restrictive myopathy from constrictive pericarditis (increased pericardial thickness). Thallium scans may be abnormal in restrictive myopathy but should not be ordered as a diagnostic test for this disorder.
    Cardiac catheterization reveals high mean diastolic filling pressures, from the high teens to low twenties. A deep steep *y* descent is seen in the atrial tracing, while a dip and plateau are seen in the ventricular tracing.[31]

## Differential Diagnosis

Hemochromatosis may produce a restrictive myopathy that can be reversed if the iron load can be reduced. Iron studies are abnormal.
    A physician should be highly suspicious of constrictive pericarditis in a patient with restrictive/constrictive physiology who has a history of tuberculosis or radiation therapy or an abnormal chest roentgenogram with calcifications of the pericardium.

## Treatment

No medical therapy is satisfactory. Symptoms of dyspnea may improve slightly with low-dose diuretics or calcium antagonists. Digitalis is not indicated if left ventricular systolic function is normal.

# ARRHYTHMOGENIC RIGHT VENTRICULAR CARDIOMYOPATHY

## Definition

Arrhythmogenic right ventricular cardiomyopathy is a progressive disorder beginning as fibrofatty replacement of the right ventricular myocardium that can progress to diffuse right and occasionally some left ventricular involvement.

## Etiology

Autosomal dominant inheritance with incomplete penetrance and an autosomal recessive form are both described.

## Clinical Manifestations

Arrhythmias and sudden death are common presentations.

# MYOCARDIAL INVOLVEMENT IN SYSTEMIC ILLNESS

## Amyloid Heart Disease

Amyloid heart disease is a restrictive myopathy characterized pathologically by extracellular deposition of protein in a beta-pleated sheet configuration. Recognized on electron microscopy as randomly arranged nonbranching fibers, this protein is insoluble and impervious to proteolytic digestion.

In primary amyloid, no other illness is identified. Amyloid deposits are found in the tongue, heart, muscles, and gastrointestinal tract. In secondary amyloid, there is an underlying chronic illness such as tuberculosis, rheumatoid arthritis, or familial Mediterranean fever. Amyloid infiltration in the lymph nodes, liver, and spleen is seen.[30,31] A monoclonal immunoglobulin spike is detectable in the urine or serum of most patients with primary amyloid.[1]

The majority of patients diagnosed with this disorder are dead within 2 years. The cardiovascular clinical findings have been previously described.

## Carcinoid Heart Disease

The carcinoid syndrome is due to carcinoid tissue metastatic beyond the liver, which normally breaks down the products liberated by the tumor. These products cause the characteristic symptoms of cutaneous flushing, diarrhea, and bronchoconstriction.

Endocardial plaques of fibrous tissue involve the pulmonic and tricuspid valves. Mitral valve involvement can be seen in the setting of a patent foramen ovale or metastatic disease to the lungs.

A restrictive myopathy can be seen in the carcinoid syndrome. Murmurs of tricuspid regurgitation, pulmonic regurgitation, and pulmonic stenosis are described.

The echocardiogram is characterized by tricuspid or pulmonic valve thickening. The right atrium is enlarged without right ventricular hypertrophy.

## Endomyocardial Fibroelastosis

The histology of endomyocardial fibroelastosis includes (1) an acute inflammatory eosinophilic myocarditis, (2) inflammatory changes of intramyocardial vessels with thrombosis, (3) mural thrombosis, and (4) thickening of the endocardium.[3] Tropical and nontropical (Loeffler's) forms are described.

Eosinophils are seen in the peripheral smear. The myocardial eosinophilic infiltrate is characterized by an intense myocardial necrosis.

The physical examination is characterized by tachycardia and findings suggestive of a restrictive cardiomyopathy.[31]

## Sarcoid Heart Disease

Noncaseating granulomas and fibrosis are seen in 25 to 50 percent of patients with active sarcoid on autopsy.[31] Clinical cardiac involvement in these same patients is much less evident. In patients in whom sarcoid is the cause of death, myocardial involvement is frequently the cause. Clinical manifestations of sarcoid heart disease include arrhythmias, atrioventricular or conduction abnormalities, and restrictive physiology. With clinically evident sarcoid heart disease, the prognosis is poor and sudden death is not uncommon.[31]

Management includes a trial of steroids, automatic implantable cardiac defibrillators in high-risk patients, and consideration of heart-lung transplantation.

## REFERENCES

1. Mason JW: Classification of cardiomyopathies. In: Alexander RW, Schlant RC, Fuster V, et al (eds): *Hurst's The Heart,* 9th ed. New York, McGraw-Hill, 1998:2031–2038.
2. Richardson P, McKenna W, Bristow M, et al: Report of the 1995 World Health Organization/International Society and Federation of Cardiology Task Force on the definition and classification of cardiomyopathies. *Circulation* 1996; 93:841–842.
3. Wynne J, Braunwald E: The cardiomyopathies and myocardities. In: Braunwald E (ed): *Heart Disease,* 5th ed. Philadelphia, W. B. Saunders, 1996:1404–1463.
4. Bristow MR, Bohlmeyer TJ, Gilbert EM: Dilated cardiomyopathy. In: Alexander RW, Schlant RC, Fuster V, et al (eds): *Hurst's The Heart,* 9th ed. New York, McGraw-Hill, 1998:2039–2055.
5. Ho KKL, Anderson KM, Kannel WB, et al: Survival after the onset of congestive heart failure in Framingham Heart Study patients. *Circulation* 1993; 88:107–115.

6.  Cohn JN, Johnson GR, Shabetai R, et al for the V-Heft VA Co-operative Study Group: Ejection fraction peak exercise oxygen consumption. Cardiothoracic ration, ventricular arrhythmias, and plasma norepinephrine as determinants of prognosis in heart failure. *Circulation* 1993; 87(suppl VI):VI4–VI16.

7.  Eichhorn EJ, Bristow MR: Medical therapy can improve the biologic properties of the chronically failing heart: a new era in the treatment of heart failure. *Circulation* 1996; 94:2285–2296.

8.  Elefteriades JA, Kron IL: CABG in advanced left ventricular dysfunction. *Cardiol Clin* 1995; 13:35–42.

9.  Alderman EL, Fisher LD, Litwin P, et al: Results of coronary artery surgery in patients with poor left ventricular function (CASS). *Circulation* 1983; 68:785–795.

10. The SOLVD Investigators: Effect of enalapril on survival in patients with reduced left ventricular ejection fractions and congestive heart failure. *N Engl J Med* 1991; 325:293–302.

11. The SOLVD Investigators: Effect of enalapril on mortality and the development of heart failure in asymptomatic patients with reduced left ventricular ejection fractions. *N Engl J Med* 1992; 327:685–691.

12. Olsen SL, Gilbert EM, Renlund DG, et al: Carvedilol improves left ventricular function and symptoms in chronic heart failure: A double-blind randomized study. 1995; 25: 1225–1231.

13. CIBIS Investigators and Committees: A randomized trial of β-blockade in heart failure. The Cardiac Insufficiency Bisoprolol Study. *Circulation* 1994; 90:1765–1773.

14. CIBIS-II Investigators and Committees: The Cardiac Insufficiency Bisoprolol Study II (CIBIS-II): a randomised trial. *Lancet* 1999; 353:9–13.

15. Waagstein F, Bristow MR, Swedberg K, et al: Beneficial effects of metoprolol in idiopathic dilated cardiomyopathy. *Lancet* 1993; 342:1441–1446.

16. Colucci WS, Packer M, Bristow MR, et al: Carvedilol inhibits clinical progression in patients with mild symptoms of heart failure. *Circulation* 1996; 94:2800–2806.

17. Packer M: Effects of beta-adrenergic blockade on survival of patients with chronic heart failure. *Am J Cardiol* 1997; 80(suppl 11A):46L–54L.

18. Francis GS, Chatterjee K, Prystowsky E: Should asymptomatic ventricular arrhythmias in patients with congestive heart failure be treated with antiarrhythmic drugs? *J Am Coll Cardiol* 1988; 12:274–283.

19. Cheitlin MD, Conill A, Epstein AE, et al: ACC/AHA guidelines for implantation of cardiac pacemakers and antiarrhythmic devices. *J Am Coll Cardiol* 1998; 31:1175–1209.

20. Amidon TM, Parmley WW: Is there a role for positive inotropic agents in congestive heart failure: focus on mortality. *Clin Cardiol* 1994; 17:641–647.

21. Hill AB, Chiu RC-J: Dynamic cardiomyoplasty for treatment of heart failure. *Clin Cardiol* 1989; 12:681–688.

22. Salerno TA, Bhayana J: Volume reduction surgery in the treatment of end-stage heart disease. *Adv Cardiac Surg* 1997; 9:83–95.

23. Geisterfer-Lawrence AA, Kass S, Tanigawa G, et al: A molecular basis for familial hypertrophic cardiomyopathy: A beta-cardiac myosin heavy chain missense mutation. *Cell* 1990; 62:999–1006.

24. Maron B: Hypertrophic cardiomyopathy. In: Alexander RW, Schlant RC, Fuster V, et al (eds): *Hurst's The Heart,* 9th ed. New York, McGraw-Hill, 1998:2057–2074.

25. McKenna WJ, Oakley CM, Krikler DM, Goodwin JF: Improved survival with amiodarone in patients with hypertrophic cardiomyopathy and ventricular tachycardia. *Br Heart J* 1985; 53:412–416.

26. McKenna WJ, Adams J, Polonieaki JD, et al: Long-term survival with amiodarone in patients with hypertrophic cardiomyopathy and ventricular tachycardia (abstract). *Circulation* 1998; 80(suppl II):II-7.
27. Fananapazir L, Epstein ND, Curiel RV, et al: Long-term results of dual-chamber (DDD) pacing in obstructive hypertrophic cardiomyopathy. *Circulation* 1994; 90:2731–2742.
28. Nishimura RA, Trusty JM, Hayes DL, et al: Dual-chamber pacing for hypertrophic cardiomyopathy: a randomized, double blind, crossover trial. *J Am Coll Cardiol* 1997; 29:435–441.
29. TenBerg JM, Suttorp MJ, Knaepen PJ, et al: Hypertrophic obstructive cardiomyopathy: initial results and long-term follow-up after Morrow septal myectomy. *Circulation* 1994; 90:1781–1785.
30. Colgan TK, Hurst JW: Amyloid and the heart. In: Hurst JW (ed): *Update to The Heart V*. New York, McGraw-Hill, 1981:189–204.
31. Shabetai R: Restrictive, obliterative, and infiltrative myopathies. In: Alexander RW, Schlant RC, Fuster V, et al (eds): *Hurst's the Heart,* 9th ed. New York, McGraw-Hill, 1998:2075–2088.

**CHAPTER**

# MYOCARDITIS AND CARDIAC TOXICITIES

**29**

## MYOCARDITIS

### Definition

Myocarditis is an inflammatory process involving the heart. Inflammatory changes may involve the myocytes, the interstitium, or the vascular elements. The pericardium may or may not be concomitantly involved.

### Etiology and Pathology

Virtually any infectious agent (viral, rickettsial, bacterial, protozoal, or metazoal) can cause cardiac inflammation (Table 29-1). Noninfectious causes would include allergic reactions, pharmacologic agents, and systemic vasculitides.[1] The process may be either acute or chronic. Coxsackie B enterovirus has a special affinity for myocardial membrane receptors[2] and is the most common cause of myocarditis in North America, while Chagas' disease produced by *Trypanosoma cruzi* is the most common cause in South America.[1,2]

The histologic findings vary with the stage of the disease, the mechanism of damage, and the specific etiologic agent. Myocardial involvement may be focal or diffuse. Small lesions involving the conduction system are potentially fatal.

On gross examination in severe acute myocarditis, the heart is flabby, with focal hemorrhages. Hearts which are chronically involved may be hypertrophied and dilated. On microscopic examination, cellular types may include polymorphonuclear cells (bacterial), lymphocytes (viral), macrophages, plasma cells, eosinophils (hypersensitivity), or giant cells. Findings specific to the etiologic organism may also be found. Although cardiac involvement is common pathologically in acquired immunodeficiency syndrome (AIDS) (25 to 50 percent), clinical disease is much less common (about 10 percent),[3] and human immunodeficiency virus (HIV) has rarely been isolated from the myocardium.[4] A vasculitis with periarterial interstitial infiltrate secondary to *Borrelia burgdorferi* may manifest

**TABLE 29-1.   Important Causes of Myocarditis**

I. Infection
  A. Viral
     Coxsackie (A, B)
     ECHO
     Influenza (A, B)
     Polio
     Herpes simplex
     Varicella-zoster virus
     Epstein-Barr virus
     Cytomegalovirus
     Mumps
     Rubella
     Rubeola
     Vaccinia
     Coronavirus
     Rabies
     Hepatitis B
     Hepatitis C
     Arbovirus
     Junin virus
     Human immunodeficiency virus
  B. Bacterial, rickettsial, spirochetal
     *Corynebacterium diptheriae*
     *Salmonella typhi*
     Beta-hemolytic streptococci
     *Neisseria meningitidis*
     *Legionella pneumophila*
     *Listeria monocytogenes*
     *Campylobacter jejuni*
     *Coxiella burnetii* (Q fever)
     *Chlamydia trachomatis*
     *Myocoplasma pneumoniae*
     *Chlamydia psittaci* (psittacosis)
     *Rickettsia rickettsii* (Rocky Mountain spotted fever)
     *Borrelia burgdorferi* (Lyme disease)
     *Mycobacterium tuberculosis*
  C. Protozoal
     *Trypanosoma cruzi* (Chagas' disease)
     *Toxoplasma gondii*
  D. Metazoal
     Trichinosis
     Echinococcosis
  E. Fungal
     Aspergillosis
     Blastomycosis
     Candidiasis
     Coccidioidomycosis

**TABLE 29-1.   Important Causes of Myocarditis** *(continued)*

|   |
|---|
|       Cryptococcosis<br>      Histoplasmosis<br>      Mucormyocosis<br>  II. Toxic<br>      Anthracyclines<br>      Catecholamines<br>      Interleukin-2<br>      Alpha$_2$ interferon<br> III. Hypersensitivity |

*Source:* From O'Connell JB, Renlund DG: Myocarditis and specific cardiomyopathies. In: Alexander RW, Schlant RC, Fuster V (eds): *Hurst's The Heart,* 9th ed. New York, McGraw-Hill, 1998:2090, with permission.

itself clinically as atrioventricular block in about 10 percent of patients with Lyme disease.[5,6]

## Physiology

Myocardial damage may occur by direct invasion of the myocardium, production of a myocardial toxin (diphtheria), or immunologically mediated myocardial damage.[1] Vasospasm leading to focal ischemia and infarction has also been postulated.[7] Although the precise mechanism is unknown, cell-mediated immunologic reactions to cell surface antigens related to the infection are probably involved. Antibodies against intercellular components and increased intercellular adhesion molecules (ICAM-1) are commonly found.[1]

## Clinical Manifestations

Presentations are variable, ranging from asymptomatic to fulminant congestive heart failure secondary to diffuse myocarditis. Manifestations clinically relate to myocardial dysfunction (systolic or diastolic), arrhythmias, or heart block.[1,2] Clinical characteristics from the Myocarditis Treatment Trial are included in Table 29-2.[8,9]

**SUBJECTIVE.**   Most cases are self-limited and unrecognized. Nonspecific complaints including pleurodynia, myalgia, upper respiratory symptoms, and arthralgias may predate any cardiac symptoms. Chest pain may or may not sound anginal in nature. Palpitations due to supraventricular arrhythmias are not uncommon. Syncope (atrioventricular block or ventricular tachycardia) and sudden death are rare occurrences.

**OBJECTIVE.**   Bradycardia is less common than tachycardia. Fever usually antedates cardiac findings. With severe diffuse cardiac involvement, an S$_3$ gallop or apical systolic murmur can be heard. Diastolic murmurs are rare. Noncardiac

**TABLE 29-2.**   Clinical Characteristics of Patients in the Myocarditis Treatment Trial[8,9]

| | |
|---|---|
| Age | 42 ± 14 years |
| Sex | 62% male |
| Ejection fraction | 0.24 ± 0.10 |
| Chest pain | 35% |
| Increased MB fraction of creatine kinase | 12% |
| Flulike symptoms | 59% |
| Increased erythrocyte sedimentation rate | 61% |
| Elevated white blood cell count | 24% |
| Fever | 18% |

* Data are expressed as mean ± standard deviation.

From O'Connell JB, Renlund DG: Myocarditis and specific cardiomyopathies. In: Alexander RW, Schlant RC, Fuster V (eds): *Hurst's The Heart,* 9th ed. New York, McGraw-Hill, 1998:2089–2104, with permission.

findings including rales and evidence of right heart failure are seen only in severe cases.

Romaña's sign is seen in some cases of Chagas' disease and is characterized by lateral periorbital edema and swollen eyelids. Skin lesions (chagoma) may also be seen if the *T. cruzi* infection is inoculated via the bite of the reduviid bug.[10] The physical examination may be entirely normal, however.

**ELECTROCARDIOGRAM.**   Physical findings are less common than abnormal electrocardiographic changes. Arrhythmias (atrial and ventricular), conduction defects (atrioventricular block and bundle branch block), ST–T-wave changes, and occasionally Q waves are all reported (Tables 29-3 and 29-4).[11]

**CHEST ROENTGENOGRAM.**   On the chest x-ray film, the heart size may be normal or markedly enlarged. Pulmonary congestion may be seen with fulminant involvement.

**ECHOCARDIOGRAM.**   Left ventricular wall thickness may be normal or increased. Systolic and diastolic dysfunction may also be present. Focal or diffuse wall motion abnormalities may be seen. With severe left ventricular dysfunction, ventricular thrombi may occur.

**NUCLEAR SCANS.**   Gallium, indium-111 antimyosin antibody, and technetium pyrophosphate scans may each be abnormal. These scans tend to be sensitive but not specific.

**TABLE 29-3.   Electrocardiographic Abnormalities Associated with Bacterial Infections**

| ST- and T-Wave Changes | Conduction Disturbances* | New Q Waves or Changes Mimicking Myocardial Infarction |
|---|---|---|
| Diphtheria | Diphtheria | Bacterial endocarditis |
| Typhoid fever | Typhoid fever | Melioidosis |
| Scarlet fever | Scarlet fever | Tuberculosis |
| Meningococcemia | Acute rheumatic fever | |
| Staphylococcus | Tuberculosis | |
| Pneumococcus | | |
| Brucellosis | | |
| Tetanus | | |

* Including atrioventricular block and bundle branch block.

*Source:* From Silverman BD: Electrocardiographic abnormalities in myocarditis. *J Med Assoc Ga* 1988; 67:999–1003, with permission.

**ENDOMYOCARDIAL BIOPSIES.**   In early reports, the frequency of abnormal findings varied greatly, with tremendous interobserver variation. The Dallas criteria[12] were established to provide uniformity of interpretation of biopsy results. "An inflammatory infiltrate and damage of adjacent myocytes" was required for the def-

**TABLE 29-4.   Electrocardiographic Abnormalities Associated with Viral Infections**

| ST- and T-Wave Changes | Conduction Disturbances* | Arrhythmias |
|---|---|---|
| Poliomyelitis | Poliomyelitis | Poliomyelitis |
| Coxsackie | Influenza | Coxsackie |
| Mumps | Mumps | Infectious hepatitis |
| Rubeola | Rubeola | Rubeola |
| Herpes simplex | Varicella | Herpes zoster |
| Rubella | Rubella | |
| Rabies | Infectious mononucleosis | |
| Lymphocytic choriomeningitis | | |

* Including PR prolongation, atrioventricular block, and bundle branch block.

*Source:* From Silverman BD: Electrocardiographic abnormalities in myocarditis. *J Med Assoc Ga* 1998; 67:999–1003, with permission.

inite diagnosis of myocarditis. Other specimens were labeled as showing borderline or no evidence of myocarditis. Subsequent biopsies were interpreted as persistent, resolving, or resolved.

## Natural History

The variable presentations and natural history of myocarditis are summarized in Fig. 29-1.[13] Because of difficulty in the diagnosis of asymptomatic or minimally symptomatic patients, the prognosis on a percentage basis is not possible.

## Treatment

Once the diagnosis of myocarditis is suspected, the patient should be admitted to the hospital and monitored, since the conduction system could conceivably be involved. Activity restriction is recommended for 6 months after heart size and func-

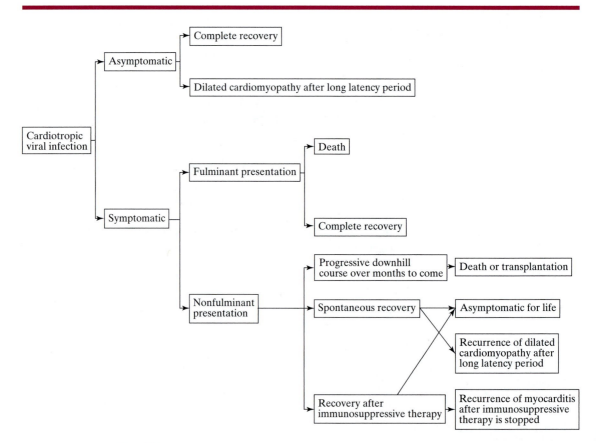

Figure 29-1    The natural history of human myocarditis. [From Herskowitz A, and Ansari AA: Myocarditis. In: Abelmann WH, and Braunwald E (eds): *Cardiomyopathies, Myocarditis, and Pericardial Disease. Atlas of Heart Disease* vol. 2. Philadelphia, Current Medicine, 1995.[13] Reproduced with permission.]

tion return to normal, since exercise may be deleterious.[14] Salt and water should be restricted until ventricular function normalizes. Cardiac toxins like cocaine and alcohol should be avoided.

Digitalis is indicated, but caution is necessary because of possible increased sensitivity. Angiotensin-converting enzyme inhibitors are indicated if left ventricular function is diminished. Diuretics are indicated for volume overload. Severe left ventricular dysfunction may require the addition of intravenous inotropes, vasodilators, an intraaortic balloon pump, and even a left ventricular assist device in advanced cases. Beta blockers should be used cautiously if at all, since there are few data on this subset of patients with congestive heart failure.

Specific antibiotic or antifungal therapy would be predicated on the specific infectious agent isolated.

Although nonsteroidal anti-inflammatory drugs (NSAIDs) may be beneficial late in the course, aspirin, NSAIDs, and cyclosporine are all contraindicated during the first few weeks because of increased myocardial damage.[2]

In the Myocarditis Treatment Trial, prednisone combined with either azathiaprine or cyclosporine did not significantly improve left ventricular function,[15] and so routine use of this combination cannot be recommended. Since no patient deteriorated on the immunosuppressives, however, these medications could be added to the regimen of those patients with severe myocarditis who are worsening on conventional therapy.[2]

# CARDIAC TOXICITIES

## Definition

Substances other than infectious agents may act on the heart to damage the myocardium. If the damage is acute, inflammatory infiltrates and myocyte necrosis may occur.[1]

## Abusable Substances and Toxins

**ALCOHOL.**   Acute and chronic myocardial damage due to alcohol is related to the dose and rate of exposure; the type of alcohol is irrelevant. The mecha-nism appears to be impaired or accelerated degradation of the contractile proteins.[16] Abnormal diastolic relaxation is an early manifestation of alcoholic heart disease, but this can progress first to left ventricular hypertrophy and subsequently to dilatation of the left ventricle, decreased systolic function, low cardiac output, and pulmonary congestion. Arrhythmias including atrial fibrillation, atrial flutter, premature atrial contractions, ventricular ectopy, and sudden death are all common. Prognosis is poor, especially if the patient continues to consume alcohol.

**COCAINE.**   Cocaine use can be associated with myocardial ischemia and infarction, toxic myopathy, acute myocarditis, and chronic dilated cardiomyopathy.[17]

Vasoconstriction can lead to platelet aggregation, endothelial dysfunction, and focal myocarditis.[18,19] Smoking of crystal methamphetamine is also associated with vasospasm and toxic myopathy.[20]

Empirical therapy for acute infarction or ischemia due to cocaine includes nitrates, α-adrenoreceptor blockers, calcium antagonists, and lytic therapy. All are advocated, but none have been proven effective.[17] Beta blockers may stimulate vasoconstriction (thus increasing myocardial damage) and suppress conduction.

### Psychotropic Agents

Arrhythmias (including sinus tachycardia), orthostatic hypotension, Q-T prolongation, and hypersensitivity myocarditis are all associated with tricyclic antidepressants.

### Phenothiazines

Q-T prolongation, torsades de pointes, and sudden death may occur secondary to phenothiazines. Deposition of acid mucopolysaccharides between muscle bundles may be seen on pathology specimens.[1]

### Lithium

T-wave inversion, U waves, Q-T prolongation, ventricular ectopy, and sinus node and atrioventricular node dysfunction can occur with lithium toxicity. Congestive heart failure and sudden death are rare. Lymphocytic infiltration and fibrosis can be seen on pathologic specimens.[1]

### Antiparasitic Agents

With emetine, which is used in the treatment of amebiasis and schistosomiasis, myocyte degeneration and mononuclear infiltrates may be seen. Chloroquine is associated with conduction disturbances and a restrictive myopathy. Whereas patients on antimony compounds may exhibit Q-T prolongation and T-wave inversion on the ECG, most exhibit no changes.

### Antineoplastic Agents

Cardiac toxicity from anthracycline antineoplastics may become manifest during or after completion of therapy. Electrocardiographic changes including ST–T-wave changes, decreasing QRS voltage, Q-T prolongation, and ectopy are all reported; however, early electrocardiographic changes are not indicative of incipient or long-term left ventricular dysfunction and are therefore not an indication to discontinue therapy.[21] A drop in ejection fraction of 10 percent or a drop in ejection fraction to less than 50 percent (normal is 54 to 65 percent) is an indication to discontinue anthracycline therapy. Left ventricular dysfunction is usually manifest within 1 year of completion of antineoplastic therapy;

however, late cardiac abnormalities in long-term survivors of pediatric malignancy treated with anthracyclines are unfortunately becoming more prevalent.[22] Mitoxantrone, high-dose cyclophosphamide, 5-fluorouracil, amsacrine, paclitaxel, interleukin-2, and α interferon have all been associated with cardiac toxicities.

## Venoms

Scorpion venom has been associated with electrocardiographic changes and myocardial damage. Wasp stings and spider bites are associated with myocardial toxicity either from direct effects or indirectly secondary to hypertension. Although snake venoms are neurotoxic rather than cardiotoxic, ECG changes have been rarely described.

## Medications

Although methysergide toxicity has been associated with fibrotic endocardial lesions leading to a restrictive myopathy, and catecholamine infusions can be associated with focal myocardial necrosis and arrhythmias, the most frequent cardiac abnormality associated with medications is a hypersensitivity vasculitis. The principal drugs associated with the disorder are listed in Table 29-5.[23]

**TABLE 29-5.   Principal Drugs Capable of Causing Hypersensitivity Myocarditis**

| | |
|---|---|
| **Antibiotics** | **Anti-inflammatory** |
| Amphotericin B | Indomethacin |
| Ampicillin | Oxyphenbutazone |
| Chloramphenicol | Phenylbutazone |
| Penicillin | |
| Tetracycline | **Diuretics** |
| Streptomycin | Acetazolamide |
| | Chlorthalidone |
| **Sulfonamides** | Hydrochlorothiazide |
| Sulfadiazine | Spironolactone |
| Sulfisoxazole | |
| | **Others** |
| **Anticonvulsants** | Amitriptyline |
| Phenindione | Methyldopa |
| Phenytoin | Sulfonylureas |
| Carbamazepine | Tetanus toxoid |
| | |
| **Antituberculous** | |
| Isoniazid | |
| Paraaminosalicylic acid | |

*Source:* From Kounis NG, Zavras GM, Soufras GD, Kitrou MP: Hypersensitivity myocarditis. *Ann Allergy* 1989; 62:71–74, Copyright 1989; with permission.

## Organophosphates

Commercially available pesticides containing organophosphates have been associated with Q-T prolongation, torsades de pointes, atrioventricular conduction disturbances, and ST–T-wave changes.

## Halogenated Hydrocarbons

Solvents, refrigerants, and fluid from fire extinguishers contain halogenated hydrocarbons, which depress myocardial contraction and can lead to arrhythmias.

## Radiation

A wide variety of cardiac abnormalities can result from radiation exposure, including pericardial disease (acute, chronic, or constriction), restrictive myopathy (radiation fibrosis), premature coronary artery disease, conduction system disease, and valvular heart disease (fibrous thickening leading to aortic or mitral valve regurgitation).

### REFERENCES

1. Wynne J, Braunwald E: The cardiomyopathies and myocarditides. In: Braunwald E (ed): *Heart Disease*, 5th ed. Philadelphia, W. B. Saunders, 1996:1435–1451.
2. O'Connell JB, Renlund DG: Myocarditis and specific cardiomyopathies. In: Alexander RW, Schlant RC, Fuster V, et al (eds): *Hurst's The Heart,* 9th ed. New York, McGraw-Hill, 1998:2089–2104.
3. Acierno LJ: Cardiac complications in acquired immunodeficiency syndrome: A review. *J Am Coll Cardiol* 1989; 13:1144–1154.
4. Grody WW, Cheng L, Lewis W: Infection of the heart by the human immunodeficiency virus. *Am J Cardiol* 1990; 66:203–206.
5. Asch ES, Bujak DL, Weiss M, et al: Lyme disease: An infectious and postinfection syndrome. *J Rheumatol* 1994; 21:454–461.
6. Cary NRB, Fox B, Wright DJM, et al: Fatal lyme carditis and endodermal heterotopia of the atrioventricular node. *Postgrad Med J* 1990; 66:134–136.
7. Ferguson DW, Farwell AP, Bradley WA, Rollings RC: Coronary artery vasospasm complicating acute myocarditis. *West J Med* 1988; 148:664–669.
8. Myocarditis Treatment Trial Investigators: Incidence and characteristics of myocarditis (Abstract). *Circulation* 1991; 84(suppl II):II-2.
9. Hahn EA, Hartz VL, Moon RE, et al: The myocarditis treatment trial: Design methods and patient enrollment. *Eur Heart J* 1995; 16(suppl 0):162–167.
10. Bestetti RB, Freites OC, Mucillo G, Oliveira JS: Clinical and morphologic characteristics associated with sudden cardiac death in patients with Chagas disease. *Eur Heart J* 1990; 14:1610–1614.
11. Silverman BD: Electrocardiographic abnormalities in myocarditis. *J Med Assoc Ga* 1988; 67:999–1003.
12. Aretz TA: The Dallas criteria. *Hum Pathol* 1987; 18:619–624.
13. Herskowitz A, Ansari AA: Myocarditis. In: Abelman WH, Braunwald E (eds): *Car-

*diomyopathies, Myocarditis and Pericardial Disease. Atlas of Heart Disease* vol. 2. Philadelphia, Current Medicine, 1995.

14. Friman G, Larrson E, Rolf C: Interaction between infection and exercise with special reference to myocarditis and the increased frequency of sudden deaths among young Swedish Orienteers. *Scand J Infect Dis* 1997; 104(suppl):41–49.

15. Mason JW, O'Connell JB, Herskowitz A, et al: Clinical trial of immunosuppressive therapy for myocarditis. *N Engl J Med* 1995; 333:269–275.

16. Regan TJ: Alcohol and nutrition. In: Alexander RW, Schlant RC, Fuster V, et al (eds): *Hurst's The Heart*, 9th ed. New York, McGraw-Hill, 1998:2109–2115.

17. Kloner RA, Hale S, Alker K, Rezkalla S: The effects of acute and chronic cocaine use on the heart. *Circulation* 1992; 85:407–419.

18. Smith AL, Schlant RC: Effect of noncardiac drugs, electricity, poisons, and radiation on the heart. In: Alexander RW, Schlant RC, Fuster V, et al (eds): *Hurst's The Heart*, 9th ed. New York, McGraw-Hill, 1998:2153–2166.

19. Willens HJ, Chakko SC, Kessler KM: Cardiovascular manifestations of cocaine abuse. *Chest* 1994; 106:594–599.

20. Hong R, Matsuyama E, Nur K: Cardiomyopathy associated with the smoking of crystal methamphetamine. *JAMA* 1991; 265:1152–1154.

21. Frishman WH, Sune HM, Yee HCM, et al: Cardiovascular toxicity with cancer chemotherapy. *Curr Probl Cardiol* 1996; 21:225–288.

22. Singal PK, Iliskovie N, Timso LI, Kumar D: Adriamycin cardiomyopathy: Pathophysiology and prevention. *FASEB J* 1997; 11:931–936.

23. Kounis NG, Zavras GM, Soufas GD, Kitrou MP: Hypersensitivity myocarditis. *Ann Allergy* 1989; 62:71–74.

JOYCE P. DOYLE / W. DALLAS HALL

CHAPTER

# 30

# HYPERTENSION: ASSESSMENT AND MANAGEMENT OF THE USUAL CASE

Hypertension, currently defined as a confirmed systolic blood pressure ≥140 or a diastolic blood pressure ≥90, is a major health problem in the United States. Trends indicate that hypertension has become the number one reason for a physician visit as well as the leading indication for prescription drugs in this country. National data from 1988 to 1991[1] estimate an overall prevalence of 24 percent for hypertension in adults, translating to approximately 43 million Americans. An additional 7 percent, or 13 million, of the normotensive adult population (not receiving a prescription medication for hypertension) report a prior history of hypertension; half of this group reported adherence to lifestyle changes for control of blood pressure.

Increasing age is a significant risk factor for the development of hypertension. By age 60, hypertension is present in approximately 60 percent of non-Hispanic whites, 71 percent of non-Hispanic blacks, and 61 percent of Mexican Americans.[1] Although the overall prevalence of hypertension is greater in males than in females, by age 60 the prevalence in women exceeds that in men for both African Americans and Mexican Americans, and by age 70 the prevalence in women exceeds that in men for whites. In African Americans, the age-adjusted prevalence of hypertension is 32.4 percent, among the highest in the world. In comparison, the prevalence of hypertension is 23.3 percent in non-Hispanic whites and 22.6 percent in Mexican Americans. African Americans have not only a higher prevalence of hypertension but also more severe hypertension with a higher complication rate.

Hypertension is a major risk factor for cardiovascular and cerebrovascular disease, leading causes of death in the United States. A direct relationship exists between hypertension and stroke, congestive heart failure (CHF), myocardial infarction (MI), and end-stage renal disease. Since the first randomized controlled hypertension treatment trial in 1967, multiple large clinical trials[2-4] have demonstrated that the pharmacologic treatment of hypertension significantly reduces cardiovascular complications. As treatment is both widely available and effective, hypertension is considered one of the most important modifiable cardiovascular risk factors.

413

Referred to as "the silent killer," hypertension is generally an asymptomatic disease, even when severe. Most patients are diagnosed by routine screening; however, in some cases, hypertension may be discovered only after significant target organ damage has occurred. Increasing the population's awareness of hypertension, encouraging routine screening, and providing continuity of care for hypertensives are of paramount importance. National data indicate that approximately 69 percent of hypertensive adults are aware of their diagnosis, but only 27 percent of *all* hypertensives are controlled (an improvement over the 11 percent control rate reported from 1976 to 1980). Of pharmacologically *treated* hypertensives, approximately 50 percent are controlled.[1]

The diagnosis of hypertension should not be made on the basis of a single elevated blood pressure reading. Elevated blood pressure readings—average systolic blood pressures ≥140 mmHg or diastolic blood pressures ≥90 mmHg—must be confirmed on at least two subsequent visits separated by one to several weeks. Exceptions include systolic levels ≥210 mmHg, diastolic levels ≥120 mmHg, or the presence of significant target organ damage at the time of the first reading. Many factors may transiently increase a patient's blood pressure, including pain, fear, physical activity, and exogenous substances. Incorrect labeling of patients as hypertensive can have serious consequences, such as increased health insurance premiums, work limitations imposed by employers, and increased health care costs. For these reasons, a standardized approach to blood pressure measurement must be followed, taking into consideration patient comfort and appropriate use of blood pressure measuring equipment (Table 30-1).

Hypertension, often defined in the past as an average blood pressure ≥160/95 mmHg, was recently redefined as an average systolic blood pressure ≥140 mmHg or diastolic blood pressure ≥90 mmHg. Population data indicate an increased cardiovascular risk even at systolic pressures <160 mmHg or diastolic pressures <100 mmHg. The results of the Treatment of Mild Hypertension Study, published in 1993, demonstrated decreased cardiovascular and other clinical end points with treatment of "mild" hypertension (defined as diastolic blood pressures ≤100 mmHg).[4]

Although previously used to classify the severity of hypertension, the terms *mild, moderate,* and *severe* are no longer recommended by hypertension experts because of concern that the term *mild hypertension* conveys a lack of seriousness to both health care providers and patients. A new system, proposed in the Sixth Report of the Joint National Committee,[5] classifies hypertension into stages, with higher stages indicating higher blood pressure values and risks. In this system, systolic and diastolic blood pressure elevations are given equal weight (Table 30-2). In the past, diastolic blood pressure elevations were considered clinically more significant than systolic elevations, and control of diastolic hypertension was the goal of treatment. Current evidence, however, indicates that systolic blood pressure is as least as important a determinant of cardiovascular risk as diastolic blood pressure.[6]

Isolated systolic hypertension is a common form of hypertension in the elderly, the segment of the population at highest risk for cardiovascular disease. The Systolic Hypertension in the Elderly Program (SHEP)[7] demonstrated a reduction in strokes

TABLE 30-1.   Blood Pressure Measurement Checklist

Patient seated/resting for at least 5 min

No caffeine or tobacco for ≥30 min

Choose correct cuff size (adults with midarm circumference ≥33 cm require a large cuff)

Support arm at level of the heart (on table or shoulder)

Palpate radial pulse and quickly inflate cuff to 20 mmHg above disappearance of pulse

Deflate slowly (~3 mmHg/s)

Record systolic pressure, mmHg (first sound)

Record diastolic pressure, mmHg (disappearance of sound)

Completely deflate cuff and repeat

Take average of 2 values

Initially record blood pressure in both arms; use the higher value

Assess the 2-min standing BP (particularly in the elderly, or diabetics) with arm support as above

and MIs in patients over 60 years old treated pharmacologically for isolated systolic hypertension. In this study, a low-dose diuretic (chlorthalidone) with the addition of a low-dose beta blocker (atenolol) as needed was effective and well tolerated. Data on Stage 1 isolated systolic hypertension are unavailable, as SHEP included only patients with Stage 2 isolated systolic hypertension or greater (systolic blood pressure

TABLE 30-2.   Classification of Blood Pressure for Adults Aged 18 Years and Older*

| Category | Systolic, mmHg | | Diastolic, mmHg |
|---|---|---|---|
| Normal | <130 | | <85 |
| High normal | 130–139 | | 85–89 |
| Hypertension** | | | |
| Stage 1 | 140–159 | or | 90–99 |
| Stage 2 | 160–179 | or | 100–109 |
| Stage 3 | ≥180 | or | ≥110 |

* Not taking antihypertensive drugs and not acutely ill.
** Based on the average of two or more readings taken at each of two or more visits after an initial screening.

≥160 mmHg and diastolic blood pressure <90 mmHg). The natural history of Stage 1 isolated hypertension, however, was illustrated by the Framingham Heart Study, in which 80 percent of untreated patients progressed to more severe blood pressure elevations over a 20-year follow-up period. As a group, these patients had an increased cardiovascular morbidity and mortality.

Once the diagnosis of hypertension is made, four main questions must be addressed: (1) Is this primary (essential) or secondary hypertension? (2) How many other cardiovascular risk factors are present? (3) Is there evidence of target organ damage? and (4) Are there comorbid illnesses that influence the choice of therapy?

Over 95 percent of patients have essential hypertension. If possible secondary causes of hypertension are suggested by the initial evaluation, additional testing for such causes may be indicated. Features suggestive of secondary hypertension include early or late age of onset of hypertension (<20 years or >50 years); an associated history of episodic tachycardia, sweating, and headache; a history or family history of renal disease; an abdominal bruit; an abnormal urinalysis; unprovoked hypokalemia; or resistant hypertension in an adherent patient prescribed multiple antihypertensive drugs.

The hypertensive patient's overall cardiovascular risk increases with the presence of additional cardiovascular risk factors: sedentary lifestyle, dyslipidemia, diabetes mellitus, tobacco use, obesity, and a family history of premature heart disease. Each of these risk factors should be investigated. Uncontrolled hypertension often leads to clinically significant damage of the cardiovascular, cerebrovascular, and renal systems. Evidence of target organ damage at these sites is obtained through the clinical history, physical examination, laboratory evaluation, and electrocardiographic assessment during the initial evaluation and as indicated on subsequent visits.

The presence of comorbid illnesses such as asthma or gout influences the type of treatment. A thorough past medical history during the initial visit may prevent adverse effects caused by an inappropriate drug choice.

Formulate an initial approach to treatment, and understand the individual patient's beliefs about hypertension. Provide a strategy that minimizes the negative impact of treatment on the patient's life, giving close attention to treatment-related adverse effects, convenience of medication dosing, convenience of appointments, and the cost of treatment in both time and money. For most patients with Stage 1 hypertension, 3 to 6 months of aggressive lifestyle modifications are recommended as first-line therapy.[5]

The five main lifestyle modifications that can lead to blood pressure reductions are weight loss, salt restriction, limiting alcohol to ≤1 oz of ethanol/day, regular aerobic exercise, and increased potassium intake (Table 30-3). Address other modifiable cardiovascular risk factors such as smoking, dyslipidemia, and diabetes. Remind the patient of the dangers associated with untreated hypertension and the benefits of treatment because hypertension is a chronic, asymptomatic disease.

In patients with Stage 2 or 3 hypertension, pharmacologic treatment is recommended. Selective use of pharmacologic agents based on patient characteristics and comorbidity helps maximize benefits and minimize adverse effects. There are currently six classes of antihypertensive drugs available, with different mechanisms of

**TABLE 30-3.    Lifestyle Modifications and Blood Pressure Control**

| Lifestyle Issues | When | Recommendation | Average Blood Pressure Effect |
|---|---|---|---|
| Salt restriction | All | Limit to <100 mmol/day or 2.3 g/day sodium (≤6 g/day sodium chloride) | −5 mmHg/−3 mmHg |
| Aerobic exercise | Check with doctor | At least 30 min/day moderate activity (e.g., brisk walking) | −7 mmHg/−7 mmHg |
| Weight loss | >10% overweight | Caloric restriction and exercise | −11 mmHg (diastolic) for 4.5-kg (10 lb) weight loss |
| Alcohol use | All | Limit daily intake to <8 oz wine, 24 oz beer, or 2 oz whiskey | |
| Increased dietary potassium | Check with doctor | Maintain adequate dietary intake of 50 to 90 mEq daily (preferably from food sources) | −3 mmHg/−2 mmHg (potassium supplementation trials of ≥60 mEq daily) |

action and class-specific and drug-specific advantages and disadvantages. Drugs considered appropriate include diuretics, beta blockers, angiotensin-converting enzyme inhibitors, calcium channel antagonists, alpha$_1$ blockers, alpha-beta blockers, and angiotensin II receptor blockers. Of these drugs, only diuretics and beta blockers have been adequately studied and documented in randomized controlled trials to decrease cardiovascular morbidity and mortality in the treatment of hypertension.

Unless patients are experiencing acute target organ damage, there is no reason to abruptly lower blood pressure to normal. Use a low starting dose of the chosen drug with upward titration as needed because some antihypertensives will achieve blood pressure control at low doses.

# PATIENT ASSESSMENT

## Clinical

Once the diagnosis of hypertension has been confirmed, the initial evaluation consists of a careful medical history, physical examination, and standard laboratory and electrocardiographic assessment. The goal of the initial evaluation is to determine if the patient has features suggestive of a secondary cause of hypertension, to assess the patient's overall cardiovascular risk, to identify any target organ damage, and to detect illnesses or factors that may influence the treatment approach.

A history of previous blood pressure measurements should be sought in an attempt to determine the onset of hypertension. In patients with a prior history of hypertension, reasons for discontinuing treatment may give useful information. For example, if the patient discontinued treatment because of adverse effects of medication or cost of treatment, these issues must be addressed.

Make note of drug allergies and current medications, including nonprescription medications. Question the patient specifically about the use of other medications that can increase blood pressure, such as cold preparations containing vasoconstrictors, diet pills or other stimulants, nonsteroidal anti-inflammatory drugs (NSAIDs), and oral contraceptives. Discuss diet and other personal habits that may be modifiable (e.g., level of physical activity; use of tobacco, alcohol, and illicit substances such as cocaine). In women, address the possibility of current or future pregnancy, as it may influence your treatment strategy. Ask about sexual dysfunction at baseline because antihypertensive therapy may be associated with impotence in men or changes of libido in women. Obtain a family history of hypertension, premature cardiovascular disease, renal disease, or endocrine disorders.

Measure the blood pressure, heart rate, height, and weight. Do a funduscopic examination looking for soft exudates, retinal hemorrhages, or papilledema, all indicative of a poor prognosis. Examine the neck for carotid bruits, jugular venous pulsations, and thyromegaly. Examine the heart for presence of a sustained or displaced apical impulse, ejection click, murmur, or $S_3$ or $S_4$. Note the presence of rales or wheezing on lung examination and bruits, masses, or abnormal pulsations on abdominal examination. Examine the extremities for the presence or absence of peripheral pulses and edema. Do a baseline neurologic examination, particularly in patients reporting weakness or symptoms suggestive of transient ischemic attacks.

## Laboratory

The pretreatment laboratory assessment recommended for newly diagnosed hypertensives includes fasting serum glucose, potassium, creatinine, cholesterol, high-density lipoprotein (HDL) cholesterol, and urinalysis. An elevated fasting serum glucose warrants further investigation for diabetes mellitus, if not already diagnosed. Unprovoked hypokalemia ($<3.5$ mEq/L) can indicate a high-renin, high-aldosterone state seen in renovascular hypertension, or a high-aldosterone state due to primary or secondary hyperaldosteronism. An elevated creatinine can be secondary to hypertensive nephrosclerosis or may suggest an underlying renal cause of hypertension such as renoparenchymal, renovascular, or polycystic kidney disease. On urinalysis, proteinuria may indicate nephrosclerosis, but this rarely reaches the nephrotic range. The presence of red blood cells, white blood cells, or casts warrants further evaluation, such as ultrasonography. Cholesterol measurement and an electrocardiogram (ECG) (primarily to assess for silent infarction or severe left ventricular hypertrophy) are part of the cardiovascular risk assessment. Although the ECG is insensitive for left ventricular hypertrophy when compared with echocardiography, ECG evidence of left ventricular hypertrophy is an ominous harbinger of cardiovascular sequelae.

Other laboratory tests that have been recommended during the initial evaluation include a serum calcium, uric acid, and complete blood count. Hypercalcemia is a rare cause of hypertension and may preclude the use of thiazide diuretics. Hyperuricemia is associated directly with hypertension and indirectly with renal blood flow; however, treatment of asymptomatic hyperuricemia is not indicated, nor is avoidance of diuretics, if needed. A complete blood count should be checked if otherwise indicated by the history or physical examination, but is typically normal with uncomplicated hypertension.

## MANAGEMENT

Once the diagnosis of hypertension has been made (systolic blood pressure ≥140 or diastolic blood pressure ≥90 mmHg on two or more consecutive occasions), begin treatment. Individualize the approach, taking into account patient characteristics, existing cardiovascular risk factors, and comorbidity. Minimizing adverse effects of treatment is of paramount importance because hypertension is a chronic disease, asymptomatic until target organ damage has occurred. Long-term compliance with prescribed antihypertensive therapy may be improved by involving patients in treatment decisions and educating patients on the asymptomatic nature of the disease, the dangers of untreated hypertension, and the benefits of treatment (Table 30-4).

### Lifestyle Modifications

Recommend lifestyle modifications for all hypertensive patients. Lifestyle modifications often are the initial treatment strategy for patients with Stage 1 hypertension. Recommendations include sodium restriction, weight reduction, aerobic exercise, limiting alcohol intake, and increasing dietary potassium.[5] Although the majority of patients will not become normotensive with lifestyle modifications alone, this approach will be effective in approximately 10 percent of patients and may offer overall health benefits. If after 3 to 6 months of lifestyle modification the blood pressure remains elevated, add antihypertensive drugs, with continued lifestyle modification as adjunctive therapy.

**SODIUM RESTRICTION.**   The average American adult consumes a large quantity of sodium, about 4 g daily. High intake of dietary sodium contributes to the risk of developing hypertension and may blunt the effect of antihypertensive therapy. Population data from the INTERSALT study[8] support sodium reduction as a means to prevent and control hypertension. Randomized controlled trials have shown that moderate sodium reduction can lower blood pressure in both hypertensive and normotensive persons. Some 40 to 50 percent of hypertensives are salt resistant, but the rest (particularly African Americans and the elderly) are sensitive to changes in dietary salt. Recommend reducing sodium intake to <100 mmol/day (<2.3 g/day of sodium or <6 g/day of sodium chloride). Avoid the salt shaker and processed foods, as a large proportion of dietary sodium is added during food manufacturing or at the table.

**TABLE 30-4.    Patient Education: Hypertension (High Blood Pressure)**

Defined as blood pressure >140/90 mmHg on ≥2 consecutive occasions (off medicines). The only way to know your blood pressure is to have it measured with a blood pressure cuff!!

**Hypertension**

Can lead to a stroke, heart attack, heart failure, or kidney failure
Generally has no symptoms even when the blood pressure is very high

**Treatment for hypertension**

Decreases strokes, heart disease, heart failure, and kidney failure
Requires active involvement of the patient

**All of the following can lower blood pressure** (discuss with your doctor first):

1.  *Aerobic exercise:* can improve overall health and decrease blood pressure. Recommended: at least 30 min of moderate physical activity (brisk walking) on most days.
2.  *Weight loss:* can improve overall health and decrease blood pressure. Recommended: if you are overweight by 10% or more, decrease calories and increase exercise.
3.  *Low-salt diet:* can reduce blood pressure and increase the action of blood pressure medicines. Recommended: avoid canned foods, fast foods, and adding salt to food. Read food labels; look for the terms *sodium* and *sodium chloride*. The goal is <100 mmol/day or <2.3 g/day for sodium (≤6 g/day for NaCl).
4.  *Limiting alcohol intake:* limit daily intake to less than 8 oz of wine, 24 oz of beer, or 2 oz of whiskey.
5.  *Dietary potassium:* maintain adequate dietary intake of 50 to 90 mEq daily (preferably from food sources), but check with your doctor first.
6.  *Blood pressure medicines:* must be taken as prescribed *everyday.**

* There are many different kinds of blood pressure medicines. The goal of hypertension treatment is to find the one that works best for you. If your hypertension medicine doesn't agree with you, tell your doctor.

**WEIGHT REDUCTION.**    For patients who are more than 10 percent above ideal body weight, weight reduction decreases blood pressure. Advise all hypertensive patients who are overweight to lose weight through a combination of caloric restriction and increased physical activity. Excessive weight, particularly centripetal obesity (truncal or abdominal distribution of excess fat), correlates with hypertension, dyslipidemia, insulin resistance, and increased cardiovascular mortality. Weight loss, therefore, is a vital part of overall cardiovascular risk reduction.

**EXERCISE.**    National surveillance programs indicate that about one in four adults have sedentary lifestyles with no leisure-time physical activities, and an additional one-third have a level of activity inadequate for physical fitness. Inactivity correlates with a 20 to 50 percent increased risk of developing hypertension, and regular exercise has been shown to reduce blood pressure in multiple clinical trials. Two meta-analyses of controlled trials (on physical activity and blood pressure) independently concluded that regular aerobic exercise resulted in a reduction of 6 to 7 mmHg systolic and 6 to 7 mmHg diastolic.[9,10] Most of these studies used moderate aerobic exercise for 30- to 60-min sessions three to four times per week. Current recommendations from the Surgeon General's Report on Physical Activity and Health (1996)[11] are a minimum of 30 min of physical activity of moderate intensity (such as brisk walking) on most, if not all, days of the week. Patients with known or suspected atherosclerotic heart disease usually require further evaluation prior to starting a vigorous exercise plan.

**LIMITING ALCOHOL INTAKE.**   Moderate to heavy alcohol use can both increase blood pressure and decrease a hypertensive patient's response to antihypertensive therapy. Withdrawal from alcohol may transiently increase blood pressure because of the associated hyperadrenergic state. Although alcohol in low doses has been associated with an increase in HDL cholesterol levels and may have a cardioprotective effect, heavy use should be discouraged. Limit alcohol consumption to <1 oz/day of ethanol, equivalent to 24 oz of beer, 8 oz of wine, or 2 oz of 100 proof whiskey.

**INCREASING DIETARY POTASSIUM.**   Since evidence suggests that a high dietary potassium may protect against hypertension, and since blood pressure may increase with hypokalemia, maintaining a normal serum potassium level and an adequate potassium intake (i.e., 50 to 90 mEq daily) are recommended.[12]

## Pharmacologic Treatment

In patients in whom lifestyle modification alone inadequately controls blood pressure, in patients with Stage 2 or 3 hypertension (systolic blood pressure ≥160 mmHg or diastolic blood pressure ≥100 mmHg), and in those with evidence of target organ damage, start pharmacologic therapy. Management of hypertensive patients with acute target organ damage or hypertensive emergencies is discussed in Chap. 31.

Considerations in the initial choice of drug therapy include comorbid illnesses, personal characteristics of the patient, and the adverse effect profile, cost, and convenience of dosing of the agent. To improve adherence to therapy, drugs requiring more than twice-daily dosing should be avoided if possible. Most drugs are currently available in once-daily preparations. Educating the patient on the asymptomatic nature of the disease, the benefits of treatment, and the importance of daily medication adherence is crucial. Encourage patients to actively participate in their care and to report any adverse treatment effects.

Six classes of antihypertensive drugs are currently available for individualization of treatment: (1) diuretics, (2) adrenergic inhibitors, (3) angiotensin-converting enzyme inhibitors, (4) calcium channel antagonists, (5) direct vasodilators, and (6) angiotensin II receptor antagonists. Of these drugs, only diuretics and beta blockers have been documented to decrease cardiovascular morbidity and mortality in large, randomized, controlled clinical trials.[2] Large treatment trials such as the Antihypertensive and Lipid Lowering Treatment to Prevent Heart Attack Trial (ALLHAT) are currently underway to assess morbidity and mortality reduction with use of the newer antihypertensive drugs. Pending the results of these trials, thiazide diuretics or beta blockers are often used for initial therapy unless contraindicated or unless there is a clear indication for use of another agent. Available antihypertensive drugs that are not usually considered appropriate for initial therapy include the centrally acting drugs clonidine and alpha-methyldopa and the smooth muscle relaxants hydralazine and minoxidil.

Once the initial drug is chosen, begin at the lowest starting dosage, because cost and adverse effects of antihypertensive drugs generally increase with increasing dose. The range of dosages recommended and the cost of available drugs are summarized in Table 30-5. About 40 to 50 percent of adherent patients' blood pressures will be adequately controlled with initial drug therapy. Precipitous lowering of blood pressure can result in acute adverse effects, such as dizziness, weakness, and fatigue, that can be unpleasant or dangerous, particularly in the elderly. These experiences can interfere with a patient's willingness to comply with future treatment.

Initiating low-dose monotherapy is the current standard. However, initiating therapy with single-tablet combinations of two low-dose drugs (e.g., a combination of low-dose angiotensin-converting enzyme inhibitor and diuretic, low-dose beta blocker and diuretic, etc.) is being done more frequently. Many such combination preparations are currently available, and many more will be available in the near future. The rationale for low-dose combination therapy includes minimizing dose-dependent adverse effects of individual drugs, providing additive effects of the two drugs, and potentially reducing the frequency of office visits. The major goals of initial therapy are control of blood pressure with convenient dosing and few adverse effects (including high cost), rather than the use of a single drug class per se.

### FACTORS INFLUENCING INITIAL DRUG CHOICE.

*Age.*    There are special considerations in the treatment of hypertension in the young and in the old, including increased attention to the possibility of a secondary cause. The 1996 Task Force on Blood Pressure Control in Children provides a comprehensive approach to the detection, evaluation, and treatment of hypertension in children.[13] Hypertension is defined as average systolic or diastolic blood pressure > the 95th percentile for the child's age, sex, and height, measured on at least three separate occasions. Standard blood pressure measurement techniques are similar to those in adults. After years of controversy over which Korotkoff phase to use to define diastolic blood pressure, the American Heart Association now recommends the fifth Korotkoff phase (disappearance of Korotkoff sounds) as the definition of diastolic pressure. Hypertensive values based on age, sex, and percentile height are presented in Table 30-6. For the treatment of hypertension in children, dietary intervention to control obesity can benefit blood pressure, but there is no clear evidence supporting salt restriction. Drug therapy for hypertension is similar to that for adults (with dosage adjustments as needed), although clinical trials are limited. Particularly in adolescents, abuse of alcohol, cocaine, other stimulants or appetite suppressants, chewing tobacco, or anabolic steroids should be considered.

Hypertension is prevalent in the elderly, as is comorbid disease. Secondary causes of hypertension, particularly renal artery stenosis, must be considered in elderly in-

**TABLE 30-5.   Oral/Transdermal Antihypertensive Agents: Dosage Range and Average Monthly Cost for Lowest Recommended Dosage**

| Drug | Usual Adult Dosage Range/Day | Cost for 30 Days* |
|---|---|---|
| **Diuretics** | | |
| Thiazide type | | |
| Hydrochlorothiazide (Esidrix) | 12.5–50 mg in 1 dose | 1.88 |
| Metolazone (Zaroxolyn) | 1.25–5mg in 1 dose | 6.69 |
| (Mykrox) | 0.5–1 mg in 1 dose | 22.09 |
| Trichlormethiazide (Naqua) | 2–4 mg in 1 dose | 9.24 |
| Chlorthalidone (Hygroton) | 12.5–50 mg in 1 dose | 10.37 |
| Bendroflumethiazide (Naturetin) | 2.5–5 mg in 1 dose | 12.23 |
| Indapamide (Lozol) | 1.25–2.5 mg in 1 dose | 20.55 |
| Loop | | |
| Furosemide (Lasix) | 40–80 mg in 2 doses | 9.53 |
| Bumetanide (Bumex) | 0.5–2 mg in 1 dose | 9.34 |
| Torsemide (Demadex) | 5–20 mg in 1 dose | 13.13 |
| Potassium-sparing | | |
| Triamterene (Dyrenium) | 50–150 mg in 1 or 2 doses | 10.65 |
| Amiloride (Midamor) | 5–10 mg in 1 or 2 doses | 13.82 |
| Spironolactone (Aldactone) | 25–100 mg in 1 or 2 doses | 12.06 |
| Potassium-sparing combinations | | |
| Hydrochlorothiazide/Triamterene | | |
| 25 mg/37.5 mg (Maxzide) | 1/2–1 tablet in 1 dose | 6.49 |
| 25 mg/37.5 mg (Dyazide) | 1/2–1 tablet in 1 dose | 6.61 |
| Hydrochlorothiazide/Spironolactone | 1 tablet in 1 dose | 13.00 |
| 25 mg/25 mg (Aldactazide) | | |
| Hydrochlorothiazide/Amiloride | 1/2 tablet in 1 dose | 8.12 |
| 50 mg/5 mg (Moduretic) | | |
| **Adrenergic inhibitors** | | |
| Beta blockers | | |
| Metoprolol (Toprol XL) | 50–200 mg in 1 dose | 14.03 |
| (Lopressor) | 50–200 mg in 2 doses | 32.80 |
| Propranolol (Inderal) | 80–240 mg in 2 doses | 24.86 |
| (Inderal LA) | 60–240 mg in 1 dose | 24.15 |
| Timolol (Blocadren) | 10–40 mg in 2 doses | 25.64 |
| Atenolol (Tenormin) | 25–100 mg in 1 or 2 doses | 27.58 |
| Bisoprolol (Zebeta) | 5–20 mg in 1 dose | 27.89 |
| Acebutolol (Sectral) | 200–800 mg in 1 or 2 doses | 29.45 |
| Nadolol (Corgard) | 40–240 mg in 1 dose | 31.69 |
| Alpha-adrenergic blockers | All: first day, 1 mg at bedtime | |
| Doxazosin (Cardura) | Maintenance: 1–16 mg in 1 dose | 27.53 |
| Prazosin (Minipress) | Maintenance: 2–20 mg in 2 doses | 24.85 |
| Terazosin (Hytrin) | Maintenance: 1–20 mg in 1 dose | 36.67 |
| Central alpha$_2$-antagonists | | |
| Methyldopa (Aldomet) | 250–2000 mg in 2 doses | 16.13 |

*(continues)*

**TABLE 30-5.** *(continued)*

| Drug | Usual Adult Dosage Range/Day | Cost for 30 Days* |
|---|---|---|
| Guanfacine (Tenex) | 1–3 mg in 1 dose | 26.13 |
| Clonidine (Catapres) | 0.2–1.0 mg in 2 doses | 34.04 |
| Transdermal (Catapres TTS) | 0.1–0.3 mg/day (1 patch/week) | 30.49 (4 weeks) |
| Peripheral adrenergic antagonists | | |
| Reserpine | 0.1–0.2 mg in 1 dose | 1.67 |
| Guanethidine (Ismelin) | 10–100 mg in 1 dose | 15.50 |
| Guanadrel (Hylorel) | 10–75 mg in 2 doses | 22.46 |
| Combined alpha and beta blockers | | |
| Labetalol (Normodyne) | 200–1200 mg in 2 doses | 26.66 |
| **ACE inhibitors** | | |
| Lisinopril (Prinivil) (Zestril) | 5–40 mg in 1 dose | 23.59 |
| | 5–40 mg in 1 dose | 23.59 |
| Ramipril (Altace) | 1.25–20 mg in 1 dose | 17.87 |
| Benazepril (Lotensin)** | 5–40 mg in 1 dose | 20.04 |
| Fosinopril (Monopril) | 10–40 mg in 1 dose | 21.90 |
| Quinapril (Accupril) | 5–80 mg in 1 or 2 doses | 24.54 |
| Captopril (Capoten) | 25–150 mg in 2 or 3 doses | 40.25 |
| Enalapril (Vasotec) | 2.5–40 mg in 2 doses | 44.87 |
| **Angiotensin receptor antagonist** | | |
| Losartan (Cozaar) | 25–100 mg in 1 or 2 doses | 33.00 |
| **Calcium channel antagonists** | | |
| Nondihydropyridine | | |
| Verapamil (Isoptin SR) | 120–480 mg in 1 dose | 26.72 |
| (Calan SR) | 120–480 mg in 1 dose | 27.78 |
| (Verelan) | 120–480 mg in 1 dose | 33.88 |
| Diltiazem (Dilacor XR) | 120–360 mg in 1 dose | 27.79 |
| (Cardizem CD) | 120–360 mg in 1 dose | 30.60 |
| Dihydropyridine | | |
| Felodipine (Plendil) | 2.5–20 mg in 1 dose | 25.61 |
| Nifedipine (Adalat CC) | 30–90 mg in 1 dose | 26.11 |
| (Procardia XL) | 30–90 mg in 1 dose | 38.25 |
| Isradipine (DynaCirc) | 5–10 mg in 2 doses | 33.62 |
| Amlodipine (Norvasc)** | 2.5–10 mg in 1 dose | 36.60 |
| **Direct vasodilators** | | |
| Minoxidil (Loniten) | 2.5–40 mg in 1 dose | 14.06 |
| Hydralazine (Apresoline) | 50–200 mg in 2 doses | 18.37 |
| **Beta blockers/diuretics** | | |
| Bisoprolol 2.5, 5, or 10 mg plus hydrochlorothiazide 6.25 mg (Ziac)** | In 1 dose | 27.89 |
| Propranolol 40 or 80 mg plus hydrochlorothiazide 25 mg (Inderide) | In 1 dose | 29.45 |
| Propranolol 80, 120, or 160 mg plus hydrochlorothiazide 50 mg (Inderide LA) | In 1 dose | 42.13 |

**TABLE 30-5.** *(continued)*

| Drug | Usual Adult Dosage Range/Day | Cost for 30 Days* |
|---|---|---|
| Atenolol 50 or 100 mg plus chlorothalidone 25 mg (Tenoretic) | In 1 dose | 30.89 |
| Metoprolol 50 or 100 mg plus hydrochlorothiazide 25 or 50 mg (Lopressor HCT) | In 2 doses | 37.63 |
| Timolol 10 mg plus hydrochlorothiazide 25 mg (Timolide) | In 2 doses | 38.70 |
| Nadolol 40 or 80 mg plus bendroflumethiazide 5 mg (Corzide) | In 1 dose | 39.53 |
| **ACE inhibitors/diuretics** | | |
| Benazepril 5, 10, or 20 mg plus hydrochlorothiazide 6.25, 12.5, or 25 mg (Lotensin HCT) | In 1 dose | 20.04 |
| Captopril 25 or 50 mg plus hydrochlorothiazide 15 or 25 mg (Capozide) | In 2 or 3 doses | 44.25 |

* Cost to the pharmacist for 30 days' treatment with the lowest recommended dosage, based on wholesale price (AWP) listings in *Drug Topics Red Book* 1996 (may require breaking scored tablets in half).
** Same price per tablet for increasing dosage.

**TABLE 30-6.** Hypertension in Children and Adolescents Based on Age, Sex, and Percentile Height*

| Age (years) | Percentile Height | Blood Pressure (mmHg) | |
|---|---|---|---|
| | | Boys | Girls |
| 6 | 50th | 114/74 | 111/73 |
| | 75th | 115/75 | 112/73 |
| | 90th | 117/76 | 114/74 |
| 10 | 50th | 119/80 | 119/78 |
| | 75th | 121/80 | 120/79 |
| | 90th | 122/81 | 121/80 |
| 13 | 50th | 126/82 | 125/82 |
| | 75th | 128/83 | 126/82 |
| | 90th | 129/83 | 127/83 |
| 17 | 50th | 136/87 | 129/84 |
| | 75th | 138/88 | 130/85 |
| | 90th | 140/89 | 131/86 |

* Defined as blood pressure in the 95th percentile.

dividuals with new-onset or difficult-to-control hypertension. Renal artery stenosis is more common in those with evidence of coronary heart disease, peripheral vascular disease, carotid disease, or concomitant diabetes. Elderly hypertensives typically have increased peripheral vascular resistance, reduced plasma renin activity, and more left ventricular hypertrophy than younger patients. All classes of drugs exhibit similar blood pressure lowering effects. However, drugs that tend to induce postural hypotension should be avoided or used cautiously if otherwise indicated (e.g., an alpha$_1$ blocking agent in men with concomitant prostatic hypertrophy). Start therapy with the lowest available dose, and titrate upward at longer intervals.

*Gender.*    At this time, recommended treatment strategies for hypertension are similar for both men and women.[5] Although data supporting treatment of hypertension are convincing in men, fewer data exist in women.[13] Of the seven large studies that have shown a reduction in cardiovascular morbidity and mortality with treatment of hypertension, three included no women.

In women of child-bearing years, discuss plans for pregnancy or contraception. Choose antihypertensive drugs only after weighing their risks and benefits. Current evidence argues against drug treatment of chronic hypertension in pregnancy for diastolic pressures below 100 mmHg because treatment has not been proven to improve maternal or fetal outcomes.[14] Angiotensin-converting enzyme inhibitor use is contraindicated during pregnancy and is associated with fetal hypocalvaria, renal abnormalities, and fetal and neonatal death. Women who conceive while on these agents should be advised to discontinue them immediately. If antihypertensive drugs are to be started during pregnancy, alpha-methyldopa should be considered first-line because of documented fetal safety. Labetalol and atenolol, considered reasonable alternatives, have been associated with intrauterine growth retardation when used in early pregnancy; they require careful fetal monitoring. Because of the theoretical dangers of plasma volume loss, diuretics should not be initiated during pregnancy unless blood pressure cannot be controlled with other drugs. Women with hypertension who become pregnant should be instructed to notify their physicians immediately.

*Race.*    In comparison with Caucasian patients, African American hypertensives are more likely to have a high plasma volume and a low renin profile. Their hypertension is generally more responsive to monotherapy with diuretics or calcium channel antagonists than with beta blockers, angiotensin-converting enzyme inhibitors, or angiotensin II receptor blockers. The addition of a low dosage of a diuretic, however, equalizes the blood pressure lowering efficacy of beta blockers, angiotensin-converting enzyme inhibitors, and angiotensin II receptor blockers in African Americans.

*Comorbid Illness.*    Although hypertension can occur in isolation, many patients have comorbid illnesses. These illnesses may be present at the time of initial diagnosis of hypertension or may develop with time. Comorbid illnesses typically pose significant limitations on the choice of antihypertensive drugs. Comorbid illnesses encountered commonly in clinical practice are presented in Table 30-7, with comments on the advantages and disadvantages of using particular drugs.

**TABLE 30-7. Commonly Encountered Comorbidity and the Treatment of Hypertension**

| Comorbidity | Drugs Offering Possible Advantages | Drugs Used with Caution* |
|---|---|---|
| **Cardiac disease** | | |
| Systolic dysfunction | ACE-I, diuretics, hydralazine | Beta blockers, ND-CCA |
| Diastolic dysfunction | Beta blockers, ND-CCA, ACE-I | |
| Angina | Beta blockers, ND-CCA | Peripheral vasodilators |
| SVT | Beta blockers, ND-CCA | Peripheral vasodilators |
| **Pulmonary disease** | | |
| Asthma | CCA | Beta blockers |
| COPD | CCA; cardioselective beta blockers are generally tolerated | Noncardioselective beta blockers |
| **Kidney disease** | | |
| Diabetic nephropathy | ACE-I | None |
| Chronic renal failure | Loop diuretics | Thiazide ineffective |
| Renal artery stenosis | ACE-I in unilateral disease | ACE-I in bilateral disease |
| Diabetes mellitus | Diuretics in elderly; ACE-I | Beta blockers in diabetics prone to hypoglycemic events (e.g., on insulin) |
| Prostatic hypertrophy | Alpha$_1$ blockers | Diuretics, particularly loop |
| Depression | None | Relationship between lipid-soluble beta blockers (i.e., propranolol) and depression suggested, but no good data |
| Migraine headache | Beta blockers, CCA | Peripheral vasodilators |
| Osteoarthritis | None | NSAIDs may blunt treatment effect and lead to fluid retention |
| Constipation | None | CCA (particularly verapamil) |
| Liver disease | Spironolactone in cirrhotic edema | |
| Impotence | ACE-I, CCA, ARB may have lower incidence | Any agent may worsen impotence, beta blockers and diuretics may be worse |

* The drugs are to be used with caution, if used at all. ACE-I = angiotensin-converting enzyme inhibitor; ND-CCA = nondihydropyridine calcium channel antagonist (e.g., verapamil, diltiazem); SVT = supraventricular tachycardia; CCA = calcium channel antagonist; COPD = chronic obstructive pulmonary disease; ARB = angiotensin-II receptor blocker.

**ANTIHYPERTENSIVE DRUGS.** Like other drugs, all antihypertensives can cause adverse effects, some more frequently than others. Strategies for assessment and management of commonly encountered adverse effects are presented in Table 30-8.

*Diuretics.* Diuretics inhibit renal sodium absorption and reduce plasma and extracellular volume. There is a secondary decrease in peripheral vascular resistance associated with blunted responsiveness of the vascular wall to endogenous vasoconstrictors by unclear mechanisms. Diuretics, like beta blockers, have been shown to decrease cardiovascular mortality in hypertensive patients. They are widely used for monotherapy and will enhance the effectiveness of all other drug classes, although there is some disagreement as to whether the combination of diuretics and calcium channel antagonists is additive. Large doses (the equivalent of 100 mg of hydrochlorothiazide) were used previously in many of the large treatment trials, but most patients can be treated successfully with doses equivalent to 12.5 to 25 mg of hydrochlorothiazide daily while minimizing adverse effects. In support of low-dose diuretics, one study reported an association between diuretics and sudden death that was not present with lower doses or with potassium-sparing diuretics.[16]

1. *Thiazides and related sulfonamide compounds.* Thiazides are more effective antihypertensive drugs than loop diuretics or potassium-sparing diuretics, but they are not effective in patients with significant renal impairment (glomerular filtration rate <25 mL/min, a serum creatinine approximately 2 to 2.5 mg/dL in most patients, or a serum creatinine 1.5 to 2 mg/dL in the elderly). Although most of the antihypertensive effect of thiazides is seen within 2 weeks, additional lowering of blood pressure can continue for several weeks. Unlike those taking loop diuretics, patients taking thiazide-like diuretics generally do not experience any noticeable increase in urine output and do not usually need to modify their daily activities. Because the adverse metabolic effects (hypokalemia, hyperglycemia, metabolic alkalosis, hypercalcemia, and hyperuricemia) appear to be dose-dependent, use a low starting dose (i.e., the equivalent of 12.5 to 25 mg of hydrochlorothiazide per day). Doses as low as 6.25 mg have been used successfully to potentiate the blood pressure lowering effect of some of the beta blockers (e.g., bisoprolol) and angiotensin-converting enzyme inhibitors (e.g., benazepril).

2. *Loop diuretics.* When compared with thiazides, in patients with normal renal function, loop diuretics are somewhat less effective antihypertensives. In hypertensive patients with significant renal impairment (glomerular filtration rate <25 mL/min), however, they are the diuretics of choice. Furosemide, the most widely used agent, requires twice-daily dosing because of its short half-life. The usual starting dose is 20 to 40 mg twice daily. Diuresis can be expected to begin about 30 to 90 min after the oral dose. In patients with renal insufficiency, the dose should be increased until a response occurs. Concomitant use of NSAIDs competitively interferes with the delivery of a loop diuretic to its site of action. The adverse metabolic effects are similar to those seen with thiazides; however, unlike thiazides, loop diuretics promote rather than inhibit calcium excretion.

**3.** *Potassium-sparing agents.* The potassium-sparing drugs are weak antihypertensives, so they are often used as once-daily combinations with a thiazide-like diuretic. Spironolactone, an aldosterone antagonist, is useful in cirrhotic patients, in whom hemodynamic alterations lead to high aldosterone levels and fluid accumulation. High doses, however, are often accompanied by gynecomastia or impotence in men and by menometrorrhagia in women. Amiloride and triamterene directly inhibit potassium secretion in the distal tubule of the kidney. Uncommonly, patients may develop hyperkalemia while on these drugs, especially if used in conjunction with supplemental oral potassium, NSAIDs, or an angiotensin-converting enzyme inhibitor.

*Recommended Laboratory Follow-Up.*   Most data on the adverse metabolic effects of thiazide diuretics are based on large clinical trials that used doses higher than those currently recommended. At lower doses these effects are less common, but can still occur.

1. *Potassium:* Repeat the potassium level within 2 weeks or less in patients in whom hypokalemia is more likely or poses a particular danger (e.g., with digoxin use, a history of arrhythmia, etc.). In patients who are at relatively low risk for developing arrhythmia or hypokalemia (e.g., usual hypertensives or those prescribed a potassium-sparing diuretic), the serum potassium level can be rechecked after 3 months or at the next follow-up blood pressure visit.
2. *Glucose:* Repeat the glucose with the potassium check in patients with glucose intolerance or diabetes, and in those who have risk factors for diabetes (i.e., positive family history or obesity).
3. *Lipids:* Obtain follow-up lipid measurements after approximately 3 months of therapy. Compare the results with the values obtained prior to the institution of the diuretic.
4. *Uric acid:* Although both thiazides and loop diuretics may raise serum uric acid levels, we do not recommend routine follow-up of the uric acid level in the absence of clinical gout.

### Antiadrenergics.

**1.** *Beta-adrenergic antagonists.* The proposed antihypertensive action of beta blockers includes a reduction of heart rate and cardiac output, a decrease in plasma renin activity, and modulation of peripheral efferent sympathetic nervous activity. In most large randomized clinical trials on the treatment of hypertension, beta blockers decreased cardiovascular mortality. Beta-blocker use after MI has demonstrated a significant reduction in cardiovascular mortality in multiple clinical trials, and beta blockers are the preferred first-line drugs in patients with atherosclerotic heart disease if no contraindications exist. They must be used with caution in most patients with depressed systolic function, as they can precipitate CHF. They also should be avoided in patients with conduction distur-

**TABLE 30-8.  Approach to Commonly Encountered Adverse Effects**

| Symptom/ Laboratory Abnormality | Possible Inciting Drugs | Further Assessment | Management Strategies |
|---|---|---|---|
| Cough | ACE-I | Verify temporal association; consider confirming by the usual disappearance of cough <4 days off ACE-I; consider other etiologies (i.e., URI, postnasal drip, CHF); weigh benefits of ACE-I vs. severity of symptoms. | Switch agents if no clear advantage of ACE-I or severe symptoms; continue for mild/moderate symptoms and clear advantage of ACE-I; consider 50% dose reduction; consider angiotensin-II receptor antagonist |
| Angioedema | ACE-I | Evaluate need for emergency services (e.g., airway compromise); consider other possible inciting agents (e.g., foods, other drugs) or settings (e.g., C-1 esterase deficiency, multiple myeloma, dialysis) | Discontinue ACE-I; acutely treat with antihistamine (i.e., diphenhydramine 25 mg PO q6h) or, if needed, subcutaneous epinephrine or oral/intravenous corticosteroids |
| Hyperkalemia | ACE-I; potassium-sparing diuretics | Evaluate renal function with serum creatinine; ask about use of supplemental potassium and potassium-containing salt substitutes | Discontinue exogenous potassium; for $K^+$ >6.0 mEq/L, stop ACE-I; add or increase dose of thiazide or loop diuretic |
| Hypokalemia | Diuretics | Consider other etiologies (diarrhea, vomiting, chewing tobacco, occult alcohol abuse, low $Mg^{2+}$); if severe, consider secondary causes of HTN (renal artery stenosis, hyperaldosteronism); assess for increased risk of arrhythmia (e.g., digoxin use) | Supplement potassium orally; consider the addition of a potassium-sparing diuretic; encourage sodium restriction |

| Condition | Drug class | Evaluation | Management |
|---|---|---|---|
| Hyperglycemia | Diuretics | Reevaluate adherence to diet and drug therapy; recheck serum $K^+$ | Reinforce compliance with diabetic diet/medications; consider reducing diuretic dose; keep serum >3.5 mEq/L $K^+$ (hypokalemia suppresses insulin release) |
| Gout | Diuretics | Joint aspiration to document urate crystals in newly diagnosed gout; assess factors that may provoke gout (e.g., alcohol use, caloric binges, renal failure); assess need for diuretic vs. frequency of attacks | Discontinue diuretic if possible; acute treatment with colchicine and NSAIDs (for normal renal function) or intraarticular corticosteroid injection for single joint; use systemic corticosteroids for severe symptoms and renal insufficiency |
| Impotence | All are possible; relatively rare with ACE-I, ARB, CCA, hydralazine, or minoxidil | All antihypertensive agents have been associated with impotence; verify temporal association between impotence and antihypertensive agents; consider other etiologies (diabetes, aortoiliac disease, alcohol) | Consider switching antihypertensive therapy to classes that are less frequently associated with impotence |
| Peripheral edema | CCA (dihydropyridine class); direct vasodilators (minoxidil, hydralazine) | Evaluate for evidence of CHF, renal or liver disease; if unilateral, consider venous disease | Sodium restriction and avoidance of NSAIDs; add loop diuretic for significant edema; consider adding ACE-I |

* ACE-I = angiotensin-converting enzyme inhibitor; URI = upper respiratory infection; CHF = congestive heart failure; HTN = hypertension; NSAID = nonsteroidal anti-inflammatory drug; CCA = calcium channel antagonist; ARB = angiotensin-II receptor blocker.

bances or heart rates less than 50 beats per minute. As monotherapy, their efficacy may be blunted in African American patients.

From a clinical perspective, beta blockers differ mainly in the degree of cardioselectivity. Nonselective beta blockade could lead to bronchospasm (via blockade of beta$_2$ receptors) in patients with reactive airway disease, unrecognized hypoglycemia in treated diabetics, or pressor responses in hypertension associated with elevated catecholamines and exaggerated alpha stimulation (e.g., pheochromocytoma, cocaine abuse). Cardioselective or beta$_1$-selective beta blockers have a lower risk of these responses. Many beta blockers (without intrinsic sympathomimetic activity) have been shown to decrease reinfarction and related mortality when used after MI. Exertional fatigue, depression, insomnia, and nightmares are other potential adverse effects of beta blockers. Both hypertension and depression are common clinical entities, and the causal relationship between beta-blocker use and depression has been refuted. However, in hypertensive patients who develop depression after beta blockers are instituted, tapering the beta blocker and switching to another class of drugs is reasonable. If a depressed patient has a clear indication for beta-blocker use (i.e., recent MI), a more water-soluble drug (e.g., atenolol) with decreased entry into the central nervous system may be preferred.

*Recommended Laboratory Follow-Up.*    *Lipids:* Beta blockers without intrinsic sympathomimetic activity can increase triglycerides and decrease HDL levels. Obtain follow-up lipid measurements after 3 to 6 months of therapy. Compare the results with values obtained prior to beta-blocker use.

**2.**    *Alpha$_1$-adrenergic antagonists.* Alpha$_1$ receptor antagonists (i.e., doxazosin, prazosin, terazosin) produce arterial and venous dilatation through blockade of postsynaptic alpha$_1$ receptors. Postural hypotension and dizziness can occur with any of these drugs, particularly after the first dose, and are more frequent in the elderly or in patients (such as many diabetics) with autonomic dysfunction. These effects are minimized by beginning with the lowest starting dosage, then proceeding with slow upward titration. Alpha$_1$ blockers have a modestly favorable effect on lipids, increasing the HDL/total cholesterol ratio.[17] In men with obstructive voiding symptoms due to benign prostatic hypertrophy, alpha$_1$ blockers often provide significant relief by relaxing smooth muscle at the bladder neck and prostate. These same effects, however, can worsen symptoms of stress incontinence in women.

*Recommended Laboratory Follow-Up.*    No laboratory follow-up is necessary.

**3.**    *Peripherally acting adrenergic antagonists.* This class of drugs (e.g., reserpine, guanethidine, guanadrel) is seldom used because of their adverse effects. Reserpine, effective and inexpensive, was previously associated with severe depression and stuffy nose at doses much higher than those now recommended. Guanethidine and guanadrel reduce cardiac output and are associated with postural and exertional hypotension, worsened by exercise, alcohol, or a hot climate.

*Recommended Laboratory Follow-Up.*   No laboratory follow-up is necessary.

**4.**   *Centrally acting adrenergic antagonists.* These drugs (e.g., clonidine, methyl-dopa) are effective, but are not considered appropriate first-line agents as a result of their adverse effect profile. Adverse effects include sedation, dry mouth, and depression. The central nervous system effects may be particularly problematic in the elderly. Bradycardia can be induced or potentiated, especially in patients already taking drugs that tend to slow heart rate. Rebound hypertension can occur with abrupt discontinuation of higher doses of clonidine, which should generally be avoided in noncompliant patients. The problem with rebound hypertension and compliance is averted by use of the once-weekly clonidine patch.

***Calcium Channel Antagonists.***   Calcium channel antagonists decrease blood pressure through vasodilatation and a decreased peripheral resistance. An initial reflex tachycardia can occur with the dihydropyridine types (e.g., nifedipine, amlodipine, felodipine). Diltiazem and verapamil slow heart rate and can cause significant bradycardia, particularly in the setting of underlying conduction disturbances or use with other heart rate–slowing drugs such as beta blockers. Verapamil and diltiazem are useful in the treatment of diastolic dysfunction, but because of their negative inotropic effects can provoke CHF in patients with systolic dysfunction.

As a class, calcium channel antagonists do not adversely affect serum lipids, glucose, or electrolytes. However, a number of investigators have recently questioned their overall safety, particularly with regard to use in coronary artery disease (CAD). In one case-control study, hypertensive patients that had been prescribed short-acting nifedipine, verapamil, or diltiazem were 1.6 times more likely to have a MI than those taking other agents.[18] A randomized controlled trial of 883 hypertensive patients comparing treatment with immediate-release isradipine with hydrochlorothiazide showed a trend toward a higher incidence of serious vascular events (MI, angina, sudden death, CHF, or stroke) in the isradipine group (5.65 percent versus 3.17 percent, $p = .07$).[19] However, these concerns relate primarily to the short-acting types of calcium antagonists, now used very infrequently in clinical practice. There are no current data on which to convey concern about the long-acting, once-daily forms of calcium channel antagonists. In a recent case-control study, when compared with beta-blocker monotherapy, patients on long-acting calcium channel antagonists had no increased risk of cardiovascular events.[20]

*Recommended Laboratory Follow-Up.*   No specific laboratory follow-up is necessary.

***Direct Vasodilators.***   The direct vasodilators, hydralazine and minoxidil, are potent antihypertensives but are not considered first-line agents because of adverse effects. They typically cause reflex tachycardia and fluid retention and usually require concomitant use of a rate-slowing drug and a loop diuretic. In patients with congestive heart failure due to systolic dysfunction, hydralazine used in combination with nitrates has been shown to decrease mortality. This combination may be used in heart failure patients who cannot tolerate angiotensin-converting enzyme inhibitors. Hydralazine can cause drug-induced systemic lupus with arthralgias, pleuritis, rash, and a positive antinuclear antibody (ANA), typically antihistone. Minoxidil causes hirsutism and, rarely, pericardial effusion.

*Recommended Laboratory Follow-Up.*    No specific laboratory follow-up is indicated for these drugs other than that indicated for the concomitant use of a diuretic.

***Angiotensin-Converting Enzyme Inhibitors.***    These drugs inhibit the production of angiotensin II, a potent vasoconstrictor, by blocking conversion of angiotensin I to angiotensin II. This blockade also indirectly decreases aldosterone production and can rarely cause hyperkalemia. Angiotensin-converting enzyme inhibitors are effective and generally well tolerated. They have no apparent adverse effect on lipids and may even improve glycemic control. They have been shown to reduce mortality in patients with CHF due to systolic dysfunction. In Type I diabetic patients with proteinuria and early-stage renal failure, angiotensin-converting enzyme inhibitors slow the progression of renal disease. They decrease glomerular perfusion pressure (through dilatation of efferent arterioles) and decrease proteinuria in both hypertensive and normotensive diabetics. The blood pressure lowering effect of monotherapy is blunted in African Americans but is potentiated with the addition of a diuretic.

Cough is the most common adverse effect (10 to 15 percent). Another uncommon adverse effect is hyperkalemia, due mainly to inhibition of aldosterone. This occurs most often in patients who are receiving supplemental potassium, have renal insufficiency, or have type IV renal tubular acidosis (more common in diabetics). Patients with bilateral renal artery stenosis or unilateral stenosis in a solitary kidney can develop acute renal failure due to an abrupt decrease in renal perfusion. Angioedema, an infrequent (1 in 500 to 1000) but life-threatening adverse effect, may relate to an accumulation of inflammatory mediators (e.g., bradykinins, substance P) whose breakdown is inhibited by the angiotensin-converting enzyme inhibitor. These drugs should not be used in pregnancy and should be used with caution in women of childbearing years, as they are associated with fetal injury and death.

*Recommended Laboratory Follow-Up.*

1. *Potassium:* In patients with normal renal function, repeat the potassium level at the next routine visit. In patients with renal insufficiency or a baseline potassium between 5 and 5.5 mEq/L, recheck the potassium level within 1 week of instituting or increasing the angiotensin-converting enzyme inhibitor dose.
2. *Creatinine:* In patients with known or suspected renal artery stenosis, recheck the creatinine level within 1 week (or less) of instituting the angiotensin-converting enzyme inhibitor or increasing the dose.

***Angiotensin-II Receptor Antagonists.*** The recently available angiotensin-II receptor antagonists interfere with binding of angiotensin II to angiotensin type I receptors. They are often useful in patients with angiotensin-converting enzyme inhibitor–induced cough. A recent 1-year trial of losartan (50 mg/day) versus captopril (50 mg three times/day) reported a significant decrease in mortality (9 versus 13 percent, respectively) in elderly patients with congestive heart failure.[21] Like the angiotensin-converting enzyme inhibitors, these drugs should not be used in pregnancy.

*Recommended Laboratory Follow-Up.* Same as those for angiotensin-converting enzyme inhibitors.

## SUMMARY

Although significant strides have been made in the detection, evaluation, and treatment of hypertension, its incidence and prevalence in the United States remain very high. Moreover, only 27 percent of hypertensive patients (or their physicians) have achieved adequate blood pressure control. Framingham data indicate that 20 percent of hypertension occurs in isolation, whereas 80 percent occurs in combination with obesity, hyperlipidemia, insulin resistance, and glucose intolerance, indicating an urgent need for primary prevention with weight control, exercise, and reduced salt and alcohol intake. In the treatment of hypertension, greater focus has now been placed on aggressive lifestyle modification as both initial and adjunctive therapy. The current approach to the hypertensive patient is that of risk profiling and cardiovascular risk factor reduction. The national goal of the U.S. Department of Health and Human Services is to achieve control of hypertension in at least 50 percent of the hypertensive population within the year 2000. Attaining this goal will be a great challenge to both health care providers and patients.

## REFERENCES

1. Burt VL, Whelton P, Roccella EJ, et al: Prevalence of hypertension in the U.S. adult population: results from the Third National Health and Nutrition Examination Survey, 1988–1991. *Hypertension* 1995; 25:305–313.
2. MacMahon S, Peto R, Cutler J, et al: Blood pressure, stroke, and coronary heart disease: I. Prolonged differences in blood pressure: prospective observational studies corrected for the regression dilution bias. *Lancet* 1990; 335:765–774.
3. Psaty BM, Smith NL, Siscovick DS, et al: Health outcomes associated with antihypertensive therapies used as first-line agents. *JAMA* 1997; 277:739–745.
4. Neaton JD, Grimm RH, Prineas RJ, et al: Treatment of Mild Hypertension Study. *JAMA* 1993; 270:713–724.
5. The Sixth Report of the Joint National Committee on Detection, Evaluation, and Treatment of High Blood Pressure (JNC VI). *Arch Intern Med* 1997; 157:2413–2446.

6. Stamler J, Stamler R, Neaton JD: Blood pressure, systolic and diastolic, and cardiovascular risks: U.S. population data. *Arch Intern Med* 1993; 153:598–615.

7. SHEP Cooperative Research Group: Prevention of stroke by antihypertensive drug treatment in older persons with isolated systolic hypertension: final results of the Systolic Hypertension in the Elderly Program. *JAMA* 1991; 266:3255–3264.

8. Elliott P, Stamler J, Nichols R, et al: INTERSALT revisited: further analysis of 24-hour sodium excretion and blood pressure within and across populations: INTERSALT Cooperative Research Group. *Br Med J* 1996; 312:1249–1253.

9. Arroll B, Beaglehole R: Does physical activity lower blood pressure? A critical review of the clinical trials. *J Clin Epidemiol* 1992; 45:439–447.

10. Kelley G, McClellan P: Antihypertensive effects of aerobic exercise: a brief meta-analytic review of randomized controlled trials. *Am J Hypertens* 1994; 7:115–119.

11. U.S. Department of Health and Human Services: *Physical Activity and Health: A Report of the Surgeon General.* Atlanta, GA, U.S. Department of Health and Human Services, Centers for Disease Control and Prevention, National Center for Chronic Disease Prevention and Health Promotion, 1996.

12. Whelton PK, He J, Cutler JA, et al: Effects of oral potassium on blood pressure. Meta-analysis of randomized controlled clinical trials. *JAMA* 1997; 277:1624–1632.

13. Update on the 1987 Task Force Report on High Blood Pressure in Children and Adolescents: A Working Group Report from the National High Blood Pressure Education Program. *Pediatrics* 1996; 98:649–658.

14. Anastos K, Charney P, Charon RA, et al: Hypertension in women: what is really known? *Ann Intern Med* 1991; 115:287–293.

15. Committee on Technical Bulletins of the American College of Obstetricians and Gynecologists: Hypertension in pregnancy. *Int J Gynaecol Obstet* 1996; 53:175–183.

16. Siscovick DS, Raghunathan T, Psaty B, et al: Diuretic therapy for hypertension and the risk of primary cardiac arrest. *N Engl J Med* 1994; 330:1852–1857.

17. Kasiske BL, Ma JZ, Kalil RS, Louis TA: Effects of antihypertensive therapy on serum lipids. *Ann Intern Med* 1995; 122:133–141.

18. Psaty BM, Heckbert SR, Koepsell TD, et al: The risk of myocardial infarction associated with antihypertensive drug therapies. *JAMA* 1995; 274:620–625.

19. Borhani NO, Mercuri M, Borhani PA, et al: Final outcome results of the Multicenter Isradipine Diuretic Atherosclerosis Study (MIDAS). A randomized controlled trial. *JAMA* 1996; 276:785–791.

20. Alderman MH, Cohen H, Roque R, Madhavan S: Effect of long-acting and short-acting calcium antagonists on cardiovascular outcomes in hypertensive patients. *Lancet* 1997; 349:594–598.

21. Pitt B, Segal R, Martinez FA, et al: Randomized trial of losartan versus captopril in patients over 65 with heart failure (Evaluation of Losartan in the Elderly Study, ELITE). *Lancet* 1997; 349:747–752.

W. DALLAS HALL / JOYCE P. DOYLE

# CHAPTER 31

# HYPERTENSION: ASSESSMENT AND MANAGEMENT OF THE DIFFICULT CASE

## UNCONTROLLED HYPERTENSION

"Uncontrolled" hypertension is *not* synonymous with "resistant" hypertension. Recall from Chap. 30 that 73 percent of *all* U.S. hypertensives (and 50 percent of *treated* hypertensives) are uncontrolled, defined as a diastolic blood pressure that remains ≥90 mmHg *or* a systolic blood pressure that remains ≥140 mmHg.[1] Yet data from clinical trials document that 40 to 50 percent of patients can be controlled with monotherapy, 65 to 90 percent with two-drug therapy, and 91 to 96 percent with three-drug therapy. Why is there such a discrepancy between the relatively easy control achieved in clinical trials and the terribly low control rates (about 27 percent) in surveys of the community at risk?[2]

The answer is fairly obvious. In clinical trials on hypertension, special attention is given to assure medication adherence and compliance to protocol visits; study medications are free. Patients who are overtly nonadherent to medications and those who are alcoholic or have psychiatric problems are not usually enrolled. The levels of blood pressure cannot be severe at baseline (a typical average study entry level would be 150 to 160 mmHg systolic and 98 to 102 mmHg diastolic). Marked obesity is often an exclusion because of the difficulty in obtaining accurate casual or ambulatory blood pressure measurements. Moreover, the vast majority of clinical trials on hypertension have defined control as a diastolic blood pressure below 90 mmHg *or* a systolic blood pressure below 160 mmHg, which is not the current definition of control (i.e., diastolic blood pressure <90 mmHg *and* systolic blood pressure <140 mmHg). In simple terms, it is more difficult than clinical trials suggest to achieve control of blood pressure in the *usual* patient with hypertension.

**TABLE 31-1.   Usual Causes of "Uncontrolled" Hypertension in Treated Patients**

1. Noncompliance with appointments

2. Not getting prescriptions filled

3. Nonadherence to medication
   a. Forgetfulness
   b. Inconvenience
   c. Cost
   d. Adverse effects
   e. Lack of patient involvement in attaining goal/target blood pressure

4. Dietary indiscretion (calories, salt)

5. Inadequate or inappropriate therapy

Table 31-1 provides an outline of the usual causes of uncontrolled hypertension. Most cases are due to problems with visit compliance and medication adherence. To improve control of blood pressure, focus your attention first on ways to improve or assure visit compliance, prescription refills, and adherence to therapy. *After* these problems are addressed, consider altering the drug dose or class.

# RESISTANT HYPERTENSION

By definition, all cases of resistant hypertension are uncontrolled. However, as discussed previously, *most* cases of uncontrolled hypertension are not resistant to therapy. Resistant hypertension can be defined as a blood pressure that remains above goal (i.e., 140/90 mmHg or more) in patients who are *compliant* with a triple-drug regimen (used in near-maximal or full doses) where one of the three (or more) drugs is at least low doses of a diuretic. For elderly patients with isolated systolic hypertension, resistance can be defined as a systolic blood pressure consistently above 160 mmHg despite the above treatment criteria. Patients should not, however, be labeled as having resistant hypertension until the possibility of medication nonadherence is assessed thoroughly. Table 31-2 provides an outline of common causes of resistant hypertension. The order is ranked roughly from the most to the least likely explanations (in the authors' experience).

# PATIENT ASSESSMENT

## Clinical

Because 90 percent or more of compliant hypertensive patients *can* be controlled with three or more drugs, the relatively small proportion of patients who are resistant to therapy requires special attention, particularly in the context of their inordinate risk of AMI, heart failure, stroke, and renal failure. Special attention begins

**TABLE 31-2.  Usual Causes of "Resistant" Hypertension**

1. Inadequate (or no) diuretic therapy

2. Inadequate dose or inappropriate dosing schedule of antihypertensive drug(s)

3. Unblocked alpha receptors

4. Alcohol abuse

5. White coat effect

6. Drug interaction interfering with blood pressure response
   a. Nonsteroidal anti-inflammatory drugs
   b. Steroid therapy
   c. Diphenylhydantoin[3]

7. Undetected secondary cause
   a. Renovascular hypertension
   b. Sleep apnea
   c. Primary aldosteronism
   d. Cushing's disease/syndrome
   e. Pheochromocytoma

8. Measurement artifacts
   a. Use of regular cuff in an obese arm
   b. Pseudohypertension

9. Cocaine abuse

with a "revamp" of the clinical evaluation. Table 31-3 provides useful hints for the clinical assessment of the patient with resistant hypertension.

## Laboratory

Table 31-4 provides an outline of the laboratory or other special diagnostic screening tests that should be considered in the evaluation (or reevaluation) of patients with resistant hypertension. The table is divided into tests that relate to control of blood pressure and tests that relate to screening for secondary causes.

**TESTS FOR CONTROL OF BLOOD PRESSURE.**
*24-h Ambulatory Blood Pressure Monitoring.*  Ambulatory blood pressure monitoring is not indicated for either the diagnosis or the management of the vast majority of hypertensive patients. In those few with resistant hypertension, however, it is often useful to assure that the office levels of blood pressure are representative of those outside of the office setting.[4] As many as 20 percent of hypertensive patients have "white coat hypertension," an impressive pressor effect associated with the office visit. Approximately 2 percent of patients who appear to have resistant hypertension will have ambulatory blood pressure monitoring levels indicating

**TABLE 31-3.   The Revamped Clinical Assessment of Patients with Resistant Hypertension**

*History*

1. Are your home measurements just as bad?

2. Just how high is your salt intake? Do you use the shaker? Do you ever eat potato chips, dill pickles, or pizza?

3. Did you really take each of the medications yesterday *and* this morning?

4. Should you be drinking less alcohol?

5. How often do you use Advil, Motrin, or Aleve?

6. Do others complain that you snore terribly, have "gaspy" breathing at night, and seem sleepy all day?

7. You don't chew tobacco, do you?

8. Do you have "spells" where your blood pressure shoots up and your heart races?

*Physical*

1. Measure the circumference of the upper arm halfway between the olecranon and the acromion. Switch to an adult obese cuff if it exceeds 33 cm.

2. Look again for facial plethora, truncal obesity, and supraclavicular fat pads (Cushing's syndrome).

3. Look at the neck veins (with the patient at a 30° to 45° angle) for evidence of distention or overactivity (volume expansion).

4. Listen for at least 2 min around the epigastrium, RUQ, LUQ, and umbilicus for a bruit that radiates laterally (renovascular hypertension).

5. Firmly indent the lower pretibial area for subtle evidence of edema (volume expansion).

RUQ = right upper quadrant; LUQ = left upper quadrant.

excellent control, with more than 85 percent of readings in the normotensive range outside the office.[5,6] Figure 31-1 shows a dramatic example of a compliant, symptomatic (i.e., dizzy, weak) patient whose office blood pressures were consistently uncontrolled, but whose ambulatory blood pressure monitoring demonstrated that the out-of-office blood pressures were all low. The drug treatment was reduced (rather than increased), and her symptoms resolved. We quit taking the office blood pressure and managed her according to her home blood pressure values. Ambulatory blood pressure monitoring may be cost-effective if it prevents unwarranted additional chronic drug therapy.[7]

***Serum Creatinine.***   Serum creatinine levels above 2 to 2.5 mg/dL (or above 1.4 mg/dL in the elderly) usually indicate that the patient needs a diuretic as part of

**TABLE 31-4.   Selected Laboratory and Other Diagnostic Test Considerations in Patients with Resistant Hypertension**

For Control of Blood Pressure:

1. 24-h ambulatory blood pressure

2. Serum creatinine

3. Serum potassium

4. 24-h urine sodium and creatinine

5. Urinary drug screen

6. Echocardiography

For Detection of Secondary Causes:

| | | |
|---|---|---|
| 7. | Renoparenchymal disease | Renal ultrasonography |
| 8. | Renovascular hypertension | Captopril renal scan |
| 9. | Sleep apnea | Home oximetry monitoring |
| 10. | Primary aldosteronism | Saline infusion test |
| 11. | Cushing's disease/syndrome | Overnight dexamethasone suppression test |
| 12. | Pheochromocytoma | 24-h urine metanephrine and creatinine |

the antihypertensive regimen. At this level of renal dysfunction, thiazide-like diuretics begin to fail and should generally be switched to loop diuretics. Furosemide should be prescribed in a twice-daily dose.

***Serum Potassium.***   The serum potassium level should be rechecked because if it is below 3.5 mEq/L, supplemental oral potassium therapy per se (in a dose adequate to raise the potassium level by about 0.5 mEq/L) can lead to a significant improvement in blood pressure.[8]

***24-h Urine Sodium and Creatinine.***   Inordinate amounts of dietary salt intake can override the blood pressure lowering efficacy of almost all antihypertensive drugs. In a steady state (including patients who have been taking diuretics for at least a month), the 24-h urinary sodium excretion is an estimate of dietary sodium intake. Always also obtain a simultaneous 24-h urine creatinine level to assure that there is reasonable accuracy in the sample collection, as reflected by a total creatinine output between 1000 and 3000 mg daily. Values of urinary sodium above 176 mEq per day indicate a sodium intake of 4000 mg or more, whereas the recommended level of sodium intake is 2400 mg or less (i.e., 106 mEq per day or less) for hypertensive patients. Some patients with resistant hypertension have 24-h urine sodium excretions of 300 mEq per day or more, reflecting a sodium intake of at least 6800 mg, equivalent to 17 g of salt daily.

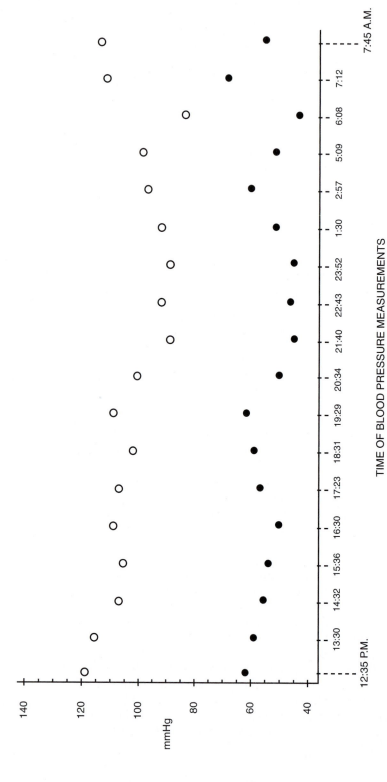

**Figure 31-1** Low 24-h ambulatory systolic and diastolic blood pressure readings in a patient with apparent uncontrolled "resistant" hypertension on office visit readings. ○ = systolic blood pressure. ● = diastolic blood pressure.

*Urinary Drug Screen.*    Although the majority of cocaine-dependent hypertensives are normotensive, cocaine abuse can induce markedly exacerbated levels of blood pressure in known hypertensives. A urinary drug screen for cocaine metabolites (i.e., benzoylecgonine) should be considered in patients with resistant hypertension. This is especially true for relatively young patients with unexplained sinus tachycardia, intermittent chest pain, or a past history of unexplained seizures. Screening tests can usually detect cocaine metabolites for about 2 days following use, and more sensitive tests (gas chromatography or mass spectroscopy) can detect significant benzoylecgonine levels for 5 to 6 days or more.

*Echocardiography.*    Echocardiography is not indicated for either the diagnosis or the management of most hypertensive patients. In those with resistant hypertension, however, limited echocardiography can provide useful information and remain "cost-tolerable."[9] For example, the finding of an unexpected low ejection fraction (e.g., 25 percent) might encourage the physician to reduce therapy with beta blockers and substitute a drug without cardiodepressant properties, especially if the patient had vague complaints that might be attributed to nonspecific effects of the beta blocker. In contrast, the finding of a hyperdynamic left ventricle with a relatively high ejection fraction might encourage the use of drugs with cardiodepressant properties (e.g., beta blockers, labetalol, or clonidine), especially if the patient was already receiving direct vasodilators such as hydralazine or minoxidil, which can further worsen the hyperdynamic state. The absence of echocardiographic left ventricular hypertrophy in a patient with long-standing, severe, resistant hypertension would lead to reevaluation of the representativeness of the usual office blood pressure, including review of the appropriate blood pressure cuff size, consideration of intraarterial blood pressure measurement if the patient is markedly obese, and probably a request for a 24-h ambulatory blood pressure monitoring.

## TESTS FOR DETECTION OF SECONDARY CAUSES.

*Renoparenchymal Hypertension.*    Renal ultrasonography is a relatively inexpensive test that provides information about kidney size. In essential hypertension, with or without related chronic renal damage, the kidneys are usually symmetric. In advanced hypertensive nephrosclerosis, they may be small, in the range of 9 to 11 cm. The presence of one small, shrunken kidney, however, suggests the possibility of atherosclerotic renal artery stenosis, unilateral pyelonephritis (e.g., due to ureteral reflux), or past renal trauma with atrophy. Each of these conditions can be associated with renin-mediated hypertension. Rarely, renal ultrasonography reveals unsuspected polycystic kidney disease or hydronephrosis.

*Renovascular Hypertension.*    Renovascular disease is by far the most common reversible secondary cause of hypertension. With narrowing of the renal artery, decreased renal blood flow stimulates the renin-angiotensin system, thereby driving the hypertension. This narrowing can occur in the main renal artery or in a smaller branch; *branch stenosis* represents up to 30 percent of cases. In elderly men and women the etiology is atherosclerotic narrowing of the renal artery, whereas in young persons (especially women) the cause is typically fibrous dysplasia of the renal artery. Fibrous dysplasia of the renal and other (e.g., carotid) arteries is occasionally hereditary with an autosomal dominant pattern (i.e., mother-daughter or sister-sister). Resistant hypertension is not uncommon in patients with either the fibrous or the atherosclerotic type of renal artery stenosis. Other clinical clues that lead an astute clinician to suspect the diagnosis are outlined in Table 31-5.

If a young woman has resistant hypertension and an abdominal bruit, one should proceed directly to renal arteriography without risking a false-negative screening test result. In most other suspicious clinical settings, however, a screening test is appropriate in order to decide whether to proceed with the more expensive and potentially more risky angiography. The captopril renal scan [or angiotensin-converting enzyme inhibitor (ACE-I) scintigraphy, using intravenous enalapril] is an excellent screening test with a sensitivity (about 95 percent if the patient is not taking diuretics and 87 percent if the patient is taking diuretics) superior to that of other options, such as other types of renal scans or a random peripheral renin activity (usually obtained on multiple medications that cannot be safely discontinued). The standard protocol requires that the patient discontinue ACE-I for 3 to 5 days prior to the scan. On the day of the study, baseline radionuclide images of the kidneys are obtained, 25 to 50 mg of captopril is administered orally (or a maximum of 2.5 mg of enalaprilat intravenously), and the radionuclide images are repeated. Post-captopril radionuclide changes compatible with renal artery stenosis include a significant decrease in glomerular filtration rate and (in more severe cases) renal plasma flow on the stenotic side. Specific criteria are complex and depend on the individual nuclear medicine techniques (e.g., the postinjection imaging intervals or the selection of regions of interest for counting), as well as the particular tracer used to estimate glomerular filtration rate (e.g., Tc 99m pentetate) or renal plasma flow [e.g., $^{131}$I or $^{123}$I orthoiodohippurate (OIH) versus Tc 99m mercaptoacetyltriglycine (MAG-3)]. If the patient cannot safely withhold the ACE-I prior to the scan, one can continue the ACE-I and request only a post-ACE-I scan, although in this set-

## TABLE 31-5.   Clinical Clues to the Diagnosis of Renovascular Hypertension

1. Resistant hypertension, especially in a previously well-controlled patient

2. Initial onset of hypertension below age 30 or above age 50

3. Abdominal bruit that radiates laterally

4. Carotid bruit in a young woman

5. Nonobesity

6. Accelerated or malignant hypertension

7. Marked short-term blood pressure decrease with ACE-I (in absence of dehydration)

8. Unexplained recurrent acute pulmonary edema

ting the sensitivity of the test is reduced to 75 to 80 percent. False-positive captopril scans, however, are not unusual in patients with primary renoparenchymal disease.

Duplex ultrasound scanning is very operator-dependent and is limited technically by excess bowel gas and obesity and anatomically by multiple renal arteries or branch stenoses. Magnetic resonance angiography is noninvasive and uses no radiation, but also has limitations in the detection of branch stenoses. Magnetic resonance angiography also tends to overestimate the severity of any stenosis.

***Sleep Apnea.***    Sleep apnea is a recently recognized secondary cause of hypertension and can cause resistant hypertension. It occurs most often in men and in patients with marked obesity. Table 31-6 lists the clinical clues to the diagnosis.

Once sleep apnea is suspected clinically, the simplest and least expensive initial ($100 to $200) screening test is nocturnal home oximetry monitoring to detect significant transient desaturations (i.e., below 90 percent).[10] A negative test is very sensitive in excluding sleep apnea, but a positive test is not very specific and often requires confirmation by the more expensive ($1000 or more) polysomnography in a sleep laboratory. Control of hypertension often improves markedly following effective therapy with continuous positive airway pressure or uvulopalatopharyngoplasty.[11]

***Primary Aldosteronism.***    Primary aldosteronism is a rare but sneaky secondary cause of hypertension. It is sneaky because the most direct clinical hint is hypokalemia, which is often attributed to other, more common causes such as diuretic therapy, heavy alcohol intake, poor nutrition, vomiting, or diarrhea. The true clue is that the hypokalemia keeps happening and never seems to normalize despite what seems to be more than adequate replacement therapy. Table 31-7 provides other helpful clues to the diagnosis.

Simple initial screening tests include a low or undetectable level of plasma renin activity or elevated levels of either plasma aldosterone or the 24-h urinary excretion of aldosterone. These tests, however, are not very sensitive or specific. For example, the plasma aldosterone level may not be elevated in 20 to 30 percent of patients with adrenal adenoma because the secretion of aldosterone from the contralateral adrenal gland may be suppressed, or because hypokalemia per se inhibits aldo-

## TABLE 31-6.  Clinical Clues to the Diagnosis of Sleep Apnea

1. Hypertension

2. Obesity

3. Male gender (90%)

4. History (usually from others) of nocturnal snoring and "gaspy" breathing

5. Daytime somnolence

6. Patient who goes to sleep/snores in your office

**TABLE 31-7.　Clinical Clues to the Diagnosis of Primary Aldosteronism**

1. Hypertension

2. Hypokalemia (serum potassium < 3.5 mEq/L)

3. Persistence of hypokalemia despite oral potassium supplements (≥60 mEq/day)

4. Hypernatremia (144–148 mEq/L)

5. Family history of hypokalemia

6. Amelioration of hypertension during pregnancy

sterone production. Moreover, 10 to 30 percent of patients with essential hypertension have low levels of plasma renin activity.

If the diagnosis is suspected strongly, a more direct and efficient initial screening test is the saline infusion test. However, this requires that the patient (if not already hospitalized) remain in the office setting for 4 to 5 h for monitoring of the blood pressure and saline infusion. Insert a heparin lock and have the patient supine for at least 20 min. Then draw a baseline plasma aldosterone and renin level and begin a 4-h infusion of 2 L of normal saline, monitoring blood pressure every 30 to 60 min for safety. After 4 h, repeat the plasma aldosterone level. Patients with primary aldosteronism will not suppress their postsaline plasma aldosterone level to below 10 ng/dL. In addition, the baseline aldosterone level is usually (but not always) elevated, and the renin activity is low. An unsuppressed aldosterone level (i.e., ≥10 ng/dL) is an indication for thin-cut (0.5-mm) adrenal computed tomography (CT) or adrenal magnetic resonance imaging (MRI), which will detect unilateral adrenal adenoma or bilateral adrenal hyperplasia in 70 to 80 percent of cases. Detection of a unilateral adrenal adenoma is an indication for referral to a surgeon. A negative CT scan or MRI in this setting is an indication for referral to a specialist in hypertension.

***Cushing's Disease/Syndrome.***　In recent years, advances in imaging technology have made it apparent that both Cushing's disease (i.e., due to a pituitary microadenoma) and Cushing's syndrome (i.e., due to adrenal adenoma, adrenal hyperplasia, or ectopic ACTH syndrome) are not as rare as thought previously. The classic clinical clues to the diagnosis, however, remain the same as we all learned in medical school (Table 31-8).

Once Cushing's disease/syndrome is suspected clinically, the overnight dexamethasone suppression test is a simple and cheap way to proceed with initial screening. Give the patient a prescription for one 1-mg tablet of dexamethasone. Have him or her take it at exactly 11 P.M. and come in for a plasma cortisol level at 8 A.M. the next morning. Most patients (about 95 percent) without Cushing's disease/syndrome will suppress the plasma cortisol to below 5 $\mu$g/dL. Those who do not suppress require further pursuit, often beginning with high-resolution pituitary MRI before and after gadolinium pentetic acid, which will detect (only) 70 percent (or

**TABLE 31-8.  Clinical Clues to the Diagnosis of Cushing's Disease/Syndrome**

1. Hypertension

2. Truncal obesity ("thin" extremities)

3. Rapid weight gain

4. Moon face with plethora

5. Palpable supraclavicular fat pads

6. Acne, especially extrafacial

7. Hirsutism

8. Premenopausal amenorrhea or oligomenorrhea

9. Glucose intolerance, especially if difficult to control

10. Hypokalemia

less) of microadenomas; CT is not helpful. A positive pituitary MRI is an indication for referral to a neurosurgeon. A negative pituitary MRI (and subsequent adrenal CT) in this setting is an indication for referral to an endocrinologist. The single largest problem with use of the overnight dexamethasone suppression test is a false-positive result in patients with major depression, alcoholism, or acute illness.

*Pheochromocytoma.*    Pheochromocytoma is rare, occurring in about 1 out of 1000 or more hypertensive patients. This is why it is usually missed despite abundant symptoms that suggest the diagnosis retrospectively. Any clinician who suspects and then diagnoses a pheochromocytoma should get a gold star and an honorary plaque on the wall because he or she has probably saved the patient from unexpected death. Table 31-9 outlines the clinical tipoffs to the diagnosis. The problem is that there are many clinical settings that mimic the diagnosis, including occult alcoholism, sporadic drug compliance, clonidine rebound hypertension, and cocaine-related hypertension. In the "usual" suspicious patient, however, the strongest hint that pheochromocytoma is *not* present may be the absence of marked heart rate increases during the periods of marked rises in blood pressure.

In a patient suspected of pheochromocytoma, an excellent screening test (90 to 96 percent sensitive) is the urinary metanephrine excretion. Order a 24-h urine for metanephrine *and* creatinine. The test is positive if the ratio of total metanephrine (expressed in micrograms) to creatinine (expressed in milligrams) is above 2.2. Most patients with essential hypertension have a ratio below 1, and most with pheochromocytoma have a ratio above 5. Do *not* also order a urinary vanillylmandelic acid or "total catecholamines" unless you are just curious or want to be confused. The reason is that both of these tests are less sensitive, less specific, and more likely to give false results because of interference from blood pressure medications or other substances. Very few things interfere with the metanephrines except for a true rise

TABLE 31-9.   Clinical Clues to the Diagnosis of Pheochromocytoma

1. Hypertension

2. Triad of headaches (often migraine-like), palpitation, and sweating (90%)

3. "Yo-yo" blood pressure and blood pressure control

4. Sinus tachycardia

5. History of supraventricular tachycardia or ventricular ectopy

6. History of unexplained catastrophic surgery or anesthesia

7. Orthostatic hypotension

8. Neurofibromatosis, café-au-lait spots, von Hippel-Lindau disease, tuberous sclerosis, Sturge-Weber disease

9. Family history of pheochromocytoma, medullary thyroid carcinoma, or hyperparathyroidism

(of about 40 percent but not usually above the normal range) in patients receiving alpha blockers (e.g., doxazosin, terazosin) and a false low for 24 to 72 h after intravenous methylglucamine contrast material.

If the urine metanephrines are positive, obtain an adrenal CT scan, which will reveal the tumor in 90 percent of cases of pheochromocytoma. A positive adrenal CT scan is an indication for referral to a surgeon with experience with pheochromocytomas. A negative adrenal CT in this setting is an indication for referral to a specialist in hypertension. Plasma catecholamine levels are sometimes useful but are plagued by the occurrence of modest elevations (800 to 1500 pg/mL), which can occur if the samples are obtained in a stressful setting (intensive care unit, etc.) or without the patient resting supine in a quiet room for at least 20 min after the needle is inserted. Plasma catecholamines also may be elevated to these levels in some patients with the hyperadrenergic type of essential hypertension, during panic attacks or hypoglycemia, and in occasional elderly individuals.

# MANAGEMENT

## Lifestyle Modifications

The lifestyle modifications discussed in Chap. 30 (see Table 30-3) are even more important for management of the difficult case receiving multiple antihypertensive drugs.

## Adherence Counseling

Adherence counseling often requires a personal review of the number or color of pills taken that day, yesterday, etc.[12] Physicians are not very good at predicting who is and is not adherent to medications. Therefore, a direct but nonthreatening approach to assessment of compliance is recommended for all patients. A simple four-item questionnaire provides an excellent indicator of medication adherence (Table 31-10).[13] An adherence score (0 to 4) is obtained by adding the "yes" answers. Estimates of high, medium, and low adherence are indicated by scores of 0, 1–2, and 3–4, respectively. Morisky et al[13] reported that these scores correlated significantly ($p < .01$) with the likelihood of both current and future blood pressure control. Try having your hypertensive patients complete this simple questionnaire in the waiting room. Provide special counseling for those with scores of 3 or more.

## Pharmacologic Treatment

Table 31-11 provides a listing of several pharmacologic "tricks" to improve the control of blood pressure in patients with resistant hypertension. In a review of 91 patients referred for resistant hypertension, Yakovlevitch and Black[14] reported that the cause in 39 patients (43 percent) was a suboptimal medical regimen, primarily due to inadequate diuretic therapy. Graves and associates[15] reached similar conclusions in a study of nine patients with resistant hypertension. Blood pressures were in the142 to 185/94 to 120 mmHg range despite compliance to three or more antihypertensive drugs; seven of the nine patients weighed between 223 and 266 lb, and six had serum creatinine levels of 1.4 mg/dL or less. Eight (of the nine) patients had a markedly expanded plasma volume ($^{125}$I radiolabeled albumin) *despite* diuretic therapy. Addition of aggressive loop diuretic therapy (e.g., mean daily furosemide dose of 272 mg) led to an average decrease in blood pressure of 34/20 mmHg, with a subsequent reduction of total antihypertensive medications from an average of 3.8 to 2.6 drugs daily. Data such as these provide the scientific evidence for the first three pharmacologic "tricks" in Table 31-11. Of course, caution must be used in following the levels of serum potassium during such regimens. Also, some patients may need more aggressive control of their hyperlipidemia or gout prior to implementing the regimen.

## TABLE 31-10.   Medication Adherence Questionnaire

|  | Yes | No |
|---|---|---|
| 1. Do you ever forget to take your blood pressure medicine? | ☐ | ☐ |
| 2. Are you careless at times about taking your blood pressure medicine? | ☐ | ☐ |
| 3. When you feel better, do you sometimes quit taking your blood pressure medicine? | ☐ | ☐ |
| 4. Sometimes, if you feel worse when you take your blood pressure medicine, do you stop taking it? | ☐ | ☐ |

*Source:* Adapted from Morisky DE, Green LW, Levine DM: Concurrent and predictive validity of a self-reported measure of medication adherence. *Med Care* 1986; 24:67–74, with permission.

**TABLE 31-11.   Pharmacologic "Tricks" for the Management of the Patient with Resistant Hypertension**

1. Add a diuretic (e.g., 12.5 to 25 mg hydrochlorothiazide daily) if the patient is on no diuretic.

2. Switch a thiazide or thiazide-like diuretic to a loop diuretic (furosemide, bumetanide, torsemide) if the serum creatinine is 2 mg/dL or more (or 1.4 mg/dL or more in the elderly). Consider subsequent increases in the doses of the loop diuretic (see text).

3. Switch any once-daily furosemide dose to twice daily (e.g., 40 mg once daily to 40 mg twice daily), or switch the furosemide to a once-daily loop diuretic (e.g., bumetanide or torsemide).

4. Block excessive alpha-adrenergic activity.
   a. Add an alpha blocker (e.g., doxazosin, terazosin) and gradually titrate upward to at least 8 mg daily.
   b. Add clonidine, 0.1 mg orally twice daily, increasing to 0.4 mg orally twice daily if tolerated. Adverse effects are sometimes lessened by switching to the once-weekly transdermal patch.

5. In elderly patients whose level of systolic blood pressure remains recalcitrant to multiple therapies, try the addition of nitrates (even in those without angina) such as isosorbide dinitrate (20 to 40 mg twice daily).

Once the diuretic and presumed volume expansion issues have been adequately addressed, the next consideration is whether the alpha-adrenergic system has been blocked adequately. Vasodilators (such as the calcium channel antagonists and ACE inhibitors), diuretics, and beta blockers do not inhibit the alpha-adrenergic system, which may actually be activated in patients receiving multiple medications. The use of alpha receptor blockers (e.g., doxazosin, terazosin) and inhibition of central catecholamine release (e.g., with clonidine) are sometimes very useful in this particular setting.

# HYPERTENSIVE URGENCIES AND EMERGENCIES[16–19]

## Diagnosis

A *hypertensive emergency* is a situation in which blood pressure must be reduced within 15 to 60 min. Examples include accelerated and malignant hypertension, hypertensive encephalopathy, and severe hypertension (usually in the range of 240 to 300/120 to 160 mmHg) that is associated with acute pulmonary edema, ischemic chest pain, dissecting aortic aneurysm, or intracerebral hemorrhage.

A *hypertensive urgency* is a situation in which severe elevations of blood pressure are not causing acute end organ damage but should be lowered within 24 h to reduce potential risk to the patient. An example would be a patient with a blood pressure of 220/132 mmHg with minimal or no symptoms.

## Management

Hypertensive emergencies are treated by hospitalization for intravenous antihypertensive therapy. Hypertensive urgencies are generally treated by short-term or overnight observation with use of oral antihypertensive therapy. Almost all newly discovered cases of urgent hypertension will require hospitalization, whereas known patients can sometimes be managed in the office setting if there is a relatively recent update on their laboratory values (i.e., electrolytes, blood urea nitrogen, and creatinine) and absence of microscopic hematuria (i.e., more than five red blood cells per high-power field).

**HYPERTENSIVE EMERGENCIES.**  Table 31-12 provides an outline of the drugs used most often for the treatment of hypertensive emergencies. Included are the recommended starting dose, the infusion rate, the duration of action, and adverse effects.

*Sodium Nitroprusside.*  Intravenous therapy with sodium nitroprusside allows minute-to-minute titration of blood pressure to a desired level. The usual starting dose is 0.3 to 0.5 $\mu$g/kg/min, followed by increases of 0.5 to 1.0 $\mu$g/kg/min as necessary. The maximum infusion rate should not exceed 8 $\mu$g/kg/min. Sodium nitroprusside must be protected from light by wrapping the infusion bottle with tinfoil, and the solution must be renewed every 12 h. Administration of sodium nitroprusside requires careful monitoring by experienced staff in an intensive care setting.

The goal of initial therapy is often a reduction of diastolic blood pressure toward 110 to 120 mmHg, or a reduction of the mean arterial blood pressure (i.e., diastolic blood pressure plus one-third of the pulse pressure) toward 120 mmHg, depending on the clinical setting and the course of the individual patient. For example, the reduction should be slower in patients with acute cerebral thrombosis, where the goal is often to maintain a blood pressure of 170 to 180/90 to 100 mmHg or more. Oral antihypertensive therapy can often be started once the severely elevated blood pressure has improved, typically within less than 24 h after beginning sodium nitroprusside. Choices for use during the transition period include labetalol (200 mg PO q12h), clonidine (0.1 mg PO q12h), or captopril (12.5 mg PO q12h).

Serum thiocyanate or cyanide levels should be monitored in patients with renal insufficiency or whenever therapy with sodium nitroprusside is continued for 3 days or more. Thiocyanate levels above 12 mg/dL suggest toxicity and require discontinuation or downward titration of the sodium nitroprusside. Acute toxicity is indicated most readily by metabolic acidosis or vomiting and can be treated with a vitamin $B_{12}$ derivative (i.e., hydroxycobalamin) that binds cyanide. Sodium nitroprusside therapy is associated with sodium retention and activation of the sympathetic nervous system. The latter is reflected clinically by tachycardia. What may ap-

**TABLE 31-12.  Hypertensive Emergency: Intravenous Therapies**

| Drug (Route) | Mixture | Initial Adult Dose | Onset | Duration | Major Adverse Effects | Comments |
|---|---|---|---|---|---|---|
| Sodium Nitroprusside (continuous infusion) | 50 mg dissolved in 250 mL D5W provides a solution of 200 $\mu$g/mL. Protect from light and change q12h | 20–50 $\mu$g/min (0.3–0.5 $\mu$g/kg/min) | Immediate | 2–5 min | Thiocyanate toxicity, acidosis, vomiting, seizures | Infusion rates greater than 8 $\mu$g/kg/min should be avoided. Monitor SCN levels in presence of renal failure or with prolonged infusions. |
| Nitroglycerin (continuous infusion) | 32 $\mu$g/mL often constituted by adding 50–250 mg into 250 mL D5W in a special delivery system | 32 $\mu$g/min (0.5 $\mu$g/kg/min) | Immediate | 2–5 min | Headache, tachycardia, methemoglobinemia, alcohol intoxication (prolonged high-dose infusion) | Infusion rates above 50 $\mu$g/min are often necessary to achieve reduction in blood pressure. |
| Labetalol (IV minibolus) | 5 mg/mL in 20-mL ampule | 20 mg (4 mL) in 2 min, then 40–80 mg (8–16 mL) at 15-min intervals | 10 min | 4–6 h (variable) | Dizziness, scalp tingling, orthostasis, bradycardia | Contraindicated in patients with bronchospasm, CHF, bradycardia, or heart block greater than first degree. |

| Drug | Preparation | Dose | | | Adverse Effects | Special Considerations |
|---|---|---|---|---|---|---|
| Labetalol (continuous infusion) | 100–200 mg in 1000 mL D5W | 0.5 mg/min; increase as necessary to a maximum of 2.0 mg/min | As above | As above | As above | As above |
| Enalaprilat (IV minibolus) | 1.25 mg/mL in a 2-mL Vasotec IV vial. Can be mixed with either dextrose or saline | 1.25 mg (1 mL) in 5 min, followed by 1.25 mg q6h if effective. Total daily dosages should not exceed 20 mg | 5–15 min | 6 hr or more | Excessive hypotension; rarely, angioedema, hyperkalemia, or acute renal failure | Initial dose should be reduced to 0.625 mg (0.5 mL) if the patient has active CHF, is receiving diuretic therapy, or has a serum creatinine level >3 mg/dL. |
| Nicardipine (continuous infusion) | Each 10-mL (25-mg) ampule must be diluted with 240 mL of IV fluids (dextrose or saline, but not lactated Ringer's) | 5.0–7.5 mg/h depending on body weight | 5–60 min | 20–40 min | Headache, flushing, phlebitis at infusion site | Contraindicated in patients with tight aortic stenosis. |

SCN = thiocyanate; CHF = congestive heart failure.

pear to be development of tolerance to the blood pressure lowering effect of sodium nitroprusside can usually be overcome after effective diuresis with furosemide or sometimes by concomitant therapy with an ACE-I or beta blocker.

Intravenous nitroglycerin may have advantages over sodium nitroprusside in some patients with chest pain and/or myocardial ischemia, but when the elevation of blood pressure is severe, sodium nitroprusside or labetalol is more potent than nitroglycerin.

*Labetalol Minibolus.*   Minibolus therapy with labetalol is sometimes preferable to continuous infusion of sodium nitroprusside, particularly in an emergency room or perioperative setting where it is not always possible to monitor blood pressure on a minute-to-minute basis. Intravenous labelatol, however, is contraindicated in the presence of sinus bradycardia, sick sinus syndrome, second- or-third degree heart block, bronchospasm, or left ventricular dysfunction. The appropriate initial dose of intravenous labetalol is 20 mg (4 mL), given over a 2-min period. After 15 min, a second bolus of 40 mg is given, increasing to 80 mg 15 to 20 min later as necessary. Once blood pressure is improved (usually within 2 to 3 h), following a total labetalol dose of 180 to 300 mg, therapy can be maintained by continuous infusion of 0.5 to 2 mg/min labetalol. Transition to oral therapy is best accomplished after 12 to 48 h, beginning with an oral labetalol dose of 200 mg every 12 h with titration to 400 mg orally twice a day as needed. Low-dose diuretic therapy is additive for control of blood pressure.

**HYPERTENSIVE URGENCIES.**   Table 31-13 provides an outline of several oral antihypertensive regimens used for the management of hypertensive urgencies.

*Clonidine Loading.*[20,21]   The clonidine loading regimen is often effective when it is desirable to gradually reduce blood pressure over a 6- to 24-h period, especially if intensive care unit monitoring is neither desirable nor judged necessary. An initial oral dose of 0.2 mg is followed by a dose of 0.1 mg once every hour until diastolic blood pressure is below 110 mmHg or a total dose of 0.8 mg clonidine is reached. Therapy is effective in 80 to 90 percent of patients, and maintenance therapy can then be initiated at approximately 75 percent of the total loading dose, given in divided doses twice daily.

*Labetalol Loading.*[21]   Labetalol loading is another effective oral antihypertensive regimen, when not contraindicated. Give a single dose of 200 to 300 mg, followed by 100 to 200 mg every 8 h. The onset of blood pressure lowering usually occurs within 2 h.

*Resume Previous Therapy.*   Reinstitution of previous antihypertensive therapy (that the patient had not been taking) is often effective within 6 h or less for improvement of "urgent" hypertension. Use caution, however, because some patients may never have taken *all* their medications. To avoid "overshoot" in patients previously on multiple medications, it is sometimes advisable to restart the medications

**TABLE 31-13.  Hypertensive Urgency: Oral Therapies**

| Drug | Initial Adult Dose | Onset | Duration | Major Adverse Effects | Comments |
|------|--------------------|-------|----------|------------------------|----------|
| Clonidine loading | 0.2 mg PO then 0.1 mg q1h to a maximum total dose of 0.8 mg or until diastolic BP is reduced 20 mm or more (or below 110 mmHg) | 30–120 min | 8–12 h | Sedation, dry mouth, dizziness, orthostasis | Contraindicated in patients with sinus bradycardia, sick sinus syndrome, or heart block. Excess hypotension can be counteracted with IV saline plus 5 mg IV tolazoline |
| Labetalol | 200–300 mg single oral dose followed by 100–200 mg q8h | 60–120 min | 12–24 min | Bradycardia | Contraindicated in patients with bronchospasm, congestive heart failure, bradycardia, or heart block greater than first degree |
| Hospitalize and resume previous therapy for 24 h | Previous medications and dosage | NA | NA | Excessive hypotension | This plan will control BP within 3–6 h in 25–50% of patients seemingly resistant to outpatient therapy. Occasional quasicompliant patients can experience excessive hypotension |

at half dose. For example, a patient previously on 200 mg/day metoprolol, 20 mg/day minoxidil, 80 mg twice-daily furosemide, and 0.4 mg twice-daily clonidine might initially receive each of these four medications on the same schedule but with half the dose of each drug.

***Short-Acting Calcium Channel Antagonists.***   Although effective in rapidly lowering marked elevations of blood pressure, short-acting calcium channel antagonists, such as nifedipine, are not indicated for hypertensive urgencies because of concern about precipitous decreases in blood pressure and reflex sympathetic stimulation. Alternative therapies include the clonidine or labetalol loading regimens, each of which has an onset within 3 h or less.

## SPECIALTY REFERRAL

Table 31-14 provides a guideline for when referral to a specialist in hypertension should be considered for patients who need either further diagnostic tests, improved level of blood pressure control, or both.

### TABLE 31-14.   Indications for Referral to a Specialist in Hypertension

For Diagnosis of Secondary Causes:

| | | |
|---|---|---|
| 1. | Renovascular hypertension | If the captopril renal scan is positive, or if renal angiography (with or without angioplasty) seems indicated |
| 2. | Sleep apnea | If the nocturnal home oximetry monitoring is positive |
| 3. | Primary aldosteronism | If the plasma aldosterone level is 10 ng/dL or more 4 h after a 2-L saline infusion, but the adrenal CT or MRI is normal |
| 4. | Cushing's disease/syndrome | If the 8 A.M. plasma cortisol is 5 $\mu$g/dL or more after 1 mg dexamethasone at 11 P.M. the previous evening |
| 5. | Pheochromocytoma | If the 24-h urinary metanephrine ($\mu$g) to creatinine (mg) ratio exceeds 2.2 and the adrenal CT or MRI is normal |

For Pharmacologic Control of Blood Pressure:

1. Patients with resistant hypertension, defined as a blood pressure that remains above goal (i.e., 140/90 mmHg or more) despite compliance to a triple-drug regimen (used in near-maximal or full doses) where one of the three (or more) drugs is at least low doses of a diuretic.
2. Patients whose blood pressure has been so poorly controlled that extremely potent drugs such as minoxidil are being considered.

## REFERENCES

1. Burt VL, Whelton P, Roccella EJ, et al: Prevalence of hypertension in the U.S. adult population. Results from the Third National Health and Nutrition Examination Survey, 1988–1991. *Hypertension* 1995; 25:305–313.
2. Thurmer HL, Lund-Larsen PG, Tverdal A: Is blood pressure treatment as effective in a population setting as in controlled trials? Results from a prospective study. *J Hypertens* 1994; 12:481–490.
3. Ahmed S: Renal insensitivity to furosemide caused by chronic anticonvulsant therapy. *Br Med J* 1974; 3:657–659.
4. Mejia AD, Egan BM, Schork NJ, Zweifler AJ: Artifacts in measurement of blood pressure and lack of target organ involvement in the assessment of patients with treatment-resistant hypertension. *Ann Intern Med* 1990; 112:270–277.
5. Setaro JF, Black HR: Refractory hypertension. *N Engl J Med* 1992; 327:543–547.
6. Mancia G, Sega R, Milesi C, et al: Blood-pressure control in the hypertensive population. *Lancet* 1997; 349:454–457.
7. Yarows SP, Khoury S, Sowers JR: Cost effectiveness of 24-hour ambulatory blood pressure monitoring in evaluation and treatment of hypertension. *Am J Hypertens* 1994; 7:464–468.
8. Kaplan NM, Carnegie A, Raskin P, et al: Potassium supplementation in hypertensive patients with diuretic-induced hypokalemia. *N Engl J Med* 1985; 312:746–749.
9. Sheps SG, Frohlich ED: Limited echocardiography for hypertensive left ventricular hypertrophy. *Hypertension* 1997; 29:560–563.
10. Series F, Marc I, Cormier Y, LaForge J: Utility of nocturnal home oximetry for case finding in patients with suspected sleep apnea hypopnea syndrome. *Ann Intern Med* 1993; 119:449–453.
11. He J, Kryger MH, Zorick FJ, et al: Mortality and apnea index in obstructive sleep apnea: experience in 385 male patients. *Chest* 1988; 94:9–14.
12. Eisen KA, Miller DK, Woodward RS, et al: The effect of prescribed daily dose frequency on patient medication compliance. *Arch Intern Med* 1990; 150:1881–1884.
13. Morisky DE, Green LW, Levine DM: Concurrent and predictive validity of a self-reported measure of medication adherence. *Med Care* 1986; 24:67–74.
14. Yakovlevitch M, Black HR: Resistant hypertension in a tertiary care clinic. *Arch Intern Med* 1991; 151:1786–1792.
15. Graves JW, Bloomfield RL, Buckalew VM Jr: Plasma volume in resistant hypertension: guide to pathophysiology and therapy. *Am J Med Sci* 1989; 298:361–365.
16. Ram CVS: Hypertensive crisis. In: Hurst JW (ed): *Medicine for the Practicing Physician*, 4th ed. Stamford, CT, Appleton & Lange, 1996:1086–1092.
17. Kaplan NM: Hypertensive crisis. In: Kaplan NM (ed): *Clinical Hypertension*, 6th ed. Baltimore, Williams & Wilkins, 1994:281–297.
18. Hall WD: Hypertensive crisis. In: Kassirer JP (ed): *Current Therapy in Adult Medicine*, 4th ed. St. Louis, Mosby-YearBook, 1997:587–590.
19. Fagan TC: Acute reduction of blood pressure in asymptomatic patients with severe hypertension. An idea whose time has come—and gone. *Arch Intern Med* 1989; 149:2169–2170.
20. Houston MC: Treatment of hypertensive emergencies and urgencies with oral clonidine loading and titration. A review. *Arch Intern Med* 1986; 146:586–589.
21. Atkin SH, Jaker MA, Beaty P, et al: Oral labetalol versus oral clonidine in the emergency treatment of severe hypertension. *Am J Med Sci* 1992; 303:9–15.

LOUIS L. BATTEY

DONALD ST. CLAIRE, JR.

CHAPTER

# MITRAL AND AORTIC VALVE DISEASE

32

## MITRAL STENOSIS

Mitral stenosis is the obstruction of blood flow from the left atrium into the left ventricle caused by a narrowed mitral orifice. The most common etiology of mitral stenosis is rheumatic heart disease. Rare causes of mitral stenosis are congenital deformities, atrial myxoma, large thrombus, vegetations, calcified mitral annulus and leaflets, chronic methylsergide therapy, and appetite-suppressing drugs.[1,2] Mitral stenosis occurs more often in females than in males by a 2:1 ratio.

### Pathophysiology

Rheumatic fever results in scarring and contracture of the leaflets and chordae tendineae. Adhesion and fusion of the commissure and shortening of the chordae restrict motion of the two leaflets and cause them to be tethered in a downward position. The leaflets become thickened and may calcify, further restricting their mobility.[1]

The normal mitral valve area in the adult is 4 to 6 $cm^2$. A pressure gradient across the mitral valve is produced as the mitral valve area falls below 2 $cm^2$. Left atrial pressure rises and will continue to increase as the valve area decreases. The increased left atrial pressure is transmitted to the pulmonary vasculature, leading to pulmonary hypertension. Right ventricular pressure overload may occur and cause right ventricular failure.[1,3]

Heart rate and cardiac output influence the hemodynamics of mitral stenosis. An increase in heart rate reduces the time for left ventricular filling and increases left atrial pressure. Therefore, symptoms usually occur with physical activity and may worsen during conditions such as rapid atrial fibrillation, pregnancy, fever, or emotional upset.[1]

Left ventricular size is normal in patients with isolated mitral stenosis. Left ventricular enlargement suggests coexisting mitral regurgitation, aortic valve disease, or cardiomyopathy. Left ventricular contractility is usually normal in mitral stenosis, but some patients have a reduced ejection fraction.[3] Contributing factors include extension of the rheumatic scarring process into the myocardium, ischemic heart disease, and leftward displacement of the interventricular septum caused by the overloaded right ventricle.[1,2] In addition, the ejection fraction may be impaired by the chronic reduction in preload and an increased afterload resulting from a reduced cardiac output and a reflex increase in systemic vascular resistance.[3]

## Symptoms

The average age at the time of the initial attack of rheumatic fever is 12 years old.[1] In the United States and Europe, symptoms occur 15 to 20 years later, and it takes approximately 3 years for patients to progress from class II to class III or IV symptoms.[2] The age at onset of symptoms may be younger and the rate of progression of symptoms much faster in underdeveloped areas, for unexplained reasons.[1,2] Approximately 50 percent of patients develop symptoms gradually, while others experience a much more rapid onset of symptoms, often precipitated by atrial fibrillation.[1]

Dyspnea is the most prominent symptom of mitral stenosis. Orthopnea, paroxysmal nocturnal dyspnea, and congestive heart failure (CHF) develop as the stenosis worsens. Angina pectoris is uncommon in mitral stenosis and may be due to right ventricular ischemia or coronary atherosclerosis.[1,2] Systemic thromboembolism can occur in the setting of chronic or paroxysmal atrial fibrillation and may be the initial manifestation of mitral stenosis. Hemoptysis is caused by rupture of thin-walled bronchial veins and may occur with sudden rises in pulmonary venous pressure.[2] Hoarseness may result from compression of the left recurrent laryngeal nerve by an enlarged left atrium.[1,2]

## Physical Examination

The apical impulse is unremarkable, but a right ventricular lift in the left parasternal area may be felt if pulmonary hypertension is present. The peripheral pulses are normal except in patients with low cardiac output, where the amplitude is small.[1] Patients in sinus rhythm have a prominent a wave in the jugular pulse, whereas those in atrial fibrillation have a prominent v or c-v wave.[2] A prominent v wave may also be present in patients with tricuspid regurgitation.

The principal auscultatory findings in mitral stenosis are an accentuated first heart sound ($S_1$), an opening snap, and a diastolic murmur (rumble).[1–3] Accentuation of $S_1$ occurs if the leaflets are flexible; however, as the leaflets calcify and become rigid, the first sound diminishes in intensity. $S_1$ is loud because the valve leaflets are held open by the transmittal gradient until the force of ventricular systole closes the valve.[3]

The opening snap is a high-pitched sound in early diastole, heard best at the left lower sternal border and cardiac apex with the diaphragm of the stethoscope. It is produced by sudden tensing of the valve leaflets as the valve cusps reach their maximum excursion within the left ventricle.[1,2] The higher the left atrial pressure, the shorter the interval between the second heart sound and the opening snap.

The diastolic rumble is a low-pitched murmur, heard best at the cardiac apex with the bell of the stethoscope. The murmur may be accentuated by exercise or by turning the patient in the left lateral decubitus position. The severity of the mitral obstruction correlates with the duration of the murmur, rather than its intensity. The murmur becomes accentuated in late diastole as transvalvular blood flow is accentuated by atrial contraction.[1,2]

Pulmonary hypertension that develops as a result of severe mitral stenosis may result in elevated neck veins, ascites, and edema.[1–3] Auscultatory findings associated with pulmonary hypertension include accentuation of the pulmonic component of the second heart sound, a pulmonic ejection sound caused by dilatation of the pulmonary artery, a diastolic decrescendo murmur of pulmonary regurgitation (Graham Steell's murmur), a systolic murmur of tricuspid regurgitation, and a right atrial gallop.[1–3]

## Electrocardiogram

A left atrial abnormality is present if the patient is in sinus rhythm. Atrial fibrillation eventually occurs in approximately 50 percent of patients. A vertical or rightward mean QRS axis and right ventricular hypertrophy occur as pulmonary hypertension develops (Fig. 32-1).

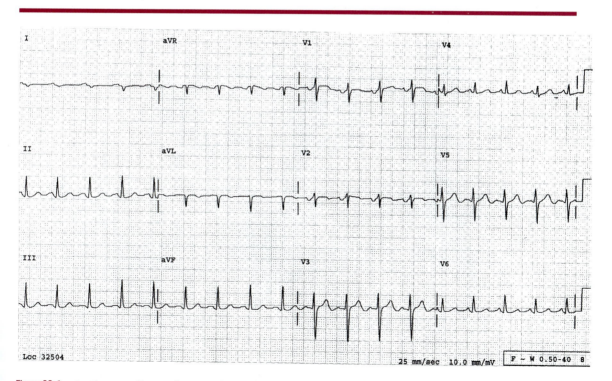

Figure 32-1　An electrocardiogram from a patient with severe mitral stenosis. There is sinus rhythm, left atrial abnormality, and a rightward mean QRS axis. The R wave in lead $V_1$ is 4 mm, which is greater than usual.

## Chest Roentgenogram

The major radiologic findings are left atrial enlargement and pulmonary venous hypertension. Pulmonary hypertension causes enlargement of the pulmonary arteries and right ventricle. Right ventricular enlargement is best seen on the lateral x-ray. The left ventricle is normal in size in isolated mitral stenosis. Calcium may be seen in the area of the mitral valve (Fig. 32-2).

## Diagnosis

Two-dimensional echocardiography with Doppler is the diagnostic test of choice and reveals diastolic doming of the thickened leaflets as well as restriction of leaflet motion. The mitral orifice size can be measured and the mitral apparatus evaluated for suitability for mitral balloon valvuloplasty.[1–3] Doppler studies accurately determine the transvalvular gradient, mitral valve area, and pulmonary artery pressure. Color-flow imaging provides further information on other valve lesions, especially mitral regurgitation. Cardiac catheterization provides data on the mitral valve gradient, cardiac output, and mitral valve area. There is usually good correlation between echocardiographic data and catheterization findings, and cardiac catheterization may not be needed in younger patients unless coronary angiography is required.

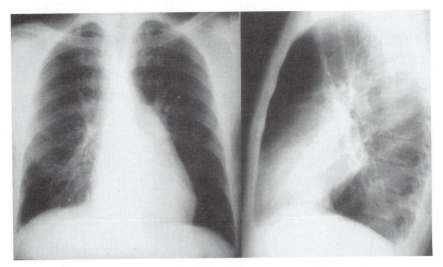

A

B

**Figure 32-2**    Posteroanterior (*A*) and lateral (*B*) chest x-ray films from a patient with mitral stenosis. The left atrial appendage is enlarged and causes a straight left heart border in *A* and protrusion of the large left atrium toward the thoracic vertebrae in *B*. Left ventricular size is normal.

## Treatment

Rheumatic fever prophylaxis is indicated for patients with rheumatic mitral stenosis. All patients with mitral stenosis should also receive endocarditis prophylaxis.[1-3] (See Chaps. 24 and 38.)

Conditions that cause tachycardia, such as fever or anemia, should be treated promptly. Diuretics and sodium restriction are indicated for symptoms of pulmonary congestion.[2] The onset of atrial fibrillation usually results in a worsening of symptoms and often leads to congestive heart failure. Control of the ventricular response is very important. Digoxin is widely used, and the combination of digoxin and a beta blocker is especially effective in blunting exercise-induced tachycardia.[1] The calcium antagonists diltiazem and verapamil may also be used intravenously or orally for rate control. A reasonable goal is a resting heart rate of 60 to 70 beats per minute.[1,2] Every effort should be made to restore and maintain normal sinus rhythm after the onset of atrial fibrillation, but 3 to 4 weeks of oral anticoagulation is indicated both before and after electrical or pharmacologic cardioversion to prevent systemic embolization. Oral anticoagulation with warfarin is indicated in all patients with mitral stenosis and either chronic or paroxysmal atrial fibrillation.[1-3]

Asymptomatic patients or those with minimal physical limitations can be observed. Patients with more than mild symptoms or evidence of pulmonary hypertension should be offered mechanical relief of the mitral valve obstruction. Echocardiography is extremely helpful in determining which type of procedure is most appropriate. Patients with rigid, thickened, calcified valves; extensive subvalvular fibrosis; or significant mitral regurgitation usually require mitral valve replacement. Open mitral commissurotomy (valvulotomy) using cardiopulmonary bypass or mitral balloon valvuloplasty is a reasonable approach in patients with pliable, less-calcified valves and no significant mitral regurgitation. Mitral balloon valvuloplasty is now widely used in patients with these valvular characteristics and no left atrial thrombus seen by transesophageal echocardiography. During mitral balloon valvuloplasty, a catheter is inserted into the femoral vein and advanced into the right atrium. The interatrial septum is punctured and the opening enlarged. One large or two small balloons are advanced across the mitral orifice and inflated.[1,2] The procedure results in improved hemodynamics, a reduction in symptoms, and improved exercise tolerance. The 3-year restenosis rate is approximately 10 percent.[2] Potential complications include a small atrial septal defect, embolic events, significant mitral regurgitation, and cardiac perforation.

# MITRAL REGURGITATION

## Definition

Mitral regurgitation is the retrograde flow of blood from the left ventricle into the left atrium as a result of inadequate closure of the mitral valve leaflets.[1]

## Chronic Mitral Regurgitation

**PATHOPHYSIOLOGY.**[4] Chronic mitral regurgitation results in volume overload to the left ventricle and the left atrium. As the mitral regurgitation slowly progresses, the left atrium dilates, becomes more compliant, and blunts the rise in left atrial pressure. Pulmonary venous hypertension develops late in the course of this disease, and patients are often asymptomatic for years. Eventually the atrium may become thin-walled with increased amounts of fibrous tissue, and atrial fibrillation may occur. The left ventricle enlarges through a combination of dilatation and hypertrophy to accommodate a larger end-diastolic volume. Initially, contractility and ejection fraction remain normal as the low-pressure left atrium reduces impedance to the ventricular ejection. Eventually, however, left ventricular contractility declines and left ventricular end-diastolic pressure increases. This further contributes to the elevated left atrial pressure and leads to an increase in pulmonary artery pressure.

Mitral regurgitation causes structural changes within the left atrium, left ventricle, and mitral apparatus that lead to progressive regurgitation. The left atrium is continuous with the posterior leaflet, and the posterior cusp becomes distorted as the left atrium dilates. Enlargement of the left ventricle results in dilatation of the mitral annulus and lateral displacement of the papillary muscles. Traction on the chordae tendineae and leaflets is abnormal, and the regurgitation worsens.

**ETIOLOGY.** The mitral valve apparatus is a complex structure; it is composed of the valve leaflets, annulus, chordae tendineae, papillary muscles, and adjacent atrial and ventricular myocardium. Mitral valve competence depends on the normal function of these structures, and any abnormality in one of these components may cause mitral regurgitation.[1]

Mitral regurgitation, both acute and chronic, is caused by a diverse group of disease processes (Table 32-1). The most common causes of chronic mitral regurgitation are

- *Mitral valve prolapse* (see the section on Mitral Valve Prolapse). This is the most common cause of pure mitral regurgitation in the western world.[5]
- *Left ventricular dilatation*. This condition occurs in dilated cardiomyopathy, hypertensive heart disease, coronary artery disease (CAD), and valvular heart disease. As the left ventricle dilates, the normal relationship between the papillary muscles, chordae tendineae, and mitral leaflets is altered, and mitral regurgitation results.
- *Coronary artery disease*. Acute myocardial infarction (AMI) may result in papillary muscle rupture, leading to acute mitral regurgitation. More commonly, myocardial infarction (MI) or ischemia causes papillary muscle dysfunction and hypokinesis or akinesis of the adjacent left ventricular myocardium. This altered left ventricular geometry may also cause mitral annular dilatation.[6] Enlargement of the annulus and distortion of the alignment of the papillary muscles and the chordae tendineae produce the regurgitation.[1]

**TABLE 32-1.   Common Etiologies of Mitral Regurgitation**

| Chronic Regurgitation | Acute Regurgitation |
|---|---|
| Myxomatous degeneration (mitral valve prolapse) | Myxomatous degeneration (mitral valve prolapse) |
| Left ventricular dilatation | Acute myocardial ischemia or infarction |
| Coronary artery disease | Acute infective endocarditis |
| Rheumatic heart disease | Trauma |
| Mitral annular calcification | |
| Infective endocarditis | |

- *Rheumatic heart disease.* This remains the leading cause of chronic mitral regurgitation in many underdeveloped countries. The rheumatic process results in fusion and calcification of the commissure and deformity and retraction of the leaflets.[1] In addition, there may be shortening and fusion of chordae tendineae and papillary muscles, infiltration of the papillary muscles, and annular dilatation.[6]
- *Calcification of the mitral annulus.* The elderly, especially females, are often affected. Other predisposing conditions include chronic renal failure, diabetes mellitus, hypertension, aortic stenosis, and rheumatic heart disease. The annular calcification is mostly subvalvular and prevents the normal constriction of the annulus during systole. In addition, the basal portion of the leaflets may be immobile, which prevents normal diastolic excursion and normal systolic coaptation.[6] On rare occasions, mitral annular calcification may cause mitral stenosis.
- *Infective endocarditis.* This may result in acute or chronic mitral regurgitation as a result of perforation of a valve leaflet or rupture of chordae tendineae. Large vegetations may interfere with normal coaptation of the leaflets. The healing process in endocarditis may cause retraction of the mitral cusps, leading to regurgitation.[6]

**SYMPTOMS.**   Patients with chronic mitral regurgitation are often asymptomatic for many years. When symptoms develop, exertional dyspnea and fatigue are common. Orthopnea and paroxysmal nocturnal dyspnea imply severe mitral regurgitation with left ventricular dysfunction. Angina pectoris is an uncommon symptom, and its presence suggests coexisting coronary artery disease or aortic valve disease. Patients with atrial fibrillation may experience palpitations. Sudden worsening of symptoms may occur with the onset of atrial fibrillation, chordal rupture, or myocardial ischemia.[7]

**PHYSICAL EXAMINATION.**   The carotid pulsation in chronic severe mitral regurgitation is sharp, unlike the delayed carotid upstroke in aortic stenosis, and this finding can be helpful in differentiating these two valvular lesions.[2] The apical impulse is diffuse, hyperdynamic, and displaced laterally and inferiorly. A right ventricular impulse may be palpitated along the left sternal border.

The intensity of the first heart sound is diminished. There is increased splitting of the second sound as a result of shortened left ventricular ejection and early aortic valve closure. The third heart sound is often present and suggests that the mitral regurgitation is severe. The third heart sound is caused by rapid ventricular filling and does not necessarily imply CHF.[3] A diastolic rumble may be present as a result of increased flow across the mitral valve. A fourth heart sound is not usually present in chronic mitral regurgitation but can occur in acute mitral regurgitation.

The primary auscultatory finding is a high-pitched, blowing, holosystolic murmur, heard best at the cardiac apex with the diaphragm of the stethoscope. The murmur usually radiates to the axilla and to the left infrascapular area, but abnormalities of the posterior leaflet may cause the murmur to radiate to the sternum or aortic area. The murmur is usually constant in intensity and is not affected by respiration, the cycle length variations of atrial fibrillation, or a premature beat.[1,2,4] This contrasts with aortic outflow tract murmurs, which increase in intensity after a premature beat. The severity of the regurgitation does not correlate with the intensity of the murmur. Patients with mitral regurgitation caused by mitral valve prolapse, papillary muscle dysfunction, or hypertrophic cardiomyopathy often have murmurs only in late systole.[1,2,4]

**ELECTROCARDIOGRAM.**   Atrial fibrillation is common, and left ventricular hypertrophy is seen in approximately 50 percent of cases.[2] Patients in sinus rhythm will have left atrial enlargement. ST-segment changes are nonspecific and may be due to hypertrophy, coronary artery disease, cardiomyopathy, or mitral valve prolapse.[1]

**CHEST ROENTGENOGRAM.**   Enlargement of the left ventricle and left atrium are the characteristic findings in chronic mitral regurgitation. Left atrial enlargement results in elevation of the left main stem bronchus, double density along the right heart border, and a straight left heart border. A calcified mitral annulus may be present, especially in the elderly (Fig. 32-3).

**DIAGNOSIS.**   Two-dimensional echocardiography with Doppler examination is the diagnostic modality of choice in the evaluation of mitral regurgitation. Echocardiography can evaluate the size and function of the cardiac chambers, as well as the structure and integrity of the leaflets, chordae tendineae, papillary muscles, and annulus. Color-flow Doppler examination can estimate the severity of the mitral regurgitation and the degree of pulmonary hypertension. Transesophageal echocardiography provides a more accurate assessment of the severity of mitral regurgitation, especially in the presence of a mechanical prosthetic valve, and is also very useful in the operating room in assessing the adequacy of mitral valve repair. Left ventricular cineangiography is also used to assess the degree of mitral regurgitation as well as left ventricular size and function.[1]

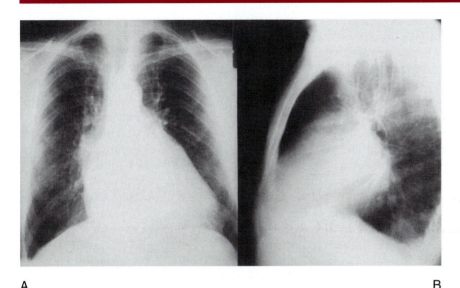

A                                                                        B

Figure 32-3    Posteroanterior (*A*) and lateral (*B*) chest x-rays from a patient with chronic severe mitral regurgitation. Both the left ventricle and the left atrium are enlarged.

**MEDICAL THERAPY.**    Asymptomatic patients with chronic mitral regurgitation may benefit from the use of vasodilators such as hydralazine or angiotensin-converting enzyme inhibitors.[1,3] These drugs reduce the impedance to ejection into the aorta and decrease the volume of blood that is ejected into the left atrium.[2] However, it has not been proved that these drugs slow the progressive deterioration of left ventricular function or delay the need for surgical intervention.[1,3]

Symptomatic patients with chronic mitral regurgitation should be treated with digitalis, diuretics, and vasodilators. Digitalis is especially useful for slowing the ventricular response if atrial fibrillation is present. Beta-adrenergic blocking drugs, diltiazem, and verapamil may also be used to slow the ventricular response if left ventricular function is adequate. Patients with atrial fibrillation should receive anticoagulation with warfarin to reduce the risk of systemic embolization. Endocarditis prophylaxis is indicated in all patients with mitral regurgitation, and rheumatic fever prophylaxis is indicated in patients with rheumatic heart disease.[1,2]

**SURGICAL TREATMENT.**    Advances in surgical techniques and the increasing use of mitral valve reconstructive procedures have resulted in a more aggressive approach to the surgical therapy of chronic mitral regurgitation. Mitral valve repair is now possible in the majority of patients with chronic mitral regurgitation and results in improved postoperative left ventricular function and reduced operative mortality compared with mitral valve replacement.[8] Valve repair is more successful in patients with mitral regurgitation caused by myxomatous transformation, annular dilatation, and papillary muscle dysfunction resulting from coronary disease. Patients with rigid, calcified valves of rheumatic heart disease or a history of infective endocarditis usually require valve replacement.[1,2]

The timing of mitral valve surgery in chronic mitral regurgitation is difficult. Preoperative left ventricular function is the main determinant of postoperative outcome, and surgery is indicated before any irreversible left ventricular dysfunction occurs. Mitral valve surgery is recommended for patients with chronic severe mitral regurgitation and class II symptoms, i.e., symptoms with heavy exertion.[2]

Asymptomatic patients with moderate to severe mitral regurgitation are more problematic. They should be followed with serial echocardiography every 6 to 12 months, and mitral valve surgery should be considered when echocardiographic studies indicate progressive left ventricular enlargement and/or systolic dysfunction.[8] An ejection fraction below 60 percent or a left ventricular end-systolic dimension of >45 mm should prompt consideration of mitral valve surgery.[2,3,7,8] Patients older than 75 years should be considered for mitral valve surgery only for symptoms.[2] Cardiac catheterization and left ventriculography are usually needed prior to mitral valve surgery to confirm the severity of the mitral regurgitation, assess left ventricular function, determine the presence of coronary artery disease, and look for coexistent valve lesions.[2]

## Acute Mitral Regurgitation

Acute mitral regurgitation is distinctly different from chronic mitral regurgitation with respect to pathophysiology, clinical presentation, physical examination, and treatment. However, acute mitral regurgitation is caused by the same disease processes that under other circumstances cause chronic mitral regurgitation.[2]

**ETIOLOGY.**

- *Myxomatous transformation* may result in spontaneous rupture of one or more chordae tendineae. This is most commonly seen in middle-aged and older men. (See the section on Mitral Valve Prolapse.)
- *Infective endocarditis* may cause destruction of a valve leaflet or rupture of chordae tendineae. Large vegetations may interfere with normal coaptation of the leaflets.
- *Acute myocardial infarction* may result in severe papillary muscle dysfunction or rupture of a portion of the papillary muscle. Papillary muscle rupture is more common in inferoposterior infarctions and involves the posteromedial papillary muscle more commonly than the anterior papillary muscle by a ratio of 4:1.[1] Papillary muscle rupture complicates 1 to 5 percent of acute infarctions and usually appears 2 to 7 days after the acute event.[6]
- *Trauma* may cause rupture of a papillary muscle, the chordae tendineae, or a valve leaflet.

**PATHOPHYSIOLOGY.**   The left ventricle and left atrium are usually unable to handle the sudden volume overload of acute mitral regurgitation. The acute regurgitant flow rapidly increases left atrial pressure, and the noncompliant left atrium cannot dilate to prevent this large increase in atrial pressure. The increased pressure is transmitted back into the pulmonary vasculature, resulting in dyspnea and pulmonary edema.[6]

**CLINICAL PRESENTATION.**   Patients with acute mitral regurgitation are usually very ill. Severe dyspnea is the major symptom, and tachycardia and hypotension are often present. The chest x-ray demonstrates a relatively normal-sized cardiac silhouette and pulmonary edema. The electrocardiogram may show nonspecific changes, but evidence of a recent AMI should be sought. Fever and/or evidence of systemic embolization suggest bacterial endocarditis.

The cardiac examination is often subtle and may be hindered by the patient's tachycardia and tachypnea. The apical impulse is hyperdynamic but not displaced. The markedly elevated left atrial pressure reduces the pressure gradient between the left ventricle and left atrium in late systole. Therefore, the murmur is usually not holosystolic but decrescendo, ending before the second heart sound, and it is lower-pitched and softer than the murmur of chronic mitral regurgitation.[2] The murmur may radiate to the base if the posterior mitral valve leaflet is affected. Atrial gallops ($S_4$) and ventricular gallops ($S_3$) are common.

**DIAGNOSIS.**   Two-dimensional echocardiography with color-flow Doppler examination is the diagnostic modality of choice. The integrity and function of the mitral valve leaflets, chordae tendineae, papillary muscles, and left ventricle can be evaluated. Vegetations can be visualized, and the severity of the mitral regurgitation can be estimated. Transesophageal echocardiography may be helpful if the severity of the mitral regurgitation is in question, to exclude the presence of small vegetations and to further evaluate the functional integrity of the mitral valve apparatus.

The severity of the mitral regurgitation and left ventricular function can be confirmed by left ventricular cineangiography. Coronary anatomy can be evaluated at this time, and this is especially important in patients with acute mitral regurgitation following an acute myocardial infarction.

**TREATMENT.**   The initial medical management of acute mitral regurgitation is afterload reduction and diuresis. Afterload reduction with vasodilators such as sodium nitroprusside, angiotensin-converting enzyme inhibitors, or hydralazine lowers the impedance to ejection into the aorta and reduces the volume of blood ejected into the left atrium. In addition, diuretics and vasodilators decrease left ventricular volume and reduce the diameter of the mitral annulus.[1,2] Patients with infective endocarditis should receive appropriate antibiotics. (See Chap. 24.)

Intraaortic balloon counterpulsation may be very effective in stabilizing patients with acute mitral regurgitation. Pulmonary edema refractory to medical therapy, hemodynamic instability, and ongoing myocardial ischemia are indications for intraaortic balloon counterpulsation. Urgent mitral valve surgery, usually valve replacement, is necessary if patients cannot be stabilized with medical therapy or intraaortic balloon counterpulsation.

# MITRAL VALVE PROLAPSE

Mitral valve prolapse is the abnormal systolic billowing of one or both of the mitral valve leaflets into the left atrium. It is the most common valvular abnormality in industrialized nations, with a prevalence of 3 to 5 percent of adults.[1,2] Females are affected twice as often as males.

Mitral valve prolapse is usually a primary condition and is not associated with other diseases. Inheritance is autosomal dominant with varying penetrance, but isolated cases also occur. Mitral valve prolapse is very common in inherited connective tissue diseases such as Marfan syndrome, Ehlers-Danlos syndrome, pseudoxanthoma elasticum, and osteogenesis imperfecta.

The principal pathologic defect in primary mitral valve prolapse is the abnormal synthesis and breakdown of valvular elastic fibers.[5] This leads to a loss of fibrous and elastic tissue and marked proliferation of the acid mucopolysaccharide-containing spongiosa layer of the leaflets (myxomatous proliferation).[1,9,10] The basic support of the leaflets is weakened, and they become thickened and redundant. This process may also result in thinning and elongation of the chordae tendineae and an increase in the size of the mitral annulus.[9] (See Fig. 32-4.)

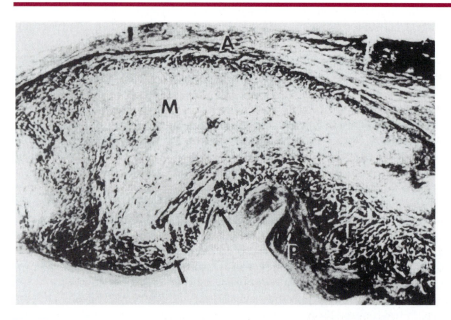

Figure 32-4   Histopathology of a myxomatous valve. Atrial surface at the top, ventricular surface at the bottom. Histologic levels, top to bottom: A = atrialis, with fibrosis; M = large zone of loose myxomatous tissue; F = valve fibrosa, disrupted by myxomatous tissue, at arrows; P = fibrous pads of ventricular endocardium. (Reproduced with permission from Fontana ME, Sparks EA, Boudoulas H, Wooley CF: Mitral valve prolapse and the mitral valve prolapse syndrome. *Curr Probl Cardiol* 1991; 16:327.)

Secondary mitral valve prolapse occurs in the absence of myxomatous proliferation. The valve leaflets are functionally, rather than morphologically, abnormal. Coronary artery disease, rheumatic heart disease, hypertrophic cardiomyopathy, low body weight, atrial septal defect, and low intravascular volume may cause mitral valve prolapse by a variety of mechanisms, especially if the left ventricle is small in relation to the mitral apparatus.[1,2,5]

## Associated Conditions

Tricuspid valve prolapse occurs in 40 percent of patients with mitral valve prolapse. Prolapse of the pulmonic and aortic valves is much less common. Patients with mitral valve prolapse have an increased incidence of atrioventricular bypass tracts and secundum atrial septal defects.[1,2,11]

There is an increased incidence of mitral valve prolapse in patients with asthenic body habitus and a variety of thoracic skeletal abnormalities, such as straight thoracic spine, scoliosis, pectus excavatum, and a narrowed anteroposterior chest diameter. This association suggests that mitral valve prolapse may be the cardiovascular manifestation of a generalized developmental disorder of connective tissue, as the mitral and tricuspid valves, the thoracic vertebrae, and the sternum and ribs develop in the seventh week of embryonic life.[11]

## Symptoms

Most patients with mitral valve prolapse are asymptomatic. Many patients, however, complain of a variety of symptoms, including palpitations, nonanginal chest pain, dyspnea, fatigability, and panic attacks. Controlled studies, however, have demonstrated that these symptoms, with the exception of palpitations, are not truly linked to mitral valve prolapse.[5,10] Autonomic nervous system dysfunction appears to be weakly associated with mitral valve prolapse. This phenomenon may result in low blood volume, leading to syncope or presyncope, and may explain the low resting blood pressure in some patients with mitral valve prolapse.[5]

## Physical Examination

The characteristic auscultatory feature of mitral valve prolapse is a mid-systolic click. This high-pitched sound is heard best with the diaphragm of the stethoscope at the left lower sternal border or cardiac apex. Multiple clicks may be present. Sudden tensing of the chordae tendineae and the prolapsing of the mitral leaflets produce the click.[1,2,11] The click is often followed by an apical late systolic murmur that is crescendo to the second heart sound. The murmur may have a musical or honking quality.[11] The systolic murmur is produced by mitral regurgitation due to failure of the mitral leaflets to coapt properly.

The auscultatory features of mitral valve prolapse are variable. Some 20 to 30 percent of patients will not have a click or a murmur on a single examination.[5] Reexaminations may reveal an isolated click, multiple clicks, and/or a systolic murmur.

The diagnosis of mitral valve prolapse can be confirmed by dynamic ausculta-tion—changes in the timing of the click and murmur with various physiologic and pharmacologic maneuvers. For this reason, patients should be examined supine, sit-ting, standing, and squatting.

The timing in systole and the intensity of the click and/or murmur are determined by the left ventricular end-diastolic volume and ventricular contractility.[1,2,11] Ma-neuvers that decrease left ventricular end-diastolic volume, increase myocardial contractility, or decrease resistance to left ventricular ejection cause the mitral leaflets to prolapse earlier in systole, and the click and murmur move closer to the first heart sound. Such maneuvers include standing from the supine position, the Valsalva maneuver, and inhalation of amyl nitrate. Maneuvers that increase left ven-tricular volume, reduce myocardial contractility, or increase left ventricular after-load cause the click and/or murmur to move closer to the second heart sound. This occurs with squatting, handgrip, or slowing of the heart rate.[1,2,11] (See Fig. 32-5.)

## Electrocardiogram

Most patients with mitral valve prolapse have a normal resting electrocardiogram. The most common electrocardiographic abnormalities are T-wave inversion and/or ST-segment depression in the inferior leads. These repolarization changes are more common in mitral valve prolapse patients with ventricular arrhythmias.[1,2]

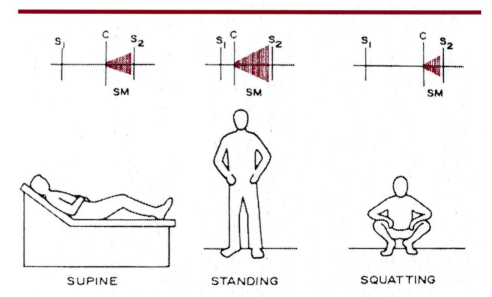

**Figure 32-5**   Schematic diagram showing the effects of standing and squatting on the mid-systolic click–late systolic murmur in a patient with mitral valve prolapse. Standing causes the click to move closer to the first heart sound ($S_1$) and the murmur to get longer and louder. Squatting causes the click to move closer to the second heart sound ($S_2$) and the murmur to get shorter and softer. (Reproduced with permission from Schlant RC, Felner JM, Mikolzek CL, et al: Mitral valve prolapse. *Dis Mon* 1980; 26:25.)

## Echocardiogram

Two-dimensional echocardiography is very helpful in confirming the diagnosis, but strict criteria should be used. Echocardiography is highly specific for mitral valve prolapse but may have a false-negative rate of 10 to 20 percent.[11] Color-flow Doppler examination provides an excellent estimate of the degree of mitral regurgitation. Echocardiography also provides important prognostic information. Complications such as infective endocarditis and significant mitral regurgitation are most common in patients with thickened, redundant leaflets, and serial examinations can be used to follow the progression of mitral regurgitation.[1,2,5]

## Complications

Mitral valve prolapse is a benign condition in the great majority of patients. Serious complications, however, may occur and are more common in men, older patients, and those with thickened, redundant leaflets. The cumulative risk for all complications of mitral valve prolapse by age 75 is 2 to 5 percent for women and 5 to 10 percent for men.[5]

**MITRAL REGURGITATION.**   Mitral valve prolapse is now the most common valvular cause of severe mitral regurgitation in industrialized countries.[5] The incidence of severe mitral regurgitation increases with age; it is more common in men and in patients with thickened, redundant leaflets. By age 75, 1 to 2 percent of women and 5 to 6 percent of men with mitral valve prolapse will develop mitral regurgitation severe enough to warrant valve surgery.[5] Hypertension and obesity may contribute to the progression of the mitral regurgitation.[5] The mechanism of the progressive regurgitation is rupture of chordae tendineae and/or stretching and distortion of the leaflets and annulus. Some patients exhibit a slow progression of their mitral regurgitation, while others abruptly worsen as chordae tendineae rupture. Progressive mitral regurgitation causes enlargement of the left atrium, and atrial fibrillation may occur.

**INFECTIVE ENDOCARDITIS.**   Some 1 percent of patients with mitral valve prolapse will develop this complication by age 75.[5] Predisposing conditions include male gender, the presence of mitral regurgitation, and age greater than 45 years.[1,2,5]

**NEUROLOGIC EVENTS.**   Transient ischemic attacks, amaurosis fugax, and cerebral infarction are more common in patients with mitral valve prolapse, especially women under 45 years of age. However, these events occur in less than 1 percent of the population with mitral valve prolapse.[9] Smoking and the use of oral contraceptives may be contributing factors.[1] Platelet-fibrin complexes that form on denuded areas of endothelium have been identified pathologically in patients with mitral valve prolapse who have cerebral ischemic events.[5] Embolic events are more frequent in patients with significant mitral regurgitation, an enlarged left atrium and left ventricle, atrial arrhythmias, and CHF.[6]

**ARRHYTHMIAS.**   The incidence of arrhythmias in patients with mitral valve prolapse varies between 40 and 75 percent.[1] Most of the arrhythmias are benign and consist of sinus tachycardia and isolated premature atrial and ventricular contractions. Serious supraventricular and ventricular arrhythmias may occur. Complex ventricular arrhythmias appear to be more common in patients with inferior ST-T-wave changes on the resting electrocardiogram. There is an increased incidence of atrioventricular bypass tracts in patients with mitral valve prolapse.[1,2]

**SUDDEN DEATH.**   Mitral valve prolapse appears to very slightly increase the risk of sudden death.[1,2,5] Risk factors for this catastrophic event include severe mitral regurgitation, severe valve deformity, left ventricular dysfunction, complex ventricular ectopy, Q-T-interval prolongation, and a history of syncope.[2] The presumed etiology of sudden death is ventricular fibrillation, but bradyarrhythmias and asystole have been reported.[1,2]

## Management

The severity of mitral regurgitation determines the need for active treatment and more frequent follow-up.[5] Younger women with only a mid-systolic click and a late systolic murmur or no murmur are at particularly low risk for complications.[11] Such low-risk patients require only reassurance and infrequent follow-up. Older patients, especially men and patients with significant mitral regurgitation, have an increased risk of complications and should be evaluated clinically and with Doppler echocardiography more frequently (Table 32-2).

Patients with severe mitral regurgitation require mitral valve surgery at a rate of 10 percent per year.[8] Mitral valve repair is often possible. The timing of mitral valve surgery is difficult, but it should be performed before any decline in left ventricular function occurs.

Endocarditis prophylaxis for dental or surgical procedures is indicated in patients with an audible murmur or evidence of mitral regurgitation by Doppler echocardiography. Patients with an isolated systolic click and no murmur and no evidence of mitral regurgitation by Doppler echocardiography do not appear to need antibiotic prophylaxis, although this is controversial (Fig. 32-6).[12]

Patients with symptoms of distressing palpitations, presyncope, or syncope should be evaluated for serious arrhythmias by ambulatory electrocardiography or electrophysiological testing. Symptomatic isolated premature supraventricular or ventricular complexes or nonsustained episodes of supraventricular tachycardia may be controlled with beta-blocker therapy, which usually can be low-dose. Beta-blocker therapy may also improve the symptoms of chest pain, anxiety, and fatigue. Orthostatic symptoms may be improved by liberalizing fluid and salt intake, but support stockings and/or mineralocorticoid therapy may be needed.[1]

Aspirin therapy (80 to 325 mg/day) is indicated for patients with mitral valve prolapse and suspected cerebral emboli. Cigarettes and oral contraceptives should be avoided. Anticoagulant therapy with warfarin may be needed if focal cerebral symptoms occur despite aspirin therapy.[1]

**TABLE 32-2.   Matching Risk and Management in Patients with Mitral Valve Prolapse**

| Risk Level | Patients | Management |
|---|---|---|
| Lowest | Subjects without mitral regurgitant murmurs or regurgitation revealed by Doppler echocardiography, especially women younger than age 45 | Reassurance; periodontal antibiotics not clearly necessary and if used should not include medication with risk of allergic reaction; reevaluation and echocardiography at moderate intervals (5 years) |
| Moderate | Subjects with intermittent or persistent mitral murmurs and mild regurgitation revealed by Doppler echocardiography | Antibiotic prophylaxis with amoxicillin (unless allergic); treatment of even mild established hypertension; reevaluation and echocardiography more frequently (2 to 3 years) |
| High | Subjects with moderate or severe mitral regurgitation | Antibiotic prophylaxis with amoxicillin (unless allergic); optimization of afterload (arterial pressure); reevaluation with Doppler echocardiography and other tests if needed annually; consider valve repair or replacement for exertional dyspnea or decline of left ventricular function into low-normal range |

*Source:* Adapted with permission from Devereux RB, Kligfield P: Mitral valve prolapse. In Rakel RE (ed): *Current Therapy 1992.* Philadelphia, Saunders, 1992:237–241.

# AORTIC STENOSIS

Aortic stenosis is the obstruction of blood flow from the left ventricle into the aorta caused by narrowing of the aortic valve orifice. Impedance to left ventricular outflow may also result from supravalvular obstruction due to congenital heart disease or from subvalvular obstruction as occurs with hypertrophic obstructive cardiomyopathy or congenital membranous subaortic stenosis. These entities need to be considered during the evaluation and treatment of the patient with suspected aortic stenosis, but are much less common. Calcific aortic stenosis is currently the most common valve lesion for which valve replacement surgery is performed.[13] Nearly 30,000 patients, over 60 percent of whom are age 65 or older, undergo aortic valve replacement annually in the United States.[14] The prevalence of clinically significant aortic stenosis will almost certainly increase as the population of America continues to age. Some 25 percent of Americans are over the age of 65, and the age group over

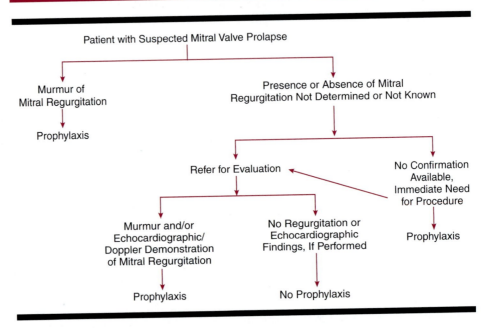

**Figure 32-6**    Clinical approach to determine the need for endocarditis prophylaxis in a patient with suspected mitral valve prolapse. (Reproduced with permission from Dajani AS, Taubert KA, Wilson W, et al: Prevention of bacterial endocarditis: Recommendations by the American Heart Association. *JAMA* 1997; 277:1796. Copyright 1997, American Medical Association.)

80 is the fastest-growing segment of the population. Fortunately, technologic advances in the diagnosis and treatment of aortic stenosis have kept pace with the growing population burdened with the disease.

## Etiology

The most common etiologies for valvular aortic stenosis are calcific disease of the elderly, congenital malformation, and rheumatic disease. The most frequently seen congenital abnormality is a bicuspid valve, which is the most common cause of aortic stenosis in young adults. Older patients most often have calcific disease of the elderly.[15] Calcific aortic valve disease of the elderly evolves from aortic valve sclerosis.[16] This condition, as well as calcific aortic stenosis, is now considered by many experts to be caused by the same process that causes atherosclerosis.

## Pathophysiology

The normal aortic valve is a three-leaflet structure with an orifice size of approximately 3.0 to 4.0 square centimeters ($cm^2$). Significant changes in circulation do not generally occur until the valve area is reduced to less than one-forth its normal size.[13,17] The degree of aortic stenosis is graded as mild if the valve area is greater than 1.5 cm$^2$, moderate for valve areas between 1.0 and 1.5 cm$^2$, and severe if the valve area is less than 1.0 cm$^2$. A valve area less than 0.75 cm$^2$ is generally considered critical.[13,17]

The development of outflow obstruction with aortic stenosis is a gradual, usually decades-long process. During this time, the left ventricle adapts to the pressure overload by increasing wall thickness while maintaining normal chamber size. This adaptive process of concentric hypertrophy allows the left ventricle to maintain a normal ejection fraction, stroke volume, and systolic wall stress despite very high intracavity systolic pressure.[13] While the progressive hypertrophy initially maintains normal systolic function, however, the left ventricle becomes less compliant and diastolic filling becomes impaired. As a consequence, the end-diastolic component of ventricular filling that is contributed by atrial contraction becomes increasingly important. Atrial contraction briefly raises left ventricular end-diastolic pressure to the higher level needed to maintain a normal stroke volume, while allowing the mean left atrial pressure to remain near normal. Loss of this atrial "booster pump" function, as in atrial fibrillation, can lead to sudden decompensation.[18] The thickened heart muscle may also be more prone to ischemia, even in the presence of normal epicardial coronary arteries. Eventually, the afterload burden imposed by severe aortic stenosis leads to a fall in stroke volume and cardiac output, ventricular dilation, elevation of diastolic filling pressures, and finally, in the terminal stages, right heart failure.[13,18,19]

## Symptoms

Aortic stenosis is characterized by a prolonged latent period, during which time the aortic valve area gradually decreases, but patients remain asymptomatic and mortality rates are very low. Long-term follow-up of patients with mild aortic stenosis shows progression to severe disease in 8 percent of patients at 10 years, 22 percent at 20 years, and 38 percent at 25 years.[20] In studies of patients with baseline moderate aortic stenosis, the average rate of decline in valve area is about 0.1 cm$^2$ per year with a concomitant increase in transvalvular gradient of about 10 to 15 mmHg per year.[13,17] The development of symptoms may be quite insidious, and the initial diagnosis is often made by the serendipitous discovery of a systolic murmur. A more abrupt onset of symptoms may occur with the development of atrial fibrillation or the imposition of a hemodynamic load such as fever, anemia, or pregnancy.[14]

The classic triad of symptoms of aortic stenosis is heart failure, angina, and syncope. Heart failure, manifested as exercise intolerance or exertional dyspnea, is the most common initial complaint. Angina may occur in the absence of obstructive coronary disease, owing to an imbalance of myocardial oxygen supply and demand. Oxygen demand is increased as a result of left ventricular hypertrophy and increased wall stress, while the capacity to increase oxygen supply is diminished as a result of reduced coronary perfusion pressure and abnormal vasomotor function.[13,14,17] Syncope, either orthostatic or exertional, may occur as a consequence of arrhythmias or inappropriate peripheral vasodilatation and consequent cerebral hypoperfusion.[14]

The onset of symptoms heralds a critical change in the natural history of aortic stenosis. While the prolonged latent period is characterized by very low morbidity and mortality, average survival after the onset of symptoms is less than 2 to 3 years.[17]

## Physical Examination

The manifestations of aortic stenosis found on physical examination depend upon the etiology of the valvular pathology, the severity of stenosis, and the contractile function of the left ventricle. The murmur of aortic stenosis can be distinguished from systolic murmurs from other causes on the basis of a number of associated features (see Table 32-3).[18]

In severe aortic stenosis, systolic blood pressure is low, with a narrow pulse pressure. The arterial pulse has a slow and sustained rise (pulsus parvus et tardus). In elderly patients with reduced peripheral arterial compliance, however, this finding may be absent or less pronounced. Conversely, severe left ventricular dysfunction may result in a diminished arterial pulse in the absence of significant aortic stenosis.[13,18] The jugular venous pulse is usually normal until the most advanced stage of disease, when severe left heart failure leads to right ventricular decompensation accompanied by tricuspid regurgitation. Precordial palpation usually demonstrates a forceful and sustained left ventricular apical impulse. A presystolic impulse of forceful left atrial filling of the left ventricle may also be felt, corresponding to a fourth heart sound heard on auscultation. When stenosis is severe, a systolic thrill may be felt over the aortic area at the upper right sternal edge.

Auscultation generally reveals a normal or accentuated first heart sound ($S_1$). In

## TABLE 32-3.   Differential Diagnosis of Systolic Murmurs

| Parameter | Aortic Stenosis | Aortic Sclerosis | IHSS | Mitral Regurgitation |
|---|---|---|---|---|
| Location | Upper RSB | Upper RSB | Apex/lower LSB | Apex |
| Radiation | Neck and apex | None | None | Left axillae and base |
| Quality | Harsh diamond-shaped | Medium pitch and intensity | Harsh diamond-shape | Blowing, holosystolic |
| Associated findings | ↓$S_2$, Sustained PMI, ↓carotid upstroke | Normal $S_2$, normal PMI, normal carotid | Normal $S_2$ loud $S_4$, ↑carotid upstroke or bisferiens | ↓$S_1$ widely split $S_2$ |
| Effect of maneuvers on murmur | ↓Valsalva, ↓squatting | Little change | ↑Valsalva, ↓squatting | ↑Squatting, ↑handgrip |

IHSS = idiopathic hypertrophic subaortic stenosis; RSB = right sternal border; LSB = left sternal border; PMI = point of maximal left ventricular impulse.

*Source:* St. Claire DA Jr, Hollenberg M: Valvular heart disease. In: Longergan ET (ed): *Geriatrics.* Stamford, CT: Appleton & Lange 1996:59–78. Used with permission.

patients with a congenital bicuspid valve, an aortic ejection sound (click) may be heard at the cardiac apex shortly after $S_1$, but this usually disappears with age as the valve becomes calcified and less mobile. When aortic stenosis is mild, the second heart sound ($S_2$) is normal and is physiologically split into the aortic ($A_2$) and pulmonic ($P_2$) components. In severe aortic stenosis, $S_2$ may be a single sound or paradoxically split ($A_2$ after $P_2$, widening in expiration) as a result of prolongation of left ventricular systolic ejection time and delayed aortic valve closure. $A_2$ may become inaudible when leaflet excursion is severely impaired. Some 90 percent of patients with severe aortic stenosis and sinus rhythm will have a fourth heart sound ($S_4$) as a result of vigorous atrial contraction against a noncompliant left ventricle.[17] The cardinal auscultatory finding in aortic stenosis is a harsh crescendo-decrescendo (diamond-shaped) systolic murmur. It is usually heard best at the base, with radiation to the carotid vessels and apex. The murmur may also be heard at the apex, where it is higher-pitched. Although the murmur is typically quite loud, its intensity does not correlate well with the degree of stenosis. In fact, as left ventricular stroke volume falls with very severe stenosis, the murmur may become quite soft. On the other hand, the duration of the murmur does correlate fairly well with stenosis severity, a more prolonged crescendo being associated with more severe stenosis.

## Electrocardiogram

The electrocardiogram in aortic stenosis reflects the development of left ventricular hypertrophy in nearly 90 percent of patients.[21] In addition to the increase in QRS amplitude, there may also be depression of the ST segment and T-wave inversion in lead I and in the left percordial leads. About 80 percent of patients will have evidence of left atrial abnormality, manifested as prolongation of the P-wave duration in lead II ($>120$ ms) and a prominent negative deflection of the terminal portion of the P-wave in lead $V_1$.[13] Extension of calcification into conduction system may result in atrioventricular nodal block in a small percentage of patients. Atrial fibrillation may be present, particularly in the elderly.

## Chest Roentgenogram

Heart size is usually normal, although the apex may become prominent with rounding of the left heart border. The ascending aorta is sometimes enlarged as a result of poststenotic dilatation. Calcification of the aortic valve is not usually apparent on a posteroanterior x-ray film of the chest, but is often seen in lateral x-ray film of the chest.

## Diagnosis

When aortic stenosis is suspected on clinical grounds, the initial diagnostic test should be an echocardiogram. Two-dimensional imaging usually permits good visualization of the aortic valve, permitting assessment of its morphology, its mobility, and the presence of calcification. Masquerading conditions such as hypertrophic obstructive cardiomyopathy, aortic sclerosis, or mitral regurgitation are readily distinguished. Left ventricular chamber size, wall thickness, and systolic function can be assessed, and the presence of other valve disease or structural heart disease can be determined. Doppler techniques permit measurement of flow velocity across the aortic valve, which can be used to calculate a pressure gradient and derive an aortic valve area. Occasionally, adequate images cannot be obtained on a routine transthoracic echocardiogram. In this circumstance, transesophageal echocardiography or cardiac catheterization may be necessary.

Cardiac catherterization permits direct measurement of the pressure gradient and cardiac output to yield a calculated aortic valve area. Coronary angiography is necessary prior to valve surgery in patients over the age of 40 or in those with risk factors for CAD.[17]

Once the diagnosis of aortic stenosis is established, periodic reevaluation with clinical examination and echocardiography is indicated to assess for progression of disease. Echocardiography is generally recommended every year in asymptomatic patients with severe aortic stenosis; less frequently if the degree of stenosis is mild or moderate. Repeat examination is also indicated whenever there is a change in clinical findings or symptoms.[13,17] An algorithm for the serial assessment of patients with aortic stenosis is shown in Fig. 32-7.[18]

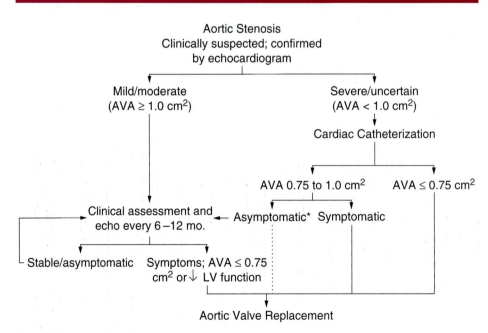

Figure 32-7   Management algorithm in aortic stenosis. When symptoms are uncertain, exercise stress testing may be helpful.
*Asymptomatic patients with valve areas between 0.75 and 1.0 $cm^2$ should be considered for surgery if they have decreased LV systolic function, significant coronary artery disease, exercise-induced hypotension, or significant arrhythmias. AVA = aortic valve area; LV = left ventricle.

## Treatment

Aortic valve replacement should be contemplated in all patients with symptomatic severe aortic stenosis, regardless of age. Asymptomatic patients should be considered for surgery if they have critical aortic stenosis (valve area less than 0.75 cm$^2$) or severe stenosis (valve are 0.76 to 1.0 cm$^2$) associated with left ventricular systolic dysfunction, significant obstructive coronary disease, or a fall in blood pressure during exercise stress testing (Fig. 32-7).[13,17] The survival of symptomatic patients without surgery is dismal, averaging less than 3 years with an 80 to 90 percent mortality after 10 years.[13] While medical therapy may palliate symptoms, it does not improve prognosis. In the absence of serious comorbid conditions or severe left ventricular dysfunction, operative morbidity and mortality are quite low. Surgical mortality in experienced centers is less than 2 percent for isolated valve replacement and less than 5 percent when valve replacement is combined with coronary bypass grafting. Mortality is considerably higher in the extreme elderly (age >80 years), averaging 8 percent for isolated valve replacement and 13 percent for combined valve replacement and coronary bypass grafting.[19]

The type of valve prosthesis used at operation depends on a number of patient-specific considerations. Mechanical valves have the advantage of longevity, but are associated with a higher risk for thromboembolism and require anticoagulation with warfarin. Tissue valves have a lower risk of thromboembolism, but tend to degenerate sooner. Patients with extensive annular calcification or aortic root disease may require a composite valve–aortic root graft. Autotransplant of the pulmonic valve to the aortic position with replacement of the pulmonic valve using a tissue prosthesis (Ross procedure) may be particularly advantageous in young patients.[13,17,19]

Aortic balloon valvuloplasty may be an effective alternative in young patients with congenital aortic stenosis.[17] One or more balloons are placed across the aortic valve by percutaneous insertion and retrograde advancement from the femoral artery. Inflation of the balloon(s) causes splitting of the fused valve commissures and relief of obstruction. This technique has an extremely limited role in older patients with degenerative calcific disease, as improvements in valve area are usually very small and short-lived, and serious complications are frequent. The only indication for balloon valvuloplasty in older patients is to serve as a bridge to future valve replacement in patients at excessively high immediate surgical risk as a result of serious comorbid conditions or cardiogenic shock.[22]

Medical therapy assumes only a palliative role in the management of aortic stenosis and should not be considered a substitute for definitive surgical treatment.[13,14,17–19] Antibiotic prophylaxis is indicated in all patients for prevention of infective endocarditis.[23] Patients with associated hypertension should be treated cautiously, generally avoiding medications with negative inotropic effect. Diuretics are helpful for pulmonary congestion but need to be used cautiously. Patients with severe aortic stenosis should be advised to limit their activity to relatively low levels. Those with moderate stenosis should avoid strenuous competitive sports, while patients with mild stenosis require no restriction in activity.[24]

Calcific aortic valve stenosis is a powerful risk factor for coronary atherosclerosis. In fact, the condition may be due to the atheromatous process.

# AORTIC REGURGITATION

Aortic regurgitation results from incompetence of the aortic valve during diastole, resulting in regurgitation of a portion of the stroke volume ejected during systole back into the left ventricle. Valve incompetence may be due to disease affecting the aortic valve leaflets, the aortic root, or both. The etiology, pathophysiology, clinical presentation, and treatment of acute and chronic aortic regurgitation are quite distinct and will be discussed separately.

# CHRONIC AORTIC REGURGITATION

## Etiology

The most common causes of primary valve disease leading to chronic aortic regurgitation are calcific degeneration, rheumatic disease, congenital bicuspid valve, and myxomatous proliferation (Table 32-4). Less common etiologies include ankylosing

**TABLE 32-4.   Causes of Chronic Aortic Regurgitation**

Common
 Aortic root/annular dilatation
 Rheumatic disease
 Biscuspid aortic valve
 Calcific degeneration
 Systemic hypertension
 Myxomatous proliferation

Less common
 Marfan syndrome
 Ankylosing spondylitis
 Rheumatoid arthritis
 Syphilitic aortitis
 Use of anorectic drugs

Unusual
 VSD with prolapse of an aortic cusp
 Reiter's syndrome
 Ehlers-Danlos syndrome
 Osteogenesis imperfecta
 Giant cell aortitis
 Takayasu's arteritis

VSD = ventricular septal defect.

spondylitis, rheumatoid arthritis, systemic lupus erythematosus, discrete subaortic stenosis, and ventricular septal defects with prolapse of an aortic cusp. Recently, anorectic drugs have been implicated as a cause of aortic regurgitation. Aortic regurgitation may also result from dilatation of the aortic root and valve annulus in disorders such as annuloaortic ectasia, Marfan syndrome, systemic hypertension, syphilitic aortitis, and aortitis associated with a variety of collagen vascular diseases.[17,19]

## Pathophysiology

Aortic regurgitation results in volume and pressure overload of the left ventricle. A portion of the blood ejected during systole regurgitates into the left ventricle during diastole, thus reducing the effective forward stroke volume. The left ventricle responds with progressive dilation and compensatory eccentric and concentric hypertrophy. Eccentric hypertrophy permits maintenance of normal preload and contractile performance, while concentric hypertrophy permits adaptation to increased afterload, resulting in overall maintenance of forward stroke volume and systolic performance.[17] In this compensated phase, measurements of systolic function such as ejection fraction remain normal, although left ventricular chamber size is increased. As the disease progresses, however, the capacity of these compensatory mechanisms is exceeded, and systolic function declines, with a fall in ejection fraction and a progressive increase in end-systolic and end-diastolic volume. Unfortunately, the transition from a compensated to a decompensated state is often insidious, and patients may remain asymptomatic until severe and potentially irreversible left ventricular dysfunction has developed.[17,25,26] The understanding of this pathophysiologic process forms the basis of recommendations regarding surveillance and treatment of patients with chronic aortic insufficiency.

## Symptoms

Most patients with chronic aortic regurgitation remain remarkably symptom-free for many years. The only complaint may be an uncomfortable awareness of their heartbeat, especially when lying down at night. Palpitations may be unusually symptomatic because of the very large stroke volume of the postpremature beat. A peculiar symptom of excessive upper body sweating is sometimes reported.[18,27]

When the left ventricle begins to fail, patients experience fatigue, shortness of breath, orthopnea, and paroxysmal nocturnal dyspnea. Chest pain of an anginal character may occur in the absence of obstructive coronary disease.

## Physical Examination

Findings of mild aortic regurgitation are often quite subtle, while those of severe regurgitation are rather dramatic. The pulse pressure is wide as a result of a high systolic and an abnormally low diastolic pressure. In fact, a diastolic pressure above 70 strongly argues against severe aortic regurgitation.[27] The large rise and abrupt diastolic collapse of the arterial pulse produces a number of eponymous peripheral manifestations (Table 32-5). The vigor of the arterial pulse abnormalities correlates

**TABLE 32-5.**   Eponyms Associated with Peripheral Arterial Manifestations of Chronic Aortic Regurgitation

| Eponym | Physical Finding |
| --- | --- |
| Corrigan's pulse | Bounding "water-hammer" femoral pulses |
| Musset's sign | Systolic head bobbing |
| Duroziez's sign | To-and-fro systolic and diastolic murmurs heard upon auscultation with light pressure of the stethoscope over the femoral artery |
| Muller's sign | Systolic pulsation of the uvula |
| Quincke's pulse | Visible capillary pulsations in the nail beds |
| Traube's sign | Pistol-shot pulses heard over the femoral artery |

quite well with the extent of valvular leak.[27] The left ventricular apical impulse is hyperdynamic, enlarged, and laterally displaced. A pulsus bisferiens may be noted.

Auscultation may reveal a faint $S_1$ as a result of premature closure of the mitral valve. $A_2$ may be soft or absent, and $P_2$ is often obscured by the early diastolic murmur. An $S_3$ gallop correlates well with the presence of severe regurgitation. Aortic insufficiency produces a decrescendo diastolic murmur, high in frequency and blowing in quality, that is usually heard best over the mid-left sternal border or apex with the diaphragm of the stethoscope. Clinical experience has shown that when the murmur is best heard along the right sternal edge, the etiology of valvular incompetence is most likely related to dilation of the aortic root.[27] When the leak is mild, it may be audible only with the patient sitting up and leaning forward, with the breath held at end-expiration. The severity of chronic aortic regurgitation correlates better with the duration than with the intensity of the murmur. The murmur of mild regurgitation usually ends early in diastole, whereas that of severe regurgitation is typically holo-diastolic. Severe aortic regurgitation may also produce a separate apical, late diastolic rumble (Austin Flint murmur) due to functional narrowing of the mitral orifice caused by a rapid rise in left ventricular diastolic pressure and regurgitant flow against the anterior mitral valve leaflet.[18,27] Finally, a midsystolic aortic murmur due to turbulent flow associated with the high forward stroke volume is commonly heard.

## Electrocardiogram

Left ventricular hypertrophy is usually present in patients with moderately severe aortic valve regurgitation. Patients usually remain in sinus rhythm except in far advanced cases with secondary mitral regurgitation in whom atrial fibrillation may occur.[21]

## Chest Roentgenogram

Left ventricular enlargement is characteristic of chronic severe aortic regurgitation. The aortic root and ascending aorta may be dilated, sometimes quite dramatically, as in the case of annuloaortic ectasia and Marfan syndrome.

## Diagnosis

Echocardiography is the diagnostic study of choice for confirming the clinical suspicion of aortic regurgitation and evaluating its etiology and severity. Two-dimensional and M-mode imaging permit visualization of the aortic valve, aortic root, and proximal ascending aorta and quantitative measurement of left ventricular chamber size, wall thickness, and systolic function. Doppler techniques permit a semiquantitative assessment of the severity of regurgitation. In the serial assessment of asymptomatic patients, the left ventricular chamber measurements (end-diastolic dimension, end-systolic dimension, and ejection fraction) are useful in determining the need for surgical intervention (Fig. 32-8). In some circumstances, radionuclide angiography or cardiac magnetic resonance imaging can be used to obtain these same measurements, but these modalities are less widely available.[17]

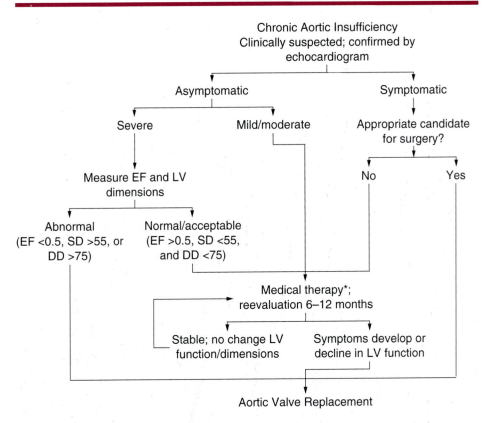

Figure 32-8    Management algorithm in aortic regurgitation. When symptoms are uncertain, stress testing may be appropriate. NYHA class II or greater symptoms are considered significant. *See text for discussion of medical therapy. EF = ejection fraction; SD = end-systolic dimension; DD = end-diastolic dimension; LV = left ventricle.

Exercise testing is generally not necessary, but it may be useful for evaluating patients with equivocal symptoms or to assess patients' symptoms and functional capacity prior to their participation in athletic activities.

Cardiac catheterization is indicated if other techniques are of insufficient quality to assess left ventricular function or the severity of aortic regurgitation. Coronary angiography is indicated before aortic valve surgery in patients at risk for coronary artery disease.[17,19,21,25]

## Treatment

The cornerstone of management of chronic aortic regurgitation is the detection of a decline in left ventricular function before significant symptoms develop, allowing aortic valve replacement to occur at a time when postoperative ventricular function will remain good.[18] Patients with chronic severe aortic regurgitation should be evaluated clinically every 6 to 12 months and undergo annual echocardiographic assessment of left ventricular dimensions and ejection fraction (Fig. 32-8). More frequent assessment is indicated when there is a change in symptoms or evidence of left ventricular chamber enlargement. Less frequent assessment is needed in patients with mild or moderate aortic regurgitation and initially normal chamber measurements.[17]

Medical therapy with vasodilating agents may improve forward stroke volume and reduce regurgitant volume. Beneficial acute hemodynamic effects have been demonstrated with angiotensin-converting enzyme inhibitors, hydralazine, and nifedipine.[17,19,25,26,28,29] However, long-term clinical benefit has been demonstrated only with long-acting nifedipine, which has been shown to delay the onset of symptoms and/or development of left ventricular dysfunction and reduce the need for aortic valve replacement.[25] Vasodilator therapy is indicated for (1) patients with moderate to severe aortic regurgitation but normal systolic function, (2) short-term improvement of symptomatic patients awaiting aortic valve replacement, or (3) long-term treatment of patients who are not surgical candidates.[17,19,29] Vasodilators are not necessary in asymptomatic patients with mild regurgitation and normal blood pressure. Antibiotic prophylaxis is indicated in all patients for prevention of infective endocarditis.

Surgical therapy should be considered in all symptomatic patients or when there is evidence of left ventricular systolic dysfunction. An ejection fraction of <0.5, an end-systolic dimension >55 mm, or an end-diastolic dimension >75 mm should prompt evaluation for aortic valve replacement regardless of symptoms. Once left ventricular dysfunction is advanced (ejection fraction <0.25 and/or end-systolic dimension >60 mm), myocardial function my not improve after operation and surgical mortality is high. Patients with concomitant aortic root disease may require surgery based on the primary disease of the aorta. Aortic valve replacement and aortic root reconstruction are usually indicated when the aortic root dimension exceeds 50 mm.[17,19,25,29]

# ACUTE AORTIC REGURGITATION

## Etiology

Acute aortic regurgitation most often results from infective endocarditis, dissection of the aorta, or trauma (Table 32-6). Endocarditis usually occurs in patients with a predisposing valvular lesion such as rheumatic disease or a bicuspid valve. Dissection may occur spontaneously in patients with severe hypertension or diseases affecting the aortic root, or as a consequence of trauma. The risk of aortic dissection is also increased in pregnancy, particularly in the third trimester and peripartum period.

## Pathophysiology

In contrast to chronic aortic regurgitation, in severe acute aortic insufficiency the left ventricle has not had an opportunity to undergo adaptive remodeling. The sudden volume overload results in an abrupt increase in end-diastolic pressure and a decrease in forward stroke volume. The hemodynamic changes are particularly pronounced in patients with preexisting hypertension, in which case the small, hypertrophied, and noncompliant left ventricle is particularly poorly adapted to an acute volume overload. This is often the case in patients with acute aortic dissection.[17–19]

## Symptoms

The hemodynamic consequences of acute severe aortic insufficiency present clinically as pulmonary edema and cardiogenic shock. Patients appear gravely ill, with severe dyspnea, weakness, and evidence of cardiovascular collapse. In the case of endocarditis, patients may describe an antecedent febrile illness or other symptoms of systemic infection. Aortic dissection may present with severe chest and/or back pain.

TABLE 32-6.  Causes of Acute Aortic Regurgitation

| |
|---|
| Infective endocarditis |
| Dissecting aneurysm |
| Marfan syndrome |
| Traumatic leaflet repture |
| Following aortic valve replacement |
| Rheumatic |

## Physical Examination

Patients will present with evidence of cardiovascular collapse, including tachycardia, hypotension, peripheral vasoconstriction, tachypnea, and cyanosis. The left ventricular apical impulse is usually normal or slightly enlarged. Unlike the hyperdynamic arterial pulses and wide pulse pressure characteristic of chronic severe aortic regurgitation, the peripheral pulse in acute aortic insufficiency is often weak and thready, with a normal or narrow pulse pressure. The diastolic murmur of acute aortic insufficiency may be deceptively inconspicuous. It is typically grade 3 or less in intensity and is often quite short in duration as a result of rapid diastolic equalization of pressure between the aorta and the left ventricle. An $S_3$ gallop is commonly present.[18,19]

## Electrocardiogram

There are no distinguishing electrocardiographic findings, although nonspecific ST-segment and T-wave changes are common.

## Chest Roentgenogram

Cardiac size is most often normal. If aortic regurgitation is severe, there is usually evidence of pulmonary edema. When aortic insufficiency is due to dissection of the aorta, there may be enlargement of the ascending aorta or separation of calcification in the aortic knob.[21]

## Diagnosis

Acute aortic insufficiency, particularly if due to aortic dissection, is a surgical emergency that requires prompt definitive diagnosis. The diagnosis depends first and foremost on a high clinical index of suspicion. Once this is established, the initial diagnostic study is usually a transthoracic echocardiogram. If adequate images cannot be obtained or uncertainty persists, transesophageal echocardiography is indicated. The diagnostic accuracy of transesophageal echocardiography is excellent, and it has the advantage of being feasible in most patients, even those who are critically ill and hemodynamically unstable. If transesophageal echocardiography is not available, aortography should be performed. Computed tomography or magnetic resonance imaging (MRI) may be helpful when aortic dissection is suspected. When appropriate diagnostic imaging modalities and/or cardiothoracic surgery capability is not available, transfer to an appropriate facility should not be delayed.[18,19,21]

## Treatment

Mortality from acute severe aortic regurgitation is extremely high, and early surgical intervention is recommended. The role of medical therapy is to stabilize the patient until surgery can be performed; in no way should it delay surgery. If the patient has an adequate blood pressure level, sodium nitroprusside should be given to reduce afterload. Hypotension requires inotropic support with dobutamine, dopamine, or both. Use of intraaortic balloon pump counterpulsation for circulatory support is contraindicated, as it will worsen aortic regurgitation. When acute aortic insufficiency is due to endocarditis and is only mild to moderate in severity, surgery may be delayed and appropriate antibiotic treatment instituted. If patients become hemodynamically unstable, however, surgery should not be delayed.[17–19,21]

## REFERENCES

1. Rahimtoola SH, Enriquez-Sarano M, Schaff HV, Frye RL: Mitral valve disease. In: Alexander RW, Schlant RC, Fuster V, et al (eds): *Hurst's The Heart*, 9th ed. New York, McGraw-Hill, 1998:1789–1819.
2. Braunwald E: Valvular heart disease. In: Braunwald E (ed): *Heart Disease*, 5th ed. Philadelphia, W. B. Saunders, 1996: 1007–1076.
3. Carabello BA, Crawford FA: Valvular heart disease. *N Engl J Med* 1997; 337:32–41.
4. Morris DC: Mitral valve regurgitation. In: Hurst JW (ed): *Medicine for the Practicing Physician*, 4th ed. Stamford, CT, Appleton and Lange, 1996:1230–1232.
5. Devereux RB: Recent developments in the diagnosis and management of mitral valve prolapse. *Curr Opinion Cardiol* 1995; 10:107–116.
6. Fenster MS, Feldman MD: Mitral regurgitation: An overview. *Curr Probl Cardiol* 1995; 20:193–280.
7. Carabello BA: Management of valvular regurgitation. *Curr Opinion Cardiol* 1995; 10:124–127.
8. Gaasch WM, Eisenhauer AC: The management of mitral valve disease. *Curr Opinion Cardiol* 1996; 11:114–119.
9. Fontana ME, Sparks EA, Boudoulas H, Wooley CF: Mitral valve prolapse and the mitral valve prolapse syndrome. *Curr Probl Cardiol* 1991; 16:315–375.
10. Hancock E: Valvular heart disease. In: Dale DC, Federman DD (eds): *Scientific American Medicine*. New York, Scientific American Inc., 1996.
11. Felner JM, Schlant RC: Mitral valve prolapse. In: Hurst JW (ed): *Medicine for the Practicing Physician*, 4th ed. Stamford, CT, Appleton and Lange, 1996:1232–1236.
12. Dajani AS, Taubert KA, Wilson W, et al: Prevention of bacterial endocarditis: Recommendations by the American Heart Association. *JAMA* 1997; 277:1794–1801.
13. O'Rourke RA: Aortic valve stenosis: a common clinical entity. *Curr Probl Cardiol* 1998; 23:429–476.
14. Otto CM: Aortic stenosis: clinical evaluation and optimal timing of surgery. In: Zoghbi WA (ed): Valvular heart disease. *Cardiol Clin* 1998; 16:353–373.
15. Passik CS, Ackerman DM, Piuth JR, Edwards WD: Temporal changes in the causes of aortic stenosis: a surgical pathologic study of 646 cases. *Mayo Clin Proc* 1987; 62:119–123.
16. Otto CM, Lind BK, Kitzman DW, et al: Association of aortic-valve sclerosis with cardiovascular mortality and morbidity in the elderly. *N Engl J Med* 1999; 341:142–147.
17. Bonow RO and Committee: ACC/AHA guidelines for the management of patients with valvular heart disease. *J Am Coll Cardiol* 1998; 32:1486–1558.
18. St.Claire DA Jr, Hollenberg M: Valvular heart disease. In Lonergan ET (ed): *Geriatrics*. Stamford, CT, Appleton & Lange, 1996;59–78.

19. Rahimtoola SH: Aortic valve disease. In: Alexander RW, Schlant RC, Fuster V, et al (eds): *Hurst's The Heart,* 9th ed. New York, McGraw-Hill, 1998;1759–1787.

20. Horskotte D, Loogen F: The natural history of aortic valve stenosis. *Eur Heart J* 1998; 9 (suppl E):57–64.

21. Braunwald E: Valvular heart disease. In: Braunwald E (ed): *Heart Disease: A Textbook of Cardiovascular Medicine,* 4th ed. Philadelphia, W. B. Saunders, 1992;1007–1077.

22. Rahimtoola SA: Catheter balloon valvuloplasty for severe calcific aortic stenosis: a limited role. *J Am Coll Cardiol* 1994; 23:1076–1078.

23. Dajani AS, Taubert KA, Wilson W, et al: Prevention of bacterial endocarditis: recommendations by the American Heart Association. *Circulation* 1997; 96:358–366.

24. Cheitlin MD, Douglas PS, Parmley WW: 26th Bethesda conference: recommendations for determining eligibility for competition in athletes with cardiovascular abnormalities. Task Force 2: acquired valvular heart disease. *J Am Coll Cardiol* 1994; 24:874–880.

25. Cheitlin MD: Valvular heart disease: management and intervention. *Circulation* 1991; 84(suppl I):1259.

26. Bonow RO, Lakatos E, Maron BJ, Epstein SE: Serial long-term assessment of the natural history of asymptomatic patients with chronic aortic regurgitation and normal left ventricular systolic function. *Circulation* 1991; 84:1625–1635.

27. Stapleton JF: Clinical aspects of nonrheumatic valvular disease. In: Chizner MA (ed): *Classic Teachings in Clinical Cardiology: A Tribute to W. Proctor Harvey.* Cedar Grove, NJ, Laennec Publishing, 1996;1017–1048.

28. Scognamiglio R, Rahimtoola SH, Fasoli G, et al: Nifedipine in asymptomatic patients with severe aortic regurgitation and normal left ventricular function. *N Engl J Med* 1994; 331:689–694.

29. Bonow RO: Chronic aortic regurgitation: role of medical therapy and optimal timing for surgery. In: Zoghbi WA (ed): Valvular heart disease. *Cardiol Clin* 1998; 16:449–461.

WENDY M. BOOK /
ROBERT H. FRANCH

# CONGENITAL HEART DISEASE

The introduction of open surgical repair of congenital heart defects in the late 1950s permitted long-term survival for patients with congenital heart defects that had previously been fatal in childhood.[1] Since then, surgical techniques have improved considerably, with 85 percent of children with congenital heart disease now expected to survive to adulthood.[1] Worldwide, an estimated 1.5 million children are born each year with congenital heart defects, an incidence of 7 to 8 per 1000 live births.[2] Currently, there are more than 500,000 adults in the United States with congenital heart disease.[1,2]

Congenital heart defects can be divided into common malformations with expected adult survival, uncommon malformations with expected adult survival, and malformations where survival without surgical repair is exceptional (see Table 33-1). For the purposes of this chapter, we shall focus primarily on common congenital heart defects, with mention of uncommon defects that may present in adolescence and adulthood.

Surgeries for congenital heart disease may be "curative" (as for an atrial septal defect), "corrective" (as for tetralogy of Fallot), or "palliative" (as in the Fontan operation for tricuspid atresia). Table 33-2 describes common operations performed for congenital heart disease. Therefore, sequelae of surgical repairs in childhood may become evident in adolescence and adulthood.

## SHUNTS

### Ventricular Septal Defect

**INCIDENCE.**   Ventricular septal defect (VSD), as well as mitral valve prolapse and bicuspid aortic valve, are common cardiac malformations at birth. Approximately 30 to 40 percent of VSDs close spontaneously in childhood.[2] The majority of the remaining VSDs are surgically closed by 4 years of age.[3] Thus, the practitioner will see few open VSDs in children beyond grade school age.

**TABLE 33-1.    Survival Patterns in Unoperated Patients with Congenital Heart Disease**

| | |
|---|---|
| Common defects with expected adult survival | Bicuspid aortic valve<br>Coarctation of the aorta<br>Pulmonary valve stenosis<br>Atrial septal defect<br>Hypertrophic cardiomyopathy<br>Patent ductus arteriosus |
| Common defects with exceptional adult survival | Ventricular septal defect<br>Tetralogy of Fallot |
| Uncommon defects with expected adult survival | Situs inversus with dextrocardia<br>Congenital complete heart block<br>Congenitally corrected transposition of the great arteries<br>Congenital mitral regurgitation<br>Discrete subaortic stenosis<br>Ebstein's anomaly of the tricuspid valve<br>Quadricuspid aortic valve<br>Uhl's anomaly<br>Pulmonary artery branch stenosis<br>Pulmonary valve regurgitation isolated<br>Partial anomalous pulmonary venous return<br>Sinus of Valsalva aneurysm<br>Coronary arterial fistula<br>Pulmonary arteriovenous fistula |
| Uncommon defects with exceptional adult survival | Unicuspid aortic valves<br>Supravalvular aortic stenosis<br>Double-outlet ventricle<br>Left coronary artery originating from the pulmonary artery<br>Truncus arteriosus<br>Aortopulmonary window<br>Univentricular heart<br>Complete transposition of the great arteries<br>Total anomalous pulmonary venous return<br>Common atrium<br>Tetralogy of Fallot with absent pulmonary valve<br>Tricuspid atresia |

*Source:* Data obtained from Perloff JK, Child JS: *Congenital Heart Disease in Adults,* 2d ed. Philadelphia, W. B. Saunders, 1998.

**ANATOMY.**    The perimembranous VSD is the most common, accounting for 75 percent of VSDs.[1,3] This defect lies immediately beneath the aortic valve, in proximity to the septal leaflet of the tricuspid valve. Muscular VSDs (frequently multiple), posterior or inlet VSDs, and supracristal (outlet) defects are less common. Supracristal (subpulmonary) VSDs may underlie the aortic valve in the region of the right and noncoronary cusps. The aortic leaflet may be pulled into the defect, partially sealing off the VSD. These generally require repair when diagnosed to prevent progressive aortic insufficiency, however.[3]

**PHYSIOLOGY.**   Defect size and the relative resistances of the pulmonary and systemic vascular beds determine the physiologic consequences of the defect. Small VSDs provide high resistance to flow, thus maintaining normal right-sided pressures. Large defects, however, permit equilibration of right- and left-sided pressures, with large left-to-right shunting and volume overload of the left atrium and ventricle. When pulmonary vascular resistance becomes elevated, right-to-left shunting occurs (Eisenmenger's syndrome), resulting in cyanosis.[2]

**CLINICAL PRESENTATION AND DIAGNOSIS.**   The majority of VSDs will be detected in infancy or early childhood by the characteristic loud holosystolic murmur, which is often associated with a parasternal thrill. Infants with large VSDs may present with signs and symptoms of congestive heart failure and an $S_3$ gallop. The electrocardiogram (ECG) and chest radiograph are generally normal in small VSDs. Left atrial enlargement and left ventricular hypertrophy develop with larger defects, and right axis deviation in the ECG and right ventricular hypertrophy are seen with elevated pulmonary vascular resistance and Eisenmenger's syndrome. Echocardiography is particularly useful in the diagnosis and follow-up of VSDs.[1,2]

**MANAGEMENT.**   Small VSDs with a ratio of pulmonary to systemic blood flows $(Q_p:Q_s)$ of <1.5:1 can be followed medically with attention to endocarditis prophylaxis. The exception is the supracristal VSD with aortic insufficiency, which should be surgically repaired to prevent progressive aortic insufficiency.[3,4] Spontaneous closure of the VSD is more likely to occur with smaller defects, in females, and in the first decade of life. Spontaneous closure may occur in adulthood, although less frequently. Approximately 15 percent of medically managed VSDs in adults will close spontaneously.[1,3] A percutaneous closure device for muscular VSDs, which are difficult to close surgically, is under development.[5] Larger shunts should be closed in childhood if they have not spontaneously closed.[3,4] Management of the patient with Eisenmenger's syndrome will be discussed later in this chapter.

**PROGNOSIS.**   Approximately 5 percent of patients who have had a VSD surgically closed require reoperation.[4] The incidence of serious ventricular arrhythmias is higher than for the general population, with ventricular tachycardia occurring in 3 percent of medically managed and 5 percent of surgically closed VSDs.[4] Development of aortic regurgitation after repair is rare, occurring in less than 1 percent of patients in the Natural History Study-2 (NHS-2).[4] Pulmonary hypertension developed in patients with both surgically treated (13.8 percent) and medically managed (18.2 percent) VSDs in the NHS-2 study, indicating the need for routine scheduled follow-up even after surgical closure.[4] The probability of survival at 20 years in the

**TABLE 33-2. Glossary of Some Operative Procedures for Cyanotic Congenital Heart Disease**

| Name of Procedure | Purpose | Description | Use |
|---|---|---|---|
| Blalock-Taussig shunt | To increase pulmonary blood flow | Anastomoses of the subclavian artery to the PA | Tetralogy of Fallot with severe pulmonary stenosis or atresia |
| Pott's procedure | To increase pulmonary blood flow | Anastomoses of the descending aorta, side to side, to proximal left PA (done in the past) | Tetralogy of Fallot with severe pulmonary stenosis or atresia |
| Waterston shunt | To increase pulmonary blood flow | Anastomoses of the descending aorta to the right PA, side to side (done infrequently now) | Tetralogy of Fallot with severe pulmonary stenosis or atresia |
| Glenn procedure | To increase pulmonary blood flow and to decrease systemic ventricular work | Anastomoses of the end of the SVC to the end of the right PA. Now modified by joining the SVC to the side of the right pulmonary artery. | Univentricular heart Tricuspid atresia |
| Muller-Damman pulmonary artery banding | To reduce pulmonary artery pressure and blood flow | Annular constriction (banding) of the main pulmonary artery (done infrequently now) | Large VSD |
| Rashkind's procedure | To increase intracardiac mixing or flow | At catheterization, an ASD is created by rupture of the fossa ovale membrane with a balloon or blade catheter (medical septostomy) | TGA |

494

| Procedure | Purpose | Description | Indication |
|---|---|---|---|
| Mustard (baffle) procedure | To direct both systemic and pulmonary venous blood to the proper ventricle | Insertion of an interatrial baffle of pericardium or prosthetic material to direct systemic venous blood to the pulmonary ventricle and pulmonary venous blood to the systemic ventricle. Senning modification—baffle is made from the right atrial wall, atrial septum, and if needed a small piece of pericardium | TGA |
| Jantene operation (arterial switch procedure) | To direct systemic and pulmonary blood flow to the proper great artery | The ascending aorta and the main pulmonary artery are switched to serve the proper ventricle and the coronary arteries are reimplanted above the pulmonic valve, which acts as the systemic semilunar valve | TGA |
| Rastelli conduit procedure | To connect the right ventricular blood flow to the pulmonary tree | A new outflow channel from the right ventricle to the pulmonary artery is made using a woven Dacron conduit containing a semilunar valve | TGA with pulmonary stenosis, truncus arteriosus, pulmonary atresia with VSD |
| Fontan procedure | To direct caval or right atrial blood flow to the pulmonary artery | The modified procedure directs the entire systemic venous return from the cavae or the right atrium to the PA by using a nonvalved conduit or direct anastomosis of the right atrium to the PA or an SVC to right PA anastomosis combined with an inferior vena cava to right PA intraatrial tunnel anastomosis | Univentricular heart or tricuspid atresia |

PA = pulmonary artery; SVC = superior vena cava; VSD = ventricular septal defect; ASD = atrial septal defect; TGA = transposition of the great arteries.

NHS-2 cohort was 87 percent, with the highest risk of death in the group with large VSDs and the lowest risk in the group with small VSDs managed medically.[4]

## Atrial Septal Defect

Atrial septal defect (ASD) is the most common congenital heart defect in adults. ASD is more common in females than in males (2 to 1).[2] Diagnosis may be delayed well into adulthood because symptoms are frequently absent until the third or fourth decade and physical findings are subtle and often overlooked. Although adults with unrepaired ASD often survive to adulthood, their life expectancy is shortened to 40 to 50 years of age if pulmonary hypertension is present.[1]

**ANATOMY.**   Ostium secundum ASD is the most common type of atrial septal defect, involving the fossa ovalis in the midseptum. Sinus venosus ASDs are located high in the atrial septum near the superior vena cava and are often associated with anomalous pulmonary veins. Ostium primum defects (partial endocardial cushion defects) are located in the lower part of the atrial septum near the atrioventricular valves. This defect is often associated with cleft mitral and occasionally tricuspid valves.

**PHYSIOLOGY.**   In addition to size, the relative compliance and resistance of the pulmonary and systemic circulations determine the magnitude of the shunt across the ASD. The left-to-right shunt across the defect results in volume overload of the right ventricle and increased pulmonary blood flow. Eisenmenger's syndrome may occur in patients with large defects that go unrepaired.

**CLINICAL PRESENTATION.**   Most children with ASD are asymptomatic and therefore may go undetected until adulthood. Symptoms often develop in the third or fourth decade of life. Dyspnea on exertion, palpitations, and atrial arrhythmias are the most common presenting symptoms. Unfortunately, the patient and physician often attribute these symptoms to other disease processes, such as asthma or upper respiratory illness.

Physical examination may reveal a right ventricular heave, fixed splitting of the second heart sound, and an early systolic flow murmur from increased flow across the pulmonary valve. With progressive pulmonary hypertension, the pulmonary valve closure sound increases in intensity, and pulmonic and tricuspid insufficiency may develop. Atrial fibrillation becomes more common with increasing age. A right intraventricular conduction delay with rSR' in lead $V_1$ is common in ostium secundum ASD (Fig. 33-1). The ECG in ostium primum ASD characteristically shows left anterior fascicular block, first-degree atrioventricular block, and right bundle branch block. Cardiomegaly may be present on chest radiography, with further increases in the size of the pulmonary arteries as pulmonary hypertension develops. In Eisenmenger's syndrome, pruning of the distal pulmonary arteries and enlarged main pulmonary arteries can be seen (Fig. 33-2). The majority of ASDs are readily

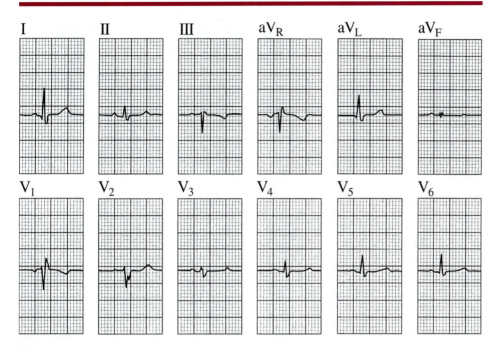

**Figure 33-1**   Electrocardiogram from a 40-year-old woman with a previously unrecognized ostium secundum atrial septal defect. Lead $V_1$ shows rSR' configuration consistent with right intraventricular conduction delay.

diagnosed with transthoracic echocardiography; however, transesophageal echocardiography may be necessary to determine the location of the ASD and any anomalies of the pulmonary veins.

**MANAGEMENT AND PROGNOSIS.**   Surgical closure of all ASDs, regardless of symptoms, with a pulmonary to systemic flow ratio greater than 1.5 to 1.0 is recommended to prevent the development of pulmonary hypertension and atrial arrhythmias.[3,6–8] If repair is performed before age 25 and pulmonary resistance is low, long-term survival is the same as that for age-matched controls.[9] With repair after age 25, survival is still good if pulmonary vascular disease is absent.[1,9] Older patients have more atrial rhythm disturbances, right ventricular dysfunction, and pulmonary hypertension. Transcatheter closure of ASDs is currently being performed in experimental trials. Isolated ostium secundum ASD does not require endocarditis prophylaxis; however, these patients do remain at risk for paradoxical emboli. If the ASD remains undiagnosed, Eisenmenger's syndrome may develop in the third or fourth decade of life in 15 percent of large ASDs. The management of the patient with Eisenmenger's syndrome will be discussed later in this chapter.

**Figure 33-2**  Frontal chest radiograph of a 33-year-old with a previously unrecognized atrial septal defect who subsequently developed pulmonary hypertension and Eisenmenger's physiology. Note the marked dilatation of the proximal pulmonary arteries and distal pruning.

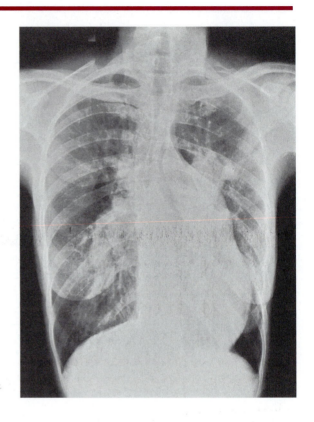

## Patent Ductus Arteriosus

Patent ductus arteriosus (PDA) accounts for 5 to 10 percent of congenital heart defects.[2] The ductus arteriosus connecting the pulmonary artery and aorta is a normal fetal structure that closes within several days after birth. Premature infants commonly have delayed closure of the ductus, with PDA present in 45 to 80 percent of these infants. High altitude, female gender, and maternal exposure to rubella all increase the incidence of PDA.[2,3]

**ANATOMY AND PHYSIOLOGY.**   Failure of the ductus to close normally initially produces a left-to-right shunt. When the shunt is large, there is increased pulmonary blood flow, with subsequent development of pulmonary hypertension. If Eisenmenger's syndrome develops, the upper extremities may be oxygenated while the lower extremities are cyanotic.

**CLINICAL PRESENTATION.**   Symptoms depend on the size of the shunt, from no symptoms in the presence of a small shunt to congestive heart failure (CHF) with a large shunt. Recurrent pneumonia may also be present in children with large shunts.

The classic physical examination finding is the continuous "machinery murmur," heard best at the upper left sternal border. Because of the runoff into the pulmonary circulation, peripheral pulses are bounding and the pulse pressure is wide (with large shunts). If pulmonary hypertension develops, the pulmonary closure sound increases in intensity. The ECG findings are similar to those with VSD. There is volume overload of the left atrium and ventricle, with left atrial abnormality and left ventricular hypertrophy on the ECG. With smaller shunts, the ECG may be normal. Similarly, chest radiography will be normal with smaller shunts. Cardiomegaly and increased pulmonary blood flow are present with larger shunts. Color Doppler interrogation with transthoracic echocardiography is usually diagnostic in both children and adults.

**MANAGEMENT.**   Closure at the time of diagnosis is indicated for all PDAs with a murmur.[1] PDAs are unlikely to close spontaneously in term infants.[2] The development of sensitive echocardiographic techniques has allowed for the detection of silent PDAs, whose management is controversial. Surgical closure is the current standard for repair; however, transcatheter closure with coils has been successful in small PDAs.[10]

PDAs left unoperated place the patient at risk for endocarditis and, if large, subsequent development of pulmonary hypertension. Long-term outcome following early closure of the PDA is excellent.

## Complete Endocardial Cushion Defect (Atrioventricular Canal)

Atrioventricular canal defects are found in 2 percent of patients with congenital heart disease, with a third of these defects occurring in children with Down syndrome.[2] The defect results in the absence of the lower portion of the atrial septum (ostium primum ASD) and the inlet portion of the ventricular septum (VSD). The mitral and tricuspid valves are often abnormal, with a common atrioventricular valve. Patients with atrioventricular canal defects present early with congestive heart failure and failure to thrive. Surgical correction with valve reconstruction is performed in early childhood.[11] Endocarditis prophylaxis is required after surgical repair. Without surgical intervention, most patients die within 2 to 3 years.[11]

## Anomalous Pulmonary Venous Return

The four pulmonary veins normally carry oxygenated blood to the left atrium. Anomalous pulmonary veins account for less than 1 percent of congenital heart defects.[1,2] One or more of the pulmonary veins may drain abnormally into the right atrium, superior vena cava, inferior vena cava, coronary sinus, or innominate vein. The majority of patients with partial anomalous pulmonary venous return are asymptomatic. Evidence of right ventricular volume overload may develop on ECG and chest radiography. Untreated significant shunts may result in pulmonary hypertension in the third or fourth decade of life.[1,2] Surgical repair is preferable and should be carried out before grade school.[1-3] Endocarditis prophylaxis is not necessary.

## Eisenmenger's Syndrome

Eisenmenger's syndrome can occur in any shunt lesion with initial left-to-right shunting. Pulmonary arteriolar occlusive disease may eventually develop after years of increased flow and pressure in the pulmonary circulation. Those with large left-to-right shunts are most likely to develop Eisenmenger's physiology. Once pulmonary vascular resistance becomes elevated, the shunt will reverse and become right to left. Cyanosis and clubbing develop as a consequence of the reversal of blood flow through the shunt.

The patient with Eisenmenger's physiology will notice fatigue, dyspnea, and occasionally syncope. Cyanosis, clubbing, polycythemia, and signs of right heart failure will be present on examination. The chest x-ray will show large pulmonary arteries with distal pruning, cardiomegaly, and enlargement of the right heart structures. On ECG, supraventricular arrhythmias may be evident. Right ventricular hypertrophy, right atrial abnormality, and right axis deviation are often present.

Once Eisenmenger's physiology develops, the prognosis is poor.[12] The majority of patients die within 15 years from progressive arrhythmias or right heart failure.[1,12]

**MANAGEMENT.**　Endocarditis risk is high; therefore, prophylaxis is mandatory. Any change in systemic venous return or systemic vascular resistance can alter shunt hemodynamics and cause death. Surgery, pregnancy, dehydration, hemorrhage, and fever may all be life-threatening to the patient with Eisenmenger's syndrome.[12,13] A fall in systemic blood pressure results in increased right-to-left shunting and cyanosis; thus sudden or prolonged standing should be avoided.

In the adult with pulmonary vascular occlusive disease, hemoptysis may occur. This does not require bronchoscopy or special studies and is nearly always self-limited. If there is exertional faintness or severe hypoxia, a handicapped vehicle or wheelchair is prescribed.

Flying at an altitude of 40,000 feet produces a cabin $P_{O_2}$ of 118 mmHg, giving an arterial $P_{O_2}$ of 58 mmHg in the normal patient. Home oxygen therapy may be offered continuously for a $Pa_{O_2}$ less than 55 mmHg ($Sa_{O_2} < 88$ percent) or intermittently for a $Pa_{O_2}$ of 56 to 59 mmHg, especially with exertion, straining at stool, or nocturnally.

The patient with Eisenmenger's syndrome should be managed in conjunction with a center specially trained in caring for these patients. Pregnancy is contraindicated and carries a >50 percent maternal mortality rate.[12] Oral contraceptives should also be avoided because of the risk of progressive pulmonary vascular obstruction and thrombosis. Intrauterine devices may increase the risk of infection and endocarditis. Phlebotomy is indicated *only* for patients with hematocrit >65 percent *and* symptoms of hyperviscosity (headache, dizziness, blurred vision).[12] Indiscriminate use of phlebotomy may lead to iron deficiency anemia, worsening symptoms, and eventual death of the patient. Phlebotomy should be carried out by or in consultation with physicians trained in the care of Eisenmenger's patients, as death may occur. Heart-lung transplant is the only definitive treatment for suitable candidates. Both intravenous and subcutaneous prostacyclins are currently under investigation for treatment of Eisenmenger's patients.

# LEFT-SIDED LESIONS

## Coarctation of the Aorta

**INCIDENCE.**   Coarctation of the aorta accounts for 8 to 10 percent of congenital heart defects (it is the fourth most common defect) and has a 2.5:1 male preponderance.[14] Associated defects include bicuspid aortic valve, PDA, VSD, mitral valve abnormalities, cerebral aneurysms (usually around the circle of Willis), and Turner's syndrome (XO chromosomal abnormality).[2]

**ANATOMY AND PHYSIOLOGY.**   Coarctation occurs at the junction of the distal arch and the descending aorta, with its location defined as either preductal (usually associated with PDA), juxtaductal (at the level of the ductus), or postductal. The coarctation is usually focal or a diffuse narrowing, although there may be distal arch hypoplasia. Collateral circulation via the intercostal arteries develops to supply adequate circulation to the lower extremities. A bicuspid aortic valve is found in 50 to 85 percent of patients with coarctation of the aorta.

Hypertension occurs in patients with coarctation as a result of loss of aortic compliance, stimulation of the renin-angiotensin system, and resetting of the carotid sinus baroreceptors. Systemic or exercise-induced hypertension may persist after repair, even in the absence of a residual gradient. Premature coronary disease may also develop.[14,15]

**CLINICAL PRESENTATION AND DIAGNOSIS.**   Presentation depends on the degree of obstruction and collateral development. Approximately 10 percent of patients will present in infancy with heart failure, renal failure, and failure to thrive.[2] Older children and young adults may present with upper-extremity hypertension or lower-extremity claudication. If coarctation is not corrected surgically, life expectancy is significantly shortened (median survival 30 years).[1,14] Rupture of the aorta or dissection may occur in the third or fourth decade. Endocarditis also occurs more frequently with age.

On physical examination, the lower-extremity pulses are absent or delayed. Blood pressure is higher in the arm than in the leg. In all young patients with unexplained hypertension, both brachial and femoral pulses should be palpated, as well as measuring arm-leg blood pressures. An ejection click indicates the presence of a bicuspid aortic valve. A systolic ejection murmur is also present. The ECG may be normal or show left ventricular hypertrophy. The chest radiograph may show a mildly enlarged heart and rib notching from intercostal collateral vessels. Echocardiography with Doppler will confirm the diagnosis and document the gradient across the obstruction. Magnetic resonance imaging (MRI) can also be used to identify the presence and extent of the coarctation.

**MANAGEMENT AND PROGNOSIS.**   A 20-mmHg systolic blood pressure difference between the upper and lower extremities indicates the need for further evaluation. A 50-mmHg difference indicates the need for intervention. Generally, open surgical repair is recommended, although balloon angioplasty has been used experimentally for native coarctation.[16] The risks of surgical repair include lower-extremity paralysis related to cross-clamping of the aorta. Aortic rupture, dissection, or aneurysm formation may complicate balloon angioplasty.[16] Hypertension may persist postoperatively and is effectively treated with beta blockers or angiotensin-converting enzyme inhibitors.[14,15] Recommendations regarding endocarditis prophylaxis, pregnancy, and sports participation are detailed in Tables 33-3 to 33-5. Exercise testing should be performed in all patients with repaired coarctation prior to participation in sports to evaluate for exercise-induced hypertension.[17]

Earlier repair is associated with the best long-term survival rates (92 percent at 25 years), with survival declining the later the procedure is performed.[1,15] The incidence of recurrence of the coarctation varies, depending on the surgical procedure used. Recurrence is most common with end-to-end anastomoses and least common with a subclavian flap repair.[14] Balloon angioplasty has been used successfully for recurrent coarctation.[18]

The use of patch aortoplasty has largely been abandoned because of the high incidence of aortic aneurysm formation (25 percent).[19] Patients who have had their coarctation repaired by this method require regular surveillance with either MRI or computed tomography (CT) to detect the presence of aneurysms.[19] Annual chest radiographs may be utilized initially to screen for the development of aneurysms.

## Congenital Aortic Stenosis—Bicuspid and Unicuspid Aortic Valves

A bicuspid aortic valve is the most common congenital cause of aortic stenosis, accounting for nearly 5 percent of congenital heart defects.[20] Bicuspid aortic valves

TABLE 33-3.   Antibiotic Prophylaxis Guidelines

| **Dental/Upper Respiratory Tract Procedures** | |
| --- | --- |
| Low to moderate risk, no penicillin allergy | Amoxicillin 2 g PO 1 h before procedure |
| Penicillin allergy | Clindamycin 600 mg or cephalexin 2 g or azithromycin 500 mg PO 1 h before procedure |
| **Genitourinary/Gastrointestinal Procedures** | |
| Low to moderate risk, no penicillin allergy | Amoxicillin 2 g PO 1 h before procedure |
| High risk, no penicillin allergy | Ampicillin 2 g IV plus gentamicin 1.5 mg/kg IV 30 min prior to procedure; in 6 h, amoxicillin 1 g PO or ampicillin 1 g IM/IV |
| Penicillin allergy | Vancomycin 1 g IV 1 h before procedure, plus gentamicin 1.5 mg/kg IV; repeat in 8 h |

*Source:* Data obtained from Prevention of Bacterial Endocarditis: Recommendations by the American Heart Association by the Committee on Rheumatic Fever, Endocarditis, and Kawasaki Disease. *Circulation* 1997; 96:358–366. Adapted and used with permission.

**TABLE 33-4.   Pregnancy Risks in Congenital Heart Disease**

| | |
|---|---|
| Low risk (maternal mortality <1%) | ASD, VSD, PDA, small shunt, without pulmonary hypertension<br>Surgically repaired tetralogy of Fallot (normal RV function, no arrhythmia, no symptoms)<br>Mild pulmonary valve stenosis |
| Moderate risk (mortality 5–15%) | Prosthetic valves<br>Aortic stenosis (mild–moderate)<br>Coarctation of the aorta without hypertension<br>Marfan syndrome with normal aortic root (<4 cm, no aortic insufficiency) |
| High risk (prohibitive, maternal and/or fetal mortality >25%) | NYHA class III or IV symptoms<br>Any cyanotic congenital heart disease<br>Coarctation of the aorta with systemic hypertension, any corrected or uncorrected coarctation<br>Any shunt lesion with moderate to severe pulmonary hypertension<br>Severe aortic stenosis or other left heart obstruction<br>Marfan syndrome with enlarged aortic root (>4 cm)<br>Myocardial dysfunction |

ASD = atrial septal defect; VSD = ventricular septal defect; PDA = patent ductus arteriosus; RV = right ventricle; NYHA = New York Heart Association.

*Source:* Data obtained from Siu SC, Sermer M, Harrison DA, et al: Risk and predictors for pregnancy-related complications in women with heart disease. *Circulation* 1997; 96:2789–2794; Pitkin RM, Perloff JK, Koos BJ, et al: Pregnancy and congenital heart disease. *Ann Intern Med* 1990; 112:445–454; Ramin SM, Maberry MC, Gilstrap LC: Congenital heart disease. *Clin Obstet Gynecol* 1989; 32:41–47.

are more common in males and are associated most frequently with coarctation of the aorta.[20] Unicuspid aortic valves are rare and are often detected in infancy or early childhood.[2] A systolic ejection click and systolic murmur are present in most patients with bicuspid aortic valves.

The bicuspid aortic valve becomes scarred and calcified with time as a result of turbulence across the abnormal valve. Eventually aortic stenosis and insufficiency develop. Aortic valve replacement can be performed in adults with an operative mortality of less than 5 percent.[20,21]

The diagnosis, management, and prognosis of patients with aortic valve stenosis and regurgitation are described in detail in Chap. 32.

## Subaortic Stenosis

**INCIDENCE, ANATOMY, AND PHYSIOLOGY.**   Subaortic stenosis is uncommon, accounting for 0.5 percent of congenital heart defects in childhood.[22] Clinical manifestations are rarely present before age 10 and are much more common in adolescence.

**TABLE 33-5.**   Athletic Participation in Congenital Heart Disease

| | |
|---|---|
| **Atrial Septal Defect—Unoperated** | |
| Unoperated, no pulmonary hypertension | May participate in all competitive sports |
| Pulmonary hypertension (mean pulmonary pressure >20 mmHg) | Individual assessment |
| | |
| **Atrial Septal Defect—Operated** | |
| >6 months postoperative | All competitive sports |
| Pulmonary pressure >20 mmHg (mean), or sinus node dysfunction, or complete atrioventricular block or cardiomegaly on chest radiograph | Individual assessment |
| | |
| **Ventricular Septal Defect—Unoperated** | |
| Small (pulmonary to systemic flow <1.5 : 1.0) or moderate (1.5–1.9 : 1.0) defect | All competitive sports |
| Large defect (pulmonary to systemic flow >2.0 : 1.0) | Some low-intensity sports |
| | |
| **Ventricular Septal Defect—Operated** | |
| >6 months from operation, no residual defect, none of the following: pulmonary hypertension, ventricular arrhythmias on 24-h ambulatory monitoring, abnormal exercise tolerance test (ventricular arrhythmias), hypertrophy on electrocardiogram | All competitive sports |
| One or more of the above | Low-intensity sports |
| | Consider repair of residual defects |
| | |
| **Patent Ductus Arteriosus—Unoperated** | |
| Small | All competitive sports |
| Moderate to large | Low-intensity sports. Ligation recommended prior to unrestricted participation |
| | |
| **Patent Ductus Arteriosus—Operated** | |
| >3 months postoperative, normal cardiac examination, normal chest radiograph | All competitive sports |
| Persistent pulmonary hypertension | Individual assessment |
| | |
| **Pulmonary Valve Stenosis—Unoperated** | |
| Peak gradient <50 mmHg, normal right ventricular function, no symptoms | All competitive sports |
| Peak gradient >50 mmHg or right ventricular dysfunction | Low-intensity sports; consider referral for balloon valvuloplasty |
| | |
| **Pulmonary Stenosis—Operated** | |
| Normal right ventricular function, adequate relief of obstruction | All competitive sports |
| Persistent gradient >50 mmHg for balloon | Low-intensity sports; consider referral for balloon valvuloplasty |
| Severe pulmonary insufficiency | Individual assessment |

**TABLE 33-5.** *(continued)*

| | |
|---|---|
| **Aortic Valve Stenosis—Unoperated** | |
| Mild aortic stenosis, normal electrocardiogram, no history of syncope, arrhythmia, or chest pain (peak gradient <20 mmHg) | All competitive sports |
| Moderate aortic stenosis, asymptomatic, normal ECG, no hypertrophy on echocardiogram (gradient 21–49 mmHg), no arrhythmia, normal exercise test | Low-static, low-moderate dynamic, and moderate-static, low-dynamic sports |
| All others | Restricted until repaired High risk for sudden death |
| **Coarctation of the Aorta—Unoperated** | |
| Mild coarctation, no collateral vessels, normal exercise test, small gradient at rest | All competitive sports |
| Arm/leg gradient >20 mmHg, exercise-induced hypertension (>230 mmHg systolic) | Low-intensity sports |
| **Coarctation of the Aorta—Operated** | |
| Gradient <20 mmHg, >6 months postoperative, normal blood pressure at rest and during exercise | All competitive sports, except weight lifting, high-intensity static exercises |
| **Tetralogy of Fallot** | |
| Postoperative with normal right heart pressure, no residual shunt, no arrhythmias on 24-h ambulatory monitoring, no history of syncope, normal exercise test | All competitive sports |
| Significant pulmonary valve regurgitation, elevated right heart pressures, arrhythmias, syncope, abnormal exercise test | Individual assessment |
| **Ebsteins's Anomaly** | |
| Mild Ebstein's, no cyanosis, normal heart size, no arrhythmias | All competitive sports |
| All others | Individual assessment |
| **Congenital coronary anomalies** | Excluded from all sports—high risk of sudden death without surgery |
| Postoperative, normal exercise test | All competitive sports |

Examples of low-intensity sports include billiards, bowling, cricket, curling, and golf.

*Source:* Data obtained from Graham TP, Bricker JT, James FW, Strong WB: Task Force 1: congenital heart disease. *J Am Coll Cardiol* 1994; 24:867–873.

Discrete subaortic stenosis is defined by the presence of a discrete obstructing membrane along the left ventricular outflow tract. The membrane may be weblike or made of dense, fibrous connective tissue. Other cardiac anomalies may also be present. The high-velocity turbulent flow may lead to aortic valve thickening and aortic insufficiency if not corrected.[22] Endocarditis is also a risk.

Tunnel aortic stenosis is a rare form of subaortic stenosis that presents in child-hood.[2] This is characterized by tubular narrowing of the aortic outflow tract and marked left ventricular hypertrophy, with associated abnormalities of the intra-mural coronaries and aortic valve annulus..

**CLINICAL PRESENTATION AND DIAGNOSIS.**   The most common present-ing symptoms (similar to those in valvular aortic stenosis) are dyspnea, chest pain, and syncope. The presence of symptoms correlates with more significant outflow tract obstruction. The majority of patients present during adolescence or young adulthood. On examination, the left ventricular impulse is sustained and prominent. A harsh systolic ejection murmur is present at the second to fourth intercostal spaces. A diastolic blowing murmur of aortic insufficiency is also often present. Paroxysmal splitting of the second heart sound may occur.

The ECG may show left ventricular hypertrophy. First-degree atrioventricular block may also be present. The chest radiograph may show cardiomegaly. A transthoracic echocardiogram is generally diagnostic. Occasionally in adult patients, a transesophageal echocardiogram may be necessary to visualize the subaortic membrane.

**MANAGEMENT AND PROGNOSIS.**   Discrete subaortic stenosis is a progres-sive disease, with increasing outflow tract obstruction and aortic insufficiency over time. Surgical correction is therefore recommended at the time of diagnosis, re-gardless of the outflow tract gradient, to prevent progressive aortic insufficiency.[22] Complete excision of the membrane is necessary to prevent restenosis. Higher residual gradients postoperatively predict lower long-term survival rates.[22] Recur-rence of the subaortic stenosis as a result of fibromuscular hyperplasia is common. The lesion is more complex than was previously thought. Repeat subaortic surgery and aortic valve replacement may be needed.

## Congenital Mitral Anomalies

Congenital obstructive mitral valve lesions include parachute mitral valve with a single papillary muscle, supravalvular mitral ring, and hypoplastic annulus. Congen-ital mitral stenosis is uncommon and may be associated with other defects, includ-ing coarctation of the aorta, hypoplastic left heart syndrome, atrioventricular canal defects, aortic outflow obstruction, and double-outlet right ventricle.

The presentation and physical findings are similar to those of acquired mitral stenosis. Presentation may be in childhood or adolescence. Surgical repair or valve replacement is required in order to correct the obstruction. Management of mitral stenosis is discussed in detail in Chap. 32.

Congenital abnormalities of the leaflets or chordal attachments can produce mi-tral regurgitation. Congenital mitral regurgitation is managed in a similar manner to acquired mitral regurgitation (see Chap. 32). Mitral prolapse is also discussed in de-tail in Chap. 32. Echocardiography is diagnostic.

## Pulmonary Valve Stenosis

**INCIDENCE, ANATOMY, AND PATHOPHYSIOLOGY.**   Congenital valvular pulmonic stenosis (VPS) makes up 10 percent of cases of congenital heart disease. Symmetric fusion of the commissures of the valve results in a circular central orifice. The valve diaphragm is mobile and inflexible, doming in systole. Usually, there is no significant pulmonary valve incompetence. In less than 15 percent of cases, the valve is dysplastic. The myxomatous leaflets are not fused but are thick, folded, and immobile. This condition is associated with small stature and mild mental retardation (Noonan's syndrome).

In cases of moderate to severe VPS, right ventricular hypertrophy is present. A patent foramen ovale may be a site for right-to-left atrial shunting, especially if the hypertrophied right ventricle offers increased resistance to filling. Calcification of the stenotic pulmonary valve is uncommon but may occur in middle age.

**DIAGNOSIS.**   Symptoms are usually absent in patients with mild to moderate VPS. With severe stenosis, dyspnea on exertion and fatigue are progressive, especially in the adult. Exercise tolerance and working capacity are also abnormal. Auscultation is a valuable tool in the diagnosis of VPS. A systolic ejection murmur that is maximal in the second left interspace at the sternal edge is always present. An early systolic ejection click, caused by sudden doming of the valve, is diagnostic (see Fig. 33-3A). A large a wave related to decreased compliance of the thick right ventricle may be seen in the internal jugular venous pulse.

The ECG in moderate and severe valvular pulmonic stenosis shows right ventricular hypertrophy. A qR complex in lead $V_1$ correlates with a gradient greater than 80 mmHg, while a tall R wave in lead $V_1$ with T-wave inversion suggests systemic or suprasystemic pressure in the right ventricle (Fig. 33-4). Tall, peaked P waves in leads II and $V_1$ reflect right atrial abnormality.

The chest x-ray usually shows a normal cardiothoracic ratio. In severe VPS, there is right atrial and right ventricular prominence. An important feature in all cases of VPS is marked poststenotic dilation of the main and left pulmonary arteries but not the right pulmonary artery (see Fig. 33-5). The left pulmonary artery at fluoroscopy pulsates vigorously, whereas the right pulmonary artery is quiet. The direction of the stenotic jet passes from the main pulmonary artery directly into the left pulmonary artery. Though the diagnosis and severity of VPS are assessed quite well clinically, echocardiography yields close agreement with the pulmonary valve gradient obtained at right heart catheterization.

In VPS, the right ventricular systolic pressure is mildly (35 to 59 mmHg), moderately (60 to 89 mmHg), or severely (greater than 90 mmHg) elevated and may exceed twice systemic pressure.

**MANAGEMENT.**   The procedure of choice in the treatment of valvular pulmonic stenosis in both children and adults is balloon valvuloplasty, a safe and effective interventional procedure with excellent short- and long-term results.[23] Ideally, balloon valvuloplasty should be performed after the severity of VPS has been established by

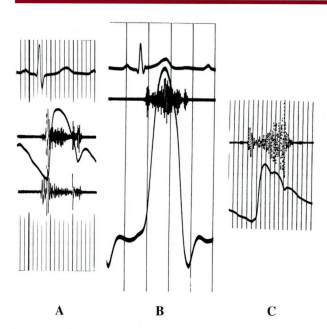

**A**                    **B**                    **C**

**Figure 33-3**  Phonocardiograms from three patients with various degrees of valvular pulmonic stenosis (VPS). *A*. Mild VPS. The right ventricular (RV) pressure is 32/5 mmHg, and the peak systolic gradient is 17 mmHg. The systolic ejection murmur peaks early, stopping before the aortic valve closure sound and before the dicrotic notch of the carotid pulse. An ejection click (EC) is noted, and the second heart sound is split. A & P indicate aortic and pulmonary valve closure, respectively; and LICS, left intercostal space. *B*. Moderate VPS. The RV systolic pressure is 80/5 mmHg, and the peak systolic gradient is 60 mmHg. The triangular peak on the RV systolic pressure tracing is characteristic in VPS. The systolic ejection murmur peaks in midsystole and is diamond-shaped. *C*. Severe VPS. The RV systolic pressure is 208/10 mmHg, and the peak systolic gradient is 194 mmHg. Note the late-peaking long systolic murmur extending past the aortic valve closure sound ($A_2$) and past the dicrotic notch of the carotid artery pulse tracing. $S_1$ indicates. (From Franch RH: Recognition and management of valvular pulmonary stenosis. In: Hurst JW (ed): *Heart Dis Stroke* 1994;3(No. 6):367. Used with permission.)

clinical means and Doppler echocardiography. Balloon dilatation produces a tear in the fused pulmonary valve commissure, reducing the right ventricular/pulmonary artery gradient by 70 to 90 percent.[24] As the subvalvular hypertrophy regresses gradually over weeks, the gradient declines further. Rarely, in a small percentage of patients, severe hypoplasia of the annulus or a dysplastic valve may preclude successful balloon valvuloplasty.[24]

**PROGNOSIS.**   Untreated mild VPS rarely progresses over the years, whereas moderate or severe VPS is likely to progress if untreated. Despite concern about the regression of right ventricular muscle mass and infundibular hypertrophy, and the presence of residual mild to moderate pulmonary regurgitation after treatment, the relief of moderate and severe VPS improves symptoms and the quality of life.[23]

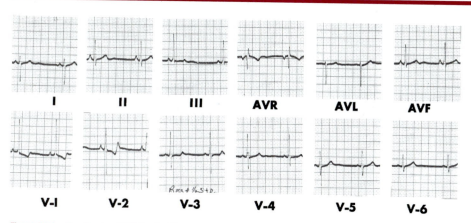

**Figure 33-4**   Twelve-lead ECG of a 17-year-old male with severe valvular pulmonic stenosis. Note the tall R wave in lead $V_1$ and the T-wave inversion; this is consistent with severe right ventricular hypertrophy. (From Franch RH: Recognition and management of valvular pulmonary stenosis. In: Hurst JW (ed): *Heart Dis Stroke* 1994;3(No. 6):367. Used with permission.)

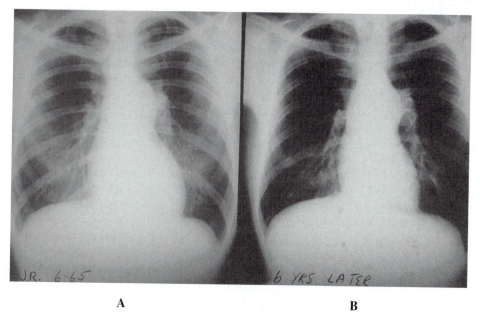

**Figure 33-5**   Frontal chest radiographs of an asymptomatic 27-year-old mechanic taken before (*A*) and 6 years after (*B*) surgery for severe valvular pulmonic stenosis. Preoperative right ventricular systolic pressure was 160/5 mmHg. Note the decrease in heart size after surgery. Dilatation of the main and left pulmonary arteries persists, but the right atrium and right ventricle are smaller. (From Franch RH: Recognition and management of valvular pulmonary stenosis. In: Hurst JW (ed): *Heart Dis Stroke* 1994;3(No. 6):368. Used with permission.)

## Tetralogy of Fallot

**INCIDENCE, ANATOMY, AND PATHOPHYSIOLOGY.**   Tetralogy of Fallot is the most common cyanotic congenital heart defect. A large VSD lies below the right aortic cusp, with the aorta overriding the ventricular septum. One-fifth of these patients have a right aortic arch. There is variable obstruction of the right ventricular outflow tract. The pulmonary valve may also be bicuspid and stenotic. Right ventricular hypertrophy is always present. Tetralogy of Fallot is a clinical and hemodynamic spectrum based on the severity of right ventricular outflow obstruction. Most commonly, right ventricular outflow obstruction is severe, resulting in a cyanotic child. Severely cyanotic adults may be seen who have a large VSD and pulmonary atresia with multiple systemic collateral arteries supplying pulmonary blood flow. Moderate right ventricular outflow obstruction and VSD result in mild or absent resting cyanosis—the so-called acyanotic tetralogy of Fallot ("pink tet").

**DIAGNOSIS AND MANAGEMENT.**   The patient with tetralogy of Fallot will usually have cyanosis and clubbing. The murmur from the right ventricular outflow tract obstruction is heard at the left upper and mid-lower sternal border. On the chest radiograph, heart size is not increased in the anterior-posterior view; the apex is upturned, and the mid-pulmonary artery area is concave, resulting in a boot-shaped heart. Pulmonary vasculature is diminished bilaterally. The aortic arch may be right-sided (see Fig. 33-6). The ECG shows right ventricular hypertrophy and right axis deviation. Transthoracic echocardiography is diagnostic.
   Only rarely will tetralogy of Fallot escape diagnosis until adult life. Usually patients who are seen as adults will present having undergone prior surgical repair. These patients require a clinical examination, chest radiograph, and ECG to evaluate for residual VSD and/or right ventricular outflow tract obstruction as well as right ventricular size and function. Moderate to severe pulmonary regurgitation is common postrepair.[25] Systolic and diastolic murmurs of outflow obstruction and pulmonary valve regurgitation are frequently heard. The chest radiograph shows prominence of the right ventricular outflow tract marking the site of the right ventricular outflow tract patch. The ECG shows right bundle branch block in nearly all, left axis deviation in 20 percent, and complete heart block in 1.2 percent. The late appearance of 2 : 1 atrioventricular block indicates the need for an immediate pacemaker. Generally, right ventricular size and function are abnormal in those who required a large outflow tract patch. Replacement of the regurgitant pulmonary valve may improve right ventricular failure. Malignant ventricular arrhythmias, particularly ventricular tachycardia, may occur late after repair of tetralogy of Fallot[25] (see Fig. 33-7). Therefore, prompt evaluation of the patient with palpitations or syncope should be performed.

## Ebstein's Anomaly

**INCIDENCE, ANATOMY, AND PATHOPHYSIOLOGY.**   In Ebstein's anomaly, the anterior tricuspid valve leaflet is attached normally to the annulus, but the septal and posterior leaflets of the tricuspid valve originate in the right ventricular

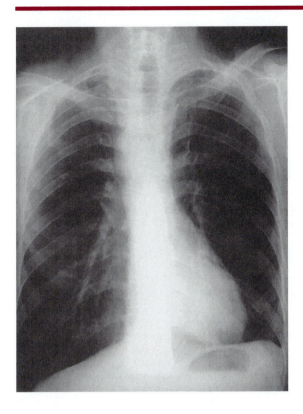

Figure 33-6   Chest radiograph frontal view. Blalock-Taussig anastomosis of 13 years' duration in a 38-year-old man. The aortic arch is on the right. The arterial blood oxygen saturation was 82 percent. Heart size is normal.

wall below the annulus. Thus the functioning right ventricle is made smaller and the atrial cavity (now made up of the right atrium proper and the thin-walled atrialized portion of the right ventricle) is made larger than normal. The abnormal tricuspid valve is often incompetent. A patent foramen ovale or an ASD is nearly always present, permitting right-to-left shunting of varying degree.

**DIAGNOSIS.**   A broad spectrum of signs and symptoms is related to the severity of the deformity of the tricuspid valve, the amount of displacement of the leaflets, and the amount of the right-to-left atrial shunt. Bouts of supraventricular dysrhythmias may prompt referral as well. A large heart is noted on routine chest radiograph. Cyanosis and clubbing may be present. A systolic regurgitant v wave occurs in the jugular veins if tricuspid valve regurgitation is significant. A systolic murmur at the lower left sternal border is common. The first and second heart sounds are split, with a faint pulmonary valve closure sound. An $S_4$ gallop is commonly heard.

The ECG has large peaked P waves, consistent with right atrial abnormality. The right precordial leads show low QRS voltage and right bundle branch block. In 10 percent, a short P-R interval and preexcitation (Wolff-Parkinson-White syndrome) is noted, with slurring of the initial QRS forces. The chest radiograph shows an enlarged, flask-shaped heart with a convex, prominent right atrial bor-

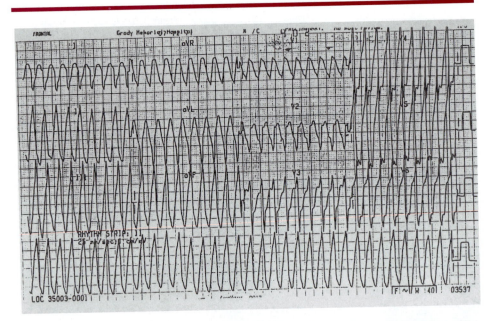

Figure 33-7   Twelve-lead ECG of a 16-year-old male who had total intracardiac repair of tetralogy of Fallot at age 4. The ECG shows ventricular tachycardia at a rate of 214. At catheterization, the right ventricular pressure was 63/7 and pulmonary artery pressure was 37/10(19) with severe pulmonary regurgitation and dilated right ventricle. He is now well controlled on an antiarrhythmic therapy.

der. Pulmonary vascularity is decreased, and the main pulmonary artery segment is not prominent.

Transthoracic echocardiography is diagnostic, showing the apical displacement of posterior and septal leaflets and an elongated tethered anterior leaflet. Color flow imaging detects the ASD.

**MANAGEMENT.**   Pregnancy in women with mild Ebstein's (sinus rhythm, mild cyanosis, and mild cardiomegaly) is well tolerated, and outcome is excellent.

Many adult patients with Ebstein's anomaly have not had surgery. Continued clinical follow-up is needed. If right ventricular failure occurs or increasing cyanosis is observed, surgical referral is then considered.[26] If the patient also has troublesome atrial dysrhythmias, ablation of an accessory pathway can be done at the time of tricuspid valve surgery and ASD closure.

## Dextrocardia (Heart to the Right)

**INCIDENCE, ANATOMY, AND PATHOPHYSIOLOGY.**   Dextrocardia usually presents to the clinician as one of three types:

1.  In mirror-image dextrocardia, with situs inversus of the abdominal and thoracic viscera, the incidence of congenital heart disease is less than 3 percent. The P

wave and the QRS complex are inverted in lead I. Kartagener 's syndrome, occurring in 20 percent, includes the most common noncardiac anomalies: situs inversus, bronchiectasis, and sinusitis. A congenital defect in the motion of the ciliary epithelium is present.

2. In dextrocardia with normal position of the abdominal viscera, the incidence of heart disease is greater than 90 percent, and the majority have complex cyanotic heart disease. The P wave in lead I is upright.

3. One-third of all patients with dextrocardia have uncertain (ambiguous) situs of the viscera and splenic anomaly syndrome. Dextrocardia occurs in well over one-half of all patients with asplenia, but less in those with polysplenia. Severe complex cyanotic heart disease is nearly always present in this subset of dextrocardia.

**DIAGNOSIS.**   To detect dextrocardia at the bedside, one should simultaneously palpate the right and left precordium with the right and left hands in order to compare and detect all anterior chest impulses. In dextrocardia, the apical impulse is in the right precordium. Heart sounds and murmurs tend to be maximum to the right of the sternum. The chest x-ray shows the apex of the heart pointing rightward. The ECG is diagnostic.

**MANAGEMENT AND PROGNOSIS.**   Further evaluation and treatment for dextrocardia depend on coexisting cardiac and noncardiac anomalies.

## Pulmonary Arteriovenous Fistula

**INCIDENCE, ANATOMY, AND PATHOPHYSIOLOGY.**   Congenital pulmonary arteriovenous fistula may be single or multiple, unilateral or bilateral, small or large. It may be beneath the pleural surface or deep within the lung, and tends to occur in the lower lobes.

Approximately 20 percent of patients with hereditary (autosomal dominant) hemorrhagic telangiectasia (Rendu-Osler-Weber syndrome) have pulmonary arteriovenous fistula associated with hemoptysis or gastrointestinal or cerebral bleeding. On examination, telangiectasias are noted on the skin and mucous membranes. Pulmonary arteriovenous fistulas are preferably treated with embolic therapy. Multiple small acquired pulmonary arteriovenous fistulas may occur in association with cirrhosis or metastatic thyroid carcinoma and following caval to pulmonary artery anastomosis (Glenn and Fontan procedures).

**DIAGNOSIS.**   Many patients are asymptomatic. Brain abscess, cerebrovascular thrombosis, transient vertigo, and motor and sensory symptoms may occur, however. Rupture of the fistula may result in hemoptysis or hemothorax. The degree of cyanosis depends on the size of the fistula. A continuous murmur increasing with inspiration is often heard. The ECG is within normal limits. Chest radiography shows the heart to be of normal size. A large fistula typically appears as a round or lobulated shadow near the costophrenic sulcus or behind the heart and diaphragm. Pulmonary angiography is diagnostic with ultrasound; microbubbles injected into the pulmonary artery appear in the left heart, bypassing the lung capillary bed.

## Adults with Cyanosis and Complex Congenital Heart Disease

The examiner should be aware that a patient may have a congenital heart anomaly that is associated with right-to-left shunting; however, clinical cyanosis may not be evident or may be overloaded. Medical treatment is primarily supportive and palliative; surgical treatment may be palliative or anatomically or physiologically corrective. The adult with cyanotic congenital heart disease has certain problems regardless of the underlying anatomy.

The cyanotic adult may have symptoms of hyperviscosity syndrome, including headache, dizziness, visual disturbance, fatigue, muscle pains, paresthesias, and slow thinking. These symptoms usually appear with a hematocrit of 70 percent or greater. The hematocrit should be lowered only to the level that relieves symptoms, which is usually 65 percent. Ordinarily 500 mL of blood is withdrawn and replaced with an equal volume of normal saline, using an air trap or filter on the intravenous line. Iron deficiency should be avoided to prevent increased rigidity and decreased deformability of red blood cells, thus increasing resistance to capillary blood flow. Iron supplementation should be limited to 200 mg daily for 1 week because the hematocrit will rapidly rise. Symptoms and hematocrit are then reassessed. In severe erythrocytosis, spontaneous thrombotic events and bleeding may occur. The cyanotic patient with erythrocytosis may have problematic bleeding intra- or postoperatively. Hyperuricemia tends to be present in the cyanotic patient. Indomethacin may be used to treat the occasional acute case of gout. A CT scan should be considered for the cyanotic patient with fever, headache, lethargy, and visual defect or other focal neurologic signs to exclude brain abscess.

The patient with congenital asplenia and complex cyanotic heart disease has the potential for sepsis due to the encapsulated bacteria. Pneumococcal vaccines should therefore be given. The febrile patient with asplenia requires cultures and prompt attention to a febrile illness.

The cyanotic adult is also susceptible to endocarditis. Unexplained fever demands blood cultures; endocarditis prophylaxis is mandatory.

## Other Congenital Heart Anomalies

**CONGENITALLY CORRECTED TRANSPOSITION OF THE GREAT ARTERIES.** Patients with isolated congenitally corrected transposition of the great arteries may go undetected until adulthood. In congenitally corrected transposition, the great arteries are transposed, but the ventricles are inverted as well, thus "correcting" the circulation. The child therefore will not be cyanotic. The right ventricle becomes the systemic ventricle, however. Symptoms and the timing of presentation depend largely on associated anomalies. The adolescent or adult may present with systemic atrioventricular valve regurgitation or with varying degrees of heart block. The systemic atrioventricular valve may be abnormal and regurgitant in childhood, with a classic Ebstein's anomaly seen in some. The diagnosis should be suspected in the adolescent or young adult with unexplained systemic atrioventricular valve regurgitation.

The electrocardiogram demonstrates a normal P-wave axis, but ventricular activation is right to left, producing Q waves in the right precordial leads and the absence of Q waves in the left precordial leads. Supraventricular arrhythmias may be present. Echocardiography is diagnostic.[2]

Eventually, the morphologic right ventricle fails as a systemic ventricle, producing classic signs and symptoms of congestive heart failure. Progressive systemic atrioventricular valve regurgitation is also problematic, requiring valve replacement in some patients. Complete heart block also occurs at a rate of approximately 2 percent per year. For patients with intractable heart failure, transplantation may be necessary.[2]

**RIGHT VENTRICULAR DYSPLASIA.**   Arrhythmogenic right ventricular dysplasia appears to be a genetically determined disorder resulting in infiltration of the right ventricular myocardium with fat. The clinical presentation is generally ventricular arrhythmias (ventricular tachycardia) originating from the right ventricle. The incidence of sudden death is approximately 1 percent per year. Less commonly, right ventricular failure may occur. Epsilon waves may be seen in the ECG. Suspicion of the diagnosis should prompt referral to a cardiologist specializing in electrophysiology.

**OPERATED COMPLEX CONGENITAL HEART DISEASE.**   The adult with complex congenital heart disease is a survivor of surgical advances over the past 50 years. The need for specialized care and follow-up has led to the formation of regional adult congenital heart centers that offer follow-up and medical, surgical, and catheter-based interventional treatments to these adults. A review of all past medical records, including diagnostic studies and all operative notes, is mandatory. Patients' complaints are the results of ventricular dysfunction, arrhythmias, or pulmonary vascular obstructive disease.

The most frequent reoperation in the adult who has complex congenital heart disease is replacement of a right ventricular outflow valve conduit or aortic valve replacement. In the cyanotic adult with congenital heart disease, surgical creation of a shunt and total repair of tetralogy of Fallot are the commonest operations performed. These patients have the greatest risk related to postoperative bleeding and renal failure. Occasionally a cyanotic adult may be seen who has had a palliative aortic-to-pulmonary shunt (Blalock-Taussig, Potts, or Waterston) to increase pulmonary blood flow and may now require dilatation of the old shunt or placement of an additional new shunt. Total correction, if feasible, is preferred, in an effort to eliminate the social and economic duress of multiple hospitalizations and surgical procedures.

Two groups defy surgical anatomic correction at present: those with inadequate pulmonary arteries as a result of congenital diffuse or segmental hypoplasia or atresia, and those with absence or severe hypoplasia of one ventricle (single-ventricle physiology). In the latter, however, physiologic correction is possible by anastomosis of the vena cava to the pulmonary artery (Fontan procedure modification), provided pulmonary vascular resistance is normal and left ventricular function is good.

Recurrent long-term atrial dysrhythmias are a problem in 40 percent of patients with Fontan circulation.

In transposition of the great arteries, a baffle procedure was used in the past to switch the atrial flow. These patients are susceptible to CHF, as the right ventricle may eventually fail as a systemic ventricle.[27] Currently, the great arteries are switched in infancy along with the origin of both coronary arteries.

One must possess a missionary zeal for ensuring the smooth passage of young congenital heart patients from the pediatric to the adult cardiologist interested in and knowledgeable about congenital heart disease. The care of these patients must not be left to chance, but requires systematic follow-up in a center of expertise. These centers offer comprehensive care and planning for adult congenital heart disease patients and their caregivers. They furnish consultation and teaching for the interested referring physician

## ENDOCARDITIS

Congenital heart disease is a significant predisposing risk factor for bacterial endocarditis, accounting for 20 percent of cases of endocarditis in adults. Most patients with congenital heart defects, with few exceptions, require endocarditis prophylaxis. Surgical advances have permitted the survival of patients with many types of complex congenital heart disease. Many of these operations, however, involve prosthetic conduits or valves or repairs of native valves that leave the individual at risk for endocarditis. All patients with congenital heart disease (repaired or unrepaired) who have abnormal native valves, prosthetic valves, repaired valves, conduits, or shunts require endocarditis prophylaxis.[28,29] Exceptions include isolated ostium secundum ASD; surgically corrected ASD, VSD, or PDA; and anomalous pulmonary veins.[29] Patients with a prior history of endocarditis, mechanical valves, and bicuspid aortic valves are at particularly high risk.[28,29] Table 33-3 outlines current recommendations for prophylaxis. At each visit, the physician and the patient with congenital heart disease should review endocarditis prophylaxis recommendations.

## PREGNANCY

### Normal Changes during Pregnancy

During pregnancy, many changes occur that affect the mother's cardiovascular system. Cardiac output increases 30 to 50 percent, plasma volume increases 40 to 50 percent, heart rate increases 20 percent, pulse pressure increases, both systolic and diastolic blood pressures decrease, systemic vascular resistance decreases, and pulmonary vascular resistance decreases. Respiratory changes occur as well, including an increase in minute ventilation, oxygen consumption, and tidal volume. During the last trimester and at delivery, a hypercoagulable state develops. For women with prosthetic heart valves, this can be a difficult management problem, which is discussed further in Chap. 47.

## Pregnancy in Congenital Heart Disease

Labor and delivery increase myocardial contractility, systemic vascular resistance, and venous return. Oxygen consumption may increase by as much as threefold. Hemodynamic fluctuations are minimized in the lateral decubitus position, as the pressure of the gravid uterus is off of the aorta and inferior vena cava. Therefore, in women with heart disease, laboring in the lateral decubitus position is preferred. Blood loss with a normal vaginal delivery is approximately 500 mL; a cesarean delivery can double the blood loss. Therefore, cesarean delivery should be reserved for accepted obstetric indications. Arrhythmias may be more pronounced during labor and immediately postpartum; therefore, women with cardiac disease should deliver in a monitored setting.[30] Cardiac output, heart rate, and blood volume fall after delivery.

The functional state of the mother is a major determinant of fetal and maternal outcome. Women who are symptomatic at rest have a maternal mortality and fetal loss of greater than 30 percent. Maternal cyanosis inhibits fetal development and promotes fetal loss or prematurity. Eisenmenger's syndrome presents a high risk to the mother and fetus. Sudden changes in pulmonary or systemic vascular resistance can reduce cardiac output and cause maternal death. Therefore, pregnancy should be considered to be contraindicated in women with Eisenmenger's syndrome.[31]

Regurgitant lesions are generally well tolerated during pregnancy, whereas stenotic lesions are not.[32,33] Similarly, left-to-right shunts but not right-to-left shunts are tolerated. Ideally, the woman with congenital heart disease who desires pregnancy should have surgical repair of the defect prior to becoming pregnant. The relative risks of pregnancy to the mother and fetus posed by specific conditions are shown in Table 33-4.

Women with congenital heart disease may choose from a variety of contraceptive methods. Fluid retention may accompany hormonal methods but should not be a problem except for the patient with severe heart failure. Intrauterine devices carry a risk of infection and may increase menstrual bleeding; therefore, these should generally be avoided in women with cyanotic heart disease.

The woman with congenital heart disease who desires pregnancy should be counseled regarding the maternal and fetal risks, including the risk of transmission of congenital heart defects. Should she become pregnant, a team approach with a high-risk obstetrician and a cardiologist knowledgeable in congenital heart disease is necessary to manage the patient.

# SPORTS PARTICIPATION

In general, the recommendations for sports participation are similar to those for pregnancy. Patients with severe aortic stenosis, Eisenmenger's syndrome, pulmonary hypertension, cyanotic heart disease, and Marfan syndrome with dilated aortic root and unoperated coarctation of the aorta with hypertension are at high risk for sudden death while participating in anything but low-intensity sports. Table 33-5 describes recommendations based on specific congenital heart defect and intensity of sport.

## NONCARDIAC SURGERY AND CONGENITAL HEART DISEASE

In general, surgery should be carried out at a specialty center with anesthesiologists trained in cardiac anesthesia.[34] Any patient with a shunt is at risk for paradoxical emboli; therefore, careful attention to eliminate air from all venous lines is essential.[35–37] Patients with surgically corrected ASD, VSD, or PDA or repaired coarctation of the aorta who have no sequelae may be treated similarly to noncardiac patients. Those patients with pulmonary hypertension, cyanosis, or CHF should be considered at high risk for complications.

### REFERENCES

1. Perloff JK, Child JS: *Congenital Heart Disease in Adults,* 2d ed. Philadelphia, W. B. Saunders, 1998.
2. Emmanouilides GC, Riemenschneider TA, Allen HD, Gutgesell HP: *Moss and Adams: Heart Disease in Infants, Children, and Adolescents; Including the Fetus and Young Adult,* 5th ed: Vols. I and II. Baltimore, Williams & Wilkins, 1995.
3. Mahoney LT: Acyanotic congenital heart disease: atrial and ventricular septal defects, atrioventricular canal, patent ductus arteriosus, pulmonis stenosis. *Cardiol Clin* 1993; 11:603–616.
4. Kidd L, Driscoll DJ, Gersony WM, et al: Second natural history study of congenital heart defects: results of treatment of patients with ventricular septal defects. *Circulation* 1993; 87(suppl I):I-38–I-51.
5. Amin Zahid, Gu Xiaoping, Berry JM, et al: New device for closure of muscular ventricular septal defects in a canine model. *Circulation* 1999; 100:320–328.
6. Groundstroem KWE, Livainent TE, Talvensaari T, Lahtela JT: Late postoperative follow-up of ostium secundum defect. *Eur Heart J* 1999; 20:904–909.
7. Gatzoulei MA, Freeman MA, Siu SC, et al: Atrial arrhythmia after surgical closure of atrial septal defects in adults. *N Engl J Med* 1999; 340:339–346.
8. Ryan T: Atrial septal defect in the adult. *ACC Current Journal Review* January/February 1996; 39–42.
9. Shah D, Azhar M, Oakley CM, et al: Natural history of secundum atrial septal defect in adults after medical or surgical treatment: a historical prospective study. *Br Heart J* 1994; 71:224–228.
10. Fisher EG, Moodie DS, Sterba R, Gill CC: Patent ductus arteriosus in adults—long-term follow-up: nonsurgical versus surgical treatment. *J Am Coll Cardiol* 1986; 8:280–284.
11. Najm HK, Coles JG, Endo M, et al: Complete atrioventricular septal defects: results of repair, risk factors, and freedom from reoperation. *Circulation* 1997; 961(suppl II):II-311–II-315.
12. Vongpatausin W, Brickner ME, Hiller LD, et al: The Eisenmenger syndrome in adults. *Ann Intern Med* 1998; 128:745–755.
13. Niwa K, Perloff JK, Kaplan S, et al: Eisenmenger syndrome adults: ventricular septal defect, truncus arteriosus, univentricular heart. *J Am Coll Cardiol* 1999; 34:223–232.
14. Bashore TM, Lieberman EB: Aortic/mitral obstruction and coarctation of the aorta. *Cardiol Clin* 1993; 11:617–641.
15. Stewart AB, Ahmed R, Travill CM, Newman CGH: Coarctation of the aorta: life and health 20–44 years after surgical repair. *Br Heart J* 1993; 69:65–70.

16.  Waldman JD, Karp RB: How should we treat coarctation of the aorta? *Circulation* 1993; 87: 1043–1045.

17.  Graham TP, Bricker JT, James FW, Strong WB: Task Force 1: congenital heart disease. *J Am Coll Cardiol* 1994; 24:867–873.

18.  Hijazi ZM, Fahey JT, Kleinman CS, Hellenbrand WE: Balloon angioplasty for recurrent coarctation of aorta: immediate and long-term results. *Circulation* 1991; 84:1150–1156.

19.  Mendelsohn AM, Crowley DC, Lindauer A, Beekman RH: Rapid progression of aortic aneurysm after patch aortoplasty repair of coarctation of the aorta. *J Am Coll Cardiol* 1992; 20:381–385.

20.  Sabet HY, Edwards WD, Tazelaor HD, et al: Congenitally bicuspid valves: a surgical pathology study of 542 cases (1991 through 1996) and a literature review of 2,715 additional cases. *Mayo Clin Proc* 1999; 74:14–26.

21.  Keane JF, Driscoll J, Gersony WM, et al: Second natural history study of congenital heart defects: results of treatment of patients with aortic valvular stenosis. *Circulation* 1993; 87(suppl I):I-16–I-27.

22.  Brauner R, Laks H, Drinkwater DC Jr, et al: Benefits of early surgical repair in fixed subaortic stenosis. *J Am Coll Cardiol* 1997; 30:1835–1842.

23.  Hayes CJ, Gersony WM, Driscoll DJ, et al: Second natural history study of congenital heart defects: results of treatment of patients with pulmonary valvular stenosis. *Circulation* 1993; 87(suppl I):I-28–I-37.

24.  Chen C-R, Cheng TO, Huang T, et al: Percutaneous balloon valvuloplasty for pulmonic stenosis in adolescents and adults. *N Engl J Med* 1996; 335:21–25.

25.  Foster E, Webb G, Human D, et al: The adult with tetralogy of Fallot. *J Am Coll Cardiol* 1998; 7:62–66.

26.  Celernager DS, Biell C, Till JA, et al: Ebstein anomaly presentation and outcome from fetus to adult. *J Am Coll Cardiol* 1994; 23:170–176.

27.  Puley G, Siu S, Connelly M, et al: Arrhythmia and survival in patients >18 years of age after the Mustard procedure for complete transposition of the great arteries. *Am J Cardiol* 1999; 83:1080–1084.

28.  Morris CD, Reller MD, Menashe VD: Thirty-year incidence of infective endocarditis after surgery for congenital heart defect. *JAMA* 1998; 279:599–603.

29.  Freed MD: Infective endocarditis in the adult with congenital heart disease. *Cardiol Clin* 1993; 11:589–602.

30.  Siu SC, Sermer M, Harrison DA, et al: Risk and predictors for pregnancy-related complications in women with heart disease. *Circulation* 1997; 96:2789–2794.

31.  Pitkin RM, Perloff JK, Koos BJ, et al: Pregnancy and congenital heart disease. *Ann Intern Med* 1990; 112:445–454.

32.  Perloff JK: Pregnancy and congenital heart disease. *J Am Coll Cardiol* 1991; 18:340–342.

33.  Ramin SM, Maberry MC, Gilstrap LC: Congenital heart disease. *Clin Obstet Gynecol* 1989; 32:41–47.

34.  Warner MA, Lunn RJ, O'Leary PW, et al: Outcomes of noncardiac surgical procedures in children and adults with congenital heart disease. *Mayo Clin Proc* 1998; 73:728–734.

35.  Mulhern KM, Mahoney LT, Bjornsen KD, Skorton DJ: Management of adults with congenital heart disease undergoing noncardiac surgery. *ACC Current Journal Review* May/June 1997; 51–54.

36.  Baum VC, Perloff JK: Anesthetic implications of adults with congenital heart disease. *Anesth Analg* 1993; 76:1342–1358.

37.  Ammosh NM, Connolly HM, Abel MD, et al: Noncardiac surgery in Eisenmenger syndrome. *J Am Coll Cardiol* 1999; 33:222–227.

STEPHEN FROHWEIN

CHAPTER

# PERICARDITIS

34

Diseases of the pericardium are becoming increasingly more common as patients live longer with chronic disorders such as neoplasm and end-stage renal disease. Acute pericarditis is the most common disorder of the pericardium and is a syndrome characterized by positional chest pain that commonly varies with changes in respiration and/or the physical finding of a pericardial friction rub. There are many etiologies, but the pathophysiologic basis is one of inflammation of the visceral pericardium, the parietal pericardium, and in some instances the superficial aspect of the myocardium. In reaction to the acute inflammation, the visceral pericardium may exude fluid to form a pericardial effusion, and there is potential for fibrinous adhesions to form between the pericardium and epicardium and produce constrictive pericardial disease.

The diagnosis is predominantly clinical and there is usually a paucity of laboratory findings; specific electrocardiographic (ECG) criteria have been developed.[1] The most common cause of acute pericarditis is metastatic carcinoma, viral inflammation, or an idiopathic presentation.[2] A list of the most common etiologies of acute pericarditis can be found in Table 34-1. Among the secondary forms of pericarditis, the primary disorder is usually evident before pericardial involvement; the most common of these primary disorders are metastatic carcinoma and uremic pericardial disease secondary to end-stage renal disease. By contrast, most cases of acute pericarditis without an initial apparent cause are idiopathic in origin, although presumably viral. The incidence of a specific etiology in acute pericarditis often depends on the clinical scenario and whether the patient presents to a local primary care physician or to a tertiary referral clinic.

Acute pericarditis is a common cause of chest pain in the primary care setting. In young and otherwise healthy patients presenting to a primary care physician with chest pain, pericarditis should be seriously considered given the proper clinical scenario. Almost all patients present with a combination of positional or pleuritic chest pain and shortness of breath. The discomfort may be attributable to inflammation of both the pericardium and the surrounding pleura, hence contributing to the pleuritic nature of the pain. The shortness of breath associated with pericarditis is in part due to the need to breathe shallowly in order to avoid discomfort. Other nonspecific

**TABLE 34-1.   Common Causes of Acute Pericarditis**

Idiopathic pericarditis

Metastatic tumor

Uremia

Viral or bacterial infection

Postmyocardial infarction

Postpericardiotomy syndrome

Connective tissue disease

Trauma, including proximal aortic dissection

Radiation

Anticoagulant therapy

Myxedema

AIDS-related pericarditis

Tuberculosis

Drugs

symptoms such as fever, weight loss, or cough may be due to an underlying condition that has acute pericarditis as a manifestation. The line distinguishing primary from secondary pericarditis is often difficult to find, and the history is often the most important diagnostic tool in making this determination. Uncommonly, patients with acute pericarditis can present with hypotension, dyspnea, and neck vein distention and by clinical as well as echocardiographic data have cardiac tamponade. These patients may or may not have a chest pain syndrome.

# DIAGNOSIS

## History

All that may be required for an accurate diagnosis are a thorough history and physical examination, an ECG, and a chest x-ray. There is usually a characteristic chest pain syndrome. It is usually sharp and pleuritic, or less commonly dull and oppressive, and is increased by breathing or rotating the thorax. The location of the pain is usually precordial or along the trapezius ridge and may radiate to the neck or left arm. The typical duration is hours or days, and there can be a rather abrupt or sudden onset. There is no specific relation to effort, such as walking, but there is often a relation to positional change in that changing the posture and leaning forward seems to relieve the pain and recumbency tends to exacerbate the discomfort.

## Pericardial Rub

A pericardial friction rub is the pathognomonic finding on the physical examination. The most common description of the rub is that it is a three-component rub.[3] Each component of the rub is related to either atrial systole (presystolic), ventricular systole, or the rapid phase of early ventricular filling (diastole), which is about the same timing as a third heart sound. The rub is thought to be due to the friction created by the inflamed pericardium moving up against the epicardium. There is commonly a hemodynamically insignificant pericardial effusion, identified by echocardiography, that may not affect the loudness of the rub. The rub is most commonly diphasic (systolic and diastolic) or triphasic (systolic, diastolic, and presystolic). The component associated with ventricular systole is almost always present and is the most easily appreciated and often the loudest. The presystolic component was present in nearly 70 percent of cases in one large analysis.[4] The component associated with the rapid early phase of ventricular diastole is the least common and may be confused with the sound attributable to atrial systole. A three-component rub is heard more than 50 percent of the time, and a one-component rub is the least common unless the patient is in atrial fibrillation.[4] The sound of the rub may be exaggerated by making the patient lean forward or by inspiration. A rub can be transient, lasting a few hours, or persist for days. Although the rub is present in 50 to 75 percent of cases, one does not need it to diagnose pericarditis. Because of the fleeting and transient nature of the pericardial friction rub, relying on its presence to make the diagnosis will lead to the underdiagnosis of pericarditis.

## 12-Lead Electrocardiogram

The most common laboratory study utilized in the diagnosis of acute pericarditis is the 12-lead ECG. There are several typical changes that can be found in the majority of cases, and these are listed in Table 34-2. Characteristic ECG changes often follow a serial pattern. Spodick[1] described the typical serial ECG pattern as having the following four stages (Table 34-2): (1) concordant ST-segment elevation without reciprocal depression (Fig. 34-1), (2) return of the ST segment to baseline with later

### TABLE 34-2.    Stages of Electrocardiographic Changes in Acute Pericarditis

| | |
|---|---|
| Stage 1 | Concordant ST-segment elevation without reciprocal depression (mean ST vector directed to left and inferiorly) |
| Stage 2 | Return of ST segment toward baseline |
| Stage 3 | T-wave inversion with minimal ST-segment changes |
| Stage 4 | Return of ST segment to baseline; normalization of T-wave changes |

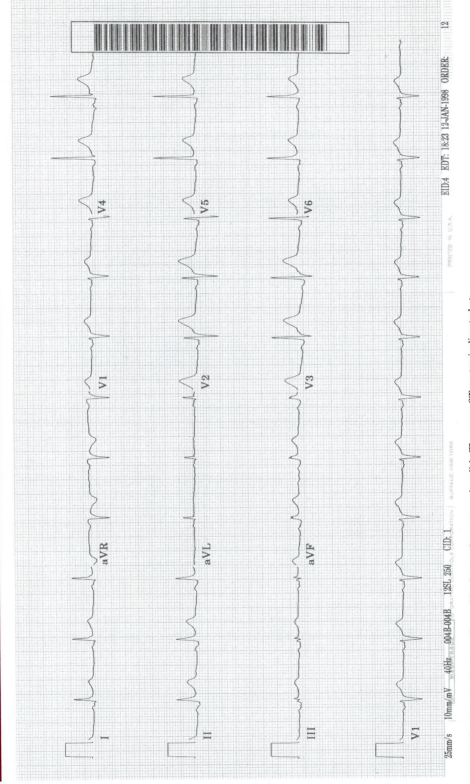

**Figure 34-1** Stage 1 electrocardiographic changes in acute pericarditis. The mean ST vector is directed at +60° in the frontal plane. This produces concordant ST-segment elevations in all extremity leads except lead a$V_R$. P-R-segment elevation is seen in lead a$V_R$, and P-R-segment depression is seen in the inferior leads.

T-wave change, (3) T-wave negativity, and (4) return to normal; patients may present during any one of these stages. In the Spodick study, just over 40 percent of the patients had atypical ECG changes and did not exhibit the aforementioned serial pattern. Over 80 percent of patients exhibited some ECG abnormalities, however, and typical Stage 1 changes or serial ECG changes may be diagnostic even if other characteristics of pericarditis are absent. Other ECG changes involving the P-R segment occur in about 80 percent of patients with acute pericarditis. P-R-segment depression usually occurs in the inferior limb leads and can be seen in the precordial leads; it is primarily seen during the early stages of ST-segment elevation or T-wave inversion (see Fig. 34-1). P-R-segment changes are thought to be due to atrial inflammation and the subsequent effect on atrial repolarization. The sensitivity of serial ECG changes in diagnosing pericarditis is somewhat low, and the lack of ECG changes does not rule out the diagnosis of pericarditis. In fact, the ECG abnormalities attributed to pericarditis are seldom seen in patients with uremic pericarditis. ST-segment elevation is also present in other common cardiac conditions. The presence of ST-segment elevation may be indicative of early repolarization. Young and otherwise healthy patients may have an early repolarization pattern on the ECG that can be confused with pericarditis (Fig. 34-2). In early repolarization, the ST segment is usually elevated no more than 1 to 2 mm in the limb leads or 2 to 3 mm in the precordial leads. Serial ECGs can help sort out these differences, as patients with an early repolarization pattern will show no evolution of ST-segment changes like that seen in patients with acute pericarditis. Acute myocardial injury produces ST-segment elevation that may resemble acute pericarditis. There are, however, significant differences between the ECG changes of acute myocardial infarction (MI) and those of acute pericarditis. Most importantly, the changes in acute MI are often localized, and reciprocal ST-segment depression may be present. The serial ST-segment and T-wave changes in acute MI differ from those seen in pericarditis. In acute MI, the T waves tend to become negative while the ST segments are still elevated, and Q waves may develop. In pericarditis, the T wave does not invert until the ST segment has settled back to baseline.

A large pericardial effusion may depress the size of the QRS complex in the limb leads and/or the precordial leads, and on the ECG this appears as "low voltage" (Fig. 34-3). Low voltage of the QRS complex in the limb leads is usually defined as less than 5 mm in height. In the precordial leads, the normal QRS complex is usually at least 10 mm in height.[5] If the voltage of the QRS varies from beat to beat in the same lead, a large pericardial effusion and possible cardiac tamponade should be suspected. In this setting, the heart is "swinging" within the large effusion with each heartbeat. The swinging action causes beat-to-beat shifting of the electrical axis of the heart, thus shifting the axis and size of the QRS complex on the ECG. The descriptive term for these ECG findings is *electrical alternans* (see Fig. 34-3). The common ECG changes are listed in Table 34-3.

The presence of a previous baseline ECG is very important when evaluating a patient with suspected pericarditis. In determining whether or not there is "low voltage" on the ECG, the previously described measurements are relative. One must take into account the baseline size of the QRS complex. If the patient has a base-

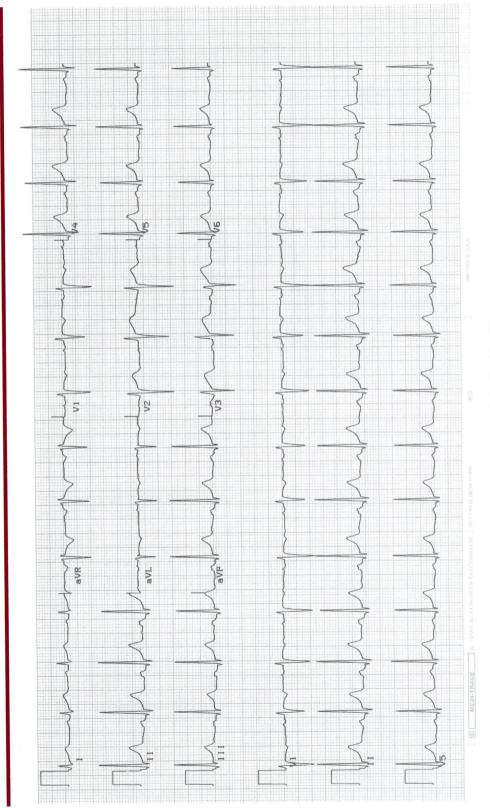

**Figure 34-2** Example of a 12-lead electrocardiogram in a patient with early repolarization. The ST-segment elevation noted in many leads can be misinterpreted as heavy due to pericarditis. This patient's electrocardiogram was not changed from a previous one performed one year earlier.

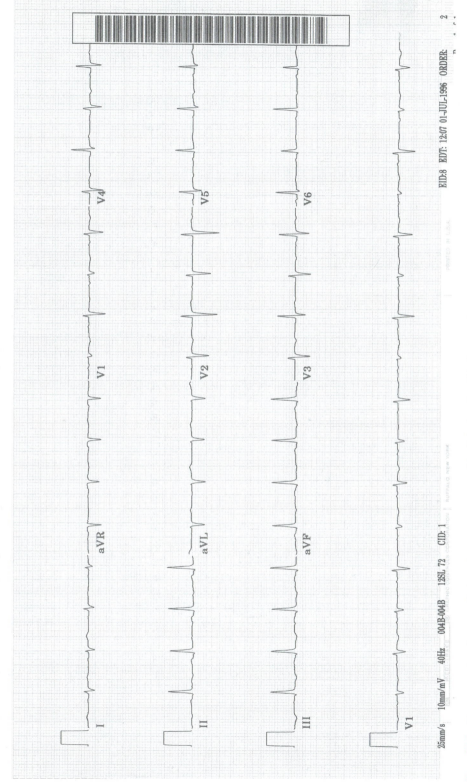

**Figure 34-3** Representative electrocardiogram from a young man with clinical pericarditis, hypotension, and enlarged cardiac silhouette. Note the alternating size of the QRS complexes. This is an example of electrical alternans.

**TABLE 34-3.   Electrocardiographic Changes in Acute Pericarditis**

1. Concordant ST-segment elevation in most leads except lead $aV_R$.

2. T waves become negative only after ST segment has returned to baseline.

3. PR-segment depression seen predominantly in inferior leads.

4. Usually sinus rhythm; atrial fibrillation, atrial flutter occasionally.

5. Absence of ST-segment depression, except in lead $aV_R$.

6. Low voltage: seen with large pericardial effusions.

7. Occasional electrical alternans: seen with pericardial effusion.

line high-voltage QRS, such as that in hypertensive patients, a significant diminution in the height of the QRS complex may be sufficient to label the ECG "low voltage" even though the previously described criteria may not have been met.

## Chest X-ray

The chest x-ray in acute pericarditis is often normal. Cardiac enlargement will be seen as the size of the pericardial effusion increases. If large, the pericardial effusion may cause the cardiac silhouette to assume a "water bottle" configuration. Not uncommonly pleural effusions are present, either on the left or bilateral.

## Echocardiography

Echocardiography has become the diagnostic study of choice in the complete evaluation of the patient with pericardial disease. Although not uncommonly found in patients with acute pericarditis, pericardial effusions may represent an incidental finding. In fact, a number of common problems such as congestive heart failure (CHF), thyroid abnormalities, and AIDS have a pericardial effusion as a common echocardiographic finding. In acute pericarditis, the pericardium often appears normal. In some cases there may be a coarse rub and a scant amount of fluid present. The echocardiogram can identify as little as 15 mL of fluid in the pericardium. The fluid is usually located posterior and may be a normal finding. If the acute inflammatory process of the pericarditis secretes increased amounts of fluid, the effusion tends to extend laterally and anterior around the heart. A larger effusion that extends anterior is not usually a normal finding. In patients with acute pericarditis, the effusion may be either due to the acute inflammatory process or secondary to an underlying disease state that is involving the pericardium and leading to the secretion of increased pericardial fluid as well as the signs and symptoms of acute pericarditis. Echocardiography can often aid in identifying the etiology of the fluid. Metastatic tumors, mass lesions, thrombus, and fibrinous strands within the pericardium can all be accurately assessed with a combination of transthoracic and, if necessary, transesophageal echocardiography.[6] Using a combination of M-mode, two-dimensional, and Doppler echocardiography, one can assess the hemodynamic effect of a pericardial effusion on cardiac function. If cardiac tamponade is suspected, echocardiography not only will aid in making the diagnosis but can be used to help guide needle placement during a diagnostic or therapeutic pericardiocentesis.[7] One must keep in mind that not all patients with acute pericarditis have effusions and not all effusions seen in patients with acute pericarditis are related solely to the pericarditis but may be indicative of another underlying condition.

Certain echocardiographic features of the pericardium may aid in the diagnosis. Fibrinous strands can be seen in patients with metastatic disease, uremic pericarditis, and infectious pericardial diseases. Thrombus within the pericardium can be seen in postpericardotomy patients or in patients who may have bled into the pericardium. The thrombus can cause a localized compression of one of the cardiac chambers and can present with either tamponade or constrictive physiology.[8] The differentiation of these scenarios can be defined by echocardiography.

# SPECIFIC CLINICAL SETTINGS OF PERICARDITIS

## Metastatic Disease

Metastatic involvement of the pericardium can produce a specific variety of pericarditis. With improved treatment plans, patients are living longer and involvement of the pericardium is becoming more frequent. The most common types of cancer that metastasize to the pericardium include lung, breast, lymphoma, and leukemia. Lung cancer is responsible for a third of the cases, with breast cancer accounting for one-quarter and lymphoma involvement in 15 percent.[9] Patients may present with direct invasion of the tumor, causing pericardial inflammation and pain as well as a pericardial effusion. However, over one-half of the pericardial effusions present in patients with cancer are not due to direct invasion of the tumor into the pericardium. In these instances, there may be other antecedent etiologies for the syndrome, such as radiation injury, drug therapy, or infection. Evaluation of these patients is often based on echocardiography, computed tomography (CT) scan, or magnetic resonance imaging results. As previously mentioned, these patients can present initially with large effusions and the presence of cardiac tamponade. Echocardiography can guide needle aspiration for both diagnostic and therapeutic purposes.

## Idiopathic Pericarditis

Pericarditis of unknown etiology is often called idiopathic pericarditis, and in the outpatient primary care setting this is probably the most common variety of pericarditis. In a hospital setting it is probably the second most common variety. The most probable etiology is a virus, but a viral cause can be identified less than 15 percent of the time.[10] Patients present with a combination of chest pain, dyspnea, fever, and malaise. A common finding is an antecedent upper respiratory infection. Clinically the patients may have pulmonary infiltrates on chest x-ray as well as "cardiac shadow enlargement" secondary to a pericardial effusion. Some patients may have myocardial involvement and can develop signs and symptoms of myocarditis, such as arrhythmia and CHF. In patients who have an enlarged cardiac silhouette on chest x-ray or who are hemodynamically unstable, cardiac tamponade should be considered. In one small series, 6 of 54 patients who developed cardiac tamponade had idiopathic pericarditis.[3] The sedimentation rate is almost always significantly elevated; it is normal in less than 10 percent of cases.[10]

The common viral etiologies include Coxsackie A and B viruses, echovirus, and influenza virus.[2] Cytomegalovirus is a relatively rare causative agent.[11] Idiopathic pericarditis can last from 1 to 3 weeks, and occasionally up to 2 months, and is usually self-limited and responsive to conventional therapy. The recurrence rate is approximately 25 percent.[12]

## Postinfarction Pericarditis

Pericarditic pain is a common cause of recurrent pain in postmyocardial infarction patients, but the diagnosis is often missed because the pain is often attributed to recurrent ischemia and the diagnosis is often not entertained unless a pericardial friction rub is present. Pericardial rubs may be fleeting, and therefore the lack of a rub should not rule out the diagnosis.

In 1956, Dressler[13] described a syndrome commonly seen in patients within 2 to 10 weeks postinfarct. This *postinfarction pericarditis syndrome* comprised recurrent positional pleuritic chest pain, pulmonary infiltrates, fever, and a pericardial friction rub. The general incidence is dependent on the type of infarct. In a prospective study of over 700 patients with acute myocardial infarction (AMI), pericarditis occurred in 25 percent of patients with a transmural infarct and 9 percent of patients with a subendocardial infarction.[14] The general incidence of Dressler's syndrome appears to be declining. Thrombolytic therapy for AMI provides early restoration of coronary blood flow, leading to smaller infarct size, better left ventricular function, and improved survival. In the GISSI[15] trial, the incidence of pericardial involvement in patients treated with thrombolytic therapy was approximately 6.7 percent, which was nearly half of that in the control group (12 percent). Also, this trial demonstrated that the presence of pericardial involvement was strongly associated with infarct size as evaluated by ECG criteria, creatinine kinase peak, and echocardiographic determinants of regional wall motion abnormalities. The presence of pericardial involvement was associated with a higher long-term mortality.

In fatal transmural infarctions, pericarditis can be found on postmortem examination nearly 40 percent of the time.[16] If serial echocardiograms are routinely performed following a nonfatal transmural infarction, pericardial effusions are detected more frequently than clinically recognized pericarditis.[17] In a small study of 43 postinfarct patients, 28 percent had clinically recognized pericarditis manifested by typical pleuritic chest pain and/or a pericardial friction rub, and of these only 5 had a pericardial effusion. Of the 43, 16 (37 percent) had a pericardial effusion, and only 5 of these patients had a clinical diagnosis of pericarditis.[18] Therefore, there is not a close clinical association between the echocardiographic recognition of a pericardial effusion postmyocardial infarction and the clinical syndrome of pericarditis.

## Infectious Pericardial Diseases

A number of infectious diseases can involve the pericardium. Some infections that involve the pericardium may do so because of septicemia, whereas others may reach the pericardium through contiguous extension from infection in nearby organs (e.g., pneumococcal pneumonia). Immunocompromised patients are at risk for not only bacterial infections of the pericardium but also fungal and viral infections. People who live or travel to endemic regions may be exposed to various forms of parasitic infections that may involve the pericardium, most commonly trichinosis, microfilaremia, and echinococcosis. Patients who are infected with the AIDS virus can develop a variety of abnormalities involving the pericardium. Pericardial effusion is one of the most common clinical syndromes of cardiac involvement in patients with AIDS, and cardiac tamponade in these patients has a reported incidence of nearly 30 percent.[19] They can have direct invasion of the HIV virus into the myocardium as well as the pericardium, causing myocarditis. They are also at risk for other viral infections and a variety of bacterial and fungal infections if they have low CD4 counts. Finally, tuberculous pericarditis has had a resurgence, especially among AIDS patients and other immunocompromised patients, and not uncommonly the pericardium may be the organ first recognized as being affected by the mycobacterium organism.[20] Interestingly, in AIDS patients who present with tuberculous pericarditis, the CD4 count is usually higher than in AIDS patients who have other cardiac manifestations such as dilated cardiomyopathy, suggesting that tuberculous pericarditis may be an earlier manifestation of AIDS. In tuberculous pericarditis there is always evidence of infection elsewhere in the body, although it may be clinically silent. In at least one-third of the cases pulmonary infection is absent, and therefore pericardial biopsy may be the best test to establish the diagnosis.

## Collagen Vascular Disorders and Pericarditis

Pericarditis is commonly seen in certain collagen vascular disorders. The common syndromes associated with pericarditis are systemic lupus erythematosus, rhematoid arthritis, Wegener's granulomatosis, scleroderma, and polyarteritis nodosa. In systemic lupus erythematosus, pericarditis is the most common cardiac manifestation and has a reported incidence of 25 percent. Clinically silent pericardial fluid is apparently an even more common finding than clinical pericarditis and in one study occurred in nearly 36 percent of the patients.[21] The presence of pericarditis did not correlate with the presence of the lupus anticoagulant, however, which has become a clinical marker of cardiac disease in lupus.[22] Rarely, pericarditis may be the presenting symptom, and not uncommonly pericarditis was recurrent. In scleroderma, pericarditis has been described as a common pathologic finding but a rather unusual clinical manifestation. In one small series, the presence of pericarditis with pericardial effusion was indicative of a poor prognosis, as these patients had a higher incidence of pericardial constriction or restrictive cardiomyopathy.[23] In rheumatoid arthritis, pericarditis is a common extraarticular manifestation. The presence of a silent pericardial effusion is even more common. Although most cases of rheumatoid pericarditis have a benign course and a favorable outcome, a small number exhibit a complicated course, and these patients are at risk for not only chronic pericarditis but also cardiac tamponade. In Wegener's granulomatosis, pericarditis is the most common cardiac manifestation both clinically and pathologically.[24] Pathologically it has been found nearly 50 percent of the time, and the incidence clinically is difficult to ascertain, as Wegener's granulomatosis is an uncommon clinical entity. Other systemic vasculitides and connective tissue diseases that may cause pericarditis include dermatomyositis, ankylosing spondylitis, Reiter's syndrome, Behçet's disease, and familial Mediterranean fever.

## Uremic Pericarditis

Uremic pericarditis is one of the most common causes of acute pericarditis in hospital patients and those referred to a tertiary care facility. In one series, uremic pericardial disease was responsible for 7 of 65 cases of cardiac tamponade.[3] Uremic pericarditis has been found in as many as 20 percent of patients on hemodialysis or peritoneal dialysis. In patients with end-stage renal disease, pleuritic chest pain appears to be less common than in those with idiopathic pericarditis, being found in only 37 percent of patients in one series. The course is variable and depends on the patient's response to treatment, which usually entails aggressive dialysis, antiinflammatory treatment, and pericardiocentesis if necessary.[25] In one small series, 4 of 25 patients developed cardiac tamponade, 3 required pericardiectomy, and 3 others developed constrictive pericardial disease. Patients with end-stage renal disease who develop signs and symptoms of pericardial disease should undergo echocardiography to evaluate the extent of pericardial involvement and define the size of a pericardial effusion if present. It is important to remember that the ECG signs of pericarditis are uncommon in patients with uremic pericarditis.

## Iatrogenic Pericarditis

Several drugs and therapeutic procedures can produce acute pericarditis, and the clinician should always be aware that pericarditis may be a side effect. The anticoagulant warfarin and thrombolytic agents can lead to spontaneous pericardial bleeding in patients who have had a previous MI. Spontaneous bleeding into the pericardium has been reported for patients on warfarin for other therapeutic reasons. These patients are at high risk for developing cardiac tamponade but usually present with the characteristic pleuritic chest pain with a pericardial friction rub. Drugs that cause a lupus-like syndrome can produce acute pericarditis. The common medicines responsible for this syndrome include procainamide and hydralazine.

Methysergide has been causally related to pericardial diseases, and there are many drugs for which a case report exists attributing pericarditis to the specific medication.

Finally, in the hospital setting, pericarditis is a potential complication among patients undergoing diagnostic or therapeutic procedures. Central venous catheter placement, Swan-Ganz catheter placement, cardiac pacemaker and automatic defibrillator placement, and transcatheter coronary interventions have all been associated with pericarditis. Presumably, the pericarditis in these cases is due to possible cardiac perforation and blood in the pericardium. Therefore, these patients are also at risk for cardiac tamponade. As previously mentioned, patients undergoing direct pericardial incision are at risk for developing pericarditis as well as tamponade or constriction. Blood can collect in the pericardium and compress cardiac chambers as well as producing pain and dyspnea. Rarely, patients undergoing abdominal or laparoscopic surgery may experience a syndrome not dissimilar from pericarditis.

## EVALUATION AND TREATMENT

The initial step in the management of patients with acute pericarditis is to determine if the pericarditis is related to an underlying disorder that requires specific therapy. A complete history and physical examination will not only ensure a proper diagnosis but also help in determining if further testing to rule out secondary causes of pericarditis is necessary. Baseline studies that should be obtained in all patients include an ECG and a chest roentgenogram. Echocardiography should not be routinely employed, as the demonstration of a pericardial effusion is often of no clinical usefulness unless the patient is hemodynamically unstable, there is a markedly enlarged cardiac silhouette on chest x-ray, or the proper clinical scenario exists. The presence of a pericardial rub or ECG changes of acute pericarditis are not in themselves absolute indications to obtain an echocardiogram.

The need to obtain laboratory studies to rule out an infectious etiology or collagen vascular disorder will depend on clinical data obtained from the history and physical examination. If there is a chance that a viral infection is present, acute and convalescent serum markers are helpful in making a diagnosis, but often treatment is initiated and symptomatic improvement is realized long before the results of these studies are available. They are often expensive and contribute insignificantly to the management of these patients. On the other hand, patients that may suffer from a bacterial infection or tuberculosis require additional testing to make an accurate diagnosis to ensure proper treatment. In patients suspected of these infections, pericardial drainage of the fluid for adequate culture and evaluation is necessary. Often pericardial tissue biopsy is required in order to make the diagnosis of tuberculous pericardial disease, as there is a very low yield from laboratory evaluation of the fluid.

Patients who have had pericardial incisional surgery, trauma, or percutaneous procedures that can injure the pericardium should undergo echocardiography if the symptoms of pericarditis are present. Postmyocardial infarction patients and patients who have received thrombolytic therapy or anticoagulants who complain of pericarditis should also have a diagnostic echocardiogram to ensure that there is no significant effusion and no signs of cardiac tamponade.

In general, most patients with acute pericarditis need to be closely observed initially to ensure that they are not having an MI and that they are not at risk for developing a large pericardial effusion and cardiac tamponade. Patients who have idiopathic pericarditis of postpericardotomy syndrome and who have a normal-size cardiac silhouette on chest x-ray and no evidence of hemodynamic instability can probably be managed as outpatients as long as they are reliable and will follow up on a regular basis to ensure that treatment has been effective. In some published reports the incidence of cardiac tamponade is as high as 15 percent, and therefore close clinical follow-up is necessary if an outpatient treatment regimen is attempted.[26]

Treatment options are directed not only at reducing the discomfort of pericarditis but also at reducing the inflammation that is the pathophysiologic basis of the syndrome. Acceptable initial treatment options include aspirin, 650 mg every 4 to 6 h; indomethacin, 25 to 50 mg three times daily; or ibuprofen, 200 to 600 mg every 6 h. If the pain is severe, a small dose of a narcotic analgesic may be given until the anti-inflammatory effect of the treatment has taken effect. If the initial trial of medicines is ineffective or the pain lingers for more than 2 to 3 weeks, a course of parenteral steroids may be indicated; however, because of the potential side effects of steroids, these drugs should be avoided. If necessary, prednisone should be given at an initial dose of 20 mg three times daily for 4 to 5 days and then reduced to twice daily for 4 to 5 days, to 10 mg twice daily for 4 to 5 days, and finally to 5 mg twice daily for 4 to 5 days. Antibiotics should be given only to those patients who have documented purulent pericarditis. It should be emphasized that purulent pericardial fluid must be surgically drained. Tuberculous pericarditis is treated with the standard doses of isoniazid, rifampin, and ethambutol for 9 months. Patients who have documented evidence that their acute pericarditis is due to a collagen vascular disorder should be treated with adrenal corticosteroids, such as the prednisone therapy described above. Anticoagulants should be avoided if possible in order to avoid the potential side effect of developing cardiac tamponade from pericardial bleeding. If needed, as in patients who have prosthetic valves, heparin should be started and serial examinations, chest x-rays, and, if needed, echocardiograms should be performed to ensure that no significant effusion has developed.

# RELAPSING PERICARDITIS

The majority of cases of acute pericarditis are usually self-limited, with symptoms predominantly improved over 2 to 6 weeks. Unfortunately, there is a high incidence of recurrence, with up to 25 percent of patients experiencing some form of relapse in signs and symptoms of pericarditis.[12] A large percentage of these patients will respond to reinstitution of high-dose anti-inflammatory drugs or corticosteroids. The treatment, however, will need to be extended for a longer period than the initial treatment and therefore will require tapering over several months to discontinuation or alternate-dose therapy. Rarely, the pain will be persistent over months or years and will not respond to conventional therapy. Alternative medical regimens have been utilized. Colchicine has shown some promise in a small group of patients who have had recurrent pericarditis not responsive to the above-mentioned conventional therapies.[27] Immunosuppressive therapy has been effective in a cohort of refractory patients.[28] In this study, 11 of 12 patients demonstrated no recurrence in symptoms at a mean follow-up period of 42 months after receiving a 3-month course of prednisone at immunosuppressive doses. The one refractory patient then received azathioprine in addition to prednisone and achieved no evidence of recurrence. Three patients in this study suffered severe steroid-related side effects that required additional therapy. Some investigators have attempted pericardiectomy in these unfortunate cases, but with mixed results.[29,30] In these studies, only approximately 50 percent of the patients were pain-free after the recovery period.

One devastating complication of not only recurrent pericarditis but also pericarditis in general is constrictive pericarditis (see Chap. 39). In this syndrome, the pericardium adheres to the epicardial surface of the heart and produces a compressive effect on the ability of both the right and left ventricles to properly expand and fill during diastole. These patients present with evidence of right-sided congestion and dyspnea. The incidence of constriction after acute pericarditis is low, and it is more common in the setting of pericarditis in which blood or some form of infection was present within the pericardium. The possibility of developing this complication should alert the clinician to the importance of the proper diagnosis and treatment of pericarditis.

Even more serious, is development of cardiac tamponade in patients with pericardial effusion. This condition is discussed in Chap. 14.

## REFERENCES

1. Spodick DH: Electrocardiogram in acute pericarditis: distributions of morphologic and axial changes by stages. *Am J Cardiol* 1974; 33:470–474.
2. Shabetai R: Diseases of the pericardium. In: Alexander RW, Schlant RC, Fuster V, et al (eds): *Hurst's The Heart,* 9th ed. New York, McGraw-Hill, 1998:2169–2203.
3. Fowler NO: Pericardial disease. *Heart Disease and Stroke* 1992; 1:85–94.
4. Spodick DH: Pericardial rub: prospective, multiple observer investigation of pericardial friction rub in 100 patients. *Am J Cardiol* 1975; 35:357–362.
5. Chou TC (ed): *Electrocardiography in Clinical Practice,* 3d ed. Philadelphia, W. B. Saunders, 1991:219–233.
6. Chandraratna P, Aronow WS: Detection of pericardial metastases by cross-sectional echocardiography. *Circulation* 1981; 63:197–199.
7. Callahan JA, Seward JB, Nishimura RA, et al: Two dimensional echocardiographically guided pericardiocentesis: experience in 117 consecutive patients. *Am J Cardiol* 1985; 55:476–479.
8. Beppu S, Nakatani S, Ikegami K, et al: Pericardial clot after open heart surgery: its specific localization and haemodynamics. *Eur Heart J* 1993; 14:230–234.

9.   Hancock EW: Neoplastic pericardial disease. *Cardiac Clin* 1990; 8:673–682.

10.  Carmichael DB, Spraque HB, Wyman SM, et al: Acute nonspecific pericarditis: clinical, laboratory, and follow up considerations. *Circulation* 1951; 2:321–331.

11.  Campbell PT, Li JS, Wall TC, et al: Cytomegalovirus pericarditis: a case series and review of the literature. *Am J Med Sci* 1995; 309:229–234.

12.  Sagrista-Sauleda J, Permanyer-Miralda G, Candell-Riera J, et al. Transient cardiac constriction: an unrecognized pattern of evolution in effusive acute idiopathic pericarditis. *Am J Cardiol* 1987; 59:961–966.

13.  Dressler W: A postmyocardial infarction syndrome. Preliminary report of a complication resembling idiopathic recurrent benign pericarditis. *JAMA* 1956; 160:1379–1383.

14.  Tofler GH, Muller JA, Stone PH, et al: Pericarditis in acute myocardial infarction: characterization and clinical significance. *Am Heart J* 1989; 117:86–92.

15.  Gruppo Italiano per lo Studio della Streptochinasi nell'Infarto Miocardico (GISSI): Effectiveness of intravenous thrombolytic treatment in acute myocardial infarction. *Lancet* 1986; 1:397–402.

16.  Roeske WR, Savage RM, O'Rourke RA, Bloor CM: Clinico-pathologic correlations in patients after myocardial infarction. *Circulation* 1981; 63:36–45.

17.  Pierard LA, Albert A, Henrard L, et al: Incidence and significance of pericardial effusion in acute myocardial infarction as determined by two dimensional echocardiography. *J Am Coll Cardiol* 1988; 8:517–520.

18.  Kaplan K, Davison R, Parker M, et al: Frequency of pericardial effusion as determined by M-mode echocardiography in acute myocardial infarction. *Am J Cardiol* 1985; 55:335–337.

19.  Anderson DW, Virmani R: Emerging patterns of heart disease in human immunodeficiency virus infection. *Hum Pathol* 1990; 21:253–259.

20.  Pedro-Botet J, Auguet T, Coll J, et al: Tuberculous pericarditis as the first manifestation of AIDS. *Infection* 1993; 21:334–335.

21.  Ong ML, Veerapen K, Chambers JB, et al: Cardiac abnormalities in systemic lupus erythematosus: prevalence and relationship to disease activity. *Int J Cardiol* 1992; 34:69–74.

22.  Jouhikainen T, Pohjola-Sintonen S, Stephansson E: Lupus anticoagulant and cardiac manifestations in systemic lupus erythematosus. *Lupus* 1994; 3:167–172.

23.  Wefuan J, Aaron SL. Pericardial disease in scleroderma: prognosis and clinical associations. *Clin Exp Rheumatol* 1993; 11:582–583.

24.  Grant SCD, Levy RD, Venning MC, et al: Wegener's granulomatosis and the heart. *Br Heart J* 1994; 71:82–86.

25.  De Pace NL, Nestico PF, Schwartz AB, et al: Predicting success of intensive dialysis in the treatment of uremic pericarditis. *Am J Med* 1984; 76:38–46.

26.  Permanyer-Miralda G, Sagrista-Sauleda J, Soler-Soler J: Primary acute pericardial disease: a prospective series of 231 consecutive patients. *Am J Cardiol* 1985; 56:623–630.

27.  Adler Y, Zandman-Goddard G, Ravid M, et al: Usefulness of colchicine in preventing recurrences of pericarditis. *Am J Cardiol* 1994; 73:916–917.

28.  Marcolongo R, Russo R, Laveder F, et al: Immunosuppressive therapy prevents recurrent pericarditis. *J Am Coll Cardiol* 1995; 26:1276–1279.

29.  Fowler NO, Harbin AD: Recurrent pericarditis: follow-up of 31 patients. *J Am Coll Cardiol* 1986; 7:300–305.

30.  Hatcher CR, Logue RB, Logan WD, et al: Pericardiectomy for recurrent pericarditis. *J Thorac Cardiovasc Surg* 1971; 62:371–378.

THOMAS F. DODSON

# CHAPTER 35

# THE MANAGEMENT OF PERIPHERAL VASCULAR DISEASE

The busy primary care physician will frequently be called upon to evaluate patients with peripheral vascular disease. In this chapter, for the sake of simplicity, we will consider only patients with vascular disease of the lower extremities. Other texts are available to guide the physician who is confronted with uncommon or unusual vascular presentations. It should be emphasized that vascular disease of the lower extremities is an important marker for underlying cardiovascular disease, especially coronary artery disease. An evaluation of 565 men and women with an average age of 66 years by measurement of segmental blood pressures and determination of flow velocity by Doppler ultrasound identified 67 subjects with peripheral arterial disease, and these were followed prospectively for 10 years. Even those patients with lower-extremity vascular disease who would not ordinarily come to clinical attention had a three- to sixfold increase in risk of death from coronary heart disease and cardiovascular disease. Those patients who had symptomatic or severe lower-extremity disease had an even greater risk of death, one 10 to 15 times greater than that of patients who were free of disease.[1] These alarming statistics were confirmed and emphasized a year later when investigators from the University of Pittsburgh evaluated 1492 white women who were 65 years of age or older by means of analysis of their ankle/arm blood pressure index and their mortality over time. When these women had an ankle/arm index of 0.9 or less, their crude overall mortality was about five times greater than that of women with higher ankle/arm index values.[2]

This information is analogous to data obtained over a decade ago concerning the risks of having an asymptomatic carotid bruit.[3] While it was falsely intuitive that such patients would be at greatest risk of cerebral ischemic events, more patients died of *cardiac* ischemic events than of cerebral events. The alert clinician will recognize that the presence of diminished or absent flow in the lower extremities is a call for heightened concern about underlying cardiovascular disease.

Patients with peripheral vascular symptoms of the lower extremities classically present in one of two manners: (1) pain with exercise which is relieved by rest (claudication) or (2) pain at rest (rest pain) or the presence of a nonhealing lesion or even gangrene. It is well worthwhile during the initial evaluation to obtain a detailed history of not only the primary symptomatology, but also the past medical history, family history, medications, and, perhaps most importantly, risk factors for the presence of vascular disease. Are the patient's parents still alive, and if not, what did they die of? Grandparents, brothers, sisters: Do they have any history of vascular or cardiovascular disease? Has the patient ever had a stroke or a heart attack? Is the patient on medications for heart disease or for circulatory problems? Does the patient have diabetes, high blood pressure, elevated cholesterol, or angina, and, probably most importantly, *does he or she smoke*? It has been estimated that this last factor, smoking, is present in almost 100 percent of patients who experience claudication and that it is similarly present in a high percentage of patients who undergo lower-extremity amputation for ischemia.[4] Currently, while cigarette companies seem to be "on the run," about 25 to 30 percent of the population continues to smoke, even in the face of increasingly dire information about the relationship between smoking and premature morbidity and mortality. Interestingly, investigators at the School of Public Health in Berkeley recently published information about smokers from the Health and Retirement Survey which was sponsored by the National Institute on Aging. They found that while smokers recognized that smoking reduces their chances of reaching age 75, the heavy smokers "significantly" underestimated the magnitude of this effect and were overall more optimistic about reaching "old age" than the data would warrant. The authors concluded that dissemination of this information might be another important factor in persuading patients to reduce or stop cigarette consumption.[5] In those patients who smoke, have peripheral vascular disease, and will need a surgical procedure, it has also recently been reported that the surgical hospitalization provides an excellent opportunity to stop smoking. While the results are modest (15 percent in the intervention group and 8 percent in the comparison group stopped), this twofold improvement is a step in the right direction.[6]

Cholesterol reduction has increasingly become a mainstay of the treatment of cardiac and cardiovascular disease. Not surprisingly, effective treatment of patients with elevated cholesterol also led to "statistically significant differences" between the control and intervention groups in the development of clinically evident peripheral vascular disease. Interestingly, while the clinical examination and ankle/arm index were improved in the treatment group, the arteriograms in these two groups of patients showed "no appreciable differences."[7] Given that other investigators have shown a reduction in the carotid artery wall thickness in patients on lipid-lowering therapy,[8] the lack of an effect on an arteriogram in this study might be unexpected. Arteriograms, however, visualize the vessels under study in only one plane and are able to detect only the channel of blood flow and not the thickness of the arterial wall. It could be that if femoral and/or superficial femoral vessels were also assessed by ultrasound technology, as they could easily be, they might show the same salubrious effect after treatment with lipid-lowering agents.

The final leg of the three-legged stool of risk modification (smoking and dietary therapy being the other two) is exercise. This is often the most difficult of the three subjects to discuss with the patient, for although cigarette smoking is addictive, there are treatments [nicotine gum, nicotine patches, bupropion (Wellbutrin)]. Diets can be changed or adjusted, and medication can be added to treat those patients with elevated cholesterol and/or triglycerides. Lack of exercise, however, seems to be the factor that is most resistant to the physician's attempt to modify risks. A recent study confirmed that "low fitness" is an important precursor of mortality. It also confirmed that "moderate fitness" is protective against premature mortality. The investigators' admonitions bear repeating:

> Whether our subjects were unhealthy or healthy, smokers or nonsmokers, had elevated blood pressure or increased cholesterol levels or normal values for these variables, were obese or had normal weights, did or did not have a family history of coronary heart disease or had combinations of other mortality predictors or were at low risk by standard criteria, *all seemed to benefit from being moderately or highly fit compared with low fit men and women of like risk profile*. We believe that physicians should counsel all of their sedentary patients to become more physically active and improve their cardiorespiratory fitness.[9]

Let us now try to put a "face" on two typical patients with peripheral vascular disease: first Mary with claudication, and then Joe with rest pain.

# CLAUDICATION

Mary is a 65-year-old retired Wall Street broker who has been bothered with right leg pain after walking two blocks. She first noticed this pain about 2 months ago during one of her infrequent morning walks, and she also noticed that the pain would go away when she stopped and rested. She has been a long-time smoker, having started in college, and she smokes about one pack per day. Her cholesterol is mildly elevated (as yet untreated), and she is a reluctant exerciser ("I never found the time").

On examination, she has easily palpable femoral pulses, weakly palpable popliteal pulses, and no pulses in her right foot. She has $1+/4+$ posterior tibial and dorsalis pedis pulses in the left foot. Her right foot is warm and pink, with no lesions and a capillary filling time of less than 2 s.

Mary has claudication and, based on information recounted earlier in this chapter, is at increased risk of cardiovascular disease and resultant premature mortality. Her first question to you is the most common one: "Will I lose my leg?" You can reassure her that that outcome is unlikely. Based on information obtained more than two decades ago, in an analysis of more than 600 patients seen for claudication and not primarily considered for surgery, only 5.8 percent of patients came to amputation over a mean follow-up of 2.5 years.[10] Although Mary's claudication would be classified as "moderate" (one to two blocks before onset of pain), only 15 percent of the most severely symptomatic group (less than one block before onset of pain) underwent amputation during the observation period.

Next, it is important to determine how disabling Mary's claudication is to her lifestyle. As vascular surgeons, we are taught to be "conservative" in treating patients with claudication.[11] The reasons for this frequently nonsurgical approach are several and persuasive: (1) The risk of limb loss is relatively low; (2) the incidence of underlying cardiovascular disease, with its attendant increased mortality, is high; (3) patients who are able to stop smoking and participate in an exercise rehabilitation program often improve walking distance; and (4) operation, while often successful, is not always so.

The critical issue is the effect that the claudication has on Mary's life. It can be argued that inability to work as a result of claudication or inability to have an adequate quality of life because of limitations on walking is a reason for consideration of operative intervention. In Mary's case, neither situation is extant. She is retired, she is able to do her gardening and work around the house without difficulty, and she notices the discomfort in her leg only when she is trying to "push" herself. She does plan to travel to Europe with her husband and is looking forward to a lot of sightseeing, but you should not factor that into the equation for or against further intervention.

Mary seems willing to embark on a program of smoking cessation, and you refer her to a program that utilizes nicotine patches and antidepressants. She seems resistant to advice about exercise, however, and asks for "the data." Fortunately, there are two recent studies that support your advice. A meta-analysis of 21 studies showed an increase of 179 percent in mean walking distance before the onset of pain after adherence to a program of exercise rehabilitation.[12] This effect came after participation for a period of at least 6 months in a program with intermittent walking to near-maximal pain as an end point.

A more recent study evaluated 47 patients with claudication who were randomized to either a 12-week supervised exercise program or a home exercise group which received weekly exercise instruction.[13] Although each group improved, it is no surprise that the supervised exercise program provided "superior" increased walking ability. The authors concluded that a supervised program was "optimal" but that the home-based program was a "satisfactory alternative."

Pulse volume recordings, both at rest and during exercise, ideally would be done to provide documentation of the degree of Mary's vascular disease and to provide a baseline for further comparison. In my practice, at this point Mary would be sent on her way with treatment of all three risk factors: a smoking-cessation program, dietary modification and cholesterol-lowering agents, and an exercise program. She would be advised to return in 3 months for an examination and a report on her progress, along with another attempt to give positive reinforcement on these important and difficult changes in her life. Exercise pulse-volume recordings would be repeated at 6 months and perhaps at 1 year to document any changes in arterial perfusion both at rest and after exercise. The outlook for Mary would be somewhat guarded: The loss of her right limb would be unusual, but unless she made a stringent effort to adhere to the new guidelines, her life would be at increased risk.

For completeness' sake, the only other issue in Mary's care would be consideration of the drug pentoxifylline (Trental). This issue was addressed by Radack and

Wyderski, who noted that in 9 of 12 randomized controlled trials, pentoxifylline was found to be "more effective than placebo" in improving walking distance.[11] They further noted, however, that the actual increase in walking distance was unpredictable, and it is this feature of the drug, along with its substantial cost, that makes its use infrequent in our patient population. It does seem reasonable, however, to consider this medication in patients with severe claudication who are not candidates for exercise programs or operative intervention either for anatomic reasons or because of concurrent illness.

Although I am comfortable with the above scenario, it must be acknowledged that not everyone would agree with such an approach. Ambiguity is a constant part of a physician's life, and the treatment of vascular disease is no exception. The British seem to be the most provocative with respect to the use of angioplasty in patients with mild[14] or stable[15] claudication, but Fraser et al., from St. Mary's Hospital in London, recently warned against "treating the lesion rather than the patient."[16] An even more aggressive approach, although for "severe" claudication, not for mild or stable claudication, was put forth by the vascular surgery team from the Brigham and Women's Hospital in their presentation on "femorotibial bypass for claudication." In 53 patients undergoing 57 tibial reconstructions, they had no perioperative deaths, but 9 percent of patients did have "major complications." The overall 5-year survival was 54 percent, and no major amputations were performed.[17] These are excellent results, and since they were performed in patients at "low risk who [were] severely limited by claudication," they seem—in general—in keeping with my own conservative bent.

## REST PAIN

Joe is a 75-year-old man in poor health who had onset of left foot pain about 1 month ago. He was a heavy smoker for "many years," but stopped about 5 years ago when he had a myocardial infarction. About 2 weeks ago, he noticed a "blister" on his left great toe, and several days later, he noticed that the blister had broken, leaving a raw area on the distal one-half of the toe. His son noticed "drainage" on his father's sock and found pus seeping from under the toenail.

The patient has no history of diabetes, does not know his cholesterol level, and has not exercised for many years. He lives alone and has cared for himself since the death of his wife several years ago.

On examination, he has an easily palpable femoral pulse in the left groin, but no distal pulses. He has erythema of the distal one-half of his foot, and foul-smelling drainage from his great toenail.

Joe has a limb-threatening problem and needs urgent attention. He will need admission to the hospital, intravenous antibiotics, and possibly removal of the toenail to allow better drainage of the infected focus. He will need an operation to deal with his ischemic foot and leg, and he will also need an evaluation of his cardiac status to determine the risk of operative intervention, and perhaps even an improvement in his cardiac status prior to either an attempt at revascularization or amputation. The question is how to evaluate his cardiac status in the most efficient and most effective manner. This question is, to me, still open and unanswered. Two recent studies address this issue; the first of these, by a group from Iowa, stated, "The optimal approach to the evaluation and treatment of coronary artery disease in the patient with peripheral vascular disease remains undefined." As they pointed out in their discussion, nonsurgical therapy is often not an option for the geriatric patient with severe peripheral vascular disease, and the risks of screening and prophylactic treatment of coronary artery disease may often outweigh the benefits of such therapy.[18] The vascular surgery team from Worcester, Massachusetts, came to similar conclusions in a review of 70 consecutive patients who underwent coronary angiography because of "redistribution" on a Persantine-thallium scan compared to 70 other patients who were matched for age, gender, peripheral vascular operation, and the number of segments of redistribution who did *not* undergo additional cardiac evaluation. Although the patients who underwent coronary angiography and were considered for coronary revascularization had fewer cardiac events, the positive results were canceled by three deaths and two myocardial infarctions in the more carefully studied group. This team concluded that "the risks of extended cardiac evaluation and treatment did not produce any improvement in either the perioperative or the long-term survival rate."[19] I suspect that in our institution, Joe would undergo either dobutamine stress echocardiography or a Persantine-thallium scan, and it would be hoped that he would not require cardiac catheterization prior to operative intervention on his leg.

The next step for Joe is an arteriogram to allow some assessment of the feasibility of arterial revascularization. His blood urea nitrogen and creatinine would need to be checked to determine the risk of renal dysfunction secondary to the nephrotoxicity of the angiogram dye load. Fortunately, his renal function is found to be normal. An arteriogram is performed and shows lesions both above the knee and below the knee: He has a block in his superficial femoral artery and one vessel runoff to his foot, a dorsalis pedis artery which reconstitutes about at his mid-calf and goes down to the dorsum of the foot.

At this point, Joe's son asks to see you on your afternoon rounds, and asks you the following question: "Doc, why not just amputate his leg? He's an old man, and I'm worried that his heart just can't take it." He has asked an important question and one that would be very difficult to answer if you had no data. Several studies, however, have looked at this very question, and, perhaps surprisingly, the results of revascularization are equal to or even better than those of amputation. In 1991, Taylor and colleagues reviewed 498 patients with critically ischemic legs. Only 14 of these patients underwent amputation as an initial procedure. Amputations were done only when there were no graftable distal vessels, the patient was neurologically impaired, or the patient was hopelessly nonambulatory. Of the 484 remaining patients, the mortality for revascularization was only 2.3 percent, and the median hospital stay was 11 days.[20] The vascular group from Hershey, Pennsylvania, reviewed 211 patients who underwent infrainguinal vascular reconstructions and 98 patients who had 122 major amputations. Procedure-specific mortality was 2.1 percent for primary revascularization and 4.9 percent for amputation. As the authors stated,

"Although the mortality rate of amputation was more than twice that of revascularization, this difference did not achieve statistical significance."[21]

Thus, you can confidently answer that revascularization would be preferable in his father and would have the added benefit that, if it were successful, the patient would probably be able to ambulate postoperatively, something that would be unlikely for this frail man after an amputation. Joe will need to have pulse volume recordings performed preoperatively and postoperatively to document the perfusion to his legs, and he will need continuing antibiotic therapy for several days postoperatively. Because of his history of a previous myocardial infarction, arrangements should be made for a bed in the intensive care unit for a day or two postoperatively.

The night before Joe is to go to the operating room, you meet his son on your evening rounds, and he asks, "What can we expect from this operation?" You can give him good news in that in the largest series of "in situ" bypasses in the literature, 91 percent of which were done for limb-threatening ischemia, limb salvage rates were 97 percent and 95 percent at 1 and 5 years, respectively.[22] The operative mortality in this large series of over 2000 patients was 3.7 percent. You can further tell him that the outlook for Joe's being able to return to his home is hopeful as well. In a recent study of patients' functional outcome after infrainguinal bypass, 99 percent of survivors who lived independently before developing the need for a limb salvage procedure remained independent 6 months after surgery, and 97 percent of those who were ambulatory preoperatively were ambulatory 6 months after surgery.[23]

## SUMMARY

Vascular disease is endemic in our population. With the aging of the "baby boom" generation, vascular problems seem even more likely in the coming years. Primary care physicians are the front-line troops in this battle, and their recognition of lower-extremity ischemia, whether acute or chronic, will aid in the timely diagnosis and treatment of this ailment. It should be remembered that evidence of distal vascular disease is not only an indicator of that limb's perfusion but, more importantly, a marker for systemic vascular disease. Conservative therapy is often effective in patients with claudication or pain after exercise, but surgical intervention is required in the patient with pain at rest or a nonhealing lesion. In the patient with distal vessels seen on arteriogram and a venous conduit, the outlook is both promising and hopeful.

## REFERENCES

1. Criqui MH, Langer RD, Fronek A, et al: Mortality over a period of 10 years in patients with peripheral arterial disease. *N Engl J Med* 1992; 326:381–386.
2. Vogt MT, Cauley JA, Newman AB, et al: Decreased ankle/arm blood pressure index and mortality in elderly women. *JAMA* 1993; 270:465–469.

3.  Chambers BR, Norris JW: Outcome in patients with asymptomatic neck bruits. *N Engl J Med* 1996; 315:860–865.

4.  Krupski WC: The peripheral vascular consequences of smoking. *Ann Vasc Surg* 1991; 5:291–304.

5.  Schoenbawm M: Do smokers understand the mortality effects of smoking? Evidence from the health and retirement survey. *Am J Public Health* 1997; 87:755–759.

6.  Simon JE, Solkowitz SN, Carmody TP, Browner WS: Smoking cessation after surgery. *Arch Intern Med* 1997; 157:1371–1376.

7.  Buchwald H, Bourdages HR, Campos CT, et al: Impact of cholesterol reduction on peripheral arterial disease in the Program on the Surgical Control of the Hyperlipidemias (POSCH). *Surgery* 1996; 120:672–679.

8.  Hodis HN, Mack WJ, LaBree L, et al: Reduction in carotid arterial wall thickness using Lovastatin and dietary therapy. A randomized, controlled clinical trial. *Ann Intern Med* 1996; 124:548–556.

9.  Blair SN, Kampert JB, Kohl HW III, et al: Influences of cardiorespiratory fitness and other precursors on cardiovascular disease and all-cause mortality in men and women. *JAMA* 1996; 276:205–210.

10. Imparato AM, Kim GE, Davidson T, Crowley JG: Intermittent claudication: Its natural course. *Surgery* 1975; 78:795–799.

11. Radack K, Wyderski RJ: Conservative management of intermittent claudication. *Ann Intern Med* 1990; 113:135–146.

12. Gardner AW, Poehlman ET: Exercise rehabilitation programs for the treatment of claudication pain. A meta-analysis. *JAMA* 1995; 274:975–980.

13. Patterson RB, Pinto B, Marcus B, et al: Value of a supervised exercise program for the therapy of arterial claudication. *J Vasc Surg* 1997; 25:312–319.

14. Whyman MR, Ruckley CV, Fowkes FGR: Angioplasty for mild intermittent claudication. *Br J Surg* 1991; 78:643–645.

15. Perkins JTM, Collin JC, Morris PJM: Angioplasty versus exercise for stable claudication: Long term results of a prospective randomized trial. *Br J Surg* 1995; 82:557–558.

16. Fraser SCA, Al-Kutoubi MA, Wolfe JHN: Percutaneous transluminal angioplasty of the infrapopliteal vessels: The evidence. *Radiology* 1996; 200:33–43.

17. Conte MS, Belkin M, Donaldson MC, et al: Femorotibial bypass for claudication: Do results justify an aggressive approach? *J Vasc Surg* 1995; 21:873–881.

18. Kresowik TF, Hoballah JJ, Sharp WJ, Corson JD: Cardiac screening tests prior to lower extremity revascularization: Routine versus selective application. *Semin Vasc Surg* 1997; 10:55–60.

19. Massie MT, Rohrer MJ, Leppo JA, Cutler BS: Is coronary angiography necessary for vascular surgery patients who have positive results of dipyridamole thallium scans? *J Vasc Surg* 1997; 25:975–983.

20. Taylor LM Jr, Hamre D, Dalman RL, Porter JM: Limb salvage versus amputation for critical ischemia. *Arch Surg* 1991; 126:1251–1258.

21. Schina MJ Jr, Atnip RG, Healy DA, Thiele BL: Relative risks of limb revascularization and amputation in the modern era. *Cardiovasc Surg* 1994; 2:754–759.

22. Shah DM, Darling RC III, Chang BJ, et al: Long-term results of in situ saphenous vein bypass. Analysis of 2058 cases. *Ann Surg* 1995; 222:438–448.

23. Abou-Zamzam AM Jr, Lee RW, Moneta GL, et al: Functional outcome after infrainguinal bypass for limb salvage. *J Vasc Surg* 1997; 25:287–297.

ANGEL R. LEÓN

# SUDDEN CARDIAC DEATH

Sudden cardiac death (SCD) refers to the abrupt termination of vital signs leading to irreversible death, usually from loss of cardiac output due to ventricular asystole, ventricular tachycardia (VT), or ventricular fibrillation (VF). More than 300,000 Americans suffer a sudden cardiac death each year. Some deaths classified as sudden reflect the natural end of life in the ill or elderly person. Most deaths classified as sudden, however, involve an unexpected premature end of life.

Management of SCD consists of prompt resuscitation by reestablishing cardiac output. Physicians do not usually arrive at the scene of cardiac arrest, since most SCD occurs outside the hospital or clinic. Emergency medical units and technicians following the Advanced Cardiac Life Support protocols bring survivors to the hospital. The initial management of the SCD survivor consists of achieving hemodynamic and respiratory stability. The physician should proceed immediately with diagnostic testing to identify the underlying cause of the aborted SCD. Recognition and correction of acute problems such as conduction block, ischemia, electrolyte disturbance, and medication-induced arrhythmia can prevent early recurrence of SCD. The primary physician should understand that coronary artery disease (CAD), nonischemic dilated cardiomyopathy, myocarditis, hypertrophic cardiomyopathy, and the long QT syndrome are the most common causes of SCD in our population. Prevention of SCD depends on identifying the individual at risk for sudden death by recognizing the acquired and congenital diseases that lead to ventricular dysrhythmia. The management of SCD involves interaction with the cardiologist or electrophysiologist to definitively treat the survivor, as well as to identify individuals at high risk and refer them for preventive therapy.

## EPIDEMIOLOGY OF SUDDEN CARDIAC DEATH

The *cause* of SCD in the U.S. population varies with the patient's age. Data from autopsy series show that congenital heart anomalies, viral myocarditis, hypertrophic cardiomyopathy, and the long QT syndrome cause the majority of SCD prior to age

30. Atherosclerotic CAD becomes the leading cause of SCD beyond age 30, followed by idiopathic dilated cardiomyopathy, myocarditis, hypertrophic cardiomyopathy, and congenital coronary anomalies. Gender differences in SCD rates reflect the difference in prevalence of CAD among men and women in the United States. SCD rates in women lag behind those in age-matched males but quickly accelerate after menopause. Analyses of race as a factor in SCD rates fail to detect any difference between Caucasian and non-Caucasian men, but non-Caucasian women have a higher SCD rate than Caucasian women.[1]

Approximately 20 to 30 percent of cases of SCD associated with CAD result from the electrical instability produced by ongoing acute myocardial injury or ischemia. Chest pain often precedes loss of consciousness, and the ECG demonstrates acute changes associated with coronary artery occlusion. The remaining cases of SCD probably result from VT or VF originating from a substrate of chronic myocardial infarction (MI) without fresh coronary occlusion. Chronic MI with ventricular scar containing islets of viable myocardium produces areas of relatively slow myocardial conduction, which leads to VT and eventually to VF. Autopsy findings in cases of SCD reflect the prevalence of coronary disease in developed countries, with over 80 percent of individuals demonstrating atherosclerotic plaque in one or more coronary arteries. The incidence of healed MI approaches 80 percent in individuals with CAD.[2]

Congenital coronary artery anomalies, such as the single coronary syndrome, anomalous origin of the left or right coronary artery, coronary artery fistulas, and coronary artery spasm, can cause SCD by producing acute ischemia and electrical instability. SCD due to hypertrophic cardiomyopathy exhibits a bimodal age distribution, with an early peak in the second decade of life followed by another peak in the sixth decade. Coxsackie A or B viral infection of the heart produces myofiber scarring, creating a substrate for VF and VT. Viral myocarditis during childhood usually resolves with consequences. Viral myocarditis in the adult often leads to cardiomyopathy, however, with high risk for recurrent VT or VF. The long QT syndrome and right ventricular dysplasia cause a small percentage of SCD at all ages. Mitral valve prolapse alone rarely causes SCD.[3]

The *genetically linked causes* of SCD include hypertrophic cardiomyopathy with autosomal dominant inheritance and variable penetrance; the autosomal dominant long QT syndrome, resulting from genetically coded ionic channel abnormalities; and right ventricular dysplasia with a polygenic transmission pattern. Brugada recently described another genetically mediated cause of SCD typified by ST-segment elevation at the terminal portion of a right bundle branch complex in the anterior precordial leads on the ECG. Familial dyslipidemia leading to premature CAD and MI may be associated with familial clustering of SCD. Understanding of the genetic link in specific causes of SCD can be used by the clinician obtaining a family history of SCD as a guide to diagnostic testing to determine the underlying cause of SCD and a guide to treatment and counseling of affected family members.

*Temporal trends* in SCD suggest that individuals who suffer SCD most commonly die in the morning hours. Data from clinical trials of the implantable defibrillator

(ICD) with 24-h data storage counters show a peak in arrhythmic activity between 6 A.M. and 12 noon consisting of 60 percent of all stored episodes. A second peak may occur between 5:00 and 6:00 P.M. Roughly 20 percent of episodes occur during routine sleeping hours. Myocardial infarction and coronary spasm occur most often in the early morning hours. Temporal distribution of SCD appears to follow the circadian variation in sympathetic tone.[4]

# MECHANISMS OF SUDDEN CARDIAC DEATH

Most SCD in the United States and other industrial nations occurs as a result of ventricular tachyarrhythmia, VT, or VF. VT in patients with CAD accounts for the majority of SCD, primarily because of the prevalence of CAD in these populations. Asystole from atrioventricular block may produce SCD, but often those individuals have a slow ventricular escape rhythm that prevents death. Asystolic cardiac arrest usually represents an agonal rhythm following a deterioration from VT to VF to asystole in a dying heart. True asystolic arrest therefore carries a severe prognosis, with almost zero probability of survival to hospital discharge.[5]

Some 20 to 30 percent of individuals suffering out-of-hospital SCD survive to hospital discharge. Individuals likely to survive SCD include those with VT or VF. Persons suffering asystolic cardiac arrest rarely survive to hospital discharge. Prompt restoration of sinus rhythm and systemic circulation limits end-organ damage and improves survival chances. Historically, widespread use of bystander cardiopulmonary resuscitation (CPR) marginally improves survival to hospital discharge. Mobile emergency units with defibrillators have had the greatest impact in improving survival. CPR serves as a bridge until cardioversion or defibrillation can be performed. CPR alone cannot be expected to provide major benefit. Survival from SCD drops by 50 percent after only 6 min of loss of circulation and decreases geometrically beyond that time. The introduction of automatic external defibrillators (AEDs) throughout the community provides the potential for more prompt restoration of sinus rhythm and may further improve survival in SCD.[6]

Underlying reversible causes of SCD include acute myocardial ischemia or infarction, electrolyte disturbance, proarrhythmia by various medications, high-degree atrioventricular block producing asystole, or bradycardia resulting in pause-induced VT or VF. Acute coronary insufficiency or occlusion producing myocardial ischemia causes partial depolarization in ischemic tissue, leading to electrical instability and arrhythmia. VT or VF may complicate acute myocardial infarction (AMI) or unstable coronary syndromes. Reversal of the coronary supply-demand imbalance restores normal tissue perfusion and may prevent recurrence of arrhythmia. Therefore, recognition of any underlying unstable coronary syndromes in the patient resuscitated from VT or VF may be crucial to treating aborted SCD. The physician should search for a history of angina prior to cardiac arrest or syncope. Electrocardiographic evidence of acute subepicardial injury (ST-segment elevation) or subendocardial ischemia (ST-segment depression) suggests reduced myocardial perfusion and should lead the physician to consider referral for emergency cardiac catherization or administration of thrombolytic agents.

With rare exceptions, every survivor of SCD should undergo cardiac catheterization and coronary angiography as part of the diagnostic effort to detect underlying structural heart disease. Coronary spasm with dynamic obstruction to flow produces VT and VF in patients with minimal or no obstructive coronary disease. The absence of obstructive plaque on coronary angiography in the patient with a history of angina preceding collapse suggests coronary spasm as a mechanism of ischemia leading to VT or VF. Provocative testing with Methergine (methylergonovine maleate) to detect spasm should routinely follow coronary angiography in patients with otherwise normal or nonobstructed coronary arteries.[7]

Hypokalemia or hypomagnesemia leads to polymorphic VT, which may resemble self-terminating VF on the electrocardiogram (ECG). When these electrolyte disturbances occur in the patient with aborted SCD, swift administration of potassium and/or magnesium may be necessary to prevent arrhythmia recurrence. One should take note that a large release of catecholamines leads to hypokalemia by beta-receptor-mediated intracellular shifting of potassium. Therefore, many patients with aborted SCD present with initial hypokalemia. The low serum potassium concentration results from the sympathetic discharge associated with resuscitation and defibrillation. Total body potassium may be normal. In such cases, hypokalemia most likely did not cause VT or VF; the arrest caused the hypokalemia. Prominent U waves and T-wave/U-wave fusion on the ECG signal the hypokalemic effect on cardiac repolarization. One should suspect hypokalemia as the cause of VT or VF in patients taking potassium-wasting diuretics and in those with disease states that produce hypokalemia. Hypokalemia and hypomagnesemia also increase the proarrhythmic effect of medications that prolong the QT interval on the ECG.

A number of drugs prolong the QT interval on the ECG and have an adverse, proarrhythmic effect on the heart. A history of medication use in the patient with aborted SCD may reveal a proarrhythmic drug effect. Phenothiazine derivatives, erythromycin-class antibiotics, certain antifungal drugs, class Ia antiarrhythmic drugs, and certain antihistamines delay repolarization and prolong the QT interval. Tricyclic antidepressants prolong the action potential, the QRS duration, and the QT segment.[8]

The *anatomic substrate* for chronic VT or VF consists mainly of focal ventricular myocardial scars from previous MI, aneurysm, infiltrative processes such as sarcoid, or the diffuse cardiac conduction abnormalities seen in dilated cardiomyopathy. Hypertrophic cardiomyopathy produces diffuse microscopic scarring consistent with myocardial necrosis and infarction, which lead to electrical instability and VT or VF. The presence of structural heart disease, particularly ventricular enlargement, focal damage, or segmental wall abnormalities, identifies patients at risk for SCD. The probability of SCD increases with progressive ventricular dysfunction. A left ventricular ejection fraction less than 30 percent identifies a greatly increased risk of SCD.

# IDENTIFICATION OF THE PATIENT AT RISK FOR SCD

Recognition of the risk factors and symptoms suggesting an increased risk of SCD before it occurs provides individuals with the best chance of survival. Even the most effective resuscitative techniques still fail to rescue most victims of out-of-hospital cardiac arrest. The primary physician can intervene to reduce SCD by identifying those persons at greatest risk and referring them to the cardiologist or electrophysiologist for appropriate therapy or preventive measures.

Most patients surviving SCD provide a history of antecedent structural heart disease such as MI, valvular heart disease, or cardiomyopathy. A history of snycope or near-syncope is often the only preceding symptom. A family history of premature sudden cardiac death points to one of the genetically mediated causes of SCD mentioned above. The physician should also review the history for medications implicated as direct proarrhythmic agents, potassium-wasting diuretics, drugs that prolong the QT segment, or any combination of such drugs. Individuals with structural heart disease who survive SCD have the greatest probability of recurrent SCD if left untreated.

The primary care physician should also interview and examine family members when the family history suggests a genetically mediated cause of SCD. Genetic screening and mapping that may better identify relatives at risk may be available at tertiary care centers.

*Diagnostic modalities* that help identify individuals at risk for SCD include evidence of MI, repolarization abnormalities, conduction block, or chamber enlargement of the ECG. Exercise radionuclide scans may detect underlying ischemia or infarction. The chest radiograph, echocardiogram, or contrast ventriculogram detects left ventricular enlargement or dysfunction.

Echocardiographic evidence of severe mitral valve prolapse with a thickened valve and dual leaflet prolapse in the presence of QT abnormalities or nonsustained VT (NSVT) may herald a potentially malignant form of the syndrome. The echocardiogram may also detect hypertrophic cardiomyopathy with or without left ventricular outflow tract obstruction. Techniques that poorly image the right ventricle may fail to detect right ventricular dysplasia. Special echocardiographic windows or magnetic resonance imaging may provide a better look at right ventricular anatomy.

Complex ventricular ectopy including NSVT in the presence of left ventricular dysfunction clearly suggests an increased risk of SCD. Continuous 24- to 48-h ECG monitoring of patients with left ventricular ejection fraction less than 35 percent due to previous MI in order to detect NSVT may identify a group at risk for SCD. The signal-averaged ECG, a  noninvasive tool, detects the presence of delayed, low-amplitude cardiac depolarization, which is associated with a high probability of VT or VF within 1 year after detection. Programmed ventricular stimulation during invasive electrophysiologic testing identifies which individuals in each group have the greatest risk of SCD and would benefit from ICD implant.[9]

Invasive and noninvasive tests do not estimate the risk of SCD as accurately in patients with cardiomyopathy or left ventricular dysfunction not due to MI as they do in patients with left ventricular dysfunction due to coronary disease. Newer techniques such as assessment of heart rate variability, detection of T-wave alternans, and T-wave dispersion may better identify patients at risk for SCD.

Recognition of risk factors and symptoms suggesting an increased risk of SCD provides patients with the best chance of survival. Even the best resuscitative techniques still fail to rescue most individuals stricken out of the hospital. The SCD survivor should undergo extensive evaluation to detect any of the underlying causes listed in this chapter. Numerous clinical studies suggest that unless a clearly reversible problem produced the cardiac arrest, the patient remains at risk for SCD. The ICD provides individuals at risk for recurrent SCD with a superior therapy to enable them to survive recurrent events. Ongoing investigations will determine whether prophylactic ICD implant in individuals with severe left ventricular dysfunction will improve survival in the cardiomyopathy population. Family members of SCD victims who demonstrate a high-risk profile by genetic mapping, multiple deaths in close relatives, or familial cardiomyopathy may also benefit from prophylactic ICD implant.[10]

## REFERENCES

1. Gillum RF: Sudden coronary death in the United States, 1980–1985. *Circulation* 1989; 79:756–765.
2. Goldberg RJ, Gore JM, Alpert JS, et al: Incidence and case fatality rates of acute myocardial infarction (1975–1984): the Worcester Heart Attack Study. *Am Heart J* 1988; 115:751–767.
3. Devereaux RB, Kramer-Fox R, Kligfield P: Mitral valve prolapse: causes, clinical manifestations, and management. *Ann Intern Med* 1989; 111:305–311.
4. Muller JE, Ludmer PL, Willich SN, et al: Circadian variation in the frequency of sudden cardiac death. *Circulation* 1987; 75:131–138.
5. Myerburg RJ, Conde CA, Sung RJ, et al: Clinical, electrophysiologic and hemodynamic profile of patients resuscitated from prehospital cardiac arrest. *Am J Med* 1980; 68: 568–577.
6. Cummins RO, Ornato JP, Thies WH, et al: Improving survival from sudden cardiac arrest: the "chain of survival" concept. *Circulation* 1991; 83:1832–1847.
7. Myerburg RJ, Kessler KM, Mallon SM, et al: Potentially fatal arrhythmia in patients with silent myocardial ischemia due to coronary artery spasm. *N Engl J Med* 1992; 326:1451–1455.
8. Jackman WM, Friday KJ, Anderson JL, et al: The long QT syndromes: a critical review. New clinical observations and a unifying hypothesis. *Prog Cardiovasc Dis* 1988; 31: 115–132.
9. Bigger JT, Fleiss JL, Steinman RC, et al: Frequency domain measures of heart period variability and mortality after myocardial infarction. *Circulation* 1992; 85:164–171.
10. Bardy GH, Hofer B, Johnson G, et al: Implantable transvenous cardioverter-defibrillators. *Circulation* 1993; 87:1152–1168.

ANGEL R. LEÓN

# CARDIAC ARRHYTHMIA: OUTPATIENT AND INPATIENT MANAGEMENT

## 37

This chapter reviews the recognition and management of supraventricular and ventricular arrhythmia. Any discussion of the treatment of cardiac rhythm disorders should begin with a review of antiarrhythmic agents. Traditionally, drug therapy served as the primary treatment modality for life-threatening ventricular arrhythmia. The results of numerous investigations over the last 10 years, however, have shifted the choice of therapy away from drugs and toward catheter ablation and implantable arrhythmia control devices. Catheter ablation has revolutionized therapy for supraventricular arrhythmias. Drug therapy still plays a role in management of some less dangerous supraventricular arrhythmias, however. The primary care physician should learn how to differentiate ventricular from supraventricular arrhythmia and how to recognize disease states associated with rhythm disorders, the circumstances under which drugs help patients, and when to proceed to hospitalization and ask consultation to aid with the management of complex cardiac rhythm problems.

## THE ELECTROCARDIOGRAPHIC DIFFERENTIATION OF SUPRAVENTRICULAR ARRHYTHMIA

The surface 12-lead electrocardiogram (ECG) provides clues that help identify the origin of supraventricular tachycardia. One should begin the ECG interpretation by identifying P waves or atrial depolarization waves and noting their relationship to the QRS complex.

A chaotic baseline without any organized atrial activity and irregular intervals between QRS complexes makes atrial fibrillation (AF) the likely diagnosis. The presence of typical "sawtooth" waves, with no isoelectric segments, at rates of 280 to 320 beats per minute in the inferior ECG leads suggests atrial flutter (AFL). Atrial rates between 200 and 280 beats per minute suggest atrial tachycardia. A variable atrial to QRS interval suggests atrial tachycardia or flutter with variable atrioventricular(AV) block at the AV node (Fig. 37-1).

When the atrial to QRS interval does not vary, the duration of the interval between each P wave and the preceding QRS complex (the R-P interval) often leads to the diagnosis. When the P wave has morphology similar to that of the P wave in sinus rhythm and the R-P interval exceeds 200 ms, one should consider sinus tachycardia as the cause of supraventricular tachycardia (SVT). The absence of P waves during a regular, narrow QRS tachycardia suggests simultaneous activation of the atria and ven-

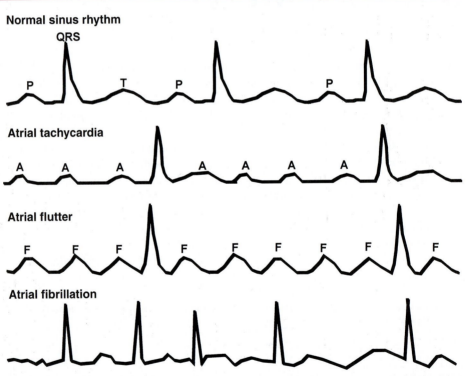

**Figure 37-1**   Differences between baseline patterns on a rhythm strip of different supraventricular tachycardias. Distinct P waves appear on the baseline ECG during normal sinus rhythm. Atrial tachycardia inscribes atrial waves, which appear different from the P waves caused by sinus rhythm, reflecting an ectopic origin of the atrial rhythm. The ECG during atrial tachycardia usually contains an isoelectric interval between atrial waves. The ECG in classic atrial flutter contains a "sawtooth" pattern with no isoelectric interval between the flutter waves. Atrial fibrillation shows no organized atrial activity, with its hallmark of irregularly irregular QRS complexes.

tricles by AV node reentry. The QRS complex obliterates the P wave, or the ultrashort ventriculoatrial activation time creates new S waves in the inferior leads or an rSr' pattern in the first precordial lead. The deflections represent retrograde atrial activation during tachycardia, not a ventricular conduction delay. R-P intervals between 100 and 200 ms suggest longer ventriculoatrial activation intervals, such as those associated with reciprocating atrioventricular tachycardia mediated by an accessory atrioventricular connection. R-P intervals exceeding 200 ms with large negative P waves in the inferior leads strongly suggest that the patient has the atypical form of AV node reentry in which retrograde conduction occurs across the "slow" AV node pathway, with decremental conduction properties. Incessant tachycardia with similar giant negative P waves in the inferior ECG leads points to the rare but easily identified syndrome of permanent junctional reciprocating tachycardia.

# A REVIEW OF ANTIARRHYTHMIC DRUGS

The widely accepted Vaughan Williams classification categorizes drugs as sodium channel blockers (class I), beta-receptor blockers (class II), potassium channel blockers (class III), and calcium channel antagonists (class IV). Although many drugs may inhibit or antagonize more than a single channel or receptor, the class each drug falls into depends on its primary pharmacologic effect.[1]

The *class I drugs* include agents that block the inward sodium current, leading to depolarization of the cardiac cell membrane. Sodium channels control primarily conduction velocity. Secondary effects of these drugs on potassium channels affect repolarization and refractoriness. There are three subclassifications of the class I drugs.

Quinidine, procainamide, and disopyramide make up the first subset (Ia) of this group; these drugs block the sodium channels involved in the earliest phase of cardiac depolarization as well as prolong the duration of the cardiac action potential by delaying repolarization mediated by specific potassium currents. Lack of efficacy, proarrhythmia, and noncardiac side effects greatly reduce the use of these drugs today. The drug effect delaying cardiac repolarization manifests itself as prolongation of the QRS and QT segments of the surface ECG.

Lidocaine, mexiletine, and tocainide form the second subset (Ib); they primarily slow depolarization and conduction velocity, with little effect on repolarization or refractoriness. Lidocaine, a local parenteral anesthetic agent, has no oral form. Although similar in classification, the oral agents mexiletine and tocainide do not possess the same pharmacologic properties as lidocaine. The hematologic side effects of tocainide severely limit its use. The class Ib drugs produce little effect on the surface ECG.

Flecainide, encainide, and propafenone form the class Ic subset. These drugs markedly slow conduction velocity and prolong cardiac refractoriness to a lesser degree. Pharmacologists occasionally classify moricizine in this subset, although it does not have the same pharmacologic properties as the other three agents. Cardiologists and electrophysiologists have almost totally stopped using moricizine. Adverse events resulting from the use of encainide in patients with structural heart disease led to its removal from the market. The class Ic drugs produce little effect on the normal ECG. Flecainide and propafenone may worsen preexisting intraventricular conduction block and widen the QRS complex.

The *class II drugs* include competitive inhibitors of the beta-adrenergic receptors in vascular and cardiac muscle tissue. Distinctions among members of this class include beta$_1$-specific blockade (metoprolol, atenolol, timolol), hydrophilic properties preventing crossing of the blood-brain barrier (atenolol, nadolol), duration of action (ultrashort, esmolol; short, propranolol; medium, metoprolol; long, nadolol), and combined intrinsic sympathomimetic activity that stimulates beta$_1$ and blocks beta$_2$ receptors simultaneously (pindolol and acebutolol). The beta blockers primarily slow the sinus rate on ECG and may also prolong the P-R interval.

The *class III drugs* represent the most vague category of the Vaughan Williams classification. Inhibition of one or various potassium channels during cardiac depolarization or repolarization primarily characterizes the action of amiodarone, sotalol, ibutilide, bretylium, and the newly introduced class III drugs dofetilide, azimilide, and trecetilide. Amiodarone also exhibits beta-blocking properties and antagonizes calcium channels. The levorotatory isomer of sotalol (L-sotalol) has strong beta-blocking activity. Only the racemic version of sotalol has government approval for general use in the United States, however. Ibutilide, as yet only an intravenous agent for cardioversion of AF and AFL, has short-acting class III properties. Bretylium not only blocks potassium channels but also depletes sympathetic ganglia of neurotransmitter, producing delayed chronotropic and hemodynamic depression. Class III drugs slow the sinus rate and may produce first-degree AV block on the surface ECG. Increasing doses of sotalol progressively lengthen the QT segment.

The *class IV drugs* include the calcium channel antagonists, whose primary electrophysiologic effect consists of blocking sinus node and AV node conduction. Verapamil and diltiazem strongly inhibit the calcium fluxes that promote automaticity and therefore slow the firing of cardiac pacemaker tissue. They also inhibit slow channel–dependent AV nodal conduction. The dihydropyridine inhibitors (nifedipine, nicardipine, amlodipine, etc.) have little or no electrophysiologic effect.

Standard classifications of antiarrhythmic drugs do not include adenosine. Adenosine, a naturally occurring carrier of high-energy phosphate groups during cellular metabolism, increases cyclic AMP levels in cell membranes via G protein interaction. Intravenous administration of adenosine relaxes vascular smooth muscle, constricts bronchial smooth muscle, and strongly inhibits calcium channel–mediated conduction in specialized cardiac tissue such as the sinus and AV nodes. Clinically, adenosine (6 to 12 mg intravenous bolus) produces transient AV block.

## PROARRHYTHMIA

Administration of an antiarrhythmic medication may incite a new arrhythmia, worsen the frequency or severity of an existing tachycardia, or turn a nonsustained tachycardia into an incessant one. Most often proarrhythmia results from the use of a class I or III drug. A beta blocker or calcium channel antagonist may rarely worsen a supraventricular arrhythmia, particularly AV node reentry, however. Proarrhythmia most often strikes the patient with structural heart disease and left ventricular dysfunction. Hepatic or renal dysfunction leading to unexpectedly high drug levels as a result of low clearance also increases the risk. Proarrhythmia can occur in *any* patient, however; therefore, the primary care physician should consult a cardiologist or cardiac electrophysiologist *before initiating class I or III therapy in any patient.*

The clinician should understand that *any antiarrhythmic drug* may potentially worsen an arrhythmia. Proarrhythmia may occur after a few doses or after months to years of chronic therapy. Proarrhythmia early after onset of treatment may occur with a drug such as quinidine, sotalol, or dofetilide. Each drug prolongs repolarization and may promote the onset of a polymorphic ventricular tachycardia called torsades de pointes in a small percentage of patients. Prolongation of the corrected QT interval beyond 500 ms on the ECG serves as the hallmark of this type of proarrhythmia. Factors contributing to the likelihood of prolonged QT proarrhythmia include hypokalemia, hypomagnesemia, hypocalcemia, cardiac hypertrophy, and bradycardia. Recognizing the cause of QT prolongation and discontinuing the offending drug eliminate the problem. Treating this form of proarrhythmia with another antiarrhythmic agent, such as lidocaine, fails; using other drugs, such as procainamide, worsens the problem. Many authors suggest that one should initiate class Ia or III antiarrhythmic therapy *only* during telemetry monitoring of hospitalized patients.

Changes in serum electrolytes, unrecognized drug interactions, decreased metabolism or clearance of a drug, and progression of myocardial disease change the electrophysiologic milieu of the heart and may facilitate onset of a previously absent arrhythmia in a patient taking antiarrhythmic agents. A potent antiarrhythmic drug such as flecainide may enhance disparities in electrophysiologic characteristics between adjacent segments of myocardium in the diseased heart and cause ventricular tachycardia. Cardiac hypertrophy due to chronic hypertension may increase the risk of torsades de pointes after the administration of class III agents as a result of physiologic abnormalities induced by myocardial fiber stretch. Potassium-wasting diuretics, phenothiazine derivatives, decongestants, or tetracycline antibiotics may facilitate proarrhythmia when given to patients on antiarrhythmic drugs.

Late proarrhythmia presents a difficult problem, since it most often occurs outside the hospital. The clinician should see it as a warning sign when a patient taking an antiarrhythmic drug reports syncope, near syncope, or increased palpitations. The physician should monitor the patient, either in the hospital or with ambulatory monitoring (depending on the level of concern about the severity of symptoms), while discontinuing the drug. Failure to detect the cause of worsening symptoms during ambulatory monitoring should prompt hospitalization, discontinuation of the drug, and cardiology consultation.

# THERAPY FOR SUPRAVENTRICULAR ARRHYTHMIA

Clinically relevant supraventricular arrhythmias include atrial ectopy, atrial tachycardia, AF, AFL, and AV node reentry that occur with enough frequency or severity to produce symptoms, prompt trips to the emergency room, or increase the risk of end organ damage such as thromboembolism. Tachycardia mediated by accessory atrioventricular connections, as seen in the Wolff-Parkinson-White syndrome, utilizes ventricular tissue as part of the tachycardia circuit. Therefore, in the strict anatomic sense, one cannot classify this as supraventricular. However, for purposes of outlining therapy, this chapter will include it with the true supraventricular arrhythmias.

*Acute management of SVT* includes termination of the rapid, narrow QRS tachycardia commonly referred to as paroxysmal atrial tachycardia (PAT) or paroxysmal supraventricular tachycardia (PSVT), slowing atrioventricular conduction during AFL flutter or AF, and cardioversion of AF or AFL to sinus rhythm in the compromised patient.

When confronted with a patient with a regular, narrow QRS tachycardia without obvious AFL waves in the inferior leads of the ECG, the clinician should administer adenosine 6 to 12 mg by rapid intravenous infusion with immediate saline flush. Adenosine will terminate AV node reentry and AV reciprocating tachycardia associated with accessory atrioventricular connections by producing AV block. Peripheral effects of adenosine are chest pressure and flushing. AV block or asystole usually resolves in less than 10 s and does not require treatment. One should avoid administering adenosine to the asthmatic patient, in whom it may trigger a bronchospastic crisis.

Adenosine infusion blocks conduction across the AV node and also provides the clinician with valuable diagnostic information in the patient with tachycardia. Interruption of tachycardia suggests the presence of either AV node reentry or a tachycardia mediated by conduction down the AV node and up an accessory AV pathway. When adenosine infusion does not terminate tachycardia, the AV block may unmask the underlying atrial waves of AFL, atrial tachycardia, or sinus tachycardia with AV block. Failure to produce any effect on a wide-complex tachycardia establishes the diagnosis of ventricular tachycardia.

Repeated recurrences of tachycardia after obvious termination with adenosine require continuous pharmacologic suppression with intravenous agents such as the short-acting beta blocker esmolol (130 μg/min) or diltiazem (0.25 mg/kg bolus, then 10 mg/h infusion). Atrial tachycardia or flutter with AV block diagnosed during adenosine infusion may require an intravenous calcium channel antagonist or beta blocker for adequate ventricular rate control. When adenosine infusion unmasks sinus tachycardia, one should consider an underlying cause for the arrhythmia, such as thyrotoxicosis, pulmonary embolism, hypovolemia, or other metabolic disturbances.

Rapid AV conduction during AF or AFL occasionally produces hypotension, ischemia, congestive heart failure (CHF), or shock in the patient with poor left ventricular function. The compromised patient may not tolerate the hypotensive and negative inotropic effects of calcium antagonists or beta blockers. Intravenous digoxin (1 to 1.5 mg in 12 h) usually takes hours to effectively reduce ventricular rates. In the emergency setting, immediate direct-current cardioversion is the best option for terminating AF or AFL. Without prior anticoagulation, one has to weigh the risk of thromboembolism against the hemodynamic benefit of restoring sinus rhythm. When the patient's condition permits, and in the presence of adequate left ventricular function, the use of intravenous calcium channel antagonists or beta blockers often provides excellent rate control until oral agents have time to work. Orally administered verapamil (120 to 360 mg daily), diltiazem (120 to 480 mg daily), atenolol (25 to 100 mg daily), or metoprolol (25 to 200 mg daily) provides excellent rate control for the patient with AF or AFL. Digoxin (0.125 to 0.5 mg daily) offers less adequate rate control. Increased circulating catecholamines during exercise or stress rapidly overcome the effect of digoxin on atrioventricular conduction and limit its effectiveness as chronic therapy. Failure to adequately control atrioventricular conduction during AF or AFL despite high doses of calcium channel antagonists or beta blockers suggests the presence of underlying thyrotoxicosis, pulmonary embolism, or, rarely, pheochromocytoma.

The *chronic management of patients with SVT* changed dramatically with the advent of catheter ablation techniques. Radiofrequency ablation of the slow pathway limb of AV node reentry eliminates the arrhythmia with greater than 95 percent success. Catheter ablation of the accessory pathway cures the Wolff-Parkinson-White syndrome as well as reciprocating tachycardia mediated by concealed bypass tracts, with efficacy rates well over 95 percent. Furthermore, radiofrequency ablation can eliminate classic AFL, with its characteristic negative "sawtooth" pattern on the ECG, in over 75 percent of patients. Catheter ablation can also eliminate most ectopic atrial tachycardia. The low risk and complication rates of these procedures permit their performance on an ambulatory basis.[2]

Clinicians should consider referral for catheter ablation as the primary treatment for patients with PSVT, the Wolff-Parkinson-White syndrome, ectopic atrial tachycardia, and pure AFL without AF. Individuals with infrequent arrhythmia or tachycardia of short duration and minimal clinical symptoms probably require no chronic treatment. When symptoms trigger emergency room visits for tachycardia termination, when patients have syncope or near syncope due to tachycardia, or when symptoms occur frequently enough to interfere with the patient's lifestyle, however, catheter ablation offers an excellent alternative to chronic medical therapy, with its side effects and uncertain efficacy. Catheter ablation ultimately results in lower overall costs than medical therapy in patients with frequent episodes of SVT.[3]

Class Ic and III drugs effectively suppress AV node reentry, atrial tachycardia, and conduction across accessory AV pathways. Flecainide (100 to 200 mg bid), propafenone (150 to 300 mg tid), sotalol (80 to 160 mg bid), or amiodarone (200 mg daily) can serve as an alternative for patients who are not considered proper candidates for ablation, who refuse ablation, or in whom catheter ablation failed to cure tachycardia. Calcium channel and beta blockers may not completely suppress sustained SVT, although these agents usually slow the frequency of attacks and diminish the severity by slowing the heart rate during tachycardia.

Recurrent atrial ectopic beats occur in many individuals, yet produce symptoms in few. When severe symptoms produce discomfort or anxiety, low doses of beta blockers or calcium antagonists may suffice. In the absence of structural heart disease, flecainide (50 to 100 mg bid) or propafenone (150 to 300 mg tid) may suppress ectopy in the extremely symptomatic patient. One should think strongly, however, before prescribing a drug with potentially lethal side effects for an arrhythmia associated with little morbidity and no mortality.

The primary care physician may use calcium channel antagonists and beta blockers to provide safe, somewhat effective symptomatic relief for supraventricular ectopy. In cases of supraventricular arrhythmia, the primary care physician should defer initiation of antiarrhythmic therapy with class I or III drugs to the cardiologist or electrophysiologist.

*Chronic antiarrhythmic management of AF* consists primarily of restoring normal sinus rhythm or, when that fails, ventricular rate control. The presence of structural heart disease or age greater than 60 years dictates the need for warfarin anticoagulation in patients with chronic or paroxysmal AF. Multiple large trials identify chronic warfarin anticoagulation [international normalized rate (INR) 2.0 to 2.5] as the only pharmacologic therapy that prevents long-term mortality and morbidity in patients with atrial fibrillation and structural heart disease.[4] Rate control and anticoagulation should precede the decision to convert AF to sinus rhythm.

Factors for the clinician to consider when deciding whether to proceed with cardioversion include the age of the patient, degree of structural heart disease, degree of symptoms, duration of AF, and number of previous attempted cardioversions. Physically active patients who develop symptoms during exertion may not tolerate AF. Elderly patients or patients with ventricular dysfunction may depend greatly upon atrial contribution to cardiac output. Symptomatic patients with new-onset AF probably deserve at least one attempt at cardioversion. The likelihood of successful cardioversion drops when AF has been present longer than 1 year. Persistent AF decreases the probability of successful cardioversion and maintenance of sinus rhythm. Patients with recurrent or chronic AF under adequate rate control who have minimal or no symptoms may not benefit from cardioversion. Traditionally, rate control and anticoagulation suffice in many patients. The patient avoids the expense and side effects of cardioversion and antiarrhythmic drugs.

Recent experimental and clinical evidence suggests that inducing sustained AF produces electrical changes in atrial muscle that favor the persistence of AF. Conversely, prompt restoration of sinus rhythm after the onset of AF may reverse this "electrical remodeling" and diminish the probability of recurrent AF. Such evidence supports an aggressive approach using repeated cardioversion in any patient with newly discovered AF. Sequential cardioversions that restore sinus rhythm may prolong each interval after cardioversion, thereby diminishing the total time spent in atrial fibrillation.[5]

The primary care physician who refers a patient with recent-onset AF for cardioversion should first consider the possibility of underlying thyroid dysfunction, pulmonary disease, or occult cardiac disease. Each may contribute to the onset of AF. Thyroid function studies, chest radiograph, oxygen saturation determination, ECG, and possibly echocardiography support the history and physical examination to complete the evaluation of the patient with AF prior to referral.

Echocardiographic examination in select patient groups suggests the presence of atrial thrombus formation as early as 24 to 48 h following the onset of atrial fibrillation.[6] Therefore, unless contraindicated by active bleeding or recent hemorrhagic stroke, any patient considered for *elective* cardioversion of AF greater than 24 h duration should receive 4 weeks of therapeutic anticoagulation (warfarin, INR 2.0 to 2.5) prior to attempted cardioversion. The stroke rate following cardioversion without anticoagulation approaches 10 percent, but this rate falls to nearly zero after therapeutic warfarin anticoagulation for 4 weeks. Transesophageal echocardiographic visualization of the left atrium and its appendage identifies patients at low risk for stroke following cardioversion without antecedent anticoagulation. The absence of echocardiographic risk factors during transesophageal echocardiography does not totally eliminate the risk of stroke associated with cardioversion, however.[7] One still must weigh the risk of stroke versus the expediency of avoiding warfarin anticoagulation for 4 weeks prior to cardioversion. Anticoagulation should continue for 4 weeks *after* cardioversion even in patients not requiring chronic anticoagulation. Mechanical atrial activity may not begin for up to 2 weeks following cardioversion, and unless protected, the patient may suffer stroke late after a cardioversion that restores sinus rhythm.

Direct-current cardioversion (DCC) has very high efficacy, no proarrhythmia, and, if performed with proper preparation, few side effects. Delivery of synchronized direct current across anterior/posterior adhesive electrodes at 200 to 360 J restores sinus rhythm in most patients with AF. Increasing defibrillation energy to 720 J by using two external defibrillators simultaneously cardioverts more than 80 percent of those who fail DCC at 360 J. Internal cardioversion across electrodes positioned in the right atrium and coronary sinus may work in the most resistant cases. Premedication with class I or III antiarrhythmic agents increases the success rate and lowers the energy requirements of DCC.[8] Complications of DCC include sinus arrest and bradycardia, skin burns, pain, and, extremely rarely, induction of ventricular fibrillation by failure to synchronize the DCC pulse with the QRS. We recommend that physicians perform DCC in the hospital, preferably under the supervision of a cardiologist.

Pharmacologic cardioversion occurs mainly with administration of class Ia, Ic, or III drugs. Intravenous short-acting class III agents may have the greatest efficacy in restoring sinus rhythm. Digoxin, calcium channel antagonists, and beta blockers do not increase the rate of conversion to sinus rhythm above the spontaneous cardioversion rate seen in placebo-controlled comparisons. Beta blockers may promote conversion to sinus rhythm in patients with sympathetic overload such as that produced by thyrotoxicosis.

Table 37-1 lists the characteristics and efficacy rates of various antiarrhythmic agents for converting AF and AFL to sinus rhythm. Pharmacologic cardioversion

**TABLE 37-1.** Efficacy of Various Antiarrhythmic Drugs in the Acute Conversion of Paroxysmal Atrial Fibrillation to Sinus Rhythm

| Drug | Dose | Half-Life | Success (%) |
|------|------|-----------|-------------|
| Procainamide (IV) | 1 g (30 min) | 1.5–3 h | 25–30 |
| Ibutilide (IV) | 1–2 mg (20 min) | <1 h | 30–40 |
| Flecainide (PO) | 200 mg (single) | 24 h | 25–30 |
| Propafenone (PO) | 600 mg (single) | 6–10 h | 20–30 |

*Source:* Created from data appearing in Podrid PJ: Oral antiarrhythmic drugs used for atrial fibrillation; Clinical pharmacology. In: Podrid PJ (ed): *Atrial Fibrillation Mechanisms and Management.* New York, Raven Press 1992:197–231.

should take place only in a monitored setting to maximize safety by detecting early proarrhythmia or bradycardia following conversion to sinus rhythm.

Maintaining sinus rhythm following cardioversion succeeds more often with continued use of antiarrhythmic drugs (refer to Table 37-2). Depending upon the underlying cardiac pathology, up to 70 percent of patients with recurrent AF prior to cardioversion relapse within the first year if not treated with class I or III antiarrhythmic drugs. Quinidine or procainamide given before and after DCC increases the probability of maintaining sinus rhythm for 1 year to 40 percent. Flecainide, propafenone, and sotalol may further increase maintenance of sinus rhythm to 50 percent in select groups. Low doses of amiodarone (100 to 200 mg daily) maintain sinus rhythm after cardioversion more effectively than any other drug, including sotalol. Amiodarone maintains sinus rhythm in up to 65 percent of patients during the first year and 60 percent at 3 years after DCC.[9] Recent trials of the new class III drugs dofetilide and azimilide show suppression of up to 60 percent of recurrent AF.

**TABLE 37-2.** Efficacy of Various Antiarrhythmic Drugs in the Maintenance of Sinus Rhythm-One Year after Cardioversion from Atrial Fibrillation (Multiple Studies)

| Drug | Dose | Metabolism | Success (%) |
|------|------|------------|-------------|
| Placebo | | | 30 |
| Quinidine | 300 mg tid | 90% hepatic | 25–45 |
| Disopyramide | 100 mg tid | 70% renal | 40–50 |
| Propafenone | 300 mg tid | Hepatic | 40–75 |
| Flecainide | 100 mg bid | 75% hepatic | 45–75 |
| Sotalol | 120 mg bid | Renal | 35–45 |
| Amiodarone | 200 mg qd | Hepatic | 40–85 |

*Source:* Created from data appearing in Podrid PJ: Oral antiarrhythmic drugs used for atrial fibrillation; Clinical pharmacology. In: Podrid PJ (ed): *Atrial Fibrillation Mechanisms and Management.* New York, Raven Press 1992:197–231.

Ventricular rate control improves symptoms in most patients with AF who fail repeat attempts at cardioversion. Rapid ventricular rates and irregular ventricular filling intervals contribute to inefficient cardiac output and patient symptoms. Drugs
that slow atrioventricular conduction in AF and AFL do so by prolonging AV node
refractoriness. Vagal stimulation by digoxin and antagonism of circulating catecholamines by beta blockers indirectly prolong AV node refractoriness. Calcium
channel antagonists and modulators of cyclic AMP activity in the AV node (adenosine, beta blockers) slow conduction by directly prolonging refractoriness.

*Catheter ablation of the AV junction* creates complete AV block and eliminates
rapid ventricular rates during atrial arrhythmia. Ablation of the AV junction eliminates the need for drugs that control AV node conduction in patients with refractory AF, AFL, or atrial tachycardia. Patients do require a ventricular pacing system
implant to maintain adequate ventricular rates even during rest, and particularly
during physical activity. Patients undergoing catheter ablation of the AV node experience improvement in symptoms and quality of life through complete elimination of rapid and irregular ventricular rates and through elimination of side effects
attributable to the multiple medications previously used to slow AV node conduction.[10] Modification of AV node conduction by catheter ablation may slow the ventricular response to AF without the need for permanent pacing. The development
of late AV block and failure to completely regularize the ventricular response limit
the appeal of AV node modification.

Catheter ablation or modification of the AV node does not eliminate AF; therefore patients should remain on therapeutic warfarin anticoagulation to prevent
thromboembolic complications.

The *creation of linear lesions in the atria* that disrupt the multiple rotating
wavelets in the atria that produce AF may cure AF in selected patients. The open-
chest "maze" surgical procedure creates segments of atrial myocardium that are too
narrow to allow macroreentrant wavelets, and therefore may effectively terminate
AF. Complications of the procedure include sinus node dysfunction requiring permanent pacing, questionable transport by the reconstructed atrium, and the usual
side effects of cardiopulmonary bypass.

An *endocardial transcatheter technique* utilizes special tools, currently in the infancy of their development, to mimic the cuts made by the open heart procedure.
Complications of the catheter maze procedure include stroke, pericardial effusion
or cardiac tamponade, and pulmonary vein stricture producing pulmonary venous
hypertension. An increasing, yet undetermined, number of patients with AF have
been found to have a focus of atrial tachycardia originating from the inlet of pulmonary veins into the left atrium which triggers the AF. Ablation of the focus may
diminish or eliminate this specific form of AF. Primary catheter ablation of AF remains an experimental procedure with significant risks.[11]

The *implantable atrial defibrillator* effectively restores sinus rhythm by delivering
relatively low-energy shocks from the right atrium to the coronary sinus. Selected
patients with intermittent AF who convert to sinus rhythm by low-energy shocks
may benefit from this innovative therapy. Disadvantages of the atrial defibrillator
include the need for uncomfortable shocks and the early recurrence of AF immediately following apparently successful cardioversion.

# MANAGEMENT OF VENTRICULAR TACHYCARDIA

*Ventricular tachycardia (VT)* denotes a rhythm originating below the AV ring, greater than three consecutive depolarizations, and at rates faster than 120 to 300 beats per minute. Ventricular tachyarrhythmia producing hemodynamic instability usually deteriorates into ventricular fibrillation (VF) and cardiac arrest. The widely accepted definition of nonsustained VT begins at four consecutive beats. The classification of sustained VT in this chapter includes tachycardia lasting longer than 30 s.

VT may produce cardiac arrest, syncope, mildly symptomatic hypotension, or no symptoms other than the sensation of tachycardia. The rate of tachycardia and the extent of underlying structural heart disease usually determine the degree of symptoms. Patients with VT in the absence of structural heart disease may tolerate tachycardia even at rates approaching 200 beats per minute. VT at much lower rates may produce hypotension and syncope in the patient with reduced ventricular function, however.

# THE ELECTROCARDIOGRAPHIC DISTINCTION BETWEEN VT AND SVT

Algorithms for the interpretation of the 12-lead ECG during a wide-complex tachycardia accurately identify the rhythm as originating below or above the AV ring based upon the pattern of ventricular activation. Utilization of a stepwise approach to interpreting the ECG (Fig. 37-2) directs the clinician to select the proper treat-

1. Is there a QS pattern on the complex (no R wave) from leads $V_1$ to $V_6$?
   If true: Ventricular tachycardia
   If not, and there is an rS pattern, $\longrightarrow$ step 2
   If the ECG has a dominant R or RsR′ in $V_1$ to $V_6$, $\longrightarrow$ step 3
2. What is the duration from the onset of the R to the nadir of the S?
   If >100 ms: Ventricular tachycardia
   If <100 ms: Supraventricular tachycardia
3. Can you distinguish P waves and AV dissociation?
   If yes: Ventricular tachycardia
   If no: Analyze the R-to-S ratio in $V_1$ and $V_6$ (step 4)
4. Large R wave or RsR′ in $V_1$ and R > s in $V_6$: Supraventricular tachycardia
   Large R wave in $V_1$ with R < S in $V_6$: Ventricular tachycardia

**Figure 37-2**  Stepwise approach to the diagnosis of a wide-complex tachycardia (how to distinguish VT from SVT on the basis of QRS morphology). (Adapted from data from Brugada P, Brugada J, Mont L, Smeets J, Andries E: A new approach to the differential diagnosis of a regular tachycardia with a wide QRS complex. *Circulation* 1991; 83:1649–1659.)

ment for VT or SVT. The systematic use of this approach succeeds in over 98 percent of cases.[12]

Clinical history always supports the electrocardiographic criteria that identify VT. The presence or absence of structural heart disease adds helpful clues as to the origin of the wide-complex rhythm. VT occurs most often, but not exclusively, in patients with underlying heart disease. Wide-complex tachycardia occurring in a patient with a history of myocardial infarction (MI), CHF, valve disease, cardiomyopathy, or complex congenital heart disease should lead the physician to consider VT as the cause of the rhythm disturbance. Absence of structural heart disease more often than not points to SVT as the cause.

The *acute management of sustained VT* depends most on the hemodynamic and symptomatic condition of the patient. The physician should immediately apply synchronized direct-current shocks (50 to 360 J) to cardiovert the unconscious patient or the patient in extreme cardiorespiratory distress. The awake patient who tolerates sustained VT with minimal hypotension or angina can receive pharmacologic agents to terminate VT without direct-current shock. The widely adopted Advanced Cardiac Life Support (ACLS) algorithm provides guidelines for the emergency management of VT and VF.

Lidocaine (75 to 150 mg by intravenous bolus followed by infusion at 1 to 3 mg/min) may terminate VT. Procainamide (500 to 1000 mg infusion at <50 mg/min followed by 1 to 3 mg/min) also effectively terminates many episodes of VT. Each drug produces side effects. Lidocaine affects the sensorium of the elderly patient up to the point of producing seizure. The neurotoxic effect worsens in patients with reduced cardiac output. Procainamide dilates arterioles, producing hypotension, and directly suppresses ventricular function, further compromising the patient's hemodynamic status if it fails to terminate VT. Procainamide lengthens repolarization, lengthening the QT segment, which may lead to induction of torsades de pointes. Failure of intravenous adminstration of a class I drug should prompt the physician to sedate the patient appropriately as preparation for elective DCC. Administration of synchronized direct current at 50 to 360 J effectively terminates VT without further side effects of antiarrhythmic drugs.

Recurrence of VT following DCC and lidocaine or procainamide infusion should prompt intravenous administration of a class III drug. Amiodarone (150 mg bolus over 10 min with constant infusion at 1 mg/min) effectively suppresses recurrence of VT. The introduction of amiodarone has greatly reduced the use of intravenous bretylium in the management of VT.

The presence of VT in any patient calls for hospital admission and consultation with a cardiologist or cardiac electrophysiologist. Along with termination and immediate suppression of the VT, the consultant may guide the primary physician in identifying and treating the underlying cause of the VT and treating potentially reversible causes.

Most VT results from electrical instability in ventricular myocardium. Reversible abnormalities, such as drug toxicity producing prolongation of the corrected QT segment on the ECG, electrolyte abnormalities, or ischemia, usually produce polymorphic, irregular wide-complex tachycardia. Chronic scarring following myocardial injury creates stable reentry circuits in ventricular myocardium that produce regular, monomorphic VT. Myocardial infarction produces the most common substrate for VT. Less common causes of ventricular scarring that produce VT include myocarditis, infiltrative myocardial processes, scars from previous surgical intervention, and stretching of components of the normal conduction system by dilated cardiomyopathy. Some rare episodes of VT result from the abnormal firing of a single cell or group of cells with abnormal membrane activity. This arrhythmia usually occurs in patients with grossly normal hearts.

The patient with VT should undergo an in-hospital evaluation to determine its cause. The history and physical examination usually reveal previous myocardial infarction, a cardiac surgical history, use of proarrhythmic drugs and diuretics, or findings suggestive of myocarditis or infiltrative diseases. Laboratory studies may detect hypokalemia, hypocalcemia, or hypomagnesemia. The assessment of ventricular function by echocardiography, contrast ventriculography, or radionuclide imaging yields diagnostic and prognostic information. The presence of segmental wall motion abnormalities suggests previous infarction. Global hypokinesis of the left ventricle suggests nonischemic cardiomyopathy. Isolated focal or diffuse right ventricular enlargement points to arrhythmogenic right ventricular dysplasia, a rare cause of VT. The absence of any structural abnormality in the heart leads to the diagnosis of idiopathic VT originating in the left ventricle (right bundle branch block pattern on ECG) or in the right ventricular outflow tract (left bundle branch block, normal axis on ECG). The degree of left ventricular dysfunction predicts patient prognosis more accurately than any other factor for patients with VT. Patients with VT in normal ventricles very rarely die from arrhythmia. Marked ventricular dysfunction (ejection fraction <20 percent and NYHA class III or IV) leads to a poor long-term outcome without aggressive intervention, however.[13]

Cardiac catherization with coronary angiography provides important information in the evaluation of almost all patients with VT. In the patient with a structurally normal heart and with no history to suggest ischemia or coronary disease, however, a noninvasive assessment of coronary reserve, such as exercise radionuclide scans, provides adequate data without the need for invasive testing.

The *chronic management of sustained VT* includes drug therapy to suppress reentry, surgical resection of the arrhythmia circuit, catheter ablation of the focus of tachycardia, and implantation of automatic pacing defibrillators to treat recurrent VT. The primary care physician should involve a cardiologist or cardiac electrophysiologist for assistance in the management of these patients.

Widespread drug therapy for VT began with the use of the class Ia antiarrhythmic agents. Quinidine, procainamide, and disopyramide have yielded disappointing results over the past 30 years. Failure to suppress VT, proarrhythmia, and intolerable side effects have limited their indication to the point where physicians should rarely use them today. Multiple studies have demonstrated efficacy rates as low as 10 percent for suppressing VT, discontinuation because of side effects in up to 40 percent of patients, and proarrhythmia in up to 10 percent of cases.[14]

Results from the CAST, CAST II, and CASH multicenter trials suggest that use of the class Ic agents flecainide, encainide, moricizine, and propafenone increases mortality in patients with left ventricular dysfunction and ventricular arrhythmia.[15–17] Consequently, one should avoid these drugs in treating ventricular arrhythmia in patients with structural heart disease. Only the class III antiarrhythmic drugs sotalol and amiodarone appear to show adequate efficacy and acceptable risk for treating VT. However, sotalol and amiodarone produce powerful electrophysiologic effects in the heart and effects in other organs that limit their use to selected patients.

Catheter ablation of VT due to coronary disease eliminates exit sites from zones of slow conduction in ventricular myocardium. Catheter ablation also cures less common forms of VT originating in otherwise normal myocardium. A small minority of patients with VT have a tachycardia that is amenable to catheter ablation, however. Endocardial resection guided by intraoperative electrophysiologic evaluation eliminates VT in selected patients; however, mortality, morbidity, and technical difficulty, combined with refinements in the implantable cardiac defibrillator, greatly limit the widespread utilization of surgical resection.

The development of small implantable cardioverter defibrillators (ICDs) with transvenous electrodes for endocardial defibrillation revolutionized the treatment of ventricular arrhythmia. Direct comparisons between medical therapy and ICD implantation for management of VT clearly demonstrate the superiority of the ICD. Therefore, antiarrhythmic drugs now serve mostly as adjunctive therapy to ICDs for reducing the number and rate of VT/VF episodes that trigger ICD discharges. The ability to terminate VT by rapid ventricular pacing without shocking the patient provides an excellent alternative to drug therapy, catheter ablation, or surgery. Electrophysiologists can implant the device in the electrophysiology laboratory under local anesthesia with low complications. The great initial expense of the ICD often discourages its use, however. Preliminary economic analysis of ICD utilization supports its long-term cost-effectiveness when compared to drug therapy in patients with VT and VF.[18]

The *treatment of nonsustained VT and ventricular ectopy* has created tremendous controversy during the past 15 years. Data from observational studies during the 1970s and 1980s suggest that complex ventricular ectopy independently predicts a poor outcome in patients with structural heart disease. The assumption that suppression of ventricular ectopy would improve survival in those patients, however, led to numerous studies that demonstrated that antiarrhythmic drugs suppressed ectopy but increased mortality in the treated groups. Proarrhythmia and deterioration in ventricular function produced by class I drugs led to early termination of the studies. Amiodarone eliminates ectopy and improves ventricular function, yet controlled studies consistently fail to prove improvement in patient survival.[18] Antiarrhythmic drugs may produce adverse noncardiac effects and proarrhythmia even in patients without structural heart disease. Therefore, the detrimental effects of antiarrhythmic drugs should discourage the physician from prescribing them to any patient with simple ventricular ectopy. The association between ventricular ectopy, left ventricular dysfunction, and sudden death has led to trials to determine which patients benefit from aggressive intervention, including prophylactic ICD implant.

The primary care physician may acquire a growing number of patients with ICDs for management of VT or cardiac arrest. Recognition of ICD-related problems by the primary care physician may be the first step in appropriate intervention to help the patient. ICD-sensing lead failure produces inaccurate arrhythmia detection and causes multiple shocks during sinus rhythm. Slower than expected VT with rates below the rate threshold programmed into the ICD fails to trigger the ICD and leads to no therapy. Sinus tachycardia during vigorous physical activity may trigger ICD firing when the sinus rate exceeds the VT detection threshold. Device infection or erosion produces local pain, fever, or systemic infection. Failure of appropriate ICD firing to restore sinus rhythm suggests myocardial ischemia, electrolyte imbalance, or a drug effect that has increased the defibrillation threshold in the patient. Any of these situations requires immediate attention and consultation with a cardiac electrophysiologist to correct the underlying problem. Familiarity with ICD systems may help the primary care physician recognize problems and deal with them more effectively.

## REFERENCES

1. Vaughan Williams EM: Classification of antiarrhythmic drugs. In: Sandoe EM, Flensted-Jensen T, Olsen E (eds): *Symposium on Cardiac Arrhythmias*. Sodertalje, Sweden, AB Astra, 1970:449–472.
2. Kalbfleisch SJ, Calkins H, Langberg JJ, et al: Comparison of the cost of radiofrequency catheter modification of the atrioventricular nodal and medical therapy for drug-refractory atrioventricular node reentrant tachycardia. *J Am Coll Cardiol* 1992; 19:1583–1587.
3. Langberg JJ, Chin MC, Rosenqvist M, et al: Catheter-induced ablation of the atrioventricular junction with radiofrequency energy. *Circulation* 1989; 80:1527–1535.
4. Stroke Prevention in Atrial Fibrillation II Investigators: Warfarin versus aspirin for prevention of thromboembolism in atrial fibrillation. *Lancet* 1994; 19:687–691.
5. Rodriguez LM: Are electrophysiological changes induced by longer lasting atrial fibrillation reversible? Observations using the atrial defibrillator. *Circulation* 1999; 100:113–116.
6. The Stroke Prevention in Atrial Fibrillation Investigators: Predictors of thromboembolism in atrial fibrillation: I. Clinical features of patients at risk. *Ann Intern Med* 1992; 116:1–5.
7. ELAT Study Group: Transesophageal echocardiography to assess embolic risk in patients with atrial fibrillation. *Ann Intern Med* 1998; 128:630–638.
8. Oral H: Facilitating transthoracic cardioversion of atrial fibrillation with ibutilide pretreatment. *N Engl J Med* 1999; 340:1849–1854.
9. Podrid PJ: Oral antiarrhythmic drugs used for atrial fibrillation; clinical pharmacology. In: Podrid PJ (ed): *Atrial Fibrillation Mechanisms and Management*. New York, Raven Press, 1992:197–231.
10. APT Investigators: The Ablate and Pace Trial: a prospective study of catheter ablation of the AV conduction system and permanent pacemaker implantation for treatment of atrial fibrillation. *J Interv Card Electrophysiol* 1998; 2:121–135.
11. Stevenson WG, Ellison KE, Lefroy DC, Friedman PL: Ablation therapy for cardiac arrhythmias. *Am J Cardiol* 1997; 80:56G–66G.
12. Brugada P, Brugada J, Mont L, et al: A new approach to the differential diagnosis of a regular tachycardia with a wide QRS complex. *Circulation* 1991; 83:1649–1659.

13. Wilber D, Garan H, Finkelstein D, et al: Out of hospital cardiac arrest: use of electrophysiologic testing in the prediction of long-term outcome. *N Engl J Med* 1988; 318:19–24.
14. Echt DS, Liebson PR, Mitchell LB, et al: Mortality and morbidity in patients receiving encainide, flecainide, or placebo: the Cardiac Arrhythmia Suppression Trial. *N Engl J Med* 1991; 324:781–788.
15. Cardiac Arrhythmia Suppression Trial II Investigators: Ethmozine exerts an adverse effect on mortality in survivors of acute myocardial infarction. *N Engl J Med* 1989; 327:227–233.
16. Siebels J, Cappato R, Ruppel R, et al: Preliminary results of the Cardiac Arrest Study Hamburg (CASH). *Am J Cardiol* 1993; 72:109F–113F.
17. Moss AJ, Hall WJ, Cannom DS, et al: Improved survival with an implanted defibrillator in patients with coronary disease at high risk for ventricular arrhythmia: Multicenter Automatic Defibrillator Implantation Trial Investigators. *N Engl J Med* 1996; 335:1933–1940.
18. AVID Investigators: The Antiarrhythmic versus Implantable Defibrillator Trial in ventricular arrhythmia. *N Engl J Med* 1997; 337:1576–1583.

WILLIAM H. PLAUTH, JR. /
HARRY R. FOSTER, JR.

**CHAPTER**

# ACUTE RHEUMATIC FEVER

**38**

## ACUTE RHEUMATIC FEVER

### Definition and Etiology

Acute rheumatic fever (ARF) is an acute, self-limited, nonsuppurative inflammatory process involving the connective tissues of specific target organs, among them the joints, blood vessels, subcutaneous tissues, serous surfaces, and heart. This inflammation is responsible for the fever, migratory polyarthritis or polyarthralgia, chorea, erythema marginatum, subcutaneous nodules, and carditis characteristic of this disease. All manifestations except those involving the heart subside spontaneously and, although troublesome at the time, eventually disappear without sequelae. Inflammation of the heart, or carditis, involves all three layers of the heart, namely, the pericardium, myocardium, and endocardium, but it is the endocardial inflammation, with its potential for serious acute and long-term injury to the heart valves, particularly the mitral and aortic valves, that makes ARF important.[1–3]

ARF is invariably preceded by an untreated or inadequately treated pharyngitis caused by the group A beta-hemolytic streptococcus (GABHS). GABHS infections in the pharyngeal area and other tissues such as the skin (i.e., impetigo) can produce acute glomerulonephritis and scarlet fever, but ARF follows only GABHS pharyngitis.

The precise mechanism linking GABHS pharyngitis to ARF is unknown, but it appears to involve an autoimmune inflammatory response that makes its clinical appearance anywhere from 1 to 4 weeks (average 18 days) after the onset of the acute infection.[4] The attack rate varies from 0.9 percent among untreated children in an outpatient setting to 3 percent or higher among young military recruits housed under crowded conditions.[5,6]

## NATURAL HISTORY

Unfortunately, there is no direct relationship between the ability of GABHS to produce ARF and its ability to produce symptoms. Approximately one-half to two-thirds of these infections produce so little discomfort or symptoms that the individual and the family are unaware of the illness or do not seek medical attention.[7,8] Untreated, the patient typically becomes asymptomatic in 2 to 3 days. The "latent period," averaging about 18 days, ensues, during which the patient feels well but the suspected immunopathologic process has its inception.[1,4] This is also the time when streptococcal antibodies begin to rise, signaling the body's recognition of the active infection. These antibodies include, among others, antistreptolysin (ASO), anti-deoxyribonuclease B (anti-DNase B), and antihyaluronidase (AH). Appropriate antibiotic treatment during the first 9 days of the pharyngitis avoids the risk of acute rheumatic fever and prevents or significantly attenuates the rise of these antibodies.[1]

The onset of the inflammatory phase of ARF is heralded, most commonly, by joint pain. Acute migratory polyarthritis or arthralgia, occurring in anywhere from 60 to 85 percent of patients with the acute attack, is almost invariably accompanied by fever and characteristically involves the larger joints. It is self-limited and subsides, as does the fever, in 2 to 4 weeks, leaving no sequelae.[1,9] Anywhere from 50 to 85 percent of these patients can be expected to show evidence of carditis either when first seen or shortly thereafter. In approximately 70 percent, this will take the form of an isolated, apical, systolic blowing murmur of mitral regurgitation. In perhaps 25 percent, mitral regurgitation will be accompanied by the blowing decrescendo murmur of aortic regurgitation. Isolated aortic regurgitation is very uncommon (2 to 7 percent of patients).[9,10] If a murmur is to be heard in the setting of joint pain, it will be evident in approximately 76 percent of patients during the first week of the attack. It will appear in another 11 percent of patients in the 3 weeks that follow. In approximately 7 percent of patients, a murmur is heard for the first time between the fourth and sixth weeks of the attack. Between 6 and 10 percent of patients can be expected to show clinical evidence of pericarditis (chest pain and/or precordial friction rub). Carditis is judged mild if only the mitral valve is involved and there is no cardiac enlargement, moderate if both the mitral and aortic valves are involved and/or there is only mild to moderate cardiac enlargement, and severe when valve involvement is associated with marked cardiac enlargement, pericarditis, or congestive heart failure (CHF).[1,8] Between 20 and 30 percent of untreated patients will develop severe carditis, and a small number, perhaps 15 percent of this group, may require acute surgical valve repair or replacement.[10,11]

Carditis will be the presenting manifestation in 20 to 30 percent of patients with ARF.[12] It may be discovered only after 1 or more weeks of intermittent low-grade fever, malaise, poor appetite, pallor, progressive fatigue, palpitations, and shortness of breath, at a point when mitral and/or aortic valve injury may be well established and CHF present.

Carditis, whether associated with joint pain or chorea or as an isolated manifestation, occurs in anywhere from a low of 40 percent to a high of 78 percent of patients with ARF in the United States.[1,11] If patients with silent mitral regurgitation, demonstrated only by Doppler echocardiography, are included, cardiac involvement may exceed 90 percent.[8,13]

Sydenham's chorea, or St. Vitus' Dance, will be the presenting feature in the remaining 20 to 30 percent of patients. This central nervous system disorder tends to occur late in the natural history of the acute attack, when acute-phase reactants and streptococcal antibody titers have returned to normal. Concurrent arthritis is rare but may precede chorea by a matter of weeks. Somewhere between 30 and 40 percent of patients will have a murmur characteristic of rheumatic involvement when chorea is first recognized. Chorea without joint involvement or carditis is termed "pure chorea." The long-term outlook for the development of rheumatic heart disease does not differ between these two groups. After 20 years, without antibiotic prophylaxis, approximately 25 percent of patients will be found to have valvular disease, usually mitral regurgitation and/or stenosis, often without intervening rheumatic manifestations.[1] The average duration of chorea is approximately 3 months, with mild cases subsiding within a few weeks and more protracted cases lasting 6 months or longer. There are no long-term neurologic sequelae.

Multiple subcutaneous nodules occur in about 10 percent of patients and seldom appear before the third week of the illness. They are almost invariably associated with active carditis, usually severe. They are never a sole manifestation, are confirmatory rather than diagnostic in value, and usually take many weeks to disappear. Erythema marginatum also occurs in approximately 10 percent of patients. It, too, tends to occur relatively late and never appears without arthritis or carditis. Neither nodules nor erythema marginatum is a presenting sign.[1,7,9,10]

Abdominal pain may be the earliest presenting symptom, occurring toward the end of the latent period. The precise cause of this pain is unclear, but it may be difficult to distinguish from that of early acute appendicitis. Nonimprovement may lead to surgical exploration of the abdomen, only to have other, more characteristic signs of ARF appear during the early postoperative period.[1,2]

The duration of untreated ARF can be as short as 6 weeks in those patients in whom arthritis is the sole manifestation but usually extends into the 9- to 12-week range when carditis is present. In a very few patients, particularly those with severe carditis, CHF, and/or previous attacks, the illness may continue for 6 months or longer and is termed "chronic" rheumatic fever.[1,7]

Recurrences of ARF are the result of inadequate protection from subsequent GABHS pharyngitis. The attack rate of ARF following a GABHS pharyngitis is far higher in those individuals who have had ARF than in those who have not. The younger the child, the greater the severity of residual heart disease, the shorter the interval since the previous attack, and the greater the number of preceding attacks, the more likely it will be that ARF will follow any given episode of GABHS pharyngitis.[1,7] Approximately 70 percent of patients can be expected to have a recurrence within 3 years of the initial attack if left without antibiotic prophylaxis.[1,7]

The severity of residual heart disease depends on the severity of cardiac injury during the initial attack and the number of recurrences thereafter. Although individuals without carditis during their initial attack are less likely to develop carditis during a second attack than those who experienced cardiac involvement initially, approximately 25 percent of this group will develop carditis if a second attack occurs. If recurrences can be prevented, 80 percent of patients with mild carditis and as many as 35 percent of patients with severe carditis at the onset can expect to have the murmur of mitral regurgitation disappear over a 10-year period. Without antibiotic prophylaxis, only 20 percent of patients with mild carditis will have such a favorable outcome. Aortic regurgitation is more persistent under the best of circumstances, but disappearance is observed in approximately 25 percent of patients over the same interval.[14] Aortic stenosis is rare in the absence of prominent aortic regurgitation. Before the advent of antibiotic prophylaxis, approximately 40 percent of patients who appeared to have escaped their initial attack of ARF without residual cardiac injury developed mitral stenosis over the following 20 years. Diligent prophylaxis can reduce this complication to the vanishing point.[14] Late development of tricuspid stenosis or regurgitation is described but is rare, and late involvement of the pulmonary valve is extremely rare. Infective endocarditis remains a persistent danger, as it does for all individuals with structural heart disease.[15]

# EPIDEMIOLOGY

ARF is, by and large, an illness of children and adolescents, with the average age of onset being between 8 and 10 years. The majority of patients present between 5 and 15 years of age. It is very rare in children less than 3 years of age (0.5 to 2.0 percent) and is uncommon beyond 20 years, except among young military recruits housed in crowded barracks. In the latter, ARF may reach epidemic proportions, with an incidence of between 25 and 100 per 1000 troops.[1,8,16] In the United States, ARF occurs most frequently in the spring months, with a peak in March and April, and follows the peak incidence of GABHS pharyngitis.[8,16] There is no sex predilection with the exception of chorea, where females are afflicted twice as frequently as males. Racial differences are difficult to distinguish from the effects of poverty, crowded living conditions, and differences in access to or utilization of medical care. Nevertheless, the Maoris of New Zealand and Polynesian children appear to have a disproportionately high incidence of ARF.[17] A predisposition for family members to develop ARF and a higher incidence among monozygotic compared to dizygotic twins is compatible with a genetic factor, but the specific genetic pattern or marker has yet to be identified with certainty.

The incidence of ARF declined in the United States, Western European countries, and Japan from approximately 200 per 100,000 in 1900 to 50 per 100,000 by the mid-1940s.[7] This decline has been attributed to the overall improvement in the standard of living, with better nutrition, better sanitation, and less crowding at home and in schools. The discovery of penicillin during World War II and the recognition that it could eradicate as well as prevent GABHS pharyngitis no doubt contributed to the acceleration in the decline in incidence and mortality during the 1950s, but the most dramatic improvement occurred during the late 1960s and 1970s, when there was a 50-fold decrease in incidence, from 24 to 0.5 cases per 100,000 population.[18] Although the standard of living continued to improve, as did access to medical care, the explanation for this dramatic change is not altogether clear. The incidence of ARF has remained relatively low (estimated at 0.5 to 3.1 per 100,000 population)[19] in most areas of the United States, but beginning in the mid-

1980s, reports of significant localized outbreaks of ARF began to appear, along with descriptions of regions in which the incidence of ARF had not fallen to the low levels experienced by the country as a whole.[8,11,20,21] A reason for this resurgence or persistence of ARF is not readily apparent. The reappearance of streptococcal M-protein serotypes historically linked to ARF (i.e., "rheumatogenic" serotypes) and/or an increase in the virulence of the streptococcus by virtue of its ability to produce a protective hyaluronic acid capsule are two of several possible explanations.[8,11,20]

Despite its low incidence today in the United States and other economically developed countries, ARF and its sequela, rheumatic heart disease, remain a scourge for four-fifths of the world's population. This combination is responsible for 30 to 50 percent of all hospital cardiac admissions in developing countries,[6,17] and, worldwide, it is the leading cause of death from heart disease in the first 50 years of life.[10] The incidence of ARF remains anywhere from 300 to 1000 per 100,000 population in many areas of Africa and Asia, while the prevalence of rheumatic heart disease among school-age children is reported as being anywhere from 5 per 1000 in Egypt, India, and Turkey to 10 per 1000 in the Sudan and Morocco.[17] The prevalence in the United States is between 0.7 and 1.6 per 1000.[17]

# DIAGNOSIS AND THE JONES CRITERIA

In 1944, T. Duckett Jones proposed a set of clinical and laboratory criteria to aid in the diagnosis of ARF. These criteria have been revised several times, with the most recent revision being in 1992.[22] If there is laboratory evidence of a preceding GABHS infection, the presence of two major manifestations, or one major and two minor manifestations, indicates a high likelihood of an initial attack of ARF. Abdominal pain, rapid heart rate, epistaxis, precordial pain, and a family history of rheumatic fever may heighten one's suspicions but are not criteria.

## The Jones Criteria, 1992 Update

Supporting evidence of an antecedent group A streptococcal infection:

1. Positive or rising streptococcal antibody test. The onset of ARF characteristically coincides with a significant streptococcal antibody response. The two most commonly employed measures of this response are the antistreptolysin O (ASO) and antideoxyribonuclease B (anti-DNase B) titers. An ASO titer, expressed in Todd units, of 340 in a child or 240 in an adult is generally considered a modest elevation.[22] The titers of anti-DNaseB, also in Todd units, that would carry the same interpretation are somewhat less clear. In the Jones criteria, 1992 update,[22] titers of 240 for a child and 120 for an adult were proposed as representing a moderate elevation. More recent data[23] indicate that for a child the upper limit of normal is closer to 640 Todd units, with 800 Todd units

representing an elevation.[22] An elevated titer of at least one of these antibodies can be demonstrated in approximately 90 percent of all patients with ARF, excluding those with Sydenham's chorea. Use of a third antibody test, anti-hyaluronidase (AH), raises this figure to 95 percent, but laboratory facilities for this test are less commonly available. The Streptozyme test is not recommended. To demonstrate a rise in antibody titer, acute and convalescent serum samples should be obtained at 2- to 4-week intervals. The ASO titer usually peaks at 3 to 6 weeks and the anti-DNase B titer at 6 to 8 weeks after the onset of the acute infection. A significant antibody rise is defined as a rise in titer of two or more dilution increments between the acute- and convalescent-phase specimens.

2. Positive throat culture or positive rapid antigen test for GABHS. Neither distinguishes, unfortunately, between a current infection and chronic pharyngeal carriage of GABHS. A negative rapid antigen test should be confirmed by throat culture. The yield of cultures in this setting is relatively low (25 percent), presumably because of the delay engendered by the latent period, perhaps compounded by the administration of an antibiotic prior to the culture. Without evidence of a preceding streptococcal infection, one should be reluctant to make the diagnosis of rheumatic fever. Exceptions are instances of chorea or indolent carditis where supporting laboratory evidence of preceding streptococcal infection has already disappeared.

Two major or one major and two minor criteria are required for diagnosis.

**MAJOR MANIFESTATIONS.**

1. *Carditis.* The confirmation of carditis, the only serious element of ARF, rests on the recognition of mitral regurgitation and/or aortic regurgitation. Myocarditis and pericarditis are never present in the absence of valvular involvement. The murmur of mitral regurgitation is a pansystolic, blowing murmur heard best at the apex, with radiation into the axilla. When the murmur is very soft, it may be best heard with the patient lying in the left lateral position holding his or her breath in deep exhalation. This murmur must be distinguished from a functional or flow murmur and that associated with mitral valve prolapse or congenital heart disease. A low-pitched, diastolic murmur may be heard at the apex in the presence of significant mitral regurgitation. This will not be the murmur of mitral stenosis but is the result of increased flow across the mitral valve in diastole as a consequence of the left atrial volume overload produced by the mitral regurgitation.

   The murmur of aortic regurgitation is much less common, is more difficult to hear, and almost always is heard in conjunction with the murmur of mitral regurgitation. It is a high-pitched, blowing decrescendo murmur beginning immediately after the aortic second heart sound ($S_2$) and usually is heard best at the left mid or upper sternal border with the patient sitting upright, leaning forward, and holding his or her breath in deep exhalation. This murmur should be distinguished from that caused by a congenital bicuspid aortic valve with isolated aortic regurgitation.[1,7]

The scratchy, to and fro sound of a friction rub may be heard in the small number of patients, approximately 10 percent, who develop clinical pericarditis.[10] This may be accompanied by chest pain and usually signals severe carditis. Accumulation of pericardial fluid and/or the friction rub may possibly obscure the murmurs of mitral and/or aortic regurgitation, and in these instances echocardiographic interrogation will be helpful.

Two-D echocardiography with color flow Doppler and M-mode assessment plays an important role in identifying the nonrheumatic causes of valvular regurgitation, detecting the presence of pericardial effusion or chamber enlargement, and assessing ventricular function. Its role in identifying pathologic but inaudible mitral regurgitation ("silent" mitral regurgitation), particularly as it applies to the diagnosis of carditis in instances of suspected ARF, has not, to date, been universally accepted.[22] It has been proposed that Doppler-identified silent mitral regurgitation be added to the Jones criteria as a minor manifestation if (1) the color Doppler jet of mitral regurgitation (*a*) is greater than 1 cm in length, (*b*) can be demonstrated in at least two echocardiographic planes, (*c*) has a posterolateral orientation within the left atrium, and (*d*) has a mosaic pattern characteristic of chaotic flow, and (2) the continuous-wave or pulsed Doppler signal persists throughout systole.[13,24]

2. *Polyarthritis.* Polyarthritis is the most common major manifestation of ARF (75 percent) and frequently the earliest. It is distinguished from polyarthralgia, a minor criterion, by the presence of heat, redness, and tenderness to touch. The pain is usually intense and aggravated by the slightest touch or motion—the latter resulting in such guarding that the patient may present as pseudoparalysis. It is characteristically migratory and generally involves the larger joints, particularly the knees, ankles, elbows, and wrists. Involvement of the hips and small joints of the hands and feet is uncommon. Involvement is usually asymmetrical, with inflammation of each joint lasting anywhere from 1 to 5 days and new joints becoming involved as those previously involved improve. In this fashion, several joints may be involved at once, with each at a different stage of inflammation. This process usually lasts 2 to 4 weeks, if untreated. Arthritis is very sensitive to treatment with salicylates, and the response characteristically is dramatic, with resolution of pain, swelling, and tenderness within 48 h.[25]

Arthritis persisting beyond this time despite salicylate therapy suggests a different diagnosis. Synovial fluid in joints affected by ARF contains between 10,000 and 100,000 white blood cells per cubic millimeter, with the majority being neutrophils. The protein concentration is approximately 4 g/dL, the glucose is normal, the Gram stain shows no bacteria, and the culture is normal. Permanent joint deformities almost never occur, although a chronic process referred to as Jaccoud's arthritis, which causes deformities of the fingers and toes, has been described in rare instances.[19] The differential diagnosis might include infectious arthritis, as seen with the gonococcus and other pyogenic organisms; infective endocarditis; trauma; Lyme disease; Henoch-Schönlein purpura; systemic lupus erythematosus; serum sickness; viral infections; malignant diseases such as leukemia; sickle cell anemia and other hemoglobinopathies; chondromalacia of the patella; osteochondroses of the hip and upper end to the tibia; the reactive arthritis associated with *Shigella, Salmonella,* and *Yersinia enterocolitica;* and, finally, rheumatoid arthritis. The entity termed poststreptococcal reactive arthritis may also follow GABHS pharyngitis. The latent period between the streptococcal infection and the onset of arthritis is usually shorter (1 to 2 weeks) than with classic ARF, the arthritis is more severe and less likely to be migratory, the response to aspirin and other anti-inflammatory medications is much less dramatic, and carditis is unusual during the initial episode. Evidence of cardiac involvement has been described, however, with recurrences, and at present it is recommended that these patients receive the same antibiotic prophylaxis as patients with ARF.[24,26]

3. *Chorea.* Sydenham's chorea, or St. Vitus' dance, is a neurologic disorder characterized by involuntary, purposeless movements of the extremities and trunk. It may be ushered in by what appears to be clumsiness or indistinct speech. Behavioral changes such as moodiness, fretfulness, or being easily provoked or easily made to cry are common. Spasmatic movements, usually jerky and rapid, interfere with voluntary acts. Any muscle group may be involved, but those in the upper part of the body, particularly the muscles of the face and upper extremities, are involved most frequently. Movements may be limited to one side of the body (hemichorea). All abnormal movements disappear with sleep. Other characteristics are explosive speech, flexion of the wrists with hyperextension of the fingers when the arms are held out straight horizontally, and pronation of the arms when extended overhead. Although chorea may occur at a point in the course in the illness when it is the sole manifestation of ARF and the acute-phase reactants and streptococcal antibody titers have returned to normal, this is not always the case, and a careful examination on repeated occasions for signs of rheumatic activity, such as carditis and/or erythema marginatum, is essential. Chorea should be differentiated from tics or habit spasms, choreoathetosis, Wilson's disease, Huntington's chorea, cerebral palsy, lupus erythematosus, and the antiphospholipid syndrome.[1,7,19,27,28]

4. *Erythema marginatum.* Erythema marginatum is a transient, nonpruritic, slightly red rash, usually seen on the trunk and sometimes the upper arms. It never involves the face. It starts as small, pink, slightly raised macules, which gradually extend outward. The outermost margins are sharp and usually continuous, while the inner margins become blurry, and the skin at the center returns to normal. It may occur at any time during the course of the illness, appearing and disappearing within a few hours and then returning and disappearing again. A hot bath or shower may bring out the rash for the first time or accentuate it if it is already present. It is an uncommon manifestation and often appears in the company of subcutaneous nodules. The lesions are not specific for acute ARF and may be seen in drug reactions and glomerulonephritis.[1,7,9]

5. *Subcutaneous nodules.* These firm, nontender, mobile nodules characteristically occur after the first few weeks of illness and in most instances only in patients

with carditis. If they are found in the absence of carditis, the diagnosis of ARF should be suspect. They may be seen or felt over the extensor surfaces of joints, notably the elbows, knuckles, knees, and ankles, and over the spine. They also are found on the scalp, where they may be somewhat less firm. They vary in size from 3 to 4 mm to 1 to 2 cm. They are never transient and usually take several weeks to resolve.[1,9]

## MINOR MANIFESTATIONS

1. *Arthralgia.* Like arthritis, this joint pain is usually migratory and involves the large joints, but objective signs of inflammation are lacking. It can be severe and incapacitating. Care should be taken to distinguish joint pain from that arising from periarticular or muscular tissues. When arthritis is present, arthralgia cannot be used as a supporting criterion.

2. *Fever.* An elevated temperature is almost always present with the onset of polyarthritis, is often present with isolated carditis, and characteristically is absent with isolated chorea. It rarely exceeds 39°C and returns to normal or near-normal in 2 to 3 weeks, even without treatment. It has no characteristic pattern. Continued temperature elevations exceeding 39°C should suggest other diagnoses, such as rheumatoid arthritis, systemic lupus erythematosus, or bacterial sepsis.[28]

3. *Elevated acute-phase reactants.* The erythrocyte sedimentation rate (ESR) and the C-reactive protein are nonspecific but reflect the presence of an inflammatory process. They are almost invariably elevated at the onset of ARF but often are normal in patients with isolated chorea. The ESR may be suppressed by congestive heart failure and become elevated when failure is brought under control. The C-reactive protein is not affected by heart failure and tends to return to normal more quickly than the ESR.[1,7]

4. *Prolonged PR interval.* This abnormality of atrioventricular conduction is nonspecific. It does not reflect carditis, nor does it correlate with the development of subsequent rheumatic heart disease. First-degree atrioventricular block is the most common abnormality, but second-degree and third-degree block may be observed. Atrioventricular conduction eventually returns to normal, but it can be brought to normal quite readily with atropine, if so desired.

## Exceptions to the Jones Criteria

The diagnosis of ARF can be made without strictly adhering to the Jones criteria under three circumstances, provided other illnesses have been excluded. These are (1) in the presence of chorea, the diagnosis can be made despite the absence of laboratory evidence of preceding streptococcal infection or other manifestations of ARF; (2) the diagnosis can be made in the presence of "indolent carditis," defined as a new murmur of mitral or aortic regurgitation without evidence of a recent streptococcal infection or of acute rheumatic activity, and (3) in the case of a patient with a well-documented history of previous ARF, a presumptive diagnosis of new ARF (a recurrence) can be made if a single major or several minor manifestations are present, provided there is supporting evidence of a recent group A streptococcal infection.[22]

## MANAGEMENT AND TREATMENT

The first priority should be to establish the correct diagnosis as firmly and as expeditiously as possible.[19] This will involve, ideally, a very careful initial history and physical examination; daily or twice-daily reexaminations over the course of at least a week; laboratory tests, the results of which are timely and reliable; and, almost certainly, consultation with an experienced cardiologist and, in the case of the patient with chorea, a neurologist as well. The above usually is best accomplished in a hospital setting. Once the diagnosis is established and treatment begun, continued close observation and reexamination will be necessary in order to assess the efficacy of medications and any significant or intolerable side effects of these medications. It will be important to document that carditis has not made a later-than-expected appearance, is not progressing despite therapy, and is not more severe now than it was originally judged. At the same time, the patient's home situation should be assessed in terms of the responsibilities that will fall upon the patient, parents, siblings, and others for the giving of the medications, observations, transportation, school work, and all the other adjustments made necessary by a period of convalescence at home.

Treatment to eradicate GABHS from the pharynx should be initiated even if the rapid streptococcal antigen test and throat cultures are negative. This is accomplished best, in the absence of a history of allergy to penicillin, by either a single intramuscular injection of 600,000 U of benzathine penicillin G (BPG) for a child weighing less than 27 kg (60 lb) or 1,200,000 U for a larger child or adult. The pain of the injection is less if the BPG is brought to room temperature before injection. Another alternative is oral phenoxymethyl penicillin (penicillin V potassium) in a dose of 250 mg 2 to 3 times daily for 10 days for a child and 500 mg 2 to 3 times daily for 10 days for an adolescent and adult. Oral penicillin V potassium should be taken 1 h before or 2 h after meals. For the patient allergic to penicillin, erythromycin estolate 20 to 40 mg/kg in 2 to 4 divided doses daily or erythromycin ethylsuccinate 40 mg/kg in 2 to 4 divided doses daily (maximum of 1 g/day) for a total of 10 days is recommended. If gastrointestinal side effects make erythromycin therapy untenable, oral azithromycin in a dose of 500 mg as a single dose the first day followed by 250 mg once daily for 4 days is an effective alternative. Continuous antistreptococcal antibiotic prophylaxis should be instituted 3 weeks after the BPG injection or at the end of the oral regime.[12,29] Siblings and all the household contacts of the patient, symptomatic or not, should be cultured and, if positive, should be treated. Follow-up cultures are indicated to identify treatment failures or a carrier state and appropriate therapy undertaken.[29]

The arthritis of ARF is treated with aspirin and rest. The response to aspirin usually is dramatic, with symptoms disappearing within 24 to 48 h. Absence of such a response casts doubt on the diagnosis of ARF as the cause of the arthritis. Salicylate therapy should be withheld initially to provide an opportunity for the distinctive pattern of migratory polyarthritis to emerge. In the interim, acetaminophen (Tylenol) or, if necessary, ibuprofen (Advil) may be used to provide relief. The therapeutic dose of oral aspirin is 90 to 100 mg/kg/day divided into 4 doses given at 6-h intervals. It should be given with meals or a snack to circumvent gastric irritation. At some point after 48 and 72 h of therapy, a blood sample to check the salicylate level should be drawn, 2 h after the last dose. The therapeutic range for salicylate lies between 15 and 25 mg/100 dL, and if the latter figure is exceeded, the dose should be reduced. This would be an appropriate time to switch from every 6-h dosing to four times daily during waking hours. At the end of 1 week, if the response is good, the aspirin dose can be reduced by 25 percent and continued for 6 to 8 weeks with monitoring of the ESR. When the ESR has been normal for 2 weeks, the aspirin dose may be tapered over the following 2 weeks and discontinued.[1,2,7] The patient should be observed for nausea, vomiting, tinnitus, hearing loss, or hyperpnea during the course of therapy. These signs of salicylate intoxication warrant prompt assay of the blood salicylate level and appropriate adjustment of the dose. Urticaria, asthma, or angioedema may signal an allergic response to aspirin. This is very uncommon but serious and should be managed by immediate discontinuation of aspirin and, if necessary, treatment with epinephrine. The return of clinical or laboratory evidence of activity after cessation of therapy is termed a *rebound* and is more likely to occur the shorter the duration of treatment and the more abrupt its termination. Retreatment is seldom required if the ESR has been normal for 2 weeks before therapy is discontinued.[1,2,7]

While aspirin is effective in suppressing rheumatic arthritis, it is far less effective in controlling rheumatic pancarditis. If carditis is mild, defined here as either a soft murmur of mitral regurgitation or "silent" mitral regurgitation detected by Doppler echocardiography without cardiac enlargement, it may be managed with aspirin alone, using the regime described above for arthritis but extending the initial 90- to 100-mg/kg/day regime to 2 weeks and the slightly lower dose (usually 75 mg/kg/day) to 8 to 10 weeks, again following the ESR as a guide for tapering and discontinuing therapy. The patient should be observed carefully to be certain that no signs or symptoms appear that would suggest increasing severity of the carditis while on this regime.

Patients with cardiac enlargement on x-ray film, a more impressive murmur of mitral regurgitation, the presence or the appearance of aortic regurgitation, pericarditis, or signs or symptoms of congestive heart failure such as shortness of breath or a gallop rhythm should be treated with prednisone. It is important that there be no confusion between the lack of evidence of the superiority of steroid therapy over aspirin therapy in terms of the incidence and severity of residual heart disease among patients examined years after the initial attack, on the one hand, and the efficacy and speed of steroid therapy compared to aspirin in reducing acute cardiac inflammation, on the other. The dose of prednisone is 2 mg/kg/day with a maximum of 60 mg/day, given in 2 or 4 divided doses. This is maintained for 2 to 3 weeks, during which time one can expect an encouraging or even marked improvement in clinical and laboratory signs of activity.[30] It is recommended that ranitidine (Zantac) 4 to

6 mg/kg/day in 2 divided doses orally be given to reduce the likelihood of peptic ulcer, and dietary counseling directed at controlling salt and caloric intake should coincide with the onset of steroid therapy. If, after 2 to 3 weeks of therapy, the ESR is falling, the dose of prednisone usually can be reduced to 50 percent of the original dose without interrupting the course of improvement. When the ESR has been normal for 2 weeks, further tapering can proceed over the next 4 to 6 weeks, with smaller decreases toward the end to permit the return of adrenocortical function. An option, aimed at shortening the length of prednisone therapy, is to add aspirin at 75 mg/kg/day once the ESR is approaching normal and then taper the prednisone more rapidly. If the ESR continues to fall as the prednisone is tapered and after it is discontinued, the aspirin is maintained until the ESR has been normal for at least 2 weeks and then is tapered off over a 2-week interval.[1,2]

Physical rest is indicated for those patients with active rheumatic carditis and/or heart failure until signs or symptoms have resolved.[2,19] Advice regarding subsequent activity is guided by the degree of residual heart disease. Other measures that reduce the work of the heart in the face of mitral and/or aortic regurgitation, such as diuretics and afterload reducing agents, may be used as indicated. Digoxin probably has little to offer during the acute illness in view of the absence of evidence of systolic ventricular dysfunction.[10,31] Traditionally, its use has been accompanied by the caution that it be used in smaller doses than usual lest dangerous rhythm problems be precipitated. A small number of patients will progress to severe congestive failure during the acute attack, despite steroid therapy and other supportive therapies. The problem appears to lie almost entirely with the severity of the valvular regurgitation; the contribution of myocardial inflammation or dysfunction is minimal. Continued or increased levels of steroid therapy have little or nothing to offer these patients, and valve repair or replacement, even during the acute illness, is indicated.[10,31] Rheumatic pericardial effusion tends to accumulate slowly, rarely causes tamponade, responds to steroid therapy, and never goes on to constriction.[1,7,9]

Although the onset of chorea is characteristically late in the course of the acute illness, carditis may be present, and this should be managed as described above. The patient with mild chorea usually will respond satisfactorily to rest, reassurance, a temporary home teacher, and other measures to reduce stress. Light sedation with phenobarbital may be of benefit. If chorea is more severe, hospitalization may be needed in order to provide adequate hydration and nutrition, continuous supervision, and precautions such as padded side rails on the bed to prevent injury. A variety of medications, each with its own benefits and hazards, have been recommended to control or diminish choreiform movements.[19,28] It would seem wise to ask the advice of an experienced neurologist familiar with the use of these medications and their potential side effects for this aspect of therapy.

## PRIMARY PREVENTION

The treatment for GABHS pharyngitis has been described already under "Management and Treatment." Suffice it to say here that many different regimes using many different antibiotics have been proposed and tested, but, to date, the most effective therapy in the individual who is not allergic to penicillin is intramuscular BPG.[29] Oral regimens run the risk of unreliable compliance, which, in turn, is directly related to the number of times a day the medication needs to be taken and the duration of the regimen.[32,33] Additional problems are the expense of the newer antibiotics and the development of resistance on the part of other bacteria to these relatively broad-spectrum agents. One very encouraging development has been the demonstration that 750 mg of amoxicillin suspension given once daily for 10 days is as effective as 250 mg of penicillin V potassium suspension given 3 times a day for 10 days.[34]

# SECONDARY PREVENTION

It is absolutely essential that patients with ARF be protected from GABHS pharyngitis. Continuous antibiotic prophylaxis makes this possible. An injection of long-acting benzathine penicillin G 1,200,000 U every 3 to 4 weeks is the most effective protection for the individual without penicillin allergy. The 3-week interval is recommended for the patient with significant residual heart disease in whom a recurrence might be disastrous and for patients in developing countries. The advantages of BPG are its effectiveness and documented compliance, while its disadvantages are the pain of injection and allergic reactions (3.2 percent). The latter are more common in adults than in children and include a serum sickness–like reaction and, rarely, anaphylaxis (0.2 percent).[35] Skin testing provides a means of identifying those individuals with a false-positive history of penicillin allergy and possibly (by skin testing at the time of the injections) an opportunity to reduce the already small but worrisome incidence of anaphylactic reactions in high-risk patients, such as those older than 12 years with advanced heart disease and those with a strong history of atopy.[35] Oral penicillin 250 mg twice daily is more convenient, is acceptably effective (95 percent), is inexpensive, and is associated with fewer serious allergic reactions, but has the disadvantage of undependable compliance. Sulfadiazine 0.5 g once daily for patients 27 kg (60 lb) or less and 1.0 g once daily for patients over 27 kg is as effective as oral penicillin for prophylaxis, is inexpensive, and does not encourage the emergence of resistant alpha-hemolytic streptococci in the mouth. Sulfisoxazole (Gantrisin) is equally effective when given in the same doses. Although effective in prophylaxis against GABHS pharyngitis, the sulfonamides are not bactericidal and are useless for the treatment of the established GABHS infection. They are also contraindicated during the third trimester of pregnancy because of placental transmission with potential hyperbilirubinemia in the newborn. For the patient allergic to penicillin and the sulfonamides, erythromycin 250 mg twice daily by mouth is recommended.[12,29]

For the patient who has had no evidence of carditis, it is proposed that prophylaxis be discontinued at age 21 or 5 years after the last attack, whichever is longer. Since late recurrences do occur, however, and rheumatic heart disease can develop in the fourth and fifth decades with no history of recurrences in the interval, it would seem wise to have a low threshold for continuing prophylaxis indefinitely. This would be particularly true for the patient at relatively high risk of exposure to GABHS, such as a parent of young children, a teacher, a physician, a nurse, an allied health provider, or a military recruit. For patients with residual heart disease, we would recommend prophylaxis at least until 40 years of age and perhaps for life. Prophylaxis should continue after valve repair or replacement.[12]

## INFECTIVE ENDOCARDITIS

Infective endocarditis does not occur during the initial attack of ARF but is a constant threat thereafter to those who have valve involvement. The antibiotic regimens that are used to prevent recurrences of ARF are inadequate for the prevention of bacterial endocarditis. In addition, patients receiving penicillin as prophylaxis are likely to have alpha-hemolytic streptococci, the most common cause of endocarditis following dental or oral procedures, in their oral cavities that are resistant to penicillin, amoxicillin, or ampicillin. For patients undergoing dental, oral, respiratory tract, or esophageal procedures that might involve bleeding and/or bacteremia, the following regimes are recommended: clindamycin 20 mg/kg orally in children and 600 mg orally in adults 1 h before the procedure or either azithromycin or clarithromycin 15 mg/kg IV in children and 600 mg IV in adults within 30 min prior to the procedure. For individuals undergoing genitourinary or gastrointestinal (excluding esophageal) procedures, the following are recommended: High-risk patients, defined as those with prosthetic heart valves and/or a previous history of endocarditis, should receive an infusion of vancomycin 20 mg/kg IV for children and 1.0 g IV for adults over 1 to 2 h plus gentamicin 1.5 mg/kg IV/IM (not to exceed 120 mg), with completion of the injection/infusion within 30 min of starting the procedure. Less than high-risk patients may receive only the vancomycin infusion in the doses described above.[15]

## SUMMARY

ARF and its consequence, rheumatic heart disease, are far less common today in the United States and other economically developed countries than they were 50 years ago, but they continue to be a plague in all other areas of the world. Regardless of these regional and global considerations, for the specific individual afflicted, ARF represents a life-altering and sometimes life-threatening event.

ARF should be suspected whenever one is confronted with arthritis or arthralgia, recent-onset easy fatigue or shortness of breath, chest pain, a friction rub, an unexplained heart murmur, or a fever of unknown origin in a child, adolescent, or young adult. Resources necessary to establish a diagnosis should be marshaled early in the course of the illness, when distinctive symptoms, signs, and laboratory tests are still helpful. Hospitalization and/or consultations usually are needed at that point. The plan for management and treatment should include frequent serial observations and reexaminations designed to detect unanticipated problems during the course of the illness, such as the development or progression of carditis or intolerance of or allergies to medications. The plan for home care should include the support of the family, health care providers, school, and other resources. The importance of the prevention of recurrences cannot be overemphasized to the patient and all concerned. Finally, a follow-up arrangement that is reliable, encouraging, and accessible for the months and years to come is essential.

## REFERENCES

1. Markowitz M, Gordis L: *Rheumatic Fever,* 2d ed. Philadelphia, W. B. Saunders, 1972.
2. Fyler DC: Rheumatic fever. In: Fyler DC (ed): *Nadas' Pediatric Cardiology*. Philadelphia, Hanley & Belfus, 1992:305–318.
3. Dajani AS: Rheumatic fever. In: Braunwald E (ed): *Heart Disease,* 5th ed. Philadelphia, W. B. Saunders, 1997:1769–1775.
4. Veasy LG, Hill HR: Immunologic and clinical correlations in rheumatic fever and rheumatic heart disease. *Pediatr Infect Dis J* 1997; 16:400–407.
5. Siegel AC, Johnson EE, Stollerman GH: Controlled studies of streptococcal pharyngitis in a pediatric population. *N Engl J Med* 1961; 265:559–566.
6. Gunzenhauser JD, Longfield JN, Brundage JF, et al: Epidemic streptococcal disease among Army trainees, July 1989 through June 1991. *J Infect Dis* 1995; 172:124–131.
7. Taranta A, Markowitz M: *Rheumatic Fever,* 2d ed. Boston, Kluwer Academic Publishers, 1989.
8. Veasy LG, Wiedmeier SE, Orsmond GS, et al: Resurgence of acute rheumatic fever in the intermountain area of the United States. *N Engl J Med* 1987; 316:421–427.
9. Massell BF, Fyler DC, Roy SB: The clinical picture of rheumatic fever: diagnosis, immediate prognosis, course, and therapeutic implications. *Am J Cardiol* 1958; 1:436–449.
10. Tani LY, Veasy LG, Minich LL, et al: Is rheumatic fever still a problem in the United States? Experience with 411 consecutive cases. *Pediatrics* 1998; 102(Suppl):685.
11. Tolaymat A, Goudarzi T, Soler GP, et al: Acute rheumatic fever in North Florida. *South Med J* 1984; 77:819–823.
12. Dajani A, Taubert K, Ferrieri P, et al: Treatment of acute streptococcal pharyngitis and prevention of rheumatic fever: a statement for health professionals. *Pediatrics* 1995; 96:758–764.
13. Minich LL, Tani LY, Pagotto LT, et al: Doppler echocardiography distinguishes between physiological and pathologic "silent" mitral regurgitation in patients with rheumatic fever. *Clin Cardiol* 1997; 20:924–926.
14. Tompkins DG, Boxerbaum B, Liebman J: Long-term prognosis of rheumatic fever patients receiving regular intramuscular benzathine penicillin. *Circulation* 1972; 45:543–551.
15. Dajani AS, Taubert KA, Wilson W, et al: Prevention of bacterial endocarditis: recommendations by the American Heart Association. *JAMA* 1997; 277:1794–1801.
16. Denny FW Jr: A 45-year prospective on the streptococcus and rheumatic fever: The Edward H. Kass lecture on infectious disease history. *Clin Infect Dis* 1994; 19:1110–1122.

17. Fraser GE: A review of the epidemiology and prevention of rheumatic heart disease. Parts I and II. *Cardiovasc Reviews and Reports* 1996; 17(3):10–26; (4):7–23.

18. Markowitz M: Rheumatic fever—a half-century perspective. *Pediatrics* 1998; 102: 272–274.

19. Ayoub EM: Acute rheumatic fever. In: Emmanouilides GC, Riemenschneider TA, Allen HD, Gutgesell HP (eds): *Moss and Adams Heart Disease in Infants, Children, and Adolescents,* 5th ed. Baltimore, Williams & Wilkins, 1995:1400–1416.

20. Bronze MS, Dale JB: The reemergence of serious group A streptococcal infections and acute rheumatic fever. *Am J Med Sci* 1996; 311:41–54.

21. Wald ER, Dashefsky B, Feidt C, et al: Acute rheumatic fever in western Pennsylvania and the tristate area. *Pediatrics* 1987; 80:371–374.

22. Special Writing Group of the Committee on Rheumatic Fever, Endocarditis, and Kawasaki Disease of the Council on Cardiovascular Disease in the Young of the American Heart Association: Guidelines for the diagnosis of rheumatic fever; Jones criteria, 1992 update. *JAMA* 1992; 268:2069–2073.

23. Kaplan EL, Rothermel CD, Johnson DR: Antistreptolysin O and antideoxyribonuclease B titers: normal values for children ages 2 to 12 in the United States. *Pediatrics* 1998; 101:86–88.

24. Veasy LG (editorial): Rheumatic fever—T. Duckett Jones and the rest of the story. *Cardiol Young* 1995; 5:293–301.

25. Massell BF, Narula J: Rheumatic fever and rheumatic carditis. In: Braunwald E (ed): *Essential Atlas of Heart Diseases,* vol II. Philadelphia, Current Medicine, 1997:10.1–10.19.

26. Gibofsky A, Zabriskie JB: Rheumatic fever and post-streptococcal reactive arthritis. *Curr Opin Rheumatol* 1995; 7:299–305.

27. Cervera R, Asherson RA, Font J, et al: Chorea in the antiphospholipid syndrome. *Medicine* 1997; 76:203–212.

28. Homer C, Shulman ST: Clinical aspects of acute rheumatic fever. *J Rheumatol* 1991; 18(suppl 29):2–13.

29. Committee on Infectious Diseases, American Academy of Pediatrics: Group A streptococcal infections. In: 1997 *Red Book Report of the Committee on Infectious Diseases,* 24th ed. Elk Grove Village, IL, American Academy of Pediatrics, 1997:486–494.

30. Bland EF (ed): The way it was. *Circulation* 1987; 6:1190–1195.

31. Marcus RH, Sareli P, Pocock WA, Barlow JB: The spectrum of severe rheumatic mitral valve disease in a developing country. *Ann Intern Med* 1994; 120:177–183.

32. Barlow JB: Aspects of active rheumatic carditis. *Aust N Z J Med* 1992; 22:592–600.

33. Dajani AS: Adherence to physicians' instructions as a factor in managing streptococcal pharyngitis. *Pediatrics* 1996; 97:976–980.

34. Feder HM Jr, Gerber MA, Randolph MF, et al: Once-daily therapy for streptococcal pharyngitis with amoxicillin. *Pediatrics* 1999; 103:47–51.

35. Markowitz M, Fue H-C: Allergic reactions in rheumatic fever patients on long-term benzathine penicillin G: the role of skin testing for penicillin allergy. *Pediatrics* 1996; 97(suppl):981–983.

STEVEN V. MANOUKIAN

CHAPTER

# CONSTRICTIVE PERICARDITIS

# 39

Constrictive pericarditis is a fibrotic disease of the pericardium which results in encasement of the heart and impaired diastolic ventricular filling. Though the disease has been known for centuries, Churchill's description in 1929 is one of the most vivid and enlightening. He noted that "in these cases of *concretio pericardii* the heart becomes so throttled by the unyielding wall of scar tissue that its chambers can no longer expand in diastole to receive the inflowing blood."[1] The impairment in diastolic filling is therefore due not to a myocardial abnormality, but to cardiac compression from pericardial scarring and loss of pericardial compliance, which imprisons the heart in "stone." Both the primary care physician and the cardiologist will have difficulty in diagnosing constriction by clinical evaluation alone. This is in part due to the overlap among constrictive pericarditis, restrictive cardiomyopathy, and cardiac tamponade. Echocardiography and cardiac catheterization are needed in the majority of patients. In occasional cases, definitive diagnosis may require pericardial biopsy, endomyocardial biopsy, and/or pericardiocentesis. Though medical therapy may help patients with mild symptoms, surgical pericardiectomy is usually performed for significant symptomatology. Relief of symptoms is achieved in the majority of patients, the surgical risk is acceptable, and the long-term outlook is good.

## HISTORY OF CONSTRICTIVE PERICARDITIS

The history of constrictive pericarditis has been summarized in detail in recent reviews by Fowler[2] and Brockington et al[3] and will be reported here in brief. Descriptions of diseases of the pericardium date back two thousand years to Galen, who described a pericardial tumor in a monkey. Serofibrinous pericarditis was described by Avenzoar (1113–1162), and constrictive pericarditis was reported by Lower in 1669. Important descriptions of physical findings include those of the pericardial knock by Corrigan in 1842; the paradoxical pulse by Kussmaul in 1873; and the syndrome of ascites, hepatomegaly, and constrictive pericarditis (Pick's disease) in 1896. Cardiac decortication was pioneered by Weill, in 1895; Delorme, in 1898; and Churchill, who in 1929 performed the first successful pericardiectomy for constriction in the United States. Surgical series of pericardiectomy include the Emory experience, reported by Miller et al[4] in 1982, and the Mayo Clinic experience,[5] reported in 1990. Hemodynamic findings include elevated right atrial pressure and elevated right ventricular diastolic pressure with an early diastolic dip. The utility of Doppler echocardiography for the accurate diagnosis of pericardial constriction and differentiation from restrictive cardiomyopathy has been reported by Hatle et al[6] in 1989 and by Oh et al[7] in 1994. Evaluation of these two diseases with radionuclide angiography has also been described by Aroney et al[8] in 1989, and evaluation with magnetic resonance imaging was described by Masui et al[9] in 1992.

# ETIOLOGY

As the prevalence of the diseases that can cause constrictive pericarditis changes, so too does the etiologic spectrum of this disease. In one of the largest surgical series, the Mayo Clinic[5] described 313 patients who underwent pericardiectomy for pericardial constriction since 1936. In this series, the cause was unknown in 83 percent, tuberculosis in 6 percent, postirradiation in 5 percent, postsurgical in 4 percent, and "other" in 4 percent. Another surgical series of 95 patients from Stanford[10] compared the etiologies of the disease before and after the year 1980. It was found that although idiopathic and postirradiation continued to be leading causes of pericardial constriction, previously common causes such as tuberculosis had declined. This study also found that the percentage of cases of pericardial constriction following heart surgery increased after 1980. In a series of postsurgical constrictions, Killian et al[11] reported that patients presented an average of 2 years following open-heart surgery. The etiologies in four large series are summarized in Table 39-1. In addition, the reader is referred to the excellent text on the pericardium by Spodick[12] for an exhaustive etiological list. "Eccentric" cases are always interesting and include case reports of self-mutilation with sewing needles[13] and ingestion of a toothpick.[14]

# PATHOPHYSIOLOGY

The normal pericardium is a thin and somewhat inelastic sac that has significant mechanical and membranous functions.[12] Despite its relative noncompliance, under normal circumstances the pericardium does not have a major direct effect on the size and pressures of the cardiac chambers. During cardiac stresses such as volume and/or pressure overload, acute cardiac dilatation, and valvular regurgitation, the normal pericardium exerts a greater effect in order to maintain cardiac size, shape, and efficiency. In constriction, the relatively passive but inelastic pericardium becomes a rigid shell of fibrotic and usually thickened pericardium. The primary abnormality in constrictive pericarditis is impaired right and left ventricular diastolic

TABLE 39-1.   Etiology of Constrictive Pericarditis

| | Emory[4] 26 Patients, 1974–1980 | Johns Hopkins[15] 36 Patients, 1980–1989 | Mayo[5] 313 Patients, 1936–1990 | Stanford[10] 95 Patients, 1970–1985 |
|---|---|---|---|---|
| Idiopathic | 8% | 47% | 83% | 42% |
| Postsurgical | 73% | 22% | 2% | 11% |
| Tuberculosis | 8% | 6% | 6% | |
| Postirradiation | 0% | 11% | 5% | 31% |
| Neoplastic | 0% | 3% | | 3% |
| Infectious | 0% | | | 6% |
| Other | 12% | 11% | 4% | 7% |

filling as a result of a reduction in the distensibility of the pericardium. Systolic ventricular function is usually unaffected to a significant degree. When the heart fills in diastole and reaches the unyielding pericardium, further filling is abruptly halted, resulting in the characteristic "pericardial knock." In terms of the cardiac cycle, the greatest reduction is in late diastolic filling, but characteristic changes in early diastole also occur. Impaired cardiac filling is not unique to this disease, and there is significant overlap in the physical and diagnostic findings with restrictive cardiomyopathy, cardiac tamponade, and other disorders. Restrictive cardiomyopathy is a heart muscle disease that impairs diastolic ventricular filling.[16] Systolic ventricular function is usually normal. Cardiac tamponade is a disease in which the pericardial contents (usually effusion) impair the filling of all cardiac chambers. Though the unifying aspect of these diseases is impaired cardiac filling, the cause is the abnormal myocardium in restriction and the effusion in tamponade, rather than the pericardium as in constriction.

# CLINICAL FEATURES

## History

A valuable clue to the diagnosis of constrictive pericarditis is a previous history of pericarditis or a potential cause of constriction (e.g., radiation, tuberculosis, or open-heart surgery). Since the majority of cases are idiopathic, even the best obtained history may be negative. There is variability in the time from the initial pericardial injury to presentation with constriction, which is divided into acute, subacute, and chronic forms. Acute constriction occurs at the end of an episode of acute pericarditis and is often associated with a pericardial effusion or overt cardiac tamponade. Subacute constriction is the most common form, occurring 3 to 12 months after pericardial injury. Chronic constriction occurs later and is associated with more pericardial fibrosis and less inflammation. Symptoms are variable with regard to severity and may relate to the degree of constriction. Since there is impaired ventricular filling, the disease may resemble heart failure, particularly right heart failure. Similarly, the symptoms may suggest the diagnosis of hepatic failure or other noncardiac diseases. Common symptoms include peripheral edema, abdominal swelling and pain, and fatigue. These are in part due to reduction in venous return to the right heart. Chest pain may occur but is not characteristic and is nondiagnostic. Further elevation in filling pressures causes worsening fatigue, dyspnea, orthopnea, and cough. These findings reflect impaired filling of the left heart, with resultant elevation of pulmonary pressures (usually pulmonary artery diastolic and pulmonary capillary wedge pressures).

## Physical Examination

The physical examination mirrors the pathophysiology of the disease and the history. Findings on examination may suggest right and/or left heart failure or liver disease. Vital signs may include fever, mild tachycardia, and normal to low blood pressure. Commonly seen are jugular venous distention, hepatomegaly, splenomegaly, edema, and ascites. Once again, these reflect reduction in return to the right heart. Jugular venous distention is a near-universal finding and should exclude liver disease as a potential diagnosis. Neck veins may show sharp *x* and *y* descents. Cardiac palpation may be negative or may reveal an early diastolic sharp thrust (early diastolic filling). There may be systolic retraction of the apex impulse. Murmurs are not a characteristic finding in constriction. If present, murmurs should raise the possibility of an alternative diagnosis (possibly restrictive cardiomyopathy) or coexistent cardiac disease. A pericardial knock may be present. On the basis of the physical examination, the primary care physician may have clues to the diagnosis of constriction, but the diagnosis will seldom be definitive without additional testing. The other classical findings mentioned below were originally thought to be diagnostic but may actually be somewhat variable.

**PULSUS PARADOXUS.**   Pulsus paradoxus is a variable finding in studies of constriction and occurs in 14 to 84 percent of patients.[2] Pulsus was originally described by Kussmaul as a transient loss of the radial pulse during inspiration despite continued heart sounds. Today it is defined as an exaggerated drop in systolic blood pressure of >10 mmHg with normal inspiration. In the normal heart, inspiration causes a drop in pleural pressure, which is transmitted to the cardiac chambers but does not impair ventricular filling or output. The mechanism of pulsus paradoxus is complex and in part involves the concept of ventricular coupling. Ventricular coupling or interdependence is the inverse relationship between the filling of one ventricle and the filling of the other. In general, as the filling of one ventricle increases, the interventricular septum shifts toward the other ventricle and decreases its filling. This is in part due to the pericardium, which does not allow unrestricted dilation of the chambers. Inspiration causes an increase in right ventricular filling and dilation of the right ventricle, which shifts the interventricular septum toward the left ventricle. This results in impaired left ventricular filling, a fall in left ventricular output, and therefore a drop in blood pressure. This is mild in the normal heart, and pulsus is usually <10 mmHg. Pulsus occurs in tamponade because the pericardial fluid is able to transmit the inspiratory drop in pleural pressure to the cardiac chambers. The effusion under pressure exaggerates this mechanism, and pulsus is usually >10 mmHg. This is a characteristic finding in cardiac tamponade. The variability of pulsus in constriction may be due to the relative inability of the fibrotic, thickened, and scarred pericardium to transmit the changes in pleural pressure to the heart, thus preventing pulsus from manifesting itself. When seen in constriction, it usually is 10 to 15 mmHg.

**KUSSMAUL'S SIGN.**   Kussmaul's sign is paroxysmal inspiratory distention of the neck veins. The normal response to inspiration is increased venous return, due in part to the 3- to 7-mmHg drop in right atrial pressure. The mechanism of Kussmaul's sign in constriction involves the failure of the diseased pericardium to transmit the inspiratory drop in intrathoracic pressure to the heart. This prevents the inspiratory drop in right atrial pressure, restricts the accelerated venous return during inspiration, and results in neck vein distention. This finding is variable in constriction, occurring in only 13 percent of patients in one series. It is nonspecific and may also occur in restrictive cardiomyopathy, right ventricular failure, right ventricular infarction, and other disorders.

**PERICARDIAL KNOCK.**   The pericardial knock is very specific for constrictive pericarditis but is not highly sensitive. It occurs in 5 to 58 percent of patients in various series.[2] This finding heralds the abrupt halt of diastolic ventricular filling by the fibrotic pericardium. It is an early diastolic sound likened to an $S_3$ with a knocking quality that is often palpable. It can be mistaken for the opening snap of mitral or tricuspid stenosis. The pericardial knock tends to occur earlier than other pathologic $S_3$ sounds.

## Chest Radiography

Findings on the radiograph relate more to the sequelae of constriction than to changes in the cardiac chambers themselves. Therefore, the heart (and pericardium) size is usually normal or mildly increased in the absence of other significant cardiac pathology. The pericardium may be thickened, but this does not generally enlarge the silhouette. Pericardial calcification is seen less frequently than formerly. Marked pericardial calcification, when present, does not always imply constriction. Calcification is best seen on the lateral film, especially over the right heart. Chamber enlargement is infrequent but most commonly involves the left atrium. Other findings include dilation of the superior vena cava and azygous vein, pleural effusions, and diaphragmatic irregularities (pleuropericardial adhesions).

## Electrocardiography

The electrocardiogram is usually abnormal, but unfortunately it is not diagnostic of constriction. The rhythm is usually sinus, but atrial arrhythmias including atrial fibrillation may occur. Ventricular arrhythmias may also be noted. Abnormalities of P waves include findings compatible with left and/or right atrial abnormality. The QRS complex may show low voltage as a result of pericardial fibrosis, myocardial atrophy, or pleural effusions. T waves may be low in amplitude, flat, or inverted.

# DIAGNOSTIC TESTING

## Differential Diagnosis

There is a lengthy differential diagnosis in the patient who presents with nonspecific symptoms and signs of constrictive pericarditis. The history may be negative for previous pericarditis or clues to the initial pericardial insult. The patient with fever, fatigue, abdominal swelling and pain, hepatomegaly, splenomegaly, ascites, and edema on examination may require a lengthy differential. When elevated jugular venous pressure, abnormal neck vein waveforms, pulsus paradoxus, Kussmaul's venous sign, or a pericardial knock is found, the differential diagnosis becomes more limited. There are a few notable noncardiac and cardiac diagnoses to be considered in patients with suspected constriction. Noncardiac etiologies often confused with constriction include liver failure/cirrhosis, nephrotic syndrome, venous obstruction syndromes, and ovarian carcinoma. Constriction should be suspected if elevated central venous pressure (neck veins), abnormal diastolic filling (neck vein waveforms, Kussmaul's sign, pulsus paradoxus), or a pericardial knock is found. Cardiac etiologies in the differential diagnosis of constriction include congestive heart failure (CHF) from any cause, restrictive cardiomyopathy, and cardiac tamponade. Even with the best history, physical examination, chest radiograph, and electrocardiogram, the diagnosis may be elusive to the primary care physician or cardiologist. Computed tomography (CT) scanning and/or cardiac MRI may be helpful in imaging the pericardium in selected cases. Nearly all patients will require cardiology consultation and/or testing for what might appear to be congestive heart failure, restrictive cardiomyopathy, or cardiac tamponade. The definitive diagnosis of constriction usually requires echocardiography and cardiac catheterization. Even after such testing, some patients undergo pericardiocentesis or biopsy (pericardial and/or myocardial) because of overlap in the echocardiographic and hemodynamic findings among constrictive pericarditis, restrictive cardiomyopathy, and cardiac tamponade.

## Echocardiography

Echocardiography is arguably the most valuable test in diagnosis of this disease. It is likely to be performed in every patient with heart failure or suspected constriction. Advances in technique (two-dimensional, Doppler, and transesophageal) have simplified the diagnosis.[7,8,17] The detection of constriction is an advanced technique and will usually require an experienced echocardiographer. The major echocardiographic findings in constriction are pericardial thickening, normal right and left ventricular systolic function, and abnormal diastolic flow patterns. Pericardial thickening (usually on two-dimensional echocardiography) may be seen but does not define constriction. Normal systolic function excludes systolic cardiomyopathy as a cause for unexplained heart failure. Doppler findings are the diagnostic component of the echocardiogram in constriction. Though there are several Doppler findings, two have been described by Oh et al for the diagnosis of constriction and its differentiation from restrictive cardiomyopathy.[7] With the use of these criteria, constriction was accurately diagnosed in 88 percent of patients, although restrictive cardiomyopathy was incorrectly suggested in 12 percent. The first criterion is accentuated left ventricular filling, detected by transmitral flow velocity during expiration. Stated differently, this is impaired left ventricular filling with inspiration, caused by the septal shift toward the left ventricle with inspiration. This is in part the mechanism of pulsus paradoxus. The second criterion is augmented diastolic reversal of flow in the hepatic vein with expiration. Again, stated differently, this is impaired venous return to the right heart with expiration, caused by septal shift toward the right ventricle with expiration. These findings will accurately detect constriction in most patients, but a small number will require invasive testing to make the diagnosis.

## Cardiac Catheterization

Cardiac catheterization will usually be performed in cases of suspected or known constriction. Catheterization is useful in detecting or confirming the diagnosis, assessing severity, performing endomyocardial biopsy, and evaluating coronary anatomy prior to surgery. The findings are hemodynamic, and therefore right and left heart catheterization is required. Even with many of the characteristic hemodynamics, differentiation of constriction from restrictive cardiomyopathy may require endomyocardial biopsy.[18] Like the echocardiographic findings, the hemodynamic findings in constriction are an extension of the pathophysiology. Right atrial pressure is elevated, rises with inspiration, and has prominent $x$ and $y$ descents. These findings correlate with neck vein distention, Kussmaul's sign, and abnormal neck vein waves seen on physical examination (respectively). Right ventricular diastolic pressure is elevated, generally to the same degree as right atrial pressure. Right ventricular systolic pressure is usually normal to mildly elevated (generally 30 to 45 mmHg), and since right ventricular diastolic pressure is elevated, the ratio of right ventricular diastolic to right ventricular systolic pressure is usually >1:3. By contrast, in restrictive cardiomyopathy, right ventricular systolic pressure is usually >45 mmHg and the ratio of right ventricular diastolic to right ventricular systolic pressure is usually <1:3. Left ventricular diastolic pressure is elevated. In both constriction and restriction, the characteristic "dip and plateau" or "square root sign" will be noted in the right and left ventricular diastolic pressure tracings. This reflects rapid early diastolic filling followed by an abrupt cessation of flow as a result of the constricting pericardium or restrictive myocardium. In general, constriction has a more abrupt cessation than restriction, and therefore the "dip and plateau" may be sharper in the former. In constriction, right and left ventricular diastolic pressures are equal; however, in restriction, right ventricular diastolic pressure is less than left ventricular diastolic pressure because of the more severe restrictive involvement of the left ventricular myocardium than of the right ventricular myocardium.

## TREATMENT

Once constriction is diagnosed, medical management with diuretics and/or anti-inflammatory drugs has only a limited role in mild constriction, patients who cannot undergo surgery, or cases with an inflammatory component. Definitive treatment is surgical pericardiectomy, which is best performed early in the disease. Since there is a calcified, fibrotic, thickened pericardial shell adherent to the myocardium, the procedure involves intense dissection and stripping. Pericardiectomy has been likened to peeling an orange and attempting to remove all the rind without tearing the fruit. Even incomplete removal of pericardium may offer clinical benefit. Improvement is immediate in most patients, while in others it may take weeks to months. Surgical series vary in mortality rates and response to the procedure.[11,15,19,20] Mortality rates range from 0 to 11 percent, and clinical improvement is seen in 76 to 100 percent. Most patients have resolution of New York Heart Association symptoms. Long-term survival following surgery is high, but is in part related to the underlying process, especially if coexistent coronary, valvular, or myocardial disease exists.

## SUMMARY

Constrictive pericarditis is a disease resulting in a fibrotic and scarred pericardium that is often thickened and calcified.[21] Most cases are idiopathic, although common causes are postsurgical, postirradiation, and tuberculosis. The history may be unrevealing or may include previous pericarditis or pericardial injury. Symptoms may include edema, abdominal swelling and pain, fatigue, chest pain, dyspnea, orthopnea, and cough. The physical examination may confirm the symptoms and also reveal pulsus paradoxus, Kussmaul's sign, and a pericardial knock. Murmurs are uncommon in isolated constriction. The chest x-ray and ECG are nonspecific. Presenting patients may simulate heart failure or liver disease. Most cases require echocardiography to exclude abnormal systolic ventricular function and reveal impaired diastolic flow (filling) patterns, and catheterization to reveal characteristic hemodynamics. Despite testing, some patients' symptoms continue to resemble those of restrictive cardiomyopathy or cardiac tamponade because of the overlap in findings (Table 39-2). Once constriction is diagnosed, the treatment is usually surgical pericardiectomy, which has acceptable mortality and offers good clinical improvement and long-term survival.

**TABLE 39-2.   Differentiation of Constrictive Pericarditis, Restrictive Cardiomyopathy, and Cardiac Tamponade**

|  | Constriction | Restriction | Tamponade |
|---|---|---|---|
| Source of problem | Pericardium | Myocardium | Pericardial effusion |
| Atrial findings |  |  |  |
| RA pressure | Elevated | Elevated | Elevated |
| LA pressure | Elevated | Elevated | Elevated |
| RA waveform shape | "M or W" | "M or W" | No "M or W" |
| Ventricular findings |  |  |  |
| RVd | Elevated | Elevated | Elevated |
| LVd | Elevated | Elevated | Elevated |
| RVd : LVd | RVd = LVd | RVd + 5 <LVd | RVd = LVd |
| RVd : RVs | >1:3 | <1:3 |  |
| Ventricular diastolic waveform shape | "Dip and plateau" | "Dip and plateau" | No "dip and plateau" |
| Other findings |  |  |  |
| Kussmaul's sign | May be present | May be present | Usually absent |
| Pulsus paradoxus | Usually absent | Usually absent | Usually present |

RA = right atrium; LA = left atrium; RVd = right ventricular end-diastolic pressure; LVd = left ventricular end-diastolic pressure; RVs = right ventricular systolic pressure.

## REFERENCES

1. Churchill E: Decortication of the heart (Delorme) for adhesive pericarditis. *Arch Surg* 1929; 19:1457.
2. Fowler NO: Constrictive pericarditis: Its history and current status. *Clin Cardiol* 1995; 18:341–350.
3. Brockington GM, Zebede J, Pandian NG: Constrictive pericarditis. In: Shabetai R (ed): *Diseases of the Pericardium.* Philadelphia, W. B. Saunders, 1990, *Cardiol Clin* 8(4): 645–661.
4. Miller JI, Mansour KA, Hatcher CR: Pericardiectomy: Current indications, concepts, and results in a university center. *Ann Thorac Surg* 1982; 34:40–45.
5. Tuna IC, Danielson GK: Surgical management of pericardial diseases. In: Shabetai R (ed): *Diseases of the Pericardium.* Philadelphia, W. B. Saunders, 1990, *Cardiol Clin* 8(4): 683–696.
6. Hatle LK, Appleton CP, Popp RL: Differentiation of constrictive pericarditis and restrictive cardiomyopathy by Doppler echocardiography. *Circulation* 1989; 79:357–370.
7. Oh JK, Hatle LK, Seward JB, et al: Diagnostic role of Doppler echocardiography in constrictive pericarditis. *J Am Coll Cardiol* 1994; 23:154–162.
8. Aroney CN, Ruddy TD, Dighero H, et al: Differentiation of restrictive cardiomyopathy from pericardial constriction: Assessment of diastolic function by radionuclide angiography. *J Am Coll Cardiol* 1989; 13:1007–1014.

9.  Masui T, Finck S, Higgins CB: Constrictive pericarditis and restrictive cardiomyopathy: Evaluation with MR imaging. *Radiology* 1992; 182:369–373.
10. Cameron J, Oesterle SN, Baldwin JC, Hancock EW: The etiologic spectrum of constrictive pericarditis. *Am Heart J* 1987; 113:354–360.
11. Killian DM, Furiasse JG, Scanlon PJ, et al: Constrictive pericarditis after cardiac surgery. *Am Heart J* 1989; 118:563–568.
12. Spodick DH: *The Pericardium. A Comprehensive Textbook*. New York, Marcel Dekker, 1997.
13. Keogh BE, Oakley CM, Taylor KM: Chronic constrictive pericarditis caused by self-mutilation with sewing needles. *Br Heart J* 1988; 59:77–80.
14. Meyns BP, Faveere BC, Van de Werf FJ, et al: Constrictive pericarditis due to ingestion of a toothpick. *Ann Thorac Surg* 1994; 57:489–490.
15. DeValeria PA, Baumgartner WA, Casale AS, et al: Current indications, risks, and outcome after pericardiectomy. *Ann Thorac Surg* 1991; 52:219–224.
16. Kushwaha SS, Fallon JT, Fuster V: Restrictive cardiomyopathy. *N Engl J Med* 1997; 336:267–276.
17. Klein AL, Cohen GI, Pietrolungo JF, et al: Differentiation of constrictive pericarditis from restrictive cardiomyopathy by Doppler transesophageal echocardiographic measurements of respiratory variations in pulmonary venous flow. *J Am Coll Cardiol* 1993; 22:1935–1943.
18. Schoenfeld MH, Supple EW, Dec GW Jr, et al: Restrictive cardiomyopathy versus constrictive pericarditis: Role of endomyocardial biopsy in avoiding unnecessary thoracotomy. *Circulation* 1987; 75:1012–1017.
19. Seifert FC, Miller DC, Oesterle SN, et al: Surgical treatment of constrictive pericarditis: Analysis of outcome and diagnostic error. *Circulation* 1975; 72(suppl II):II-264–II-273.
20. Trotter MC, Chung KC, Ochsner JL, McFadden PM: Pericardiectomy for pericardial constriction. *Am Surg* 1996; 62:304–307.
21. Shabetai R: Diseases of the pericardium. In: Alexander RW, Schlant RC, Fuster V, et al (eds): *Hurst's The Heart*, 9th ed. New York, McGraw-Hill, 1998; 2169–2203.

JOEL M. FELNER / MICHAEL MOLLOD

CHAPTER

# INFECTIVE ENDOCARDITIS

# 40

Infective endocarditis is a microbial infection of the heart that may affect the heart valves, valve rings, chordae tendineae, intracardiac septal defects, or mural endocardium. The fundamental pathophysiologic features usually include predisposing heart disease, persistent bacteremia, vascular embolic phenomena, and evidence of active endocardial pathology. It can be divided into sub-acute bacterial endocarditis (SBE), an *indolent* illness that evolves over several weeks and is caused by organisms of low virulence, and acute bacterial endocarditis (ABE), a *fulminant* disease that evolves over days, is caused by highly virulent organisms, and has more frequent complications. Infective endocarditis, however, is best categorized by naming the offending organism, e.g., *Streptococcus viridans,* and the heart valve infected. The mitral valve is involved in 28 percent of cases, the aortic valve in up to 35 percent, the tricuspid valve in 6 percent, and the pulmonic valve in less than 1 percent.[1]

Infective endocarditis has "changed" since the initial description by William Osler, when the disease was almost uniformly fatal within 3 months of presentation. These changes are best explained by earlier diagnosis, in large part due to advances in echocardiography, the widespread use of antibiotics, the reduction in the incidence of rheumatic heart disease, the general aging of the population, the rise in the number of acute cases, and differences in the susceptible patient population, i.e., individuals with prosthetic valves and intravenous drug abusers (IVDA). Successful treatment, however, has recently become more difficult because of the emergence of resistant organisms, drug abuse, and the increase in nosocomial endocarditis. The cooperation of the primary care physician, the cardiologist, the microbiologist, and occasionally the cardiac surgeon is instrumental in managing these patients successfully.

## EPIDEMIOLOGY

The estimated incidence of infective endocarditis is 5 to 10 per 100,000, with 0.16 to 5.4 cases per 1000 hospital admissions.[2] The second Natural History Study of Congenital Heart Defects evaluated the risk of endocarditis in over 4000 patients. The overall incidence was 13.5 per 10,000 person-years, indicating that the additional risk for patients with congenital heart defects is at least 35 times greater (Table

TABLE 40-1.   Congenital Heart Disease and Relative Risk of Endocarditis

| Lesion | Incidence per 10,000 Person-Years | Increase over the General Population |
|---|---|---|
| Mitral valve prolapse | 0.5 | |
| Aortic stenosis | | |
|   Mild | 4.5 | |
|   Moderate | 27.1 | 70-fold |
|   Severe | 54.4 | |
| Bicuspid aortic valve | ≤ 4.5 | |
| Ventricular septal defect | | |
|   Unoperated | 18.7 | |
|   Surgical closure | 7.3 | 50-fold |
|   Plus aortic regurgitation | 34.8 | |
| Coarctation of the aorta | 10.0 | |
| Tetralogy of Fallot | 180.0 | |
| Prosthetic valve | ? | 400-fold |
| Pulmonary stenosis | 0.9 | |
| Overall incidence (CHD) | 13.5 | 35-fold |
| General population | 0.4 | |

*Source:* From Gersony WM, Hayes CJ, Driscoll DJ, et al: Bacterial endocarditis in patients with aortic stenosis, pulmonary stenosis or ventricular septal defect. *Circulation* 1993; 87(suppl 1): 121–126, with permission.[3]

40-1). Despite advanced antimicrobial therapy and sophisticated diagnostic modalities, the mortality from endocarditis has remained high.[4]

Patient groups at greatest risk for endocarditis include those with acquired or congenital heart disease, those who abuse intravenous drugs, and the elderly. Almost 70 percent of cases involve elderly individuals, who, because of their impaired immune systems and because of prolonged hospitalizations, are susceptible to nosocomial endocarditis.[5,6] These hospital-acquired cases (approximately 25 percent) frequently follow iatrogenic endocardial damage, e.g., surgery or catheters for monitoring and hyperalimentation. The prognosis for these cases is worse than that for other forms of native valve infection.[7]

# ETIOLOGY

Though a large number of organisms can cause infective endocarditis, streptococci and staphylococci account for 60 to 80 percent of cases of native valve endocarditis, and gram-negative bacilli (*Haemophilus aphrophilus, Actinobacillus actino-*

*mycetemcomitans, Cardiobacterium hominis, Eikenella corrodens,* and *Kingella kingae*—the HACEK organisms) account for 5 to 10 percent. No organisms are cultured in 5 percent of cases. *Streptococcus viridans* is a low-grade pathogen that causes most of the cases of native valve endocarditis, and group D streptococci (e.g., *S. bovis*) account for 20 percent of the streptococcal cases.

*Staphylococcus aureus* is the most common cause of ABE. Coagulase-positive *S. aureus* and coagulase-negative *S. epidermidis* account for 50 to 75 percent of cases of IVDA-associated endocarditis; methicillin resistance is common in both strains. Microorganisms unique to IVDA-associated endocarditis include *Pseudomonas* species, contracted by washing shared needles in contaminated water; *Neisseria sicca*, contracted by licking shared needles; and *Candida parapsilosis*. Although the incidence of right-sided valvular infection is higher among IVDA, infection occurs on left-sided valves in about 50 percent of addicts with endocarditis.

Culture-negative endocarditis, that is, clinical evidence of infective endocarditis with persistently negative blood cultures, can be divided into three categories. In the first category, bacteria that typically cause endocarditis are not detected on blood cultures. The main cause of this is prior antibiotic therapy, but cultures are usually negative no longer than 36 h after hospitalization. Another cause is deposition of bacteria on sterile thrombi in patients with transvenous pacemakers. The second category consists of slow-growing bacteria, including the HACEK group, *Brucella* and *Neisseria* species, and anaerobes as well as mycobacteria, *Nocardia*, and *Bartonella*. The third category is nonbacterial pathogens, such as *Candida albicans, Aspergillus* species, and *Coxiella burnetii* that causes Q fever. Other considerations include noninfectious endocarditis—e.g., nonbacterial thrombotic endocarditis and systemic lupus erythematosus—and masses, e.g., myxoma.

## PATHOGENESIS

Most cases of infective endocarditis develop spontaneously (probably after occult bacteremias), usually in individuals with congenital, degenerative, or postsurgical cardiac abnormalities. Bacteremia occurs whenever a mucosal membrane heavily colonized with bacteria is traumatized. The oral cavity produces the highest risk of bacteremia. Some medical conditions (e.g., colon cancer) and IVDA may result in bacteremia and increase the risk of endocarditis even on normal heart valves. The incidence of bacteremia after various procedures is shown in Table 40-2.

Subacute infective endocarditis usually requires a predisposing intracardiac lesion, usually a damaged vascular endothelium, on which pathogens flourish, since the normal vascular endothelium is relatively resistant to bacterial infection. High-velocity intravascular jets from pressure gradients between two cardiac chambers create turbulent flow that damages the endothelial surface of the heart or great vessel and makes it attractive to microorganisms. This promotes platelet and fibrin deposition on the altered endothelial surface of the lower-pressure chamber (i.e., the atrial side of a mitral valve infection and the ventricular side of an aortic valve infection), forming a nonbacterial thrombotic endocarditis lesion. During conditions

**TABLE 40-2.    Incidence of Bacteremia after Various Procedures**

| Procedure | Percent |
|---|---|
| A.  Dental | |
| Periodontal surgery | 88 |
| Tooth extraction | 60 |
| Tooth brushing | 40 |
| B.  Genitourinary | |
| Prostatectomy: | |
| Infected urine | 60 |
| Sterile urine | 12 |
| C.  Gastroenterologic | |
| Esophageal insertion | 45 |
| Barium enema | 10 |
| Colonoscopy | 5 |
| D.  Respiratory | |
| Nasotracheal suctioning | 16 |
| Rigid bronchoscopy | 15 |
| Endotracheal intubation | < 10 |

*Source:* Adapted and modified from Durack DT: Infective endocarditis. In: Alexander RW, Schlant RC, Fuster V, et al (eds): *Hurst's The Heart,* 9th ed. New York, McGraw-Hill, 1998:2205–2239.[2]

that produce bacteremia, the offending microorganism is deposited into this sterile lesion, resulting in an infected vegetation. After initial bacterial colonization, additional layers of platelets and fibrin coat the vegetation, protecting it from the host's defenses and allowing further growth of the vegetation at a lower metabolic rate. This accounts for the poor antimicrobial efficacy of bacteriostatic agents in patients with endocarditis, since these drugs require active cell multiplication for their effect.

## CLINICAL MANIFESTATIONS

The clinical features of endocarditis depend on the infecting organism, the valve affected, the patient's age and associated medical problems, resultant complications, and the host's immune response. They can be grouped under four headings: (1) *bacteremia,* which results in fever and chills; (2) *local invasion by the pathogen,* which causes leaflet perforation, regurgitation, and heart failure; (3) *emboli,* which produce brain, kidney, and splenic infarctions; and (4) *circulating immune complexes,* which result in blood vessel, skin, and renal damage.

*General symptoms* such as fever, malaise, and anorexia are likely with SBE, whereas shaking chills, high fever, and symptoms suggestive of a rapidly progressing illness are seen with ABE. Fever is present in 80 to 90 percent of cases, but its absence does not rule out endocarditis, since patients over age 70 may be afebrile on initial presentation. Fever may also be blunted by partial antibiotic treatment, renal failure, congestive heart failure, or cerebral hemorrhage, or in the debilitated patient.

*Cardiac murmurs* are present at some stage of the illness in virtually every patient. They are usually regurgitant and are due to preexisting structural heart disease or the destructive effects of the infection. Only in ABE, however, does the murmur quality usually change. It is important to identify clinically significant regurgitant murmurs by *auscultation,* since Doppler echocardiography may identify valvular regurgitation, especially in the elderly, that may not be clinically significant. In addition, endocarditis may occur in patients with aortic stenosis and rarely in mitral stenosis. Murmurs may never be heard, however, in cardiac transplantation patients with infections at the atrial suture line or in immunocompromised patients with infection on the lead of a permanently implanted cardiac pacemaker.

Additional physical findings include *cutaneous manifestations,* e.g., Osler's nodes, Janeway lesions, petechiae, splinter hemorrhages, and digital clubbing; *ophthalmologic manifestations,* e.g., hemorrhages, petechiae, and Roth's spots; *splenomegaly* that is painless, in contrast to splenic infarction or abscess formation; *renal manifestations,* e.g., flank pain and hematuria, the result of embolic renal infarction with subsequent abscess formation, and microscopic hematuria, red blood cell casts, proteinuria, and renal insufficiency secondary to deposition of circulating immune complexes in the glomerular basement membrane; and *neurologic manifestations* secondary to cerebral hemorrhage, embolization, meningitis, or mycotic aneurysm.

# LABORATORY STUDIES

## Blood Cultures

Blood cultures should be drawn in all patients in whom the diagnosis of endocarditis is suspected. Since bacteremia is usually continuous, most cultures are positive when endocarditis is present. The following scheme is recommended for optimal isolation of the causative organism: Collect at least 10 mL of blood in each of three venous cultures drawn 1 h apart on the first day of admission. If the cultures are persistently negative on the second or third day and the diagnosis is in question, draw two additional venous and one arterial culture.

If culture-negative endocarditis is suspected because of prior antibiotic therapy, draw fresh blood and have the laboratory use a culture medium containing an antibiotic-binding resin. Cultures must be kept for 3 weeks to exclude slowly growing organisms. Appropriate serologic tests can help identify *Chlamydia, Brucella, Legionella* species, and *Coxiella burnetii.* If cultures continue to be negative and the suspicion of endocarditis is high, (1) check for teichoic acid antibodies, usually found in patients with disseminated staphylococcal disease, (2) obtain bone marrow or urine cultures, (3) discontinue antibiotics if the patient is stable, and repeat blood cultures as soon as fever occurs, (4) search for a valve ring abscess or a noninfectious cause (e.g., atrial myxoma or metastatic tumor), and (5) consider empiric treatment for the most likely organism.[5]

## Routine Tests

A normochromic, normocytic hypoproliferative anemia is often present in ABE, but is expected in SBE. The white blood cell count is frequently elevated in SBE, but may be normal or only slightly elevated in ABE. If the white blood cell count is greater than 15,000 to 20,000, a valve ring or myocardial abscess should be suspected; *Staphylococcus,* rather than *S. viridans,* should also be considered. Urinalysis may reveal microscopic hematuria, red blood cell casts, and proteinuria even in the absence of overt renal involvement.

## Echocardiography

Currently, except for cardiac surgery, two-dimensional echocardiography is the only widely available technique that can visualize a vegetation. It provides information for diagnosis, detection of complications, and assessment of ventricular function. Infective vegetations have been described on each of the four cardiac valves; they must be greater than 1 to 2 mm in diameter to be recognized. They are generally irregular in shape, mildly reflective, and attached to the valve leaflets, and they move chaotically, often in a direction and at a speed different from that of the valve leaflets.

There is substantial controversy as to the meaning of a vegetation when it is detected by echocardiography, since it may be difficult to determine whether the vegetation is from an acute illness or is sterile—i.e., from a healed infection. Neither the presence of a vegetation nor its size is an indication for surgery. A vegetation greater than 10 mm on the mitral valve, however, may be an independent predictor of embolic complications. The absence of a vegetation on transthoracic echocardiography does not rule out endocarditis, since the sensitivity of transthoracic echocardiography is 60 to 65 percent, although its specificity is 95 to 100 percent.[8,9]

Transesophageal echocardiography improves the sensitivity for visualization of vegetations to over 95 percent and should be performed on all patients with suspected endocarditis, since it makes detection of vegetations as small as 1 to 2 mm easier.[10] For example, all vegetations over 10 mm are usually detected by transthoracic echocardiography, but only 69 percent of vegetations 6 to 10 mm and 25 percent of vegetations less than 5 mm are visualized. Even a negative result in a patient with clinically suspected endocarditis is helpful in management, since transesophageal echocardiography virtually excludes the diagnosis if a vegetation is not seen or mandates a repeat study 5 to 7 days later if suspicion persists. The superior image quality of transesophageal echocardiography makes this technique more suitable than transthoracic echocardiography for the evaluation of suspected prosthetic valve endocarditis.[11]

Echocardiography is not indicated in patients whose clinical probability of having endocarditis is low. The threshold for performing echocardiography, however, should be lower in elderly patients who present with fever that has no easily identifiable source. Echocardiography has a low yield in children in the absence of physical findings or persistently positive blood cultures. In those patients with either an intermediate or high clinical probability of endocarditis, transthoracic echocardiography is the diagnostic procedure of choice. If a thorough transthoracic echocardiogram is able to image all four valves and they appear normal, transesophageal echocardiography does not appear to provide an incremental gain. Since transesophageal echocardiography can identify small vegetations and pathologic changes of the cardiac structures better than transthoracic echocardiography, its early use offers the advantage of enabling the institution of therapy prior to serious complications. Serial transesophageal echocardiographic studies during the course of the illness are advisable because they are extremely useful in assessing the extent of valvular damage and complications and may assist in determining the necessity for, and timing of, surgery.

# NATURAL HISTORY

Untreated endocarditis is uniformly fatal. The overall mortality, even with appropriate antibiotics, is high (20 to 30 percent) and approaches 100 percent with certain subgroups.[1,5] Valvular function often continues to deteriorate after endocarditis is cured.

# SPECIAL SUBGROUPS

## Prosthetic Valve Endocarditis

Prosthetic valve endocarditis complicates approximately 3 percent of valve replacements and is associated with a very high mortality rate (up to 70 percent).[11] It is classified into an early type, which occurs within 2 months of valve replacement, and a late type. Infections occur equally on bioprostheses and mechanical prostheses, with no difference in infection rates for aortic and mitral prostheses. The vegetations are difficult to visualize by transthoracic echocardiography because they are obscured by the shadows and artifacts generated by the mechanical parts of the prosthesis, and so transesophageal echocardiography is almost always required for diagnosis. Early prosthetic valve endocarditis is more common, is highly destructive, and has a poor prognosis. It is usually due to *S. epidermidis,* an organism that rarely infects native valves. Late prosthetic valve endocarditis is usually associated with the less virulent organisms, similar to those that cause native valve infection. Complications of prosthetic valve endocarditis include valve ring abscess (40 percent of cases), perivalvular regurgitation, and valve dehiscence.

## Endocarditis in the Adult Patient with Congenital Heart Disease

There is an increasing number of patients with corrected or palliated defects who have survived into adulthood. Approximately 25 to 35 percent of patients with endocarditis have preexisting congenital heart disease, and 5 percent of all patients born with a congenital heart defect will develop endocarditis at some point in their lifetime.[12]

## Endocarditis in Human Immunodeficiency Virus (HIV)–Positive Patients

Endocarditis in this subgroup is usually due to *S. aureus,* acquired by IVDA or as a complication of an indwelling central catheter. It is relatively common in HIV-infected patients who are IVDA, usually involving the tricuspid valve, but not in other HIV-positive individuals, in whom left- and right-sided valves are equally affected. The newly described entity of *Bartonella quintana* endocarditis has mainly been identified in HIV-positive patients and appears to represent a true opportunistic infection from failed cellular immunity.

## Endocarditis in the Pediatric Patient

Diagnosis and management can be more difficult in this age group, especially in infants and very small children with complex congenital heart defects. More than half of the cases follow palliative or corrective surgery for congenital heart defects.[13] Iatrogenic predisposing factors, especially central venous catheters, are commonly associated with endocarditis in children with normal anatomy. The most common pathogen isolated is *S. aureus*. It is associated with a high incidence of central nervous system complications and the need for surgical intervention.

## High-Risk Patients with Endocarditis

Patients with endocarditis who are at highest risk for death or severe complications include the elderly and those with a delayed diagnosis, staphylococcal infections, aortic valve involvement, large vegetations, congestive heart failure, central nervous system or coronary artery emboli, prosthetic valve infection, recurrent episodes, or failed antibiotic therapy.[14] With the improvement in the diagnosis of endocarditis, more patients survive the acute infection and are at risk for recurrent episodes, which carry a higher mortality rate than the initial infection. In the elderly, the prognosis is worse and the mortality is higher, not only because of these patients' advanced age, but also because mistaken or incorrect initial diagnoses are more common. The increased incidence of staphylococcal endocarditis is mainly a result of nosocomial infections and the intravenous use of illicit drugs. Staphylococcal endocarditis has a high mortality rate (40 percent) related to its destructive nature, the high frequency of delayed diagnosis and undiagnosed cases, and frequent and severe complications. The high risk associated with aortic valve endocarditis is related not only to the destruction of valve cusp tissue but to extension of the infection to the aortic ring and subaortic structures. Aortic valve endocarditis is now more frequent than mitral valve endocarditis and clearly has a worse prognosis.[6]

# DIAGNOSIS

*Endocarditis should be suspected in any patient with unexplained fever and evidence of valvular or congenital heart disease.* Investigators from Duke University have pub-

**TABLE 40-3.   Duke Criteria for the Diagnosis of Endocarditis**

---

Diagnosis: 2 major criteria, 1 major plus 3 minor criteria, or 5 minor criteria

Major criteria

 1. *Positive blood cultures:* (*a*) Typical organisms from 2 separate blood cultures; or (*b*) persistently positive cultures separated by 12 h; or (*c*) all of 3 or 3 of 4 positive cultures drawn at least 1 h apart
 2. *Evidence of endocardial involvement:* Echocardiographic confirmation or new valvular regurgitation

Minor criteria

 1. *Predisposing cardiac condition* (e.g., bicuspid aortic valve) or IVDA
 2. *Vascular phenomena:* e.g., arterial emboli, mycotic aneurysm, Janeway lesions
 3. *Fever* ($\geq 38\,^\circ$ C)
 4. *Immunologic phenomena:* e.g., rheumatoid factor, Osler's nodes
 5. *Positive blood cultures which do not meet major criteria*
 6. *Suggestive echocardiogram*

---

*Source:* Adapted from Durack DT, Lukes AS, Bright DK: The Duke Endocarditis Service. New criteria for diagnosis of infective endocarditis: Utilization of specific echocardiographic findings. *Am J Med* 1994; 96:200–209, with permission.[15]

lished major and minor criteria for the definitive diagnosis of endocarditis (Table 40-3). Echocardiographic identification of a vegetation is the cornerstone of diagnosis, especially if there is another focus of infection (e.g., a skin abscess or pneumonia), when a positive blood culture becomes a minor criterion. The value of the Duke approach, which almost doubles the number of definite cases compared with previous criteria, has been confirmed.[16] In a recent study, however, 24 percent of patients with proved endocarditis were misclassified as "possible endocarditis" despite the use of the Duke criteria, especially in cases of culture-negative and Q fever endocarditis.[16a] The differential diagnosis of infective endocarditis should include any cause of bacteremia or septicemia, fever of unknown origin, rheumatic fever, thrombotic noninfective (marantic) endocarditis, atrial myxoma, and any septic embolus.

# COMPLICATIONS

## Congestive Heart Failure

Congestive heart failure is the most common and important complication of endocarditis, occurring in 55 percent of cases. It is usually the result of perforation and destruction of valve leaflets, leading to regurgitation. It occurs more in patients with aortic valve endocarditis (75 percent) than in those with mitral valve (50 percent) or tricuspid valve (19 percent) involvement. It is the most adverse prognostic factor in endocarditis and is the leading cause of death, with an overall mortality of 30 percent. It frequently necessitates surgical intervention.[1,2]

## Systemic Emboli

Systemic emboli, the second most common complication of endocarditis, occur in 12 to 35 percent of cases of SBE and 50 to 60 percent of cases of ABE[15] Cerebral embolism occurs in up to 30 percent of cases. Rates of embolism in coronary, peripheral, and renal arteries are also high. A stroke, myocardial infarction, or cold limb may, therefore, be the first manifestation of endocarditis.

## Miscellaneous

*Mycotic aneurysms* develop in up to 15 percent of patients and usually involve the aortic root, the sinuses of Valsalva, or the cerebral arteries. *Abscess formation* complicates both native and prosthetic valve endocarditis and most often involves the aortic valve. Abscesses often develop during the course of ABE and are found in the majority of patients who die with prosthetic valve endocarditis. Clinically, they are difficult to recognize, but pericarditis or the presence of atrioventricular conduction block is a highly suggestive clue. *Intracardiac fistulae* and *valve aneurysms* are less common complications.[1, 2, 5]

# THERAPY

## Medical

High-dose parenteral antibiotics with bactericidal activity given for 4 to 6 weeks are the mainstay of therapy. Long-term therapy is needed because vegetations are avascular, and the only way antibiotics can eradicate the offending organism is by diffusing into the vegetation from the peripheral blood. In vitro susceptibility assays, including the minimal inhibitory concentration and the minimal bactericidal concentration, facilitate the selection of appropriate antibiotic therapy, whereas the serum bactericidal titer (Schlicter test) is used to monitor treatment. An isolate is considered susceptible when the mean peak serum concentration of the antibiotic being tested exceeds the minimal inhibitory concentration of the organism fourfold. Measurement of the serum bactericidal titer is most useful when treating unusual organisms, when using unconventional regimens, or when treatment is failing.

Treatment guidelines have been created by an ad hoc writing group appointed by the American Heart Association (Table 40-4). These guidelines allow for several new therapeutic regimens: (1) a 2-week inpatient treatment for susceptible streptococcal organisms or tricuspid valve endocarditis with methicillin-sensitive *S. aureus,* (2) outpatient therapy for streptococcal endocarditis, and (3) completion of the final days to weeks of therapy at home for very stable patients.

Antibiotics should be started immediately after appropriate cultures have been taken. Since staphylococcal species account for up to 60 percent of cases, when empiric therapy is necessary, an antibiotic with antistaphylococcal activity should be used. An appropriate regimen for SBE is intravenous ampicillin 2 g every 4 h plus gentamicin 1.5 mg/kg every 8 h; nafcillin 2 g every 4 h should be added for ABE.

## TABLE 40-4.   Recommended Treatment of Infective Endocarditis

| Organism | Primary Regimen | Alternative Regimen |
|---|---|---|
| Penicillin-sensitive streptococci (MIC of < 0.1 $\mu$g/mL) | Penicillin G 4 million u q6h IV × 4 weeks | Ceftriaxone 2 g IV/IM qd × 4 weeks Penicillin allergy: Vancomycin 15 mg/kg IV q12h |
| Penicillin-less-sensitive streptococci (> 0.1 MIC < 1.0 $\mu$g/mL) | Penicillin G 4 million u q4h IV × 4 weeks + Gentamicin 1.0 mg/kg q12h (1st 2 weeks) | Ceftriaxone 2 g IV qd × 4 weeks Penicillin allergy: Vancomycin 15 mg/kg IV q12h |
| Penicillin-resistant (MIC > 1.0 $\mu$g/mL)— enterococci | Penicillin G 18–30 million u/day IV continuously × 4–6 weeks + Gentamicin 1 mg/kg IV q8h × 4–6 weeks | Ampicillin 12 g/day IV continuously + Gentamicin 1 mg/kg IV qd *or* Vancomycin 15 mg/kg IV q12h + Gentamicin (as above) |
| *Staphylococcus aureus* (absence of prosthesis) | Nafcillin 2 g IV q4h × 6 weeks + Gentamicin 1 mg/kg IV q8h × 3–5 days | Cefazolin 2 g IV q8h × 4–6 weeks *or* Vancomycin 15 mg/kg IV q12h |
| Methicillin-resistant | Vancomycin 15 mg/kg IV q12h 4–6 weeks | |
| *Staphylococcus aureus* (presence of prosthesis) Methicillin-sensitive | Nafcillin 2 g IV q4h × 6 weeks + Gentamicin 1 mg/kg IV q8h × 6 weeks | |
| Methicillin-resistant | Vancomycin 15 mg/kg IV q 12h + Gentamicin 1 mg/kg IV q8h × 6 weeks + Rifampin 300 mg PO q8h | |
| HACEK group | Ceftriaxone 2 g IV qd × 4 weeks | Ampicillin 12 g/day IV continuously × 4 weeks + Gentamicin 1 mg/kg IV q12h × 4 weeks |

**TABLE 40-4.   Recommended Treatment of Infective Endocarditis** *(continued)*

| Organism | Primary Regimen | Alternative Regimen |
|---|---|---|
| Fungal species | Amphotericin B<br>1 mg/kg/day IV<br>+/− flucytosine<br>150 mg/kg | |

*Abbreviations:* MIC minimal inhibitory concentration; IV intravenous; IM = intramuscular.

*Source:* Adapted and modified from Durack DT: Infectious endocarditis. In: Alexander RW, Schlant RC, Fuster V, et al (eds): *Hurst's The Heart,* 9th ed. New York, McGraw-Hill, 1998:2205–2239;[2] and Wilson WR, Karchmer AW, Dajani AS, et al: Antibiotic treatment of adults with infective endocarditis due to streptococci, enterococci, staphylococci and HACEK microorganisms. American Heart Association. *JAMA* 1995; 274:1706–1713, with permission.[17]

When culture results become available, modify the antibiotics according to the sensitivity results. Blood cultures should be repeated during therapy to ensure that the cultures have become sterile. After antibiotic therapy is completed, continue drawing blood cultures for 2 weeks to ensure that the blood is sterilized. Persistent bacteremia is an indication for surgery.

Penicillin G sodium remains the antibiotic of choice for susceptible gram-positive organisms. Those organisms that are highly susceptible to penicillin (*S. viridans* and *S. bovis*) can be treated intravenously with a 4-week course. Ceftriaxone may also be used for these penicillin-sensitive organisms.[18] A 2-week regimen with penicillin and an aminoglycoside may be used for uncomplicated cases. Less susceptible strains of *S. viridans* and *S. bovis* require 4 weeks of therapy with penicillin plus gentamicin. The outpatient regimen for patients with strains of streptococci that are highly susceptible to penicillin consists of intravenous ceftriaxone once daily for 4 weeks. The long half-life of ceftriaxone is a major advantage in terms of cost and convenience.

Each of the regimens used to treat highly penicillin-susceptible organisms has advantages. The 2-week regimen may shorten the period of hospitalization, whereas the regimen of penicillin or ceftriaxone alone avoids the use of gentamicin, which is nephrotoxic. Vancomycin is an effective alternative in patients allergic to penicillin, but it must be infused over a period of at least 1 h to reduce the risk of the histamine-release "red man" syndrome. Prolonged use, however, may be complicated by thrombophlebitis, rash, fever, anemia, thrombocytopenia, and ototoxic reactions.

In about 5 to 20 percent of native valve endocarditis and 6 to 7 percent of prosthetic valve endocarditis, enterococci are the causative organisms. Treatment of enterococcal endocarditis is a particularly difficult problem because these organisms are relatively resistant to penicillin, expanded-spectrum penicillins, and vancomycin and uniformly resistant to cephalosporins and standard therapeutic concentrations of aminoglycosides. All strains should be screened to define antimicrobial resistance patterns, and gentamicin and streptomycin must be screened separately.[19] For organisms with high-level resistance to penicillin (minimal inhibitory concentration >

16 μg/mL), vancomycin is the agent of choice for synergistic therapy. For organisms that are definitely resistant to penicillin, combine either ampicillin-sulbactam sodium or vancomycin with an aminoglycoside. If both gentamicin and streptomycin exhibit high-level resistance, prolonged therapy (8 to 12 weeks) with high doses of penicillin or ampicillin is needed, but many of these patients require surgery for cure.[17] Serum levels should be monitored during therapy. In patients allergic to penicillin, choose between risking penicillin or ampicillin treatment and using vancomycin.

Treatment of staphylococcal endocarditis that occurs on native valves differs from that occurring on prosthetic valves. Killing of methicillin-susceptible staphylococci is accelerated by gentamicin added to nafcillin. For selected patients with methicillin-sensitive *S. aureus* endocarditis restricted to the tricuspid valve, 2 weeks of intravenous therapy appears to be adequate. This course is particularly appealing for IVDA patients, since they are difficult to keep in the hospital for prolonged periods and there is difficulty with intravenous access for longer courses. Patients treated for only 2 weeks must be carefully selected; they are appropriate candidates only if there is a clinical and bacteriologic response within 96 h of therapy and no hemodynamic compromise or embolic complications.

A high percentage of coagulase-negative staphylococci and an increasing percentage of coagulase-positive strains are resistant to nafcillin and oxacillin (methicillin-resistant staphylococci). These resistant organisms are particularly common in nosocomial and IVDA-associated endocarditis. Intravenous vancomycin is the best treatment for these patients. Coagulase-negative staphylococci causing prosthetic valve endocarditis are usually methicillin-resistant. The optimal antibiotic regimen is vancomycin combined with rifampin and gentamicin, but surgery is usually necessary for cure.

The HACEK organisms cause 5 to 10 percent of cases of native valve endocarditis. Virtually all strains are resistant to ampicillin, and recommended therapy includes 4 weeks of intravenous ceftriaxone for native valve endocarditis and 6 weeks for prosthetic valve endocarditis.

Once the patient with endocarditis is stable for 4 weeks without evidence of heart failure, it may be possible to complete the final weeks of antibiotic therapy at home. Intravenous access must be obtained with either a peripherally inserted central catheter or short-term peripheral intravenous devices that require site changes every 3 days. Complications of a peripherally inserted central catheter are uncommon, but infection, thrombophlebitis, and thrombosis have occurred. Antibiotics with long half-lives (e.g., vancomycin or ceftriaxone) permit once-daily administration.

The role of anticoagulants in endocarditis is controversial. In native valve endocarditis, heparin is contraindicated except for the immediate treatment of massive pulmonary embolus or during cardiopulmonary bypass. Heparin clearly increases the risk of cerebral hemorrhage, since mycotic aneurysms and hemorrhagic transformation of embolic infarction are common. In patients with mechanical prosthetic valve endocarditis, a retrospective study from the Mayo Clinic strongly supports continuing warfarin therapy.[20] Anticoagulants should be discontinued temporarily if cerebral embolism occurs. Bioprosthetic valve endocarditis should be treated in the same way as native valve endocarditis, with previous antithrombotic therapy continued.

**TABLE 40-5.    Surgery in Patients with Infective Endocarditis**

| Absolute Indications | Relative Indications |
| --- | --- |
| Severe congestive heart failure due to valvular dysfunction | Severe aortic regurgitation, since it results in a poorer rate of recovery |
| Intracardiac fistulae | Prosthetic valve endocarditis |
| Myocardial abscess, especially if accompanied by a conduction abnormality | Staphylococcal endocarditis |
| Persistently positive blood cultures despite several days of antibiotics | The presence of a large ($> 1$ cm) mitral vegetation associated with a single embolic event |
| Recurrent embolic events | |
| Ruptured sinus of Valsalva aneurysm | |
| Fungal infection | |

## Surgical

Valve replacement is required when medical therapy fails to clear the infection or when a serious complication occurs. The indications for surgery are listed in Table 40-5. Optimal timing of surgery is critical and depends on the hemodynamic status of the patient, the evolution and natural history of the infection, and specific problems associated with the type of endocarditis. Indications for surgery are not always clearly defined, and the decision needs to be made by the cardiologist and the cardiovascular surgeon in concert. *Although it is prudent to wait until blood cultures are sterile, surgery should not be delayed in the setting of rapid hemodynamic deterioration.*

# PREVENTION

Prevention of endocarditis is the responsibility of an informed patient with guidance from the primary care physician and dentist. The decision to use antibiotic prophylaxis in a susceptible patient should be based on the risk imposed by the existing cardiac lesion, the risk of the prophylaxis itself, and the type of procedure being performed (Table 40-6). It is estimated that less than 20 percent of cases of endocarditis can be definitely traced to a medical or dental procedure, and there are few scientific data showing that prophylaxis is actually effective in preventing endocarditis. In one retrospective study of 533 patients with prosthetic heart valves who underwent 677 dental or surgical procedures, 6 cases of endocarditis occurred in the 229 patients not receiving antibiotic prophylaxis compared to none in the 304 pa-

**TABLE 40-6.   Procedures Requiring Endocarditis Prophylaxis**

1. Dental procedures that induce gingival or mucosal bleeding

2. Tonsillectomy or adenoidectomy

3. Surgery involving gastrointestinal or upper respiratory mucosa

4. Bronchoscopy with rigid bronchoscope

5. Gallbladder surgery

6. Cystoscopy or urethral catheterization if a urinary infection is present; or urinary tract or prostate surgery

7. Incision and drainage of infected tissue

8. Vaginal hysterectomy or vaginal delivery complicated by infection

*Source:* Adapted and modified with permission from Dajani AS, Taubert KA, Wilson WR, et al: Prevention of bacterial endocarditis: Recommendations by the American Heart Association. *JAMA* 1997; 277:1794–1801. Copyright 1997, American Medical Association.[23]

tients who did.[21] Therefore, approximately 6 percent of cases of endocarditis could have been prevented with prophylaxis. Applying this figure to the United States suggests that prophylaxis could prevent 240 to 280 cases each year.[22] The estimated cost of antibiotic intervention, with only oral penicillin, using projections of the full population at risk, is about $1 million per year of life saved. The potential adverse consequences of prophylactic antibiotics are gastrointestinal distress, interaction with birth control pills and anticoagulants, allergic and anaphylactic reactions, and the development of resistant organisms.

Common procedures in which prophylaxis is usually not required include cardiac catheterization, transesophageal echocardiography, upper endoscopy, and a normal uncomplicated vaginal delivery. Atrial septal defect is one of the few cardiac lesions not requiring prophylaxis, except for the 6 months following closure of the defect. In addition, patients with flow murmurs or short-ejection murmurs are not at risk for infective endocarditis. Antibiotic prophylaxis should be given to all patients with *definite* mitral valve prolapse, whether or not a systolic murmur is audible at the time of examination.

The recommended regimens for endocarditis prophylaxis [23] are listed in Table 40-7. The ideal regimen and the efficacy of the current recommendations may never be known, but since endocarditis is a potentially fatal disease, the prevention of a small number of cases is probably worth the risk of prophylaxis (e.g., anaphylaxis) for all susceptible patients. The best advice to susceptible patients to reduce the risk of endocarditis is to encourage good oral and general body hygiene, seek medical care for any gastrointestinal or genitourinary problems, and correct any dental problems, including tooth extractions, prior to valve replacement. *Most cases of endocarditis that originate in the mouth are due to poor oral hygiene and gingivitis, not to dental procedures.*

**TABLE 40-7.**   Recommended Prophylactic Regimens for Infective Endocarditis

| Procedure | Agent | Administration Route | Administration Time | Adult | Child |
|---|---|---|---|---|---|
| **I. Dental/ oral/URT or esophageal** | | | | | |
|   A.  Standard | Amoxicillin | PO | 1 h before | 2 g | 50 mg/kg |
|   B.  Penicillin allergy | Clindamycin | PO | 1 h before | 600 mg | 20 mg/kg |
| | or | | | | |
| | Cephalexin | PO | 1 h before | 2 g | 50 mg/kg |
| | or | | | | |
| | Azithromycin | PO | 1 h before | 500 mg | 15 mg/kg |
|   C.  Unable to take PO | Ampicillin | IM/IV | ½ h before | 2 g | 50 mg/kg |
|   D.  Penicillin allergy, unable to take PO | Clindamycin | IV | ½ h before | 600 mg | 20 mg/kg |
| **II. Genitourinary/ gastrointestinal** | | | | | |
|   A.  *High risk* | Ampicillin | IM/IV | ½ h before | 2 g | 50 mg/kg |
| | | | 6 h after procedure | 1 g | 25 mg/kg |
| | + | | | | |
| | Gentamicin | IM/IV | ½ h before | 1.5 mg/kg | 1.5 mg/kg |
|     Penicillin allergy | Vancomycin | IV | ½ h before[*] | 1 g | 20 mg/kg |
| | + | | | | |
| | Gentamicin | IM/IV | ½ h before | 1.5 mg/kg | 1.5 mg/kg |
|   B.  *Moderate risk* | Amoxicillin | PO | 1 h before | 2 g | 50 mg/kg |
| | or | | | | |
| | Ampicillin | IM/IV | ½ h before | 2 g | 50 mg/kg |
|     Penicillin allergy | Vancomycin | IV | ½ h before[*] | 1 g | 20 mg/kg |

[*] Given over 1–2 h; complete infusion within 30 min of starting procedure.

URT = upper respiratory tract; PO = by mouth; IM = intramuscular; IV = intravenous.

*Source:* From Dajani AS, Taubert KA, Wilson WR, et al: Prevention of bacterial endocarditis: Recommendations by the American Heart Association. *JAMA* 1997; 277:1794–1801, with permission. Copyright 1997, American Medical Association.[23]

# SUMMARY

Infective endocarditis is a very serious illness with high morbidity and mortality. The classic signs described by Osler are now rarely seen. Improvement in the outcome of endocarditis relies mainly on early diagnosis, identification of high-risk patients, and the widespread use of antimicrobial agents. All patients with suspected endocarditis should have appropriate blood cultures drawn and a two-dimensional echocardiogram performed. If the transthoracic echocardiogram is equivocal, a transesophageal echocardiogram should be done to exclude the diagnosis. Empiric antibiotic therapy should be instituted promptly after cultures have been drawn. Surgical intervention may be life-saving, but should not be regarded as a last resort; if it is indicated, early is better. Prevention is the cornerstone of treatment, with dental hygiene at the forefront. It is critical that the primary care physician educate the patient on the need for prophylaxis. The method of prevention changes every few years, and it is useful to have the American Heart Association send the practitioner the guidelines for prevention that, in turn, can actually be given to the patient. Although cost containment measures should always be considered, diagnosis and therapy often require collaboration of a large group of highly trained workers, including the primary care physician, cardiologist, infectious disease specialist, dentist, microbiologist, and cardiovascular surgeon.

## REFERENCES

1.  Scheld WM, Sande MA: Endocarditis and intravascular infections. In: Mandell GL, Bennett JE, Dolin R (eds): *Principles and Practice of Infectious Diseases,* 4th ed. New York, Churchill Livingstone, 1992:944–964.
2.  Durack DT: Infective endocarditis. In: Alexander RW, Schlant RC, Fuster V, et al (eds): *Hurst's The Heart,* 9th ed. New York, McGraw-Hill, 1998:2205–2239.
3.  Gersony WM, Hayes CJ, Driscoll DJ, et al: Bacterial endocarditis in patients with aortic stenosis, pulmonary stenosis or ventricular septal defect. *Circulation* 1993; 87 (suppl 1):121–126.
4.  Terpenning MS, Buggy BP, Kauffman CA: Infective endocarditis: Clinical features in young and elderly patients. *Am J Med* 1987; 83:626–634.
5.  Weinstein L: Life-threatening complications of infective endocarditis and their management. *Arch Intern Med* 1986; 146:953–957.
6.  Watanakunakorn C, Burkert T: Infective endocarditis at a large community teaching hospital, 1980–1990. A review of 210 episodes. *Medicine* 1993; 72:90–102.
7.  Chen SCA, Dwyer DE, Sorrell TC: A comparison of hospital and community-acquired infective endocarditis. *Am J Cardiol* 1992; 70:1449–1452.
8.  Jaffe WM, Morgan DE, Pearlman AS, Otto CM: Infective endocarditis, 1983–1988. Echocardiographic findings and factors influencing morbidity and mortality. *J Am Coll Cardiol* 1990; 15:1227–1233.
9.  Felner JM, Martin RP: *Echocardiography.* In: Alexander RW, Schlant RC (eds): *Hurst's The Heart,* 8th ed. New York, McGraw-Hill, 1994:375–422.
10. Shively BK, Gurule FT, Roldan CA, Leggett HJ: Diagnostic value of transesophageal compared with transthoracic echocardiography in infective endocarditis. *J Am Coll Cardiol* 1991; 18:391–397.
11. Daniel WG, Mugge A, Groten J, et al: Comparison of transthoracic and transesophageal echocardiography for detection of abnormalities of prosthetic and bioprosthetic valves in the mitral and aortic positions. *Am J Cardiol* 1993; 71:210–215.
12. Freed MD: Infective endocarditis in the adult with congenital heart disease. *Cardiol Clin* 1993; 11:589–602.
13. Saiman L, Prince A, Gersony WM: Pediatric infective endocarditis in the modern era. *J Pediatr* 1993; 122:847–853.

14. Erbel R, Liu F, Ge J, et al: Identification of high-risk subgroups in infective endocarditis and the role of echocardiography. *Eur Heart J* 1995; 16:588–602.

15. Durack DT, Lukes AS, Bright DK: The Duke Endocarditis Service. New criteria for diagnosis of infective endocarditis: Utilization of specific echocardiographic findings. *Am J Med* 1994; 96:200–209.

16. Hoen B, Selton-Suty C, Danchin N, et al: Evaluation of the Duke criteria versus the Beth Israel criteria for the diagnosis of infective endocarditis. *Clin Infect Dis* 1995; 21:905–909.

16a. Habib G, Derumeaux G, Avierinos J, et al: Value and limitations of the Duke criteria for the diagnosis of infective endocarditis. *J Amer Coll Cardiol* 1999; 33:2023–2029.

17. Wilson WR, Karchmer AW, Dajani AS, et al: Antibiotic treatment of adults with infective endocarditis due to streptococci, enterococci, staphylococci and HACEK microorganisms. American Heart Association. *JAMA* 1995; 274:1706–1713.

18. Kaye D: Treatment of infective endocarditis. *Ann Intern Med* 1996; 124:606–608.

19. Eliopoulos GM: Aminoglycoside resistant enterococcal endocarditis. *Med Clin North Am* 1993; 17:117–122.

20. Wilson WR, Geraci JE, Danielson GK, et al: Anticoagulant therapy and central nervous system complications in patients with prosthetic valve endocarditis. *Circulation* 1978; 57:1004–1007.

21. Horskotte D, Rosin H, Friedrichs W, Loogan F: Contribution for choosing the optimal prophylaxis of bacterial endocarditis. *Eur Heart J* 1987; 8(suppl):379–381.

22. Durack DT: Prevention of infective endocarditis. *N Engl J Med* 1995; 332:28.

23. Dajani AS, Taubert KA, Wilson WR, et al: Prevention of bacterial endocarditis: Recommendations by the American Heart Association. *JAMA* 1997; 277:1794–1801.

ROBERT C. SCHLANT

CHAPTER

# 41

# PERIOPERATIVE EVALUATION AND MANAGEMENT OF PATIENTS WITH KNOWN OR SUSPECTED CARDIOVASCULAR DISEASE WHO UNDERGO NONCARDIAC SURGERY

## PATIENTS WITH KNOWN CARDIAC DISEASE

### Coronary Artery Disease

The risk for perioperative cardiac morbidity, which includes myocardial infarction (MI), unstable angina pectoris, congestive heart failure (CHF), serious arrhythmia, or cardiac death, is increased in patients with known coronary artery disease (CAD).

Patients with a documented history of a previous MI have a perioperative risk of about 6 percent of having a recurrent myocardial infarction. This risk is greater in patients who are operated upon less than 3 to 6 months post-MI. The perioperative mortality of a perioperative MI ranges from about 26 to 70 percent, with an average of about 50 percent. Most perioperative MIs occur within the first 4 days, with a peak incidence on the second day. Many patients have little or no cardiac ischemic pain but present with hypotension, arrhythmia, or symptoms of heart failure, and most have ST-segment changes.

Most patients with coronary artery disease should continue their medication regimens up to, during, and following surgery. In some patients, aspirin is discontinued 5 to 7 days prior to surgery in order to lessen blood loss. If such patients are not taking a beta blocker, they should be considered for this unless there is a contraindication.

There are few data to support the intraoperative administration of intravenous nitroglycerin in patients with known or suspected CAD.

## Systemic Arterial Hypertension

Patients whose systemic arterial hypertension is untreated or poorly controlled have an increased incidence of perioperative complications, including myocardial ischemia, arrhythmias, and transient neurologic symptoms. Accordingly, systemic arterial hypertension should be controlled prior to surgery, and the hypertensive medications should be continued up to, during, and following surgery. It should be noted that rebound hypertension and tachycardia can occur following the discontinuation of hypertensive medications, particularly oral clonidine or, occasionally, a beta blocker. Most internists hold diuretic therapy on the day of surgery to avoid decreasing intravascular volume.

## Valvular Heart Disease

Patients with valvular heart disease should have appropriate antibiotic prophylaxis to prevent endocarditis before either surgery likely to be associated with bacteremia or lithotripsy. For patients who are on chronic warfarin (Coumadin) therapy for a prosthetic heart valve or atrial fibrillation, the warfarin should be discontinued 3 to 5 days prior to surgery if they are of average thromboembolic risk; surgery may be performed when the international normalized ratio (INR) is $\leq$ 1.5. In general, reversal of the anticoagulation with vitamin K should be avoided, since it may increase the time needed to reinitiate oral anticoagulants postoperatively. When necessary, 1.0 to 1.5 mg vitamin K may be given subcutaneously the day prior to surgery. If the INR is lower than 2.0 for 5 days or more, intravenous heparin should be initiated together with oral anticoagulant therapy once the patient is able to take medications orally.

In patients who have a high risk of thromboembolism, oral coagulant therapy is discontinued 3 to 5 days prior to surgery on an outpatient basis. The INR is monitored daily, and the patient should be hospitalized and intravenous heparin initiated when the INR is lower than 2.0. The activated partial thromboplastin time should be 2.0 to 2.5 times the control value. The heparin should be discontinued 4 h preoperatively, and the surgery can be performed when the INR is ≤ 1.5. Postoperatively, both heparin and warfarin anticoagulation should be resumed as soon as possible, with the use of heparin maintained until the INR is ≥ 2.0.

Future studies may document the usefulness of low-molecular-weight heparin as perioperative anticoagulation; however, the appropriate randomized trials are not yet available.

Some patients with valvular heart disease are very sensitive to changes in venous return. This includes patients with severe mitral stenosis or aortic stenosis (as well as hypertrophic cardiomyopathy). During surgery that is expected to produce significant changes in intervascular volume, such patients should be monitored by a pulmonary artery balloon catheter at the discretion of the anesthesiologist.

## Congestive Heart Failure

Patients who have a history of MI, cardiac arrhythmias, or diabetes mellitus have an increased risk of postoperative CHF.

Patients who have evidence of heart failure have increased perioperative complications, and uncontrolled heart failure is the strongest predictor of perioperative cardiac morbidity and mortality. Most patients with significant CHF should be treated with triple therapy [diuretic, angiotensin-converting enzyme (ACE) inhibitor, and digoxin] prior to elective surgery. Care should be taken to avoid hypokalemia, hypomagnesemia, excess depletion of blood volume, and excess digoxin.

A more difficult group are the patients who have not been known to have CHF but who are discovered to have moderate or marked cardiomegaly on a chest film and/or significantly decreased left ventricular function by echocardiography. Such patients must be handled individually. In general, diuretics are used only if there is evidence of excess fluid on physical examination or chest film. Digoxin is used only if the left ventricular ejection fraction is less than about 40 percent and if there is enlargement of the heart, an $S_3$ gallop sound, and increased jugular venous pressure. Most patients in this situation, however, can be started on an ACE inhibitor preoperatively. Whenever possible, this should be initiated long enough before surgery to make sure that the ACE inhibitor does not cause excess elevation of the serum creatinine.

## Congenital Heart Disease

Most patients with congenital heart disease should receive antibiotic prophylaxis against endocarditis when undergoing surgery or lithotripsy likely to be associated with bacteremia. Patients with cyanotic heart disease who have a hematocrit greater than 65 percent should be considered for preoperative phlebotomy with replacement of the blood volume; this is usually indicated to lessen the chance of vascular thrombosis and postoperative bleeding.

## Arrhythmia and Conduction Disorders

In general, patients who have a history of a cardiac arrhythmia have an increased incidence of postoperative morbidity and mortality. Appropriate therapy for the arrhythmias is important preoperatively.

Since more than 60 percent of all patients have some form of perioperative arrhythmia, no therapy is usually indicated. Those patients who have very frequent or symptomatic atrial or junctional premature beats preoperatively can be treated with a beta blocker if time permits. Those patients who have known coronary artery disease who have more than about five premature ventricular contractions per minute should be considered for intravenous lidocaine, particularly if the premature ventricular contractions are multifocal or occur in runs. The lidocaine can be made up in a solution of 2 to 3 g in 1 L of 5% glucose in water and administered at a rate of approximately 1 mL/min, continuing during surgery.

Patients who have supraventricular tachyarrhythmia and who have to undergo emergency surgery could be considered for electrocardioversion or rate control with an intravenous beta blocker, diltiazem, or digoxin. Patients who have a history of Stokes-Adams attacks, complete heart block, Mobitz II atrioventricular block, or prolonged sinoatrial pause or block should be considered for a prophylactic temporary right heart pacemaker. A prophylactic pacemaker is not required prior to surgery in patients who have asymptomatic bifascicular block, with or without prolongation of the PR interval. In such patients, however, a pacing catheter should be readily available during surgery. Since the intraoperative use of electrocautery can rarely interfere with the function of a cardiac pacemaker or implantable cardioverter-defibrillator, when such conditions exist, the ground plate and electrosurgical tip should be placed as far away from the pacemaker or implantable cardioverter-defibrillator as possible. Electrosurgery should also be limited to periods of 2 to 3 s if there is any evidence of pacemaker suppression.

## Pulmonary Embolism

Patients at an increased risk of pulmonary embolism should be considered for graduated-pressure compression stockings as well as for prophylactic low-dose heparin (5000 to 10,000 units every 8 to 12 h), preferably beginning 10 to 24 h prior to surgery. Low-molecular-weight heparin or Coumadin should be used for prophylaxis of those having orthopedic surgery such as hip or knee procedures. Low-molecular-weight heparin is also a very promising modality of therapy but has not yet been shown to be cost-effective in most patients. Heparin should be avoided in patients who undergo brain, eye, or spinal cord surgery or spinal anesthesia. Such patients who have a history of previous pulmonary embolism should be started on external graduated-pressure compression stockings for 24 h preoperatively in the absence of contraindications.

## Diabetes Mellitus

There is an increased risk of asymptomatic myocardial ischemia and postoperative heart failure in patients who have diabetes mellitus. A goal of perioperative management should be to maintain the blood sugar in the range of 80 to 180 mg/dL.

# PREOPERATIVE EVALUATION OF PATIENTS WITH KNOWN OR SUSPECTED CARDIAC DISEASE

American College of Cardiology/American Heart Association guidelines for the perioperative cardiovascular evaluation for noncardiac surgery provide a useful algorithm for physicians that emphasizes the clinical markers of disease, the functional status of the patient, considerations of the type of surgery, and the selected use of noninvasive and invasive tests (Fig. 41-1). Table 41-1 lists the clinical predictors of increased perioperative cardiovascular risk, and Table 41-2 lists the cardiac risk of various noncardiac surgical procedures. It is apparent that the greatest risk is found in those patients who have recent unstable coronary ischemic syndromes, advanced or poorly controlled heart failure, or arrhythmias. Predictors of intermediate risk include diabetes mellitus, mild unstable angina pectoris, prior MI, and compensated or prior stable heart failure. These predictors are similar to those previously identified by Goldman and Detsky for cardiac complications in patients undergoing noncardiac surgery. They divide patients into those at major, intermediate, and minor risk of cardiac complications (MI, CHF, or death).

The following questions and steps correspond to the algorithm in Fig. 41-1.

*The initial evaluation asks the following five questions:*
Step 1.   What is the urgency of the noncardiac surgery?
Step 2.   Has the patient undergone coronary revascularization in the past 5 years?
Step 3.   Has the patient had a coronary evaluation in the past 2 years?
Step 4.   Does the patient have an unstable coronary ischemic syndrome or a major clinical predictor of increased risk?
Step 5.   Does the patient have major or intermediate clinical predictors of risk?

*Using the answers to the above five questions, the following determinations can be made:*
Step 6.   Patients without major but with intermediate predictors of clinical risk and with moderate or excellent functional capacity in general can undergo intermediate-risk surgery with little likelihood of perioperative death or MI. On the other hand, patients who have a poor functional ca-

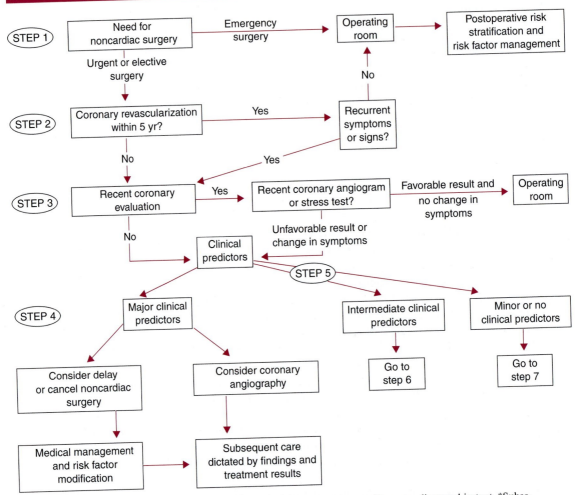

**Figure 41-1**  Stepwise approach to preoperative cardiac assessment. Steps are discussed in text. *Subsequent care may include cancellation or delay of surgery, coronary revascularization followed by noncardiac surgery, or intensified care. [Reproduced with permission from Eagle KA, Brundage BH, Chaitman BR, et al: Guidelines for perioperative cardiovascular evaluation for noncardiac surgery: Report of the American College of Cardiology/American Heart Association Task Force on Practice Guidelines (Committee on Perioperative Cardiovascular Evaluation for Noncardiac Surgery). *J Am Coll Cardiol* 1996; 27:910–948.]

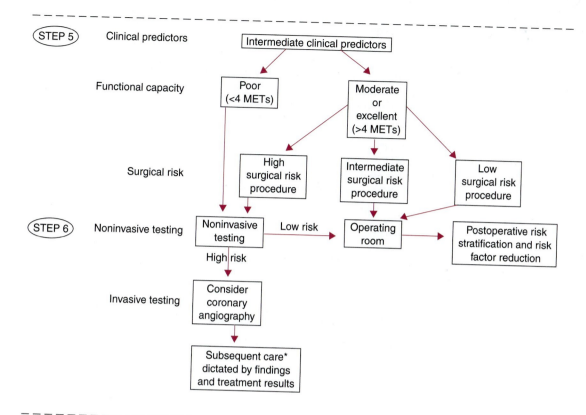

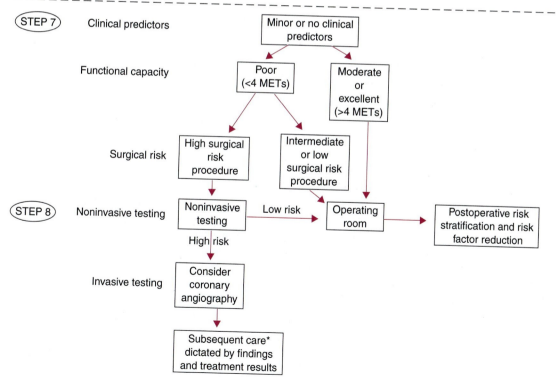

**TABLE 41-1.   Clinical Predictors of Increased Perioperative Cardiovascular Risk (Myocardial Infarction, Congestive Heart Failure, Death)**

### Major

Unstable coronary syndromes
- Recent MI* with evidence of important ischemic risk by clinical symptoms or noninvasive study
- Unstable or severe[†] angina (Canadian Class III or IV)[‡]

Decompensated CHF

Significant arrhythmias
- High-grade atrioventricular block
- Symptomatic ventricular arrhythmias in the presence of underlying heart disease
- Supraventricular arrhythmias with uncontrolled ventricular rate

Severe valvular disease

### Intermediate

Mild angina pectoris (Canadian Class I or II)

Prior MI by history or pathological Q waves

Compensated or prior CHF

Diabetes mellitus

### Minor

Advanced age

Abnormal ECG (left ventricular hypertrophy, left bundle branch block, ST-T abnormalities)

Rhythm other than sinus (e.g., atrial fibrillation)

Low functional capacity (e.g., inability to climb one flight of stairs with a bag of groceries)

History of stroke

Uncontrolled systemic hypertension

CHF = congestive heart failure; ECG = electrocardiogram; MI = myocardial infarction.

* The American College of Cardiology National Database Library defines *recent myocardial infarction* as greater than 7 days but less than or equal to 1 month (30 days).

[†] May include "stable" angina in patients who are unusually sedentary.

[‡] Campeau L: Grading of angina pectoris. *Circulation* 1976; 54:522–523.

*Source:* From Eagle KA, Brundage BH, Chaitman BR, et al: Guidelines for perioperative cardiovascular evaluation for noncardiac surgery: Report of the American College of Cardiology/American Heart Association Task Force on Practice Guidelines (Committee on Perioperative Cardiovascular Evaluation for Noncardiac Surgery). *J Am Coll Cardiol* 1996; 27:910–948, with permission.

**TABLE 41-2.    Cardiac Risk\* Stratification for Noncardiac Surgical Procedures**

| | |
|---|---|
| **High** | (Reported cardiac risk often >5%) |
| | • Emergent major operations, particularly in the elderly |
| | • Aortic and other major vascular |
| | • Peripheral vascular |
| | • Anticipated prolonged surgical procedures associated with large fluid shifts and/or blood loss |
| **Intermediate** | (Reported cardiac risk generally <5%) |
| | • Carotid endarterectomy |
| | • Head and neck |
| | • Intraperitoneal and intrathoracic |
| | • Orthopedic |
| | • Prostate |
| **Low[†]** | (Reported cardiac risk generally <1%) |
| | • Endoscopic procedures |
| | • Superficial procedure |
| | • Cataract |
| | • Breast |

\* Combined incidence of cardiac death and nonfatal myocardial infarction.

[†] Do not generally require further preoperative cardiac testing.

*Source:* From Eagle KA, Brundage BH, Chaitman BR, et al.: Guidelines for perioperative cardiovascular evaluation for noncardiac surgery: Report of the American College of Cardiology/American Heart Association Task Force on Practice Guidelines (Committee on Perioperative Cardiovascular Evaluation for Noncardiac Surgery). *J Am Coll Cardiol* 1996; 27:910–948, with permission.

pacity who are undergoing moderate- or high-risk elective surgery, especially those with two or more intermediate predictors, often need additional testing.

Step 7.    Noncardiac surgery is generally safe for patients who have moderate or excellent functional capacity (four metabolic equivalents or greater) and who have neither major nor intermediate predictors of clinical risk. Patients who have a poor functional capacity but are facing higher-risk operations, especially those with several minor predictors of risk who are to undergo vascular surgery, may require further testing.

Step 8.    Often the results of noninvasive tests can be used to determine perioperative management.

In general, the preoperative risk stratification should include a specific test only if results are likely to influence patient management, i.e., a procedure can and will be done if necessary before proceeding to surgery. Similarly, coronary revascularization before noncardiac surgery to enable the patient to "get through" the noncardiac procedure is appropriate only for a very small subset of patients who are at very high risk. Most patients who have carcinoma and in whom the chance of surgical cure would be significantly decreased by delay and most patients with lower-extremity ischemic pain at rest from peripheral vascular disease do not require testing for coronary artery disease since a delay may be riskier than proceeding directly to surgery.

Most patients who have either unstable angina pectoris or angina pectoris that is refractory to medical therapy or who are considered to be high risk based on the results of noninvasive testing should be considered for coronary arteriography in anticipation of coronary artery bypass grafting or angioplasty, particularly if they are scheduled for elective high-risk noncardiac surgery or have inconclusive noninvasive test results.

In general, the indications for revascularization by surgery or interventional cardiology should be the same as if the patient were not undergoing noncardiac surgery. If coronary angioplasty is performed, noncardiac surgery can usually be performed several days afterwards. Bypass surgery usually requires a longer interval before major surgery. Ideally, patients should be completely recovered from the bypass surgery, approximately 3 months, but, if necessary, urgent surgery could be done after a shorter interval.

# ASSESSMENT OF CARDIAC RISK

## Age

The leading cause of postoperative death in elderly patients undergoing noncardiac surgery is perioperative MI.

## Twelve-Lead Electrocardiogram (ECG)

This should be routinely obtained preoperatively in all patients over 40 years of age and in younger patients who have increased risk factors for cardiovascular disease. The ECG may identify old myocardial infarction or any arrhythmia or conduction system disease. It also serves as a baseline in case of postoperative complications.

## Chest Roentgenogram

A "routine" preoperative chest roentgenogram in patients over the age of 40 is useful primarily as a baseline for comparison with films taken after surgery, when the patient may have pneumonia, atelectasis, or pulmonary embolism. In addition, a chest film may detect unsuspected cardiomegaly, pulmonary congestion, mass, or the presence of a tortuous or calcified aorta.

## Exercise Stress Testing (EST)

The routine use of preoperative exercise stress testing is not cost-effective. On the other hand, as discussed below, it can be very useful in selected patients.

## Radionuclide Scintigraphy (RS)

Radionuclide scintigraphy employing thallium, sestimibi, or both has good sensitivity and good specificity in the identification of patients at increased risk of a perioperative complication. It can be performed utilizing treadmill exercise or the infusion of dipyridamole (Persantine) or adenosine (Adenocard). In general, it has a greater predictive value than either exercise ECG testing or the estimation of left ventricular function at risk by radionuclide angiography. Most studies have found it to be of particular value in patients with stable angina pectoris, a history of MI, or diabetes mellitus.

Either EST or RS is usually performed in patients judged to be at high risk for perioperative need. If the patient is able to exercise, EST remains the preferred method, and if combined with RS it is reasonably predictive of postoperative complications. If the patient is unable to exercise, RS using an infusion or adenosine or dipyridamole can be done.

## Radionuclide Angiography

Unfortunately, the left ventricular ejection fraction measured by radionuclide angiography either at rest or during exercise is a relatively insensitive and nonspecific predictor of perioperative complications. Clinical symptoms and signs are better identifiers of heart failure.

## Ambulatory (Continuous or Holter) Electrocardiography

To date, most studies have found that patients with evidence of myocardial ischemia on ambulatory electrocardiographic (Holter) recordings have an increase in perioperative cardiac events. At present, however, the test has a fairly low specificity and sensitivity at a relatively high cost. Accordingly, it is not recommended as a routine or frequent preoperative noninvasive test. It is likely, however, that it will be employed more frequently in the immediately postoperative period.

## Transthoracic Echocardiography

As a routine preoperative test, transthoracic echocardiography has not been well evaluated and is unlikely to be cost-effective. On the other hand, when combined with the infusion of such agents as dobutamine (Dobutrex), with or without atropine, it may identify wall-motion abnormalities Some experts believe it is as useful as RS in identifying patients with serious coronary artery disease.

## Transesophageal Echocardiography

In selected patients, transesophageal echocardiography can be very useful intraoperatively during cardiac surgery for the detection of myocardial ischemia or myocardial dysfunction. On the other hand, as a routine preoperative test, it is not cost-effective.

## Exercise and Stress Echocardiography

As noted above, exercise and pharmacologic [dobutamine (Dobutrex)] stress echocardiography can be safe and useful methods to identify patients at high or low risk of perioperative complications. Since such tests require a great deal of individual operator skill, the diagnostic accuracy, sensitivity, and specificity of the test should be determined for each institution or laboratory performing the test.

## Coronary Arteriography

A significant number of patients who undergo vascular surgery and older patients who undergo nonvascular surgery have significant CAD that can be detected on routine coronary arteriography. In general, however, the indications for coronary arteriography or revascularization by surgery or interventional cardiology should be the same as if the patient were not undergoing the noncardiac surgery; i.e., these procedures are performed in patients with poorly controlled angina or unstable coronary syndromes. Thus, in a few carefully selected patients scheduled for elective, nonurgent surgery, it may be appropriate to perform coronary arteriography and coronary revascularization by surgery or interventional cardiology before the elective surgery. It should be noted, however, that if the noncardiac surgery is urgent or necessary to prevent the spread of a malignancy or if the patient is not a candidate for coronary artery revascularization for other reasons, the result of coronary arteriography would not change patient management, and the procedure is not justified.

# POSTOPERATIVE PREDICTION OF PERIOPERATIVE CARDIAC MORBIDITY

## Postoperative Ischemia

Postoperatively, ECG evidence of myocardial ischemia in the absence of clinical symptoms is relatively frequent in men. While the majority of such patients do not progress to having ischemic events, those with ECG evidence of ischemia are much more likely to have such an event than those without it. Some patients who progress to an event develop dyspnea and/or chest discomfort, whereas others may have no symptoms and have a silent MI. The major predictors of postoperative myocardial ischemia are a history of CAD, systemic arterial hypertension, diabetes mellitus, the use of digoxin, and a finding of left ventricular hypertrophy on the electrocardiogram.

Postoperatively, most patients with known coronary artery disease or who are at significant risk of having coronary artery disease should probably have postoperative ECG monitoring using at least two leads and daily 12-lead ECGs; for selected high-risk patients, determinations of creatine kinase MB should be done every 8 h for several days following high-risk, major noncardiac surgery.

Postoperatively, patients who develop tachycardia or hypertension are usually best treated with a beta blocker in the absence of contraindications. Supraventricular tachycardia that occurs postoperatively is often related to electrolyte abnormalities, medications, infections, or hypoxia. Most patients who develop atrial fibrillation with a rapid rate postoperatively can be managed with intravenous diltiazem, a short-acting beta blocker, or cardioversion.

## ACKNOWLEDGMENT

The editors wish to thank Michael Lubin, M.D., for reviewing this chapter.

## BIBLIOGRAPHY

Abraham SA, Coles NA, Coley CM, et al: Coronary risk of noncardiac surgery. *Prog Cardiovasc Dis* 1991; 34:205–234.

Coley CM, Eagle KA: Preoperative assessment and perioperative management of cardiac ischemic risk in noncardiac surgery. *Curr Probl Cardiol* 1996; 21:291–382.

Detsky AS, Abrams HB, McLaughlin JR, et al: Predicting cardiac complications in patients undergoing noncardiac surgery. *J Gen Intern Med* 1986; 1:211–219.

Eagle KA, Brundage BH, Chaitman BR, et al: Guidelines for perioperative cardiovascular evaluation for noncardiac surgery: Report of the American College of Cardiology/American Heart Association Task Force on Practice Guidelines (Committee on Perioperative Cardiovascular Evaluation for Noncardiac Surgery). *J Am Coll Cardiol* 1996; 27:910–948, and *Circulation* 1996; 93:1276–1317.

Eagle KA, Rihal CS, Mickel MC, et al: Cardiac risk of non-cardiac surgery: Influence of coronary disease and type of surgery in 3,368 operations. *Circulation* 1997; 96:1882–1887.

Goldman L, Caldera D, Nussbaum SR, et al: Multifactorial index of cardiac risk in noncardiac surgical procedures. *N Engl J Med* 1977; 197:845–850.

Hollenberg M, Mangano DT, Browner WS, et al: Predictors of postoperative myocardial ischemia in patients undergoing noncardiac surgery. *JAMA* 1992; 268:205–209.

Kearon C, Hirsh J: Management of anticoagulation before and after elective surgery. *N Engl J Med* 1997; 336:1506–1511.

Mangano DT, Goldman L: Preoperative assessment of patients with known or suspected coronary disease. *N Engl J Med* 1995; 333:1750–1756.

Massie BM, Mangano DT: Assessment of perioperative risk: Have we put the cart before the horse? (editorial). *J Am Coll Cardiol* 1993; 21:1353–1356.

Schlant RC, Eagle KA: Perioperative evaluation and management of patients with known or suspected cardiovascular disease who undergo noncardiac surgery. In: Alexander RW, Schlant RC, Fuster V, et al (eds): *Hurst's The Heart,* 9th ed. New York, McGraw-Hill, 1998:2243–2255.

Shaw IJ, Eagle KA, Gersh BJ, et al: Meta-analysis of intravenous dipyridamole-thallium-201 imaging (1985 to 1994) and dobutamine echocardiography (1991 to 1994) for risk stratification before vascular surgery. *J Am Coll Cardiol* 1996; 27:787–798.

Tiede DJ, Nishimura RA, Gastineau DA, et al: Modern management of prosthetic valve anticoagulation. *Mayo Clin Proc* 1998; 73:665–680.

BYRON WILLIAMS /
JONATHAN J. MASOR

**CHAPTER**

# PULMONARY EMBOLISM AND DEEP VENOUS THROMBOSIS

# 42

Despite an increase in physicians' understanding of the pathophysiology of pulmonary thromboembolic disease, the diagnosis and treatment of this condition remain an important clinical challenge. Pulmonary embolism (PE) is the third most common acute cardiovascular event, after acute coronary syndrome and stroke.[1] It is estimated that approximately 500,000 pulmonary embolic events occur annually in the United States. The most serious complication of deep venous thrombosis (DVT) or PE is that the condition may be fatal.

A small randomized trial performed in 1960 suggested that the natural course of untreated PE is unfavorable.[2] Approximately 25 percent of patients with PE died, and another 25 percent had recurrent episodes of nonfatal thromboembolism. Among patients presenting with DVT or PE, the rate of fatal PE is 0.4 and 1.5 percent during anticoagulant therapy.[3] However, the case fatality rate is 8.8 and 26.4 percent, respectively, for recurrent DVT or PE during anticoagulant therapy.[3] Overall mortality approaches 10 to 15 percent. Some of these deaths can be accounted for by comorbid conditions, such as malignancy and heart failure. Fortunately, only a small percentage (0.1 to 0.2 percent) of survivors of embolism progress to chronic pulmonary hypertension. DVT and PE are manifestations of the same process, venous thromboembolic disease (VTE). The disorder typically begins with DVT, most commonly in a deep vein in the leg. The large, proximal deep veins, such as the iliofemoral and popliteal systems, manifest the most clinically apparent pulmonary emboli because of the size of the clot, whereas the small pelvic and calf veins, given their size, are seldom sources of large clots. Upper-extremity DVT is becoming more common with the increasing use of central venous catheters. "Paradoxical" arterial embolism (i.e., an embolus entering the arterial circulation via right-to-left intracardiac shunts such as patent foramen ovale) is now increasingly recognized as an important cause of embolic central nervous system events such as stroke and acute limb ischemia.

In addition to being the precursor of pulmonary embolism, DVT is a major cause of morbidity. In a recent series of 355 patients, the incidence of permanent, disabling lower-extremity postphlebitic syndrome (chronic erythema, edema, and pain) has been shown to be present in as many as 30 percent of those with diagnosed DVT. Early thrombolysis in patients with DVT may decrease the late occurrence of postphlebitic syndrome, although there are limited data to support this concept. The syndrome usually develops over many years, and its response to treatment is most often limited. In general, current initial treatments of DVT are often not effective in preventing this severe late complication.[4,5]

## PATHOPHYSIOLOGY

The classic Virchow's triad of vessel trauma, hypercoagulability, and stasis remains an important consideration in the pathophysiology of DVT. Risk factors can be divided into those that are acquired (secondary hypercoagulable states) and those associated with a genetic predisposition or thrombophilia (primary hypercoagulable states) (see Table 42-1).

Genetic predisposition apparently accounts for only 20 percent or so of first-time cases of VTE (see Table 42-1).[6] In patients with recurrent or unexplained VTE, the incidence of genetic abnormalities may approach 50 percent. The modern translation of Virchow's triad focuses on the role of traumatized endothelium and primary hypercoagulable states. The intact venous endothelium is an excellent antithrom-

### TABLE 42-1.    Risk Factors

Acquired (secondary hypercoagulable states)
  Age
  Increased body mass index
  Heavy cigarette smoking
  Hypertension
  Malignancy
  Pregnancy, especially the postpartum state
  Oral contraceptives and hormone replacement therapy
  Surgery and prolonged immobilization
  Hyperosmolar states, diabetes mellitus
  Nephrotic syndrome

Genetic Predisposition (primary hypercoagulable states—thrombophilia)
  Protein C deficiency or resistance to activated protein C
  Protein S deficiency
  Antithrombin III deficiency
  Factor V Leiden mutation
  Antiphospholipid antibodies
  Factor II (prothrombin) gene mutation
  Hyperhomocysteinemia

botic surface. When damaged by trauma, it becomes a potent prothrombic surface. Disrupted endothelium favors platelet adhesion, activation of coagulation factors, and inhibition of fibrinolysis. This contributes to a high VTE rate in orthopedic patients and trauma victims.

The genetic (primary) hypercoagulable states represent an important interface between molecular genetics and clinical epidemiology. The recently discovered factor V Leiden mutation is a single-point mutation in the gene coding for factor V. It results in a factor V that is relatively resistant to activated protein C, an important circulating anticoagulant. Factor V Leiden is associated with a 3- to 7-fold increase in DVT rates in heterozygotes and an 80-fold increase in homozygotes. The mutation (heterozygous and homozygous) is present in 5.27 percent of American Caucasians. The rates are somewhat lower in other ethnic groups in the United States (Hispanics, 2.2 percent; Native Americans, 1.25 percent; African-Americans, 1.23 percent; and Asian-Americans, 0.45 percent). Heterozygotes are much more common than homozygotes.[7,8] Resistance to activated protein C independent of the factor V Leiden mutations is also seen and is associated with an increased risk of VTE.[9] Pregnancy and oral contraceptive use appear to increase the resistance to activated protein C even in the absence of the factor V Leiden mutation.[6,10,11]

The factor II (prothrombin) gene mutation also appears to be a very important primary hypercoagulable state. In this case, another single-gene mutation is significantly more frequent in patients with unexplained or repeated VTE. A recent study shows a prevalence of the gene in 18 percent of those with VTE as compared to 1 percent in a control group.[12] In Caucasians, the carrier status is reported to vary from 0.7 to 4 percent. Heterozygous carriers are found to have a rate of DVT from three to six times that in the general population. Although these patients have elevated prothrombin levels, the exact mechanism of increased venous coagulation is still under investigation.[12,13]

Pulmonary thromboembolism runs the gamut from massive embolism with shock or sudden death to small, clinically silent embolism. In the presence of one or more of Virchow's triad, thrombi form in the deep veins of the lower extremities, upper extremities, or pelvic region. Clots may dislodge and embolize to the pulmonary arteries. This dramatic event often results in hemodynamic and physiologic consequences. First, the pulmonary artery is obstructed and vasoactive substances, such as serotonin, are released by the platelet-rich thrombus. Both pulmonary vascular obstruction and neurohormonal reflexes cause vasoconstriction and elevate the pulmonary pressure. The pulmonary consequences of thromboembolism result from reflex bronchoconstriction in the embolized lung zone, wasted ventilation with resultant increase in alveolar dead space, loss of alveolar surfactant, and changes in lung compliance.

These changes in pulmonary physiology are reflected in alveolar hypoventilation and arterial hypoxemia. In addition, pulmonary arterial pressure suddenly increases, and right ventricular wall tension and pressures rise concomitantly, with resultant right ventricular dilatation and dysfunction (which may be due to right ventricular ischemia). Such pathophysiologic alterations, in the presence of an intracardiac right-to-left shunt via a patent foramen ovale (which may be present in 20 percent of the general population) or atrial septal defect, may further impair arterial oxygen concentration. The potential for paradoxical arterial embolism also is present in the setting of intracardiac shunting; this may confuse or delay the diagnosis of pulmonary embolism. As mentioned previously, DVT and PE are really part of the same pathophysiologic process. In patients documented to have DVT but with no clinical symptoms to suggest pulmonary embolism, more than one-third will demonstrate objective evidence of pulmonary embolism by lung scan.[6,14] Also, not all patients with proven PE will have evidence of DVT by venous ultrasound or by contrast neurography.

## RISK FACTORS

Several studies[3,15–17] demonstrate that age and sex are risk factors for venous thromboembolism. For each decade of life, the incidence doubles. Men consistently seem to have a higher incidence of this problem and a higher fatality rate despite the increased risk seen in females with pregnancy and oral contraceptive use. Older women, especially if they are obese, demonstrate relatively high rates of PE.[18] Hypertension and cigarette smoking tend to add to the risk.

In the recent 25-year population-based study by Silverstein et al[16] that considered the population of Olmstead County, Minnesota, the incidence of VTE rose markedly with increasing age. By the eighth decade of life, the annual incidence of VTE exceeded 1 patient in 1000 per year. The incidence is probably even higher because of the frequent number of undiagnosed cases.[16]

In pregnant females, a leading cause of death remains pulmonary thromboembolism.[19] Oral contraceptives and female hormone replacement therapy appear to increase the risk of venous and pulmonary thromboembolism by at least two- to threefold.[20,21]

Other acquired states result in an increase in the incidence of DVT and/or PE. Numerous studies in the literature have documented that surgical procedures and other medical conditions that result in prolonged immobilization increase an individual's risk for DVT. It is clear that patients with malignancies are at increased risk for VTE. Many procoagulants have been associated with malignant cells, including increased levels of tissue factor.[22] Often, this is in the presence of advanced stages of cancer (often adenocarcinoma) with metastatic disease. The prognosis is frequently very poor with or without PE. Thus, an exhaustive search for occult malignancy in a patient with VTE rarely prolongs life.[23,24] In selected cases, however, when an explanation for the cause of the venous thrombosis is not clear, it may be wise to search for an underlying malignancy.

Detection of asymptomatic DVT in postoperative patients is seen frequently when sensitive diagnostic methods such as ultrasound, impedance plethysmography, radioactively labeled fibrinogen, or even venography are used. Early studies of DVT incidence formed the basis for the generic aggressive prophylactic strategies used in today's surgical patients. In addition, a high incidence of silent DVTs is found in medical patients, particularly when they are very ill or immobilized. Several university hospital autopsy studies show that PE is frequently either responsible for or contributory to hospital deaths. Often, in the majority of cases, PE was not suspected before death. Unfortunately, DVT prophylaxis remains underutilized in most medical centers.[16,25,26]

While the in-hospital risk of VTE cannot be overstated, it is important to note that VTE can also happen days to weeks after the patient has left the acute care setting. Typically, this occurs at 2 weeks postoperatively, but one study showed 15 percent occurring more than 1 month after surgery.[27,28]

Hypercoagulability states associated with deficiencies of protein C or S, antithrombin III, hyperhomocysteinemia, factor II mutation, and factor V Leiden mutation have been recognized in recent years to play an important role in venous thrombosis. The last, factor V Leiden, may be the most common specifically identified cause of venous hypercoagulability. The Physicians' Health Study revealed that the relative risk of DVT was 2.7 times greater if the factor V Leiden mutation was present.[28] Other researchers have documented that resistance to activated protein C and elevated plasma homocysteine levels increase the risk for VTE perhaps two- to threefold. There also appears to be a relationship between elevated homocysteine and the risk for coronary artery disease (see Table 42-1).[6,29–32]

Hyperosmolar syndromes, especially in diabetics, promote hypercoagulability and may frequently cause VTE. Nephrotic syndrome has also been associated with hypercoagulable states. Renal vein thrombosis, which can be seen in nephrotic syndrome, may be a secondary and not a primary or causal event. When antiphospholipid antibodies and lupus anticoagulant are present, there appears to be an increased risk of venous thrombosis, as well as more frequent spontaneous abortions, strokes, and pulmonary hypertension (Table 42-1).[6] In one series, the lupus anticoagulant was found in nearly 10 percent of patients with deep venous thrombosis and in no patients with normal venograms.[33]

In a recent review article, Goldhaber made recommendations for routine laboratory evaluations of patients with DVT or PE.[6] Routine assays for protein C, protein S, and antithrombin III are not recommended. Levels of all three are depressed in the acute VTE state, and treatment with heparin affects antithrombin III levels. Warfarin tends to lower protein C and S levels further. Thus, measurements of these factors during treatment may be confusing. Goldhaber recommended testing routinely for factor V Leiden mutation, hyperhomocysteinemia, and the lupus anticoagulant. In situations of recurrent VTE during adequate treatment, abnormalities of protein C, protein S, or antithrombin III should be considered.[6]

## CLINICAL FINDINGS

Most patients with acute PE present with dyspnea. However, symptoms and signs depend primarily on the size of the embolus and the patient's preexisting cardiopulmonary status. It is helpful to classify patients by clinical syndrome presented (Table 42-2).

Since PE acutely increases pulmonary artery pressures, any coexistent disorder resulting in elevated baseline pressures will increase the clinical impact of a pul-

**TABLE 42-2.   Syndromes of Clinical Presentation of Symptomatic Pulmonary Embolism**

| Characteristics of Embolus | Clinical Syndrome | Prominent Clinical Features |
|---|---|---|
| Massive | Circulatory collapse | Hypotension, acute cor pulmonale, hypoxemia |
| Moderate—central | Acute dyspnea | Variable hypotension, often hypoxemic |
| Moderate—peripheral | Pulmonary infarction | Pleuritic pain prominent, hypoxemia variable |
| Small—peripheral | Variable to none | Variable pleuritic pain, seldom hypoxemic |
| Small—intracardiac shunt (i.e., patent foramen ovale) | Paradoxical embolus | Acute stroke or limb ischemia |

monary embolic event. Examples of this would be preexisting pulmonary hypertension from any cause, especially chronic obstructive pulmonary disease, congestive heart failure, hypoxemia, previous PE, pulmonary resection, or pneumonia.

## Symptoms

If there is a massive PE, systemic arterial hypotension is almost always present. These patients may experience syncope, cyanosis, and occasionally chest discomfort. The presence of unremitting, severe pleuritic chest pain in the presence of PE usually implies pulmonary infarction, however.

Hemoptysis may be caused by pulmonary infarction. Small to moderate pulmonary emboli can have symptoms similar to those of massive PE, but patients are not usually in shock. Other unusual presentations may occur if paradoxical arterial embolism occurs while the thrombus is passing through the right heart. This uncommon event is seen when intracardiac right-to-left shunting occurs via a patent foramen ovale or atrial septal defect. Patients with paradoxical embolism may present with a devastating cerebrovascular accident or an ischemic limb, but almost always suffer from PE as well. The incidence of paradoxical embolism may be surprisingly high in younger patients with unexplained stroke or limb ischemia and should be considered, since chronic anticoagulation could be indicated.[34,35]

Nonthrombotic PE also occurs in certain situations. Air embolism from central venous catheterization is potentially lethal. This can occur after the catheter has been removed if the site of entry remains open to air. These wounds are best covered with antibiotic ointment and pressure bandage to minimize this risk. Fat emboli occur in the setting of major orthopedic trauma or surgery (usually involving pelvic, femur, tibia, or hip fractures). The timing of fat embolism is usually earlier than that of postoperative pulmonary thromboembolism, occurring 2 days after trauma versus 2 weeks for thromboembolism after most surgical procedures. Tumor embolism may occur in the setting of metastatic disease, often due to adenocarcinoma. Many other sources have been reported, including amniotic fluid, talc, hair, arthroplasty cement, and septic tissues (especially in the setting of right-sided endocarditis).

## Physical Examination

The physical examination may not always be helpful, but in patients with massive pulmonary embolism, the triad of elevated neck veins, hypotension, and cyanosis should certainly suggest the diagnosis, especially if symptomatic DVT is also present. Other physical findings to seek include an accentuated second heart sound, left parasternal lift, tachycardia, tachypnea, and a systolic murmur at the lower left sternal border that increases in intensity with inspiration, indicating acute tricuspid regurgitation. A pleural friction rub may be auscultated if pulmonary infarction is present.

## Electrocardiographic Abnormalities

Electrocardiographic findings should be included in the evaluation despite the fact that they are often nonspecific. Sinus tachycardia is probably the most consistent finding. T-wave inversions, especially in leads $V_1$ to $V_4$, are a frequent abnormality, but can be confused with acute anterior ischemia or non-Q myocardial infarction (MI).[36,37] New-onset right bundle branch block or right-axis deviation of the QRS is helpful if present, as is the $S_1, Q_3, T_3$ pattern, but these probably occur in less than 10 percent of cases.[38] (See Fig. 42-1.)

## Chest X-Ray Film

Chest roentgenography is commonly normal or the findings are nonspecific; thus, it is not helpful in the diagnosis. Some degree of atelectasis is often identified in retrospect when the chest x-ray film is reviewed carefully. Abnormal chest film findings that more specifically suggest pulmonary embolism may include focal oligemia (Westermark's sign), a wedge-shaped peripheral density above the diaphragm (Hampton's hump), elevated hemidiaphragm, pleural effusion, or a distended right descending pulmonary artery (Pallo's sign).[6,38,39] The width of the normal right pulmonary artery should be about the same as the width of the tracheal air column. (See Fig. 42-2.)

## Arterial Blood Gases

Arterial blood gases generally demonstrate arterial hypoxemia, increased alveolar-to-arterial oxygen (A-a) gradient, or hypocapnia but are by no means diagnostic. In fact, the absence of hypoxemia does not exclude the diagnosis of PE, especially in healthier patients with normal cardiopulmonary reserve. When present, arterial blood gas abnormalities should heighten one's suspicion of PE.

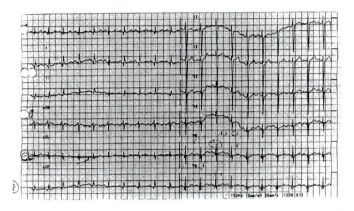

**A**

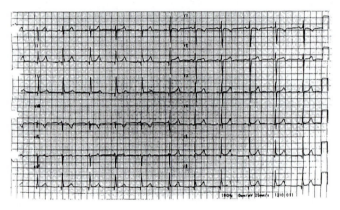

**B**

**Figure 42-1**   *A*. Electrocardiogram of a 45-year-old man who presented to the emergency room with chest pain and dyspnea. Note that tachycardia is the only significant abnormality. *B*. Electrocardiogram recorded the following day on the patient described in *A*. Note the shift in the QRS axis to +110°. The patient died of saddle embolus to the bifurcation of the pulmonary artery. *C*. Electrocardiogram of a 37-year-old man with pulmonary hypertension caused by recurrent pulmonary emboli. The tracing shows right ventricular hypertrophy. *D*. Electrocardiogram recorded on a 75-year-old female with acute pulmonary embolism proven by pulmonary angiography. Note the $S_1$, $Q_3$, and $T_3$ abnormalities. Right ventricular hypertrophy may also be present, suggesting previous emboli to the lungs. *E*. Electrocardiogram of a 70-year-old man who presented with syncope approximately 3 weeks after knee replacement surgery. Note sinus tachycardia and right ventricular conduction delay. The conduction abnormality was not present on a previous electrocardiogram.

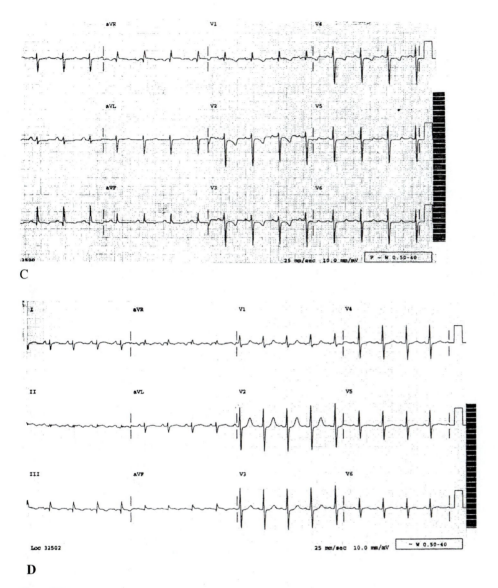

**Figure 42-1** (*Continued*)

## Echocardiography in PE

Echocardiography has evolved into an extremely helpful tool in patients with suspected or proven PE. Retrospective analysis of patients with PE has shown that a finding of significant right ventricular dysfunction correlates with an adverse outcome. This is true even in the presence of normal systemic blood pressure.[40–43] In the presence of severe right ventricular dilation and hypokinesis, patients with PE

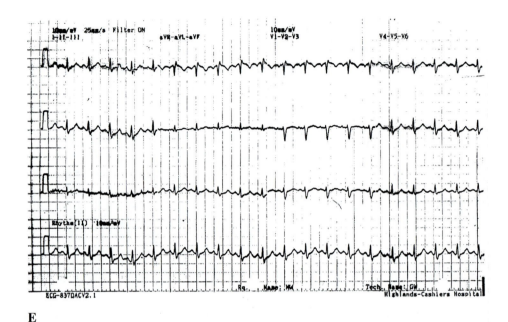

**E**

Figure 42-1   (*Continued*)

should be considered for thrombolytic therapy even in the absence of shock. If right ventricular size and function are normal, and the patient is hemodynamically stable, the prognosis remains good. This type of patient can usually be treated conservatively with intravenous heparin and then warfarin. This relatively low-risk group may be a group that in the future will be treated at home with subcutaneous low-molecular-weight heparin. (See Fig. 42-3.) Direct evidence of pulmonary thromboembolism can occasionally be detected by echocardiography. Case reports in the literature, as well as personal observations, verify that a thrombus in transit or "hung up" in the right ventricle or atrium can be visualized by echocardiography.[44,45]

## DIAGNOSIS

The differential diagnosis of pulmonary thromboembolism is quite extensive (Table 42-3). Accurate diagnosis of this disease entity remains a clinical challenge. It is a diagnosis that is frequently overlooked, especially in the setting of other chronic illnesses. The optimal approach is to suspect the diagnosis and perform a detailed history and physical examination, supplemented by selective testing to confirm or exclude the diagnosis.

Pulmonary thromboembolism can masquerade as many illnesses—pneumonia, MI, anxiety, septic shock, and hypovolemic shock, to name just a few. Once the diagnosis is seriously entertained, then a rapid sequence of events should take place.

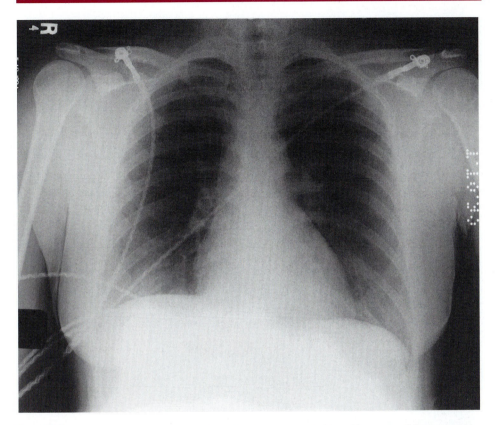

**Figure 42-2**    Chest x-ray from a 36-year-old female who presented with sudden onset of dyspnea and hypotension. The film is unremarkable except for perhaps slight elevation of the right hemidiaphragm.

Initially, a quick but guided history and physical examination should occur, with emphasis on vital signs, neck veins, lung sounds, cardiac examination (searching for right ventricular heave, loud pulmonic component of the second heart sound, sinus tachycardia, and tricuspid regurgitation), tender and enlarged liver, and the extremities (searching for cyanosis, edema, and evidence of thrombophlebitis).

Then, an assessment of arterial blood gases, electrocardiogram, and chest x-ray should be performed. After these initial diagnostic steps are completed, if the diagnosis of PE still remains a strong consideration, then therapy should be initiated unless there are definite contraindications to anticoagulation. Further diagnostic studies should then be done. (See Table 42-4.)

If clinical findings lead to suspicion of pulmonary embolism, then appropriate anticoagulation therapy should be initiated and a perfusion lung scan should be performed. In the presence of a normal lung scan, pulmonary embolism is unlikely. Normal lung scan results are almost never associated with recurrent pulmonary emboli, even if anticoagulation is withheld. In the Prospective Investigation of Pul-

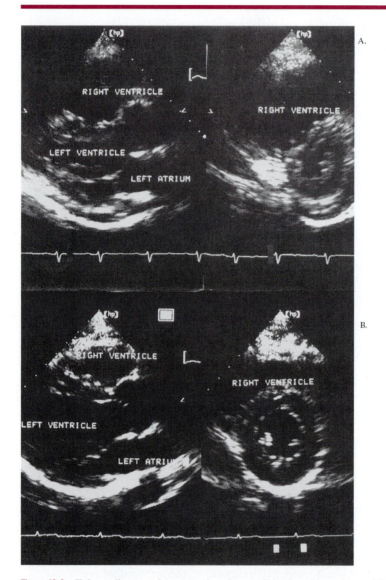

**Figure 42-3**  Echocardiograms demonstrating abnormalities found in patients with pulmonary embolism. *A.* A 35-year-old male presented with dyspnea, chest pain, and shock. Note marked right ventricular dilatation and small left ventricle with flattened or "D"-shaped interventricular septum. *B.* Contrast echocardiogram *A* and *B* in a patient with a small pulmonary embolus with normal systemic blood pressure. The right ventricular size is normal, as are left ventricular size and interventricular septal shape.

**TABLE 42-3.   Differential Diagnosis of Pulmonary Embolism**

* Pneumonia, asthma, or bronchitis

* AMI

* Pleurisy

* CHF

* COPD exacerbation

* Lung cancer

* Anxiety

* Acute pericarditis (with or without tamponade)

* Aortic dissection

* Pneumothorax

* Herpes zoster

* Neuromuscular pain (costochondritis)

* Rib fracture

* Pulmonary hypertension of other etiologies

AMI = acute myocardial infarction; CHF = congestive heart failure; COPD = chronic obstructive pulmonary disease.
*Source:* Modified From Goldhaber SZ: Pulmonary embolism. *N Engl J Med* 1998; 339:93–102, with permission.

monary Embolism Diagnosis (PIOPED) study, high-probability scans identified only 4 out of 10 patients with proven pulmonary embolism. These data indicate that most patients with pulmonary embolism have intermediate- or low-probability lung scans,[46] and only a very small percentage of patients with normal scans had pulmonary emboli. If the lung scan is low to intermediate probability, PE is still possible, however.[47,48] In fact, PIOPED further demonstrated that if the clinical probability of PE is high, angiography detects PE in 66 percent of patients with intermediate- and 40 percent of patients with low-probability ventilation-perfusion lung scans, suggesting that patients with intermediate-probability and especially those with low-probability lung scans cannot be put in the same category as patients with normal lung scans, especially if clinical suspicion is relatively strong. When the lung scan is high probability, PE is very likely. Most patients with PE have intermediate- or low-probability scans, however, and must be further investigated if strong clinical suspicions exist.[46–48] (See Fig. 42-4.)

Venous Doppler ultrasound is an excellent method for detecting clots in symptomatic outpatients with suspected DVT.[49] It can be done quickly and with reliable results. A normal venous ultrasound should not dissuade the physician from the diagnosis if clinical suspicion is moderately high, however, since in many cases the

## TABLE 42-4. Diagnostic Algorithm

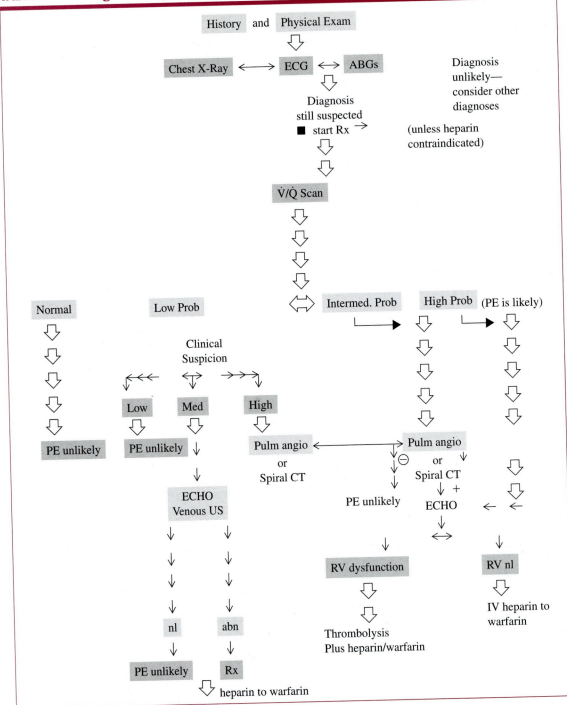

ECG = electrocardiogram; ABG = arterial blood gases; V̇/Q̇ = ventilation-perfusion; PE = pulmonary embolism; CT = computed tomography; ECHO = echocardiography; US = ultrasound; RV = right ventricular; IV = intravenous.

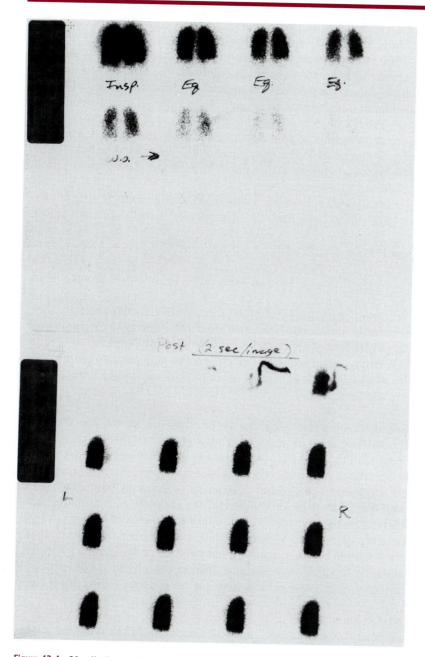

Figure 42-4   Ventilation-perfusion lung scan in a 36-year-old female showing absent perfusion to entire right lung (below) with normal ventilation (above). Read as a high-probability scan for pulmonary emboli.

potentially detectable DVT may have already embolized. In general, venous ultrasound of the lower extremities should be performed in the presence of a normal or low-probability lung scan. If the venous ultrasound is negative, then PE is not likely to be present. But if venous ultrasound is abnormal and confirms venous thrombosis, then the diagnosis of PE is likely, or at least the patient has DVT and anticoagulation should be initiated. The technique is somewhat limited for calf vein DVT. Serial Doppler ultrasonography performed over a 2-week period shows a conversion rate to positive in about 2 percent of patients with DVT as smaller clots propagate proximally up the deep venous system. Negative serial ultrasonography indicates a very low risk of subsequent VTE. The clinician should have a low threshold for performing repeat ultrasound studies, especially if initial results are normal and the symptoms of concern continue or worsen.[50,51]

Selected patients will need pulmonary angiography, usually in the setting of a low- to intermediate-probability lung scan, but a moderate to high clinical suspicion of PE.

General indications for pulmonary arteriography are

- Moderate to high clinical suspicion with low- to intermediate-probability lung scan
- Suspected recurrent pulmonary emboli on therapeutic anticoagulation
- Contraindications to anticoagulation in patients with nondiagnostic noninvasive studies, especially if venous filter placement is being considered
- When there is strong consideration of mechanical or surgical intervention
- Occasionally, when all noninvasive tests point to the diagnosis of PE but the clinical suspicion remains low

Spiral computed tomography (CT) can be used as an alternative diagnostic method to perfusion lung scans or pulmonary angiograms. Spiral CT is best utilized to identify thrombus in the proximal pulmonary vessels. A positive result is quite helpful, and the specificity is high enough to eliminate the need for angiography if a positive CT result is found. Small distal pulmonary emboli may be missed by this method, however. If clinical suspicion remains strong after a negative CT scan, then arteriography should be performed.[52–54] (See Fig. 42-5, spiral CT findings in a patient with pulmonary embolism.) It is important to remember that intravascular contrast agents are used in both CT scanning and pulmonary angiography. Risk versus benefit must be considered when using contrast in patients with a history of allergy to contrast agents or those at high risk for acute renal failure from these agents.

D-Dimer has been found to be a useful adjunct to VTE diagnosis. Elevated levels of D-dimer have been classically associated with disseminated intravascular coagulation. When VTE is present, elevated levels of D-dimer reflect systemic vascular attempts at fibrinolysis of the new clot. For the diagnosis of VTE, D-dimer is an extremely sensitive but not a specific test. A normal D-dimer value has a strong negative predictive value. The lack of specificity of the D-dimer test reflects the ability of many serious medical conditions (bleeding, sepsis, and ischemia) to also pro-

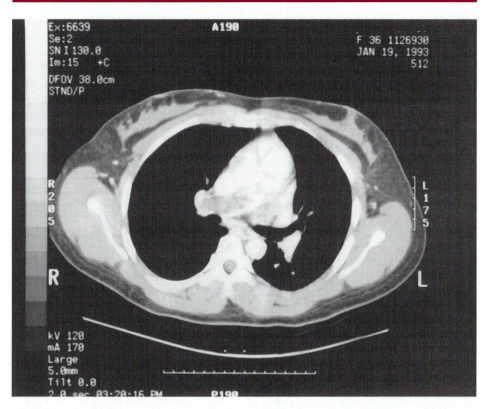

**Figure 42-5** Spiral CT scan demonstrating a large filling defect in the right main pulmonary artery in the same patient whose lung scan is seen in Fig. 42-4 and whose chest x-ray is seen in Fig. 42-2.

mote systemic fibrinolytic activity. In a recent series of 671 patients with pulmonary emboli [using less than 500 $\mu$g/L on the D-dimer enzyme-linked immunosorbent assay (ELISA) test as a normal value], D-dimer was associated with a 99 percent sensitivity for pulmonary emboli but only a 41 percent specificity. Similar studies show comparable findings when D-dimer is used as a diagnostic test in patients with DVT.[55,56] The D-dimer test may have its greatest potential use in the outpatient setting when more traditional tests yield equivocal results. Since a variety of assays now exist (whole blood, ELISA, and latex agglutination), more work on standardization of this test is needed before it can be fully implemented clinically.

Echocardiography, either transthoracic or transesophageal, can occasionally provide direct evidence of pulmonary embolism when the thrombus is identified in transit through the right heart or is visualized in the main pulmonary arteries.[44,45,57] More often, the echocardiographic findings provide indirect evidence of right ventricular dysfunction or other evidence for pulmonary hypertension. In consecutive series concerning PE, approximately 40 percent of patients will demonstrate right ventricular dilatation and/or dysfunction.[6] Just as important, evidence for acute myocardial infarction (AMI), such as new regional wall motion abnormalities, pericardial effusion with tamponade, or aortic dissection can be quickly assessed to aid in the differential diagnosis of many patients. (Note the echocardiograms shown in Fig. 42-3.) One note of caution when using echocardiography to evaluate patients when PE and AMI are being considered: Right ventricular infarction can present with clinical findings similar to those of PE (hypotension, elevated neck veins, dyspnea, chest pain), and if classic electrocardiographic changes seen with an acute inferior or posterior or RV MI are absent, other diagnostic tests (e.g., cardiac isoenzymes, serial ECG changes, cardiac catheterization, pulmonary angiography, etc.) may be needed to make the diagnosis.[58]

# THERAPY FOR PE/DVT

Patients with PE or uncomplicated DVT and no evidence of hemodynamic compromise can, in general, be treated by the primary care physician. More complicated cases, with hypotension and suspected massive pulmonary thromboembolism, should be referred to a tertiary care center for specialists' help with management decisions. A team of physicians including cardiologists, pulmonary disease experts, vascular surgeons, cardiothoracic surgeons, and interventional radiologists should be available if needed.

The gold standard for therapy in DVT and PE is heparin. One should remember that anticoagulation for established PE or DVT is mainly preventive. Heparin therapy prevents propagation of the clot but does not dissolve the thrombus. Heparin accelerates the action of antithrombin III and thereby inhibits thrombin and other clotting factors. This prevents further propagation of the thrombus and allows endogenous fibrinolysis to dissolve the clot. Many clinical studies have shown that heparin reduces the rate of recurrence of PE and the mortality associated with pulmonary thromboembolism. In the absence of contraindication to anticoagulation, patients with proven or moderate to high suspicion for DVT or PE should be given a bolus of unfractionated heparin (usually 5000 to 10,000 units) followed by a continuous weight-based infusion. The recent use of weight-based nomograms has improved the dosing accuracy and safety of intravenous heparin administration.[59] The activated partial thromboplastin time (aPTT) is monitored to assure that the desired therapeutic effect is achieved (usually 60 to 80 s or approximately two times control). If patients appear resistant to heparin, the plasma heparin level rather than the aPTT can be assayed. This approach may avoid unnecessary and potentially dangerous dose escalation.[60] In situations where oral anticoagulation cannot be used, heparin or low-molecular-weight heparin (LMWH) may be used for the duration of treatment. An example of this would be pregnancy, where warfarin is contraindicated and heparin is used for the duration of pregnancy to treat DVT or PE. Recently, studies with LMWH have shown it to be both effective and safe as treatment for patients with pulmonary embolism who are hemodynamically stable.[61,62]

Enoxaparin at a subcutaneous dose of 1 mg/kg every 12 h (with dosage adjustment in renal failure needed) is now FDA approved for the treatment of stable patients with VTE during the transition to oral anticoagulants. One advantage of this drug is that formal monitoring of the aPTT is not needed. Meta-analysis suggests that the use of LMWH is as efficacious as the use of traditional unfractionated heparin and may even be safer with regard to significant adverse bleeding complications, since there is less interaction with platelets.[63]

Oral anticoagulant therapy with warfarin should be started concurrently with heparin in most cases. Warfarin inhibits the synthesis of vitamin K–dependent procoagulants (factors II, VII, IX, and X) as well as proteins C and S. It usually takes 5 to 7 days for most patients to achieve full effectiveness from oral warfarin. Although there are no hard and fast rules, it appears that 5 mg of warfarin daily is the best approach until a therapeutic international normalized ratio (INR) (2.0 to 3.0) is achieved. Maintenance therapy will need to be adjusted up or down to maintain therapeutic anticoagulation; however, the actual maintenance dose varies widely among patients. The duration of oral anticoagulation therapy has to be individualized for each patient. Insufficient data are available to define the optimal duration of treatment for each situation. Recommendations range from 6 weeks to 6 months in incomplete cases. Most experts would agree that 3 months of therapy would be needed for patients whose predisposing risk factors can be eliminated quickly. In patients with persistent or permanent risk factors such as malignancy, protein C or S deficiency, genetic factor abnormalities, antiphospholipid syndrome, recurrent pulmonary embolism after stopping therapy, etc., intensive prolonged and possibly even lifelong treatment with oral anticoagulants will be necessary. This is especially true if the VTE was unexplained by a correctable clinical risk factor (e.g., surgery, pregnancy, or oral contraceptive therapy) or was life-threatening.

The role of thrombolytic therapy for PE and DVT remains somewhat controversial. Clearly, in situations involving shock from massive PE, thrombolysis can be lifesaving. In contrast to thrombolysis for AMI, where the window for the therapeutic efficacy appears to be limited to 6 to 12 h from the onset of symptoms, thrombolysis for acute pulmonary embolus appears to have up to a 14-day window.[64] While thrombolysis is now widely accepted as standard treatment for most AMIs, it remains unclear whether routine thrombolysis for all patients diagnosed with acute PE is appropriate therapy. It has been suggested that in patients with echocardiographic evidence of right ventricular dilatation and dysfunction, thrombolysis should be given in the absence of shock. There appears to be more rapid improvement in right ventricular function and lung perfusion with thrombolytic therapy plus heparin than with heparin alone.[65,66] One must weigh the potential risk of major bleeding complications associated with thrombolysis versus the potential benefits in situations other than cardiogenic shock. If thrombolysis is unsuccessful or contraindicated in patients with life-threatening PE, then an aggressive approach utilizing either transvenous catheter embolectomy or surgical embolectomy should be considered, despite the fact that the operative mortality is high. This group of patients should represent a very small percentage of patients with PE.

Another mechanical approach to the treatment of venous thrombosis and PE that deserves mention is the insertion of inferior vena caval filters. These filters have been demonstrated to be effective in preventing major PE in the acute setting.[67] Vena caval filters are not a permanent solution, however. First, these filters do nothing to influence the underlying condition that resulted in the formation of venous thrombi. Venous collaterals may form around the filters. If these are occluded by thrombus, vena caval thrombosis can result, causing massive leg edema that can be very difficult to control. Recurrent pulmonary emboli may again become possible, since free-floating thrombi again have unimpeded access to the pulmonary circulation. Fortunately, these complications appear to be rare. A randomized controlled trial of patients with DVT comparing inferior vena caval filters plus anticoagulation to anticoagulation alone showed that use of filters did not reduce the late mortality.[68] Having said all of the above, current clinical practice dictates the use of inferior vena caval filters in patients at risk for major PE from venous thrombosis when major contraindications to anticoagulation exist or if recurrent embolism occurs in the setting of established, prolonged therapeutic anticoagulation[6] (Table 42-1).

A final surgical approach for patients with chronic PE and severe pulmonary hypertension should be considered in selected patients: Pulmonary thromboendarterectomy may be successful in improving pulmonary hypertension and right ventricular dysfunction as well as the quality of life.[69]

The major risk of any type of anticoagulant or thrombolytic therapy is bleeding. The true incidence of major bleeding with intravenous heparin is approximately 5 percent, with a death rate of less than 1 percent. The numbers for oral anticoagulation with warfarin are similar, but serious hemorrhage is actually quite rare in patients adequately controlled in the therapeutic range (INR 2.0 to 3.0). The clinician should remember to periodically monitor platelet counts in patients on heparin to screen for heparin-associated thrombocytopenia. This condition is associated with paradoxical arterial ischemia. If thrombocytopenia develops, heparin should be discontinued and the new heparinoid (Danaparoid) should be substituted until the warfarin level is therapeutic. In patients on warfarin, especially patients with abnormalities of the protein C or S systems, very severe skin necrosis can occasionally occur. Adequate anticoagulation with heparins prior to beginning warfarin is helpful in minimizing the occurrence of this severe adverse reaction. Treatment consists of immediately withdrawing warfarin and restarting a heparin. Long-term administration of heparins is indicated in these patients, since warfarin should not be restarted.

## PREVENTION OF PE/DVT

Because of the difficulty in the diagnosis of patients with pulmonary emboli and because treatment failures are not rare, preventive strategies need to be constantly reviewed and placed high on the clinician's priority list. One must identify patients at increased risk and provide appropriate prophylactic therapy (see Table 42-5).

**TABLE 42-5.  Approaches to Prevention of Venous Thrombosis and Pulmonary Embolism**

| Patient Risk Group | Method of Prophylaxis |
|---|---|
| **General surgery** | |
| Low risk—<40 y.o., minor operation, no risk factors | Early ambulation |
| Moderate risk— >40 y.o., major operation | Elastic stockings plus low-dose heparin SQ (5000 u q12h—begin 2 h before surgery) or intermittent pneumatic compression |
| High risk— >40 y.o., major operation, additional risk factors for venous thrombosis or PE | Intermittent pneumatic compression stockings plus Low-dose SQ heparin 2–3 X daily or low-molecular-weight heparin in higher dose |
| Orthopedic surgery | Low-molecular-weight heparin<br>Enoxaparin 40 mg qd SQ<br>Dalteparin 2500 or 5000 u qd SQ |
| Total hip replacement | Warfarin (target INR 2.5)<br>Intermittent pneumatic compression<br>Enoxaparin 30 mg bid SQ<br>Danaparoid 750 u bid SQ |
| Hip fracture surgery | Low-molecular-weight heparin sq or warfarin (target INR 2.0–3.0)<br>Possibly adjuvant use of intermittent pneumatic compression |
| Total knee replacement | Enoxaparin 30 mg bid SQ<br>Ardeparin 50 u/kg bid SQ |
| High-risk patients | IVC filter only if other forms of anticoagulation therapy are not feasible |
| CABG surgery—uncomplicated | Elastic compression stockings ± low-dose heparin bid SQ |
| Thoracic surgery | Elastic compression stockings, intermittent pneumatic compression, and heparin 5000 u tid SQ |
| Neurosurgery (intracranial) | Elastic compression stockings, intermittent pneumatic compression, ± low-dose heparin bid SQ |
| Spinal cord injury with paralysis | Adjusted-dose heparin or low-molecular-weight heparin, or warfarin or the combination of low-dose heparin bid SQ, elastic compression stockings, and intermittent pneumatic compression |
| Trauma—without brain injury | Enoxaparin 30 mg bid SQ as soon as considered safe |
| Pregnancy—prior history DVT or PE | Enoxaparin 40 mg qd SQ or dalteparin 5000 u qd SQ |
| Medical ICU patients—especially with CHF or pulmonary insufficiency or pulmonary infarction | Elastic compression stockings and intermittent pneumatic compression ± low-molecular-weight low-dose heparin bid SQ or heparin |

**TABLE 42-5.  Approaches to Prevention of Venous Thrombosis and Pulmonary Embolism** *(continued)*

| Patient Risk Group | Method of Prophylaxis |
|---|---|
| Long-term central venous catheters | Warfarin (1 mg qd) |
| Ischemic stroke and lower-extremity paralysis | Low-dose heparin or low-molecular-weight heparin<br>IPC with ES may be useful if heparin contraindicated |

y.o. = years old; PE = pulmonary embolism; INR = international normalized ratio; IVC = inferior vena caval; CABG = coronary artery bypass graft; DVT = deep venous thrombosis; ICU = intensive care unit; CHF = congestive heart failure; IPC = intermittent pneumatic compression; ES = elastic compression stockings.

*Source:* Modified from Goldhaber SZ: Pulmonary embolism. *N Engl J Med* 1998; 339:93–102, and Fifth ACCP Consensus Conference on Antithrombotic Therapy: Summary recommendations. *Chest* 1998; 114 (suppl): 439S–769S, with permission.

Detection of a genetic predisposition (primary hypercoagulable state) by laboratory analysis in patients with unexplained or recurrent VTE will allow enhanced prophylactic strategies, at times including lifelong anticoagulation. Mechanical approaches to prevention include such simple maneuvers as early ambulation and the more sophisticated pneumatic compression stockings or vena caval filter insertion. Prophylactic drug therapy has historically been low-dose subcutaneous unfractionated heparin. Currently, several low-molecular-weight heparins (enoxaparin, dalteparin, and ardeparin) and one heparinoid (danaparoid) have received FDA approval for specific prophylactic indications. Oral anticoagulation with warfarin provides an alternative in some preventive strategies. Aspirin alone is not considered adequate prophylactic therapy for PE, although there is some clinical evidence for its minimal efficacy in this setting.[70] Other oral antiplatelet drugs have not been adequately studied in terms of prophylaxis for venous thrombosis. Table 42-5 lists some of the current methods accepted for prophylaxis.

## CONCLUSION

Pulmonary thromboembolism and DVT are still formidable opponents for the practicing clinician. Over the past two decades, however, we have witnessed a remarkable improvement in the understanding of the risk factors, both inherited and acquired, that lead to DVT and PE. In addition, a vast array of diagnostic tools and a therapeutic armamentarium have increased our ability to detect and treat patients with PE. A large body of knowledge has developed to give the clinician better strategies to prevent this potentially life-threatening condition. Despite these advancements, PE remains an elusive diagnosis because of its often nonspecific presentations and variable clinical course. Definitive diagnosis still requires an alert and knowledgeable physician to make the correct clinical decisions that result in good patient outcomes.

## REFERENCES

1. Giuntini C, DiRicco G, Marini C, et al: Pulmonary embolism epidemiology. *Chest* 1995; 107(suppl 1):35–95.

2. Baritt DW, Jordan SC: Anticoagulant drugs in the treatment of pulmonary embolism: a controlled study. *Lancet* 1960; 1:1309–1312.

3. Douketis JD, Kearon C, Bates S, et al: Risk of pulmonary embolism in patients with treated venous thromboembolism. *JAMA* 1998; 279:458–462.

4. Prandoni P, Lensing A, Cogo A, et al: The long-term clinical course of acute deep venous thrombosis. *Ann Intern Med* 1996; 125:1–7.

5. Bergqvist D, Jendteg S, Johansen L, et al: The long-term complications of deep venous thrombosis of the lower extremities: an analysis of a defined patient population in Sweden. *Ann Intern Med* 1997; 126:454–457.

6. Goldhaber SZ: Pulmonary embolism. *N Engl J Med* 1998; 339:93–102.

7. Ridker PM, Miletich JP, Hennekens JE, Buring JE: Ethnic distribution of factor V Leiden in 4047 men and women: implications for venous thromboembolism screening. *JAMA* 1997; 277:1305–1307.

8. Price DT, Ridker PM: Factor V Leiden mutation and the risks for thromboembolic disease: a clinical perspective. *Ann Intern Med* 1997; 127:895–903.

9. Rodeghiero F, Tosetto A: Activated protein C resistance and factor V Leiden mutation are independent risk factors for venous thromboembolism. *Ann Intern Med* 1999; 130:643–650.

10. Ridker PM, Heunekus CH, Lindpaintner K, et al: Mutation in the gene coding for coagulation factor V and risks of myocardial infarction, stroke, and venous thrombosis in apparently healthy men. *N Engl J Med* 1995; 332:912–917.

11. Oliveri O, Friso S, Maugato F, et al: Resistance to activated protein in healthy women taking oral contraceptives. *Br J Haematol* 1995; 91:465–470.

12. Poort SR, Rosendaal FR, Reitsma PH, Bertina RM: A common genetic in the 3'-untranslated region of the prothrombin gene is associated with elevated plasma, prothrombin levels and an increase in venous thrombosis. *Blood* 1996; 88:3698–3703.

13. Bertina RM, Rosendaal FR: Venous thrombosis—the interaction of genes and environment (editorial). *N Engl J Med* 1998; 338:1840–1841.

14. Moser KM, Fedullo PF, Littlejohn JK, Crawford R: Frequent asymptomatic pulmonary embolism in patients with deep venous thrombosis. *JAMA* 1994; 271:223–225.

15. Anderson FA Jr., Wheeler HB, Goldberg RJ, et al: A population based perspective of the hospital incidence and case fatality rates of deep vein thrombosis and pulmonary embolism: the Worcester DVT study. *Arch Intern Med* 1991; 151:933–938.

16. Silverstein MD, Heit JA, Mohr DN, et al: Trends in the incidence of deep vein thrombosis and pulmonary embolism: a 25-year population based study. *Arch Intern Med* 1998; 158:585–593.

17. Siddique RM, Siddique MI, Connors AF, Rimm AA: Thirty day case fatality rates for pulmonary embolism in the elderly. *Arch Intern Med* 1996; 156:2343–2347.

18. Goldhaber SZ, Grodstein F, Stamfer MJ, et al: A prospective study of risk factors for pulmonary embolism in women. *JAMA* 1997; 30:1165–1171.

19. Koonin LM, Ahash HK, Lawson HW, Smith JC: Maternal mortality surveillance: United States 1979–86. *MMWR CDC Surveill Summ* 1991; 40(sj-2):1-B.

20. WHO Collaborative Study of Cardiovascular Disease and Steroid Hormone Contraception: Venous thromboembolic disease and combined oral contraceptive: results of international multicenter case control study. *Lancet* 1995; 346:1575–1582.

21. Vaudenbrouske JP, Helmerborst FM: Risk of venous thrombosis with hormone replacement therapy. *Lancet* 1996; 348:972.

22. Kakkar AK, DeRuvo N, et al: Extrinsic-pathway activation in cancer with high factor VII a and tissue factor. *Lancet* 1995; 346:1004–1005.

23. Norstrom M, Lindblad B, Anderson H, et al: Deep venous thrombosis and occult malignancy: an epidemiological study. *Br Med J* 1994; 308:891–894.

24. Sojenson HT, Mellemkjaer L, Stefenson FH, et al: The risk of diagnosis of cancer after primary deep venous thrombosis or pulmonary embolism. *N Engl J Med* 338:1169–1173.

25. Battle RM, Pathak D, Humble CG, et al: Factors influencing discrepancies between premortem and postmortem diagnoses. *JAMA* 1987; 258:339–344.

26. Linbald B, Sternby NH, Bergqvist D: Incidence of venous thromboembolism verified by necropsy over 30 years. *Br Med J* 1991; 302:709–711.

27. Bergqvist D, Lindbald B: A 30-year survey of pulmonary embolism verified at autopsy: an analysis of 1274 surgical patients. *Br J Surg* 1985; 72:105–108.

28. Stein PD, Henry JW: Prevalence of acute pulmonary embolism among patients in a general hospital and at autopsy. *Chest* 1995; 108:978–981.

29. Hirsch DR, Mikkola KM, Marks PW, et al: Pulmonary embolism and deep venous thrombosis during pregnancy or oral contraceptive use: prevalence of factor V Leiden. *Am Heart J* 1996; 131:1145–1148.

30. Simioni P, Praudoni P, Berlina A, et al: Hyperhomocystinemia and deep vein thrombosis: a case control study. *Thromb Haemost* 1996; 76:883–886.

31. denHeijer M, Koster T, Blom HJ, et al: Hyperhomocystinemia as a risk factor for deep vein thrombosis. *N Engl J Med* 1996; 334:759–762.

32. Svensson PJ, Dahlback B: Resistance to activated protein C as a basis for venous thrombosis. *N Engl J Med* 1994; 330:517–522.

33. Simioni P, Praudoni P, Zaron E, et al: Deep venous thrombosis and lupus anticoagulant: a case control study. *Thromb Haemost* 1996; 76:187–189.

34. Stollberger C, Slany J, Schuster I, et al: The prevalence of deep venous thrombosis in patients with suspected paradoxical embolism. *Ann Intern Med* 1993; 119:461–465.

35. Nagelhout DA, Pearson AC, Labovitz AJ: Diagnosis of paradoxic embolism by transesophageal echocardiography. *Am Heart J* 1991; 121: 1552–1554.

36. Ferrari E, Imbert A, Chevalier T, et al: The ECG in pulmonary embolism: predictive value of negative T-waves in precordial leads—80 case reports. *Chest* 1997; 111:537–543.

37. Hurst JW: Important features and examples of abnormal atrial and ventricular electrocardiograms. In: *Ventricular Electrocardiography*. Philadelphia, J. B. Lippincott Co., 1991: 13.2–13.12.

38. Stein PD, Terrin ML, Hales CA, et al: Clinical laboratory, roentgenographic, and electrocardiographic findings in patients with acute pulmonary embolism and no pre-existing cardiac or pulmonary disease. *Chest* 1991; 100:598–603.

39. Pallo A, Donnamaria V, Petruzzelli S, et al: Enlargement of the right descending pulmonary artery in pulmonary embolism. *Am J Roentgenol* 1983; 141:513–517.

40. Kasper W, Konstantinides S, Geibel A, et al: Prognostic significance of light ventricular afterload stress detected by echocardiography in patients with clinically suspected pulmonary embolism. *Heart* 1997; 77:346–349.

41. Goldhaber SZ, DeRoas M, Visani L: International cooperative pulmonary embolism registry detects high mortality rate. *Circulation* 1997; 96(suppl 1):1–159; abstract.

42. Jardin F, Dunbourg O, Gueret P, et al: Quantitative two-dimensional/echocardiography in massive pulmonary embolism. *J Am Coll Cardiol* 1987; 10:1201.

43. Lualdi JC, Goldhaber SZ: Right ventricular dysfunction after acute pulmonary embolism: pathophysiologic factors, detection and therapeutic implications. *Am Heart J* 1995; 130:1276–1282.

44. Felner JF, Churchwell AL, Murphy DA: Right atrial thromboemboli: clinical echocardiographic and pathophysiologic manifestations. *J Am Coll Cardiol* 1984; 4:1041–1051.

45. Baumbach A, Erley CM: Floating right atrial thrombosis and massive PE. *N Engl J Med* 1998; 339:86.

46. PIOPED Investigators: Value of the ventilation perfusion scan in acute pulmonary embolism: results of the Prospective Investigators of Pulmonary Embolism Diagnosis (PIOPED). *JAMA* 1990; 263:2753–2759.

47. Bone RC: Ventilation perfusion scan in pulmonary embolism: the emperor is incompletely attired. *JAMA* 1990; 263:2794–2795.

48. Bone RC: The low probability lung scan: a potentially lethal reading. *Arch Intern Med* 1993; 153:2621–2622.

49. Lensing AW, Prandoni P, Brandjas D, et al: Detection of deep vein thrombosis by real time B-mode ultrasonography. *N Engl J Med* 1989; 320: 342–345.

50. Birdwell BG, Raskob GE, Whitsett TL, et al: The clinical validity of normal compression ultrasound in outpatients suspected of having deep venous thrombosis. *Ann Intern Med* 1998; 128:1–7.

51. Wells PS, Ginsberg JS, Anderson DR, et al: Use of a clinical model for safe management of patients with suspected pulmonary embolism. *Ann Intern Med* 1998; 129:997–1005.

52. Robinson PJ: Ventilation perfusion lung scanning and special CT of the lungs: Competing or complimentary modalities. *Eur J Nucl Med* 1996; 11:1547–1553.

53. Remy-Jardin M, Remy J, Deschildre F, et al: Diagnosis of pulmonary embolism with spiral CT: comparison with pulmonary angiography and scintigraphy. *Radiology* 1996; 200:699–706.

54. Goodman LR, Lipchik RJ: Diagnosis of acute pulmonary embolism: time for a new approach. *Radiology* 1996; 199:25–27.

55. Perrer A, Desmarais S, Goering C, et al: D-dimer testing for suspected pulmonary embolism in outpatients. *Am J Respir Crit Care Med* 1997; 156(2 pt 1):492–496.

56. Ginsberg JS, Kearon C, Douketis J, et al: The use of D-dimer testing and impedence plethysmographic examination in patients with clinical indications of deep venous thrombosis. *Arch Intern Med* 1997; 157:1077–1081.

57. Fishel RS, Merlino JD, Felner JM: Diagnosis of main-stem pulmonary thromboemboli by transesophageal echocardiography. *Echocardiography* 1994; 11:189–195.

58. Jugdutt BI, Sussex BA, Sivaram CA, et al: Right ventricular infarction: two-dimensional evaluation. *Am Heart J* 1984; 107:505–518.

59. Raschke RA, Reilly BM, Guidry JR, et al: The weight-based heparin dosing nomogram: a randomized controlled trial. *Ann Intern Med* 1993; 119:874–881.

60. Levine MN, Hirsh J, Gent M, et al: A randomized trial comparing activated thromboplastin time with heparin assay in patients with acute venous thromboembolism requiring large daily doses of heparin. *Arch Intern Med* 1994; 154:49–56.

61. The Columbus Investigators: Low molecular weight heparin in the treatment of patients with venous thromboembolism. *N Engl J Med* 1997; 337:657–662.

62. Callander N, Rapaport SI: Trousseau's syndrome. *West J Med* 1993; 158:364–371.

63. Weitz JI: Drug therapy: low molecular weight heparins. *N Engl J Med* 1997; 337:688–699.

64. Daniels LB, Parker JA, Patel ST, et al: Relation of duration of symptoms with repsone to thrombolytic therapy in pulmonary embolism. *Am J Cardiol* 1997; 80:184–188.

65. Goldhaber SZ, Haire WD, Feldstein ML, et al: Alteplase versus heparin in acute pulmonary embolism: randomized trial assessing right ventricular function and pulmonary perfusion. *Lancet* 1993; 341:507–511.

66. Konstantinides S, Geiberl A, Olschewski M, et al: Association between thrombolytic treatment and the prognosis of hemodynamically stable patients with major pulmonary embolism: results of a multicenter registry. *Circulation* 1997; 96:882–888.

67. Whitehill TA: Caval interruption methods: comparison of options. *Semin Vasc Surg* 1996; 9:59–69.

68. Decousus H, Leizorovicy A, Parent F, Page Y: A clinical trial of vena caval filters in the prevention of pulmonary embolism in patients with proximal deep vein thrombosis. *N Engl J Med* 1998; 338:409–415.

69. Fedullo PF, Auger WR, Channick RN, et al: A multidisciplinary approach to chronic thromboembolic pulmonary hypertension. In: Goldhaber SZ (ed.): *Cardiopulmonary Diseases and Cardiac Tumors*, vol. 3 of *Atlas of Heart Diseases*. Philadelphia, Current Medicine, 1995: 7.1–7.25.

70. Antiplatelet Trialists Collaboration: Collaborative overview of randomized trials of antiplatelet therapy: III. Reduction in venous thrombosis and pulmonary embolism by antiplatelet prophylaxis among surgical and medical patients. *Br Med J* 1994; 308:235–246.

CHARLES D. SEARLES/
LAURA C. SEEFF/PAUL H. ROBINSON

# CHAPTER

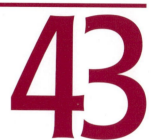

# PULMONARY HYPERTENSION AND COR PULMONALE

Pulmonary hypertension and cor pulmonale are two stages on a continuum that begins with diseases affecting ventilation and/or oxygenation and culminates in right heart failure. Cor pulmonale, or right ventricular enlargement, is invariably preceded by pulmonary hypertension and can result from any condition which leads to chronic hypoxemia and hypercapnia. This includes parenchymal pulmonary disease, pulmonary arterial disease, thoracic cage dysfunction, and defects in the centrally driven ventilatory mechanism (Table 43-1). Traditionally, the term *cor pulmonale* has been used to suggest right ventricle dysfunction specifically as a result of parenchymal pulmonary disease. While parenchymal pulmonary disease, in particular chronic obstructive pulmonary disease (COPD), is certainly the most common cause of pulmonary hypertension and cor pulmonale, this chapter will use the widely accepted World Health Organization definition of cor pulmonale:

> Hypertrophy of the right ventricle resulting from diseases affecting the function and/or structure of the lung, except when these pulmonary alterations are the result of diseases that primarily affect the left side of the heart or of congenital heart disease.[1]

It is difficult to assess the incidence of pulmonary hypertension, because it is a hemodynamic disorder and often is not clinically apparent until the right ventricle is enlarged. Cor pulmonale probably represents 5 to 10 percent of all heart diseases.[2–4] The incidence of cor pulmonale varies regionally, with higher rates in parts of the world where respiratory disease and smoking tobacco are more prevalent. Some 50 to 80 percent of cor pulmonale is caused by emphysema and chronic bronchitis.[2,3]

**TABLE 43-1.   Etiologies of Chronic Pulmonary Hypertension and Cor Pulmonale**

I. Secondary causes
  A. Chronic pulmonary parenchymal disease
    1. Chronic obstructive pulmonary disease
    2. Chronic interstitial lung disease
    3. Cystic fibrosis
    4. $\alpha_1$-antiproteinase deficiency
  B. Pulmonary vascular disease
    1. Chronic thromboembolic disease
    2. Collagen vascular disease
    3. Tumor/tumor emboli
    4. Hepatic cirrhosis/portal vein thrombosis
    5. Infection with human immunodeficiency virus
    6. Anorexic drugs
  C. Alveolar hypoventilation with normal lung parenchyma
    1. Sleep apnea
    2. Obesity
    3. Chest wall dysfunction
    4. Neuromuscular disease
    5. Central nervous system dysfunction
  D. High-altitude dwelling/chronic mountain sickness
 II. Primary pulmonary hypertension
III. Veno-occlusive disease of the lung

# PATHOGENESIS OF PULMONARY HYPERTENSION AND COR PULMONALE

Definite pulmonary artery hypertension is present when the mean pulmonary artery pressure exceeds 20 mmHg at rest. Once the pulmonary vascular bed has been reduced, exercise may cause a dramatic rise in pulmonary artery pressure.[2,5] Reduction in the pulmonary vascular bed may result from obliterative arterial diseases or from diffuse interstitial diseases that act by compression and obliteration of the small pulmonary arteries and arterioles. However, the predominant cause of pulmonary hypertension in chronic airway diseases is arteriolar constriction resulting from alveolar hypoxia.[5,6]

The normal right ventricle is a thin-walled, distensible muscular pump that is able to handle considerable variations in volume. It is less well equipped to handle the demands of increased pressure load. The response of the right ventricle to pulmonary hypertension depends on the acuteness and severity of the pressure load.

The ventricle will dilate after a sudden and severe stimulus, such as massive pulmonary emboli or severe hypoxia from an exacerbation of COPD. Chronic cor pulmonale is associated with more slowly evolving hypertension, which results in right ventricular hypertrophy.[2,5] Failure of the right ventricle is associated with salt and water retention, expansion of the plasma volume, and systemic venous congestion.[5] Relief of pulmonary hypertension diminishes the load on the right ventricle, with normalization of filling pressures and cardiac output. Recovery also reverses the water and electrolyte disturbances.

# DIAGNOSIS OF PULMONARY HYPERTENSION AND COR PULMONALE

There are few historical and physical findings related solely to pulmonary hypertension, and the diagnosis often is not clinically apparent until cor pulmonale has developed. Furthermore, the signs and symptoms of pulmonary hypertension and cor pulmonale are often masked by the symptoms of the underlying lung disease. It may be only with serial examinations that a subtle progression to cor pulmonale will become evident. The clinician must be alert to the possible development of pulmonary hypertension and cor pulmonale in predisposing diseases.

## History

The most common presenting symptoms related to pulmonary hypertension and cor pulmonale are dyspnea, fatigue, syncope, chest pain, and hemoptysis.[1,7–9] Initially, the dyspnea may be only exertional. Dyspnea at rest is more common with cor pulmonale that develops from pulmonary arterial disease.[7]

Syncope may be exertional; positional; related to coughing, as seen in COPD; or due to tachyarrhythmias. Syncope is caused by a diminished ability to increase right ventricular output with exercise, with resultant impaired exertional cerebral blood flow, and may be exacerbated by the peripheral vasodilatation that occurs normally with exertion. Coughing can cause syncope by increasing intrathoracic pressure and decreasing venous return.

Pulmonary hypertension may cause exertional chest pain ("right heart angina") that can be indistinguishable from left heart angina.[9] The mechanism is most likely right heart ischemia.[7] Both chest wall distortion and pulmonary trunk distention are probable associated mechanisms. Chest pain that is pleuritic in nature, particularly if coupled with hemoptysis and dyspnea, suggests the possibility of pulmonary embolism. Hemoptysis is frequent in bronchitis, pulmonary embolism, and advanced primary pulmonary hypertension (PPH). Hemoptysis in PPH probably occurs from ruptured alveolar capillaries under extremely high pressures.[8]

Other symptoms include edema, palpitations, early satiety, weakness, and dizziness.[4] Infrequently, patients may present with hoarseness caused by compression of the recurrent laryngeal nerve by an enlarged pulmonary artery.[5,10]

## Physical Examination

Obvious general features that should prompt the clinician to consider pulmonary hypertension include chest cage deformities, obesity, neuromuscular abnormalities, and the typical appearances associated with COPD ("pink puffers" or "blue bloaters"). Cyanosis, somnolence, plethora, and edema are also clues to the presence of pulmonary hypertension.

Vital signs may be abnormal. Both tachypnea and tachycardia are common, particularly in thromboembolic disease,[11] but will be present from any cause as the right heart fails. Patients usually have borderline systemic hypotension, except for patients with sleep apnea, in whom hypertension is more likely.[7]

**CARDIOVASCULAR EXAMINATION.**   There are numerous cardiovascular manifestations of pulmonary heart disease.[7] Jugular venous distention, from either right ventricular failure or increased intrathoracic pressure of chronic lung disease, is frequently observed. A prominent a wave may be present and suggests a noncompliant right ventricle. Abnormal c and v waves suggest tricuspid regurgitation. A right ventricular heave may be visible or palpable, most commonly in the parasternal region, but possibly in the epigastrium in patients with a vertically oriented heart seen in COPD. The ventricular lift may be more visible with the examiner standing at the foot of the bed.[7] Auscultation may reveal a prominent and delayed pulmonic component of the second heart sound. A right-sided fourth heart sound, suggesting right ventricular hypertension, or a third heart sound, suggesting right ventricular failure, may be present. Tricuspid regurgitation may be audible at the lower left sternal border. It may be augmented with inspiration (Carvallo sign) or by manual pressure on the liver. Pulmonic regurgitation (Graham Steell murmur) is an early diastolic murmur that will be heard best at the parasternal region or the second left intercostal space.

In the patient with COPD, these typical findings of cor pulmonale are often masked by a hyperinflated chest cavity and abnormal lung sounds. The epigastrium should be auscultated carefully, since the heart is vertically rotated, but the examination may be unrevealing.

**OTHER FINDINGS ON PHYSICAL EXAMINATION.**   The remainder of the physical examination may reveal findings related to the underlying disease. In thromboembolic disease, a pleural rub may be heard over an area of pulmonary infarction. In COPD, there may be wheezing, poor airway movement, a prolonged expiratory phase, or evidence of bronchitis. In interstitial lung diseases, there may be fine bibasilar crackles. In PPH, there is often a normal pulmonary examination.[5] In congestive right ventricular failure, the liver will be enlarged, and ascites and peripheral edema may be present. Tricuspid regurgitation can produce a pulsatile liver. In COPD, the diaphragm is typically low, and, consequently, the liver, while normal in size, will be much more easily palpable. Clubbing can be present in patients with chronic lung diseases, most commonly COPD, but it is unusual in PPH or thromboembolic disease.[7] Asterixis from hypercarbia may be present, most often in patients with COPD.

## Electrocardiogram

Patients with cor pulmonale due to pulmonary hypertension as defined above may develop signs of systolic pressure overload of the right ventricle (Fig. 43-1). These electrocardiographic abnormalities include:[12,13]

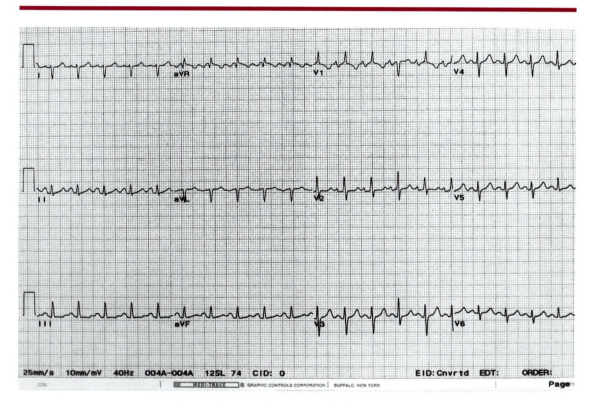

**Figure 43-1**   Electrocardiogram of a patient with primary pulmonary hypertension, showing prominent P waves, a mean QRS axis of about +125° in the frontal plane and directed at 20° anteriorly, producing a large S wave in lead I and a tall R wave in lead $V_1$. This signifies a hypertrophied right ventricle. The mean T-wave axis is +10° in the frontal plane and parallel to the frontal plane.

- A right atrial abnormality in which the amplitude of the P wave in lead II is >2.5 mm. The first half of the P wave, which represents right atrial depolarization, is commonly larger than normal in lead $V_1$.
- The electrical forces representing the QRS complex may shift to the right and anteriorly toward the right ventricle, producing an S wave in lead I and a tall initial R wave in lead $V_1$. This shift does not develop initially because such patients have normal left ventricular dominance before they develop right ventricular disease. Accordingly, the mean QRS axis is usually directed inferiorly and posteriorly before it is directed to the right and anteriorly. During the early stages of cor pulmonale the initial R wave in lead $V_1$ may be greater than 3 mm and may be larger than the S wave.
- Right bundle branch block or right ventricular conduction delay may develop in patients with chronic cor pulmonale.
- The mean T axis may eventually be directed away from the right ventricle. Accordingly, it may be directed to the left and posteriorly.

There are two electrocardiographic abnormalities that deserve special attention.

- Acute pulmonary emboli may produce no electrocardiographic changes or may precipitate atrial fibrillation. A large pulmonary embolus may precipitate the development of an S wave in lead I and a Q wave in lead III.[13a] The abnormal Q wave may be misinterpreted as being due to inferior MI. In such patients the mean T axis may shift to the left and posteriorly. Right bundle branch block may develop acutely or may evolve after the electrocardiogram reveals chronic systolic pressure overload of the right ventricle.
- The electrocardiographic abnormalities produced by cor pulmonale related to COPD and emphysema are an atrial arrhythmia may be present; when P waves are seen, the P-wave axis is directed more than $+70°$ in the frontal plane,[13b] low amplitude of the QRS complexes (the total 12-lead QRS amplitude is commonly on the low side of the normal range which is 80 to 185 mm); low amplitude of the P and T waves may also present; right ventricular delay or right bundle branch block may be present; and the uncommon $S_1$, $S_2$, $S_3$ abnormality may develop. Many of the abnormalities are due to emphysema, low diaphragm, and alteration of the location of the heart in the chest.

## Roentgenographic Findings

A posteroanterior and lateral chest roentgenogram can be helpful in the diagnosis of pulmonary hypertension and cor pulmonale. As pulmonary hypertension increases, the arteries in the superior aspect of the lung are recruited. Normal vascular distribution is a function of gravity. When a person is standing upright, blood flows preferentially to the lower lung fields, and vascular markings normally are much more prominent in the bases. One of the earliest signs of pulmonary hypertension is increased arterial vascularity in the upper lung fields.[14] Pulmonary emboli, which tend to occur more frequently in the bases because of the increased basilar flow, also can cause increased flow and increased lung markings in the upper fields. With further increasing pulmonary pressures, the central pulmonary arteries begin to dilate. This can be seen on the posteroanterior film, where the hilum appears full, and verified on the lateral film, where the vessels can easily be seen and distinguished from soft tissue masses.[15] The enlarged vessels appear to taper abruptly, with a relative diminution of the distal vessels, creating a pruning effect typical of pulmonary hypertension (Fig. 43-2).[14] Once cor pulmonale develops, enlargement of the right ventricle may be evident on the lateral view, where the retrosternal air space appears filled in (Fig. 43-3).

## Echocardiography

Echocardiography is useful in helping to rule out primary cardiac diseases, including valvular disease and congenital heart disease, as the etiology of pulmonary hypertension. It is also used to assess the degree of pulmonary hypertension, right ventricular hypertrophy and/or dilatation, and right ventricular function. It accurately detects cor pulmonale in patients with COPD twice as often as clinical methods.[16] Its most important use, however, may be in longitudinal follow-up of diseases causing pulmonary hypertension and cor pulmonale and in documenting the effects of pharmacologic treatment.

## Right Heart Catheterization

For the diagnosis of pulmonary hypertension and cor pulmonale, right heart catheterization is the gold standard diagnostic technique, but it is invasive and may

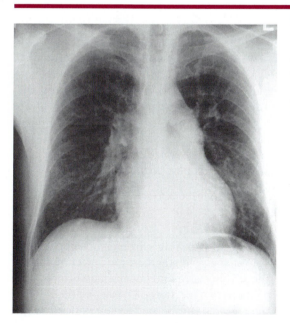

Figure 43-2  Posteroanterior roentgenogram of patient with long-standing sleep apnea. Note the enlarged main pulmonary artery, seen bulging on the left heart border. The right pulmonary artery is also enlarged, and there is abrupt tapering of the branches of this vessel, reflecting pulmonary hypertension.

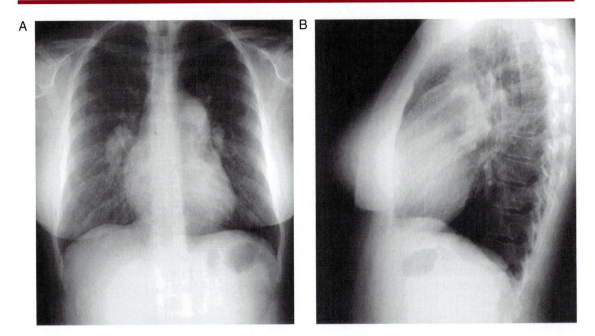

**Figure 43-3**   Posteroanterior (PA) and lateral chest roentgenogram of a patient with primary pulmonary hypertension. *A.* On the PA film, the main pulmonary artery is enlarged, as seen by its bulging beyond the left border of the heart. The right and left pulmonary arteries are also enlarged, as seen on the PA film. On the PA film, the right heart border is prominent, indicating right atrial enlargement, and the apex is upwardly displaced, suggesting right ventricular enlargement. *B.* On the lateral film, the retrosternal air space is filled in by right ventricular enlargement.

carry an increased risk of death in patients with severe pulmonary hypertension.[5,17] It is the only technique that can reliably detect early pulmonary hypertension or cor pulmonale. It enables direct determination of pulmonary artery pressures, pulmonary artery wedge pressure, and cardiac output at rest and in response to various interventions, such as exercise, oxygen, and vasodilators. Despite its sensitivity, cardiac catheterization may be superfluous when the diagnosis can be made by less invasive tests. Once the diagnosis of PPH has been made, however, right heart catheterization is essential for establishing the response to vasodilator agents.

## Lung Scans and Pulmonary Angiography

Ventilation-perfusion scans are useful in distinguishing chronic thromboembolic disease from PPH and are discussed below. The gold standard for detecting thromboemboli is pulmonary angiography, but it is invasive and has been associated with sudden death in patients with severe pulmonary hypertension.[3] Despite this, several studies have shown that pulmonary angiograms can be performed without major complications in the majority of patients,[18] particularly if selective or subselective injections of small volumes of contrast media are used.[19]

# CAUSES OF SECONDARY PULMONARY HYPERTENSION

## Chronic Obstructive Pulmonary Disease

Chronic obstructive pulmonary disease, which includes both emphysema and chronic bronchitis, is the most common cause of pulmonary hypertension and cor pulmonale.[20,21] There are approximately 15 million cases of COPD in the United States, with 70,000 yearly deaths related directly to COPD.[2] The common link among all forms of COPD is increased airway resistance during expiration. There has been some debate over the definitions of the terms used to denote these diseases. For the current discussion, the term COPD will include chronic bronchitis and emphysema, and where clinical distinctions are important, they will be emphasized.

While chronic bronchitis and emphysema are clinically and pathologically distinct, most patients have a combination of the two entities. During an exacerbation, it may be difficult to distinguish them, but at baseline, they behave differently.[22] Patients with chronic bronchitis have increased mucus production, cough, and airway resistance, which predisposes them to recurrent lung infections.[21] They are often overweight, plethoric, and cyanotic. These patients progress to pulmonary hypertension and cor pulmonale more rapidly than patients with pure emphysema because they are relatively more hypoxemic and hypercapnic.[20,21] Pulmonary pressures are persistently high, but worsen periodically with increased hypoxemia from frequent superimposed infections.[20] The clinical course is generally progressive and downhill, with periods of exacerbations and remissions. Right heart failure from sustained hypoxemia is generally the cause of death.

Patients with pure emphysema differ clinically and pathologically from those with pure bronchitis. They often appear cachectic and dyspneic, with less of a productive cough than those with pure bronchitis. They have a more pronounced barrel chest and more hyperinflation on lung examination. Anatomically, there is dilatation and destruction of the terminal airways, which leads to air trapping and eventually to bullous formation.[21] At baseline, there is less hypoxemia and, consequently, lower pulmonary vascular pressures than in patients with pure bronchitis.[20] Pulmonary hypertension is episodic as a result of acute exacerbations from an infection.[20] The physical findings and electrocardiographic signs of pulmonary hypertension and cor pulmonale may become evident only with exacerbations of the disease. The patient eventually progresses from exertional dyspnea to dyspnea at rest and, like the bronchitic patient, generally becomes oxygen-dependent. The life expectancy of emphysemic patients is somewhat longer than that of patients with bronchitis because of better baseline oxygenation.

Diagnosis of COPD is made by a combination of history and physical examination, typical ECG and x-ray findings, and pulmonary function testing. The hallmark on pulmonary function testing is a decreased $FEV_1$ and a decreased $FEV_1/FVC$. Pulmonary hypertension is usually suspected based on clinical findings, but if necessary, an echocardiogram can be performed to evaluate right-sided chambers and estimate pulmonary pressures. Close monitoring of the hematocrit, arterial blood gases, and signs of cor pulmonale will allow oxygen supplementation to be initiated before the development of right ventricular failure.

## Interstitial Lung Diseases

Interstitial lung diseases can lead to severe pulmonary hypertension and cor pulmonale, although usually only after extensive lung dysfunction. These disorders have in common the destruction of functioning pulmonary parenchyma with restriction of the pulmonary vascular bed. Interstitial lung disease can result from a wide variety of diffuse inflammatory processes, such as sarcoidosis, radiation fibrosis, connective tissue disorders, asbestosis, fibrosing alveolitis, alveolar proteinosis, and progressive massive fibrosis.

Initially, pulmonary hypertension occurs only when cardiac output is increased, as during exercise.[5] As the vascular bed becomes restricted, pulmonary hypertension persists at rest and intensifies with increased blood flow. As long as arterial hypoxemia remains mild, pulmonary hypertension is modest and is tolerated well, but as arterial hypoxemia intensifies, pulmonary hypertension worsens, and cor pulmonale evolves.[5] Eucapnia or hypocapnia, which is present early in the disease, is replaced with hypercapnia as right ventricular failure develops.[5,20] In most patients, the pathologic process can be stabilized relatively early in the course of the disease, and the development of right ventricular failure is avoided.

## Alveolar Hypoventilation with Normal Lung Parenchyma

Disorders of global alveolar hypoventilation with normal lung parenchyma can occur as a result of an abnormal ventilatory drive or of dysfunction of the muscles of respiration, the thoracic cage, or the upper airway.[23] Disorders that fall into the first category include functional depression of the ventilatory drive, as in sleep, with sedatives, and in myxedema; respiratory neuron disease secondary to stroke, bulbar poliomyelitis, or encephalitis; and organic central depression of ventilatory drive (Ondine's curse). Disorders in the second category include those involving neuromuscular impairment, as in poliomyelitis, Guillain-Barré syndrome, myasthenia gravis, polymyositis, and muscular dystrophy; disorders of the chest cage, including obesity-hypoventilation syndrome and kyphoscoliosis; and disorders of the upper airway, including tracheal stenosis and obstructive sleep apnea. Pulmonary hypertension develops from pulmonary vasoconstriction secondary to long-standing hypoxemia, hypercapnia, and respiratory acidosis.

In neuromuscular disorders, the diaphragm becomes paralyzed, and thus the respiratory pump is impaired. Physical examination will demonstrate paradoxical movement of the abdomen with respiration. Patients may complain of disturbed sleep, daytime somnolence, headache, and breathlessness when supine, but the problem may not be recognized until acute respiratory failure occurs as a result of an intercurrent infection. Kyphoscoliosis, or any severely deforming skeletal abnormality of the thoracic cage, leads to chronic alveolar hypoventilation because of impaired mechanics of breathing. The chest wall loses its elastic resistance and the lungs remain very small, leading to chronic hypoxia and eventually cor pulmonale.

In obstructive sleep apnea, arterial hypoxemia and hypercapnia are initially manifested only during sleep.[24] The patient has frequent nocturnal awakenings, with resultant morning headaches, irritability, intellectual deterioration, and daytime somnolence. Impotence and arrhythmias may develop. Systemic hypertension develops initially at night, but may become persistent. Three factors seem to be most important in the pathogenesis of the syndrome: upper airway anatomy, neural control of respiration, and hormonal balance. Progesterone is a respiratory stimulant, whereas testosterone reduces respiratory drive. Without correction of the hypoxemia, pulmonary hypertension and ultimately cor pulmonale develop.

Polysomnography is diagnostic for sleep apnea.[24] Parameters measured include sleep stage, ventilation, respiratory effort, and gas exchange. Treatment options include weight loss, nasal continuous positive airway pressure, and uvulopalatopharyngeoplasty.

## Thromboembolic Disease

Pulmonary hypertension with ensuing cor pulmonale can develop from either acute or chronic thromboembolism. Generally, thromboembolic disease is categorized according to the size of the involved vessels; pathogenesis and treatment are distinct in the different groups.[20,25]

**OCCLUSION OF SMALL ARTERIES AND ARTERIOLES.**   Pulmonary hypertension has been associated with thrombosis of the small muscular arteries. While these lesions were once felt to arise from showers of microemboli to the small vessels, they are now felt to be the result of in situ thrombosis.[20,25] Endothelial dysfunction and disruption in the coagulation and fibrinolysis balance is the proposed mechanism of action. Clinically, these patients present with chronic breathlessness, nondescript chest pain, and often anxiety.

In patients suspected of having chronic thromboembolic disease, ventilation-perfusion scanning is necessary to exclude chronic proximal or large-vessel thromboembolism, because the treatment differs.[26] Treatment for small-vessel thrombosis consists of anticoagulation with warfarin or antiplatelet agents.

**OCCLUSION OF INTERMEDIATE-SIZED VESSELS.**   These are the most common pulmonary vessel occlusions.[22] A source of peripheral embolization is usually identifiable (i.e., deep venous thrombosis), and there are generally multiple emboli, with some leading to pulmonary infarction. These patients have persistent or paroxysmal dyspnea, tachycardia, and tachypnea, the latter two persisting during sleep. The patient may have pleuritic chest pain with or without pulmonary infarction, and there may be localized rales or wheezing over the area of the embolus. Chest radiography may be normal or may reveal Westermark's sign (an area of avascularity beyond the site of the embolus) or Hamptom's hump (a wedge-shaped peripheral infiltrate representing an infarct). Both ventilation-perfusion scanning and angiography are helpful diagnostically, with level of clinical suspicion playing a significant role.[27]

**PROXIMAL PULMONARY THROMBOEMBOLISM.**   Thromboembolism in the central or proximal pulmonary arteries can be either acute or chronic, with each having a distinct clinical presentation.[20] Massive acute proximal pulmonary embolism is often fatal when a saddle embolus obstructs at least two lobar arteries. These patients will present with listlessness, hypotension, confusion, and oliguria. The physical findings of pulmonary hypertension and cor pulmonale are striking, because the massive pulmonary embolus causes an acute rise in pulmonary pressures. More commonly, large emboli compromise less than two lobar arteries and will not be fatal. The degree of the compromise dictates the clinical presentation. The patient may be tachypneic, tachycardic, febrile, and anxious, with hypotension depending on the degree of arterial compromise. Some 10 percent of emboli will cause infarction. Pulmonary infarction is associated with pleuritic pain, hemoptysis, and a pleuritic friction rub.

In most patients who survive a massive proximal embolism, radiographic abnormalities resolve as the clot is destroyed and resorbed. Occasionally, the clot is not dissolved and becomes incorporated into the walls of the vessel. In chronic proximal thromboembolism, the organized clot may propagate and obstruct a wide area of arterial supply, leading to pulmonary hypertension. A high index of suspicion is required for diagnosis of chronic proximal thromboembolism; the lesion can be mistaken clinically and radiographically for a carcinoma. Clinically, the patient complains of significant dyspnea and often has a history of a previous embolus, but there may be few clues on physical examination other than an accentuated pulmonic component of the second heart sound.

Ventilation-perfusion scanning is essential to the diagnosis of chronic proximal pulmonary embolism. The benefit of making this diagnosis is that pulmonary hypertension can be relieved surgically by pulmonary thromboendarterectomy. Medical treatment with thrombolytic agents can be an alternative. Proximal pulmonary thromboembolism will usually show two or more segmental perfusion defects. A scan showing segmental-sized defects requires selective contrast pulmonary angiography.[20,22] Angiography is necessary in this situation because ventilation-perfusion scans often underestimate the severity of central pulmonary obstruction, and angiography helps identify the extent and location of the clot for surgical removal.[20,26] In addition, there are a number of nonembolic causes of ventilation-perfusion mismatch that can be ruled out by angiography, including various forms of vasculitis and interstitial fibrous and pulmonary vascular compression.

Thromboendarterectomy is advocated in selected patients who have had a persistent embolus for more than 6 months despite adequate anticoagulation.[20] Immediately following the procedure, there is often significant localized reperfusion pulmonary edema. Hemodynamic recovery occurs rapidly, however, and the patient generally has remarkable improvement in the original symptomatology. Patients require lifelong anticoagulation.

## Pulmonary Vascular Diseases

Pulmonary vascular disease is an important component of many collagen vascular diseases, in addition to its effects on the lung parenchyma. In many of these patients, the interstitium appears uninvolved, and abnormalities are localized to the pulmonary vessels.[20] There is a high incidence of pulmonary hypertension in patients with systemic lupus erythematosus, many of whom exhibit Raynaud's phenomenon.[28] There is also a high incidence of pulmonary vascular disease in systemic sclerosis, CREST syndrome, and the overlap syndromes.[20,29]

Pulmonary hypertension has been described in patients with other forms of pulmonary vasculitis, including isolated Raynaud's phenomenon, dermatomyositis, rheumatoid arthritis, and sarcoidosis.[30] Diffuse lymphatic spread of carcinoma may also cause pulmonary hypertension and right heart failure.[30,31] In many cases, vascular obstruction may be the result of tumor microemboli that have produced a thrombotic and fibrotic reaction in the pulmonary vasculature. In addition, the major pulmonary arteries may be obstructed by tumor and thus cause right ventricular and main pulmonary artery hypertension.[32] In rare instances, left atrial tumors may result in pulmonary venous occlusive disease and pulmonary hypertension.

Residence at high altitude is associated with pulmonary hypertension and right ventricular hypertrophy. The higher the altitude, the more marked the pulmonary hypertension, mostly as a result of alveolar hypoxia.[5] In addition, certain individuals appear to have a genetic predisposition to inordinate pulmonary pressor effects when they are exposed to hypoxia.[2,5] The pulmonary hypertensive response to high-altitude hypoxia is greater in men than in women.[2]

Acute and chronic mountain sickness are more severe manifestations of failure to adapt to the hypoxic conditions of high altitude. Acute mountain sickness affects the newcomer at high altitude and affects most people at altitudes over 12,000 ft.[5] It is associated with headache, weakness, nausea, vomiting, palpitations, cyanosis, and Cheyne-Stokes breathing. Chronic mountain sickness affects native residents at high altitude and is uncommon.[2,5]

Hepatic cirrhosis and portal vein thrombosis have been associated with pulmonary hypertension and obliterative changes in the pulmonary arteriolar bed.[33] The clinical and pathologic features of this form of pulmonary hypertension are similar to those of PPH. The mechanisms responsible for the changes in the pulmonary vasculature are unclear, but portal hypertension, rather than cirrhosis itself, appears to be the prerequisite for development of pulmonary hypertension

(Figs. 43-4 and 43-5), and this may be magnified and accelerated by portal-systemic anastomoses.[33,34]

Infection with HIV can be associated with pulmonary hypertension; clinical and pathologic features are similar to those of PPH.[34] However, the number of patients described with HIV infection and pulmonary arteriopathy has been small compared to the overall population of patients with HIV infection, suggesting that a genetic predisposition must be present to permit the development of severe pulmonary hypertension.[35]

A recent study showed that the use of appetite suppressants was associated with an increased risk of PPH.[36] This study estimates the absolute risk for obese persons who use anorexic agents for more than 3 months to be more than 30 times higher than that for nonusers (from an annual incidence of 1 case per 500,000 European inhabitants to 30 cases per 500,000). Fenfluramine and dexfenfluramine, inhibitors of

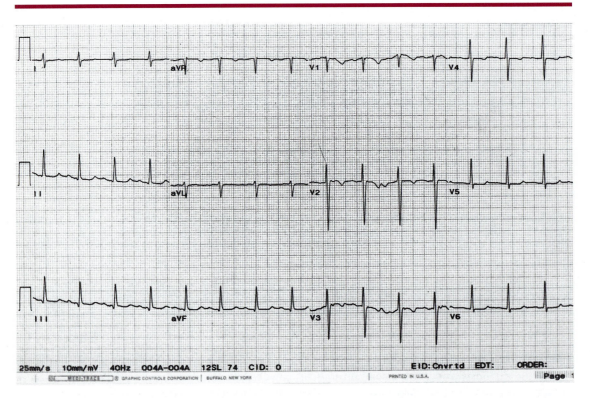

**Figure 43-4**　Electrocardiogram of a patient with hepatic cirrhosis, portal hypertension, and pulmonary hypertension. The mean QRS axis is directed at +90° in the frontal plane and 50° posteriorly. The mean T axis is about +60° in the frontal plane and 45° posteriorly. The vertical QRS axis is the only clue to possible right ventricular hypertrophy. The patient had undergone coronary bypass surgery in the past, and the left ventricle was large (see x-ray of chest in Fig. 43-5). Therefore, definite electrocardiographic signs of right ventricular hypertrophy would be prevented or delayed.

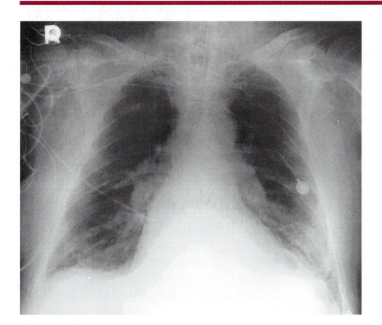

**Figure 43-5**   Anteroposterior roentgenogram of a patient with hepatic cirrhosis, portal hypertension, and pulmonary hypertension. The film shows sternotomy wires from prior bypass surgery for coronary atherosclerosis. The main, right, and left pulmonary arteries are enlarged, indicating pulmonary hypertension. There is left ventricular enlargement.

serotonin uptake, were the drugs most commonly associated with pulmonary hypertension, but amphetamines were also implicated.

# PRIMARY PULMONARY HYPERTENSION

Primary pulmonary hypertension is a disease characterized by sustained elevation of pulmonary artery pressure without a demonstrable cause. This definition entails a normal wedge pressure with a mean pulmonary artery pressure of more than 25 mmHg at rest and the exclusion of any significant underlying cardiac or pulmonary disease.

There are a number of theories regarding the etiology of PPH, but none has yet gained clear ascendancy. The pathologic changes are in the small muscular arteries and arterioles, with medial hypertrophy as the earliest pathologic feature.[5,37] Various defects in coagulation, including abnormal platelet function and defective fibrinolysis, have been demonstrated in patients with PPH, leading to the theory that in situ thrombosis in the small pulmonary arteries may be an important component of increased pulmonary vascular resistance in these patients.[30,38] Furthermore, it has been argued that at least one type of PPH may result from recurrent episodes of asymptomatic pulmonary embolism.[17,38]

PPH is an uncommon disorder, with an incidence estimated at 1 to 2 cases per million people in the general population.[34,37] Symptoms are usually first manifested in early adulthood, although the onset may occur at any age. In adults, the female-male ratio has ranged from 1.7:1 to 5:1 in different studies, and this female-male predominance is higher among blacks.[20] There are usually 2 years between the time of first onset of symptoms to the time of clinical and hemodynamic diagnosis of PPH.[18]

The most common presenting symptoms at the time of diagnosis are dyspnea (60 percent), fatigue (19 percent), and syncope or near syncope (13 percent).[18] The chest x-ray film is commonly abnormal (see Fig. 43-3) and electrocardiographic abnormalities such as right ventricular hypertrophy, right axis deviation, and/or right atrial abnormality may be present (see Fig. 43-1). Approximately 10 percent of patients, usually women, have symptoms of Raynaud's phenomenon.[18] There is also a familial form of PPH whose histopathological and clinical features are identical to those of the sporadic form.[37] The familial form is inherited as an autosomal dominant trait and is associated with a pattern of worsening of disease in subsequent generations.

Early in the disease, symptoms and clinical findings are nonspecific. As the disease progresses, findings on physical examination are consistent with pulmonary hypertension and right ventricular pressure overload. Cardiac catheterization and pulmonary angiography carry an increased risk of death,[17,30] but these procedures may be needed for confirmation of the diagnosis. Right heart catheterization reveals elevated pulmonary arterial and right ventricular systolic pressures that approach, equal, or sometimes exceed systemic arterial levels. The calculated pulmonary vascular resistance is extremely high. Left ventricular diastolic, left atrial, and wedge pressures are low or normal.

The average period of survival after diagnosis is 3 years, although with newer therapies, patients may survive much longer.[39] Predictors of survival include hemodynamic parameters (mean pulmonary artery pressure, mean right atrial pressure, cardiac index), New York Heart Association functional class, exercise tolerance, anticoagulant therapy, and response to vasodilators.[17,39] Prognosis in PPH has also been strongly correlated with the presence and severity of pericardial effusion, possibly because pericardial effusion serves as an indicator of the presence of severe, sustained right heart failure.[40]

The mode of death in patients with PPH is variable, but most patients die of progressive right-sided heart failure.[17,39] Patients with severe pulmonary hypertension are prone to sudden death. In a few instances, bradycardia leading to cardiac arrest has preceded sudden death.[5]

Patients with PPH may not tolerate diagnostic procedures well. They can experience sudden cardiovascular collapse and even death during cardiac catheterization and angiography, during or shortly after the induction of general anesthesia for surgical procedures, and even following ventilation-perfusion scanning.[30] Why these interventions result in cardiovascular collapse and sudden death is not clearly defined, but they may act as stimuli for further constriction of the pulmonary vascular bed. This can lead to sudden development or exacerbation of right heart failure, decreased cardiac output, and arrhythmias.

# TREATMENT OF PULMONARY HYPERTENSION AND COR PULMONALE

## When to Refer to a Specialist

The majority of patients with pulmonary hypertension and cor pulmonale have COPD. These patients may be successfully managed by a primary care physician who is able to treat the underlying disease, and who recognizes that chronic hypoxemia will lead to pulmonary hypertension and cor pulmonale (Fig. 43-6). Patients with other causes of cor pulmonale, including interstitial lung diseases, alveolar hypoventilation, and thromboembolic disease, often will have been referred to a specialist during their initial evaluation, and they may continue to be followed by both their primary care physician and a specialist. In many cases, long-term care can be delivered by a primary care physician, but a specialist may be required to assist with complications of therapy, as well as to introduce new medical and surgical therapies as they become available.

Primary pulmonary hypertension requires the expertise of a specialist familiar with the disease process. Often the patient is referred to a specialist once a thorough evaluation by a primary care physician has revealed no clear diagnosis. Once the diagnosis is made, the necessary medications, particularly vasodilators, are better administered by a physician familiar with their use and side effects. If the patient is a transplantation candidate, he or she will need to be referred to a transplantation center, where a transplantation team will manage his or her care. The primary care physician should maintain a role in the patient's care, since she or he often knows the patient best and can better assess long-term progress.

## Treatment of Underlying Disease

The cornerstone of treatment for pulmonary hypertension and cor pulmonale is treatment of the underlying disease, with the hope of slowing the development of right ventricular failure. It is imperative that the physician recognize diseases that are associated with pulmonary hypertension and recognize that apparent progression of the disease process may be a signal that cor pulmonale is developing. It is also important to recognize that there is considerable individual variability in the development of pulmonary hypertension in the different disease states. In many cases of pulmonary hypertension, the underlying disease process can be stabilized,

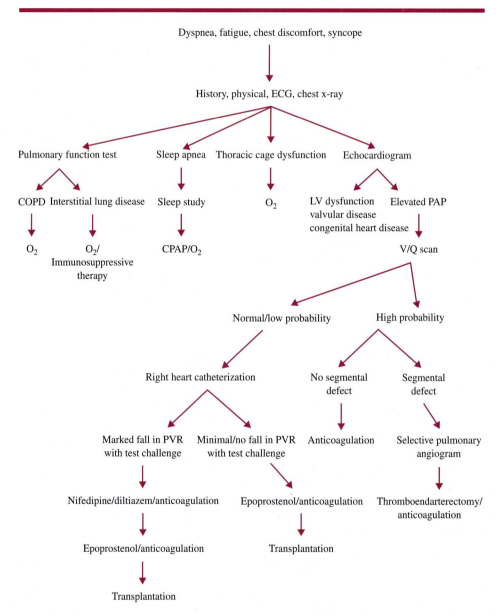

**Figure 43-6**   Evaluation and primary therapy for pulmonary hypertension. Evaluation of pulmonary hypertension starts with a thorough history and physical examination, ECG, and chest x-ray. Based on findings from this initial evaluation, the work-up turns to investigation of primary versus secondary causes of pulmonary hypertension.

and the patient is left with a modest elevation of pulmonary artery pressure that may be tolerated for a long time.

## Oxygen Therapy

In all the disease states in which chronic alveolar hypoxia and hypoxemia is involved in the development of pulmonary hypertension, oxygen therapy can reduce pulmonary pressures and delay progression to right ventricular failure.[41] Most patients will need oxygen for life, as withdrawal of oxygen therapy is associated with a return of hypoxemia.

Several studies have clearly shown a survival benefit associated with supplemental oxygen and also an improvement in exercise tolerance, pulmonary hemodynamics, and neuropsychiatric performance.[42–44] Improved survival is directly correlated with hours per day on oxygen.

In general, oxygen supplementation is indicated in patients with $Pa_{O_2}$ less than 55 mmHg and/or $O_2$ saturation less than 88 percent, or with a $Pa_{O_2}$ of 56 to 59 mmHg and concomitant erythrocytosis or right heart failure. Patients who become hypoxemic with exercise or during sleep should receive oxygen supplementation at those designated times. In general, $Pa_{O_2}$ should be maintained between 60 and 65 mmHg. Arterial blood gases should be obtained initially to document oxygen and carbon dioxide levels. Patients who are hypercapnic need arterial blood gases to guide titration of the oxygen, but pulse oximetry can be used to monitor non-$CO_2$ retainers. Airline travel is generally safe for people on supplemental oxygen, but the flow of oxygen often needs to be increased by 1 to 2 L/min. Patients need to be informed that oxygen is highly combustible and that they must never smoke while using oxygen.

## Pharmacotherapy

**ANTICOAGULATION.**   Patients with chronic thromboembolic disease require lifelong anticoagulation therapy, but chronic anticoagulation therapy is more controversial in patients with other forms of secondary pulmonary hypertension and cor pulmonale. There is evidence that severe pulmonary hypertension itself predisposes to in situ thrombosis in the pulmonary microvascular beds.[45] Low-blood-flow states resulting from poor cardiac output also predispose to pulmonary thromboembolism. In addition, once the patient experiences right heart failure, venous thrombosis and pulmonary embolism are frequent complications of venous stasis, dilated right heart chambers, and decreased physical activity. For these reasons, some have recommended anticoagulation for any patient with cor pulmonale whether or not overt right heart failure is present.[20]

Chronic anticoagulation therapy is generally indicated in patients with PPH. Histologically, the presence of thrombosis in the small pulmonary arteries and arterioles is common in patients with PPH. Both a retrospective analysis[17] and a small, nonrandomized prospective study[46] suggest that anticoagulation prolongs life in patients with PPH. Warfarin is the drug of choice, and it is used in doses adjusted to obtain an international normalized ratio of approximately 2.0.[37] Since right-sided heart failure may impair hepatic function, these patients must be monitored closely. In addition, caution is indicated in using anticoagulants in patients who manifest syncope or hemoptysis.

**DIURETICS, DIGITALIS, AND PHLEBOTOMY.**   Diuretics can be useful in relieving the volume overload state and hepatic congestion associated with right ventricular failure, but they should be given with care. The right ventricle is highly dependent on preload, and care should be taken to avoid excessive diuresis, which can lead to a fall in cardiac output. Contraction alkalosis aggravates respiratory insufficiency by depressing the effectiveness of carbon dioxide as a stimulus to breathing. In addition, diuresis may increase blood viscosity by increasing the hematocrit. Meticulous monitoring of serum electrolytes is mandatory.

The use of digitalis in patients with right ventricular dysfunction has been controversial. The risk of digitalis toxicity is enhanced in the setting of hypoxemia and diuretic-induced hypokalemia, and arrhythmias caused by digitalis may occur at relatively low serum levels in patients with pulmonary disease.[2] Despite this, studies have shown that digitalis can improve right ventricular function in cor pulmonale when given cautiously and carefully.[2,34] It should be given only when hypoxemia has been stabilized. It is also appropriate to give this drug when there is concurrent left ventricular systolic dysfunction.

Phlebotomy to decrease the circulating blood volume and reduce pulmonary artery pressure and pulmonary vascular resistance (PVR) may improve right ventricular function.[2,47] The benefit of phlebotomy is usually apparent only when polycythemia is severe and the hematocrit is above 60 to 65 percent. Repeated phlebotomies in small volumes (200 to 300 mL) may be necessary to sustain the benefit. In patients with precarious volume status, cell separator techniques with reinfusion of plasma are better tolerated.

**VASODILATORS.**   Vasodilator agents have been tried for various types of secondary pulmonary hypertension without much success. Unfortunately, vasodilator agents may aggravate arterial hypoxemia by exaggerating ventilation-perfusion abnormalities and can cause systemic hypotension.[22] At present, there is no justification for the long-term use of vasodilators in patients with COPD, interstitial fibrosis, or chronic thromboembolic disease. In alveolar hypoventilation syndromes, pharmacologic therapy is rarely needed because of the efficiency of oxygen therapy and assisted ventilation in promoting pulmonary vasodilatation. In systemic diseases associated with Raynaud's phenomenon, such as the CREST syndrome, there are potential beneficial effects of vasodilator therapy, but to date no long-term benefit has been proven.[22]

The use of vasodilator therapy for PPH has been more successful than its use for secondary causes of pulmonary hypertension. The goal of vasodilator therapy in PPH is to reduce pulmonary artery pressure and increase cardiac output without symptomatic systemic hypotension. This is successful in approximately one-fourth of PPH patients, a response that may be sustained indefinitely.[34,48] In approximately one-half of PPH patients, vasodilators will increase cardiac output without a reduction in mean pulmonary artery pressure, which may improve symptoms, but does not improve survival. In the remaining one-fourth of patients, vasodilators either lower systemic pressure without improvement in pulmonary artery pressure or cardiac output, or increase pulmonary artery pressure as a result of increased cardiac output. These patients probably have fixed pulmonary vasoconstriction and should not receive vasodilator therapy.

Before initiation of oral vasodilator therapy in patients with PPH, a pharmacologic challenge is required in order to identify patients who are likely to respond to long-term oral therapy. Typically, a potent, short-acting titratable vasodilator such as nitric oxide, epoprostenol (prostacyclin), or adenosine is acutely infused intravenously during right heart catheterization. Patients with a favorable response to this challenge are likely to have a sustained hemodynamic and symptomatic improvement and prolonged survival.[46,49] These patients may then be tried on long-term therapy.

The calcium channel blockers nifedipine and diltiazem have been the drugs most widely used for long-term therapy in PPH. Doses higher than those used to treat systemic hypertension (120 to 240 mg/day for nifedipine and up to 900 mg/day of diltiazem) are often necessary.[46,49] Empiric treatment is strongly discouraged. The major side effects of long-term vasodilator therapy include systemic hypotension, edema, and hypoxemia. Verapamil, oral nitrates, angiotensin-converting enzyme inhibitors, hydralazine, and beta-adrenergic agonists are not recommended.[22,34]

Epoprostenol, or prostacyclin, is an arachidonic acid metabolite that is continuously released by the vascular endothelium. It is a potent vasodilator, an inhibitor of platelet aggregation, and an inhibitor of smooth muscle proliferation. It is currently being used for long-term therapy in patients with PPH and has been shown to produce sustained hemodynamic and symptomatic improvement.[50,51] Epoprostenol must be given by continuous intravenous infusion because it has a very short half-life (2 to 3 min) and is inactivated by the low pH of the stomach. The drug is delivered with a portable infusion pump attached to a permanent indwelling central venous catheter. Dose requirements tend to increase over time.[37] Interruption of the infusion may lead to an immediate return of symptoms, which may be severe and life-threatening.[37] Drug-induced side effects are common and include jaw pain, cutaneous erythema, diarrhea, and arthralgias.

Epoprostenol may produce sustained hemodynamic responses even in patients who have insignificant responses to acute infusion of the drug.[51] This may be explained by actions of the drug other than vasodilatation, such as inhibition of platelet aggregation and smooth muscle proliferation. For this reason, epoprostenol can be initiated without a challenge. Epoprostenol has been used as primary therapy or as a bridge to transplantation in patients with PPH.[37]

Nitric oxide is an endothelial cell–derived relaxing factor that contributes to the low tone of the pulmonary circulation. It is synthesized from the amino acid L-arginine by the enzyme nitric oxide synthase. As a vasodilator, it has the advantage of selectively relaxing the pulmonary vasculature without affecting systemic arterial pressure. It is currently being tested in a wide variety of pulmonary hypertensive states, including PPH.[22,37]

## Transplantation

Single-lung, double-lung, and heart-lung transplantation have been used for the treatment of end-stage lung disease associated with right-sided heart failure in several pulmonary diseases, including primary pulmonary hypertension, emphysema, idiopathic pulmonary fibrosis, and cystic fibrosis.[2] Patients with severe right-sided heart failure, hepatomegaly, hyperbilirubinemia, and ascites are not suitable candidates for transplantation because these conditions have been associated with excessive mortality.[34] The widespread use of transplantation is limited by the number of specialized transplantation centers and the availability of suitable donor organs. Combined heart-lung transplantation has been the procedure of choice for many bilateral pulmonary disorders, although single- and double-lung transplantations are becoming more widely performed. Survival rates for heart-lung and lung transplantation are similar, and the waiting time for a lung transplant is one-half that for a combined heart-lung transplant.[34,37] Even markedly depressed right ventricular function can improve after lung transplantion.[52]

One-year survival rates after lung transplantation for PPH range from 65 to 70 percent.[53] The operative mortality rates for lung transplantation in patients with PPH are significantly higher than those in patients who have other indications for transplantation.[53] Recurrence of PPH after transplantation has not been reported.[37]

The major posttransplantation problems are acute organ rejection, bronchiolitis obliterans, and opportunistic infection. The incidence of bronchiolitis obliterans is high (25 to 40 percent), and it is higher in heart-lung transplantation than in single-lung transplantation.[34] Bronchiolitis obliterans is more frequent in patients with PPH.[54]

Transplantation is considered the treatment of last resort. This is particularly true in PPH, where there has been ever-improving success with the use of medical therapy, particularly epoprostenol. In patients with PPH, transplantation is considered for patients with New York Heart Association functional class III or IV who are refractory to medical management.[34]

## REFERENCES

1. World Health Organization: Chronic cor pulmonale: Report of an expert committee. *Circulation* 1963; 27:594–615.
2. Newman JH, Ross JC: Chronic cor pulmonale. In: Alexander RW, Schlant RC, Fuster V, et al. (eds): *Hurst's The Heart*, 9th ed. New York, McGraw-Hill, 1998:1739–1749.
3. Murphy ML, Dinh H, Nicholson D: Chronic cor pulmonale. *Dis-A-Month* 1989; 35(10):653–718.
4. Rubin LJ (ed): *Pulmonary Heart Disease*. Boston, Martinus Nijhoff, 1984.

5.  Fishman AP: Pulmonary hypertension and cor pulmonale. In: Fishman AP (ed): *Pulmonary Diseases and Disorders,* 2d ed. New York, McGraw-Hill, 1988:999–1048.

6.  Bohr DF: The pulmonary hypoxic response. State of field. *Chest* 1977; 71:244–246.

7.  Rubin LJ: Clinical evaluation. In: Rubin LJ (ed): *Pulmonary Heart Disease.* Boston, Martinus Nijhoff, 1984:107–116.

8.  Voelkel N, Reeves JT: Primary pulmonary hypertension. In: Moser KM (ed): *Pulmonary Vascular Diseases.* New York, Marcel Dekker, 1979:609–611.

9.  Flint FJ: Cor pulmonale. *Lancet* 1954; 2:51–58.

10. Wilmshurst PT, Webb-Peploe MM, Cohen RS: Left recurrent laryngeal nerve palsy associated with primary pulmonary hypertension and recurrent pulmonary embolism. *Br Heart J* 1983; 49:141–143.

11. Fanta CH, Wright R, McFadden ER: Differentiation of recurrent pulmonary emboli from chronic obstructive lung disease as a cause of cor pulmonale. *Chest* 1981; 79:92–95.

12. Padmavati S, Raizada V: Electrocardiogram in chronic cor pulmonale. *Br Heart J* 1972; 34:658–667.

13. Hurst JW: *Ventricular Electrocardiography.* New York, Gower, 1991:9.3.

13a. McGinn S, White PD: Acute cor pulmonale resulting from pulmonary embolism: Its clinical recognition. *JAMA* 1935; 104(17):1475.

13b. Baljepally R, Spodick DH: Electrocardiographic screening for emphysema: The frontal plane P axis. *Clin Cardiol* 1999; 22:226–228.

14. Ravin CE, Greenspan RH, McLond TL, et al: Redistribution of pulmonary blood flow secondary to pulmonary arterial hypertension. *Invest Radiol* 1980; 15:29–33.

15. Ravin CE: Roentgenographic evaluation of pulmonary heart disease. In: Rubin LJ (ed): *Pulmonary Heart Disease.* Boston, Martinus Nijhoff, 1984:135–136.

16. Himelman RB, Struve SN, Brown JK, et al: Improved recognition of cor pulmonale in patients with severe chronic obstructive pulmonary disease. *Am J Med* 1988; 84:891–898.

17. Fuster V, Steele PM, Edwards WD, et al: Primary pulmonary hypertension: Natural history and importance of thrombosis. *Circulation* 1984; 70:580–587.

18. Rich S, Dantzker DR, Ayers SM, et al: Primary pulmonary hypertension: A national prospective study. *Ann Intern Med* 1987; 107:216–223.

19. Nicod P, Peterson K, Levine M, et al: Pulmonry angiography in severe chronic pulmonary hypertension. *Ann Intern Med* 1987; 107:565–568.

20. Palevsky HI, Fishman AP: Chronic cor pulmonale. *JAMA* 1990; 263:2347–2353.

21. Reid LM: Chronic obstructive pulmonary disease. In: Fishman AP (ed): *Pulmonary Diseases and Disorders,* 2d ed. New York, McGraw-Hill, 1988:1247–1472.

22. Fishman AP: Pulmonary hypertension. In: Alexander RW, Schlant RC, Fuster V, et al (eds): *Hurst's The Heart,* 9th ed. New York, McGraw-Hill, 1998:1699–1717.

23. Millman RP, Fishman AP: Disorders of alveolar ventilation. In: Fishman AP (ed): *Pulmonary Diseases and Disorders,* 2d ed. New York, McGraw-Hill, 1988:1335–1346.

24. Millman RP, Fishman AP: Sleep apnea syndromes. In: Fishman AP (ed): *Pulmonary Diseases and Disorders,* 2d ed. New York, McGraw-Hill, 1988:1347–1362.

25. Kelley MA, Fishman AP: Pulmonary thromboembolic disease. In: Fishman AP (ed): *Pulmonary Diseases and Disorders,* 2d ed. New York, McGraw-Hill, 1988:1059–1086.

26. Powe JE, Palevsky HI, McCarthy KE, Alavi A: Usefulness of lung scanning in the evaluation of patients with pulmonary arterial hypertension. *Radiology* 1987; 164:727–730.

27. PIOPED Investigators: Value of ventilation perfusion scan in acute pulmonary embolism. Results of the prospective investigation of pulmonary embolism diagnosis. *JAMA* 1990; 263:2753–2759.

28.  Asherson RA, Oakley CM: Pulmonary hypertension and systemic lupus erythematosus. *J Rheumatol* 1986; 13:1–5.

29.  Stapi AM, Steen VD, Owens GD, et al: Pulmonary hypertension in CREST syndrome variant of systemic sclerosis (scleroderma). *Arthritis Rheum* 1986; 29:515–524.

30.  Rich S, Grossman W, Braunwald E: Pulmonary hypertension. In: Braunwald E (ed): *Heart Disease*, 5th ed. Philadelphia, W. B. Saunders Company, 1997:780–806.

31.  Kane RD, Hawkins HK, Miller JA, Noce PS: Microscopic pulmonary tumor emboli associated with dyspnea. *Cancer* 1975; 36:1473.

32.  Jacques JE, Barclay R: The solid sarcomatous pulmonary artery. *Br J Dis Chest* 1974; 11:123.

33.  McDonnell PJ, Toye PA, Hutchins GM: Primary pulmonary hypertension and cirrhosis: Are they related? *Am Rev Respir Dis* 1983; 127:437–441.

34.  Rubin LJ: ACCP Consensus statement: Primary pulmonary hypertension. *Chest* 1993; 104:236–250.

35.  Rubin LJ: Pathology and pathophysiology of primary pulmonary hypertension. *Am J Cardiol* 1995; 75:51A–54A.

36.  Abenhaim L, Moride Y, Brenot F, et al: Appetite-suppressant drugs and the risk of primary pulmonary hypertension. *N Engl J Med* 1996; 335:609–616.

37.  Rubin LJ: Primary pulmonary hypertension. *N Engl J Med* 1997; 336:111–117.

38.  Rich S, Brundage BH: Pulmonary hypertension: A cellular basis for understanding the pathophysiology and treatment. *J Am Coll Cardiol* 1989; 14:545.

39.  D'Alonzo GE, Barst RJ, Ayers SM, et al: Survival in patients with primary pulmonary hypertension: Results from a national prospective registry. *Ann Intern Med* 1991; 115:343–349.

40.  Eysmann SB, Palevsky HI, Reicheck N, et al: Two-dimension and Doppler-echocardiographic and cardiac catheterization correlates of survival in primary pulmonary hypertension. *Circulation* 1989; 80:353.

41.  Tarpy SP, Celli BR: Long-term oxygen therapy. *N Engl J Med* 1995; 333:710–714.

42.  Weitzenblum E, Sautegeau A, Ehrhart M, et al: Long-term oxygen therapy can reverse the progression of pulmonary hypertension in patients with chronic obstructive pulmonary disease. *Am Rev Respir Dis* 1985; 131:493–498.

43.  Nocturnal Oxygen Therapy Trial Group: Continuous or nocturnal oxygen therapy in hypoxemic chronic obstructive lung disease: A clinical trial. *Ann Intern Med* 1980; 93:391–398.

44.  Levi-Valensi P, Weitzenblum E, Rida Z, et al: Sleep-related oxygen desaturation and daytime pulmonary haemodynamics in COPD patients. *Eur Respir J* 1992; 5:301–307.

45.  Chaouat A, Weitzenblum E, Higgenbottam T: The role of thrombosis in severe pulmonary hypertension. *Eur Respir J* 1996; 9:356–363.

46.  Rich S, Kaufman E, Levy PS: The effect of high doses of calcium-channel blockers on survival in primary pulmonary hypertension. *N Engl J Med* 1992; 327:76–81.

47.  Weisse AB, Moshcos CB, Frank MJ, et al.: Hemodynamic effects of staged hematocrit reduction in patients with stable cor pulmonale and severely elevated hematocrit levels. *Am J Med* 1975; 58:92–98.

48.  Rich S: Medical treatment of primary pulmonary hypertension: A bridge to transplantation? *Am J Cardiol* 1995; 75:63A–66A.

49.  Rich S, Brundage BH: High-dose calcium channel-blocking therapy for primary pulmonary hypertension: Evidence for long-term reduction in pulmonary arterial pressure and regression of right ventricular hypertrophy. *Circulation* 1987; 76:135–141.

50.  Rubin LJ, Mendoza J, Hood M, et al: Treatment of primary pulmonary hypertension with continuous intravenous prostacyclin (epoprostenol). *Ann Intern Med* 1990; 112:485–491.

51.  Barst RJ, Rubin LJ, Long WA, et al: A comparison of continuous intravenous epoprostenol (prostacyclin) with conventional therapy for primary pulmonary hypertension. *N Engl J Med* 1996; 334:296–301.

52.  Pasque MK, Trulock EP, Kaiser LR, Cooper JD: Single-lung transplantation for pulmonary hypertension: Three-month hemodynamic follow-up. *Circulation* 1991; 84:2275–2279.

53.  Hosenpud JD, Novick RJ, Bennett LE, et al: The Registry of the International Society for Heart and Lung Transplantation: Thirteenth official report—1996. *J Heart Lung Transplant* 1996; 15:655–674.

54.  Kshettry VR, Kroshus TJ, Savik K, et al: Primary pulmonary hypertension as a risk factor for the development of obliterative bronchiolitis in lung allograft recipients. *Chest* 1996; 110:704–709.

# PART

# 4

# CARDIOVASCULAR TOPICS OF SPECIAL INTEREST FOR PRIMARY CARE PRACTICE

WILLIAM S. WEINTRAUB /
KIMBERLY RASK

CHAPTER

# COST-EFFECTIVE CARDIOVASCULAR CARE

# 44

In the recent past, it was sufficient for physicians to show that a therapy was effective or that a particular diagnostic strategy provided clinical information. Thereafter, providers could charge the usual and customary charge and expect insurance companies and Medicare to pay for it. Escalating medical care costs as well as other pressures within our society have made this untenable. New forms of diagnostic testing and therapies, and existing ones as well, will have to be justified on economic grounds as well as on efficacy grounds. When diagnostic or therapeutic options are being considered, both the cost and the relationship of cost to outcome are questioned. This has given birth to a new discipline called clinical microeconomics. As with many new fields, the goals of this field are, as yet, not entirely well defined, and the methods are still being developed. The problems of assessment of costs and comparison to efficacy are especially relevant when considering expensive forms of therapy that are commonly used and have multiple complex and interrelating indices of outcome. To perhaps no single area within medicine are these issues as relevant as to cardiovascular care.

## PURPOSES AND GOALS OF ECONOMIC ANALYSES

Economic analyses in medicine can involve macroeconomic policy issues or microeconomic assessment of any aspect of health care. This review will concentrate on microeconomic assessment of diagnostics and therapy. The goal may be to assess the cost of a test or therapy or to compare two tests or therapies. For instance, the goal of one study may be to quantify the direct medical costs of coronary angioplasty, whereas another study may compare the costs of coronary angioplasty (PTCA) to the costs of coronary surgery (CABG) for a particular group of patients. Two treatments or two diagnostic strategies can be compared through a prospective randomized controlled trial or, more frequently, by making use of existing databases. Randomized trials permit comparison in a matched population that is free of selection bias. Database studies, although more timely and generally less expensive, will always suffer from selection bias. One advantage of database studies is that a broader population may be considered than in a randomized trial.

There are three related forms of economic analysis that may be used to study relative efficacies and relative costs. Cost-effectiveness analysis measures the cost per unit of effectiveness.[1] This form of analysis assumes that one measure of effectiveness can be achieved, often survival or quality of life–adjusted years. This method breaks down when there are multiple measures of effectiveness. This problem may, in principle, be addressed through cost-utility analysis, in which all measures of effectiveness are incorporated into one measure called utility.[2] There are clear-cut and well-known limitations to determining utility. Different approaches to measuring utility will be addressed in the following section. A third, and somewhat less popular, form of analysis is cost-benefit analysis, in which measures of both cost and effectiveness are reduced to a single measure, generally dollars (or some other currency).[3] Clinicians often find this form of analysis to be confusing (or perhaps just more confusing than cost-effectiveness and cost-utility analysis).

How should these analyses be used? In principle, all that is needed is to choose the therapy or diagnostic strategy that costs less per unit increase in effectiveness than the alternatives. If one choice of therapy or testing can be convincingly shown to be both more effective and less expensive than the competing therapy, there can be little argument. If one choice is more effective, but at a higher cost, then the decision as to whether the therapy or test in question is worth spending money on is a societal decision. When efficacy and costs are uncertain, as is often the case, the decision is even harder. Cost-effectiveness analyses cannot in and of themselves set policy. If only effectiveness is important, then the most effective choice will be chosen, regardless of cost. If only saving money is important, then the least expensive choice will be chosen. Cost-effectiveness analyses are naturally of greatest interest to policy makers who must weigh selection of therapy or diagnostics given limited resources.

Different shareholders have different stakes in the outcome. Physicians and patients have traditionally been more concerned about effectiveness. The separation of concerns over effectiveness and costs to different stockholders has removed the normal market mechanism governed by willingness to pay.[4-7] Employers and insurance companies have been more concerned about costs. To be most useful, cost-effectiveness analysis should be performed from a societal perspective. Such a perspective attempts to measure all of the costs associated with a particular treatment—the costs incurred by the patient, the costs of medical resources that could have been used for other patients, and any loss of income that the patient sustained because of poor health. By looking at all of these costs, a policy maker could decide, for example, whether a given population's health status would be improved by allocating limited health care resources to a lipid screening program or to subsidized hypertensive medications.

Complete analyses of this type are difficult to perform and so are infrequently done. They are used most often in countries with centralized health care plans. In the United States, cost studies tend to be focused cost-effectiveness analyses that compare two alternative treatments for a single medical condition, for example, PTCA and CABG for symptomatic angina. In addition to focusing on a single clinical condition, the analyses most commonly limit the measured costs to direct and indirect medical costs. The following section will describe common strategies for measuring costs related to cardiovascular treatments.

# METHODS FOR DETERMINING COSTS

Medical costs for a procedure such as coronary surgery can be naturally broken down into three components: in-hospital direct costs, follow-up direct costs, and indirect costs. Inpatient hospital costs comprise hospital costs (e.g., room, lab testing, pharmacy, etc.) and physician professional billings. Follow-up direct costs include physician office visits, outpatient testing, medications, home health providers, and additional hospitalizations. Indirect costs reflect opportunity costs from loss of work or other economic losses to the patient, family, and business. The appropriate length of time over which to measure costs is dependent upon the procedures being studied and the outcome that is being measured. There may well be very different levels of resource consumption after hospital discharge for patients undergoing bypass surgery as opposed to those undergoing coronary angioplasty, for example.

The most common first source for hospital costs is hospital charges. Hospital charges may be gathered from line item charges of every single item consumed or from grouped charges generally prepared by hospital finance departments. The most commonly used source in nonfederal hospitals is the UB-92, in which the charges are grouped into categories. This is a uniform billing statement used by all third-party carriers. Charges are available for, but not limited to, such services as the surgical suite, the cardiac catheterization laboratory, the intensive care unit, postoperative or postprocedural floor care, respiratory therapy, physical therapy, pulmonary functions, anesthesia, the recovery room, medical and surgical supplies, laboratory costs, pharmaceutical costs, pulmonary functions, ECG, telemetry, and social services. The data elements were determined by the National Uniform Billing Committee, which included representatives from the Health Care Financing Agency (HCFA), Blue Cross, and multiple other national organizations.

However, there is a very real difference between hospital charges and costs.[8] While hospitals will generally follow the American Hospital Association guidelines in setting charges, charges are known to vary widely. Hospitals will set their charges to maximize insurance reimbursements. This does not always mean setting the highest price for a service, but it does mean that the relationship of cost to charges is tenuous. What is the economic cost of a service? From a societal perspective, the economic cost is the cost of the resources consumed to deliver the service. From an employer's or insurance company's perspective, the payment made for the service represents the cost because this is the payer's cost. Most cost studies have measured the resources consumed because the results are more generalizable. Approximating or measuring resources used is not simply "counting," since the costs of many services are shared in ways that may be very difficult to separate. For instance, how much of a pharmacist's time goes into dispensing an aspirin? Worse yet, how much of the operating room expense can be meaningfully applied to one patient undergoing a cholecystectomy? Cross subsidies are inevitable in a business that offers multiple products. When a business (hospital) offers many products, it is difficult to definitely determine the production cost of any individual product. Accountants try to allocate costs using either "top-down" or "bottom-up" methods. In top-down methods, all of the expenses or costs of a particular department, such as the operating room, are determined, and then all of the billed charges are totaled. By dividing the total costs by the total charges, a fraction is produced. For any one patient, the cost of the operating room would be the charge multiplied by this ratio. Although relatively simple, this method may be criticized as being too broad to describe differing services. For instance, a chest x-ray would not be expected to have the same cost-to-charge ratio as an intravenous pyelogram. More sophisticated bottom-up accounting approaches in which the resource utilization for each hospital procedure is directly accounted for are being developed and implemented.[9–12] The importance of determining cost accurately varies with different audiences. The health services research community may be well satisfied with approximations using departmental cost-to-charge ratios, understanding that there is considerable error. However, to hospital administrators who must set prices, the issue of defining cost more accurately becomes crucial as profit margins narrow.

Another issue when measuring hospital or procedure costs is average versus marginal cost. Average costs include all resources used, including fixed resources or overhead whose costs would not be decreased if they were not utilized. Marginal costing accepts fixed costs as a given and focuses only on variable costs, or those additional resources consumed by each additional patient. Separating fixed from variable costs is done by establishing the perspective and time frame of the analyses. For instance, the costs of facilities are often sunk or fixed costs. However, how do you determine the marginal cost of operating room staff? If coronary surgery decreases as angioplasty becomes more common, do the operating room nurses remain on staff in the operating room, or will they be assigned to other duties?

Hlatky et al[13] have developed four methods of measuring marginal costs: (1) cost of supplies, (2) cost of personnel and supplies, (3) average direct costs, and (4) average direct costs plus hospital overhead. Although each of the methods has its disadvantages, any one of them is superior to the use of hospital charges. The importance of marginal costs may also vary with the audience. For instance, policy planners may be more interested in average costs because that is what they pay. Hospital administrators may be more interested in marginal costs because it is the cost relative to reimbursement for the next patient that determines whether a patient can be operated on profitably. Given the difficulties in measuring marginal costs, most hospital cost studies use average costs.

Assessing professional costs for procedures presents additional challenges. It is not sufficient to consider the surgeon's or the angioplasty operator's fee alone, as other professionals provide services in each of these cases. The goal must be to capture all of the professional services for a procedure. For coronary surgery, this may include fees for the surgeon, his or her assistants, the consultant cardiologist, the anesthetist, the radiologist, the clinical pathologist, professionals involved in other testing, and any other consultants. It is necessary to create a profile of the professional services delivered and then assess the costs of those services. One method is to use the Medicare diagnosis-related group (DRG) reimbursement rate and the Medicare allowable physician charge to estimate cost. The disadvantages of this method are that the average DRG payment may not adequately describe an individual hospitalization, and the primary physician allowable charge does not account for the multiple other physician charges associated with a hospitalization. Simulated hospital charges may, at times, be needed when actual cost data are not available. However, the simulated estimate should be based on real data from as similar a hospitalization as possible. In any case, real data will always be more compelling than simulations based on uncertain sources.

Professional charges have not historically been subject to the same type of accounting scrutiny as hospital charges. In fact, a substantial amount of health economics literature documents the distortions in the market for physician services and the fact that this market does not satisfy the economic conditions for being reasonably competitive on physician prices.[14] If a surgeon charges $5000 for coronary surgery, is this a reasonable estimate of the charge or the costs? In 1991, the Health Insurance Association of America collected mean surgical charges for a three-vessel CABG and found that physician charges were: New York City, $8189; Philadelphia, $6118; Atlanta, $4656; Chicago, $5902; Denver, $4499; Dallas, $2461; and Los Angeles, $6375.[15] The range in physician charges for the three-vessel CABG among these seven major U.S. cities is $5728. Few health care researchers would be confident that the wide variation is due to significant cost differences. Furthermore, using physician payments rather than charges as a gauge of costs does little to improve the estimates. Given the widespread variation in insurance arrangements, physician payments are still significantly distorted and biased.

There has been an effort to rationalize physician payments by developing a set of scales for services. This system, called the resource-based relative value scale (RBRVS), was developed over a period of years and involved many physician consultants, who tried to assess the relative time and physical and cognitive efforts associated with physician services.[16,17] Each service is assigned a number called the relative value units (RVUs). If the profile of physician services for a procedure or hospitalization is known, then RVUs for each service may be used to develop a proxy for the physician costs. The total RVUs may be converted to a dollar figure by a conversion factor. The HCFA, the federal agency that administers Medicare and Medicaid, has a standard conversion factor. The appeal of the RBRVS is that it is a relative weighting system that assigns unique weights for physician work and practice costs for each physician service by CPT-4 code. As a result, after assigning a conversion factor, standardized estimates of the costs can be calculated and used as a gauge of physician costs. While there are still some problems with this approach and experience is limited, especially for the practice cost values in the RBRVS, it holds considerable promise and overcomes some of the major drawbacks in physician charge data.[18] A significant challenge in using the RBRVS is the need to get a complete and accurate profile of physician services for any hospitalization or procedure in order to generate RVUs.

Determining the costs of follow-up care presents a different set of challenges. To determine costs during follow-up, it is essential to determine patient utilization of services, including direct medical costs and indirect costs. Direct costs include medical services such as additional hospitalizations, physician office visits, medications, procedures and testing, rehabilitation, nursing home stays, and home health services. Direct nonmedical costs include out-of-pocket expenses and travel to receive medical care. While the particular services used may be assessed by mailout questionnaires or telephone interviews, patients may not know how much they spend for services. This is complicated by insurance, as patients cannot be expected to reliably report how much they paid out of pocket for services and how much the insurance company paid for services. Unless there is access to a comprehensive insurance claims database, the most reasonable approach is to have patients identify the services they have received. Costs can then be attributed to the individual services and medications. Follow-up hospitalizations may be assessed by obtaining the charges, as discussed above, or costs may be estimated from similar hospitalizations for which data are available. Costs of office visits and other medical services may be similarly estimated. Costs of medications may be estimated by compiling a list of medication prices from several pharmacies. Using these cost estimates, a partial simulation of postdischarge direct costs may be determined. In determining services utilized, random repeat sampling of some fraction of the population should be performed to determine the validity of the data set.

Indirect costs include time missed from work by the patient or family members. Follow-up indirect costs are probably the most difficult to determine and are often excluded as immeasurable. In any case, it is not possible to directly measure all of the indirect costs and to perfectly define the boundaries of these costs. For instance, if an executive in a company has coronary surgery and is out of work for 6 weeks, there may or may not be loss of pay. There is, however, an effect on the business that cannot readily be determined. Indirect costs, if measured at all, are often confined to family loss of income. There are two methods to measure indirect costs—direct survey and simulation. The direct survey will have errors in that there may be uncertainty as to income loss and patients may be uncomfortable revealing this information. If this method is used, the reported income loss should be validated through another source. At the very least, a number of patients chosen at random should be resurveyed to determine reproducibility. Alternatively, a simulation can be performed in which lost work time is estimated and a dollar cost attached based on type of job. Sources of data used to construct such a simulation will require validation. Measuring indirect costs using either method creates a bias in that time spent in higher-paying jobs becomes more valued. Although loss of work may create a bigger problem for a laborer and his or her family than for a highly paid business executive, a treatment that decreases work loss for the higher-paid employees will be more cost-effective than one that is equally effective but returns lower-paid employees to work. In any case, if indirect costs are estimated, the numbers must be examined with both interest and skepticism as to their accuracy.

In all treatment studies, the validity of underlying data is crucial. In clinical studies, the investigator is responsible for assessing and attesting to the validity of the data. This is just as important in economic studies. The methods used to assess costs from financial and self-report claims data are necessarily based on a set of assumptions. When analyses have a long time horizon, inflation becomes a consideration. Costs must be inflated or deflated by multiplying by a constant to convert from any one year to another, based on the medical inflation rate. In the same sense that effect sizes are considered subject to confidence intervals, cost estimates must be considered an attempt to estimate a value that cannot truly be measured. Sensitivity analysis, a standardized approach to varying parameters, can be used to identify which study assumptions are critical to the final cost-effectiveness results.

# COMPARING COSTS TO OUTCOME

The determination of procedure costs independent of how these costs relate to patient outcomes is not helpful for clinical decision making or policy making. Several different methods have been developed to attempt to relate costs to outcome.

## Determination of Patient Utility

In the treatment of coronary artery disease (CAD), it is unusual for one measurement of outcome to be sufficiently important clinically that all other outcome measures may be ignored for the purpose of clinical decision making. While death overwhelms other outcome measures in importance when it occurs, its relative infrequency over several years of follow-up compared to myocardial infarction, unstable angina, revascularization procedures, measures of quality of life, and return to work make it necessary to consider all outcome measures together. In principle this may be accomplished through the determination of patient utility.

The utility of a procedure is the sum of benefits, both positive and negative, that flow to a patient over time as the result of the procedure.[19–21] It is, in principle, all-encompassing. We may begin the assessment of utility with a decision tree (Fig. 44-1). In this model, nodes with squares represent choices and nodes with circles represent chance events. In the simplified model shown, a single choice is made, and for each choice there are two possible outcomes. Each outcome is called a health state. Each health state has a utility and a probability of occurrence. The utility of choice A in Fig. 44-1 is the sum of the utility of health state 1 times its probability plus the utility of health state 2 times its probability. If choices were this simple, then determining the utility of diagnostics or therapeutics would be simple. However, decision trees are almost never this simple. The decision trees for diagnostic tests tend to be much more complicated than those for therapeutics because

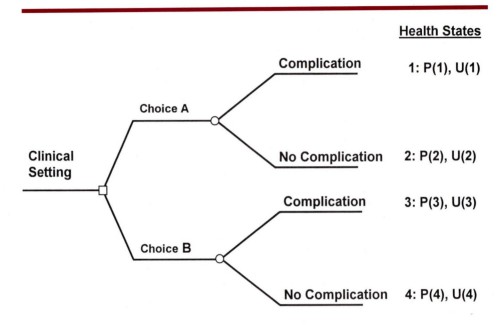

**Health States**

**Complication**    1: P(1), U(1)

**Choice A**

**Clinical Setting**

**No Complication**    2: P(2), U(2)

**Complication**    3: P(3), U(3)

**Choice B**

**No Complication**    4: P(4), U(4)

**P(x): Probability of Health State X**
**U(x): Utility of Health State X**

Figure 44-1   Idealized decision tree for a decision on diagnostic strategy or therapeutic choice.

a test can lead to additional tests or to a range of therapeutic alternatives. For any one treatment, there may be multiple possible health states, and the paucity of clinical literature may make it difficult to determine the probability of each of the different health states, much less the utility associated with each health state.

Utility, like health status, changes over time. We may compare the utility after coronary angioplasty if a patient either does or does not suffer restenosis in Fig. 44-2. After successful coronary angioplasty, the patient feels well and utility rises, but then the patient may suffer restenosis and utility falls. After successful redilatation, utility rises again. After angioplasty that is not complicated by restenosis, utility gradually rises. Ultimately, the patients get to the same point, but the patient who had the episode of restenosis suffered a period of decreased utility. Utility also cannot be aggregated across patients, as patients may value things differently. One patient may dislike chest pain sufficiently to be willing to undergo repeat procedures to relieve angina. Another patient may dislike the catheterization suite sufficiently to be willing to put up with more angina. Given this limitation, investigators may wish to try to include several measures of outcome into a summary measure called utility, recognizing that this is not "utility" in strict economic terms. The measurement of utility is a complex process that is beyond the scope of this review. The interested reader is referred to a monograph and several excellent references.[2,22–25]

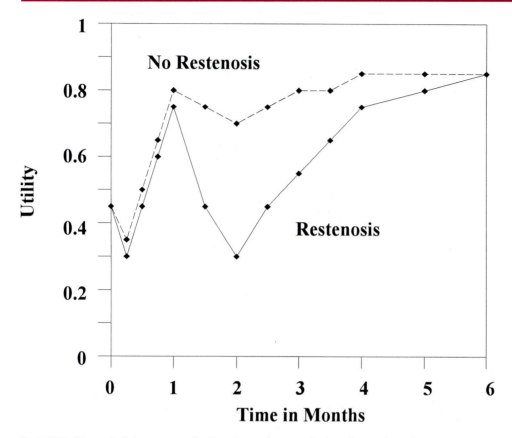

**Figure 44-2**   Theoretical time course of utility after coronary angioplasty in a patient who does not suffer restenosis (top line) and a patient who does suffer restenosis (bottom line).

Utility by itself does not provide a final summary measure of outcome because it does not include life expectancy. This may be approached through the concept of quality-adjusted life years (QALYs).[26] QALYs are calculated by combining utility and survival.[27] Median or mean survival must be estimated either from the data set under consideration or from the literature. Survival is generally discounted, which means that patients value a year of survival at the present time more than a year of survival in the future. The "true" discount rate for survival is unknown. Values in the literature for the discount rate have varied from 2 to 10 percent. Thus, with a discount rate of 3 percent, next year's survival is 3 percent less important than this year's survival. The choice of an appropriate discount rate is highly technical and beyond the scope of this review. Whatever the chosen discount rate, QALYs is the best summary measure of outcome in cost-utility analysis because it incorporates patient value, risk aversion, expected survival, and a discount rate—although each of these components is, of course, subject to error.

## Cost-Effectiveness and Cost-Utility Analysis

Many published cost-effectiveness analyses are simulations in which the medical literature is used to define the patient population and expected outcomes from procedures, and then dollar costs are estimated for the procedure. Such analyses can provide insight into the decision-making process but are not likely to have the same impact on either the clinical community or policy makers as cost-effectiveness analysis based on observed data. Cost-effectiveness analysis based on clinical data within observational databases has the limitation of selection bias when it is used to compare two therapies. Cost-effectiveness analysis conducted within a clinical trial suffers from the potentially narrow range of patients within the trial. Each type of analysis has its own place and may be used to answer somewhat different questions. Given the measurement difficulties in performing cost-utility analysis to compare one form of therapy to another—for instance, coronary angioplasty to coronary surgery—most economic studies have been based upon simulations. The following comments on cost-effectiveness or cost-utility analysis apply to simulations, observational studies, and clinical trials.

Once cost and a measure of outcome are available, it is, in principle, simple to determine cost-effectiveness. Cost-effectiveness is the change in cost per unit increase in effectiveness. If the summary measure is in QALYs, then the cost-effectiveness of procedure X compared to procedure Y is described as the dollars per quality-adjusted year of life gained. As discussed previously, however, there is uncertainty in the measurement of cost as well as in the measurement of effectiveness.

Uncertainty in clinical microeconomics is generally approached through sensitivity analysis. With sensitivity analysis, measurements in which there is uncertainty are varied across appropriate ranges and the analysis is repeated. If just one measurement of outcome, such as $X$ dollars per QALY, is reported, the uncertainty cannot be accounted for and the result would be subject to skepticism. The problem with sensitivity analysis is knowing the appropriate ranges for the variables. For measurements made using several different scales, such as the multiple models for calculating marginal costs, these different scales may be used to perform the sensitivity analysis. For measurements that are continuous, such as professional charges, one standard deviation of the charge might be appropriate. There is, however, no absolute standard for sensitivity analysis other than common sense and an intuitive feel for what is medically reasonable. For instance, Weinstein and Stason[28] used a variation in the severity of angina to decrease QALYs from 0 for no angina to 50 percent for severe disabling angina. If the results of a study vary significantly with changes in certain variables, then the outcome is said to be sensitive for those variables. Properly performed, sensitivity analysis should give insight into the medical decision-making process by identifying thresholds that result in changes in medical decision making. For instance, in the same study by Weinstein and Stason,[28] a threshold was noted for single-vessel disease such that if a patient were sufficiently bothered by angina to be willing to give up 8 percent of life expectancy, then coronary surgery was indicated, excluding concerns about cost.

Cost-effectiveness or cost-utility analysis can also be performed in patient subgroups. In comparing coronary surgery to coronary angioplasty, for example, natural subgroups could be defined by number of diseased vessels, left ventricular function, age, gender, socioeconomic group, employment status, and probably a host of other variables as well. If the cost-effectiveness analysis is performed within the context of a clinical trial, then the ability to do subgroup analysis is governed by the same limitations as a standard efficacy analysis within clinical trials, namely adequate statistical power and the danger of looking at too many subgroups in a post hoc fashion. In principle, the best practice is to set up the subgroups of interest at the outset and make sure that there is sufficient statistical power to do the analyses within the subgroups.

## Applications in Patient Care

To overcome some of the methodological problems outlined above, economists have begun to employ more sophisticated econometric methods that permit an assessment of the relationship of multiple clinical and cost variables to several indicators of outcome. A popular method is the multiple-indicator multiple-cause (MIMIC) model.[29–31] While in previous approaches certain outcome indicators would be selected and used as proxies for effectiveness or a scale would be developed to incorporate several variables into one final outcome measure, econometric methods such as MIMIC permit assessment of how multiple outcome measures interact. MIMIC is a confirmatory factor analysis that assumes that multiple causes affect multiple indicators through a latent variable (health) and estimates the relationship between the multiple causes and multiple indicators. Using such an approach, however, the true health improvement is not observed. Instead, the relationship of multiple outcome indicators, substituting for the latent health improvement, can be related to clinical variables, including choice of therapy, as well as cost. The MIMIC model has recently been successfully applied to the Energy Angioplasty versus Surgery Trial (EAST) study, which compared the outcome of coronary angioplasty and bypass surgery in the treatment of CAD.[32]

An increasingly common approach to providing optimal patient care is to develop algorithmic approaches to care, sometimes called care maps or practice guidelines. While these terms are often used to mean the same thing, care maps are generally locally derived algorithms for patient care and may be highly detailed, while practice guidelines are usually developed by professional societies or government agencies to provide an evidence-based approach to medical decision making. For instance, a care map may detail which blood tests should be drawn after angioplasty and when, while a practice guideline may provide information on appropriateness criteria for angioplasty. Properly constructed care maps and guidelines should consider contingent probability and cost-effectiveness.

First we consider contingent probability.[33] With any diagnostic test, there is uncertainty as to prior probability (the probability of disease before the test), sensitivity (the probability of a test's being positive if the disease is present), specificity (the probability of a test's being negative if the disease is absent), predictive value (the probability of a disease's being present if the test is positive), and predictive error (the probability of disease if a test is negative). Determination of sensitivity and specificity requires a reliable and, in the case of CAD, more invasive gold standard. Furthermore, there are a series of biases that limit determination of sensitivity and specificity for diagnostic tests.[34,35] We are most interested in predictive value because we seek to know if a patient has a disease, given a positive test result. If prior probability, sensitivity, and specificity are known, then the predictive value may be determined by Bayes' theorem.[36] A positive test will increase the posttest probability, while a negative one will decrease it (Fig. 44-3). The better the test (the higher the sensitivity and specificity), the more the posttest probability will be affected. Diagnostic testing will most affect predictive value if the prior probability is in the mid-range. Thus, when testing for CAD, it makes sense to perform a noninvasive test if there is real uncertainty as to the diagnosis. If instead the diagnosis is almost certain, testing will only confirm the diagnosis and rarely change the diagnosis. For example, in a middle-aged patient with chest pain, it frequently

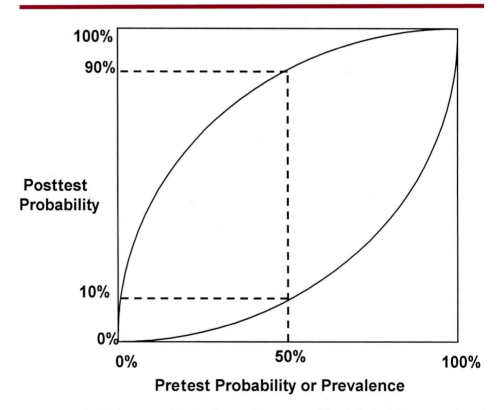

**Figure 44-3** Graphical outcome of Bayes' theorem. The top curved line is for a positive test result, and the bottom curved line is for a negative test result. If a test is performed with the prior probability (*x* axis) in the mid-range, there is the greatest effect on the posttest probability or predictive value (*y* axis).

makes sense to perform a test to diagnose coronary artery disease. This does not make sense, however, in a young woman with atypical chest pain or an older man with typical angina. This same principle applies to all diagnostic tests, including screening tests. The arguments above show that a screening test, which means a test where the risk of disease is low, cannot diagnose disease and thus should not be routinely performed. Screening tests can be reasonable if at least some of the following criteria are met: (1) the test is inexpensive, such as the test for phenylketonuria; (2) the disease is very serious, again such as phenylketonuria; (3) the screening test has high sensitivity and specificity; (4) the more invasive gold standard that would follow the screening test is not overly expensive or invasive; or (5) there is a second level of testing (e.g, cardiac imaging) that can logically follow the screening test (e.g., treadmill testing).

Next, we consider cost-effectiveness analysis. Based upon the literature and the cost-effectiveness of commonly used treatments, it is generally stated that a therapy that costs less than $50,000 per QALY is cost-effective, one that costs $50,000 to $100,000 is uncertain, and one that costs over $100,000 is not cost-effective. The cost-effectiveness of most well-established medical therapies compares well with the cost-effectiveness of other health choices, such as wearing seat belts, asbestos abatement, or toxic waste control.[37] Thus, coronary surgery for a patient with left main disease and severe angina is much more likely to be judged cost-effective by society than coronary surgery for a patient with one-vessel disease and mild angina.[28] From a societal perspective, appropriate selection of patients for a particular therapy will do more to provide cost-effective care than efforts to limit the costs of specific therapies. Clinical trials supported by registry data and practice guidelines currently offer the best approach to treatment selection. This being said, attempting to provide expensive therapy such as revascularization as inexpensively as possible without compromising care is important as well.

# CURRENT AND FUTURE TRENDS AND POLICY IMPLICATIONS

Microeconomic analyses in clinical medicine offer a powerful set of methods that may be used for clinical decision making as well as for policy. To date, most cost-effectiveness analyses have been simulations. The formidable difficulties in determining cost and utility have delayed the introduction of these tools into the clinical arena, where cost-effectiveness analyses could be part of many clinical trials or routinely applied to observational databases. Econometric methods offer potential, although unproven, ability to overcome the difficulties of traditional approaches. With the current changes in health care, accountability and cost are increasingly important, and we can expect to see more studies using these methods. Although we must maintain a level of skepticism given sources of error and theoretical limitations, clinical microeconomic analyses can help guide medical decision making. Hospitals are currently making great efforts to become more efficient, as evidenced by decreasing lengths of stay and cross-functional staffing. The impact of managed care and capitation on costs is at present unknown but presumably will result in increased efficiency. Thus, interpretation of economic data over time will require an understanding of changes in hospital and professional economic trends as well as secular inflationary trends. The real cost savings are likely to come about not through increased efficiency in performing procedures but by avoiding expensive procedures in patients for whom they are not needed.

## REFERENCES

1. Drummond MF, Stoddart GL, Torrance GW: *Cost-effectiveness analysis.* In: *Methods for the Economic Evaluation of Health Care Programmes.* Oxford, Oxford University Press, 1990:74–111.
2. Drummond MF, Stoddart GL, Torrance GW: *Cost-utility analysis.* In: *Methods for the Economic Evaluation of Health Care Programmes.* Oxford, Oxford University Press, 1990:112–148.
3. Drummond MF, Stoddart GL, Torrance GW: *Cost-benefit analysis.* In: *Methods for the Economic Evaluation of Health Care Programmes.* Oxford, Oxford University Press, 1990:149–167.
4. Machina MJ: Choice under uncertainty: problems solved and unsolved. *J Econ Perspectives* 1987; 1:121–154.
5. Cook PJ, Graham DA: The demand for insurance and protection: the case of irreplaceable commodities. *Q J Econ* 1977; 91:143–156.
6. Fuchs YR, Zeckhauser R, et al: Valuing health—a "priceless" commodity. *Am Econ Rev* 1987; 77:263–268.
7. Graham DA: Cost-benefit analysis under uncertainty. *Am Econ Rev* 1981; 71:715–725.
8. Finkler SA: The distinction between cost and charges. *Ann Intern Med* 1982; 96:102–109.
9. Finkler SA: Cost finding for high-technology, high cost services. *Health Care Manage Rev* 1980; 5:17–29.
10. Shuman J, Wolfe H, Perlman M: Model for hospital microcosting. *Industrial Engineering* 1973;39–43.
11. Cooper R, Kaplan RS: Measure costs right: make the right decisions. *Harvard Business Review* 1988; 5:96–103.
12. Dearden J: Cost accounting comes to service industries. *Harvard Business Review* Sept–Oct 1978:132–140.
13. Hlatky MA, Lipscomb J, Nelson C, et al: Resource use and cost of initial coronary revascularization: coronary angioplasty versus coronary bypass surgery. *Circulation* 1990; 82(suppl IV):IV-208–IV-213.
14. Feldstein PJ: *Health Care Economics,* 2d ed. New York, Wiley, 1983:169–197.
15. Health Insurance Association of America: *Source Book of Health Insurance Data, 1991.* Washington, DC, HIAA, 1991:55.
16. Hsiao WC, Braun P, Yntema D, Becker ER: Estimating physicians' work for a resource-based relative value scale. *N Engl J Med* 1988; 319:835–841.
17. Becker ER, Dunn D, Hsiao WC: Relative cost differences among physicians' specialty practices. *JAMA* 1988; 260:2397–2402.
18. Becker ER, Mauldin PD, Weintraub WS: CABG and PTCA physician practice profiles using the resource-based relative value scale (RBRVS): better methods for explaining the variation. *Clin Res* 1994; 42:225A.

19. Ferguson CE: *Microeconomic Theory,* 6th ed. Homewood, IL, Irwin, 1968.
20. Alchian A: The meaning of utility measurement. *Am Econ Rev* 1953; 43:26–50.
21. Harsanyi JC: Cardinal welfare, individualistic ethics, and interpersonal comparisons of utility. *J Pol Econ* 1955; 63:309–321.
22. Pliskin JS, Shepard DS, Weinstein MC: Utility functions for life years and health status. *Operations Research* 1980; 28:206–224.
23. Sackett DL, Torrance GW: The utility of different health states as perceived by the general public. *J Chronic Dis* 1978; 31:697–704.
24. Churchill DN, Morgan J, Torrance GW: Quality of life in end-stage renal disease. *Peritoneal Dialysis Bulletin* 1984; 4:20–23.
25. Kaplan RM, Bush JW, Berry CC: Health status: types of validity of the index of well-being. *Health Serv Res* 1976; 11:478–507.
26. Loomes G, McKenzie L: The use of QALYs in health care decision making. *Soc Sci Med* 1989; 28:299–308.
27. McNeil BJ, Weichselbaum R, Pauker SG: Speech and survival: tradeoffs between quality and quantity of life in laryngeal cancer. *N Engl J Med* 1981: 305:982–987.
28. Weinstein MC, Stason WB: Cost effectiveness of coronary artery bypass surgery. *Circulation* 1982; 66(suppl III):56–65.
29. Joreskog KG, Goldberger AS: Estimation of a model with multiple indicators and multiple causes of a single latent variable. *J Amer Stat Assoc* 1975; 70:631–639.
30. Van De Ven, Wynard PMM, Van Der Gaag J: Health as an unobservable: a MIMIC-model of demand for health care. *J Health Econ* 1982; 1:157–183.
31. Van De Ven, Wynard PMM, Hooijmans EM: The MIMIC health status index (what it is and what it does). In: *Economics of Health Care,* Dordrecht Kluwer Academic Publishers, 1992, 19–29.
32. Lee JS, Bailey MJ, Jeong J, et al: A study on the cost-effectiveness of coronary revascularization: introducing the simultaneous MIMIC health status model. *Health Econ* 1997;6:613–623.
33. McNeil BJ, Keeler E, Adelstein SJ: Primer on certain elements of medical decision making. *N Engl J Med* 1975; 293:211–215.
34. Ransohoff DF, Feinstein AR: Problems of spectrum and bias in evaluating the efficacy of diagnostic tests. *N Engl J Med* 1978; 299:926–930.
35. Weintraub WS, Madeira SW Jr, Bodenheimer MM, et al: Critical analysis of the application of Bayes' theorem to sequential testing in the noninvasive diagnosis of coronary artery disease. *J Am Coll Cardiol* 1984; 54:43–49.
36. Diamond GA, Forrester JS: Analysis of probability as an aid in the clinical diagnosis of coronary artery disease. *N Engl J Med* 1979; 300:1350–1358.
37. Tengs TO, Adams ME, Pliskin JS, et al: Five-hundred life-saving interventions and their cost-effectiveness. *Risk Analysis* 1995; 15:369–390.

## ADDITIONAL REFERENCES

Drummond MF, Richardson WS, O'Brien BJ, et al: How to use an article in economic analysis of clinical practice: A. Are the results valid? *JAMA* 1997; 277:1552–1557.
Drummond N, Brandt A, Luce B, Rovira J: Standardizing methodologies for economic evaluation in health care: practice, problems, and potential. *Int J Tech Assessment in Health Care* 1993; 9:26–36.

Eisenberg JM: Clinical economics: a guide to economic analysis in clinical practices. *JAMA* 1989; 262:2879–2886.

Haddix AC, Teutsch SM, Shaffer PA, Dunet DO (eds): *Prevention Effectiveness: A Guide to Decision Analysis and Economic Evaluation.* New York, Oxford University Press, 1996.

Mark DB, Hlatky MA, Califf RM, et al: Cost effectiveness of thrombolytic therapy with tissue plasminogen activator as compared with streptokinase for acute myocardial infarction. *N Engl J Med* 1995; 332:1418–1424.

O'Brien BJ, Heyland D, Richardson WS, et al: How to use an article in economic analysis of clinical practice: B. What are the results and will they help me in caring for my patients? *JAMA* 1997; 277:1802–1806.

Weinstein MC, Stason WB: Cost effectiveness of interventions to prevent or treat coronary heart disease. *Ann Rev Public Health* 1985; 6:41–63.

BARRY J. MARON

# CARDIOVASCULAR CAUSES OF SUDDEN DEATH, PREPARTICIPATION SCREENING, AND THE EVALUATION OF ATHLETIC ACTIVITIES IN YOUNG PEOPLE

Sudden deaths of competitive athletes are personal tragedies with great impact on the lay and medical communities[1] and are usually due to a variety of previously unsuspected cardiovascular diseases.[2–20] Such events, particularly in young people, often assume a high public profile because of the widely held perception that trained athletes constitute the healthiest segment of our society; the occasional deaths of well-known elite athletes exaggerate this visibility.[1,21] These athletic-field catastrophes have also substantially increased interest in the role and efficacy of preparticipation screening.[22]

Therefore, the present discussion will assess (1) the benefits and limitations of preparticipation screening for early detection of cardiovascular abnormalities in competitive athletes; (2) cost-efficiency and feasibility issues and the medical-legal implications of screening; and (3) consensus recommendations and guide-

Portions of the present text are adapted from Maron BJ, Thompson PD, Puffer JC, et al: Medical/ Scientific Statement, Cardiovascular preparticipation screening of competitive athletes. *Circulation* 1996; 94:850–856, with the permission of the American Heart Association. © American Heart Association.

lines for the most prudent, practical, and effective screening procedures and strategies, based on a recent American Heart Association consensus panel.[22] Given the large number of competitive athletes in this country and recent public health initiatives on physical activity and exercise, these issues have become particularly relevant.

## DEFINITIONS AND BACKGROUND

The present considerations focus on the competitive athlete, previously described as one who participates in an organized team or individual sport requiring systematic training and regular competition against others, while placing a high premium on athletic excellence and achievement.[20] The purpose of screening, as described here, is to provide medical clearance for participation in competitive sports through routine and systematic evaluations intended to identify clinically relevant and preexisting cardiovascular abnormalities and thereby reduce the risks associated with organized sports. It should be emphasized, however, that raising the possibility of a cardiovascular abnormality on a standard screening examination is only the first tier of recognition; after this, referral to a specialist for further diagnostic investigation will probably be required. When a definitive cardiovascular diagnosis is made, the consensus panel guidelines of Bethesda Conference 26[23] should be utilized to formulate recommendations regarding continued participation in or disqualification from competitive sports.

The American Heart Association guidelines,[22] reproduced here (see Appendix), focus primarily on the potential for population-based screening of high school and collegiate student-athletes rather than on individual clinical assessments of athletes and are designed to apply to competitors of all ages and both genders. These recommendations may also be extrapolated to athletes in youth, middle-school, masters, or professional sports and in some instances to participants in intense recreational sporting activities. It is also recognized that the overall preparticipation screening process extends well beyond the considerations described here (which are limited to the cardiovascular system) and involves many other organ systems and medical issues.

The American Heart Association screening recommendations are predicated on the probability that intense athletic training is likely to increase the risk for sudden cardiac death (or disease progression) in trained athletes with clinically important underlying structural heart disease, although presently it is not possible to quantify that risk. Certainly, the vast majority of young athletes who die suddenly do so during athletic training or competition.[3–5] These observations support the proposition that physical exertion is an important trigger for sudden death, given the presence of certain underlying cardiovascular diseases. Finally, the early detection of clinically significant cardiovascular disease through preparticipation screening may well, in many instances, permit timely therapeutic interventions that prolong life.

# CAUSES OF SUDDEN
# DEATH IN ATHLETES

A variety of cardiovascular abnormalities are the most common causes of sudden death in competitive athletes.[2–19] The precise lesions responsible differ considerably with age. For example, in youthful athletes (less than about 35 years of age), the vast majority of sudden deaths are due to a variety of largely congenital cardiac malformations (Figs. 45-1 to 45-3).[2–15] Indeed, virtually any disease capable of causing sudden death in young people may potentially do so in young competitive athletes. It should be emphasized that while these cardiovascular diseases may be relatively common among young athletes who die suddenly, each is uncommon in the general population. Also, those lesions that are responsible for sudden death do not occur with the same frequency, with most individual abnormalities responsible for ≤5 percent of all such deaths (Fig. 45-1). Such deaths occur most commonly in intense team sports, such as basketball and football, which also have high levels of participation.

The single most common cardiovascular abnormality among the causes of sudden death in young athletes is hypertrophic cardiomyopathy (HCM), usually in the nonobstructive form,[2–5,8,11,12,14,24–29] which accounts for about 35 percent (Figs. 45-1 and 45-2).[3] HCM is a primary and familial cardiac disease with heterogeneous

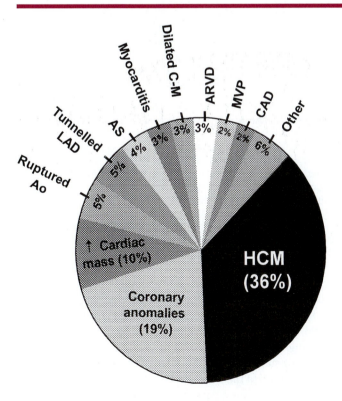

Figure 45-1   Causes of sudden cardiac death in young competitive athletes (median age, 17) based on systematic tracking of 158 athletes in the United States, primarily 1985–1995. (Adapted with permission of the American Heart Association from Maron BJ, Thompson PD, Puffer JC et al: Cardiovascular preparticipation screening of competitive athletes. *Circulation* 1996; 94:850–856.)

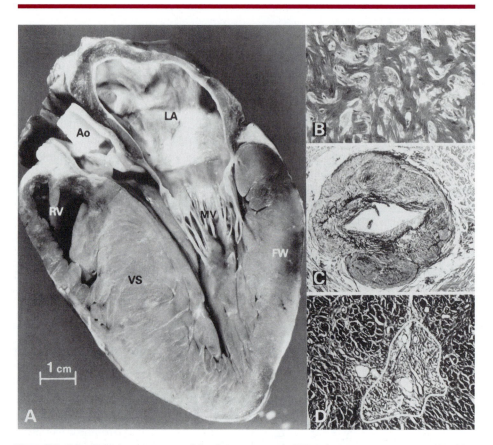

**Figure 45-2** Morphologic components of the disease process in HCM, the most common cause of sudden death in young competitive athletes. *A.* A gross heart specimen sectioned in a cross-sectional plane similar to that of the echocardiographic (parasternal) long axis; left ventricular wall thickening shows an asymmetric pattern and is confined primarily to the ventricular septum (VS), which bulges prominently into the left ventricular outflow tract. Left ventricular cavity appears reduced in size. FW = left ventricular free wall. *B, C,* and *D.* Histologic features characteristic of left ventricular myocardium in HCM. *B.* Markedly disordered architecture with adjacent hypertrophied cardiac muscle cells arranged at perpendicular and oblique angles; *C,* an intramural coronary artery with thickened wall (due primarily to medial hypertrophy) and apparently narrowed lumen; *D,* replacement fibrosis in an area of ventricular myocardium adjacent to an abnormal intramural coronary artery. Ao = aorta; LA = left atrium; RV = right ventricle. (Reproduced with permission from Maron BJ: Hypertrophic cardiomyopathy. *Lancet* 1997; 3350:127–133.)

expression, complex pathophysiology, and a diverse clinical course for which several disease-causing mutations in genes encoding proteins of the cardiac sarcomere have been reported,[27,30–34] including β-myosin heavy chain, cardiac troponin T and tropinin I, α-tropomyosin, and myosin-binding protein C. HCM is a relatively uncommon malformation, occurring in about 0.2 percent of the general population.[35]

The next most frequent cause of sudden death is a variety of congenital coronary anomalies, particularly anomalous origin of the left main coronary artery from the right (anterior) sinus of Valsalva.[36–40] Less common causes are myocarditis (Fig. 45-3), di-

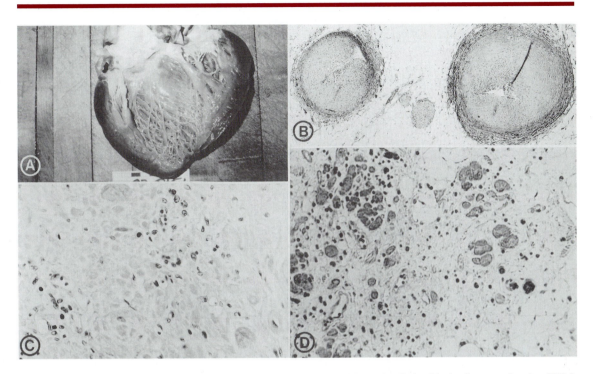

**Figure 45-3**  Cardiac morphologic findings at autopsy in four competitive athletes who died suddenly of causes other than HCM. *A.* Gross specimen from an athlete with greatly enlarged ventricular cavities, consistent with dilated cardiomyopathy. *B.* Histologic section of the left anterior descending coronary artery (left) and a diagonal branch (right), showing severe (>95 percent) cross-sectional luminal narrowing by atherosclerotic plaque. *C.* Foci inflammatory cells consistent with myocarditis. *D.* Histologic section of right ventricular wall showing islands of myocytes within a matrix of fatty and fibrous replacement, which is characteristic of arrhythmogenic right ventricular dysplasia. (Adapted with permission from Maron BJ, Shirani J, Poliac LC, et al: Sudden death in young competitive athletes: Clinical, demographic and pathological profiles. *JAMA* 1996; 276:199–204.)

lated cardiomyopathy (Fig. 45-3), Marfan syndrome with aortic rupture, arrhythmogenic right ventricular dysplasia (Fig. 45-3), sarcoidosis, mitral valve prolapse, aortic valve stenosis, atherosclerotic coronary artery disease (CAD) (Fig. 45-3), long QT syndrome, and possibly intramural (tunneled) coronary arteries.[2–9,11–15,41–44]

Occasionally, athletes who die suddenly demonstrate no evidence of structural cardiovascular disease, even after careful gross and microscopic examination of the heart. In such instances (about 2 percent of one series),[3] it may not be possible to exclude noncardiac factors (e.g., drug abuse) with certainty or to know whether careful inspection of the specialized conducting system and associated vasculature with serial sectioning (which is not part of the standard medical examiner's protocol) would have revealed occult but clinically relevant abnormalities.[9,45,46] Although one can only speculate on the potential etiologies in many such deaths, it is possible that some are due to either a primary arrhythmia in the absence of cardiac morphologic abnormalities,[47] previously unidentified Wolff-Parkinson-White syndrome, rare diseases in which structural abnormalities of the heart are characteristically

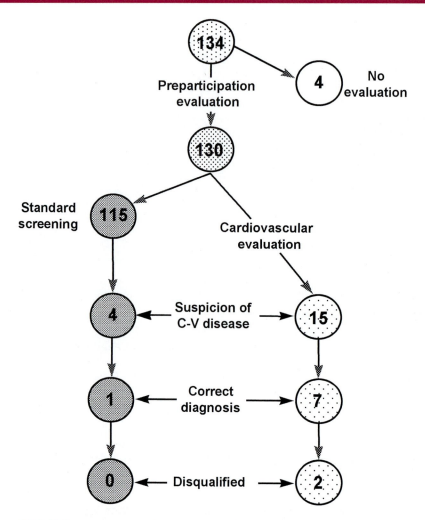

**Figure 45-4** Flow diagram showing impact of preparticipation medical history and physical examinations on the detection of structural cardiovascular disease (and causes of sudden death). * = cardiovascular evaluation with testing (independent of standard school or institutional preparticipation screening), performed in 15 athletes because of symptoms, family history, cardiac murmur, or physical findings suggestive of heart disease. (Reproduced with permission from Maron BJ, Shirani J, Poliac LC, et al: Sudden death in young competitive athletes: Clinical, demographic and pathological profiles. *JAMA* 1996; 276:199–204).

lacking at necropsy, such as long QT syndrome[41–43] or possibly exercise-induced coronary spasm, or undetected segmental forms of right ventricular dysplasia.[7]

Older athletes (over age 35) are largely involved in competitive long-distance running. The vast majority of deaths in such athletes are due to atherosclerotic coronary artery disease;[16–19] only rarely is the cause congenital cardiovascular diseases such as HCM or coronary artery anomalies.

Since this discussion focuses on the cardiovascular evaluation of athletes, other related medical problems that may occasionally cause sudden death in the young, such as cerebral aneurysm, sickle cell trait,[48] nonpenetrating blunt chest impact,[49] or bronchial asthma, have been excluded. Also, issues related to drug screening are not part of this discussion, although ingestion of agents such as cocaine may have important adverse cardiovascular consequences.[50–52] Screening for systemic hypertension has been addressed, although this disease is not regarded as an important cause of sudden unexpected death in young athletes.[53]

# PREVALENCE AND SCOPE OF THE PROBLEM

Relevant to the design of any screening strategy is the fact that sudden cardiac death in young athletes is a devastating but rather infrequent event and that only a small proportion of participants in organized sports in the United States are at risk.[54] Indeed, each of the lesions known to be responsible for sudden death in young athletes, ranging from the relatively common (i.e., HCM) to the apparently very rare (e.g., coronary artery anomalies, arrhythmogenic right ventricular dysplasia, long QT syndrome, and Marfan syndrome), occurs infrequently in the general population. It is a reasonable estimate that all congenital malformations relevant to athletic screening may have a combined prevalence of <0.5 percent in the general athlete population.

Also, the large number of competitive athletes in the United States constitutes a major obstacle to screening strategies.[4,22,54] At present, there are approximately 5 to 6 million competitive athletes at the high school level (grades 9 through 12), plus lesser numbers of collegiate (500,000) and professional (5000) athletes. This does not include an unspecified number of youth, middle school, and masters-level competitors, for which reliable estimates are not presently available. Therefore, the total number of trained athletes in the United States in any given year is probably at least 8 to 10 million.

While the prevalence of athletic-field deaths due to cardiovascular disease is not known with certainty, it would appear to be approximately 1 in 200,000 athletes of high school age per year, although it is disproportionately higher in males than in females.[54] Considering this relatively low prevalence, the heightened public awareness and intense interest in sudden deaths in athletes, often fueled by the news media, is perhaps disproportionate to the actual numerical impact of such deaths as a public health problem.

# ETHICAL CONSIDERATIONS IN SCREENING

In a benevolent society, physicians have a responsibility to initiate prudent efforts to identify life-threatening diseases in athletes in order to minimize those cardiovascular risks associated with sport and protect the health of such individuals.[1,20,22,23,55,56] Specifically, there is an implicit ethical obligation on the part of educational institutions (e.g., high schools and colleges) to implement cost-effective strategies to assure that student-athletes are not subject to unacceptable and avoidable medical risks.[22] The libertarian view, held by some, that high school- and college-aged athletes should be permitted to assume any specifically disclosed cardiovascular risk associated with sport as part of the overall uncertainty and risk of living is not ascribed to here. It is recognized that in professional sports, despite sufficient resources, the motivation to implement cardiovascular screening may not presently exist because of the economic pressures in such sports environments, where athletic participation represents a vocation and the remuneration for services is often substantial.

The extent to which preparticipation screening can be supported at any level is influenced by cost-efficiency considerations, by practical limitations, and also by the awareness that it is not possible to achieve a "zero-risk" situation in competitive sports.[56,57] Indeed, there is often an implied acceptance of risk on the part of athletes; for example, as a society, we permit or condone many sporting activities that are known to have intrinsic risks that cannot be controlled absolutely—e.g., automobile racing or mountain climbing—as well as more traditional sports, such as football, in which the possibility of serious traumatic injury exists.

## LEGAL CONSIDERATIONS

Although educational institutions and professional teams are required to use reasonable care in conducting their athletic programs, there is currently no clear legal precedent regarding their duty to conduct preparticipation screening of athletes for the purpose of detecting medically significant cardiovascular abnormalities.[56,58] Indeed, at present, it appears that there have been no lawsuits alleging that failure to either perform cardiovascular screening or diagnose cardiac disease in young competitive athletes constituted negligence. In the absence of binding requirements established by state law or athletic governing bodies, most institutions and teams presently rely on the team physician (or other medical personnel) to determine appropriate medical screening procedures.

A physician who has medically cleared an athlete to participate in competitive sports is not necessarily legally liable for an injury or death caused by an undetected cardiovascular condition. Malpractice liability for failure to discover a latent, asymptomatic cardiovascular condition requires proof that a physician deviated from customary or accepted medical practice in his or her specialty in performing preparticipation screening of athletes, and furthermore that utilization of established diagnostic criteria and techniques would have disclosed that medical condition.

It should be emphasized that the law permits the medical profession to establish the appropriate nature and scope of preparticipation screening based on the exercise of its collective medical judgment. This necessarily involves the development of reliable diagnostic procedures, taking into consideration cost-benefit and feasibility factors. The American Heart Association recommendations for cardiovascular preparticipation screening of athletes described here[22] represent evidence of the proper medical standard of care; however, these guidelines will establish the legal standard of care only if they are generally accepted or customarily followed by physicians or relied upon by courts in determining the nature and scope of the legal responsibility borne by sponsors of competitive athletes.[56–59]

While preparticipation examinations in U.S. high schools and colleges take place largely at the discretion of the examining physician or in accordance with customary practice, a considerably different situation has existed in Italy since 1971 in the form of government legislation (Medical Protection of Athletic Activities Act), unique to Italy, mandating preventive medical evaluations for all competitive athletes.[55] All Italian citizens (ages 12 to 40) who are engaged in organized sports activities must receive annual medical clearance from an approved physician, stipulating that the athlete is free of cardiovascular abnormalities that could unacceptably increase the risk of sudden cardiac death during training or competition. Since 1982, more detailed guidelines for these preparticipation examinations have been formulated; they include, as a minimum, history and physical examination, 12-lead ECG, and exercise and pulmonary function tests. Echocardiography is specifically required (since 1994) only in selected professional sports (i.e., soccer, boxing, and cycling). Under Italian law, the examining physician is primarily responsible for the accuracy of this clinical assessment and stands as the final arbitrator of eligibility for sports by issuing the official certification of medical clearance. In the event of an incorrect or incomplete medical diagnosis that leads directly to the impaired health or death of an athlete, the physician responsible for permitting athletic competition can be held accountable in criminal (as well as civil) court.

# CURRENT CUSTOMARY PRACTICE IN THE UNITED STATES

It is important to clearly acknowledge the limitations of the preparticipation screening process currently in place for student-athletes in the United States. Only in this way can an informed public be created, as many people might otherwise harbor important misconceptions regarding the principles and efficacy of athletic screening. Currently, universally accepted standards for the screening of high school and college athletes are not available, nor are there approved certification procedures for the professionals who perform such screening examinations.[60] Some form of medical clearance by a physician or other trained health care worker, usually consisting of a history and abbreviated physical examination, presently appears most common for high school athletes. Furthermore, there is no uniform agreement among the states as to the precise format of preparticipation medical evaluations. Indeed, 40 percent of all states either do not require this process, do not have recommended standard history and physical forms to serve as guides for examiners (in fact, some require only a signature to provide medical clearance), or have approved forms that are judged inadequate[60] when evaluated against the specific screening recommendations proposed by the aforementioned 1996 American Heart Association consensus panel.[22] These findings also emphasize that it is not possible at present to assume that medical clearance for sports competition precludes the possibility of underlying and potentially lethal cardiovascular disease. In a substantial proportion of states, nonphysician health care workers, including chiropractors (in 9 states) and nurse-practitioners or physician assistants (in 20 states each) are authorized to perform preparticipation screening.

# EXPECTATIONS OF SCREENING STRATEGIES

Preparticipation screening by history and physical examination alone (without noninvasive testing) does not possess sufficient power to guarantee detection of many critical cardiovascular abnormalities in large populations of young trained athletes in high school or college. Indeed, hemodynamically significant congenital aortic valve stenosis is probably the lesion most likely to be reliably detected during routine screening as a result of its characteristically loud heart murmur. Detection of HCM by the standard screening history or physical examination is unreliable because most patients have the nonobstructive form of this disease, characteristically expressed by no murmur or only a faint heart murmur.[22,24–26,29] Furthermore, the majority of athletes with HCM do not experience syncope or have a family history of premature sudden death, and therefore this disease is not easily detected by the preparticipation personal history.[22,24–26,29] When symptoms such as chest pain or impaired consciousness are involved, the standard personal history has a generally low specificity for the detection of many of the cardiovascular abnormalities that lead to sudden cardiac death in young athletes.

It should also be emphasized that most of the lesions being considered here as potentially responsible for sudden death in young athletes—e.g., a variety of congenital coronary anomalies, particularly anomalous origin of the left main coronary artery from the right sinus of Valsalva—may be particularly challenging to detect, even when echocardiography, ECG, or other noninvasive tests are incorporated into the standard screening process. Despite these major limitations, standard history and physical examination screening is theoretically of value by virtue of its capability for identifying (or raising the suspicion of) cardiovascular abnormalities in some at-risk athletes. For example, genetic diseases such as HCM, Marfan syndrome, and some cases of arrhythmogenic right ventricular dysplasia and premature atherosclerotic CAD can occasionally be suspected in athletes from the family history alone or by virtue of transient symptoms from the personal history. Physical examination may identify the stigmata of Marfan syndrome and lesions associated with left ventricular outflow obstruction (aortic valvular stenosis and some patients with HCM), which are characterized by a loud heart murmur; systemic hypertension may also be detected.

While there are no prospective data available that permit a direct assessment of the efficacy of large-scale athletic screening, a recent retrospective analysis of young athletes who died suddenly from a variety of cardiovascular diseases showed that only 3 percent of those individuals exposed to standard preparticipation screening were suspected of having cardiac disease by virtue of these examinations, and less than 1 percent ultimately received an accurate diagnosis (see Fig. 45-4).[3]

Based on these observations, the preparticipation screening process as currently structured and carried out in U.S. high schools appears to lack sufficient power to consistently recognize clinically important cardiovascular abnormalities in many athletes. It is noteworthy that preparticipation screening in Italy (which routinely includes a 12-lead ECG) reports a contrasting experience: a not inconsequential number of HCM cases were identified over a 7-year period among 33,000 consecutive athletes.[61]

# POTENTIAL EFFICACY AND LIMITATIONS OF NONINVASIVE SCREENING TESTS

The addition of noninvasive diagnostic tests to the screening process clearly has the potential to enhance the detection of certain cardiovascular defects in young athletes. For example, the two-dimensional echocardiogram is the principal diagnostic tool for clinical recognition of HCM, since it can demonstrate otherwise unexplained asymmetric left ventricular wall thickening, the sine qua non of this disease.[24–26,28,29,62] Comprehensive and routine screening for HCM by genetic testing for a variety of known disease-causing mutations is not yet practical for large populations, given the substantial genetic heterogeneity of the disease and the expensive and time-intensive methodologies involved.[27,30–34]

Echocardiography can also detect other abnormalities associated with sudden death in young athletes, such as valvular heart disease (e.g., mitral valve prolapse and aortic valvular stenosis), aortic root dilatation, and left ventricular dysfunction (associated with myocarditis or dilated cardiomyopathy). Even such diagnostic testing cannot guarantee recognition of all important lesions, however, and some relevant cardiovascular diseases may be beyond detection with any screening methodology. For example, identification of many congenital coronary artery anomalies usually requires sophisticated laboratory examination including coronary arteriography, although in selected young athletes it is possible to at least suspect important anomalies such as origin of the left main coronary artery from the right sinus of Valsalva with echocardiography.[38–40] Arrhythmogenic right ventricular dysplasia usually cannot be reliably diagnosed solely by echocardiography and ECG; the best available noninvasive test for this disease is probably magnetic resonance imaging, which unfortunately is both expensive and not universally available.[44,63]

Cost-efficiency issues are important when assessing the feasibility of applying expensive noninvasive testing to the screening of large populations of athletes.[64–68] In the vast majority of instances, adequate financial and personnel resources for such endeavors are lacking. The costs are probably prohibitive in those situations in which the full (i.e., unreduced) expense of testing would be the responsibility of administrative bodies such as schools, universities, or teams; for example, the cost of an echocardiographic study ranges from about $400 to $2000 (the average is about $600). Thus, if the occurrence of hypertrophic cardiomyopathy in a population of young athletes is assumed to be 1 in 500,[35] even at $500 per study it would theoretically cost $250,000 to detect even one previously undiagnosed case.

Screening protocols incorporating noninvasive testing at greatly reduced cost have been described.[64,66,67] These efforts, however, have involved unusual circumstances in which echocardiographic equipment was donated and professional expenses were waived for all but technician-related costs. Also, some investigators have suggested an inexpensive shortened-format echocardiogram for population screening (limited to parasternal views; about 2 min in duration).[64,67] While such individual initiatives should not be discouraged, it may also be noted that public service projects based largely on volunteerism usually cannot be sustained on a consistent basis.

An important limitation of preparticipation screening with two-dimensional echocardiography is the potential for false-positive or false-negative test results. False-positive results arise from the assignment of borderline values for left ventricular wall thicknesses (or particularly enlarged cavity size), which require formulation of a differential diagnosis between normal but extreme physiologic adaptations of athlete's heart[69–72] and pathologic conditions such as HCM or other cardiomyopathies.[73] Indeed, such clinical dilemmas (which may not always be definitively resolvable in individual athletes) generate emotional, financial, and medical burdens for the athlete, family, team, and institution by virtue of the uncertainty created and the requirement for additional testing. False-negative screening results may occur in athletes with HCM when testing by echocardiography occurs at a point of incomplete phenotypic expression during adolescence.[74] For example, in athletes of less than about age 13 to 15 years with HCM, left ventricular hypertrophy is often absent or mild, and therefore the echocardiographic findings may not yet be diagnostic at the time of preparticipation screening.

The 12-lead ECG has been proposed as a more practical and cost-efficient alternative strategy than routine echocardiography for population-based screening.[75–77] Indeed, the ECG is abnormal in about 95 percent of patients with HCM,[78] may be abnormal in patients with other potentially lethal structural lesions, and will usually identify the important (but uncommon) long QT syndrome.[41–43] Of note, however, a certain proportion of genetically affected relatives in families with long QT syndrome may not have phenotypic expression on the ECG.[41]

As a primary screening test, however, the ECG suffers in comparison to the echocardiogram because of its lack of imaging capability for recognition of structural cardiovascular malformations. Also, the ECG has relatively low specificity as a screening test in populations of athletes because of the high frequency with which

ECG alterations occur in association with the normal physiologic adaptations to training (athlete's heart).[79] Such false-positive ECG test results substantially complicate the use of the 12-lead ECG as a primary screening tool in populations of athletes. It can be anticipated that about 20 to 25 percent of athletes examined in the context of preparticipation screening will have ECG patterns that ultimately stimulate echocardiographic study.[77] Of note, elite athletes not infrequently demonstrate distinctly abnormal ECG patterns consistent with pathologic conditions,[79] even in the absence of structural heart disease and without increased cardiac dimensions due to training.

To date, there have been relatively few published reports of cardiovascular screening efforts in large populations of athletes.[61,64,65,67,68,77,80] Most of these studies have implemented noninvasive testing (i.e., conventional or limited echocardiographic examination or 12-lead ECG) in high school or collegiate athletes. The populations subjected to screening ranged in size from 250 to 2000 athletes, usually studied over a 1-year period. In general, these reports are consistent in that they describe the detection of very few definitive examples of potentially lethal cardiovascular abnormalities.

# PERSPECTIVES ON RACE AND GENDER

Hypertrophic cardiomyopathy is an important cause of sudden death in young African American athletes, and there is preliminary evidence that some such catastrophes may be more common in black athletes than in their white counterparts.[3,81] The substantial occurrence of HCM-related sudden death in young black male athletes contrasts sharply with the infrequent reporting of black patients with HCM in hospital- and clinic-based populations from tertiary referral centers.[24–29] Therefore, in African Americans, HCM is most frequently encountered when the disease results in sudden and unexpected death during competitive athletics. These data suggest that a disproportionate access to subspecialty health care between the black and white communities in the United States may make it less likely that young black male athletes will receive a relatively sophisticated cardiovascular diagnosis such as HCM. Consequently, African American athletes with HCM may be less likely to be identified or disqualified from competition to reduce their risk for sudden death, in accordance with the recommendations of Bethesda Conference 26.[23]

Sudden death of young women on the athletic field is uncommon,[3] representing only about 10 percent of all such deaths. This disproportionality in women may in some instances be explained on the basis of lower participation rates or less severe training demands and cardiac adaptation[72] and also by the fact that HCM is less commonly recognized clinically in women.[24–26,28,29] This observation also suggests the possibility that a measure of protection from sudden death is attributable in some physiologic fashion to gender itself. Nevertheless, available data do not provide a compelling justification to construct specific screening algorithms based on gender, race, or demographic subgrouping.

## APPENDIX

## AMERICAN HEART ASSOCIATION RECOMMENDATIONS FOR PREPARTICIPATION SCREENING

### Advisability

The 1996 American Heart Association consensus panel recommendations[22] state that some form of preparticipation cardiovascular screening for high school and college student-athletes is justifiable and compelling based on ethical, legal, and medical grounds. Noninvasive testing can enhance the diagnostic power of the standard history and physical examination; however, it is not prudent to recommend the routine use of tests such as 12-lead ECG, echocardiography, or graded exercise testing for the detection of cardiovascular disease in large populations of youthful or older athletes. This recommendation is based on both practical and cost-efficiency considerations, given the large number of competitive athletes in the United States, the relatively low frequency with which the cardiovascular lesions responsible for these deaths occur, and the low rate of sudden cardiac death in the athletic community. This viewpoint is not, however, intended to actively discourage all efforts at population screening that may be proposed by individual investigators. Nevertheless, there is concern that the widespread application of noninvasive testing to athletic populations could result in many false-positive results, creating unnecessary anxiety among substantial numbers of athletes and their families, as well as unjustified exclusion from competition. Indeed, in such a circumstance with a low incidence of disease in the community, a great likelihood exists that the number of false-positive results would exceed that of true positives.

Consequently, it would appear that a complete and careful personal and family history and physical examination designed to identify (or suspect) those cardiovascular lesions known to cause sudden death or disease progression in young athletes is the best available and most practical approach to screening populations of competitive sports participants regardless of age. Such cardiovascular screening is an obtainable objective and should be mandatory for all athletes. *It is recommended that both a history and physical examination be performed by a qualified examiner prior to the initial engagement in organized high school (grades 9 through 12) and collegiate sports.* In the intervening years, an interim history should be obtained. Indeed, for young competitive athletes, this recommendation is consistent with those procedures that are customary for most high school and college athletes in the United States.

However, it is important to point out that official recommendations or requirements by athletic governing bodies regarding the nature and scope of preparticipation medical evaluations of athletes are not standardized among the states, nor can they necessarily be viewed as medically sufficient in many instances. Therefore, because of this heterogeneity in the design and content of preparticipation examinations, it is also recommended that a systematic national standard for preparticipation medical evaluations be developed. Adherence to uniformly applicable guidelines would impact substantially on the health of student-athletes in a cost-effective manner by enhancing the safety of their athletic activities.

For older athletes (>35 years of age), despite the limitations of the history and physical examination in detecting CAD, a personal history of coronary risk factors or familial occurrence of premature ischemic heart disease may be useful for identification of that disease in a screening setting and therefore should be performed prior to initiating competitive exercise. In addition, it is prudent to selectively perform medically supervised exercise stress testing in men over age 40 (women over age 50) who wish to engage in habitual physical training and competitive sports when the examining physician suspects occult CAD on the basis of risk factors, either multiple (≥2, other than age and gender) or single but markedly abnormal. Older athletes should also be warned specifically about prodromal cardiovascular symptoms such as exertional chest pain.

The present guidelines should not promulgate a false sense of security on the part of medical practitioners or the general public, since the standard history and physical examination intrinsically lack the power to reliably identify many potentially lethal cardiovascular abnormalities. Indeed, it is an unrealistic expectation that large-scale standard athletic screening examinations can reliably exclude all of the important cardiac lesions.

## Methodology

Preparticipation sports examinations are presently performed by a variety of individuals, including paid or volunteer physicians or nonphysician health care workers with variable training and experience. Examiners may be associated with, or administratively independent of, the concerned institution, school, or team. Athletic screening should be performed by an appropriately trained health care worker with the requisite training, medical skills, and background to reliably perform a detailed cardiovascular history and physical examination and to recognize heart disease. While it is preferable that such an individual be a licensed physician, this may not always be feasible, and under certain circumstances it may be acceptable for an appropriately trained registered nurse or physician-assistant to perform the screening examination. In those states in which nonphysician health care workers (including chiropractors) are permitted to perform preparticipation screening, it will be necessary to establish a formal certification process to demonstrate expertise in performing cardiovascular examinations (the precise nature of which is presently undetermined). Specifically, athletic screening evaluations should comprise a complete medical history and physical examination, including brachial artery blood pressure measurement. This examination should be conducted in a physical environment conducive to optimal cardiac auscultation, whether performed individually in a private office or in a station format as part of a school program. The evaluation should also emphasize certain elements critical to the detection of those cardiovascular diseases known to be associated with morbidity or sudden cardiac death in athletes.

## Specific Recommendations

The cardiovascular history should include key questions designed to determine from the athlete (1) prior occurrence of exertional chest pain/discomfort or syncope/near-syncope as well as excessive, unexpected, and unexplained shortness of breath/fatigue associated with exercise; (2) past recognition of a heart murmur or increased systemic blood pressure; and (3) family history of premature death (sudden or otherwise), or morbidity from cardiovascular disease in close relative(s) < age 50, or specific knowledge of the occurrence of certain conditions in family members (e.g., hypertrophic cardiomyopathy, dilated cardiomyopathy, long QT syndrome, Marfan syndrome, or clinically important arrhythmias). These recommendations are offered, recognizing that the accuracy of some responses elicited from young athletes may depend on their level of compliance and historical knowledge. Indeed, parents should be responsible for completing the history form of high school athletes.

The physical examination should emphasize (but not necessarily be limited to) (1) precordial auscultation in both the supine and standing positions to identify, in particular, those heart murmurs consistent with left ventricular outflow obstruction; (2) assessment of the femoral artery pulses to exclude coarctation of the aorta; (3) recognition of the physical stigmata of Marfan syndrome; and (4) brachial blood pressure measurement in the sitting position.

## Eligibility Criteria

When a previously unsuspected cardiovascular abnormality is identified in a competitive athlete, whether by standard screening or other means, the following considerations arise: (1) the magnitude of risk for sudden cardiac death associated with continued participation in competitive sports, and (2) the criteria to be implemented for determining whether or not that athlete would benefit from disqualification from athletics. In this regard, the 26th Bethesda Conference sponsored by the American College of Cardiology offers prospective and consensus recommendations for athletic eligibility or disqualification, taking into account the severity of the cardiovascular abnormality as well as the nature of sports training and competition. The 26th Bethesda Conference recommendations are predicated on the likelihood that intense athletic training will increase the risk for sudden cardiac death (or disease progression) in trained athletes with clinically important underlying structural heart disease, although it is not presently possible to quantify that risk precisely for individual participants. Nevertheless, it is presumed that the temporary or permanent withdrawal of selected athletes from participation in certain sports is prudent and likely to diminish the perceived risk. In most instances, a cardiologist should be consulted when a previously unsuspected cardiovascular abnormality is identified in a competitive athlete.

## REFERENCES

1.  Maron BJ: Sudden death in young athletes: Lessons from the Hank Gathers affair. *N Engl J Med* 1993; 329:55–57.
2.  Burke AP, Farb V, Virmani R, et al: Sports-related and non-sports-related sudden cardiac death in young adults. *Am Heart J* 1991; 121:568–575.
3.  Maron BJ, Shirani J, Poliac LC, et al: Sudden death in young competitive athletes: Clinical, demographic and pathological profiles. *JAMA* 1996; 276:199–204.
4.  van Camp SP, Bloor CM, Mueller FO, et al: Nontraumatic sports death in high school and college athletes. *Med Sci Sports Exer* 1995; 27:641–647.
5.  Maron BJ, Roberts WC, McAllister HA, et al: Sudden death in young athletes. *Circulation* 1980; 62:218–229.
6.  Corrado D, Thiene G, Nava A, et al: Sudden death in young competitive athletes: Clinicopathologic correlations in 22 cases. *Am J Med* 1990; 89:588–596.
7.  Thiene G, Nava A, Corrado D, et al: Right ventricular cardiomyopathy and sudden death in young people. *N Engl J Med* 1988; 318:129–133.
8.  Tsung SH, Huang TY, Chang HH: Sudden death in young athletes. *Arch Pathol Lab Med* 1982; 106:168–170.
9.  James TN, Froggatt P, Marshall TK: Sudden death in young athletes. *Ann Intern Med* 1967; 67:1013–1021.
10. Furlanello F, Bettini R, Cozzi F, et al: Ventricular arrhythmias and sudden death in athletes. *Ann NY Acad Sci* 1984; 427:253–279.
11. Maron BJ, Epstein SE, Roberts WC: Causes of sudden death in competitive athletes. *J Am Coll Cardiol* 1986; 7:204–214.
12. Drory Y, Turetz Y, Hiss Y, et al: Sudden unexpected death in persons <40 years of age. *Am J Cardiol* 1991; 68:1388–1392.
13. Topaz O, Edwards JE: Pathologic features of sudden death in children, adolescents and young adults. *Chest* 1985; 87:476–482.
14. Liberthson, RR: Sudden death from cardiac causes in children and young adults. *N Engl J Med* 1996; 334:1039–1044.
15. McCaffrey FM, Braden DS, Strong WB: Sudden cardiac death in young athletes: A review. *Am J Dis Child* 1991; 145:177–183.
16. Thompson PD, Stern MP, Williams P, et al: Death during jogging or running. A study of 18 cases. *JAMA* 1979; 242:1265–1267.
17. Thompson PD, Funk EJ, Carleton RA, Sturner WQ: Incidence of death during jogging in Rhode Island from 1975 through 1980. *JAMA* 1982; 247:2535–2538.
18. Waller BF, Roberts WC: Sudden death while running in conditioned runners aged 40 years or over. *Am J Cardiol* 1980; 45:1292–1300.
19. Virmani R, Robinowitz M, McAllister HA Jr: Nontraumatic death in joggers: A series of 30 patients at autopsy. *Am J Med* 1982; 72:874–882.
20. Maron BJ, Mitchell JH: Revised eligibility recommendations for competitive athletes with cardiovascular abnormalities. (Introduction to Bethesda Conference 26.) *J Am Coll Cardiol* 1994; 24:848–850.
21. Maron BJ, Garson A: Arrhythmias and sudden cardiac death in elite athletes. *Cardiol Rev* 1994; 2:26–32.
22. Maron BJ, Thompson PD, Puffer JC, et al: Cardiovascular preparticipation screening of competitive athletes. *Circulation* 1996; 94:850–856.

23. Maron BJ, Mitchell JH (eds): 26th Bethesda Conference. Recommendations for determining eligibility for competition in athletes with cardiovascular abnormalities. *J Am Coll Cardiol* 1994; 24:845–899.

24. Wigle ED, Sasson Z, Henderson MA, et al: Hypertrophic cardiomyopathy: The importance of the site and extent of hypertrophy—A review. *Prog Cardiovasc Dis* 1985; 28:1–83.

25. Maron BJ, Bonow RO, Cannon RO, et al: Hypertrophic cardiomyopathy: Interrelation of clinical manifestations, pathophysiology, and therapy. *N Engl J Med* 1987; 316:780–789 and 844–852.

26. Louie EK, Edwards LC: Hypertrophic cardiomyopathy. *Prog Cardiovasc Dis* 1994; 36:275–308.

27. Spirito P, Seidman CE, McKenna WJ, Maron BJ: The management of hypertrophic cardiomyopathy. *N Engl J Med* 1997; 336:775–785.

28. Klues HG, Schiffers A, Maron BJ: Phenotypic spectrum and patterns of left ventricular hypertrophy in hypertrophic cardiomyopathy: Morphologic observations and significance as assessed by two-dimensional echocardiography in 600 patients. *J Am Coll Cardiol* 1995; 26:1699–1708.

29. Maron BJ: Hypertrophic cardiomyopathy. *Lancet* 1997; 3350:127–133.

30. Geisterfer-Lowrance AAT, Kass S, Tanigawa G, et al: A molecular basis for familial hypertrophic cardiomyopathy. A β-cardiac myosin heavy chain gene missense mutation. *Cell* 1990; 62:999–1006.

31. Thierfelder L, Watkins H, MacRae C, et al: α-Tropomyosin and cardiac troponin T mutations cause familial hypertrophic cardiomyopathy: A disease of the sarcomere. *Cell* 1994; 77:701–712.

32. Watkins H, Conner D, Thierfelder L, et al: Mutations in the cardiac myosin binding protein-C gene on chromosome 11 cause familial hypertrophic cardiomyopathy. *Nature Genetics* 1995; 11:434–437.

33. Schwartz K, Carrier L, Guicheney P, Komajda M: Molecular basis of familial cardiomyopathies. *Circulation* 1995; 91:532–540.

34. Marian AJ, Roberts R: Recent advances in the molecular genetics of hypertrophic cardiomyopathy. *Circulation* 1995; 91:532–540.

35. Maron BJ, Gardin JM, Flack JM, et al: Assessment of the prevalence of hypertrophic cardiomyopathy in a general population of young adults: Echocardiographic analysis of 4111 subjects in the CARDIA Study. *Circulation* 1995; 92:785–789.

36. Cheitlin MD, De Castro CM, McAllister HA: Sudden death as a complication of anomalous left coronary origin from the anterior sinus of Valsalva. A not-so-minor congenital anomaly. *Circulation* 1974; 50:780–787.

37. Roberts WC: Congenital coronary arterial anomalies unassociated with major anomalies of the heart or great vessels. In: Roberts WC (ed): *Adult Congenital Heart Disease.* Philadelphia, FA Davis Co., 1987:583.

38. Gaither NS, Rogan KM, Stajduhar K, et al: Anomalous origin and course of coronary arteries in adults: Identification and improved imaging utilizing transesophageal echocardiography. *Am Heart* J 1991; 122:69–75.

39. Maron BJ, Leon BJ, Swain JA, et al: Prospective identification by two-dimensional echocardiography of anomalous origin of the left main coronary artery from the right sinus of Valsalva. *Am J Cardiol* 1991; 68:140–142.

40. Jureidini SB, Eaton C, Williams J, et al: Transthoracic two-dimensional and color flow echocardiographic diagnosis of aberrant left coronary artery. *Am Heart J* 1994; 127:438–440.

41.  Vincent GM, Timothy KW, Leppert M, Keating M: The spectrum of symptoms and QT intervals in carriers of the gene for the long-QT syndrome. *N Engl J Med* 1992; 327:846–852.

42.  Moss AJ, Schwartz PJ, Crampton RS, et al: The long QT syndrome: Prospective longitudinal study of 328 families. *Circulation* 1991; 84:1136–1144.

43.  Roden DM, Lazzara R, Rosen M, et al: Multiple mechanisms in the long-QT syndrome: Current knowledge, gaps, and future directions. *Circulation* 1996; 94:1996–2012.

44.  McKenna WJ, Thiene G, Nava A, et al: On behalf of the Task Force of the Working Group Myocardial and Pericardial Disease of the European Society of Cardiology and of the Scientific Council on Cardiomyopathies of the International Society and Federation of Cardiology: Diagnosis of arrhythmogenic right ventricular dysplasia/cardiomyopathy. *Br Heart J* 1994; 71:215–218.

45.  Bharti S, Lev M: Congenital abnormalities of the conduction system in sudden death in young adults. *J Am Coll Cardiol* 1986; 8:1096–1104.

46.  Thiene G, Pennelli N, Rossi L: Cardiac conduction system abnormalities as a possible cause of sudden death in young athletes. *Hum Pathol* 1983; 14:706–709.

47.  Benson DW, Benditt DG, Anderson RW, et al: Cardiac arrest in young, ostensibly healthy patients: Clinical, hemodynamic and electrophysiologic findings. *Am J Cardiol* 1983; 52:65–69.

48.  Kark JA, Posey DM, Schumacher HR, Ruehle CJ: Sickle-cell as a risk factor for sudden death in physical training. *N Engl J Med* 1987; 317:781–787.

49.  Maron BJ, Poliac L, Kaplan JA, Mueller FO: Blunt impact to the chest leading to sudden death from cardiac arrest during sports activities. *N Engl J Med* 1995; 333:337–342.

50.  Virmani R, Robinowitz M, Smialek JE, Smyth DF: Cardiovascular effects of cocaine: An autopsy study of 40 patients. *Am Heart J* 1988; 115:1068–1076.

51.  Isner JM, Estes NAM III, Thompson PD, et al: Acute cardiac events temporally related to cocaine abuse. *N Engl J Med* 1986; 315:1438–1443.

52.  Kloner RA, Hale S, Alkekr K, Rezkalla S: The effects of acute and chronic cocaine use on the heart. *Circulation* 1992; 85:407–419.

53.  Kaplan NM, Deveraux RB, Miller HS Jr: Systemic hypertension. Task Force 4. In: Maron BJ, Mitchell JH (eds): 26th Bethesda Conference. Recommendations for Determining Eligibility for Competition in Athletes with Cardiovascular Abnormalities. *J Am Coll Cardiol* 1994; 24:885–888.

54.  Maron BJ, Gohman TE, Aeppli D: Prevalence of sudden cardiac death during competitive sports activities in Minnesota high school athletes. *J Am Coll Cardiol* 1998; 32:1881–1884.

55.  Pelliccia A, Maron BJ: Preparticipation cardiovascular evaluation of the competitive athlete: Perspectives from the 30-year Italian experience. *Am J Cardiol* 1995; 75:827–831.

56.  Maron BJ, Brown RW, McGrew CA, et al: Ethical, legal and practical considerations affecting medical decision-making in competitive athletes. In: Maron BJ, Mitchell JH (eds): 26th Bethesda Conference. Recommendations for Determining Eligibility for Competition in Athletes with Cardiovascular Abnormalities. *J Am Coll Cardiol* 1994; 24:854–860.

57.  Mitten MJ, Maron BJ: Legal considerations that affect medical eligibility for competitive athletes with cardiovascular abnormalities and acceptance of Bethesda Conference recommendations. *J Am Coll Cardiol* 1994; 24:861–863.

58.  Mitten MJ: Team physicians and competitive athletes: Allocating legal responsibility for athletic injuries. *U Pitt L Rev* 1993; 55:129–169.

59. U.S. Court of Appeals. *N. Knapp* v. *Northwestern University and Rick Taylor*. No. 96-3450, Nov. 22, 1996.

60. Glover DW, Maron BJ: Profile of preparticipation cardiovascular screening for high school athletes. *JAMA* 1998; 279:1817–1819.

61. Corrado D, Basso C, Schiavon M, Thiene G: Screening for hypertrophic cardiomyopathy in young athletes. *N Eng J Med* 1998; 339:364–369.

62. Maron BJ, Epstein SE: Hypertrophic cardiomyopathy: A discussion of nomenclature. *Am J Cardiol* 1979; 43:1242–1244.

63. Ricci C, Longo R, Pagnan L, et al: Magnetic resonance imaging in right ventricular dysplasia. *Am J Cardiol* 1992; 70:1589–1595.

64. Weidenbener EJ, Krauss MD, Waller BF, Taliercio CP: Incorporation of screening echocardiography in the preparticipation exam. *Clin J Sport Med* 1995; 5:86–89.

65. Feinstein RA, Colvin E, Oh MK: Echocardiographic screening as part of a preparticipation examination. *Clin J Sport Med* 1993; 3:149–152.

66. Risser WL, Hoffman HM, Gordon BG Jr, Green LW: A cost-benefit analysis of preparticipation sports examination of adolescent athletes. *J Sch Health* 1985; 55:270–273.

67. Murry PM, Cantwell JD, Heith DL, Shoop J: The role of limited echocardiography in screening athletes. *Am J Cardiol* 1995; 76:849–850.

68. Lewis JF, Maron BJ, Diggs JA, et al: Preparticipation echocardiographic screening for cardiovascular disease in a large, predominantly black population of collegiate athletes. *Am J Cardiol* 1989; 64:1029–1033.

69. Huston TP, Puffer JC, Rodney McW: The athlete heart syndrome. *N Engl J Med* 1985; 4:24–32.

70. Maron BJ: Structural features of the athlete heart as defined by echocardiography. *J Am Coll Cardiol* 1987; 7:190–203.

71. Pelliccia A, Maron BJ, Spataro A, et al: The upper limit of physiologic cardiac hypertrophy in highly trained elite athletes. *N Engl J Med* 1991; 324:295–301.

72. Pelliccia A, Maron BJ, Culasso F, et al: Athlete's heart in women: Echocardiographic characterization of highly trained elite female athletes. *JAMA* 1996; 276:211–215.

73. Maron BJ, Pelliccia A, Spirito P: Cardiac disease in young trained athletes: Insights into methods for distinguishing athlete's heart from structural heart disease with particular emphasis on hypertrophic cardiomyopathy. *Circulation* 1995; 91:1596–1601.

74. Maron BJ, Spirito P, Wesley YE, Arce J: Development and progression of left ventricular hypertrophy in children with hypertrophic cardiomyopathy. *N Engl J Med* 1986; 315:610–614.

75. Zehender M, Meinertz T, Keul J, Just H: ECG variants and cardiac arrhythmias in athletes: Clinical relevance and prognostic importance. *Am Heart J* 1990; 119:1378–1391.

76. LaCorte MA, Boxer RA, Gottesfeld IB, et al: EKG screening program for school athletes. *Clin Cardiol* 1989; 12:41–44.

77. Maron BJ, Bodison SA, Wesley YE, et al: Results of screening a large group of intercollegiate competitive athletes for cardiovascular disease. *J Am Coll Cardiol* 1987; 10:1214–1221.

78. Maron BJ, Wolfson JK, Ciró E, Spirito P: Relation of electrocardiographic abnormalities and patterns of left ventricular hypertrophy identified by two-dimensional echocardiography in patients with hypertrophic cardiomyopathy. *Am J Cardiol* 1983; 51:189–194.

79. Pelliccia A, Cullasso F, Di Paolo FM, et al: Clinical significance of abnormal electrocardiographic patterns in elite athletes: The impact of gender and cardiac morphologic adaptations to training (abstract). *Circulation* 1996; 94:I-326.

80. Fuller CM, McNulty CM, Spring DA, et al: Prospective screening of 5,615 high school athletes for risk of sudden cardiac death. *Med Sci Sports Exerc* 1997; 29:1131–1138.
81. Maron BJ, Poliac LC, Mathenge R: Hypertrophic cardiomyopathy as an important cause of sudden cardiac death on the athletic field in African-American athletes (abstract). *J Am Coll Cardiol* 1997; 29(suppl A):462A.

JAMES L. SUTHERLAND

# CHAPTER 46

# HEART DISEASE IN THE ADOLESCENT

A 1994 report on the cardiovascular status of children in the United States[1] noted that more than 600,000 children have an abnormality of the cardiovascular system. Approximately 440,000 have a cardiac malformation, an estimated 160,000 have a cardiac rhythm disturbance, and 40,000 have acquired heart disease, such as cardiomyopathy, rheumatic heart disease, or Kawasaki disease. The primary care physician is in a key position to recognize, diagnose, and often manage these disorders.

## COMMON SYMPTOM COMPLEXES IN THE ADOLESCENT

There are several common symptom complexes in adolescents that raise concerns for the patient and family regarding the possibility of cardiovascular disease. These complaints are *chest pain, syncope, palpitations,* and *arrythmias.*

### Chest Pain in the Adolescent

Chest pain is common in adolescence and prompts an estimated 650,000 office visits annually for individuals between 10 and 21 years of age.[2] After heart murmurs, it is the most common cause of referral to a pediatric cardiologist.[3] Chest pain as a symptom of cardiovascular disease in the adult is well known in the United States. Cardiovascular disease accounts for approximately 40 percent of all deaths in the United States.[4] Sudden cardiac death occurs in 300,000 to 400,000 adults each year.[5] For these reasons, there is understandable anxiety and concern on the part of the patient and family regarding chest pain.

The vast majority of chest pain in the child and adolescent is benign. The most common causes are idiopathic, musculoskeletal, psychogenic, pulmonary, and gastrointestinal.[6,7] Cardiac causes of chest pain in this age group are quite rare. Psychogenic pain is more common after the age of 12 years, while organic causes are more likely in the preadolescent.[7] The most common causes of cardiac and noncardiac chest pain are provided in Tables 46-1 and 46-2, respectively.

TABLE 46-1.   Cardiac Causes of Chest Pain in Adolescents

**Structural abnormalities**

- LV outflow tract obstruction: aortic stenosis, hypertrophic cardiomyopathy
- Coronary artery anomalies
- Aortic aneurysm (Marfan syndrome)
- Mitral valve prolapse

**Acquired cardiovascular disease**

- Pericarditis
- Myocarditis
- Kawasaki disease
- Coronary artery disease (familial hyperlipidemia)

**Primary or secondary pulmonary artery hypertension**

**Arrhythmias**

**HISTORY.**   It is important to keep in mind that although a serious cardiac or non-cardiac condition is unlikely, the patient and family must be satisfied that a careful and thorough effort to evaluate the pain has been made. This entails a detailed and empathetic history. It is very useful to have the adolescent describe the symptoms. This history should include the following information:

- How long the patient has had pain and when it started
- The location of the pain (having the patient point to the area with one finger is helpful)
- Radiation of pain
- Duration and frequency of episodes
- Severity and characteristics of the pain
- Factors that initiate, exacerbate, or relieve the pain
- Effect of deep inspiration on the pain
- General setting at the time of pain (time of day, place, and events)
- Related stresses (emotional, social, or physical)
- Associated symptoms such as shortness of breath, palpitations, dizziness, or fever
- History of trauma
- Concurrent illnesses such as cough, asthma, vomiting, or fever
- Use of drugs, specifically cocaine
- Family history of cardiac disease

TABLE 46-2.   Noncardiac Causes of Chest Pain in Adolescents

Idiopathic

Pulmonary (e.g., asthma, pneumothorax, pleurodynia, pneumonia, effusion)

Gastrointestinal (e.g., gastroesophageal reflux, esophagitis, hiatal hernia, biliary colic, pancreatitis)

Musculoskeletal

- Costochondritis

- Muscle injury

- Tietze's syndrome

- Tumor

- Trauma

Psychogenic (e.g., hyperventilation, depression, somatization)

Chest pain that is of sudden onset, sharp in nature, well localized, unassociated with exercise (onset while watching TV is all too common), and lasting only a few seconds or minutes is unlikely to be due to cardiac causes. Another common benign history is a recurring, vague chest discomfort that occurs sporadically over many months or even years. This pain may persist for several hours. A history that is of more concern is chest pain that is associated with exercise, and described as a "crushing or burning" substernal pain, and relieved quickly by stopping activity. This suggests myocardial ischemia, and further cardiac work-up should be considered.

Patients with acute, severe, and persistent chest pain, often seen in the emergency room, are more likely to have an organic cause of their pain. Cardiac causes of this type of pain include pericarditis, arrhythmias, chest trauma (hemopericardium), and cocaine intoxication.[8] Noncardiac causes of pain in the emergency setting include pneumothorax, pneumonia, pleurodynia, acute esophagitis, or foreign body in the esophagus.[8] A directed history and physical examination usually will identify the cause of this acute pain. In this acute setting, useful tests include electrocardiogram, chest x-ray, or echocardiogram. Cardiac enzymes such as creatine kinase–MB fraction, total creatine kinase, and various troponin assays may be helpful.

**PHYSICAL EXAMINATION.**   Specific features that should be identified include musculoskeletal abnormalities, such as those associated with Marfan syndrome or mitral valve prolapse (pectus excavatum or scoliosis); chest wall bruising or abrasions that suggest trauma; signs of inflammation, elicited by palpation of the costochondral junction; abnormalities of rhythm or blood pressure; abnormal or asymmetric breath sounds; murmurs or clicks, found by cardiac auscultation in the supine, sitting, or standing position; and abdominal tenderness or masses.

**LABORATORY INVESTIGATION.**   An electrocardiogram (ECG) should be obtained as a baseline. Abnormalities of rhythm, voltage, ST-T waves, and QRS axis are sought. Further tests are usually not necessary unless a specific disorder is suggested from the history, physical examination, or ECG.

**MANAGEMENT.**   In the majority of cases, the cause of the pain is benign, and reassurance is all that is indicated. The patient and family should be informed that the findings are normal, that activity restrictions are not necessary, and that though the pain will probably recur, it will eventually be outgrown. It is helpful to encourage the patient and family to maintain contact regarding any change or worsening of the symptoms, so that further investigation is available if necessary.

## Syncope in Adolescents

Adolescents seem predisposed to episodes of dizziness and fainting. It is estimated that up to 25 percent of children have had at least one episode of syncope.[9] Syncope is the abrupt and transient lost of consciousness and postural tone. Presyncope (or near-syncope) is a transient episode of altered state of consciousness (dizziness or lightheadedness), but without loss of consciousness. Syncope is a distressing experience for the patient and family. It is a common cause for emergency room visits and referrals to pediatric neurologists or cardiologists. Though this is usually a benign condition in the adolescent, the evaluation is directed at identifying disorders that might cause recurring syncope or, potentially, sudden death. The major disease categories to be ruled out are neurologic and cardiovascular. The most common causes of syncope in children and adolescents are provided in Table 46-3.

The evaluation of syncope can be an expensive endeavor. In 1982, Kapoor et al[10] found that the average cost of diagnostic evaluation of 121 adults with syncope was $2,463.00. The cause of syncope was determined in 13 patients, yielding a cost of $22,925.00 per patient with a discernible diagnosis. The diagnostic tests included electroencephalography, Holter monitoring, glucose tolerance tests, computed tomography (CT) scans, and intracardiac electrophysiologic studies. The evaluation in the adolescent is generally much more cost-effective and usually involves only a history, physical examination, and ECG.

**HISTORY.**   The crux of the evaluation of syncope is the history. This is best elicited as a somewhat tedious "frame by frame" account of the syncopal episode from initial symptoms until recovery. In addition to family history and review of systems, important historical information includes the general setting and time of day; relationship to meals, physical activity, and medications; illicit drug use; intercurrent illness; amount of sleep; social and psychological dynamics; premonitory signs, symptoms, or aura; and a description of the episode from observers (this may require telephone interviews).

*The majority of adolescents with recurring syncope have autonomic dysfunction.* Other names for this form of syncope include the common faint, vasovagal attack, vasodepressor syncope, neurocardiogenic syncope, and neurally mediated syncope.

## TABLE 46-3.   Causes of Syncope in Adolescents

Neurocardiogenic

Cardiac

- Left ventricular outflow tract obstruction (aortic stenosis)
- Hypertrophic obstructive cardiomyopathy
- Coronary artery anomalies
- Congestive (dilated) cardiomyopathy
- Myocarditis
- Pulmonary hypertension (primary, Eisenmenger's syndrome)
- Arrhythmia or conduction abnormalities (LQTS, WPW, right ventricular dysplasia, heart block)
- Mitral valve prolapse
- Intracardiac tumors or masses

Neuropsychiatric

- Seizure disorder
- Hyperventilation syndrome
- Migraine headache
- Hysterical reaction
- Panic or anxiety disorder
- Malingering

Drug related

- Antihypertesive medication
- Psychoactive medication
- Antiarrhythmic medication
- Insulin
- Diuretics
- Cocaine

Other

- Micturition syncope
- Defecation syncope
- Carotid sinus syncope
- Hypoglycemia
- Dehydration

LQTS = long QT syndrome; WPW = Wolff-Parkinson-White syndrome.

Autonomic dysfunction can generally be diagnosed from the history alone. Typically, the patient is standing at the onset. Signs and symptoms such as lightheadedness, dizziness, nausea, epigastric discomfort, pallor, cold sweats, clammy skin, and blurring, dimming, or tunneling of vision often precede the syncopal episode. If the patient does not lie down, there is loss of muscular tone, with postural collapse and unconsciousness. Consciousness is regained rapidly (usually in less than a few minutes). Dizziness may persist, and if standing is attempted too rapidly, syncope may recur. Rarely, clonic or tonic jerks may accompany the episode. Following the syncopal episode, the patient returns quickly to his or her usual state of health, although he or she may complain of headache and fatigue. Autonomic dysfunction may be associated with emotional or physical stresses, which include pain, the sight of blood, prolonged recumbency, hunger, heat and humidity, heavy meals, crowded conditions, poor ventilation, and physical exhaustion.

The exact mechanism of autonomic dysfunction remains unclear, but it is speculated that upright posture reduces preload to the ventricles, resulting in a smaller ventricular volume. In response to this, adrenergic tone is increased, resulting in excessive contractility of the ventricles. Myocardial mechanoreceptors (C fibers) are activated by this vigorous contractility and produce afferent vagal impulses, which are sent to the medulla.[11] This results in sympathetic nerve inhibition (vasodilation) and/or parasympathetic stimulation (bradycardia).[12] These responses, either singly or in combination, result in inadequate cerebral profusion and produce syncope.

It is important to distinguish syncope from seizures. Features that suggest a seizure are blue face (not pallor), frothing at the mouth, tongue biting, disorientation, sleeplessness or aching muscles after the event, and duration of unconsciousness longer than 5 min. Disorientation after the episode appears to be the best discriminatory feature and is reported more frequently in patients with seizures.[13]

Cardiac causes of syncope are suggested by a positive family history of syncope, arrhythmia, or sudden death; a previous diagnosis in the patient of cardiac abnormality or cardiac surgery; palpitations, chest pain, shortness of breath with exercise; and especially exercise-induced syncope. Syncope associated with exercise requires a very thorough cardiovascular assessment.

**PHYSICAL EXAMINATION.**   In the office evaluation for syncope, the physical examination is usually normal. Nonetheless, a complete examination focusing on the cardiac and neurologic status should be performed.

Supine and standing blood pressures should be measured to assess for orthostatic hypotension. Cardiac auscultation should be performed with the patient supine, sitting, and standing to ascertain the presence of murmurs or clicks and their change with postural position, as occurs with mitral valve prolapse or hypertrophic cardiomyopathy.

**LABORATORY INVESTIGATION.**   An ECG should be performed on all patients with syncope or seizures. Abnormalities of atrioventricular conduction (heart block), right or left ventricular hypertrophy, bundle branch block pattern, prolonged Q-T interval, presence of a delta wave (Wolff-Parkinson-White syndrome), and abnormal Q waves should be sought. Other laboratory tests are guided by the clinical impression based on the history and physical examination. Patients with syncopal episodes associated with identifiable stresses, such as being overheated or the sight of blood, usually do not require further evaluation. Patients with repeated episodes of syncope, abnormal cardiac or neurologic findings, syncope with exercise, atypical syncope, or a positive family history of sudden death require further study.

Tilt table testing has proven useful to document the cardiovascular responses in patients with recurring syncope due to suspected autonomic dysfunction.[14] Testing may be done with or without the addition of Isuprel infusion. There are many protocols for tilt table testing, and positive responses result in cardioinhibitor (bradycardia), vasodepressor (hypotension), or a combination. Occasionally, dramatic asystolic pauses are produced. A positive tilt table test suggests autonomic dysfunction, and treatment can be directed at this disorder. Patients may require repeat tilt table testing while being treated to assess the efficacy of management.

Patients with suspected structural heart disease should have an echocardiogram. A treadmill stress test is helpful in patients with exercise-related syncope to detect arrhythmias, ischemic changes, or abnormal blood pressure response. Conduction or arrhythmia problems may be screened by a 24-h Holter monitor or ambulatory event monitoring. Intracardiac or transesophageal electrophysiologic study may be indicated for patients with suspected significant arrhythmias. Patients with suspected anatomic or functional abnormalities or coronary anomalies may require cardiac catheterization. Tests for neurologic abnormalities include electroencephalogram, cranial magnetic resonance imaging (MRI), or computed tomography (CT) scans. Use of these more invasive and expensive tests is rarely necessary in the majority of children and adolescents with syncope.

**TREATMENT.**   Autonomic dysfunction as a cause of syncope does not require specific therapy unless it is a recurring problem. Therapeutic options include volume expansion with increased fluid intake and/or use of a mineralocorticoid (Florinef 0.1 mg once or twice a day); beta-blocking agents to modify the feedback loop and to prevent intense vagal output; alpha-agonist agents (e.g., pseudoephedrine hydrochloride or midodrine hydrochloride); and at times a serotonin agonist (sertraline hydrochloride).[15] Treatment is individualized and may require combination therapy. Side effects of the various medications should be monitored, including blood pressure response and electrolytes. The timing of when to wean from treatment depends on the patient's clinical response and physician judgment. Syncope in the adolescent is usually a transient problem, but it may occur intermittently for months or even years.

Identified cardiac or neurologic causes of syncope require treatment directed at the specific problem. Psychiatric referral may be necessary if other causes of syncope are ruled out or psychological disorders are contributing. Basilar artery migraine is a rare cause of syncope and should be considered when syncope is associated with severe headaches.[16]

## Palpitation and Arrhythmias

**PALPITATION IN THE ADOLESCENT.**  Palpitation is an unpleasant awareness of the heartbeat. Palpitations may be described in various terms, including "racing, fluttering, pounding, skipping, stopping, jumping, or flip-flopping." Often patients will complain of chest pain, but on careful questioning the problem is actually palpitations. Symptoms may be very transient or may cause considerable anxiety and distress. Parents may describe a visible pounding or fluttering of the shirt over the heart. Although frequently benign, palpitations may be due to potentially serious arrhythmias.

**HISTORY.**    There are important historical clues that suggest the presence of a true arrhythmia. Supraventricular tachycardia (usually heart rates greater than 200/min) is suggested by sudden onset and/or cessation of the palpitation. Gradual buildup of heart rate suggests sinus tachycardia. Complaints of skips or pauses may suggest premature atrial or ventricular contractions. The frequency and duration of symptoms should be noted. Symptoms that suggest true arrhythmias include presyncope, syncope, sudden shortness of breath, and weakness. Palpitations may be associated with anxiety or panic reactions; however, true arrhythmias may also occur at times of catecholamine excess such as emotional or physical stress. Information about drug usage (especially cocaine, amphetamines, tobacco, and antidepressants), caffeine intake, and systemic illness should be sought. Knowledge of congenital, acquired, or postoperative heart disease is helpful. The family history should include questions concerning relatives with a history of sudden death, rhythm disturbances, syncope, seizures, long Q-T syndrome, and familial cardiomyopathy.

**PHYSICAL EXAMINATION.**    The physical examination may identify previously unsuspected conditions that are associated with arrhythmias. These include mitral valve prolapse, atrial septal defects, Ebstein's anomaly of the tricuspid valve, pulmonary hypertension, hypertrophic cardiomyopathy, and L transposition of the great vessels. The examination may suggest systemic illnesses such as hyperthyroidism, neuromuscular disease, rheumatic fever, or Lyme disease (conduction abnormalities).

**LABORATORY INVESTIGATION.**    In the office setting, the adolescent with palpitations commonly has a normal cardiovascular examination, including normal rhythm. An ECG and a rhythm strip should be obtained. A practical approach in patients with very rare episodes of palpitations is to teach the patient and/or parents how to use a stethoscope to count the heart rate and rhythm during these episodes. If unusually fast rates (e.g., 180 to 200) are counted, further evaluation is indicated. The essential ingredient in diagnosis is a recording of the ECG or rhythm strip during the palpitation. A 24-h Holter monitor is of limited value unless the palpitations are occurring daily and frequently. On the other hand, transtelephonic ambulatory event monitoring has proven quite helpful. These monitors continuously record rhythm information but save the recordings only when the patient activates the monitor. These recordings show the cardiac rhythm 1 to 2 min prior to activation as well as a subsequent 1 to 2 min of data. These monitors are usually worn for 2- to 4-week periods, and patients may participate in practically all activities. Recordings can be transmitted by telephone to a remote monitoring station. This allows prompt identification of and response to any significant arrhythmia (see Fig. 46-1). Event monitors have proven more cost-effective and helpful than Holter monitors in evaluation of adults with palpitations.[17] Palpitations or symptoms associated with exercise may require a treadmill stress test. When there is concern about symptoms or a more serious arrhythmia is suspected, an electrophysiologic study may be necessary.

Palpitations do not necessarily indicate an arrhythmia, and patients with arrhythmias may not have palpitations. Reiffel et al[18] found that only 50 percent of adults with palpitations actually had arrhythmias. In adolescents, it is not uncommon to have numerous monitored tracings reveal only sinus tachycardia or sinus arrhythmias. This information can be used to reassure the patient, family, and physician alike that this form of palpitation is benign. For patients with unremarkable monitoring who continue to have recurring episodic complaints, serial event monitoring over time may be necessary in order to detect an arrhythmia. The documentation of an arrhythmia prompts further work-up and treatment. These are discussed in the section below.

**ARRHYTHMIAS IN THE ADOLESCENT.**   Sinus arrhythmias are common and benign. A wandering atrial pacemaker manifested by a change in the P-wave axis but with normal atrioventricular conduction is also benign and generally occurs during slow sinus node activity. In normal children and adolescents, 24-h Holter monitor studies reveal fairly frequent rhythm and conduction disturbances. A study of 100 healthy 14- to 16-year-old boys[19] revealed a waking heart rate range of 45 to 200 beats/min and a sleeping heart rate range of 23 to 95 beats/min. Other common findings included first- and second-degree atrioventricular block, premature atrial contractions, sinus pauses or arrests, junctional beats, and ventricular ectopy.

The ECG should be scrutinized carefully for evidence of preexcitation of the ventricles because such patients are likely to have episodes of supraventricular tachycardia or atrial fibrillation (Wolff-Parkinson-White syndrome). The ST segments at leads $V_1$ and $V_2$ must be inspected for epsilon waves, which occur in patients with right ventricular dysplasia because such patients have serious ventricular arrhythmias. The Q-T interval must be measured carefully, for such children may have the long Q-T sudden death syndrome and experience ventricular arrhythmias and sudden death. A list of medications causing a long Q-T interval is shown in Table 46-4.[20]

*Premature Atrial Complexes.*   Premature atrial complexes (PACs) are common and may be conducted normally (producing an early but normal QRS complex), conducted aberrantly (producing an early but deformed QRS complex, not infrequently mistaken for a premature beat of ventricular origin), or not conducted at all (causing an abrupt pause in the ventricular rhythm). Careful inspection of the electrical activity preceding the premature complex will usually reveal a small deflection

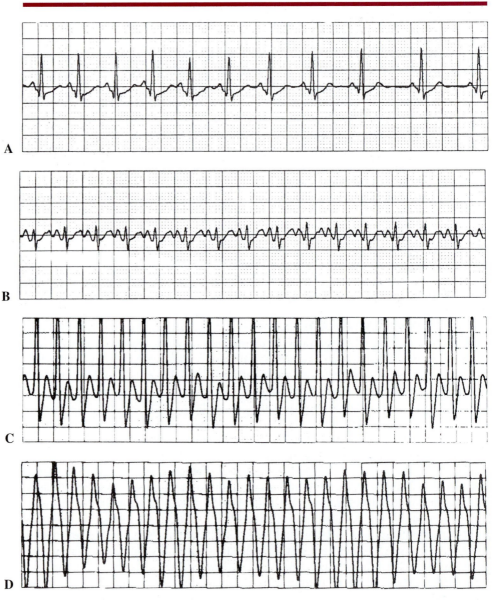

**Figure 46-1** Transtelephonic event monitor tracings from four adolescents with palpitations: A. A 17-year-old girl with "lightheadedness and pounding." Recording reveals sinus tachycardia. B. A 15-year-old girl with known Wolff-Parkinson-White syndrome with complaint of "fast heartbeat." Recording reveals sinus tachycardia at 150 beats per minute but no supraventricular tachycardia. The signs of preexcitation of the ventricles are not seen in this tracing. C. A 15-year-old boy with "racing heartbeat." Recording reveals supraventricular tachycardia at 215 beats per minute, and he was treated with oral digoxin. D. A 14-year-old boy with "fast, pounding heartbeat." Recording reveals a wide-QRS tachycardia at 240 beats per minute. He underwent electrophysiologic study, which revealed A-V nodal reentry tachycardia with aberrant conduction. He underwent radiofrequency ablation.

of the premature atrial impulse. This may require perusal of all 12 leads to identify these small waves, often buried in the preceding T wave. Premature atrial contractions are almost always benign in the face of an otherwise normal history and physical examination. PACs associated with underlying cardiac abnormalities, such as operated or unoperated congenital heart disease or cardiomyopathies or occurring in symptomatic patients, may require further scrutiny. A variety of arrhythmias and conduction disturbances are seen in well-trained adolescent athletes and are discussed in the section on the young athlete.

***Premature Ventricular Complexes.***   While atrial arrhythmias are more common in infants and young children, premature ventricular contractions (PVCs) seem to peak in adolescence, occurring in up to 50 percent of normal teenagers.[21] PVCs are identified by the following characteristics: They occur prematurely before the next expected beat; they have a bizarre morphology different from the normal QRS complex (inspection of more than one lead may be necessary to identify the abnormal morphology); they have a prolonged QRS duration of greater than 0.09 s; the T waves are commonly in a different direction than the QRS complex; and there is no preceding P wave visible. They can be differentiated from aberrantly conducted premature atrial beats by identification of a P wave preceding the premature atrial complex. Aberrantly conducted premature junctional beats can be confirmed only by electrophysiologic study.

Benign PVCs generally have the following pattern: They usually occur singly; they have a fixed R-to-R interval relationship with the preceding QRS complex; they are unifocal (all have identical morphology); they arise from the right ventricle and have a left bundle branch block pattern; they disappear with exercise or elevated heart rate; they are usually infrequent (less than 30 per hour); and the cardiovascular examination is otherwise normal. Benign PVCs may occur in a ventricular bigeminy, trigeminy, or quadrigeminy pattern or as couplets (paired PVCs). The evaluation of the adolescent with PVCs involves a history, physical examination, 12-lead ECG, and frequently an echocardiogram. Patients should be exercised in the office to determine if the PVCs disappear with increasing heart rate. Treadmill stress testing may be used to more formally assess the response to exercise. If this evaluation is normal, no further work-up is indicated and no treatment or restrictions are necessary. Complex ventricular ectopy, such as multiform PVCs, ventricular couplets, or self-limited ventricular tachycardia, has been reported in up to 12 percent of young adults with otherwise normal hearts.[21] These more complex forms of ventricular ectopy, especially sustained ventricular tachycardia, require careful investigation, however, which may include catheterization and electrophysiology study.

***Supraventricular Tachycardia.***   The adolescent with supraventricular tachycardia (SVT) may complain of palpitations, chest pains, shortness of breath, or near-syncope. It is the most common form of sustained tachycardia in children. The electrical substrates are usually an accessory atrioventricular connection or atrioventricular node reentry tachycardia.[23] The evaluation of suspected SVT is the same as that outlined above for palpitations. The physical examination is usually

**TABLE 46-4.  Drugs that Prolong the Q-T Interval and/or Induce *Torsades de Pointes***

| Drug (Brand Names) | Drug Class (Clinical Usage) | QT | TdP | Comments |
|---|---|---|---|---|
| Amiodarone (Cordarone) | Antiarrhythmic (heart rhythm) | QT | TdP | Literature References |
| Amitriptyline (Elavil, Endep) | Antidepressant (depression, pain, others) | | | Literature References |
| Astemizole (Hismanal) | Antihistamine (allergy) | QT | TdP | Off Market |
| Azelastine (Astelin) | Antihistamine | QT | | |
| Bepridil (Vascor) | Antianginal (heart pain) | QT | TdP | |
| Chlorpromazine (Thorazine) | Mental illness & nausea/vomiting | | | Literature References |
| Cisapride (Propulsid) | Stimulates intestinal motility | QT | TdP | |
| Clarithromycin (Biaxin) | Antibiotic | | | Strong/Few, Interacts with QT Drugs, Literature References |
| Clemastine (Tavist) | Antihistamine | | | Limited Data, Literature References |
| Desipramine (Norpramin) | Antidepressant (depression and others) | QT | | Literature References |
| Disopyramide (Norpace) | Antiarrhythmic (heart rhythm) | QT | TdP | Females>Males |
| Doxepin (Sinequan, Zonalon) | Antidepressant (depression, pain, others) | | | Literature References |
| Erythromycin (Akne-Mycin, E.E.S., EryDerm, Erygel, EryTab, Erythrocin, Erythromycin Base Filmtab, Erythrostatin) | Antibiotic and intestinal motility stimulant | QT | TdP | Females>Males |
| Felbamate (Felbatrol) | Anticonvulsant | | TdP | |
| Flecainide (Tambocor) | Antiarrhythmic | QT | TdP | Limited Data |
| Fluoxetine (Prozac) | Antidepressant | QT | | Reports not supported by lab data or literature reports |
| Foscarnet (Foscavir) | Antiviral | QT | | |
| Fosphenytoin (Cerebyx) | Anticonvulsant | QT | | |
| Grepafloxacin (Raxar) | Antibiotic | QT | | Off Market |
| Halofantrine | Antimalarial | QT | TdP | Females>Males |
| Haloperidol (Haldol) | Mental illness, agitation | QT | TdP | |

**TABLE 46-4.**   Drugs that Prolong the Q-T Interval and/or Induce *Torsades de Pointes (continued)*

| Drug (Brand Names) | Drug Class (Clinical Usage) | QT | TdP | Comments |
|---|---|---|---|---|
| Ibutilide (Corvert) | Antiarrhythmic | QT | TdP | Females>Males |
| Imipramine (Tofranil) | Antidepressant (depression, pain, others) | | | Literature References |
| Indapamide (Lozol) | Diuretic (stimulates water and salt loss) | QT | | Literature References, Increased QT in Animals |
| Isradipine (Dynacirc) | Cardiac drug for high blood pressure | QT | | |
| Levomethadyl (Orlaam) | Treat narcotic dependence | QT | | |
| Moexipril/HCTZ (Uniretic) | Antihypertensive agent | QT | | |
| Naratriptan (Amerge) | Migraine treatment | QT | | |
| Nicardipine (Cardene) | Cardiac drug | QT | | |
| Octreotide (Sandostatin) | Diarrhea therapy | QT | | |
| Pentamidine (Pentacarinat, Pentam, NebuPent) | Anti-infective (pneumonia, others) | QT | TdP | Females>Males |
| Pimozide (Orap) | Tourette's syndrome, seizures | QT | | Females>Males, Literature References |
| Probucol (Lorelco) | Lowers cholesterol | QT | TdP | Females>Males |
| Procainamide (Procan, Procanbid, Pronestyl) | Antiarrhythmic | | TdP | |
| Quetiapine (Seroquel) | Antipsychotic | QT | | |
| Quinidine (Cardioquin, Duraquin, Quinidex, Quinaglute) | Antiarrhythmic | QT | TdP | Females>Males |
| Risperidone (Risperdal) | Mental illness | QT | | |
| Salmeterol (Serevent) | Sympathomimetic/Adrenergic | QT | | |
| Sotalol (Betapace) | Antiarrhythmic | QT | TdP | Females>Males |
| Sparfloxacin (Zagam) | Antibiotic | QT | TdP | |
| Sumatriptan (Imitrex) | Migraine treatment | QT | | |
| Tamoxifen (Nolvadex) | Breast cancer treatment | QT | | |
| Terfenadine (Seldane) | Antihistamine (allergy) | QT | TdP | Females>Males, Off Market |
| Thioridazine (Mellaril) | Mental illness | QT | TdP | |

*(continues)*

**TABLE 46-4.   Drugs that Prolong the Q-T Interval and/or Induce *Torsades de Pointes (continued)***

| Drug (Brand Names) | Drug Class (Clinical Usage) | QT | TdP | Comments |
|---|---|---|---|---|
| Tizanidine (Zanaflex) | Muscle relaxant | QT | | Increased QT in animals, but not evaluated in humans |
| Trimethoprim Sulfamethoxazole (Bactrim, Septra, Trimeth-Sulfa) | Antibiotic | | | Questionable case report |
| Venlafaxine (Effexor) | Antidepressant | QT | | |
| Zolmitriptan (Zomig) | Migraine treatment | QT | | |

*Source:* This table was prepared in 2000 by Dr. Raymond L. Woosley of Georgetown University for *Heart to Heart*, Sudden Arrhythmia Death Syndrome Foundation, Salt Lake City, Utah, and used with his permission.

- *QT* indicates that QT prolongation is mentioned in the labeling as a potential action of the drug.
- *TdP* indicates that the labeling includes mention of cases or risk of the syndrome of torsades de pointes.
- *Limited Data* indicates that there is only limited data to suggest the drug's ability to prolong QT or induce torsades de pointes.
- *Literature References* indicates that there are reports in the medical literature of torsades de pointes.
- *Females>Males* indicates that substantial evidence indicates a greater risk (usually two-fold) of torsades de pointes in women.
- *Strong/Few* indicates that there is strong evidence for QT prolongation and/or torsades de pointes in a few cases.
- *Off Market* indicates that this drug has been removed from the U.S. market because of drug-induced torsades de pointes.

normal. The central element in the diagnosis is to record the cardiac rhythm during an episode of tachycardia. In the office setting, the patient is rarely in SVT, but an analysis of the 12-lead ECG may identify an ectopic atrial pacemaker, a delta wave indicative of Wolff-Parkinson-White syndrome, or a long Q-T interval (suggesting ventricular tachycardia). Some 2 to 4 weeks of transtelephonic monitoring is very helpful to capture the arrhythmia on paper (see Fig. 46-1). When complaints are associated with exercise, a treadmill stress test may be useful. Electrophysiologic studies are indicated for patients with more serious symptoms or poor control of rhythm.

*Acute treatment* of sustained SVT involves vagal maneuvers (e.g., Valsalva maneuvers, diving reflex, ice to the face, and headstand) or medications. Adenosine given rapidly intravenously is the drug of choice (6 to 12 mg in adult-size adolescents). It should be given while monitoring with a continuous ECG to document underlying rhythm disturbances such as atrial flutter or rhythm problems associated with the treatment itself. Other useful drugs in the acute setting are esmolol (use with caution in infants), verapamil (contraindicated in infants), amiodarone, and procainamide. If available, transesophageal electrophysiologic study with overdrive atrial pacing has proven helpful in managing SVT.[24] Electrical cardioversion should be used if the rhythm cannot be controlled and the patient is in severe congestive heart failure. Other than vagal maneuvers, the acute treatment is best performed in an emergency room or intensive care unit setting so that potential complications can be managed expediently.

The *long-term management* of supraventricular tachycardia entails the following approach. Patients with infrequent or very self-limited episodes of SVT but with an otherwise normal heart and no evidence of Wolff-Parkinson-White syndrome may be followed without treatment. Patients with problematic recurrences of SVT require daily medication. Digoxin is a common first-line drug but should be avoided in the patient with Wolff-Parkinson-White syndrome because of its potential proarrhythmic effects in Wolff-Parkinson-White syndrome. Other medications include beta blockers, calcium channel blockers, amiodarone, sotalol, and procainamide. The initiation of treatment with the last three medications should be done with telemetry monitoring in the hospital. Most of these patients are periodically seen by a cardiologist in conjunction with the primary care physician. The length of treatment is based on clinical response and physician judgment.

For patients with difficult to control arrhythmias or if medication appears to be a lifelong need or there are associated side effects, intracardiac radiofrequency ablation should be considered. Radiofrequency ablation procedures have been established as an effective and safe treatment for many forms of SVT. Success rates ranging from 85 to 95 percent are reported from experienced electrophysiologic laboratories.[25]

Additional information about supraventricular tachycardia is provided in Chap. 37.

***Ventricular Tachycardia.***    Even in the asymptomatic patient, ventricular tachycardia (VT) should be considered a marker for cardiac abnormality. Ventricular tachycardia is defined as three or more consecutive ventricular complexes, usually at a rate of >120 beats per minute.[26] The QRS complexes are wide ($\geq$0.09 s), but in some ECG leads these changes may be subtle, and inspection of several ECG leads is necessary to appreciate the abnormal complexes. The presence of atrioventricular dissociation is diagnostic of VT. The distinction between VT and SVT with aberrantly conducted QRS complexes may be difficult and may necessitate transesophageal or intracardiac electrophysiologic study. Wide QRS tachycardia in childhood and adolescence should be considered VT.

Cardiac conditions in the adolescent that are associated with VT include cardiomyopathies, myocarditis, drug ingestion, arrhythmogenic right ventricular dysplasia, cardiac tumors, and long QT syndrome. Postoperative tetralogy of Fallot patients with significant residual defects or elevated right ventricular pressures have been shown to have a relatively high risk of sudden death related to ventricular arrhythmia.[27]

The discovery of VT requires an extensive cardiac evaluation that often includes a cardiac catheterization, myocardial biopsy, and electrophysiologic study. For patients with cardiac disease, therapy includes antiarrhythmic medications, surgical or catheter ablation procedures, surgical repair of residual heart defects or removal of tumors, or implantation of a cardioverter-defibrillator device. Patients who have otherwise normal cardiac findings despite a comprehensive evaluation are usually asymptomatic and do not require treatment.

# "SILENT" CARDIAC CONDITIONS DETECTED IN ADOLESCENCE

Although most cardiac defects are detected in infancy or childhood, congenital heart disease may be first recognized in adolescence. These abnormalities usually do not produce symptoms in the young. Instead, elevated blood pressure, unusual heart sounds, or murmurs may prompt investigation leading to the diagnosis. The murmurs may be subtle and often are considered innocent. This section will briefly review four relatively common cardiac conditions that may remain "silent" throughout childhood. Mitral valve prolapse is included in this section, although it is not generally considered a congenital lesion. Hypertrophic cardiomyopathy may present in adolescence and is discussed in Chap. 28. A more detailed discussion of congenital heart lesions is presented in Chap. 33.

## Coarctation of the Aorta

Coarctation of the aorta in the adolescent is generally detected during evaluation of a heart murmur or hypertension. Coarctation is usually a discrete narrowing of the aorta, distal to the take-off of the left subclavian artery at the site of the aortic insertion of the ductus arteriosus or ligamentum arteriosum. There is an indention of the outer aortic wall, with formation of an intraluminal shelf that produces the obstruction. This obstruction tends to progress as a result of intimal proliferation. Some coarctations may have a long segment narrowing in the aortic arch or, rarely, isolated obstruction in the abdominal aorta. A bicuspid aortic valve commonly coexists with coarctation. Other associated anomalies may include ventricular septal defect, patent ductus arteriosus, mitral valve abnormalities, and subaortic obstruction. A potentially lethal coexisting though rare anomaly is a congenital aneurysm of the circle of Willis. Coarctation of the aorta is also seen in patients with Turner syndrome.

**HISTORY.**   The patients discussed in this section are usually asymptomatic.

**PHYSICAL EXAMINATION.**   Recognition of diminished or absent femoral pulses with associated brisk radial or brachial pulses allows a presumptive diagnosis of coarctation of the aorta. Blood pressure measurement in the arms and legs documents the pressure gradient across the narrowing. Systolic murmurs may arise from aortic stenosis or other associated lesions and are usually heard along the left sternal border or at the base. The coarctation itself may produce a murmur in the interscapular region. Patients with abundant collateral vessels around the coarctation site may have a continuous murmur heard over the back. A systolic ejection click heard at the apex or base suggests an associated bicuspid aortic valve.

In infancy, coarctation frequently presents with heart failure and requires early surgical intervention. Patients who escape early detection and advance, untreated, into adulthood have an average life expectancy of only 33 years.[28] The effects of chronic hypertension predispose these patients to premature coronary atherosclerosis and congestive heart failure. The aortic wall in the region of coarctation develops changes of medial necrosis that may result in aneurysm or rupture.[29] There is a risk of infective endocarditis at the coarctation site or bicuspid aortic valve.

**LABORATORY INVESTIGATION.**  The chest x-ray film may reveal rib notching and the ∍ sign. The ECG may show left ventricular hypertrophy. The diagnosis of coarctation is usually confirmed by echocardiography. The coarctation site can frequently be imaged from the suprasternal notch view. Doppler interrogation in the descending aorta reveals increased flow velocity as well as a characteristic diastolic "tailing" pattern. MRI is also helpful when the anatomy cannot be clearly seen with echocardiography. Catheterization is rarely necessary unless an interventional procedure is contemplated.

**TREATMENT.**  Surgical resection of the coarctation with end-to-end anastomosis is a time-proven method of treatment. Variations of the coarctation anatomy may necessitate other approaches, such as an interposition tubular graft, "bucket-handle" graft, or left subclavian flap aortoplasty (usually reserved for infants). The use of a patch to repair coarctation is associated with late aneurysms and aortic wall rupture and should be avoided.[30]

There is growing acceptance of balloon dilatation as an alternative treatment for native or unoperated coarctation. This procedure has been generally safe and successful in midterm follow-up studies.[31] Because balloon dilatation produces a tear through the vessel intima and media, there is concern over late aneurysm formation, and long-term results are not yet available. Balloon dilatation of a recurrent coarctation in a previously surgically repaired patient is widely accepted, however. Postoperative scar tissue surrounds the coarctation site and is felt to offer a protective encasement if there is a balloon-induced wall tear. Simultaneous balloon dilatation and implantation of a balloon expandable stent has been utilized effectively in both native and recurrent coarctation in older patients.[32]

Patients who have undergone either surgical or interventional catheterization treatment require long-term follow-up for persistent systemic arterial hypertension (despite adequate relief of obstruction), recurrent obstruction, and aneurysm formation. Antihypertensive medications are sometimes necessary. Lifelong infective endocarditis prophylaxis is indicated.

Additional information about coarctation of the aorta is provided in Chap. 33.

## Bicuspid Aortic Valve

Bicuspid aortic valve occurs in 2 percent of the population and is one of the most common congenital cardiac malformations.[33] It is more common in males and is usually detected early in life. Patients with very mild forms of stenosis or regurgitation may be detected in later childhood, usually during evaluation for a heart murmur or ejection click sound. It is important to recognize a bicuspid aortic valve because of the risk of infective endocarditis and the natural history of gradual fibrocalcific thickening with progressive obstruction and/or regurgitation.[34] Associated abnormalities include coarctation of the aorta, subaortic stenosis, and mitral valve abnormalities.

**HISTORY.**   The patients described in this section on silent cardiac conditions are asymptomatic.

**PHYSICAL EXAMINATION.**   The murmur of aortic valve stenosis is discussed in Chaps. 32 and 33. An ejection sound is heard at the cardiac apex (see Chap2. 32 and 33).

**LABORATORY INVESTIGATION.**   The chest x-ray film may show a slightly dilated aortic root, and the ECG may reveal left ventricular hypertrophy. The diagnosis and functional status of the bicuspid aortic valve are confirmed by echocardiography.

**TREATMENT.**   Patients with mild obstruction or regurgitation do not require treatment and generally do not require restriction from activities. Participation in competitive sports depends on the degree of obstruction and the intensity of activity. The 26th Bethesda Conference Guidelines[35] are very helpful in making recommendations for patients with aortic stenosis or regurgitation. Medical management requires an emphasis on infective endocarditis prophylaxis, dental hygiene, and education of the patient or family regarding the natural history of progressive stenosis or regurgitation.

Patients with significant aortic valve stenosis may be palliated with a balloon dilatation or surgical valvotomy. Eventually, these patients usually require a valve replacement. Severe aortic regurgitation necessitates surgical valvuloplasty or, more likely, valve replacement.

## Atrial Septal Defect

Atrial septal defects (ASDs) occur in 1 in 1500 live births, with a female-to-male predominance of 2 to 1.[35] Because the physical findings are often subtle and the children are usually asymptomatic, these patients may escape detection until late in life. The natural history of ASD includes the development of right ventricular fibrosis and failure, significant atrial arrhythmias, pulmonary arterial hypertension, and paradoxical emboli. Pregnancy may unmask significant pulmonary hypertension as well as right ventricular dysfunction in a woman with previously undiagnosed ASD.

Approximately 80 percent of ASDs occur in the ostium secundum or central portion of the atrial septum. Ostium primum ASDs involve the lower portion of the atrial septum and are often associated with atrioventricular canal defects such as a cleft mitral valve and left ventricular outflow tract obstruction. Sinus venosus defects occur high in the atrial septum near the junction with the superior vena cava and frequently are associated with partial anomalous pulmonary venous return. All of these defects result in left-to-right shunts, with secondary enlargement of the right atrium, right ventricle, and pulmonary artery. Small subclinical right-to-left shunting may occur and become more exaggerated if right ventricular dysfunction or pulmonary hypertension develops.

**HISTORY.**   The patients discussed in this section are asymptomatic.

**PHYSICAL EXAMINATION.**   The diagnosis of ASDs can be made from the physical examination. Careful inspection of the chest may reveal slight prominence of the left anterior thorax due to right ventricular enlargement. The precordial impulse may be mildly increased. The second heart sound is widely split, with little respiratory variation. This "fixed splitting" persists when the patient stands. A systolic murmur of grade I–III/VI intensity is heard at the left upper sternal border and is produced by excessive blood flow across the pulmonary valve. It may be confused with a normal murmur. When the patient is examined in the supine position, a diastolic flow murmur at the lower left sternal border may be heard; this corresponds to excessive flow across the tricuspid valve.

Patients with an ostium primum defect may have a systolic murmur at the apex and a large left ventricle due to a cleft mitral valve.

**LABORATORY INVESTIGATION.**   The ECG in patients with an ostium secundum defect reveals right axis deviation of the QRS complexes, an rsR' pattern over the right precordial leads ($V_3R, V_1$), and a relatively deep S wave over the left precordial leads. Patients with ostium primum ASD have a superior QRS axis of between zero and –90° that is directed anteriorly.

The chest x-ray film of a patient with an ostium secundum defect reveals large pulmonary arteries, a small aorta, and right ventricular dilatation. The left atrium and left ventricle may be enlarged in patients with an ostium primum defect.

The echocardiogram demonstrates the location and size of the ASD and helps quantify the amount of volume overload change in the right heart. Color Doppler mapping documents the direction of the shunt. In older patients, elevated pulmonary arterial pressures may be detected by the high-velocity flow of tricuspid regurgitation. Catheterization is rarely necessary.

**TREATMENT.**   The standard treatment for ASD is surgical closure with a patch or primary suture. The results are excellent. A nonsurgical option is closure of ostium secundum ASDs in the catheterization laboratory with double umbrella-type devices. Candidates for this approach require an adequate rim of atrial septal tissue around the defect to allow purchase for the device. These defects are usually less than 2 cm in diameter. Patients with an ostium secundum ASD do not require endocarditis prophylaxis. Patients with an ostium primum septal defect do require endocarditis prophylaxis because of the cleft mitral valve.

## Mitral Valve Prolapse

Mitral valve prolapse (MVP) is a relatively common disorder in the adolescent, with an estimated incidence of between 1.5 and 5 percent.[36,37] The true incidence is unclear because of the lack of unanimity on diagnostic criteria. The accuracy of diagnosis has been enhanced by the development of specific major and minor criteria utilizing cardiac auscultation, echocardiography, and nonspecific findings (e.g., ECG changes, symptoms, and body habitus).[38]

Abnormalities of any portion of the mitral valve apparatus may result in MVP; however, the anatomic substrate is usually a floppy, redundant, and thickened mitral valve leaflet. Histologic studies reveal an increase in mucopolysaccharide content of the middle or spongiosa layer, resulting in disruption and encroachment of this tissue within the valve leaflet. Prolapse occurs during systole as one or both leaflets balloon beyond the mitral annulus into the left atrium.

**HISTORY.**   Most children and adolescents with MVP are asymptomatic. The incidence of symptoms such as chest pain, palpitations, syncope, or dyspnea appears to be no different in patients with mitral valve prolapse and in the general population.[39] Symptoms tend to be more common with aging. There is concern over the association of MVP and arrhythmias, cerebral embolism, endocarditis, mitral regurgitation, and sudden death. Arrhythmias reported in association with MVP include atrial and ventricular premature beats and tachycardia. Embolic events are rare in children.[40] Infective endocarditis is related to the severity of leaflet thickening and redundancy.[41] Sudden death is extremely rare in children and adolescents with MVP; only a few cases in people under the age of 20 years have been reported, and these appear to be related to more severe mitral valve deformity and to familial forms of MVP.[42]

**PHYSICAL EXAMINATION.**   Mitral valve prolapse is appreciated on auscultation as a mid- or late systolic click (or multiple clicks) and, at times, a late systolic murmur of mitral insufficiency with the patient supine. With the patient standing, the click(s) becomes earlier and the murmur longer and louder. These findings may be labile and inconsistent in serial examinations. Mitral valve prolapse may be an isolated abnormality or associated with a wide spectrum of cardiac, connective tissue, metabolic, or genetic conditions. It is more common in females, and patients frequently have a tall, slender body habitus with pectus abnormalities, scoliosis, and kyphosis. Other findings include a high-arched palate, increased joint laxity, and hypomastia.

**LABORATORY INVESTIGATION.**   The ECG and chest x-ray film may be normal. The echocardiogram confirms the diagnosis of mitral valve prolapse. Established, rigid echo criteria should be used to avoid overdiagnosis.[38] In addition to the anatomic features, functional abnormalities of mitral regurgitation, ventricular chamber size, and ventricular function should be assessed. The ECG is normal in most children with MVP. Abnormalities of repolarization have been described as prolongation of the Q-T interval and T inversion in the inferior and lateral leads. While a prolonged Q-T interval may be implicated in patients with ventricular arrhythmias and sudden death, the Framingham Study revealed no difference in the prevalence of prolonged Q-T intervals in patients with and without mitral valve prolapse.[43]

**TREATMENT.**   The prognosis during childhood and adolescence for patients with MVP is excellent. MVP tends to be an evolving process, and these patients should be followed periodically into adulthood. Endocarditis prophylaxis is recommended in those patients with mitral regurgitation and with more than minor valve thickening or redundancy. Because of the variability of mitral regurgitation, some clinicians recommend endocarditis prophylaxis in all patients with MVP. Event or Holter monitoring should be obtained for patients with suspected arrhythmia. Beta blockers have been successful in patients with atrial and ventricular arrhythmias. Patients with anxiety and chest discomfort along with palpitations may also be helped with beta blockers. These patients should avoid caffeine, cigarettes, alcohol, and sympathomimetic medications. Patients with embolic phenomena are placed on aspirin and, at times, warfarin. Cigarettes and oral contraceptives should be avoided by these patients. Pregnancy and childbirth are generally safe with MVP. Infective endocarditis prophylaxis should be used at the time of delivery.

Guidelines regarding participation of young people with MVP in athletics were provided by the 26th Bethesda Conference.[35] Most patients with MVP will be able to participate in competitive sports. Patients with a history of syncope or presyncope, complex ventricular arrhythmia, prolonged Q-T interval, significant mitral regurgitation, Marfan syndrome, or a family history of sudden death should not participate in competitive sports.

Additional information on mitral valve prolapse is provided in Chap. 32.

# POSTOPERATIVE CONGENITAL HEART DISEASE

Early diagnosis leading to early medical and surgical treatment of congenital heart disease is now common. Precise anatomic diagnosis, improved surgical and anesthetic management, and advances in postoperative care have resulted in a remarkable survival rate for even the most complex congenital heart malformations. Some congenital heart defects seem to be permanently cured by surgery, such as repair of an ostium secundum atrial septal defect or patent ductus arteriosus. Most "repairs" and certainly most palliative procedures, however, have the potential for residual or future problems. For this reason, most postoperative patients require medical follow-up over a lifetime. Frequently this is a joint effort by the primary care physician and a pediatric or medical cardiologist.

## Complications of Cardiac Surgery

The complications of congenital cardiovascular surgery may result from the sequela or residua of the surgical procedure or be due to the progression of the underlying cardiac malformation. It is important to understand not only the specific cardiac diagnosis but also the details of the surgical repair or palliation. Knowledge regarding the site of incision (atriotomy, ventriculotomy, or aortotomy); use of prosthetic material, patches, or conduits; repair or replacement of valves; the intraoperative description of the anatomy; and hospital problems such as arrhythmias is quite helpful in diagnosing and anticipating long-term postoperative problems. In addition, review of the operative note and hospital summary can be enlightening.

It is important to realize that there are a variety of surgical approaches to the same congenital heart defect. For instance, procedures to repair coarctation of the aorta include resection of the coarcted segment and end-to-end anastomosis; use of the left subclavian artery as a flap or "bypass" conduit (generally in infants); enlargement of the area of coarctation with a prosthetic patch material (associated with late aneurysms at the repair site); and insertion of a large homograph or Dacron tube conduit in bucket-handle fashion for long-segment coarctations. Each method of repair has its unique problems. Patients with complex congenital heart defects frequently have only a single functioning ventricle and are often managed under the general philosophy of the Fontan procedure. In this concept, the systemic venous blood flow (superior and inferior vena caval flow) is channeled directly to the pulmonary arteries by a number of ingenious conduits, tunnels, or anastomoses. This allows the single ventricle to pump only the pulmonary venous blood (e.g., arterialized blood) to the systemic arterial circulation. For proper medical management, a clear understanding of the patient's Fontan "plumbing" is essential. Patients who have undergone extensive atrial surgery such as a Fontan operation, or a Mustard or Senning procedure for transposition of the great arteries are prone to have sick sinus syndrome and atrial arrhythmias such as atrial flutter.

## Follow-up Visits

Most postoperative patients are followed on an every 6-month to 2-year basis, depending on the cardiac abnormality, type of operation, and degree of residual problems. The most important concerns with these follow-up visits are listed in Table 46-5.

**PATIENTS WITH SPECIAL NEEDS.**   Additional scrutiny is necessary for patients with congestive heart failure (CHF), prosthetic valves, pacemakers, antiar-

### TABLE 46-5.   Postoperative Follow-up of Congenital Heart Disease: Areas of Concern

Arrhythmias, conduction abnormalities, and bundle branch blocks

Tricuspid or mitral valve abnormalities, especially regurgitation

Ventricular function and size

Right ventricle and/or left ventricle outflow tract obstruction

Semilunar valve regurgitation

Vascular abnormalities: pulmonary artery hypertension, systemic blood pressure, and distortion of the pulmonary arteries or aorta

Other consequences of surgery: scoliosis, chest wall deformities, limb growth, central nervous system injury, hemolysis, endocarditis risk, sudden death, activity restrictions, anticoagulation status, and protein-losing enteropathy

rhythmic medications, and chronic anticoagulation with warfarin. Ongoing patient education includes emphasis on infective endocarditis prophylaxis, review of medications and their side effects, dental hygiene, and activity restrictions. Special issues such as contraception, pregnancy, and noncardiac surgery may require input from other specialists.

It is important to update the medical history at each visit regarding palpitations, stamina, shortness of breath, dyspnea on exertion, presyncope or syncope, and chest pain.

**THE WORK-UP ON FOLLOW-UP.**  Serial physical examinations should document clearly the present physical findings as well as note any other changes in the examination. This especially applies to changes in cardiac rate and rhythm and murmurs or heart sounds. Routine office tests depend on symptoms, physical findings, and anticipated residual or new problems. These tests may include ECG, echocardiogram, chest x-ray, pulse oximetry, and hemoglobin with red blood cell indices to assess for iron deficiency.

**THE NEED FOR REOPERATION.**  Some operations performed in young children produce a predictable need for reoperation. These include insertion of conduits (especially between the right ventricle and pulmonary artery), pacemakers, and artificial or tissue valves at a young age. Surgery for left ventricular outflow tract obstruction and repair of complete atrioventricular septal defects (endocardial cushion defects) not uncommonly require further surgery. Repair of tetralogy of Fallot requiring a transannular pulmonary outflow tract patch to relieve pulmonary stenosis generally results in pulmonary regurgitation. Progressive right ventricular enlargement, right ventricular failure, arrhythmias, and secondary tricuspid regurgitation may necessitate insertion of a pulmonary valve. Repairs of coarctation in infants or young children may result in recoarctation by adolescence. This requires monitoring of arm and leg pressures, and if recoarctation occurs, a balloon dilatation procedure or repeat surgery may be offered.

**PROGNOSIS RELATED TO THE SPECIFIC DISEASE AND COMPLICATIONS OF SURGERY.**  Though the short- and mid-term prognosis for most postoperative patients with congenital heart disease is good, aged-matched population studies have demonstrated an increase in risk of late sudden cardiac death with certain abnormalities. Silka et al[44] reviewed the long-term results of surgery for atrial septal defect, ventricular septal defect, complete atrioventricular septal defect (endocardial cushion defect), patent ductus arteriosus, pulmonary stenosis, aortic stenosis, coarctation of the aorta, tetralogy of Fallot, and d transposition of the great vessels. This study found that the risk of late death in patients with left-to-right shunts or pulmonary stenosis was low, approaching that of the general population. In patients with cyanotic defects and left heart obstructive lesions, however, the risk of late sudden death markedly increased to 50 to 200 times that in the general population; these patients accounted for 90 percent of the unexpected late deaths in this series. The risk of sudden death increased primarily after the second operative decade. The causes of sudden death in this series were arrhythmias (75 percent), embolic phenomena (12 percent), ruptured aneurysm (5 percent), and acute ventricular failure (10 percent).[44] These high-risk patients should be followed jointly with a cardiologist experienced in congenital heart disease.

The most common defects along with their long-term complications or sequelae of surgery are provided in Table 46-6. The majority of patients who have undergone repair of congenital heart defects are productive and healthy. Long-term medical vigilance is required to assure optimal outcome.

## Rheumatic Fever and Rheumatic Heart Disease

Rheumatic fever and rheumatic heart disease are discussed in Chaps. 32 and 39.

## Pericarditis

Pericarditis is discussed in Chaps. 14, 34, and 39.

## Myocarditis

Myocarditis is discussed in Chap. 29.

# PREVENTIVE CARDIOLOGY IN THE ADOLESCENT

## Atherosclerosis

Atherosclerosis has its onset in the late teens and clinical expression in adulthood. The public health menace of this disease cannot be overstated. Coronary artery disease (CAD) is the leading cause of death among the U.S. adult population, and an estimated 30 to 40 percent of the current population will die of cardiovascular disease.[4] Vascular endothelial injury and dysfunction underlie the pathogenesis of atherosclerosis. Additional risk factors influencing the development of atherosclerosis in adolescents are the same as those in adults: abnormal blood levels of cholesterol and lipoproteins, systemic hypertension, obesity, lack of exercise, cigarette smoking, and diabetes mellitus. Early intervention may forestall coronary disease in the adult. This section is intended to highlight the issue of atherosclerosis in the adolescent and to present guidelines for cholesterol screening, follow-up, and management of these patients. Discussions regarding the other major risk factors are provided in other chapters of the text.

**CHOLESTEROL.** Autopsy studies on young soldiers killed in the Korean War revealed that over 70 percent of them had evidence of early coronary arterial atherosclerosis.[45] Evidence that abnormal cholesterol and lipoprotein levels influence the early development of atherosclerosis is convincing. The report of the National

## TABLE 46-6.   Common Postoperative Problems of Congenital Heart Disease

**Secundum Atrial Septal Defect**

- Atrial arrhythmias (sick sinus syndrome, supraventricular tachycardia, and atrial fibrillation)

- Persistence of preoperative pulmonary hypertension (older patients at the time of surgery)

- Endocarditis prophylaxis usually not indicated after 6 months postoperatively

**Ostium Primum Atrial Septal Defect**

- Atrial arrhythmias as above

- Residual mitral valve and/or tricuspid valve regurgitation or stenosis. These patients may require mitral valve replacement

- Subaortic left ventricular outflow tract obstruction

- Endocarditis prophylaxis usually indicated

**Patent Ductus Arteriosus**

- Recannulization of the ductus

- Aneurysm of ductus diverticulum

- Long-term problems of cath-lab device closure are not known

- Endocarditis prophylaxis not indicated with complete ductal closure

**Ventricular Septal Defect**

- Surgical heart block

- Atrial or ventricular arrhythmias (rare)

- Right bundle branch block (common)

- Residual ventricular septal defects (no reoperation necessary for small defects)

- Aortic regurgitation

- Acquired subaortic stenosis

- Persistence of preoperative pulmonary hypertension

- Endocarditis prophylaxis recommended

**Atrioventricular Septal Defect (Endocardial Cushion Defect, Complete Atrioventricular Canal)**

- First-degree atrioventricular block

- Mitral or tricuspid valve regurgitation or stenosis (may require mitral valve replacement)

- Residual cleft in the mitral valve leaflet

*(continues)*

**TABLE 46-6.**   **Common Postoperative Problems of Congenital Heart Disease** *(continued)*

- Development of subaortic stenosis

- Residual ventricular septal defect or left ventricle to right atrial shunt

- Endocarditis prophylaxis recommended

**Pulmonary Valve Stenosis**

- Residual obstruction

- Pulmonary regurgitation resulting in right ventricular enlargement and failure (may require insertion of a pulmonary valve)

**Tetralogy of Fallot**

- Ventricular ectopy (especially with ventriculotomy, late repair, or residual right ventricular hypertension)

- Distortion of pulmonary arteries related to either congenital abnormalities or secondary to surgical shunt

- Residual right ventricular outflow tract obstruction

- Pulmonary regurgitation with right ventricular enlargement and failure

- Residual ventricular septal defect

- Aortic regurgitation

- Right ventricular outflow tract aneurysm

- Repairs requiring right ventricle to pulmonary artery conduit may develop progressive obstruction and require replacement

- Right ventricular dysfunction

- Endocarditis prophylaxis recommended

**Coarctation of the Aorta**

- Aneurysm at site of repair that may rupture (this is most common with a patch repair)

- Residual systemic arterial hypertension despite relief of obstruction (usually found in older patients at the time of repair)

- Residual of obstruction or recurrent obstruction at coarctation site

- Bicuspid aortic valve that is commonly associated with coarctation may develop aortic regurgitation or stenosis

- Cerebral hemorrhage due to rupture of circle of Willis aneurysm

- Premature coronary artery disease

- Endocardial prophylaxis recommended

**TABLE 46-6.   Common Postoperative Problems of Congenital Heart Disease** *(continued)*

**Aortic Stenosis (Left Ventricular Outflow Tract Obstruction)**

- Residual atrioventricular conduction abnormalities, particularly in patients with extensive subvalvular surgery

- Residual obstruction at the subvalvular, valve, or supravalvular level

- Aortic regurgitation may be secondary to surgical or balloon dilatation procedure or native valve abnormality

- Aortic valve replacement

- Chronic anticoagulation for a prosthetic mechanical valve

- Homograph tissue valves require repeat replacement usually within 5 to 10 years because of acquired obstruction and/or regurgitation

- Ross procedure (patient's native pulmonary valve is used to replace the native aortic valve and a valve conduit is inserted between the right ventricle and pulmonary artery). Conduit deterioration requires replacement over time. The "Neo" aortic valve may develop regurgitation

- Aortic root enlargement procedure (Konno operation) may result in heart block or right ventricular outflow tract obstruction

- Endocarditis prophylaxis recommended

- Transposition of the great vessels

**Atrial Switch Operation (Mustard or Senning Operation)**

- Arrhythmias are common, particularly in the older patients; sick sinus syndrome, atrial flutter, supraventricular tachycardia

- Right ventricular (systemic ventricular) failure

- Tricuspid valve regurgitation (this is the systemic atrioventricular valve)

- Left ventricular outflow tract obstruction (subpulmonary valve obstruction)

- Venous baffle obstruction may result in inferior or superior vena cava blockage or pulmonary venous obstruction resulting in pulmonary edema

- Venous baffle leaks that may result in cyanosis

- Endocarditis prophylaxis recommended

**Arterial Switch Operation (Jantene)**

- Obstruction in the supravalvular aortic and/or pulmonary flow

- "Neo" aortic valve regurgitation

- Injury or obstruction to coronary arteries

- Endocarditis prophylaxis recommended

*(continues)*

TABLE 46-6.   Common Postoperative Problems of Congenital Heart Disease *(continued)*

**Complex Congenital Lesions (Single Ventricle)**

- Fontan operation (multiple variations of this operation: the systemic venous blood return is rerouted directly into the pulmonary arteries and the pulmonary venous return is directed into the ventricle, which pumps blood to the systemic circulation)

- Atrial arrhythmias are common: sick sinus syndrome, atrial flutter, supraventricular tachycardia, and atrial fibrillations

- Elevated central venous pressure with hepatomegaly, edema, ascites, and protein-losing enteropathy (occurs in 10% and has a high mortality)

- Atrioventricular valve regurgitation

- Ventricular dysfunction

- Cyanosis may be due to systemic vein to pulmonary venous connection, pulmonary arteriovenous malformation, or residual right-to-left atrial level shunt

- Fenestrated Fontan (a small hole purposely left between the systemic venous and pulmonary venous channels, allowing right-to-left "pop-off" shunt) can result in systemic embolus and cyanosis

- Systemic venous pathway obstruction

- Thrombosis within the low-velocity systemic venous circuit

- Residual aortic arch or ventricular outflow tract obstruction

- Endocarditis prophylaxis recommended

Cholesterol Education Program (NCEP) panel[46] summarizes the evidence of origins of atherosclerosis in childhood:

- Compared to their counterparts in many other countries, U.S. children and adolescents have higher blood cholesterol levels and higher intakes of saturated fatty acids and cholesterol, and U.S. adults have higher blood cholesterol levels and higher rates of CAD morbidity and mortality.
- Autopsy studies demonstrate that early coronary atherosclerosis or precursors of atherosclerosis often begin in childhood and adolescence.
- High serum total cholesterol, low-density lipoprotein (LDL) cholesterol, very-low-density-lipoprotein (VLDL) cholesterol levels, and high-density lipoprotein (HDL) cholesterol levels are correlated with the extent of early atherosclerotic legions in adolescents and young adults.
- Children and adolescents with elevated serum cholesterol, particularly LDL cholesterol levels, frequently come from families in which there is a high incidence of CAD among adult members.

- High blood cholesterol aggregates in families as a result of both shared environments and genetic factors.
- Children and adolescents with high cholesterol levels are more likely than the general population to have high levels as adults.

The relationship of histological severity of atherosclerotic legions to measurable risk factors in adolescents has been reported.[47,48] Elevated LDL cholesterol is directly related to atherosclerosis in youth,[47] and it is the most commonly used laboratory value in determining follow-up and treatment for hypercholesterolemia. Normative data for lipid values in adolescents are presented in Table 46-7.[49]

While the NCEP panel does not recommend universal cholesterol screening, selective screening is recommended in certain subsets of children and adolescents. These recommendations are as follows[46]:

- Screen children and adolescents whose parents or grandparents, at 55 years of age or younger, underwent diagnostic coronary arteriography and were found to have coronary atherosclerosis. This includes parents or grandparents who have undergone balloon angioplasty or coronary artery bypass surgery (CABG). The panel believes that cardiologists should make a routine practice of referring the offspring of these patients to a source of continuing health care for cholesterol testing and follow-up.
- Screen children and adolescents whose parents or grandparents, at 55 years of age or younger, suffered a documented MI, angina pectoris, peripheral vascular disease, cerebral vascular disease, or sudden death.

**TABLE 46-7.   Lipid Values for Adolescent Atherosclerosis Risk Assessment**

| Percentile | | Total Cholesterol | | | | Triglycerides | | | | LDL Cholesterol | | | | HDL Cholesterol | | | |
|---|---|---|---|---|---|---|---|---|---|---|---|---|---|---|---|---|---|
| Age (yr) | Sex | 5 | 50 | 75 | 95 | 5 | 50 | 75 | 95 | 5 | 50 | 75 | 95 | 5 | 50 | 75 | 95 |
| 10–14 | M | 119 | 158 | 173 | 202 | 32 | 66 | 74 | 125 | 64 | 97 | 109 | 133 | 37 | 55 | 61 | 74 |
|  | F | 126 | 164 | 171 | 205 | 32 | 60 | 85 | 105 | 68 | 97 | 109 | 136 | 37 | 52 | 58 | 70 |
| 15–19 | M | 113 | 150 | 168 | 197 | 32 | 66 | 88 | 125 | 62 | 94 | 109 | 130 | 30 | 46 | 52 | 63 |
|  | F | 120 | 158 | 176 | 203 | 39 | 75 | 85 | 132 | 59 | 96 | 111 | 137 | 35 | 52 | 61 | 74 |
| 20–24 | M | 118 | 159 | 179 | 197 | 44 | 78 | 107 | 165 | 66 | 101 | 118 | 147 | 30 | 45 | 51 | 63 |
|  | F | 121 | 165 | 186 | 237 | 52 | 96 | 126 | 175 | 70 | 98 | 136 | 151 | 37 | 50 | 60 | 73 |

HDL = high-density lipoprotein; LDL = low-density lipoprotein.

*Source:* Reproduced from Lipid Research Clinics: *Population Studies Data Book;* Pub. No 80-1527. Bethesda, MD, National Institutes of Health, 1980.

- Screen the offspring of a parent who has been found to have a high blood cholesterol (240 mm/dL or higher).
- For children and adolescents whose parental or grandparental history is unobtainable, particularly those with other risk factors, physicians may choose to measure cholesterol levels in order to identify those in need of individual nutritional and medical advice.

Acceptable, borderline, and high total cholesterol and LDL cholesterol levels are summarized in Table 46-8. Children who meet the criteria for testing and are above 2 years of age should undergo a measurement of nonfasting total cholesterol. If the total cholesterol is greater than 200 mg/dL, fasting lipoprotein levels should be measured. If the total cholesterol is borderline (170 to 199 mg/dL), a second total cholesterol should be obtained, and if these repeat values are borderline or high, fasting lipoprotein analysis should be measured.[46] Children or adolescents who have definite cardiovascular disease in a parent or grandparent should have a fasting lipoprotein analysis initially. Repeat values are recommended to determine the average LDL cholesterol level. An algorithm for selective cholesterol screening is provided in Fig. 46-2.[46]

Compared with those of cholesterol and lipoprotein subfractions, the role of triglycerides as a risk factor in coronary artery disease is less clear. In women, however, hypertriglyceridemia has been shown to be an independent risk factor for atherosclerosis.[50]

**ETIOLOGY OF ATHEROSCLEROSIS.** The three primary causes of elevated cholesterol in children and adolescents are single gene defects, diets high in cholesterol, and other diet-related factors such as obesity and diets lacking in fiber and antioxidants, which appear to prevent coronary arterial disease. Foods that provide antioxidants include fruits, vegetables, legumes, and complex carbohydrates. Secondary causes of elevated cholesterol should be ruled out. The major secondary causes are presented in Table 46-9.

Genetic defects result in a range of severity of type and degree of cholesterol levels. Familial hypercholesterolemia (FH) is a dominantly inherited gene abnormality on chromosome 19. Homozygotes for FH have total cholesterol levels in the

**TABLE 46-8.** Classification of Total and LDL Cholesterol Levels in Children and Adolescents from Families with Hypercholesterolemia or Premature Cardiovascular Disease

| Category | Total Cholesterol, mg/dL | LDL Cholesterol nM/dL |
|---|---|---|
| Acceptable | <170 | <110 |
| Borderline | 170–199 | 110–129 |
| High | >200 | >130 |

*Source:* Report of the Expert Panel on Blood Cholesterol Levels in Children and Adolescents. *Pediatrics* 1992; 89:525–584, with permission.

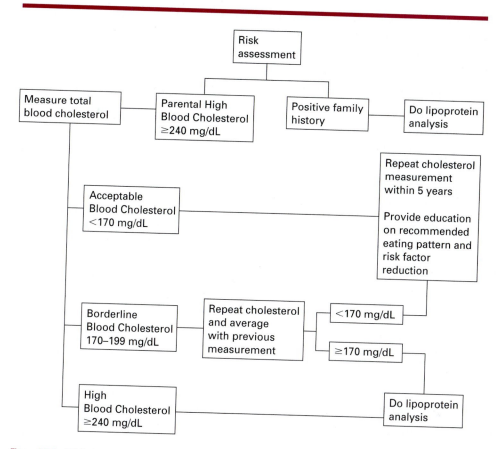

**Figure 46-2**   Risk assessment. *Positive family history is defined as a history of premature (before age 55 years) cardiovascular disease. (From Report of the Expert Panel on Blood Cholesterol Levels in Children and Adolescents. *Pediatrics* 1992; 89:525–584, with permission.)

700-mg/dL range and LDL levels in the 600-mg/dL range.[48] These patients have xanthomas, xanthelasmas, or corneal arcus due to peripheral lipid deposits. There is often a strong family history of premature coronary artery disease. Heterozygotes for FH have a total cholesterol of 250 to 400 mg/dL and normal triglyceride levels.[48] Familial combined hyperlipidemia (FCH) results in elevated total cholesterol and triglycerides due to excessive hepatic production of VLDL and abnormal catabolism of VLDL and LDL.[51] The total cholesterol in these patients is usually between 200 and 250 mg/dL, and the triglyceride level is more than 120 mg/dL. A combination of genetic predisposition and excessive dietary intake of saturated fats and cholesterol results in hyperlipidemia of a less severe form.[48]

**TREATMENT.**   The NCEP panel[46] has provided guidelines for both population and individual approaches for preventing coronary artery disease (CAD). The pop-

**TABLE 46-9.    Causes of Secondary Hypercholesterolemia**

Exogenous

- Drugs: corticosteroids, isotretinoin (Accutane), thiazides, anticonvulsants, beta blockers, anabolic steroids, certain oral contraceptives
- Alcohol
- Obesity

Endocrine and Metabolic

- Hypothyroidism
- Diabetes mellitus
- Lipodystrophy
- Pregnancy
- Idiopathic hypercalcemia

Storage Diseases

- Glycogen storage disease
- Sphingolipidoses

Obstructive Liver Disease

- Biliary atresia
- Biliary cirrhosis

Chronic Renal Disease

- Nephrotic syndrome

Others

- Anorexia nervosa
- Progeria
- Collagen disease
- Klinefelter syndrome

*Source:* Report of the Expert Panel on Blood Cholesterol Levels in Children and Adolescents. *Pediatrics* 1992; 89:525–584, with permission.

ulation approach is designed to lower blood cholesterol among all Americans by a change in nutrient intake and eating patterns. The recommendations for all healthy children and adolescents over the age of 2 years are as follows:

- Nutritional adequacy should be achieved by eating a wide variety of foods.
- Energy (calories) should be adequate to support growth and development or to reach or maintain desirable body weight.

- The following pattern of nutrient intake is recommended:
  - Saturated fatty acids should be less than 10 percent of total calories.
  - Total fat should average no more than 30 percent of total calories.
  - Dietary cholesterol should be less than 300 mg/day.

To be effective, these recommendations require a major change in present dietary patterns. To accomplish this, the NCEP has called on the cooperation of schools, health professionals, government agencies, the food industry, and mass media to support and publicize these recommendations.

The individualized approach to reducing cholesterol levels begins with identifying a child or adolescent at high risk for high cholesterol by the selective screening approach discussed above. The initial treatment for all types of hyperlipidemia involves a lifestyle change including diet modification, weight reduction (if indicated), increased physical activity, blood pressure control, and avoidance of smoking.

***Diet Therapy.***    Diet therapy is the cornerstone in managing patients with elevated blood cholesterol. The goals of dietary treatment are:[46]

- For borderline LDL cholesterol (110 to 129 mg/dL), the aim is to lower the level to <110 mg/dL.
- For high LDL cholesterol (>130 mg/dL), the aim is to lower the level to <130 mg/dL as a minimal goal and to lower the LDL to 110 mg/dL as an ideal goal.

A dietary step approach is used to reduce the intake of saturated fatty acids and cholesterol. The step I and step II diets are noted in Table 46-10. Recommendations from the step I and step II diets are based on results of LDL cholesterol testing and are outlined in Fig. 46-3. Referral to an experienced nutritionist is helpful in implementing dietary treatment. The American Heart Association has published heart-healthy diet and cookbooks.

***Drug Therapy.***    The NCEP panel recommends consideration of drug therapy in children 10 years of age or older if dietary therapy for 6 to 12 months is unsuccessful:[46]

- LDL cholesterol remains greater than or equal to 190 mg/dL; or
- LDL cholesterol remains greater than 160 mg/dL and:
  - There is a family history of premature cardiovascular disease (before 55 years of age), or
  - Two or more cardiovascular risk factors are present in the child or adolescent after vigorous attempts have been made to control these risk factors.

There is limited experience with lipid-lowering medications in young patients compared with adults. Generally approved drugs for the young include bile acid–binding resins such as colestipol and cholestyramine. One scoop of cholestyramine per day lowers LDL cholesterol approximately 40 mg/dL.[52] Gastrointestinal side effects often preclude long-term use. Niacin (nicotinic acid) reduces the synthesis

**TABLE 46-10.**  Characteristics of Step I and Step II Diets for Lowering Blood Cholesterol Levels

| Nutrient | Recommended Intake | |
| --- | --- | --- |
| | Step I Diet | Step II Diet |
| Total Fat | Average of no more than 30% of total calories | Same |
| Saturated fatty acids | Less than 10% of total calories | Less than 7% of total calories |
| Polyunsaturated fatty acids | Up to 10% of total calories | Same |
| Monounsaturated fatty acids | Remaining total fat calories | Same |
| Cholesterol | Less than 300 mg/day | Less than 200 mg/day |
| Carbohydrates | About 55% of total calories | Same |
| Protein | About 15–20% of total calories | Same |
| Calories | To promote normal growth and development and to reach or maintain desirable body weight | Same |

*Source:* Report of the Expert Panel on Blood Cholesterol Levels in Children and Adolescents. *Pediatrics* 1992; 89:525–584, with permission.

of VLDL and lowers levels of cholesterol and triglycerides. Side effects due to prostaglandin-mediated flushing may be ameliorated by pretreatment with aspirin 15 to 30 min prior to the dose.[48] Other unfavorable side effects of niacin are peptic ulcer disease, gout, and hepatic toxicity. Experience with HMG-CoA reductase inhibitors (pravastatin, simvastatin, and lovastatin), probucol, and gemfibrozil in children and adolescents is limited. These medications do have numerous side effects, and their use in the young should be monitored in an appropriate setting by clinicians with experience in the use of these agents.

Additional information about atherosclerosis is provided in Chaps. 18, 25, and 26.

## Hypertension

The measurement of blood pressure in children and adolescents has become standard office practice. While hypertension is generally an adult problem, it is estimated that 1 to 2 percent of adolescents have persistent systemic arterial hypertension.[53] During adolescence, the normal blood pressure increases gradually to adult levels. There is evidence that children and adolescents with hypertension are likely to be hypertensive as adults. Because of the cardiovascular, central nervous system, and renal consequences of chronic untreated hypertension, its detection and treatment are important. The Task Force on Blood Pressure Control in Children in 1977[54] and 1987[55] established norms for childhood blood pressure as well as the diagnostic criteria for hypertension. This work has aided the identification

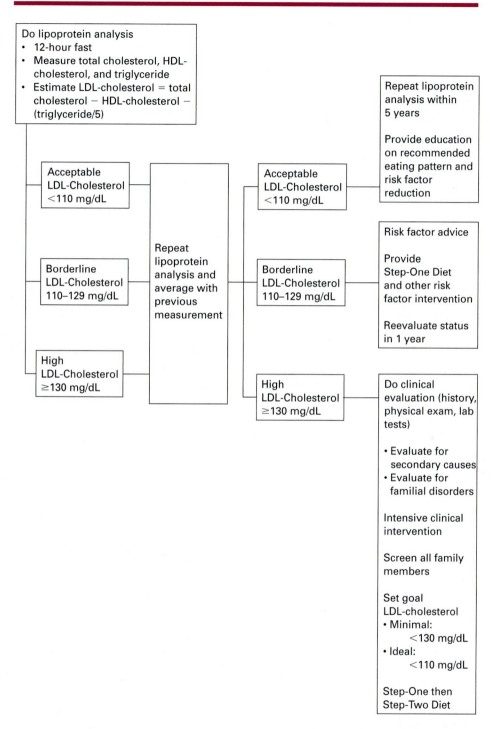

Do lipoprotein analysis
• 12-hour fast
• Measure total cholesterol, HDL-cholesterol, and triglyceride
• Estimate LDL-cholesterol = total cholesterol − HDL-cholesterol − (triglyceride/5)

Acceptable
LDL-Cholesterol
<110 mg/dL

Borderline
LDL-Cholesterol
110–129 mg/dL

High
LDL-Cholesterol
≥130 mg/dL

Repeat lipoprotein analysis and average with previous measurement

Acceptable
LDL-Cholesterol
<110 mg/dL

Borderline
LDL-Cholesterol
110–129 mg/dL

High
LDL-Cholesterol
≥130 mg/dL

Repeat lipoprotein analysis within 5 years

Provide education on recommended eating pattern and risk factor reduction

Risk factor advice

Provide Step-One Diet and other risk factor intervention

Reevaluate status in 1 year

Do clinical evaluation (history, physical exam, lab tests)

• Evaluate for secondary causes
• Evaluate for familial disorders

Intensive clinical intervention

Screen all family members

Set goal LDL-cholesterol
• Minimal:
    <130 mg/dL
• Ideal:
    <110 mg/dL

Step-One then Step-Two Diet

**Figure 46-3** Classification, education, and follow-up based on low-density-lipoprotein cholesterol. (From Report of the Expert Panel on Blood Cholesterol Levels in Children and Adolescents. *Pediatrics* 1992; 89:525–584, with permission.)

and subsequent evaluation and treatment of children and adolescents with hypertension.

A number of factors are associated with elevated blood pressure in childhood and adolescence. There is a direct relationship between weight and elevated blood pressure in adolescence.[56] Recently, recognition of height as an independent influence on blood pressure has led to revision of blood pressure guidelines in the young.[57] The slightly higher blood pressure in boys than girls during childhood becomes significantly greater during adolescence. The influence of race or ethnic group, however, is not clinically significant until adulthood.[58] Children of families with a history of hypertension are more likely to be hypertensive.[59]

**METHOD OF BLOOD PRESSURE MEASUREMENT IN THE ADOLESCENT.** The use of standardized methods to measure blood pressure is important in order to compare a patient's blood pressure to norms. Because of the wide range of body size in adolescence, a number of different size blood pressure cuffs should be available, including a large thigh cuff for leg measurements if necessary. The technique for measuring blood pressure in children and adolescents is as follows:[55]

- A mercury sphygmomanometer and auscultation with a stethoscope are the generally recommended method of choice. Automated devices have become popular, but they require frequent calibration.
- The proper size of cuff is critical. The cuff bladder should encircle the arm and be wide enough to cover 75 percent of the arm length measured from the acromion to the olecranon. Usually the largest cuff available that allows auscultation in the antecubital fossa is used.
- The blood pressure measurement should be made with the patient seated in quiet surroundings and after resting for 3 to 5 min. The antecubital fossa should be supported at the heart level.
- The cuff is inflated until the Korotkoff sounds are obliterated and then deflated at 2 to 3 mmHg/s. The first Korotkoff sound is the systolic blood pressure. The disappearance of sounds or the fifth Korotkoff sound is now used to determine the diastolic blood pressure. At least two measurements should be made and averaged.

*Ambulatory Blood Pressure Monitoring.* Ambulatory blood pressure monitoring is seldom used in children and adolescents, but it may be helpful when there is concern over "white-coat" hypertension in the office setting. Ambulatory blood pressure has been reported as being well tolerated with reproducible and accurate measurements in children.[60] As expected, there are a wide range of blood pressure measurements noted at different levels of activity and in different emotional states. More studies will be necessary for standardization of this technique.

**THE DIAGNOSIS OF HYPERTENSION.** Hypertension should not be diagnosed on a single measurement. Elevated measurements on at least three separate occasions are necessary before the diagnosis is established. Updated blood pressure tables for children and adolescents take into account the patient's height as well as age and gender and are provided in Tables 46-11 and 46-12.[57] The blood pressure is characterized in reference to these tables as follows:

- Normal blood pressure is a systolic and diastolic blood pressure less than the 90th percentile for age, sex, and height.
- Normal high blood pressure is an average systolic and/or average diastolic blood pressure between the 90th and 95th percentile for age, sex, and height.
- High blood pressure (hypertension) is an average systolic and/or average diastolic blood pressure greater or equal to the 95th percentile for age, sex, and height.
- Blood pressure may be classified severe if it is well above the 95th percentile for age, sex, and height.

**TABLE 46-11.   Blood Pressure Levels for the 90th and 95th Percentiles of Blood Pressure for Girls Aged 10 to 17 by Percentiles of Height**

| Age (yr) | Per-centile | Systolic BP (mmHg) by Percentile of Height | | | | | | | Diastolic BP (DBP5) (mmHg) by Percentile of Height | | | | | | |
|---|---|---|---|---|---|---|---|---|---|---|---|---|---|---|---|
| | | 5% | 10% | 25% | 50% | 75% | 90% | 95% | 5% | 10% | 25% | 50% | 75% | 90% | 95% |
| 10 | 90th | 112 | 113 | 114 | 115 | 116 | 118 | 118 | 75 | 75 | 76 | 77 | 77 | 78 | 78 |
| | 95th | 116 | 117 | 118 | 119 | 120 | 122 | 122 | 79 | 79 | 80 | 81 | 81 | 82 | 83 |
| 11 | 90th | 114 | 115 | 116 | 117 | 119 | 120 | 120 | 76 | 77 | 77 | 78 | 79 | 79 | 80 |
| | 95th | 118 | 119 | 120 | 121 | 122 | 124 | 124 | 81 | 81 | 81 | 82 | 83 | 83 | 84 |
| 12 | 90th | 116 | 117 | 118 | 119 | 121 | 122 | 123 | 78 | 78 | 78 | 79 | 80 | 81 | 81 |
| | 95th | 120 | 121 | 122 | 123 | 125 | 126 | 126 | 82 | 82 | 82 | 83 | 84 | 85 | 85 |
| 13 | 90th | 118 | 119 | 120 | 121 | 123 | 124 | 124 | 79 | 79 | 79 | 80 | 81 | 82 | 82 |
| | 95th | 122 | 123 | 124 | 125 | 126 | 128 | 128 | 83 | 83 | 84 | 84 | 85 | 86 | 86 |
| 14 | 90th | 120 | 121 | 122 | 123 | 124 | 125 | 126 | 80 | 80 | 80 | 81 | 82 | 83 | 83 |
| | 95th | 124 | 125 | 126 | 127 | 128 | 129 | 130 | 84 | 84 | 85 | 85 | 86 | 87 | 87 |
| 15 | 90th | 121 | 122 | 123 | 124 | 126 | 127 | 128 | 80 | 81 | 81 | 82 | 83 | 83 | 84 |
| | 95th | 125 | 126 | 127 | 128 | 130 | 131 | 131 | 85 | 85 | 85 | 86 | 87 | 88 | 88 |
| 16 | 90th | 122 | 123 | 124 | 125 | 127 | 128 | 129 | 81 | 81 | 82 | 82 | 83 | 84 | 84 |
| | 95th | 126 | 127 | 128 | 129 | 130 | 132 | 132 | 85 | 85 | 86 | 87 | 87 | 88 | 88 |
| 17 | 90th | 123 | 123 | 124 | 126 | 127 | 128 | 129 | 81 | 81 | 82 | 83 | 83 | 84 | 85 |
| | 95th | 127 | 127 | 128 | 130 | 131 | 132 | 133 | 85 | 86 | 86 | 87 | 88 | 88 | 89 |

Blood pressure percentile was determined by a single reading. Height percentile was determined by standard growth curves.

*Source:* Rosner B, Prineas RJ, Loggie JMH, Daniels SR: Blood pressure nomograms for children and adolescents, by height, sex, and age, in the United States. *J Pediatr* 1993; 123:871–886, with permission.

**TABLE 46-12.   Blood Pressure Levels for the 90th and 95th Percentiles of Blood Pressure for Boys Aged 10 to 17 by Percentiles of Height**

| Age (yr) | Percentile | Systolic BP (mmHg) by Percentile of Height | | | | | | | Diastolic BP (DBP5) (mmHg) by Percentile of Height | | | | | | |
|---|---|---|---|---|---|---|---|---|---|---|---|---|---|---|---|
| | | 5% | 10% | 25% | 50% | 75% | 90% | 95% | 5% | 10% | 25% | 50% | 75% | 90% | 95% |
| 10 | 90th | 111 | 112 | 113 | 115 | 117 | 119 | 119 | 77 | 77 | 78 | 79 | 80 | 81 | 81 |
| | 95th | 115 | 116 | 117 | 119 | 121 | 123 | 123 | 81 | 82 | 83 | 83 | 84 | 85 | 86 |
| 11 | 90th | 113 | 114 | 115 | 117 | 119 | 121 | 121 | 77 | 78 | 79 | 80 | 81 | 81 | 82 |
| | 95th | 117 | 118 | 119 | 121 | 123 | 125 | 125 | 82 | 82 | 83 | 84 | 85 | 86 | 87 |
| 12 | 90th | 115 | 116 | 118 | 120 | 121 | 123 | 124 | 78 | 78 | 79 | 80 | 81 | 82 | 83 |
| | 95th | 119 | 120 | 122 | 124 | 125 | 127 | 128 | 83 | 83 | 84 | 85 | 86 | 87 | 87 |
| 13 | 90th | 118 | 119 | 120 | 122 | 124 | 125 | 126 | 78 | 79 | 80 | 81 | 81 | 82 | 83 |
| | 95th | 121 | 122 | 124 | 126 | 128 | 129 | 130 | 83 | 83 | 84 | 85 | 86 | 87 | 88 |
| 14 | 90th | 120 | 121 | 123 | 125 | 127 | 128 | 129 | 79 | 79 | 80 | 81 | 82 | 83 | 83 |
| | 95th | 124 | 125 | 127 | 129 | 131 | 132 | 133 | 83 | 84 | 85 | 86 | 87 | 87 | 88 |
| 15 | 90th | 123 | 124 | 126 | 128 | 130 | 131 | 132 | 80 | 80 | 81 | 82 | 83 | 84 | 84 |
| | 95th | 127 | 128 | 130 | 132 | 133 | 135 | 136 | 84 | 85 | 86 | 86 | 87 | 88 | 89 |
| 16 | 90th | 126 | 127 | 129 | 131 | 132 | 134 | 134 | 81 | 82 | 82 | 83 | 84 | 85 | 86 |
| | 95th | 130 | 131 | 133 | 134 | 136 | 138 | 138 | 86 | 86 | 87 | 88 | 89 | 90 | 90 |
| 17 | 90th | 128 | 129 | 131 | 133 | 135 | 136 | 137 | 83 | 84 | 85 | 86 | 87 | 87 | 88 |
| | 95th | 132 | 133 | 135 | 137 | 139 | 140 | 141 | 88 | 88 | 89 | 90 | 91 | 92 | 93 |

Blood pressure percentile was determined by a single reading. Height percentile was determined by standard growth curves.

*Source:* Rosner B, Prineas RJ, Loggie JMH, Daniels SR: Blood pressure nomograms for children and adolescents, by height, sex, and age, in the United States. *J Pediatr* 1993; 123:871–886, with permission.

Patients with severely elevated blood pressure are more likely to have secondary causes for their hypertension. The most common secondary causes are renal parenchymal disease, renal artery stenosis, and coarctation of the aorta. The differential diagnosis of hypertension is presented in Table 46-13.

**EVALUATION OF HYPERTENSION.**   Once the blood pressure has been determined to be abnormally elevated, secondary causes must be ruled out. The diagnostic evaluation for hypertension includes a thorough history, physical examination, and laboratory investigation. The important elements of the history and physical examination are noted in Tables 46-14 and 46-15. Most cases of mild to moderate hypertension in adolescents are not due to secondary disease but are probably related to essential or primary hypertension. Patients with more severe levels of hypertension require vigorous evaluation. The initial laboratory work-up

TABLE 46-13.   Causes of Hypertension in Adolescents

| Common | Uncommon |
|---|---|
| Essential hypertension | Renal artery stenosis |
| Renal parenchymal disease | Neurogenic tumors |
| Coarctation of the aorta | • Endocrine-primary aldosteronism |
| | • Cushing syndrome |
| | • Pheochromocytoma |
| | • Hyperthyroidism |
| | • Endocrine-secreting tumors |

and subsequent tests are provided in Table 46-16. If renal disease is not identified, the additional tests are usually reserved for patients with higher levels of blood pressure.

**TREATMENT.** The office treatment of hypertension depends on the cause and severity. The step approach starts with nonpharmacologic therapies and progresses to drug treatment as necessary. Nondrug strategies include weight reduction, physical exercise, and dietary modification (generally a reduction of dietary sodium and calories). Other measures include avoidance of smoking and medications associated with cardiovascular effects. While this aspect of management may be difficult to accomplish in the adolescent, it is the foundation for long-term treatment with or without the addition of medications.

*Drug Therapy.*   Patients with persistent hypertension generally require medication. There are five classes of pharmacologic agents available for management of elevated blood pressure: angiotensin-converting enzyme inhibitors, calcium channel blocking agents, beta-adrenergic blocking agents, diuretics, and direct vasodilators. The use of a single agent once a day in the lowest effective dosage is the ideal. The goal is to reduce blood pressure to below the 95th percentile. If blood pressure control is not achieved with maximum dosage of one class of medication, then a second agent of a different class is added and increased to full dosage gradually. If adequate blood pressure control is still not achieved, a third class of antihypertensive medicine may be necessary. Consultation with a physician experienced in the management of adolescent hypertension should be sought when blood pressure control is difficult. Once satisfactory control is maintained over time, consideration should be given to gradually reducing drug therapy with careful follow-up of blood pressure.[55]

*Treatment of Hypertensive Crises.*   Hypertensive crises are rare in adolescents. Headache, vomiting, encephalopathy, CHF, and seizures may be secondary to severe

TABLE 46-14.   Historical Information to Elicit in Hypertensive Patients

| Information | Relevance |
| --- | --- |
| Family history of hypertension, preeclampsia, toxemia, renal disease, tumors | Important in essential hypertension, inherited renal disease, and some endocrine disease (e.g., familial pheochromocytoma with multiple endocrine adenopathy II) |
| Family history of early complications of hypertension and/or atherosclerosis | Suggests likely course of hypertension and/or presence of other coronary artery disease risk factors |
| Neonatal history | Use of umbilical artery catheter suggests need to evaluate renal vasculature and kidneys |
| Headaches, dizziness, epistaxis, visual problems | Nonspecific symptomatology, usually not etiologically helpful |
| Abdominal pain, dysuria, frequency, nocturia, enuresis | May suggest underlying renal disease |
| Joint pains/swelling, facial or peripheral edema | Suggests connective tissue disease and/or other forms of nephritis |
| Weight loss, failure to gain weight with good appetite, sweating, flushing, fevers, palpitations | In combination, symptoms suggest pheochromocytoma |
| Muscle cramps, weakness, constipation | May suggest hypokalemia and hyperaldosteronism |
| Age of onset of menarche, sexual development | May be helpful in suggesting hydroxylase deficiencies[61] |
| Ingestion of prescription and over-the-counter drugs, contraceptives, illicit drugs | Drug-induced hypertension[62] |

*Source:* Task Force on Blood Pressure Control in Children. Report of the Second Task Force on Blood Pressure Control in Children—1987. *Pediatrics* 1987; 79:1–25, with permission.

elevations of blood pressure. This is a medical emergency, and usually an intravenous potent antihypertensive agent such as nitroprusside, labetalol, or diazoxide is required. Oral nifedipine has been used in conscious asymptomatic patients with moderately severe hypertension. For rapid absorption, this drug must be removed from its capsule.[67]

Additional information about hypertension is provided in Chaps. 30 and 31.

**TABLE 46-15.   Findings to Look for on Physical Examination in Hypertensive Patients**

Physical Findings Relevance

| | |
|---|---|
| **General** | |
| Pale mucous membranes, facial or pretibial edema | Renal disease |
| Pallor, evanescent flushing, increased sweating at rest | Pheochromocytoma vs. hyperdynamic essential hypertension |
| Cafe´-au-lait spots, neurofibromas | Recklinghausen's disease[63] |
| Moon face, hirsutism, buffalo hump, truncal obesity, striae | Cushing's syndrome |
| Webbing of the neck, low hairline, widespaced nipples, wide carrying angle | Turner's syndrome[64] |
| Elfin facies, poor growth, retardation | William's syndrome[65] |
| Thyroid enlargement | Hyper- or hypothyroidism |
| **Cardiovascular** | |
| Absent or delayed femoral pulses, low leg pressure relative to arm pressure | Aortic coarctation |
| Heart size, rate, rhythm, murmurs, respiratory difficulty, hepatomegaly | Murmur—coarctation; tachycardia and/or arrhythmia—pheochromocytoma; large heart or heart failure—prolonged or severe hypertension |
| Bruits over great vessels | Arteritis or arteriopathy |
| **Abdomen** | |
| Epigastric bruit | Renovascular disease isolated or associated with William's or Recklinghausen's syndromes, or arteritis |
| Unilateral or bilateral masses | Wilms tumor[66] neuroblastoma, pheochromocytoma, polycystic kidneys, other tumors |
| **Neurologic** | |
| Hypertensive funduscopic changes | Chronic hypertension |
| Bell's palsy | Chronic hypertension |
| Neurologic deficits (e.g., hemiparesis) | Chronic or severe acute hypertension with stroke |

*Source:* Task Force on Blood Pressure Control in Children. Report of the Second Task Force on Blood Pressure Control in Children—1987. *Pediatrics* 1987; 79:1–25, with permission.

**TABLE 46-16.** Diagnostic Test for Hypertension in Childhood and Adolescence

**Initial Tests**

- Urinalysis
- Urine culture
- Measurement of serum electrolytes, creatinine, blood urea nitrogen, calcium, uric acid, cholesterol
- Complete blood count
- Electrocardiogram

**Additional Tests**

- Renal ultrasound
- Isotopic renography
- Measurement of urine catecholamines
- Measurement of plasma and urinary steroids
- Renal arteriography
- Renal vein renin activity

## Sudden Death in Children, Adolescents, and Young Athletes

**INCIDENCE OF SUDDEN DEATH.** Sudden death is uncommon in children. It is generally defined as death within 24 h in a child over 1 year of age following an event of sudden onset and during normal activity.[68] Sudden *cardiac* death is defined as any natural death due to cardiac causes that occur from minutes to 24 h after onset of symptoms.[69] In the age group from 1 year (beyond the age of sudden infant death syndrome) to 20 years, the estimated sudden death rate is between 1.1 and 13.8/100,000 per year,[68] accounting for approximately 5 percent of all deaths in children. Denfield and Garson related these statistics to a town of 300,000 people.[68] Approximately one-third of the town would be children, and therefore between one and thirteen young people per year would die suddenly. Sudden death in the young athlete is estimated as somewhat less, at 0.5/100,000.[70] The most common natural causes of sudden death in the young are infection and cardiovascular disease.

**CAUSES OF SUDDEN DEATH.** Sudden death of a child or adolescent has a devastating impact on the family, community, and medical establishment. Additionally, sudden death in young competitive athletes attracts extensive media coverage. Questions arise as to how these catastrophes might be prevented. Underlying cardiac abnormalities are frequently the cause of sudden death; however, these patients are often asymptomatic, and sudden cardiac death may be the initial manifestation. Suspicion of "silent" cardiac disorders depends on a careful evaluation of complaints such as chest pains, palpitations, near-syncope, or syncope. Exercise-related symptoms are especially important. A family history of sudden unexplained death in an individual less than 50 years of age, cardiac arrhythmias, syncope, or seizures may also indicate underlying familial cardiac abnormalities. When patients present with these complaints, the physical examination should focus on identifying murmurs, abnormal heart sounds, increased precordial activity, elevated blood pressure, or irregular rhythm. If cardiac disease is suspected, further evaluation should be instituted. Cardiac conditions associated with sudden death in children or adolescents are presented in Table 46-17.

Patients with known congenital, acquired, or postoperative heart disease may be at increased risk of sudden death. This is most commonly seen in patients who have left ventricular outflow tract obstruction or repair of cyanotic heart defects.[44] These

### TABLE 46-17. Cardiac Causes of Sudden Death in Children and Adolescents

**Unrecognized Heart Disease**

- Hypertrophic cardiomyopathy

- Congenital coronary anomalies

- Myocarditis

- Arrhythmogenic right ventricular dysplasia

- Rhythm disturbances:

    - Long QT syndrome, Wolff-Parkinson-White syndrome, ventricular tachycardia, and heart block

- Primary pulmonary arterial hypertension

- Commotio cordis (blunt trauma to the chest)

**Recognized Heart Disease**

- Left ventricular outflow tract obstruction (forms of aortic stenosis)

- Postoperative congenital heart disease (especially tetralogy of Fallot or Fontan operations)

- Marfan syndrome

- Kawasaki disease

- Cardiomyopathy (especially the hypertrophic variety)

- Arrhythmia:

    - Long QT syndrome, Wolff-Parkinson-White syndrome, right ventricular hypertrophy, heart block, or ventricular tachycardia.

deaths are usually due to arrhythmias and are associated with residual hemodynamic abnormalities. All of these patients require vigorous investigation when they present with symptoms.

**HEART DISEASE AND SUDDEN DEATH IN ATHLETES.**   In the United States, athletic participation is often an important part of a young person's life, and the primary care physician is often involved in preparticipation sports physical examinations. These evaluations are mandated either by school districts or by the state. Identification of cardiovascular disease should be one of the central aims of these evaluations.

In a review of 158 sudden deaths in trained U.S. athletes (median age 17 years) over a 10-year period, cardiovascular disease was identified in 134 (85 percent).[71] The most common causes were hypertrophic cardiomyopathy (36 percent) and congenital or acquired coronary artery anomalies (19 percent). A sobering aspect of this study was that despite preparticipation medical evaluation of 115 of these athletes who died, only 4 (3 percent) were suspected of having cardiovascular disease.

In a related study,[72] a review was performed of the current guidelines and requirements regarding preparticipation sports physical examinations in all 50 states and the District of Columbia. These guidelines were compared with the 1996 AHA consensus guidelines on sports screening.[73] In summary, this study concluded that 40 percent of states had no approved history or physical examination questionnaire, or had screening requirements or forms that were judged to be inadequate. In addition, various types of care providers, often with limited cardiovascular training, were allowed to administer these examinations.[72]

Despite limitations in identifying cardiovascular disease during sports examinations, the use of an itemized history and directed physical examination by qualified medical personnel should optimize the detection of cardiac conditions in the young. The salient features of the history and examination are presented in Table 46-18. The AHA consensus panel recommendations call for the history and physical examination to be performed before participation in organized high school (grades 9 to 12) and collegiate sports. Screening is to be repeated every 2 years, with an interim history recorded for each year.[73]

**CARDIAC ADAPTATION TO VIGOROUS ATHLETIC TRAINING.**   Cardiac adaptation to vigorous athletic training may result in the "athletic heart," and at times it is difficult to distinguish this from a true cardiac abnormality. Athletic training over a long period produces echocardiographically measurable increases in left ventricular wall thickness, left ventricular diastolic dimension, and myocardial mass.[74] At times the left ventricular wall thickness mimics measurements of hypertrophic cardiomyopathy, especially in rowers.[75] Differentiation between physiologic hypertrophy related to athletic training and hypertrophic cardiomyopathy may require weeks of "deconditioning" to determine if the wall thickness becomes less. While cardiac morphologic adaptations occur with exercise, the issue of whether they are truly outside the normal range has been questioned. A critical review of studies of cardiac adaption to exercise included that athletes in general have "rather" normal cardiac dimensions.[76]

TABLE 46-18.   Items Included in Recommended History and Physical Examination Forms for Preparticipation Cardiovascular Screening of High School Athletes

**History**

Past or present medications

Syncope

Prior hospitalization

Sudden death in family member <50 years

Heart murmur

Systemic hypertension

Parental verification of the history

Exertional chest pain

Excessive fatigability

Exertional dyspnea

Exertional dizziness

Prior heart problem

Palpitations

Prior limitation from sports participation

Heart disease in family

Prior rheumatic fever

Family history of Marfan syndrome

**Physical Examination**

General "cardiovascular" or "heart" section

Blood pressure

Heart rate

Peripheral (femoral) pulses

Heart murmur

Irregular heart rhythm

Marfan stigmata

*Source:* Adapted from Glover DW, Maron BJ: Profile of preparticipation cardiovascular screening for high school athletes. *JAMA* 1998; 279:1817–1819, with permission.

Other adaptations to athletic training are found in the heart rate and rhythm. Holter monitoring of elite athletes has demonstrated rates as low as 25 beats per minute and sinus pauses of more than 2 s.[77] Approximately 40 percent of athletes have single monomorphic PVCs and type I second-degree atrioventricular block.[77] Complex ventricular arrhythmias such as multiform premature ventricular contractions, nonsustained ventricular tachycardia, and ventricular couplets are rare in athletes. These complex ventricular arrhythmias require further evaluation. Athletes with uniform premature ventricular contractions and structurally normal hearts may participate in competitive sports.

While the use of screening ECGs and/or echocardiograms for athletic examinations would improve the detection of cardiovascular abnormalities, the cost of such screening is prohibitive. For example, the AHA consensus panel estimated the theoretical cost of echo screening for hypertrophic cardiomyopathy to be $250,000 to detect one previously undiagnosed case.[73]

**RECOMMENDATIONS REGARDING PARTICIPATION IN SPORTS.**   If an athlete is identified as having a cardiac condition, recommendations regarding participation in sports activities are required. These decisions are at times complex and should involve the input of the athlete, family, primary care physician, team physician, and cardiologist. The 26th Bethesda Conference (1994)[35] on eligibility recommendations for competitive athletes with cardiovascular abnormalities serves as an excellent resource. This document is an extensive review of the many factors involved in these decisions. The various types and severity of acquired, congenital, and postoperative cardiac conditions are reviewed, and guidelines for allowable athletic activity are offered. In addition, a large number of sports are classified according to the degree of peak dynamic and static exercise components during competition. These guidelines are useful in matching a patient's cardiovascular status with an appropriate sport.

It is unlikely that preparticipation sports examinations will detect all underlying cardiovascular disease. However, the use of a structured history and physical examination should help identify athletes who require further evaluation and hopefully help prevent sudden cardiac deaths.

# CARDIAC INVOLVEMENT IN ACQUIRED, GENETIC, AND SYSTEMIC DISEASES

The cardiovascular system may be involved in a wide variety of acquired, genetic, or systemic diseases of childhood and adolescence. This section will review the cardiovascular manifestation of selected illnesses that affect the young.

## Kawasaki Disease

**INCIDENCE.**   Kawasaki disease (KD) is an acute systemic vasculitis with predilection for involvement of the coronary arteries. It is the leading cause of acquired cardiovascular disease in children in the United States. It is a disease of the young child, with approximately 80 percent of cases occurring before 5 years of age and commonly before 2 years of age.[78] Onset in adolescence is rare. The importance of this illness to the adolescent is related to the long-term sequelae of coronary arterial involvement at an earlier age.

**CLINICAL CHARACTERISTICS.**   The cause of this disorder, first described by Dr. Tomasaku Kawasaki in 1967,[79] is unknown, and the diagnosis is based on clinical criteria. These criteria are provided in Table 46-19. Associated clinical and laboratory manifestations are presented in Table 46-20. Kawasaki disease may also present with atypical features that do not fully satisfy all the diagnostic criteria. Atypical KD is more common in infants less than 6 months of age, who are also at greatest risk for coronary involvement.[80]

**NATURAL HISTORY.**   Untreated, the clinical course of KD has three phases. The first day of illness is usually considered the onset of fever. The acute or first phase lasts approximately 10 days and is manifested by the features noted in Table 46-19. Cardiovascular involvement may occur in the acute phase, but more commonly it is found in the second or subacute phase. This second phase lasts from 11 to 25 days after the onset and includes desquamation of the fingers and toes and resolution of most of the acute features. It is in this phase that coronary vasculitis, coronary aneurysms, pericardial effusion, CHF, and electrocardiographic changes are more likely to appear. Thrombocytosis may occur, with platelet counts over 1 million. The convalescent or third phase extends until the acute phase reactants and platelet counts return to normal. Transverse grooves (Beau's lines) sometimes occur in the fingernails and toenails during this time.

**TABLE 46-19.   Diagnostic Criteria for Kawasaki Disease***

| |
|---|
| Fever, persisting over 5 days (frequently spiking up to 40°C) |
| Presence of at least four of the following features: |
| • Reddening and induration edema of palms and soles (subsequent periungual desquamation of fingers and toes) |
| • Changes in the mouth and lips: strawberry tongue, diffuse reddening of oral cavity, erythema and cracking of lips |
| • Polymorphous exanthem |
| • Bilateral conjunctival injection |
| • Nonsuppurative cervical lymphadenopathy |
| Exclusion of other similar diseases (see Table 46-21) |

* At least five of the six principal symptoms or with fever and less than four principal clinical features, if coronary artery involvement can be documented.

*Source:* Dajani AS, Taubert KA, Gerber MA, et al: Diagnosis and therapy of Kawasaki disease in children. *Circulation* 1993; 87:1776–1780, with permission.

**TABLE 46-20.   Associated Manifestations of Kawasaki Disease**

*Cardiovascular involvement*

- Coronary arterial vasculitis

- Myocarditis

- Pericarditis

- Aneurysms of peripheral arteries (iliac, axillary, renal)

- Aseptic meningitis

- Gallbladder hydrops

- Obstructive jaundice

- Uveitis

- Urethritis

- Joint pain and swelling

*Laboratory findings*

- Thrombocytosis (usually after 1 week)

- Elevated C-reactive protein and sedimentation rate

- Sterile pyuria and proteinuria

- Abnormal electrocardiogram: prolongation of intervals (PR, QT) and ST-T-wave abnormalities.

**DIFFERENTIAL DIAGNOSIS.**   Since there is no definitive laboratory test for KD, other conditions that produce similar clinical features may be confused with it. Table 46-21[81] lists infections and other illnesses that should be considered in the differential diagnosis.

**CARDIAC COMPLICATIONS.**   Approximately 20 to 25 percent of patients with untreated KD develop coronary aneurysms (detected by echocardiography), with a mortality rate of up to 2 percent.[82] A widespread immune-activated process is the most likely cause of the vascular injury. Although any artery may be involved, there is a predilection for coronary vessels; the reason for this is unknown. Coronary involvement occurs at approximately 2 to 4 weeks after onset of the disease. Inflammatory injury to all layers of the vascular wall occurs, and early echocardiographic changes include increased coronary arterial wall density, dilatation of coronary vessels, and aneurysm formation.[83] While most coronary aneurysms undergo remodeling and apparent regression within 2 years, structural and functional abnormalities may persist. Intravascular ultrasound studies have revealed residual intimal thickening, often with associated calcification and/or narrowed lesions at the site of the

TABLE 46-21.   Differential Diagnosis of Kawasaki's Disease

Measles

Scarlet fever

Drug reactions

Stevens-Johnson syndrome

Other febrile viral exanthems

- Epstein-Barr virus

- Adenovirus

- Enterovirus

- Parvovirus

Rocky Mountain spotted fever

Staphylococcal scalded skin syndrome

Toxic shock syndrome

Leptospirosis

Yersinia pseudotuberculosis (Izumi fever)

Juvenile rheumatoid arthritis

Polyarteritis nodosa

Mercury poisoning (acrodynia)

*Source:* Dajani AS, Taubert KA, Gerber MA, et al: Diagnosis and therapy of Kawasaki disease in children. *Circulation* 1993; 87:1776–1780, with permission.

"regressed" aneurysm.[82] Additional intravascular ultrasound studies have also revealed impaired vasoreactivity to nitroglycerin[84] and to infusion of acetylcholine.[85] These sites of residual coronary damage in previously regressed aneurysms may result in later atherosclerotic disease.

Patients with persistent coronary aneurysms are predisposed to thrombus formation and/or progressive stenosis that may occur over many years. These patients require long-term anticoagulation and monitoring. Various forms of stenoses have been described: long segment, beaded or braided, and localized or discrete forms. Frequently, these patients do not manifest ischemic symptoms despite significant luminal compromise.[86] Patients with giant coronary aneurysms (>8 mm in diameter) are at most risk for developing stenoses or thromboses.

**TREATMENT.**   In 1986, Newburger et al[82] reported the efficacy of intravenous gamma globulin (IVIG) given within 10 days of onset of the illness (marked by the first day of fever). Presently, IVIG is infused at a dose of 2 g/kg over 8 to10 h. Additionally, high-dose aspirin at 80 to 100 mg/kg/day divided into four doses is given during the acute symptoms. With defervescence of fever, the aspirin dose is reduced to 3 to 5 mg/kg/day, given once a day for its antiplatelet effect. The aspirin is continued for 6 to 8 weeks. The use of IVIG has reduced the incidence of giant coronary aneurysms to <1 percent. It also usually results in prompt resolution of acute symptoms.

During the acute phase, patients who do not respond adequately to IVIG may receive a repeat course, and at times steroids may be beneficial.[87]

Patients with persistent aneurysms, and particularly those with giant aneurysms, require long-term treatment with aspirin or Persantine and frequently the addition of warfarin. Patients with ischemic changes may require interventional catheterization with angioplasty, stent insertion, or cardiac bypass surgery.

The possibility of previous Kawasaki disease should be kept in mind when adolescents or young adults present with signs or symptoms of myocardial ischemia. Burns et al reviewed reports of 74 patients with a history of KD who presented between 12 and 39 years of age with chest pain, myocardial infarction, arrhythmias, or sudden death.[88] These symptoms were precipitated by exercise in over 80 percent of the patients. Coronary abnormalities included coronary artery aneurysms with calcification, stenoses, obstruction, and extensive collateral vessels. It is of interest that 11 of the 74 patients were thought not to have suffered coronary involvement at the time of their initial diagnosis of KD.

**LONG-TERM FOLLOW-UP.** At present, long-term follow-up of patients with Kawasaki disease is generally limited to those who have documented coronary involvement. The broad clinical outcome of KD, extending from no sequelae in the majority of patients to significant life-threatening coronary artery disease, has resulted in recommendations for treatment and long-term follow-up as presented in Table 46-22. Patients who do not have apparent coronary involvement are generally not followed after a year or two. This policy may need to change, however, if more patients who in the initial presentation have no documented coronary involvement eventually develop coronary abnormalities of clinical significance.

## Infective Endocarditis in the Adolescent

**INCIDENCE.** Infective endocarditis accounts for approximately 1 in 1000 hospital admissions in children.[89] Underlying congenital heart disease accounts for 80 percent of these patients; another 5 percent have had rheumatic heart disease. Approximately 15 percent are previously healthy children without known underlying cardiac disease.[90] Infective endocarditis (IE) has potentially severe morbidity and over 20 percent mortality.[91] The earlier it is recognized and treated, the better the outcome is likely to be. It is particularly important that the adolescent heart patient and family be educated regarding infective endocarditis prophylaxis as well as the variable manner in which IE may present. A more detailed discussion of the overall topic of infective endocarditis is covered in Chap. 40.

**TABLE 46-22. The Treatment and Investigation of Patients with Kawasaki Coronary Disease**

| Risk level | Pharmacologic therapy | Physical activity | Follow-up and diagnostic testing | Invasive testing |
|---|---|---|---|---|
| I (no coronary artery changes at any stage of illness) | None beyond initial 6 to 8 weeks | No restrictions beyond initial 6 to 8 weeks | None beyond first year unless cardiac disease suspected | None recommended |
| II (transient coronary artery ectasia that disappears during acute illness) | None beyond initial 6 to 8 weeks | No restrictions beyond initial 6 to 8 weeks | None beyond first year unless cardiac disease suspected. Physician may choose to see patient at 3- to 5-year intervals | None recommended |
| III (small to medium solitary coronary artery aneurysm) | Aspirin (3 to 5 mg/kg/day), at least until abnormalities resolve | For patients in first decade of life, no restriction beyond initial 6 to 8 weeks. For patient in second decade, physical activity guided by stress testing every other year. Competitive contact athletics with endurance training discouraged. | Annual follow-up with echocardiogram ± electrocardiogram in first decade of life | Angiography, if stress testing or echocardiography suggests stenosis |
| IV (one or more giant coronary aneurysms, or multiple small to medium aneurysms, without obstruction) | Long-term aspirin (3 to 5 mg/kg/day) ± warfarin | For patient in first decade of life, no restrictions beyond initial 6 to 8 weeks. For patients in second decade, annual stress testing guides recommendations. Strenuous athletics are | Annual follow-up with echocardiogram ± electrocardiogram ± chest x-ray ± additional electrocardiogram at 6-month intervals. For patients in first decade of life, | Angiography, if stress testing or echocardiography suggests stenosis. Elective catheterization may be done in certain circumstances. |

(*continues*)

**TABLE 46-22.    The Treatment and Investigation of Patients with Kawasaki Coronary Disease** *(continued)*

| Risk level | Pharmacologic therapy | Physical activity | Follow-up and diagnostic testing | Invasive testing |
|---|---|---|---|---|
| | | strongly discouraged. If stress test rules out ischemia, noncontact recreational sports allowed. | pharmacologic stress testing should be considered. | |
| V (coronary artery obstruction) | Long-term aspirin (3 to 5 mg/kg/day) ± warfarin. Use of calcium channel blockers should be considered to reduce myocardial oxygen consumption. | Contact sports, isometrics, and weight training should be avoided. Other physical activity recommendations guided by outcome of stress testing or myocardial perfusion scan | Echocardiogram and electro-cardiogram at 6-month intervals and annual Holter and stress testing. | Angiography recommended for some patients to aid in selecting therapeutic options. Repeat angiography with new-onset or worsening ischemia. |

*Source:* Dajani AS, Taubert KA, Takahashi M, et al: Guidelines for long-term management of patients with Kawasaki disease. Report from the Committee on Rheumatic Fever, Endocarditis, and Kawasaki Disease, Council on Cardiovascular Disease in the Young, American Heart Association. *Circulation* 1994; 89:916–922, with permission.

**RISK FACTORS FOR INFECTIVE ENDOCARDITIS.**    Risk factors for IE include congenital heart disease, rheumatic heart disease, cardiac surgery, and intracardiac or vascular devices such as prosthetic valves, transvenous pacemakers, indwelling central lines, stents, conduits, and systemic-to-pulmonary arterial shunts. Intravenous drug use, immunosuppression, and current trends such as body piercing and tattooing may predispose to IE. Acne, a very common adolescent problem, and poor dental hygiene may provide the source for infection. Infections in other sites (e.g., pneumonia, sinusitis, or pyelonephritis) that lead to bacteremia are also threats to cardiac patients. Virtually all forms of congenital heart disease have been associated with IE, but it is more common in lesions that result in a significant pressure gradient across a defect or valve. These lesions include ventricular septal defect (VSD), tetralogy of Fallot, aortic stenosis, patent ductus arteriosus (PDA), and coarctation of the aorta. On the other hand, surgical repair of VSD and PDA greatly reduces the risk of infective endocarditis.

**PATHOGENESIS.**    The essential ingredients for the development of IE are a damaged or abnormal endothelium and the presence of an infectious organism in the bloodstream. The pathologic hallmark of IE is the vegetation, which is a mesh of fibrin, platelets, red cells, leukocytes, and microorganisms. The most common bacterial causes are *Viridans streptococci* and *Staphylococcus aureus*. A wide variety of both gram-positive and gram-negative bacteria may result in IE. Fungal endocarditis is rare. Approximately 15 percent of IE cases have negative cultures.[89] The complications of infective endocarditis include destruction of valve tissue, obstruction of flow, aneurysm formation, emboli, and extension of infection into contiguous structures such as the conduction system.

**CLINICAL PRESENTATION.**   The clinical presentation and course depend on many factors, including the underlying cardiac abnormality, virulence of the infecting organism, immune status of the patient, promptness of diagnosis, and effectiveness of treatment.

*History.*   IE is often a subtle illness manifested by persistent or recurring fevers, malaise, chills, fatigue, weight loss, arthralgia, and myalgia. More acute presentation results in high fever with a toxic-like state, shock, heart failure, and peripheral embolization.

*Physical Findings.*   The physical findings of IE are noted in Table 46-23. Many of these are associated with long-standing endocarditis. By being familiar with the patient, the primary physician is positioned to appreciate many of these findings, especially changing or new heart murmurs.

*Laboratory Investigation.*   The essential element of laboratory investigation is the blood culture. At least three sets of blood cultures drawn over a 24-h period with strict aseptic technique and from different venous puncture sites are recommended. Cultures for aerobic, anaerobic, and fastidious organisms and also for fungi should be performed. Consultation with an infectious disease specialist is recommended for identifying the organism and selecting treatment. Other laboratory findings usually accompanying IE include elevated erythrocyte sedimentation rate and C-reactive protein, positive rheumatoid factor, anemia, and hematuria.

The echocardiogram is particularly useful in assessing the presence and location

**TABLE 46-23.   Endocarditis**

| Physical findings of infective endocarditis | |
| --- | --- |
| Fever | Splinter hemorrhages |
| Weight loss | Osler's nodes |
| New or changing murmur | Roth spots |
| Splenomegaly | Janeway lesions |
| Heart failure | |

of vegetations, functional status of the myocardium and valves, presence of vascular aneurysms, pericarditis, and abscess formation. Small vegetations (less than 2 mm) may not be imaged. Therefore, the absence of vegetations on echo examination does not rule out endocarditis. Serial studies are helpful in monitoring the functional status and new appearance or changes of vegetations. An ECG should be obtained to assess myocardial injury and atrioventricular conduction.

**TREATMENT.**

*Prevention.*    Prevention of IE is the best treatment. Good dental hygiene, control of acne, avoidance of unnecessary skin trauma, and prompt recognition and treatment of bacterial infections are important. Antibiotic prophylaxis for dental and surgical procedures is recommended and is discussed in Chap. 24.

*Medical and Surgical Management.*    The medical management of IE ideally involves a team of primary care physician, infection disease specialist, and cardiologist. Generally, a 4- to 6-week course of intravenous antibiotics or antifungal agents selected to provide cidal drug levels for the identified organism is necessary. In the case of culture-negative infective endocarditis, the treatment is aimed at the most likely organism. For the stable patient, insertion of a long-term intravenous line allows outpatient intravenous antibiotic management. Antibiotic peak and trough levels should be monitored carefully to avoid toxicity of these agents. Close monitoring of cardiac status is necessary in order to detect the progression of the disease. Cardiovascular surgery may be indicated for unremitting CHF, severe valve regurgitation, more than one major embolic event, persistently positive blood cultures, evidence of myocardial abscess, aneurysm of vessels, severe hemolysis, or obstruction of blood flow by large vegetations.

Additional information regarding infective endocarditis is provided in Chap. 40.

## Primary Pulmonary Artery Hypertension in the Adolescent

**INCIDENCE.**    Primary pulmonary arterial hypertension is a rare disease of the pulmonary vascular bed that primarily affects otherwise healthy young adults. It is a progressive process and is generally fatal 2 to 3 years after diagnosis.[92] In childhood it affects the sexes equally, but it becomes more common in females during adolescence.

**ETIOLOGY.**    The cause is unknown, and the diagnosis is based on excluding other illnesses. A familial form of primary pulmonary arterial hypertension accounts for 6 percent of cases.[93] A summary of the more common causes of secondary pulmonary arterial hypertension in the adolescent is provided in Table 46-24.

**HEMODYNAMIC CRITERIA.**    The hemodynamic criteria for primary pulmonary arterial hypertension are a mean pulmonary arterial pressure >25 mmHg (or >30 mmHg with exercise) or a pulmonary vascular resistance of more than 4

**TABLE 46-24.   Causes of Pulmonary Hypertension**

Cardiovascular disease

- Large left-to-right shunt lesions (e.g., ventricular septal defect, patent ductus arteriosus)

- Pulmonary venous hypertension (e.g., mitral stenosis, left ventricular failure)

Pulmonary disease

- Parenchymal lung disease (e.g., severe pneumonitis, cystic fibrosis, Hamman-Rich syndrome)

- Airway obstruction (e.g., enlarged tonsils, macroglossia, asthma, laryngotracheomalacia, micrognathia)

- Inadequate ventilatory drive (hypoxia, $CO_2$ retention)

- Chest wall deformity (e.g., kyphoscoliosis)

- Disorder of respiratory muscles

- High altitude

Thromboembolic diseases

- Hemoglobinopathies (e.g., sickle cell anemia)

- Pulmonary embolism

- Indwelling central venous lines or ventriculoperitoneal shunts for hydrocephalus

Collagen vascular diseases

Primary pulmonary hypertension

Miscellaneous causes (e.g., anorectic agents, L-tryptophan, or cocaine)

Wood units[93] in the absence of other cardiac, pulmonary, or vascular conditions. As the disease worsens, pulmonary pressures may exceed systemic pressure, and right ventricular failure may occur.

**ASSOCIATED PATHOLOGY.** Pathologically, the pulmonary vasculature demonstrates various degrees of medial wall hypertrophy, intimal cellular proliferation and fibrosis, plexiform lesions, thromboses, and venoocclusive disease.[94] The pathogenesis is considered to be a combination of abnormalities of vasoconstriction, vascular wall remodeling, thromboses in situ, and endothelial dysfunction.

**HISTORY.**   In the office setting, these patients present with a variety of symptoms, with a mean length of time from onset of symptoms to diagnosis of approximately 2 years.[93] The clinical manifestations result from the inability of the "fixed" pulmonary vascular bed to accommodate increases in cardiac output. Patients may complain of dyspnea, fatigue, palpitations, chest pain, presyncope or syncope, chronic cough, and, especially, limited exercise capacity. Sudden death may occur, especially with physical stress.

**PHYSICAL EXAMINATION.**    The physical findings include an increase in the right ventricular impulse, palpitation of the pulmonary valve closure, and diminished peripheral pulses due to a decrease in cardiac output. Cyanosis may be present if there is a patent foramen ovale allowing right-to-left atrial-level shunting. Right heart failure results in jugular venous distention, peripheral edema, and liver enlargement. Auscultation reveals a loud and frequently single second heart sound. An ejection click may be present and presumably arises from the dilated main pulmonary artery. A pansystolic murmur of tricuspid regurgitation may be heard at the lower left sternal border, and a diastolic murmur of pulmonary regurgitation at the left upper sternal border.

**LABORATORY INVESTIGATION.**    The ECG reveals right axis deviation with right ventricular and right atrial abnormality. The heart size is usually normal on the chest x-ray film, but there are enlarged main and proximal branch pulmonary arteries, with "pruning" of the peripheral pulmonary vessels. The echocardiographic findings are characterized by right ventricular enlargement and hypertrophy, right atrial enlargement, dilated main pulmonary artery, and tricuspid insufficiency. Doppler flow velocities of tricuspid regurgitation flow and pulmonary regurgitation flow are very useful in noninvasively documenting elevated pulmonary arterial pressure. The complete work-up of pulmonary arterial hypertension is extensive and includes a ventilation-perfusion scan to assess for thromboembolic phenomena, pulmonary function tests, evaluation of coagulopathies, assessment for collagen vascular disease, and cardiac catheterization with measurement of pulmonary vascular response to various vasodilators. A lung biopsy may also be indicated.

**TREATMENT.**    Recent therapeutic approaches to primary pulmonary arterial hypertension have resulted in improved quality of life and longer survival. Lifestyle changes are necessary and include avoidance of high-altitude environments; caution at times of air travel (oxygen supplements have generally made air travel safe); reduction of physical activity that aggravates the limited cardiac output; and avoidance of pregnancy, oral contraceptives, and the smoking of cigarettes. Chronic supplemental oxygen may be beneficial if there is alveolar hypoxia, especially with physical activity, during sleep, or associated with right heart failure. Digoxin and diuretics are indicated for right heart failure. Careful monitoring of electrolyte status (especially hypokalemia) and avoidance of excessive reduction of central venous pressures, which may interfere with adequate right ventricle filling, are important. These patients are susceptible to venous thromboses because of low blood flow states and dilated heart chambers. Pulmonary thrombi can exacerbate the disease process and may be fatal. In adults, chronic anticoagulation has been shown to prolong survival.[95] Oral calcium channel blockers used as pulmonary vasodilators have improved survival in patients that demonstrate acute responses to these agents in the catheterization laboratory.[96] Recent therapeutic advances that have promise are the use of chronic vasodilators such as continuous intravenous infusion of prostacyclin[97] and use of long-term inhaled nitric oxide.[98] Patients with severe right-sided failure, marked decrease in cardiac output, or syncope may benefit from an elective blade atrial septostomy in the cardiac catheterization laboratory.[99] This increases the cardiac output by allowing a right-to-left atrial shunt at the expense of some hypoxia. For patients who are unresponsive to therapy and severely symptomatic, a single or double lung transplant or heart-lung transplant remains an option.[100]

Additional information on primary pulmonary hypertension is provided in Chap. 43.

## Marfan Syndrome in the Adolescent

**DEFINITION AND INCIDENCE OF COMPLICATIONS.**   Marfan syndrome (MS) is an inborn error of connective tissue with characteristic ocular, musculoskeletal, and cardiovascular findings. Marfan syndrome is dominantly inherited and is caused by a mutation in the gene that encodes the extracellular matrix protein fibrillin-1.[101] Cardiovascular involvement is common, progressive, and the usual cause of morbidity and death in these patients. Untreated, the average age of death in MS is in the 30s and 40s[102]; death is usually secondary to aortic dissection or chronic aortic insufficiency. Below the age of 20, serious cardiovascular complications of MS occur in 4.3 percent of patients.[103] Because preventive measures have proven effective, early diagnosis of Marfan syndrome is important to permit modification of cardiovascular complications.

**PHYSICAL EXAMINATION.**   The physical findings and age at their appearance are listed in Table 46-25.

**DIAGNOSTIC CRITERIA.**   Marfan syndrome is a clinical diagnosis. A revised set of diagnostic criteria that includes family history as well as major and minor criteria is presented in Table 46-26. The role of molecular testing as a clinical tool is still limited. Young patients with only some features of MS may not merit the diagnosis; however, they should be followed over time to assess for the development of cardiovascular abnormalities.[101] Pyeritz[101] has pointed out that there are approximately 200 Mendelian disorders that involve abnormalities of connective tissue. These may have considerable phenotypic overlap with the features of Marfan syndrome. Some of the more common connective tissue disorders include Ehlers-Danlos syndrome, homocystinuria, osteogenesis imperfecta, and chondrodysplasias.

**CARDIOVASCULAR MANIFESTATIONS IN THE ADOLESCENT.**   Mitral valve prolapse is the most common cardiovascular manifestation of MS in children. Mitral regurgitation may progress to clinical significance before adulthood. Aortic root dilatation and aortic regurgitation may be present at birth but more commonly develop during adolescence or adulthood. The most serious consequences of aortic root disease include aortic regurgitation, aortic dissection in any portion of the aorta, and sudden death.

**TABLE 46-25.   Features of Marfan Syndrome and Age Dependency**

| Organ Systems | Feature | Infancy* | Childhood | Adolescence |
|---|---|---|---|---|
| Skeletal | Tall stature | + | + + | + |
| | Arachnodactyly | + + | − − | − − |
| | Anterior chest deformity | + | + + | − − |
| | Scoliosis | − − | + | + + |
| | Pes planus | + | + + | − − |
| | Joint contracture | + + | − − | − − |
| | Joint laxity | + + | + + | + |
| | Degenerative arthritis | − − | − − | − − |
| Ocular | Ectopia lentis | + + | + | + |
| | Megalocornea | + + | − − | − − |
| | Myopia | + + | + + | + |
| | Retinal detachment | − − | − − | − − |
| Cardiovascular | Mitral valve prolapse | + | + + | + |
| | Mitral regurgitation | + | + | + |
| | Aortic root dilatation | + | + + | + |
| | Aortic regurgitation | − − | − − | + |
| | Aortic dissection | − − | − − | − − |
| Pulmonary | Pneumothorax | − − | − − | + |
| Skin and integument | Striae atrophicae | − − | + | + + |
| | Inguinal herniae | + | + | + |
| | Dural ectasia | ? | ? | + |
| Other | Learning difficulties | − | + | + + |

*Likelihood of feature during this period, if it will: + + highly likely; − − somewhat likely; − + unlikely; ? undetermined.

*Source:* Pyeritz RE: The Marfan syndrome in childhood: features, natural history and differential diagnosis. *Prog Pediatr Cardiol* 1996; 5:151–157, with permission.

***Laboratory Investigation.***   Aortic root dilatation is usually monitored by serial echocardiographic measurements and indexed to the patient's body surface area. Aortic root dilatation (measured at the sinuses of Valsalva) >1.5 times the mean predicted aortic root diameter constitutes aneurysmal enlargement. MRI is helpful in assessing more distal sites of aortic dilatation, as well as in avoiding errors in measurement of an elliptical aortic root.

TABLE 46-26.  Diagnostic Criteria for the Marfan Syndrome

**Family history**

Major criteria

- Having a parent who meets diagnostic criteria *independently*

- Presence of a *FBNI* mutation known to cause Marfan syndrome

- A *FBNI* haplotype, inherited by descent, known to be associated with Marfan syndrome in the family

**Skeletal**

Major criteria *at least four of the following:*

- Pectus excavatum requiring surgery or a pectus carinatum

- Reduced upper-to-lower segment ratio or arm span-to-height ratio >1.05

- Positive wrist *and* thumb signs

- Scoliosis >20°

- Reduced extension of the elbow (170°)

- Medial displacement of the medial malleolus and pes planus

- Protrusio acetabulae of any degree

**Minor criteria**

- Pectus excavatum of moderate severity

- Scoliosis <20°

- Thoracic lordosis

- Joint hypermobility

- Highly arched palate

- Dental crowding

- "Typical" facies (dolichocephaly, malar hypoplasia, enophthalmos, retrognathia, downslanting palpebral fissures)

For the skeletal system to be "involved," at least two of the components of the Major Criteria or one of the components of the Major Criteria plus two of the Minor Criteria must be present.

**Ocular**

Major criterion

- Ectopia lentis

Minor criteria

- Flat cornea

- Increased axial length of the globe

*(continues)*

**TABLE 46-26.   Diagnostic Criteria for the Marfan Syndrome** *(continued)*

- Cataract (nucleus sclerotic, < age 50)
- Hypoplastic iris
- Miosis and hypoplastic ciliary muscle
- Glaucoma (< age 50)
- Retinal detachment

For the ocular system to be "affected," at least two of the Minor Criteria must be present.

**Cardiovascular**

Major criteria

- Aortic root dilatation (involving sinuses of Valsalva)
- Aortic dissection

Minor criteria

- Mitral valve prolapse
- Dilatation of proximal main pulmonary artery (in absence of peripheral pulmonic stenosis of other cause)
- Calcification of mitral annulus (< age 40)
- Dilatation of abdominal or descending thoracic aorta (< age 50)

For the cardiovascular system to be "involved," only one of the Minor Criteria must be present.

**Pulmonary**

No major criterion

Minor criteria

- Spontaneous pneumothorax
- Apical blebs (on the chest radiography)

For the pulmonary system to be "involved," one of the Minor Criteria must be present.

**Skin and integument**

Major criterion

- None

Minor criteria

- Striae atrophicae (in absence of marked weight changes, pregnancy, or repetitive stress)
- Recurrent or incisional hernia

For the skin and integument to be "involved," one of the minor criteria must be present.

TABLE 46-26.   Diagnostic Criteria for the Marfan Syndrome *(continued)*

**Dura**

Major criteria

- Dural ectasia (lumbosacral, by CT or MRI)

Minor criterion

- None

For the dura to be involved, dural ectasia must be present.

Requirements for diagnosis of the Marfan syndrome:

For the index case:

- At least two major criteria in different systems *and* involvement of the third system
- Exclusion of homocystinuria by plasma amino acid analysis

For a family member:

- Major criterion in family history *and* one major criterion in one system *and* involvement of a second system
- Exclusion of homocystinuria by plasma amino acid analysis

*Source*: De Paepa A, Deitz HC, Devereux RB et al: Revised diagnostic criteria for the Marfan syndrome. *Am J Med Genet* 1988; 29:581–594; Pyeritz, RE: The Marfan syndrome in childhood: features, natural history and differential diagnosis. *Prog Pediatr Cardiol* 1996, 5:151–157, with permission from Elsevier Science.

## TREATMENT.

*General Recommendations.*   The medical management of Marfan syndrome requires the interaction of primary care physicians, orthopedists, ophthalmologists, cardiologists, geneticists, and others as necessary. Once a diagnosis of MS is made, other family members should be fully evaluated. General measures for patients with cardiovascular involvement include explanations of endocarditis, education regarding IE prophylaxis, and avoidance of contact sports and weight lifting. These patients are advised to participate in only mild aerobic and noncontact exercise (e.g., golf, bowling) to minimize wall stress on the aorta. Careful follow-up of cardiovascular progression is essential in these patients.

*Drug Therapy.*   The use of chronic beta-blockade therapy has been documented to slow progression of aortic root enlargement.[104] Presumably this effect is related to the reduced aortic pulsatile wall stress secondary to the beta blocker's effect on cardiac contractility. In children or adolescents, a long-acting beta blocker is usually started at 1 mg/kg/day and slowly increased to 2 mg/kg/day or until side effects interfere with activities.[99] Effectiveness of beta blockade can be determined in the office by assessing the response to exercise. One practical method is to have the patient run up and down two flights of stairs. Adequate beta-blocker effect is assumed to be present if the maximum heart rate is 20 percent less or 40 beats slower than the pretreatment heart rate with the same exercise.[105]

Pregnancy in women with Marfan syndrome is a risk factor for two reasons: There is a 50 percent risk of transmitting the disorder to the fetus, and the risk of aortic dissection or rupture during pregnancy or shortly after delivery is increased. Patients with an aortic root of less than 4 cm and minimal aortic valve involvement have less risk at pregnancy.[106] These women should be followed very closely with serial echo measurements of the aortic root dimension throughout pregnancy and in the postpartum period. For women with significantly dilated aortic roots, pregnancy should be contraindicated. Prenatal counseling with a geneticist should be offered when either prospective parent has Marfan syndrome.

*Surgical Treatment.*   Elective surgical intervention is indicated for patients with aortic root measurements of 5.5 cm or greater. Some patients may actually have dissections or rupture with smaller measurements than this. Generally, a composite prosthetic valve and vascular graft are inserted, though valve-sparing procedures have been used in patients with MS.[107] Long-term medical management of postsurgical patients includes subacute bacterial endocarditis prophylaxis, anticoagulation with warfarin, continued use of beta blockers, and further monitoring for changes in the aortic region with echocardiography or MRI. In contrast to the relatively low mortality of elective aortic root replacement, emergency repair for dissection of the aorta or rupture has a much higher mortality.[107] Any portion of the aorta may be involved in the dissection.

Patients with MS also benefit from association with the National Marfan Foundation in Port Washington, New York, and referral to that organization is recommended.

## Anorexia Nervosa–Cardiac Implications

**INCIDENCE.**   Anorexia nervosa is almost exclusively an illness of adolescent females, with a mean age at onset of 14 years.[1] It is a clinical syndrome manifested by significant emaciation (body weight less than 85 percent of the ideal weight), accompanied by an intense fear of gaining weight and becoming fat despite being significantly underweight. It is commonly found in adolescent females from families of medium to higher socioeconomic status. It is a chronic illness with serious psychological and physiologic implications, including death in 5 to 18 percent of patients.[108]

**CARDIAC MANIFESTATIONS.**

*History.*   These patients may experience dizziness or syncope associated with exercise. These symptoms may be related to dehydration. Many of these patients have bulimic behavior, with associated binge feeding and purging. Frequent vomiting or abuse of laxatives, purgatives, and diuretics may result in severe electrolyte disorders that can produce cardiac arrhythmias.

*Physical Examination.* Cardiac findings in these patients include a low resting heart rate and low blood pressure. There also may be orthostatic hypotension.

*Laboratory Investigation.* Electrocardiographic changes in these patients are common and include bradycardia, decreased QRS amplitude, nonspecific ST–T-wave changes, and prolonged Q-T intervals. Exercise testing has revealed abnormal cardiovascular and sympathetic responses and ST-segment depression that suggest myocardial injury.[109] Echocardiographic studies have demonstrated reduced stroke volume, cardiac output, heart size, and cardiac mass.[110] Systolic ejection phase indices of left ventricular function were normal, however.[110]

*Cardiovascular Complications.* Sudden unexpected death can occur in patients with anorexia nervosa and is believed to be secondary to arrhythmias or degenerative cardiomyopathies.[111] Patients who die suddenly are usually extremely emaciated and have lost more than 40 percent of their ideal body weight.

**TREATMENT.** These patients often require very long-term psychotherapy and support. Nutritional therapy for anorexia nervosa must be carefully monitored. Generally, a gradual weight gain of 1 to 2 lb per week is the goal. Rapid weight gain may produce severe complications such as congestive heart failure, pancreatitis, and acute gastric dilatation.[108]

## Systemic Lupus Erythematosus

Systemic lupus erythematosus (SLE) is a connective tissue disease that affects all organs and is characterized by the formation of autoantibodies and immune complexes. Cardiac manifestations are reported in 31 percent of children with SLE and are serious in 10 percent.[112] The most commonly encountered cardiac abnormality is pericarditis, although the inflammatory response may cause myocarditis, Libman-Sacks endocarditis, valvulitis, and coronary arteritis. Women with collagen vascular diseases may give birth to infants with congenital complete heart block. These women may not have clinical manifestations of SLE.[113] Associated renal disease, anemia, or pulmonary involvement may complicate the cardiovascular manifestations of SLE. Cardiac management of patients with SLE depends on the type and severity of involvement.

## Juvenile Rheumatoid Arthritis

Juvenile rheumatoid arthritis (JRA) is the most common type of chronic arthritis in childhood. It is an autoimmune disorder and may be manifested by systemic illness or limited to only one or several joints. As in SLE, pericarditis is the most common form of cardiac involvement. Myocarditis is infrequent but can cause congestive heart failure and arrhythmias. Involvement of the aorta and mitral valve may cause significant valvular regurgitation. Treatment for mild involvement is with nonsteroidal anti-inflammatory agents. Corticosteroids are indicated for severe pericarditis, myocarditis, or valvulitis.

## Duchenne Muscular Dystrophy

**ETIOLOGY.**   Duchenne muscular dystrophy is a sex-linked recessive disease that presents in the first 5 years of life. A metabolic defect results in a deficiency or absence of dystrophin, which is present in a sarcolemma of skeletal muscles.[114]

**GENERAL MANIFESTATIONS.**   Involvement of skeletal muscle is progressive and ultimately fatal. Initially, pelvic muscle involvement results in a waddling gait, lordosis, protuberant abdomen, and difficulty in standing up (Gower's sign). Subsequently, the shoulders and trunk muscles are involved, leading to scoliosis, compromise of pulmonary function, and immobility. Death usually occurs in the third decade of life.

**CARDIAC MANIFESTATIONS.**   In muscular dystrophy, cardiac muscle is less severely involved than skeletal muscle. Lymphocytic and minimal fat infiltration have been described. The most severely affected areas of the heart are the posterobasal portion of the left ventricle and the posterior papillary muscle of the mitral valve.[115] Signs and symptoms of cardiac compromise appear late and may be contributed to by chronic restrictive pulmonary disease. Mitral valve prolapse with various degrees of mitral regurgitation is present in 15 percent of adolescents with muscular dystrophy. Cardiac failure occurs in approximately 20 percent and has a poor prognosis.[116]

*Laboratory Investigation.*   Electrocardiographic abnormalities are present in 90 percent of patients with muscular dystrophy. These include sinus tachycardia, short PR interval, and tall R wave over the right precordial leads, with a deep and narrow Q wave in limb leads. Flattened or inverted T waves are found in 30 percent of patients.[117] Conduction and rhythm abnormalities have been described and include atrial, ectopic, and junctional rhythm.[118]

**TREATMENT.**   Management of cardiac complications of muscular dystrophy includes anticongestive and antiarrhythmic treatment as part of the general supportive measures. Patients who require any type of surgery are at anesthetic risk for malignant hyperthermia[119] and cardiac arrest.[120] Inevitably, patients with Duchenne muscular dystrophy succumb to complications of immobility and pulmonary disease.

## Friedreich's Ataxia

**ETIOLOGY.**   Friedreich's ataxia is an autosomal recessive disease affecting the spinal cord, peripheral nerves, and heart. Diabetes can occur in approximately 20 percent of patients and is due to atrophy of pancreatic islets. The gene for Friedreich's ataxia has been localized to chromosome 9.[121]

**GENERAL MANIFESTATIONS.**   The disease generally presents in childhood with clumsiness of gait. Progressive neurologic involvement results in absence of deep tendon reflexes, proprioceptive sensory loss, dysarthria, tremors, nystagmus, and worsening of ataxia. Most patients are unable to walk by late adolescence. Scoliosis with respiratory compromise is usually severe. Patients are intellectually normal. The presentation of Friedreich's ataxia may mimic the chorea of rheumatic fever. An important clinical finding is the absence of knee and ankle reflexes in Friedreich's ataxia.

**CARDIAC MANIFESTATIONS.**   Cardiac abnormalities occur in over 90 percent of Friedreich's ataxia patients.[122] Cardiac hypertrophy, especially of the left ventricle or intraventricular septum, occurs, as well as atheromatous involvement of the coronary arteries. Dilated cardiomyopathy has been described.

*Laboratory Investigation.*   Electrocardiographic abnormalities are common, especially T-wave inversion over the left precordial leads, which is seen in more than 80 percent of cases.[122] Other findings include conduction defects, left and right ventricular hypertrophy, right axis deviation, or at times low QRS voltage.[122] Sinus tachycardia and a variety of atrial or ventricular arrhythmias may occur. Echocardiographic findings reflect the type of hypertrophic or dilated cardiomyopathy.

**TREATMENT.**   There is no specific treatment for Friedreich's ataxia. Cardiac medications are used to control arrhythmias or CHF. Hypertrophic obstructive cardiomyopathy may benefit from beta blockers. The average age at death is 28 years, and death is due to pulmonary or cardiovascular complications.

## Myotonic Dystrophy

**ETIOLOGY.**   Myotonic dystrophy is an autosomal dominant neuromuscular disease characterized by increased muscular contractility and decreased muscular relaxation. The genetic cause of myotonic dystrophy has been localized to chromosome 19.[123] Fatty infiltration and fibrosis have been found in both the myocardium and the conduction system.

**GENERAL MANIFESTATIONS.**   In a child, myotonic dystrophy is manifested by poor coordination, muscle weakness, and developmental retardation.

**CARDIAC MANIFESTATIONS.**   Cardiac abnormalities are common. Mitral valve prolapse is often present in adults and may be found in children and adolescents. A large number of patients will have cardiac conduction defects.

*Laboratory Investigation.*   The ECG may reveal long PR intervals, widened QRS complexes, and bundle branch block. Conduction abnormalities may progress to second- or third-degree atrioventricular block and result in syncope or sudden death. Arrhythmias appear as the disease progresses and include atrial fibrillation, atrial flutter, and ventricular arrhythmias.

**TREATMENT.**   Caution must be exercised with antiarrhythmic agents that affect atrioventricular conduction. Permanent pacemaker insertion may be necessary in cases of high-degree atrioventricular block.[117]

## Ehlers-Danlos Syndrome

Ehlers-Danlos syndrome comprises a group of dominantly inherited heterogeneous connective tissue disorders in which the tissues suffer abnormalities of collagen. General manifestations include hyperextensibility and fragility of skin, easy bruisability, poor wound healing, and hypermobile joints. Cardiac manifestations include tricuspid and mitral valve prolapse and regurgitation, aneurysms and dissection of the aorta, fragility of arterial walls, and venous varicosities. Treatment depends on the type and severity of involvement, though cardiovascular surgery carries increased risk because of the poor vascular integrity.[117]

## Sickle Cell Anemia

Adolescents with sickle cell anemia have cardiac findings associated with chronic anemia, compensatory increased cardiac output with low systemic vascular resistance. Symptoms of fatigue and dyspnea are also related to chronic anemia. Acute chest syndromes may present and are probably secondary to pulmonary vasoocclusive events or infection of the lungs. Myocardial infarction is rare, but myocardial fibrosis may occur. Systolic and diastolic murmurs are due to excessive blood flow across the pulmonary outflow tract and mitral valve, respectively. Cardiac enlargement is common, and the ECG often reveals left ventricular hypertrophy. Echocardiography demonstrates generalized chamber enlargement with increased stroke volume and, at times, abnormal interventricular septal motion. Adolescents may have acquired pulmonary hypertension with secondary right heart failure. High-output failure may also occur.

### REFERENCES

1. Moller JH, Taubert KA, Allen HD, et al: Cardiovascular health and disease in children: current status. *Circulation* 1994; 89:923–930.
2. Neinstein LS: Chest pain. In: Neinstein LS (ed): *Adolescent Health Care: A Practical Guide*, 3d ed. Baltimore, Williams and Wilkins, 1996:601–605.
3. Brenner JI, Berman MA: Chest pain in childhood and adolescence. *J Adolesc Health Care* 1983; 3:271–276.
4. National Heart, Lung, and Blood Institute: *NHLBI Fact Book, Fiscal Year 1995*. U.S. Department of Health and Human Services, National Institutes of Health, March 1996.
5. Gillum RF: Sudden coronary death in the United States: 1980–1985. *Circulation* 1989; 79:756–765.
6. Pantell RH, Goodman BW Jr: Adolescent chest pain: a prospective study. *Pediatrics* 1983; 71: 881–887.
7. Selbst SM, Ruddy RM, Clark BJ, et al: Pediatric chest pain: a prospective study. *Pediatrics* 1988; 82:319–323.
8. Veasy LG: Chest pain in children. In: Emmanouilides GC, Allen HD, Riemenschneider TA, Gutgesell HP (eds): *Heart Disease in Infants, Children, and Adolescents*, 5th ed. Baltimore, Williams and Wilkins, 1995:653–657.
9. Ruckman RN: Cardiac causes of syncope. *Pediatr Rev* 1987; 9:101–108.

10. Kapoor WN, Karpf M, Maher Y, et al: Syncope of unknown origin. The need for a more cost-effective approach to its diagnostic evolution. *JAMA* 1982; 247:2687–2691.

11. Abboud FM: Ventricular syncope. Is the heart a sensory organ? *N Engl J Med* 1989; 320:390–392.

12. Glick C, Yu PN: Hemodynamic changes during spontaneous vasovagal reactions. *Am J Med* 1963; 34:42–47.

13. Hoefnagels WA, Padberg GW, Overweg J, et al: Transient loss of consciousness: the value of the history for distinguishing seizure from syncope. *J Neurol* 1991; 238:39–43.

14. Lerman-Sagie T, Rechavia E, Strasberg B, et al: Head-up tilt for evaluation of syncope of unknown origin in children. *J Pediatr* 1991; 118:676–679.

15. Grubb BP, Samoil D, Kosinski D, et al: Use of sertraline hydrochloride in the treatment of refractory neurocardiogenic syncope in children and adolescents. *J Am Coll Cardiol* 1994; 24:490–494.

16. Smith MS, Glass ST: An adolescent girl with headache and syncope. *J Adolesc Health Care* 1989; 10:54–56.

17. Kinlay S, Leitch JW, Neil A, et al: Cardiac event recorders yield more diagnoses and are more cost-effective than 48-hour Holter monitoring in patients with palpitations: a controlled clinical trial. *Ann Intern Med* 1996; 124:16–20.

18. Reiffel JA, Schulhol E, Joseph B: Palpitations and dizziness: arrhythmia frequency determined by transtelephonic monitoring [abstract]. *Circulation* 1985; 72:476.

19. Dickinson DF, Scott O: Ambulatory electrographic monitoring in 100 healthy teenage boys. *Br Heart J* 1984; 51:179–183.

20. *Heart to Heart.* Sudden Arrhythmia Death Syndrome Foundation, Salt Lake City.

21. Viitasalo MT, Kala R, Eisalo A: Ambulatory electrocardiographic findings in your athletes between 14 and 16 years of age. *Eur Heart J* 1984; 5:2–6.

22. Brodsky M, Wu D, Denes P, et al: Arrhythmias detected by 24-hour continuous electrocardiographic monitoring in 50 male medical students without apparent heart disease. *Am J Cardiol* 1977; 39:390–395.

23. Ludmirsky A, Garson A Jr: Supraventricular tachycardia. In: Gillette P, Garson A Jr (eds): *Pediatric Arrhythmias: Electrophysiology and Pacing.* Philadelphia, W. B. Saunders, 1990:380–426.

24. Benson DW Jr, Dunnigan A, Sterba R, Benditt DG: Atrial pacing from the esophagus in the diagnosis and management of tachycardia and palpitations. *J Pediatr* 1983; 102:40–46.

25. Danford DA, Kugler JD, Deal B, et al: The learning curve for radiofrequency ablation of tachyarrhythmias in pediatric patients. *Am J Cardiol* 1995; 75:587–590.

26. Garson A Jr: Electrocardiographpy. In: Garson A Jr, Bricker J, Fisher DJ, Neish SR (eds): *The Science and Practice of Pediatric Cardiology,* 2nd ed. Baltimore, Williams and Wilkins, 1998:735–788.

27. Garson A Jr, Randall DC, Gillette PC, et al: Prevention of sudden death after repair of tetralogy of Fallot: treatment of ventricular arrhythmias. *J Am Coll Cardiol* 1985; 6:221–227.

28. Braimbridge MV, Yen A: Coarctation in the elderly. *Circulation* 1965; 31:209–218.

29. Campbell M: Natural history of coarctation of the aorta. *Br Heart J* 1970; 32:633–640.

30. Bromberg BI, Beckman RH, Rocchini AP, et al: Aortic aneurysm after patch aortoplasty repair of coarctation: a prospective analysis of prevalence, screening tests and risks. *J Am Coll Cardiol* 1989; 14:734–741.

31. Fletcher SE, Nihill MR, Grifka RG, et al: Balloon angioplasty of native coarctation of the aorta: midterm follow-up and prognostic factors. *J Am Coll Cardiol* 1995; 25:730–734.

32. Edeid MR, Prieto LR, Latson LA: Use of balloon-expandable stents for coarctation of the aorta: initial results and intermediate-term follow-up. *J Am Coll Cardiol* 1997; 30:1847–1852.

33. Roberts WC: The congenitally bicuspid aortic valve. A study of 85 autopsy cases. *Am J Cardiol* 1970; 26:72–83.

34. Keane JF, Driscoll DJ, Gersony WM, et al: Second natural history study of congenital heart defects. Results of treatment of patient with aortic valvar stenosis. *Circulation* 1993; 87:116–127.

35. Twenty-sixth (26th) Bethesda Conference: Revised eligibility recommendations of competitive athletes with cardiovascular abnormalities. *J Am Coll Cardiol* 1994; 24:845–899.

36. Warth DC, King ME, Cohen JM, et al: Prevalence of mitral valve prolapse in normal children. *J Am Coll Cardiol* 1985; 5:1173–1177.

37. Greenwood RD: Mitral valve prolapse: incidence and clinical course in a pediatric population. *Clin Pediatr* 1984; 23:318–320.

38. Perloff JK, Child JS: Clinical and epidemiologic issue in mitral valve prolapse: overview and perspective. *Am Heart J* 1987; 113:1324–1332.

39. Savage DD, Devereux RB, Garrison RJ, et al: Mitral valve prolapse in the general population. 2. Clinical features: the Framingham Study. *Am Heart J* 1983; 106:577–581.

40. Bisset GS III, Schwartz DC, Meyer RA, et al: Clinical spectrum and long-term follow-up of isolated mitral valve prolapse in 119 children. *Circulation* 1980; 62:423–429.

41. Marks AR, Choong CY, Sanfilippo AJ, et al: Identification of high-risk and low-risk subgroups of patients with mitral valve prolapse. *N Engl J Med* 1989; 320:1031–1036.

42. Edwards JE, Topaz O: Pathologic features of sudden death in children, adolescents, and young adults. *Chest* 1985; 87:476–482.

43. Savage DD, Levy D, Garrison RJ, et al: Mitral valve prolapse in the general population. 3. Dysrhythmias: the Framingham Study. *Am Heart J* 1983; 106:582–586.

44. Silka MJ, Hardy BG, Menashe VD, Morris DC: A population-based prospective evaluation of risk of sudden cardiac death after operation for common congenital heart defects. *J Am Coll Cardiol* 1998; 32:245–251.

45. Enos WF, Holms RH, Beyer J: Coronary disease among United States soldiers killed in action in Korea: preliminary report. *JAMA* 1953; 152:1090–1093.

46. Report of the Expert Panel on Blood Cholesterol Levels in Children and Adolescents. *Pediatrics* 1992; 89:525–584.

47. Pathological Determinants of Atherosclerosis Research Group: Relationship of atherosclerosis in young men to serum lipoprotein cholesterol concentrations and smoking: a preliminary report from the Pathological Determinants of Atherosclerosis Research Group. *JAMA* 1990; 264:3018–3024.

48. Jacobson MS: Hyperlipidemia and atherosclerosis. In: Friedman SB (ed): *Comprehensive Adolescent Health Care,* 2nd ed. St. Louis, Mosby, 1998:242–246.

49. Castelli WP: The triglyceride issue: a view from Framingham. *Am Heart J* 1986; 112:432–437.

51. Cortner JA, Coates PM, Gallagher PR: Prevalence and expression of familial combined hyperlipidemia in childhood. *J Pediatr* 1990; 116:514–519.

52. Gidding SS: Preventive pediatric cardiology. Tobacco, cholesterol, obesity, and physical activity. *Pediatr Clin North Am* 1999; 46:253–262.

53. Sinaiko AR, Gomez-Marin O, Prineas RJ: Prevalence of "significant" hypertension in junior high school-age children: the Children and Adolescent Blood Pressure Program. *J Pediatr* 1989; 114:664–669.

54. National Heart, Lung, and Blood Institute's Task Force on Blood Pressure Control in Children. Report of the Task Force on Blood Pressure Control in Children—1977. *Pediatrics* 1977; 59(suppl):797–820.

55. Task Force on Blood Pressure Control in Children. Report of the Second Task Force on Blood Pressure Control in Children—1987. *Pediatrics* 1987; 79:1–25.

56. Rocchini AP, Katch V, Anderson J, et al: Blood pressure in obese adolescents: effect of weight loss. *Pediatrics* 1988; 82:16–23.

57. Rosner B, Prineas RJ, Loggie JMH, Daniels SR: Blood pressure nomograms for children and adolescents, by height, sex, and age, in the United States. *J Pediatr* 1993; 123:871–886.

58. Update on the Task Force (1987) on High Blood Pressure in Children and Adolescents: a working group from the National High Blood Pressure Education Program. *Pediatrics* 1996; 98:649–658.

59. Munger RG, Prineas RJ, Gomez-Marin O: Persistent elevation of blood pressure among children with a family history of hypertension: the Minneapolis Children's Blood Pressure Study. *Hypertension* 1988; 6:647–653.

60. Portman RJ, Yetman RJ, West MS: Efficacy of 24-hour ambulatory blood pressure monitoring in children. *J Pediatr* 1991; 118:842–849.

61. Ingelfinger JR: Endocrine causes of hypertension. In: Ingelfinger JR (ed): *Pediatric Hypertension*. Philadelphia, W. B. Saunders, 1982:185–203.

62. Ingelfinger JR: Iatrogenic, factitious, and accidental hypertension. In: Ingelfinger JR (ed): *Pediatric Hypertension*. Philadelphia, W. B. Saunders, 1982:125–135.

63. Holt JF: 1977 Edward B.D. Newhauser Lecture: neurofibromatosis in children. *Am J Roentgenol* 1978; 130:615–639.

64. Strader WJ III, Wachtel HL, Lundberg GD Jr: Hypertension and aortic rupture in gonadal dysgenesis. *J Pediatr* 1971; 79:473–475.

65. Daniels SR, Loggie JMH, Schwartz DC, et al: Systemic hypertension secondary to peripheral vascular anomalies in patients with Williams' syndrome. *J Pediatr* 1985; 249–251.

66. Hughes JG, Rosenblum H, Horn LG: Hypertension in embryoma (Wilm's tumor). *Pediatrics* 1949; 3:201–207.

67. Sinaiko AR: Hypertension in children. *N Engl J Med* 1996; 335:1968–1973.

68. Denfield SW, Garson A Jr: Sudden death in children and young adults. *Pediatr Clin North Am* 1990; 37:215–231.

69. Oglesby P, Schatz R: On sudden death. *Circulation* 1971; 43:7–10.

70. Epstein SE, Maron BJ: Sudden death and the competitive athlete: perspectives on preparticipation screening studies. *J Am Coll Cardiol* 1986; 7:220–230.

71. Maron BJ, Shirani J, Poliac LC, et al: Sudden death in young competitive athletes. Clinical, demographic, and pathological profiles. *JAMA* 1996; 276:199–204.

72. Glover DW, Maron BJ: Profile of preparticipation cardiovascular screening for high school athletes. *JAMA* 1998; 279:1817–1819.

73. Maron BJ, Thompson PD, Puffer JC, et al: Cardiovascular preparticipation screening competitive athletes: A statement for health professionals from the Sudden Death Committee (clinical cardiology) and the Congenital Cardiac Defects Committee (cardiovascular disease in the young), American Heart Association. *Circulation* 1996; 94: 850–856.

74. Maron BJ: Structural features of the athlete's heart as defined by echocardiography. *J Am Coll Cardiol* 1986; 7:190–203.

75. Pelliccia A, Maron BJ, Spataro A, et al: The upper limits of physiologic cardiac hypertrophy in highly trained elite athletes. *N Engl J Med* 1991; 324:295–301.

76. Perrault HM, Turcotte RA: Do athletes have "the athlete heart"? *Prog Pediatr Cardiol* 1993; 2:40–50.

77. Bjornstad H, Storstein L, Meen HD, Hals O: Ambulatory electrocardiographic findings in top athletes, athletic students and control subjects. *Cardiology* 1994; 84:42–50.

78. Rauch AM: Kawasaki syndrome: issues in etiology and treatment. *Adv Pediatr Infect Dis* 1989; 4:163–182.

79. Kawasaki T: Acute febrile mucocutaneous lymph node syndrome with lymphoid involvement with specific desquamation of the fingers and toes: clinical observations of 50 cases. *Jpn J Allergy* 1967; 161:178–222.

80. Burns JC, Wiggins JW, Toews WH, et al: Clinical spectrum of Kawasaki disease in infants younger than 6 months of age. *J Pediatr* 1986; 109:759–763.

81. Dajani AS, Taubert KA, Gerber MA, et al: Diagnosis and therapy of Kawasaki disease in children. *Circulation* 1993; 87:1776–1780.

82. Newburger JW, Takahashi M, Burns JC, et al: Treatment of Kawasaki syndrome with intravenous gamma globulin. *N Engl J Med* 1986; 315:341–347.

83. Kamiya T, Suzuki A, Kijimo Y, et al: Coronary arterial lesions in Kawasaki disease—occurrence and prognosis. *Recent Adv Cardiovasc Dis* 1982; III:19–27 (in Japanese).

84. Suzuki A, Yamagishi M, Kimura K, et al: Functional behavior and morphology of the coronary artery wall in patients with Kawasaki disease assessed by intravascular ultrasound. *J Am Coll Cardiol* 1996; 27:291–296.

85. Yamakawa R, Ishii M, Sugimura T: Coronary endothelial dysfunction after Kawasaki disease: evaluation by intracoronary injection of acetylcholine. *J Am Coll Cardiol* 1998; 31:1074–1080.

86. Suzuki A, Kamiya T, Tsuda E, Tsukano S: The natural history of coronary artery lesions in Kawasaki disease. *Prog Pediatr Cardiol* 1997; 6:211–218.

87. Sundel RP, Newburger JW: Management of acute Kawasaki disease. *Prog Pediatr Cardiol* 1997; 6:203–209.

88. Burns JC, Shike H, Gordon JB, et al: Sequelae of Kawasaki disease in adolescents and young adults. *J Am Coll Cardiol* 1996; 28:253–257.

89. Berkowitz FE: Infective endocarditis. In: Nichols DG, Cameron DE, Greeley WJ, et al (eds): *Critical Heart Disease in Infants and Children.* St. Louis, Mosby, 1995:961–986.

90. Parras F, Bouza E, Romero J, et al: Infectious endocarditis in children. *Pediatr Cardiol* 1990; 11:77–81.

91. Friedman RA, Stark JR: Infective endocarditis. In: Garson A Jr, Bricker JT, Fisher DJ, Neish SR (eds): *The Science and Practice of Pediatric Cardiology,* 2nd ed. Baltimore, Williams and Wilkins, 1998:1759–1775.

92. D'Alonzo GE, Barst RJ, Ayres SM, et al: Survival in patients with primary pulmonary hypertension: results from a national prospective registry. *Ann Intern Med* 1991; 115:343–349.

93. Rich S, Dantzker DR, Ayres SM, et al: Primary pulmonary hypertension: a national prospective study. *Ann Intern Med* 1987; 107:216–223.

94. Edwards WD, Edwards JE: Clinical primary pulmonary hypertension: three pathologic types. *Circulation* 1977; 56:884–888.

95. Fuster V, Steele PM, Edwards WD, et al: Primary pulmonary hypertension: natural history and the importance of thrombosis. *Circulation* 1984; 70:580–587.

96. Barst RJ, Rubin LJ, Long WA, et al: Comparison of continuous intravenous epoprostenol (prostacyclin) with conventional therapy for primary pulmonary hypertension. *N Engl J Med* 1996; 334:296–302.

97. Rich S, Kaufman E, Levy PS: The effects of high-doses of calcium-channel blockers on survival in primary pulmonary hypertension. *N Engl J Med* 1992; 327:76–81.

98. Channick RN, Newhart JW, Johnson FW, et al: Pulsed delivery of inhaled nitric oxide to patients with primary pulmonary hypertension. An ambulatory delivery system and initial clinical tests. *Chest* 1996; 109:1545–1549.

99. Hausknecht MJ, Sims RE, Nihill MR, Cashion WR: Successful palliation of primary pulmonary hypertension by atrial septostomy. *Am J Cardiol* 1990; 65:1045–1046.

100. Sweet SC, Spray TL, Huddleston CB, et al: Pediatric lung transplantation at St. Louis Children's Hospital, 1990–1995. *Am J Resp Crit Care Med* 1997; 155:1027–1035.

101. Pyeritz RE: The Marfan syndrome in childhood: features, natural history and differential diagnosis. *Prog Pediatr Cardiol* 1996; 5:151–157.

102. Murdoch JL, Walker RA, Halpern BL, et al: Life expectancy and causes of death in the Marfan syndrome. *N Engl J Med* 1972; 286:804–808.

103. El Habbal MH: Cardiovascular manifestations of Marfan's syndrome in the young. *Am Heart J* 1992; 123:752–757.

104. Shores J, Berger KR, Murphy EA, Pyeritz RE: Progression of aortic dilatation and the benefit of long-term beta-adrenergic blockade in Marfan's syndrome. *N Engl J Med* 1994; 330:1335–1341.

105. Salinas MA, Alpert BS: Medical management of young patients with the Marfan syndrome. *Prog Pediatr Cardiol* 1996; 5:167–174.

106. Pyeritz RE: Heritable disorders of connective tissue. In: Pierpont MEM, Moller JH (eds): *The Genetics of Cardiovascular Disease.* Boston, Martinus Nijloff, 1986:265–303.

107. Gott VL, Greene PS, Alejo D, et al: Replacement of the aortic root in patients with Marfan's syndrome. *N Engl J Med* 1999; 340:1307–1313.

108. Coupey SM: Anorexia nervosa. In: Friedman SB, Fisher M, Schonberg SK, Alderman EM (eds): *Comprehensive Adolescent Health Care,* 2nd ed. St. Louis, Mosby, 1998:247–262.

109. Nudel DB, Gootman N, Nussbaum MP, Shenker IR: Altered exercise performance and abnormal sympathetic responses to exercise in patients with anorexia nervosa. *J Pediatr* 1984; 105:34–37.

110. Moodie DS: Anorexia and the heart. Results of studies to assess effects. *Postgrad Med* 1987; 81:46–55.

111. Isner JM, Roberts WC, Heymsfield SB, Yager J: Anorexia nervosa and sudden death. *Ann Intern Med* 1985; 102:49–52.

112. Fish AJ, Blau EB, Westberg NG, et al: Systemic lupus erythematosus within the first two decades of life. *Am J Med* 1977; 62:99–117.

113. Chameides L, Truex RC, Vetter V, et al: Association of maternal systemic lupus erythematosus with congenital complete heart block. *N Engl J Med* 1977; 297:1204–1207.

114. Ohlendieck K, Matsumura K, Ionasecu VV, et al: Duchenne muscular dystrophy: deficiency of dystrophin-associated protein in the sarcolemma. *Neurology* 1993; 43:795–800.

115. Sanyal SK, Johnson WW, Thapar MK, Pitner SE: An ultrasound basis for electrocardiographic alterations associated with Duchenne's progressive muscular dystrophy. *Circulation* 1978; 57:1122–1129.

116. Hunsaker RH, Fulkerson PK, Barry FJ, et al: Cardiac function in Duchenne muscular dystrophy. *Am J Med* 1982; 73:235–238.

117. Pierpont MEA, Moller JH: Cardiac manifestations of genetic disease. In: Emmanouilides GC, Allen HD, Riemenschneider TA, Gutgesell HP (eds): *Heart Disease in Infants, Children, and Adolescents,* 5th ed. Baltimore, Williams and Wilkins, 1995: 1486–1520.

118. Perloff JK: Cardiac rhythm and conduction in Duchenne's muscular dystrophy: a prospective study of 20 patients. *J Am Coll Cardiol* 1984; 3:1263–1268.

119. Heiman-Patterson TD, Natter HM, Rosenberg HR, et al: Malignant hyperthermia susceptibility in X-linked muscular dystrophies. *Pediatr Neurol* 1986; 2:235–258.

120. Seay AR, Ziter FA, Thompson JA: Cardiac arrest during induction of anesthesia in Duchenne muscular dystrophy. *J Pediatr* 1978; 93:88–90.

121. Chamberlain S, Shaw J, Rowland A, et al: Mapping of mutation causing Friedreich's ataxia to human chromosome 9. *Nature* 1988; 334:248–250.
122. Child JS, Perloff JK, Bach PM, et al: Cardiac involvement in Friedreich's ataxia: a clinical study of 75 patients. *J Am Coll Cardiol* 1986; 7:1370–1378.
123. Suthers GK, Huson SM, Davies KE: Instability versus predictability: the molecular diagnosis of myotonic dystrophy. *J Med Genet* 1992; 29:761–765.

MICHAEL A. BALK / CLYDE WATKINS

**CHAPTER**

# HEART DISEASE IN PREGNANCY

**47**

Normal pregnancy is accompanied by many hemodynamic and physiologic cardio-vascular changes. Generally, healthy women tolerate these without difficulty. The diseased heart, however, when unable to cope with these stressors, can fail, leading to increased maternal and fetal morbidity and mortality. Cardiovascular and hyper-tensive diseases are listed as common causes of maternal mortality in the United States.[1] Therefore, the primary clinician needs to be aware of common situations in which pregancy can be complicated by cardiac dysfunction or hypertension, or in which preexisting cardiac disease can lead to peripartum complications.

There are two general categories of heart disease in pregnant women. The physi-ologic changes of pregnancy impose a significant increase in the work of the heart, and the heart may fail if the stress exceeds the reserve capacity. Because more women with fully or partially corrected congenital heart defects are surviving into adulthood, primary care physicians and obstetricians are likely to see more preg-nant women with cardiac disease in the future. Diseases such as valvular or con-genital heart disease, hypertrophic cardiomyopathy, coronary disease, and hyper-tensive heart disease will be discussed in detail. The second group of patients are those who develop cardiac disease during pregnancy, but in whom there is no pre-existing cardiovascular disorder; preeclampsia, eclampsia, and peripartum car-diomyopathy are prototypical examples.

## NORMAL PHYSIOLOGY OF PREGNANCY

One must understand the anatomic, functional, and hemodynamic characteristics of normal pregnancy before attempting to understand the consequences of congenital or acquired heart disease.

The cardiac output rises early in pregnancy, and continues to rise until around 30 weeks' gestation; it then remains near this increased level until term. The heart rate increases slightly, with the peak change occurring near term. The increased heart rate and increased stroke volume lead to an increase in cardiac output of up to 30 to 50 percent over the pregravid level. The systemic vascular resistance falls during pregnancy, partially because the placenta acts like a large arteriovenous fistula. Characteristic blood pressure changes include a slight fall near the end of the first trimester; since the diastolic pressure falls more than the systolic, the pulse pressure rises, and this rise is maximal at midterm. The blood pressure returns toward normal by the third trimester. During the first 20 to 30 weeks of gestation, the blood volume increases rapidly, but the percentage increase (20 to 100 percent) varies considerably in different people.

Maternal posture becomes an important determinant of cardiac output as pregnancy advances. The supine position leads to uterine compression of the inferior vena cava and decreased venous return to the heart, so that at term, a change from the supine to the lateral position can increase the cardiac output.[2] Symptoms such as nausea, light-headedness, and faintness can often be relieved by rolling into the lateral position. This vena cava syndrome can also be relieved by pressure on the lateral abdominal wall, displacing the uterus to one side of the inferior vena cava.

Labor and delivery impose an added hemodynamic burden on the cardiovascular system. Women suffering from serious heart disease most often die of heart failure during parturition and the early puerperium. Most of the hemodynamic changes of pregnancy normalize within 2 weeks following delivery. Table 47-1 details some of the typical cardiovascular changes of pregnancy and parturition.

**TABLE 47-1.   Summary of Hemodynamic Changes Associated with Pregnancy and Parturition**

| Parameter | Pregnancy and Parturition |
| --- | --- |
| Heart rate | Slight increase between 10 and 30 weeks. Increases 50% with uterine contractions. Later, falls to bradycardia secondary to increased venous return. |
| Stroke volume | Increases. |
| Cardiac output | Increases 30% at 28–30 weeks. Remains elevated through delivery. |
| Blood volume | Increases by 40% at 30 weeks. Begins to fall to normal by 6 weeks postpartum. |
| Oxygen consumption | Increases 10–20%. |
| Systolic blood pressure | Generally falls after first trimester. Rises 10% with each uterine contraction. |
| Diastolic blood pressure | Falls to a greater degree than systolic blood pressure. |
| Systemic vascular resistance | Decreases. |
| Venous blood pressure in upper extremities | No significant change. |
| Venous blood pressure in lower extremities | Marked increase between 8 and 40 weeks. |
| Glomerular filtration rate | Increases 30–50% by 24 weeks. |

## PHYSICAL EXAMINATION

The high-output state of pregnancy resembles that of an arteriovenous fistula: The patient has warm skin, dilated arteries, and a hyperdynamic (but not sustained) apical impulse. The cardiac silhouette actually changes position and increases in size. The heart is rotated slightly anteriorly and displaced upward and to the left.[3]

More than 50 percent of pregnant women will have a soft systolic murmur over the base and precordium. The increased blood volume and hyperdynamic cardiac contractility can cause systolic ejection murmurs, and a physiologic third heart sound ($S_3$) can be heard in about 85 percent of patients. The first heart sound may increase in intensity as the heart rate and left ventricular contractility rise and may be widely split. The second heart sound does not change appreciably. A venous hum is often present during pregnancy and in late gestation. This results from the rapid downward flow of blood in the jugular veins and is best heard in the supraclavicular fossa. A systolic or continuous mammary souffle can be heard over the breasts; it is best heard in the supine position during the postpartum period and may disappear when the patient assumes the upright position.

The venous blood pressure in the upper chest and arms does not change; therefore, elevated venous pressure in the upper body on examination is suggestive of cardiac overload. Brisk $x$ and $y$ descents in the jugular tracing become evident after the 20th week. Because of the inferior vena caval compression, the lower-extremity pressure rises significantly, often leading to edema. The dependent edema of pregnancy, present in 80 percent of healthy pregnant women, requires no therapy. Basal rales that clear with coughing should not be misconstrued as congestive failure.

## SYMPTOMS OF PREGNANCY

The increased blood volume, sodium retention, and diaphragmatic elevation from a large uterus can produce orthopnea and paroxysmal nocturnal dyspnea. Ventricular and atrial extrasystoles, which are common, can lead to increased awareness of palpitations. Easy fatigability and exertional intolerance can be normal physiologic consequences of pregnancy and must be differentiated from cardiac disease.

## HYPERTENSION

Hypertension complicating pregnancy occurs infrequently but carries an increased risk of perinatal morbidity and mortality. There are four general categories of hypertensive disorders of pregnancy recognized by the American College of Obstetricians and Gynecologists:

1.   Chronic (essential) hypertension
2.   Preeclampsia–eclampsia
3.   Preeclampsia superimposed on chronic hypertension
4.   Transient hypertension

Essential hypertension (repeated blood pressures over 140 mm/90 mm), by definition, precedes pregnancy or is observed by 20 weeks' gestation, whereas preeclampsia occurs in previously normotensive women who develop a rise in blood pressure in the last trimester. A woman with essential hypertension can also develop preeclampsia if substantially increased blood pressure with proteinuria and edema develops in the last trimester.

Patients with mild hypertension without electrocardiographic, ocular, or vascular complications can be monitored and treated with rest and sodium restriction, but patients with persistently elevated diastolic blood pressure (over 100 mmHg) should receive antihypertensive therapy, even though there is little convincing evidence that this improves perinatal outcome. In addition to salt restriction, patients may be given hydralazine or methyldopa. Beta blockers have been used extensively and are discussed in detail in the section on arrhythmias. Angiotensin-converting enzyme (ACE) inhibitors are contraindicated, especially in the second and third trimesters; exposure has been associated with several fetal renal disorders, including renal insufficiency and renal tubular dysgenesis. First-trimester exposure to ACE inhibitors, however, does not appear to be teratogenic. The use of diuretics as the sole therapy for hypertension should be discouraged because they prevent adequate expansion of intravascular volume.[4]

The major obstetrical complication of chronic hypertension is the increased risk for perinatal mortality. Much of the increased risk is due to an increased incidence of intrauterine growth retardation, abruptio placenta, and prematurity. Preeclampsia develops in 10 to 20 percent of women with essential hypertension and is more common in patients with renal disease.

Preeclampsia (Table 47-2) is manifested by hypertension, edema, and proteinuria developing after 20 weeks' gestation. It occurs in about 5 percent of pregnancies. Symptoms include headache, visual disturbances, dyspnea, and right upper quadrant or epigastric pain. The pathophysiology is unknown, but the syndrome is more common in the first pregnancy, in multiple gestations, in patients with a history of preeclampsia, in obese patients, and in patients with renovascular disease and chronic hypertension.

### TABLE 47-2.   Diagnosis of Preeclampsia[*]

| |
|---|
| 1.   A rather abrupt increase in blood pressure of 30 mmHg or more systolic and 15 mmHg or more diastolic after the 20th week of pregnancy. Some authors use systolic >140 mmHg or diastolic >90 mmHg on 2 separate occasions. |
| 2.   The appearance of proteinuria of at least 300 mg/day. |
| 3.   Edema in the upper half of the body. |

[*] Requires at least two of three cardinal manifestations.

Deaths from preeclampsia are rare. In mild cases remote from term, decreased activity and salt restriction may be the sole therapy needed. This expectant management allows the fetus to mature and increases the likelihood that a successful vaginal delivery will occur. Severe preeclampsia occurs when there is marked proteinuria ($>5$ g/day), persistent elevation in blood pressure (in excess of 160 mmHg systolic or 110 mmHg diastolic), pulmonary edema, retinal hemorrhages, thrombocytopenia, oliguria, or renal failure.[5] The development of any of these complications, with the exception of dense proteinuria, is generally an indication for prompt delivery. In severe preeclampsia, the infant mortality rate is five times the normal rate.

Intravenous hydralazine 5 to 10 mg every 20 to 30 min should be administered to control hypertension. Nitroprusside is contraindicated, since it crosses the placenta and can result in fetal death. Thiazides should not be used because patients with preeclampsia have an already diminished plasma volume. Intravenous magnesium may be used to prevent convulsions during labor and postpartum when preeclampsia has been diagnosed. Once convulsions occur, the maternal mortality rate rises to 5 percent, and the fetal mortality rate rises to 20 to 25 percent. The most reliable method to prevent eclampsia is to interrupt the pregnancy once severe preeclampsia develops.

Primiparous women with eclampsia do not have an increased incidence of permanent hypertension, but multiparous women who survive eclampsia seem to have an increased incidence of cardiovascular deaths.[6] Women who have had severe preeclampsia or eclampsia are at increased risk of hypertensive disorders with subsequent pregnancies.

There is evidence that low-dose aspirin (80 mg), when started before the signs of preeclampsia, may provide prophylaxis against preeclampsia. Patients at low risk of developing preeclampsia do not seem to derive any benefit; therefore, the use of low-dose aspirin is generally limited to patients with a history of severe preeclampsia and those with a history of intrauterine growth restriction caused by uteroplacental insufficiency.[7]

Transient hypertension, or gestational hypertension, first appears late in pregnancy or during the first postpartal day in a patient without evidence of preeclampsia or chronic hypertension. These patients tend to be older and obese and may have diabetes or a family history of hypertension. Transient hypertension is not associated with fetal complications or intrauterine growth restriction, but the patients appear to be at increased risk of developing hypertension in the future.

# CONGENITAL HEART DISEASE

Untreated congenital heart disease accounts for a relatively small percentage of all cases of heart disease in pregnancy, primarily because it is now recognized and treated at a much earlier age. There are several cardiac lesions that place the pregnant woman at high risk of cardiovascular complications or death. Pregnant women with high-risk cardiac lesions often have a carefully timed induction and delivery at or near full term with adequate hemodynamic monitoring and anesthesia to decrease the maternal risk of parturition. There is an increased risk of congenital heart defects in babies born to women with congenital heart disease. Parents should receive genetic counseling prior to planning future pregnancy, and a pregnant woman should receive fetal echocardiography at 20 weeks.

Mothers with cyanotic heart disease have an increased risk of spontaneous abortion and low-birth-weight children. There is an increased incidence of prematurity and miscarriage in patients with higher hematocrits; this reflects the severity of the underlying cyanotic heart disease. Surgical correction of maternal cyanotic congenital heart disease prior to pregnancy lowers the risk of fetal congenital heart defects, suggesting that hypoxia is, at least in part, a causative factor.

Ostium secundum atrial septal defect (ASD) is a common malformation; it is more common in females and frequently does not cause symptoms until later in life. Although these patients generally tolerate the increased cardiac output and blood volume of pregnancy, there is a possibility of paradoxical embolization. The hypercoagulable state of pregnancy and decreased vena caval flow may increase the risk of venous thrombosis. Pelvic and lower-extremity emboli that travel across the septal defect into the systemic circulation can cause stroke and arterial emboli.[8]

A small or moderate-sized patent ductus arteriosus poses little risk to the pregnant woman, aside from the increased risk of infective endocarditis, because the gestational fall in systemic resistance actually decreases flow across the defect. If pulmonary hypertension is present, however, the fall in maternal systemic resistance will increase the right-to-left shunt and lead to hypoxia and fetal problems.

Coarctation of the aorta is less common in women than in men, but because of the associated connective tissue disorder and hemodynamic stress of pregnancy, there is an increased risk of aortic rupture and dissection. Women with this disorder who develop acute chest pain suggestive of aortic disease should be referred for evaluation immediately. Diagnostic testing with a transesophageal echocardiogram is preferred over computed tomography scanning because of the excellent accuracy and lack of exposure to radiation.

Patients with New York Heart Association (NYHA) class I or II symptoms and ventricular septal defects that are small to moderate-sized and restrict left-to-right shunting tolerate pregnancy with little problem. Nonrestrictive ventricular septal defects that lead to Eisenmenger's complex are associated with significant maternal mortality.

In fact, any congenital defect that results in Eisenmenger's complex results in a cumulative maternal risk estimated at 30 to 70 percent. The fixed and increased pulmonary resistance prevents any adaptive responses in cardiac output, and changes during delivery and puerperium are poorly tolerated.

Pregnant women with uncorrected tetralogy of Fallot can develop increased right-to-left shunting and decreased systemic oxygen saturation, and these changes are harmful to the developing fetus. During delivery, the hemodynamic changes in systemic resistance and venous return and the process of bearing down can be poorly tolerated. The absence of pregravid symptoms of this condition does not ensure an uncomplicated pregnancy.[9] Pregnancy after successful repair of this condition at a young age is generally tolerated with only a slightly increased risk.

**TABLE 47-3.** Cardiac Diseases Associated with Increased Maternal Mortality, in Decreasing Order of Risk[*]

| |
|---|
| Primary pulmonary hypertension |
| Marfan syndrome with aortic root dilatation |
| Secondary pulmonary hypertension (Eisenmenger's syndrome) |
| Peripartum cardiomyopathy |
| Coarctation of aorta, complicated |
| Significant mitral stenosis with atrial fibrillation |
| Corrected tetralogy of Fallot |
| Mild to moderate mitral stenosis |
| Prosthetic heart valves |

[*] Accurate numbers are not available for all cardiac diseases, so the list is incomplete.

Ebstein's anomaly of the tricuspid valve is an uncommon congenital defect in which a poorly developed right ventricle and a displaced and functionally abnormal tricuspid valve cannot handle the gestational increases in blood volume and cardiac output. Significant right-to-left shunting worsens systemic oxygen levels and carries a high risk of paradoxical emboli. Poorly tolerated atrial arrhythmias and conduction over accessory bypass tracts further complicate pregnancy.

Surgical correction of most congenital defects prior to pregnancy significantly lowers maternal and fetal risk, although there is an increased risk of infective endocarditis and arrhythmias in many conditions. Significant pulmonary hypertension of any etiology raises the maternal mortality to around 50 percent; it is the authors' opinion that pregnancy is contraindicated in this condition. Table 47-3 lists cardiac diseases associated with increased maternal mortality, in decreasing order of risk.

In summary, patients with congenital heart disease and poor functional reserve, significant pulmonary hypertension (Eisenmenger's complex), or significant risk of right-to-left shunting are at increased risk of cardiac complications of pregnancy.

# PRIMARY PULMONARY HYPERTENSION

This condition permits survival into the reproductive age; therefore, the primary care physician is likely to encounter a patient with PPH who is pregnant or wishes to become pregnant. Primary pulmonary hypertension is five times more common in women than in men. The high, fixed pulmonary vascular resistance prevents the normal hemodynamic changes required for pregnancy and places the mother at very high risk. Because roughly 50 percent of these patients do not survive pregnancy, they should be counseled on pregnancy prevention and should have a thera-peutic abortion if pregnancy occurs.

# HYPERTROPHIC CARDIOMYOPATHY

The prognosis of patients with hypertrophic cardiomyopathy is generally good. In one large study, no fetal or maternal deaths occurred.[10] Strong cardiac contractions during labor and blood loss can lead to increased dynamic left ventricular obstruc-tion, chest pain, and dyspnea, but since the diagnosis is usually recognized prior to delivery, careful attention to volume status, preload, and body position can limit the potential for complications. Esmolol, a short-acting intravenous beta blocker, has been used effectively to treat this hemodynamic deterioration.[11] Most patients will have some deterioration in symptoms during pregnancy, and sudden death has been reported.[12] Digitalis should be avoided because it increases cardiac contractility and can worsen the underlying dynamic obstruction. Patients should be advised to main-tain the left lateral position during labor to improve venous return. The use of di-uretics is controversial, because thiazides may decrease uterine and plasma blood flow. Generally, dietary restriction of salt to prevent weight gain and edema is pre-ferred.

# VALVULAR HEART DISEASE

The most severe valvular heart diseases in pregnancy are severe mitral and aortic stenoses. Pregnant women with mitral stenosis and NYHA class I/II symptoms have a low risk of maternal mortality. The presence of class III or IV symptoms in the fi-nal trimester in a patient with severe mitral stenosis is very concerning. The cardiac output in patients with severe mitral stenosis becomes fixed. As the circulating vol-ume increases during pregnancy, the left atrial pressure rises, and pulmonary edema can develop. The autotransfusion following delivery further increases the pul-monary venous congestion.

Becker reported on 101 pregnant patients, in whom closed mitral commissurot-omy resulted in no maternal deaths and the loss of only three fetuses.[13] Balloon mi-tral valvuloplasty carries with it a significant radiation exposure and the potential for marked, sudden hemodynamic changes, especially if acute, severe mitral regur-gitation complicates the procedure, but it has been used to treat hemodynamically significant mitral stenosis during pregnancy.

Significant aortic stenosis in young women is rare and typically results from a bi-cuspid valve.[14] Symptoms of angina, congestive failure, and syncope typically do not develop until late in the disease, but once symptoms develop, the risk of sudden death increases. During delivery, preload must be maintained because the cardiac output in a patient with significant aortic stenosis is essentially fixed, and even mi-nor drops in preload can lead to significantly reduced stroke volume, hypotension, and poor peripheral and uterine perfusion. Similarly, because left ventricular compliance is decreased, slight increases in volume can precipitate pulmonary edema. The primary goal during delivery is to maintain fluid balance within that narrow therapeutic window. Mild and moderate aortic stenosis, in the absence of symptoms, is usually well tolerated.

Pregnant women whose examinations suggest significant aortic stenosis (harsh murmurs, delayed carotid upstroke, soft aortic closure sound) should be referred for cardiac Doppler echocardiography. This is an accurate, noninvasive method to assess the aortic valve without maternal or fetal risk. Furthermore, since there is an increased risk of fetal congenital aortic stenosis, fetal echocardiography may be useful. Patients with NYHA class III or IV symptoms and severe mitral or aortic stenosis have a 5 to 15 percent maternal mortality.[15]

In cases of severe mitral or aortic stenosis, it is preferable to replace the valve prior to pregnancy. The use of a bioprosthetic valve obviates the need for oral anticoagulation during pregnancy but carries a significant risk of requiring reoperation in 5 to 15 years because of degeneration of the bioprosthetic valve.

Patients with previously placed mechanical valves generally tolerate pregnancy from a hemodynamic standpoint, assuming a good functional activity level and the absence of pulmonary hypertension. Since warfarin is associated with an increased risk of spontaneous abortion, stillborn fetuses, congenital abnormalities, and maternal hemorrhage, however, attempting to convert the patient to subcutaneous heparin is recommended. Nonetheless, the incidence of warfarin embryopathy is 5 percent or less, and the risk is highest during the first trimester. Although heparin does not cross the placental barrier, its use seems to be associated with an increased risk of fetal cardiac disorders and fetal loss through placental hemorrhage; this may be partially explained by the increased genetic risk to the offspring of mothers with congenital heart disease. Long-term heparin use may be associated with osteoporosis and heparin-induced thrombocytopenia; platelet levels should be monitored.

The fetal dangers of warfarin decrease during midpregnancy, and some authors recommend using heparin during the first trimester, then switching to warfarin until near term, when subcutaneous heparin is reinstituted. Guidelines published in 1995 by the Study Group of the Working Group on Valvular Heart Disease of the European Society of Cardiology recommend that the decision between continuing warfarin throughout the pregnancy and using heparin for the first trimester and switching back to warfarin thereafter be made after full discussion with the patient and her partner.[16] Antiplatelet agents alone are not effective in preventing thromboembolism of mechanical valves.

Mitral regurgitation is generally well tolerated during pregnancy. As long as there is no significant history of severe congestive failure or left ventricular dysfunction, the decreased systemic resistance allows the heart to accommodate the increased blood volume and stresses of pregnancy.

Aortic regurgitation, like mitral regurgitation, is well tolerated, and other than infective endocarditis prophylaxis, no specific intervention is usually necessary. Isolated pulmonic stenosis, if not severe, is also well tolerated, but if pulmonic stenosis is combined with other congenital defects and pulmonary hypertension, the risk rises significantly. In cases of severe pulmonic stenosis with symptoms, balloon valvuloplasty prior to pregnancy is recommended.

Although use of the cardiopulmonary bypass machine during pregnancy is associated with a low maternal mortality rate, the fetal mortality rate approaches 20 percent. Cardiac operation is not recommended during the first two trimesters, except in extreme situations. During the last trimester, one option is to deliver the baby by cesarean section at the same operation, immediately before the cardiac operation.[17]

## MITRAL VALVE PROLAPSE

This common valvular abnormality requires no special treatment or care during pregnancy. The typical mid- to late systolic click may decrease or disappear as pregnancy proceeds because the left ventricular volume increases. Many obstetricians administer antibiotic prophylaxis during procedures likely to provoke bacteremia. Significant bacteremia during normal labor and delivery is not common, and in the absence of a significantly deformed valve or significant mitral murmur, infective endocarditis is unlikely.

## MYOCARDIAL INFARCTION

In the absence of diabetes mellitus, myocardial infarction from coronary artery disease in women of childbearing age is rare. Although it has a high mortality rate, the incidence is less than 1 per 10,000 deliveries. Most cases have underlying risk factors, such as hypertension, cigarette smoking, hypercholesterolemia, or diabetes. At autopsy, underlying coronary atherosclerosis is often found.[18–20] There are reported cases of myocardial infarction during pregnancy and the puerperium among women without identifiable risk in whom subsequent coronary angiography revealed no atherosclerosis. The most likely mechanism for this is coronary spasm, and a trial with calcium channel antagonists and nitrates is recommended if coronary spasm is suspected. A diligent search for other treatable causes of myocardial infarction, such as coronary anomalies, coronary embolus from mitral valve prolapse, spontaneous coronary artery dissection,[21] paradoxical embolism through a patent foramen ovale, hypercoagulable states, cocaine abuse, and hyperhomocysteinemia, is recommended.

## PERIPARTUM CARDIOMYOPATHY

Peripartum cardiomyopathy is an idiopathic condition affecting previously healthy women during the last month of pregnancy or the first 6 months after delivery for which no other cause is found. The reported incidence is between 1 in 3000 and 1 in 8000, but a careful search for other potential causes may lower the true incidence to

1 in 15,000.[22–24] The exact etiology remains unclear, but it appears that there is an increased prevalence among women with twin gestations, with poor nutrition, from lower socioeconomic groups, with preeclampsia and eclampsia, and in tropical climates. Some cases are associated with an inflammatory response, raising the possibility of a viral etiology. Other authors have postulated a genetic predisposition or an immunologic origin, but it is likely that there are multiple etiologic factors and that a specific postpartal cardiac factor may never be found.

Presenting symptoms can include dyspnea on exertion, weakness, orthopnea, cough, palpitations, and chest pain. Since many of these are present in the healthy pregnant woman, the clinician must carefully examine the patient for clues that peripartum cardiomyopathy is present. Table 47-4 details some of the clinical findings present in peripartum cardiomyopathy.

The pathophysiologic features and clinical presentations (aside from its temporal association with pregnancy) in peripartum cardiomyopathy and other congestive cardiomyopathies are similar. Hypertension is often present at presentation, even if there is no preceding history of it. The patient usually develops biventricular failure;

**TABLE 47-4.   Clinical Features of Peripartum Cardiomyopathy**

### Physical Examination

Ventricular enlargement (left and right)
Jugular venous distention with regurgitant waves
Summation gallop
Apical murmurs of mitral regurgitation
Rales
Edema
Pulsus alternans

### ECG

Sinus tachycardia
Premature ventricular or atrial contractions
Left ventricular hypertrophy
ST- and T-wave abnormalities
Intraventricular conduction defects
Low-voltage QRS

### Radiographic

Biventricular enlargement
Pulmonary venous congestion
Pleural effusion

### Echocardiographic

Decreased left ventricular contractility
Enlarged right ventricle and left ventricle
Pericardial effusion
Biatrial enlargement

at autopsy, four-chamber dilatation with structurally normal valves and coronaries are found. Thromboembolic complications are common, and patients should be anticoagulated, as autopsy also commonly reveals mural thrombi. Arrhythmias such as atrial fibrillation occur, but they are less common than in other types of cardiomyopathy.

Therapy with digitalis, diuretics, bed rest, and afterload-reducing agents such as angiotensin-converting enzyme inhibitors (assuming delivery has already occurred) should be started as soon as possible. Some patients with cardiomyopathy are very sensitive to digitalis preparations, so serum levels should be followed. Patients should avoid excess sodium intake. In a pregnant woman without severe symptoms, a combination of bed rest, digitalis, restricted sodium intake, and adequate control of blood pressure usually suffices. Because patients who develop congestive failure during pregnancy have an increased fetal mortality rate, careful and continued examination of the fetus is indicated. Prolonged use of thiazide diuretics in late pregnancy should be avoided because of sporadic reports of severe electrolyte imbalance, neonatal jaundice, thrombocytopenia, or liver damage. On occasion, dobutamine, nitroprusside, and intraaortic balloon counterpulsation are necessary. In cases of severe pump failure and cardiogenic shock, prompt consultation and referral to a heart transplant center may be life-saving. Successful pregnancy and vaginal delivery after heart transplantation has been reported.[25]

Roughly 50 percent of patients will improve, with resolution or near resolution of the cardiac enlargement and symptoms. These patients have a favorable prognosis. Patients with continued cardiomegaly and gallop rhythms have a high risk of pulmonary emboli and death from pump failure. The survival history in peripartum cardiomyopathy correlates directly with ejection fraction and inversely with diastolic dimension. Although it appears that patients who recover fully from peripartum cardiomyopathy are still at increased risk with future pregnancies, the risk is highest in those who do not recover.[26] Therefore, future pregnancy is absolutely contraindicated in patients with persistent cardiomegaly, but it is only relatively contraindicated in those whose heart size and function have returned to normal.

## ARRHYTHMIAS

As the number of women of childbearing age who have had corrective cardiac surgery increases, the incidence of cardiac arrhythmias during pregnancy has also increased. Fortunately, most rhythm disturbances in patients with preserved cardiac function are well tolerated and do not cause severe hemodynamic consequences. The most common arrhythmias are premature atrial contractions, ectopic atrial tachycardias, and sustained paroxysmal supraventricular tachycardia. Atrial fibrillation can occur, but typically in the setting of structural heart disease; it is uncommon in otherwise healthy pregnant women without underlying heart disease. Patients with left ventricular dysfunction or congenital heart disease (even if the congenital heart disease is surgically corrected) and significant ectopy or ventricular tachycardia should be referred for consultation with a cardiologist.

Frequently, vagal maneuvers, rest, and recumbency are sufficient to control supraventricular arrhythmias. Chronic medical therapy for intermittent paroxysmal supraventricular tachycardia is usually unnecessary, but digitalis therapy is the drug of choice in the absence of preexcitation (delta wave). Oral and intravenous verapamil have been used to terminate and control paroxysmal ventricular tachycardia, and for rate control in chronic atrial fibrillation, but rapid injections can lead to maternal hypotension and fetal distress. Adenosine, administered maternally, does not appear to cause fetal bradycardia. Therefore, intravenous adenosine is preferred for the emergent conversion of paroxysmal ventricular tachycardia.[27] Other options for termination of supraventricular arrhythmias include esophageal pacing, direct-current countershock therapy, and antiarrhythmic drug therapy. Electrical cardioversion can be used for sustained atrial and ventricular arrhythmias without significant complication; however, transient fetal dysrhythmia has been reported, and fetal monitoring is recommended.

Antiarrhythmic therapy is occasionally necessary to control frequent, symptomatic arrhythmias. Therapeutic blood levels may be more difficult to achieve because of multiple interaction. First, the increased intravascular volume can increase the amount of drug needed to reach therapeutic serum concentrations. Decreased plasma protein concentration may further reduce drug-protein binding, leading to a decreased concentration. Further, the increased cardiac output and glomerular filtration rate can increase the excretion of renally metabolized drugs.

Quinidine has been used successfully for years without harmful fetal effects. For patients with atrial fibrillation, this drug may be used for maintenance therapy. For acute conversion to sinus rhythm, intravenous procainamide and electrical cardioversion have been used successfully without apparent harm to the fetus. Disopyramide, another class I antiarrhythmic, should be avoided because it has been reported to stimulate hypertonic uterine contractions. There is limited experience with flecainide and propafenone, although they appear to be relatively safe.[28]

Beta blockers have been used extensively and are generally safe. Chronic propranolol therapy should be used with caution because it is associated with intrauterine growth retardation and can both initiate premature labor by increasing uterine tone and cause neonatal bradycardia and respiratory depression. Intravenous beta blockers can be used safely to terminate certain atrial tachyarrhythmias in the emergency department. If long-term therapy is needed, one should use a cardioselective agent such as metoprolol or atenolol because these agents have less effects on uterine relaxation and $B_2$-mediated peripheral vasodilatation.

Digitalis does not appear to be teratogenic in animals or humans and does not have any detrimental fetal side effects. It has been used safely for decades, even though it is labeled as a pregnancy risk category C by the FDA. In women with heart disease, however, it may influence the time of onset and duration of labor. Spontaneous labor occurs about a week earlier and lasts about half as long in cardiac patients on digitalis compared with a control group of cardiac patients who were not taking digitalis. Nonetheless, when therapeutically indicated during pregnancy, digitalis may be used safely.

Phenytoin carries a high risk of malformations (fetal hydantoin syndrome) and should be avoided. Amiodarone can cause fetal hypothyroidism, bradycardia, and hypotonia, and should be reserved for cases of life-threatening ventricular arrhythmias when other drugs fail.

Ventricular ectopic beats are more common in pregnancy. The altered physiologic hemodynamics often lead to an increased awareness and decreased tolerance of these extra beats. In the absence of underlying structural heart disease, no therapy is indicated. Ventricular tachycardia arising from the right ventricle is the most common sustained ventricular arrhythmia occurring in pregnant women. This has a typical electrocardiographic pattern of left bundle branch block morphology and an inferior axis because it arises from the right ventricular outflow tract. Lidocaine is safe for the acute termination of ventricular arrhythmias; if this does not work, intravenous procainamide may be used, as this will treat aberrantly conducted supraventricular tachycardias as well.

## CONCLUSION

Patients with acquired or congenital cardiac disease who have minimal symptoms and a high functional class are unlikely to suffer problems during most pregnancies. Patients in whom previous pregnancy led to heart failure have an increased risk of cardiac failure in subsequent pregnancies.

As with many diseases, the sicker, more symptomatic woman is more likely to suffer an adverse cardiac consequence of pregnancy. Patients with severe mitral or aortic stenosis, severe coarctation of the aorta, primary pulmonary hypertension, Eisenmenger's syndrome, or cyanotic congenital heart disease are at highest maternal and fetal risk.

### REFERENCES

1. Rochat RW, Koonin LA, Atrash HK, et al: Maternal mortality in the United States: Report from the maternal mortality collaborative. *Obstet Gynecol* 1988; 72:91–97.
2. McAnulty JH, Metcalfe J, Ueland K: Heart disease and pregnancy. In: Alexander RW, Schlant RC, Fuster V, et al (eds): *Hurst's The Heart*, 9th ed. New York. McGraw-Hill, 1998:2389–2406.
3. Laros RK Jr: Physiology of normal pregnancy. In: Willson JR, Carrington ER, Ledger WJ, et al (eds): *Obstetrics and Gynecology*, 8th ed. St. Louis, Mosby, 1987:260–261.
4. Lowe SA, Rubin PC: The pharmacological management of hypertension in pregnancy. *J Hypertens* 1992; 94:323–330.
5. Greene MF: Hypertension in pregnancy. In: Carlson KJ, Eisenstat SA (eds): *Primary Care of Women*. St. Louis, Mosby–Year Book, 1995:354–359.
6. Chesley LC, Annitto JE, Cosgrove RA: The remote prognosis of eclamptic women. *Am J Obstet Gynecol* 1976; 124:446–459.
7. CLASP: A randomised trial of low-dose aspirin for the prevention and treatment of preeclampsia among 9364 pregnant women. *Lancet* 1994; 343:616–629.

8. Perloff JK: Congenital heart disease and pregnancy. *Clin Cardiol* 1994; 17:579–587.

9. Perloff JK: Pregnancy in congenital heart disease. In: Perloff JK, Child JS (eds): *Congenital Heart Disease in Adults*. Philadelphia, W. B. Saunders Company, 1991:129.

10. Oakley GDG, McGarry K, Limb DG, Oakley CM: Management of pregnancy in patients with hypertrophic cardiomyopathy. *Br Med J* 1979; 1:1749–1750.

11. Fairley CJ, Clarke JT: Use of esmolol in a parturient with hypertrophic obstructive cardiomyopathy. *Br J Anaesth* 1995; 75:801–804.

12. Pelliccia F, Cianfrocca C, Gaudio C, Reale A: Sudden death during pregnancy in hypertrophic cardiomyopathy. *Eur Heart J* 1992; 13:421–423.

13. Becker RM: Intracardiac surgery in pregnant women. *Ann Thorac Surg* 1983; 36:453–458.

14. Easterling TR, Chadwick HS, Otto CM, Benedetti TJ: Aortic stenosis in pregnancy. *Obstet Gynecol* 1988; 72:113–118.

15. Sullivan H: Valvular heart surgery during pregnancy. *Surg Clin North Am* 1995; 75:59–72.

16. Study Group of the Working Group on Valvular Heart Disease of the European Society of Cardiology. *Eur Heart J* 1995; 16:1320–1330.

17. Parry AJ, Westaby S: Cardiopulmonary bypass during pregnancy. *Ann Thorac Surg* 1996; 61:1865–1869.

18. Trouton TG, Sidhu H, Adgey AAJ: Myocardial infarction in pregnancy. *Int J Cardiol* 1988; 18:35–39.

19. Samra D, Samra Y, Hertz M, Maier M: Acute myocardial infarction in pregnancy and puerperium. *Cardiology* 1989; 76:455–460.

20. Hankins GDV, Wendel GD Jr, Leveno KJ, Stoneham J: Myocardial infarction during pregnancy: A review. *Obstet Gynecol* 1985; 65:139–146.

21. Coulson CC, Kuller JA, Bowes WA Jr: Myocardial infarction and coronary artery dissection in pregnancy. *Am J Perinatol* 1995; 12:328–330.

22. Veille J: Peripartum cardiomyopathies: A review. *Am J Obstet Gynecol* 1984; 148:805–818.

23. Homans DC: Peripartum cardiomyopathy. *N Engl J Med* 1985; 312:1432–1437.

24. Cunningham FG, Pritchard JA, Hankins GDV, et al: Peripartum heart failure: Idiopathic cardiomyopathy or compounding cardiovascular events? *Obstet Gynecol* 1986; 67:157–167.

25. Carvalho AC, Almeida D, Cohen M, et al: Successful pregnancy, delivery, and puerperium in a heart transplant patient with previous peripartum cardiomyopathy. *Eur Heart J* 1992; 13:1589–1591.

26. Demakis JG, Rahimtoola SH, Sutton GC, et al: Natural course of peripartum cardiomyopathy. *Circulation* 1971; 44:1053–1061.

27. Page RL: Treatment of arrhythmias during pregnancy. *Am Heart J* 1995; 130:871–876.

28. Cox JL, Gardner MJ: Treatment of cardiac arrhythmias during pregnancy. *Prog Cardiovasc Dis* 1993; 36:137–178.

WILBERT S. ARONOW /
JOSEPH G. OUSLANDER

CHAPTER

# HEART DISEASE IN THE AGED

# 48

There is a high prevalence of coronary artery disease (CAD), hypertensive heart disease, valvular heart disease, congestive heart failure (CHF), and arrhythmias in older persons. Older persons with heart disease also have a higher incidence of cardiovascular morbidity and mortality than younger persons.

There may be differences in the clinical presentation of heart disease in older persons from that in younger persons. For example, unrecognized myocardial infarction (MI) is detected by a routine electrocardiogram (ECG) more frequently in older persons than in younger persons. Chest pain as a presenting clinical manifestation of acute myocardial infarction (AMI) occurs less frequently in older persons than in younger persons. Because of limited physical activity, older persons with heart disease may be less symptomatic than younger persons. Older persons with CHF have a higher prevalence of normal systolic function than younger persons. Older persons with severe valvular aortic stenosis are less likely to have a prolonged carotid upstroke time than younger persons.

Older persons up to age 80 treated with cardiovascular drug therapy in clinical trials have had a reduction in cardiovascular events similar to or greater than that of younger persons. There is a relative lack of data on treating persons older than 80 years with cardiovascular therapy. The data that are available show that cardiovascular therapy is efficacious in treating persons with heart disease who are older than 80 years, including the frail elderly. However, one must consider the potential complications of therapy in the frail elderly. For example, they are more likely to develop digitalis toxicity, sinus node and atrioventricular node dysfunction, bleeding manifestations from warfarin, volume depletion from diuretics, orthostatic hypotension, syncope, and falls.

## CORONARY ARTERY DISEASE

CAD is the most frequent cause of death in older persons. Approximately 60 percent of hospital admissions for acute MI occur in persons older than 65 years. Morbidity and mortality from CAD are similar in men and women 75 years of age and older.

CAD is diagnosed in an older person if he or she has coronary angiographic evidence of CAD, a documented MI, a typical history of angina pectoris, or sudden cardiac death. The incidence of sudden cardiac death as the initial clinical manifestation of CAD increases with age. In a prospective study of 664 men, mean age 80 years, and 1488 women, mean age 82 years, the prevalence of CAD was 44 percent in the older men and 41 percent in the older women.[1] Prior MI was present in 97 percent of these older persons with CAD.

Table 48-1 shows the prevalence of presenting clinical manifestations of MI in a prospective study of 110 older persons, mean age 82 years, with MI.[2] The data from this study indicate the importance of obtaining an ECG routinely before and after surgery and of obtaining periodic routine ECGs in older persons.

Dyspnea on exertion is a more common clinical manifestation of CAD in an older person than is the typical exertional chest pain of angina pectoris. Because of limited physical activity, many older persons with CAD do not experience exertional angina pectoris. Substernal chest pain due to angina pectoris is less frequent in an older person than in a younger person. Myocardial ischemia due to CAD in an older person can present as pain in the back or shoulders and may be misinterpreted as degenerative joint disease. Angina pectoris in an older person may also occur as a nocturnal burning postprandial epigastric pain and be misinterpreted as peptic ulcer disease or hiatus hernia reflux. In addition, older persons describe their anginal pain as less severe and of shorter duration. Furthermore, acute pulmonary edema unassociated with an acute MI may be a clinical manifestation of unstable angina pectoris due to extensive CAD.

Many older persons with a Q-wave MI documented by an ECG do not have a history of MI. In the Framingham Study, the percentages of MI clinically unrecognized but documented by routine ECGs were 25 percent for men and 35 percent for women 65 to 74 years of age, 42 percent for men and 36 percent for women 75 to 84 years of age, and 33 percent for men and 46 percent for women 85 to 95 years of age.[3] The prevalence of unrecognized Q-wave MI in some studies of older persons was 21 percent,[2] 43 percent,[4] and 68 percent.[5]

**TABLE 48-1.   Prevalence of Presenting Clinical Manifestations of Myocardial Infarction in 110 Persons, Mean Age 82 Years**

| Clinical Manifestation | % |
|---|---|
| Dyspnea | 35 |
| Chest pain | 22 |
| Unrecognized Q-wave MI detected by routine ECG | 21 |
| Neurologic symptoms | 18 |
| Gastrointestinal symptoms | 4 |

ECG = electrocardiogram; MI= myocardial infarction.

*Source:* Adapted from Aronow WS: Prevalence of presenting symptoms of recognized acute myocardial infarction and unrecognized healed myocardial infarction in elderly patients. *Am J Cardiol* 1987; 60:1182, with permission.

**TABLE 48-2.   Independent Risk Factors for New Coronary Events in 664 Older Men and in 1488 Older Women**

| Variable | Relative Risk | |
| --- | --- | --- |
| | Men | Women |
| Age | 1.039 | 1.030 |
| Prior CAD | 1.715 | 1.909 |
| Cigarette smoking | 2.174 | 2.017 |
| Hypertension | 1.953 | 1.635 |
| Diabetes mellitus | 1.884 | 1.753 |
| Serum total cholesterol | 1.011* | 1.011* |
| Serum high-density lipoprotein cholesterol | 0.948† | 0.935‡ |
| Serum triglycerides | NS | 1.002 |

\* 1.12 for an increment of 10 mg/dL of serum total cholesterol.

† 1.70 for a decrement of 10 mg/dL of serum high-density lipoprotein cholesterol.

‡ 1.95 for a decrement of 10 mg/dL of serum high-density lipoprotein cholesterol. CAD = coronary artery disease; NS = not significant.

*Source:* Adapted from Aronow WS, Ahn C: Risk factors for new coronary events in a large cohort of very elderly patients with and without coronary artery disease. *Am J Cardiol* 1996; 77:864–866, with permission.

The incidence of new coronary events is similar in older persons with recognized or unrecognized MI.[4,6] New coronary events (MI or sudden cardiac death) developed in 45 percent of 664 older men at 40-month mean follow-up and in 43 percent of 1488 older women at 48-month mean follow-up.[1] Table 48-2 indicates independent risk factors for new coronary events in these older men and women.[1] Obesity was a risk factor for new coronary events in older men and women by univariate analysis but not by multivariate analysis. Serum triglycerides was a risk factor for new coronary events in older men by univariate analysis but not by multivariate analysis. Other studies have also shown that age,[3] prior CAD,[3] cigarette smoking,[7,8] hypertension,[3,9,10] diabetes mellitus,[3] high serum total cholesterol,[3,7,11] low serum high-density lipoprotein (HDL) cholesterol,[3,11,12] and obesity[3] are independent risk factors for new coronary events in older men and women. The Framingham Study found high serum triglycerides to be an independent risk factor for new coronary events in older women but not in older men.[11]

## Control of Coronary Risk Factors

**CIGARETTE SMOKING.**   In older persons with CAD, cigarette smoking aggravates angina pectoris, precipitates silent myocardial ischemia, increases the incidence of new coronary events, and increases mortality. At 6-year follow-up of older men and women from the Coronary Artery Surgery Study registry, the relative risk of MI or death was 1.5 for persons aged 65 to 69 years and 2.9 for persons 70 years of age or older who continued smoking compared to that for quitters during the year before study enrollment.[13] Older men and women with CAD who smoke cigarettes should be strongly encouraged to stop smoking to reduce coronary events and mortality. Studies have shown that physicians who intervene with their smoking patients have a significant impact on the patients' smoking habits, regardless of age.

**HYPERTENSION.**   Older persons with hypertension should be treated with salt restriction, weight reduction if necessary, cessation of drugs that increase blood pressure, avoidance of alcohol and tobacco, increase in physical activity, reduction of dietary saturated fat and cholesterol, and maintenance of adequate dietary potassium, calcium, and magnesium intake. The Joint National Committee on Detection, Evaluation, and Treatment of High Blood Pressure recommends diuretics or beta blockers as initial drug therapy because these drugs have been demonstrated to decrease cardiovascular morbidity and mortality in controlled clinical trials.[14] Table 48-3 shows the decrease in coronary events by antihypertensive drugs versus placebo in older persons with hypertension.[10,15–17]

Monotherapy is the best initial approach for hypertension in older patients. The drug selected should depend on associated medical conditions. Older persons with hypertension who have CAD should be treated initially with a beta blocker; those with concomitant CHF should be treated with a diuretic or an angiotensin-converting enzyme (ACE) inhibitor. The use of cardiovascular drugs in older persons is discussed extensively elsewhere.[18]

**DYSLIPIDEMIA.**   In the Scandinavian Simvastatin Survival Study, 4444 men and women with CAD and hypercholesterolemia were treated with double-blind placebo or simvastatin.[19] At 5.4-year median follow-up, simvastatin reduced serum total cho-

**TABLE 48-3.**   Decrease in Coronary Events in Older Persons with Hypertension Treated with Antihypertensive Drugs versus Placebo

| Study | Result |
| --- | --- |
| European Working Party on Hypertension in the Elderly[15] (4.7-year follow-up) | 60% reduction in fatal MIs and 47% decrease in cardiac deaths |
| Swedish Trial in Old Patients with Hypertension[18] (25-month follow-up) | 25% reduction in fatal MIs and 67% decrease in sudden deaths |
| Medical Research Council[17] (5.8-year follow-up) | 19% reduction in coronary events |
| Systolic Hypertension in the Elderly Program[10] (4.5-year follow-up) | 27% decrease in nonfatal MIs plus coronary deaths |

MIs = myocardial infarctions.

lesterol 25 percent and serum low-density lipoprotein (LDL) cholesterol 35 percent, increased serum HDL cholesterol 8 percent, and decreased major coronary events 34 percent, coronary death 42 percent, and total mortality 30 percent. The decreases in new coronary events and in total mortality in patients treated with simvastatin were similar in men and women 60 to 70 years of age at study entry and those younger.

In the Cholesterol and Recurrent Events (CARE) trial, 4159 men and women with MI and serum cholesterol levels below 240 mg/dL were randomized to pravastatin or placebo.[20] At 5-year follow-up, there was a 27 percent reduction in major coronary events in persons 60 to 75 years of age at study entry randomized to pravastatin and a 20 percent decrease in major coronary events in persons younger than 60 years of age randomized to pravastatin. The reduction in major coronary events was 35 percent in persons with LDL cholesterol levels between 150 and 175 mg/dL, 26 percent in persons with LDL cholesterol levels between 125 and 150 mg/dL, and not present in persons with LDL cholesterol levels below 125 mg/dL. On the basis of these data, older persons with CAD and serum LDL cholesterol levels of 125 mg/dL or higher despite dietary therapy should be treated with pravastatin, simvastatin, lovastatin, fluvastatin, or atorvastatin.

**OTHER CORONARY RISK FACTORS.**   Diabetes mellitus should be treated in older persons with CAD. Obese patients who have CAD must undergo weight reduction. Weight reduction is also a first approach to controlling hyperglycemia, mild hypertension, and dyslipidemia before placing persons on long-term drug therapy. Regular aerobic exercise should be added to diet in treating obesity. Exercise training programs not only are beneficial in preventing CAD[21] but also have been found to improve endurance and functional capacity in older persons after MI.[22] Moderate exercise programs suitable for older persons with CAD include walking, climbing stairs, bicycling, and swimming. Less intense exercise of longer duration is recommended. Physical therapists can help individualize exercise programs in persons with comorbidities such as degenerative joint disease or chronic obstructive pulmonary disease. Exercise training should include strategies for supervision and follow-up. A 10- to 15-min period of stretching and light activity involving the large muscle groups is appropriate for most exercise training programs with elderly cardiac patients to avoid physical injuries. There should also be an extended cooldown period following physical activity. Older patients with CAD should avoid hot showers and prolonged standing in hot and humid areas during the cooldown period. High-intensity resistance exercise training is also an effective means of counteracting muscle weakness and physical frailty in very elderly persons.

## Therapy for Coronary Artery Disease

Therapy for AMI in older persons is discussed extensively elsewhere.[23] Pooled data from five large thrombolytic trials showed that thrombolytic therapy decreased absolute mortality 3.5 percent in older persons versus 2.2 percent in younger persons.

**ASPIRIN.** Randomized trials involving 19,791 patients demonstrated at 27-month follow-up that aspirin and other antiplatelet drugs administered to patients after MI decreased the incidence of recurrent MI, stroke, or vascular death by 25 percent.[24] The benefit from aspirin was irrespective of age.[24] On the basis of the available data, older persons with CAD should receive aspirin in a dose of 160 to 325 mg daily for an indefinite period unless there is a specific contraindication to its use.

**ANTICOAGULANTS.** The American College of Chest Physicians Consensus Conference on Antithrombotic Therapy recommended long-term aspirin after MI in preference to warfarin because of its simplicity, safety, and low cost.[25] Warfarin was recommended for 1 to 3 months after MI in persons with previous emboli, severe left ventricular dysfunction, CHF, or two-dimensional echocardiographic evidence of mural thrombosis.[25] Long-term warfarin was recommended indefinitely after MI in patients who had atrial fibrillation.[25] In older persons treated with oral warfarin after MI, an international normalized ratio (INR) of 2.0 to 3.0 is recommended.

**BETA BLOCKERS.** Beta blockers are very effective antianginal and anti-ischemic agents and should be administered to all older persons with angina pectoris or silent myocardial ischemia due to CAD unless there are specific contraindications to their use. Teo et al[26] analyzed 55 randomized controlled trials comprising 53,268 patients that investigated the use of beta blockers after MI. Beta blockers significantly reduced mortality by 19 percent in these studies.[26]

Table 48-4 shows that metoprolol,[27] timolol,[28,29] and propranolol[30] caused a significant reduction in mortality after MI in older persons. This reduction in mortality

**TABLE 48-4.   Effect of Beta Blockers on Mortality in Older Persons after Myocardial Infarction**

| Study | Comment |
|---|---|
| Goteborg Trial[27] (90-day follow-up) | Compared with placebo, metoprolol caused a 45% reduction in mortality in patients aged 64–74 years |
| Norwegian Multicenter Study[28,29] (17-month mean follow-up; up to 33-month follow-up) | Compared with placebo, timolol caused a 43% decrease in mortality in persons aged 65–74 years |
| (61-month mean follow-up; up to 72-month follow-up) | Compared with placebo, timolol caused a 19% reduction in mortality in persons aged 65–74 years |
| Beta Blocker Heart Attack Trial[30] (25-month mean follow-up; up to 36-month follow-up) | Compared with placebo, propranolol caused a 33% decrease in mortality in persons aged 60–69 years |

was greater in older persons than in younger persons. A retrospective analysis also showed that MI patients aged 60 to 89 years treated with metoprolol had an age-adjusted mortality decrease of 76 percent.[31]

Beta blockers have also been found to decrease mortality in older persons with complex ventricular arrhythmias after MI and a left ventricular ejection fraction $\geq$40 percent[32] or $\leq$40 percent.[33] The decrease in mortality in older persons with CAD and complex ventricular arrhythmias caused by propranolol is due more to an anti-ischemic effect than to an antiarrhythmic effect.[34] In these older persons, propranolol also markedly reduced the circadian variation of ventricular arrhythmias,[35] abolished the circadian variation of myocardial ischemia,[36] and abolished the circadian variation of sudden cardiac death or fatal MI.[37] Beta blockers are also likely to reduce mortality and recurrent MI by 25 percent in patients with non-Q-wave MI.[38]

On the basis of the available data, older persons should be treated with beta blockers for at least 6 years after Q-wave or non-Q-wave MI unless there are specific contraindications to their use. A beta blocker with intrinsic sympathomimetic activity should not be used.

**NITRATES.** Long-acting nitrates are effective antianginal and anti-ischemic agents.[39] These drugs should be administered along with beta blockers to patients with CAD who have angina pectoris. The dose of oral isosorbide dinitrate prescribed should be gradually increased to 30 to 40 mg administered 3 times daily if tolerated. To avoid nitrate tolerance, there should be a nitrate-free interval of 12 h each day.[40] Beta blockers should be used to prevent angina pectoris and rebound myocardial ischemia during the nitrate-free interval. However, nitrates, especially when combined with beta blockers, have the potential to cause frail elderly persons to develop hypotension, syncope, and falls.

**ANGIOTENSIN-CONVERTING ENZYME INHIBITORS.** Table 48-5 shows that ACE inhibitors reduce mortality in older persons after MI.[41–44] In most studies,[41–43] ACE inhibitors caused a greater reduction in mortality in older persons than in younger persons. On the basis of the available data, ACE inhibitors should be prescribed for older persons after MI who have CHF, an anterior wall MI, or a left ventricular ejection fraction $\leq$40 percent unless there are specific contraindications to their use.

**CALCIUM CHANNEL BLOCKERS.** Teo et al[26] analyzed randomized controlled trials comprising 20,342 patients that investigated the use of calcium channel blockers after MI. Mortality was insignificantly higher (relative risk = 1.04) in patients treated with calcium channel blockers. A meta-analysis of randomized clinical trials of the use of calcium channel blockers in patients with MI, unstable angina pectoris, and stable angina pectoris showed that the relative risk for mortality in the studies using dihydropyridines such as nifedipine that increase heart rate was 1.16.[45] The calcium channel blockers diltiazem and verapamil, which decrease heart rate, had no effect on survival.[45]

TABLE 48-5.   Effect of Angiotensin-Converting Enzyme Inhibitors on Mortality in Older Persons after Myocardial Infarction

| Study | Comment |
|---|---|
| Survival and Ventricular Enlargement Trial[41] (42-month mean follow-up; up to 60-month follow-up) | In patients with MI and left ventricular ejection fraction ≤40%, compared with placebo, captopril reduced mortality 25% in patients aged ≥65 years |
| Acute Infarction Ramipril Efficacy Study[42] (15-month follow-up) | In patients with MI and clinical evidence of CHF, compared with placebo, ramipril decreased mortality 36% in patients aged ≥65 years |
| Survival of Myocardial Infarction Long-Term Evaluation Trial[43] (1-year follow-up) | In patients with anterior wall MI, compared with placebo, zofenopril reduced mortality or severe CHF 39% in patients aged ≥65 years |
| Trandolapril Cardiac Evaluation Study[44] (24 to 50 months) | In patients with MI and left ventricular ejection fraction ≤35%, compared with placebo, trandolapril decreased mortality 17% in patients aged ≥65 years |

CHF = congestive heart failure; MI = myocardial infarction.

The Multicenter Diltiazem Postinfarction Trial observed at 25-month follow-up in patients after MI that compared with placebo, diltiazem had no significant effect on mortality or recurrent MI.[46] However, in patients with pulmonary congestion at baseline or a left ventricular ejection fraction <40 percent, diltiazem caused a significant increase in new cardiac events (hazard ratios = 1.41 and 1.31, respectively).[46]

Since no calcium channel blocker has been found to improve survival after MI except for the subgroup of patients with normal left ventricular ejection fraction treated with verapamil in the Danish Verapamil Infarction Trial II,[47] calcium channel blockers should not be prescribed for older patients following MI. However, if patients with CAD have persistent angina pectoris despite therapy with beta blockers and nitrates, a nondihydropyridine calcium channel blocker such as verapamil or diltiazem can be added to the therapeutic regimen if the left ventricular ejection fraction is normal, and amlodipine or felodipine can be added if the left ventricular ejection fraction is abnormal.

**HORMONE REPLACEMENT THERAPY.**   Observational studies suggest that postmenopausal women who use estrogen/progestin regimens are at lower risk for developing CAD than those who do not use hormone replacement therapy.[48] However, on the basis of the data from the Heart Estrogen/Progestin Replacement Study (HERS) which investigated 2.763 postmenopausal women with documented

CAD the effect of hormonal therapy versus double-blind placebo on coronary events.[48a] The authors cannot recommend the use of hormonal therapy in the treatment of postmenopausal women with CAD.

**REVASCULARIZATION.**   Medical therapy alone is the preferred treatment in older persons with CAD. The two indications for revascularization in older persons with CAD are prolongation of life and relief of unacceptable symptoms despite optimal medical management. In persons older than 80 years of age, the goal is less to prolong life than to improve the quality of life. If revascularization is performed, aggressive medical therapy must be continued. If revascularization is necessary to achieve the goals of therapy, and if percutaneous transluminal coronary angioplasty can achieve these goals as well as coronary artery bypass graft surgery, then percutaneous transluminal coronary angioplasty should be performed.

# VALVULAR HEART DISEASE

In an older population, mean age 82 years, an aortic systolic ejection murmur was heard in 265 of 565 persons (47 percent).[49] In this older population, a mitral regurgitation murmur was heard in 152 of 529 persons (29 percent),[50] and a diastolic murmur resulting from mitral stenosis was heard in 31 of 529 persons (6 percent).[50] In this older population, a diastolic murmur resulting from aortic regurgitation was also heard in 113 of 450 persons (25 percent).[51] It is important to obtain a Doppler echocardiogram in all older persons with a heart murmur for an appropriate diagnosis. Older persons with mild, moderate, or severe valvular heart disease or with mitral annular calcium should be treated with prophylactic antibiotics according to American Heart Association guidelines to prevent bacterial endocarditis.

## Valvular Aortic Stenosis

Table 48-6 shows that valvular aortic stenosis was present in 14 percent of 554 unselected older men, mean age 80 years, and in 18 percent of 1243 unselected older women, mean age 82 years.[52] Valvular aortic stenosis was severe in 2 percent of the 1797 older persons.[52] In the Helsinki Aging Study, critical valvular aortic stenosis was present in 3 percent of 501 unselected persons aged 75 to 86 years.[53] Angina pectoris, CHF, or syncope was present in 89 percent of older persons with severe valvular aortic stenosis.[54] The prognosis for unoperated severe valvular aortic stenosis in older persons with CHF is poor.[55] Aortic valve replacement is the procedure of choice for symptomatic older patients with severe valvular aortic stenosis.[56] Balloon aortic valvuloplasty should be considered for older patients with symptomatic severe valvular aortic stenosis who are not candidates for aortic valve surgery and possibly for patients with severe left ventricular dysfunction as a bridge to subsequent aortic valve replacement.[56]

## Aortic Regurgitation

Table 48-6 shows that ≥1+ aortic regurgitation was present in 31 percent of 554 unselected older men and in 28 percent of 1243 unselected older women.[52] Severe or moderate aortic regurgitation was present in 16 percent of the older persons. Older persons with chronic aortic regurgitation may be asymptomatic for many years. The prognosis for older persons with CHF and unoperated severe aortic valvular regurgitation is poor, however.[57] Echocardiographic evaluation of left ventricular end-systolic dimension should be performed yearly if the measurement is less than 50 mm but every 3 to 6 months if the measurement is 50 to 54 mm.[56] Aortic valve replacement should be considered when the left ventricular end-systolic dimension exceeds 55 mm, even in the absence of cardiac symptoms.[56]

## Mitral Stenosis

Table 48-6 shows that rheumatic mitral stenosis was present in 0.4 percent of 554 unselected older men and in 2 percent of 1243 unselected older women.[52] In a prospective study of 1699 unselected older persons, the prevalence of rheumatic mitral stenosis was 6 percent in older persons with atrial fibrillation and 0.4 percent in older persons with sinus rhythm.[58]

**TABLE 48-6.**   Prevalence of Valvular Heart Disease and of Cardiomyopathies Detected by Echocardiography in 554 Unselected Older Men and in 1243 Unselected Older Women

| Variable | Men (n = 554) | Women (n = 1243) |
|---|---|---|
| Aortic stenosis | 14% | 18% |
| ≥1 + aortic regurgitation | 31% | 28% |
| Rheumatic mitral stenosis | 0.4% | 2% |
| ≥1 + mitral regurgitation | 32% | 33% |
| Mitral annular calcium | 35% | 53% |
| Hypertrophic cardiomyopathy | 3% | 4% |
| Idiopathic dilated cardiomyopathy | 1% | 1% |

*Source:* Adapted from Aronow WS, Ahn C, Kronzon I: Prevalence of echocardiographic findings in 554 men and in 1243 women aged >60 years in a long-term health care facility. *Am J Cardiol* 1997; 79:379–380, with permission.

The most common cause of mitral stenosis in older persons is mitral annular calcium. The prevalence of mitral stenosis in older persons with mitral annular calcium is 6 percent.[59] Mitral stenosis in older persons is extensively discussed elsewhere.[60]

## Mitral Regurgitation

Table 48-6 shows ≥1+ mitral regurgitation was present in 32 percent of 554 unselected older men and in 33 percent of 1243 unselected older women.[52] The most common cause of mitral regurgitation in older persons is mitral annular calcium.[50]

Other disorders causing mitral regurgitation in older persons include CAD, mitral valve prolapse, and rheumatic heart disease. The heart murmur associated with mitral regurgitation is heard as an apical holosystolic murmur, late systolic murmur, or early systolic murmur beginning with the first heart sound but ending in mid-systole. Older patients with chronic mitral regurgitation should have echocardiographic examinations every 6 to 12 months.[60] Mitral valve surgery should be considered in older patients with New York Heart Association functional class III or IV symptoms caused by mitral regurgitation or in patients with severe mitral regurgitation and a left ventricular ejection fraction less than 50 percent or a left ventricular end-systolic dimension above 45 to 50 mm.[60]

## Mitral Annular Calcium

Mitral annular calcium is a chronic degenerative process that increases with age.[61] Table 48-6 shows that mitral annular calcium was present in 35 percent of 554 unselected older men and in 53 percent of 1243 unselected older women.[52] Persons with mitral annular calcium have a high prevalence of atrial fibrillation,[58] new coronary events,[62,63] CHF,[62] bacterial endocarditis,[63] permanent pacemaker implantation,[62] thromboembolic stroke,[62–66] and transient cerebral ischemic attack.[66] Mitral annular calcium in older persons is extensively discussed elsewhere.[61]

# CARDIOMYOPATHIES

Hypertrophic cardiomyopathy is a primary myocardial disorder with a hypertrophied and nondilated left ventricle not caused by other cardiovascular disease. Table 48-6 shows that hypertrophic cardiomyopathy was present in 3 percent of 554 unselected older men and in 4 percent of 1243 unselected older women.[52] Mitral annular calcium was also present in 76 percent of older persons with hypertrophic cardiomyopathy.[67]

Idiopathic dilated cardiomyopathy is a primary disorder of ventricular muscle that can be diagnosed by echocardiography. Table 48-6 shows that idiopathic dilated cardiomyopathy was present in 1 percent of 554 unselected older men and in 1 percent of 1243 unselected older women.[52] A detailed discussion of cardiomyopathies in older persons is presented elsewhere.[68]

# CONGESTIVE HEART FAILURE

The prevalence and incidence of CHF increase with age. CHF is the most common cause of hospitalization in persons aged 65 years or older. CHF developed in 294 of 1319 older persons (22 percent), mean age 82 years.[69]

The physician must measure left ventricular ejection fraction in all patients with CHF, preferably by echocardiography, in order to determine appropriate therapy for CHF.[70,71] The prevalence of diastolic dysfunction with normal left ventricular ejection fraction causing CHF in older persons was 50 percent and increased with age.[71a] The prevalence of normal left ventricular ejection fraction associated with CHF is higher in older women than in older men.[71a] Digoxin should not be administered to older persons with CHF in sinus rhythm with normal left ventricular ejection fraction.[72] Calcium channel blockers should not be administered to older persons with CHF and abnormal left ventricular ejection fraction.[46,73]

## Therapy for Congestive Heart Failure

**DIURETICS.** Diuretics are the first-line drug in the treatment of older persons with CHF associated with abnormal or normal left ventricular ejection fraction. Persons with CHF and abnormal left ventricular ejection fraction tolerate higher doses of diuretics than do persons with CHF and normal left ventricular ejection fraction who are dependent on adequate preload to maintain an acceptable cardiac output. Older patients treated with diuretics need close monitoring of serum electrolytes. Hypokalemia and hypomagnesemia, both of which may precipitate ventricular arrhythmias and digitalis toxicity, may develop. Hyponatremia with activation of the renin-angiotensin system may also occur. Older patients with CHF are especially sensitive to volume depletion. Dehydration and prerenal azotemia may develop if excessive doses of diuretics are administered.

**ANGIOTENSIN-CONVERTING ENZYME INHIBITORS.** ACE inhibitors improve symptoms, quality of life, and exercise tolerance in older persons with CHF associated with abnormal or normal left ventricular ejection fraction. An overview of 32 randomized studies of ACE inhibitors in 7105 patients with CHF demonstrated that ACE inhibitors caused a 23 percent decrease in total mortality and a 35 percent reduction in the combined end point of mortality or hospitalization for CHF.[74] Enalapril improved New York Heart Association functional class, exercise tolerance, left ventricular ejection fraction, and left ventricular diastolic function and decreased cardiothoracic ratio and left ventricular mass in older persons with CHF associated with normal left ventricular ejection fraction.[75] Therefore, ACE inhibitors are beneficial in treating older persons with CHF associated with either abnormal or normal left ventricular ejection fraction and should be administered to all older persons with CHF unless specific contraindications to these drugs are present.

Older patients at risk for excessive hypotension should have their blood pressure monitored closely for the first 2 weeks of ACE inhibitor therapy and whenever the physician increases the dose of ACE inhibitor or diuretic. Renal function should be monitored in patients on ACE inhibitors to detect increases in blood urea nitrogen and in serum creatinine, especially in older patients with renal artery stenosis. A doubling in serum creatinine should cause the physician to consider renal dysfunction due to ACE inhibitors, a need to reduce the dose of diuretics, or exacerbation of CHF. Neither potassium-sparing diuretics nor potassium supplements should be given to patients receiving ACE inhibitors because ACE-inhibitor therapy may cause hyperkalemia by reducing the secretion of aldosterone.

Asymptomatic hypotension (systolic blood pressure between 70 and 90 mmHg) and a serum creatinine of less than 2.5 mg/dL are acceptable side effects of therapy with ACE inhibitors and should cause the physician to reduce the dose of diuretics if the jugular venous pressure is normal. Symptomatic hypotension, progressive azotemia, intolerable cough, angioneurotic edema, hyperkalemia, and rash are contraindications to treatment with ACE inhibitors.

**ORAL ISOSORBIDE DINITRATE PLUS HYDRALAZINE.**   Oral isosorbide dinitrate plus hydralazine has been demonstrated to reduce mortality in persons with CHF associated with either abnormal[76] or normal left ventricular ejection fraction.[77] Older persons with CHF associated with either abnormal or normal left ventricular ejection fraction who cannot tolerate treatment with ACE inhibitors should be treated with oral isosorbide dinitrate plus hydralazine. The physician should also consider adding isosorbide dinitrate plus hydralazine to the therapeutic regimen of older persons with abnormal left ventricular ejection fraction who have persistent CHF despite treatment with diuretics, ACE inhibitors, and digoxin and those of older persons with normal left ventricular ejection fraction who have persistent CHF despite treatment with diuretics and ACE inhibitors.

**DIGOXIN.**   Digoxin should be used in the treatment of older persons with CHF and supraventricular tachyarrhythmias such as atrial fibrillation.[72] At 37-month follow-up of 6800 patients, mean age 63 years, with a mean left ventricular ejection fraction of 29 percent, mortality was the same in patients treated with digoxin or placebo.[77a] However, digoxin reduced hospitalization for worsening CHF.[77a] On the basis of the available data, digoxin should be administered to older persons with CHF in sinus rhythm associated with abnormal left ventricular ejection fraction who do not respond to diuretics plus ACE inhibitors and to those persons who are unable to tolerate ACE inhibitors or oral isosorbide dinitrate plus hydralazine. Digoxin can often be withdrawn from older persons with compensated CHF in sinus rhythm with abnormal left ventricular ejection fraction without clinical deterioration.[78,79] Digoxin should be continued if the left ventricular ejection fraction is severely impaired. Digoxin should not be administered to older persons with CHF in sinus rhythm with normal left ventricular ejection fraction.[72]

**BETA BLOCKERS.** After 6 to 12 months of treatment, the beta blocker carvedilol was associated with a 65 percent reduction in mortality in patients with CHF and abnormal left ventricular ejection fraction also treated with diuretics, ACE inhibitors, and digoxin.[80] Older persons with prior MI and a left ventricular ejection fraction ≥40 percent treated with diuretics plus ACE inhibitors who were randomized to propranolol had a 35 percent reduction in mortality and a 37 percent decrease in mortality plus nonfatal MI.[81] The use of beta blockers in the treatment of CHF associated with abnormal or normal left ventricular ejection fraction is discussed elsewhere.[81a] If older persons with CHF associated with either abnormal or normal left ventricular ejection fraction are treated with beta blockers, the initial dose should be small (for example, 10 mg of propranolol daily), and this dose should be gradually increased, with the maintenance dose reached over 3 months.

**CALCIUM CHANNEL BLOCKERS.** Calcium channel blockers such as nifedipine, diltiazem, and verapamil exacerbate CHF in patients with CHF associated with abnormal left ventricular ejection fraction.[73] Diltiazem increased mortality in patients with pulmonary congestion associated with abnormal left ventricular ejection fraction after MI.[46] The vasoselective calcium channel blockers amlodipine[82] and felodipine[83] did not significantly affect survival in patients with CHF associated with abnormal left ventricular ejection fraction. On the basis of the available data, calcium channel blockers should not be administered to older persons with CHF associated with abnormal left ventricular ejection fraction. However, calcium channel blockers may be used in the treatment of older persons with CHF associated with normal left ventricular ejection fraction[84] which persists despite therapy with diuretics plus ACE inhibitors plus beta blockers.

# ARRHYTHMIAS

There is a high prevalence of asymptomatic arrhythmias in older persons. Table 48-7 shows the prevalence of arrhythmias detected by 24-h ambulatory ECGs in unselected older persons.[85–88] Clinical indications for obtaining a 24-h ambulatory ECG in older persons include (1) determining whether palpitations, heart pounding, skipped beats, transient cerebral ischemic attack, syncope, near-syncope, seizure disorder, unexplained dizziness, vertigo, falls, shortness of breath, or chest pain are due to ventricular or supraventricular arrhythmias, bradyarrhythmias, or conduction disturbances; (2) an arrhythmia or conduction disturbance seen on a 12-lead ECG; (3) assessment of pacemaker function; (4) assessment of the efficacy of antiarrhythmic or anti-ischemic therapy; (5) assessment of the risk of future cardiac events from arrhythmia or silent myocardial ischemia in persons with heart disease; and (6) detection of suspected arrhythmia induced by a proarrhythmic drug.

**TABLE 48-7.   Prevalence of Arrhythmias Detected by 24-Hour Ambulatory Electrocardiograms in Unselected Older Persons**

| Arrhythmia | Mean Age (years) | Prevalence |
|---|---|---|
| Nonsustained ventricular tachycardia[85] | 82 | 10% of 554 persons |
| Complex ventricular arrhythmias[86] | 82 | 55% of 843 persons |
| Simple ventricular arrhythmias[85] | 82 | 26% of 554 persons |
| Frequent atrial premature complexes[87] | 82 | 28% of 407 persons |
| Infrequent atrial premature complexes[87] | 82 | 61% of 407 persons |
| Sick sinus syndrome[87] | 82 | 13% of 453 persons |
| Atrial fibrillation[88] | 81 | 14% of 1476 persons (chronic in 195 persons and paroxysmal in 6 persons) |
| Paroxysmal supraventricular tachycardia[88] | 81 | 33% of 1476 persons |

Frequent atrial premature complexes are not associated with an increased incidence of new coronary events in older persons with or without heart disease and should not be treated with an antiarrhythmic drug. Nonsustained ventricular tachycardia and complex ventricular arrhythmias are not associated with an increased incidence of new coronary events in older persons with no clinical evidence of heart disease[86,89] and should not be treated with antiarrhythmic drugs in asymptomatic persons. Nonsustained ventricular tachycardia and complex ventricular arrhythmias are associated with an increased incidence of new coronary events in older persons with heart disease[86,90] and should be treated with beta blockers in persons without contraindications to beta blockers. Older persons with supraventricular tachyarrhythmias associated with the tachycardia-bradycardia (sick sinus) syndrome should be referred to a cardiologist for permanent ventricular pacing and should receive a beta blocker, verapamil, or diltiazem to slow a rapid ventricular rate associated with the supraventricular tachyarrhythmia.[91] Paroxysmal supraventricular tachycardia is not associated with an increased incidence of new coronary events[92] or stroke[88] in older persons with heart disease and should not be treated with antiarrhythmic drugs in asymptomatic persons. Symptomatic paroxysmal supraventricular tachycardia should be treated with a beta blocker, verapamil, or diltiazem. Atrial fibrillation in older persons is associated with an increased incidence of new coronary events and stroke[88,92] and should be treated. Therapy for atrial fibrillation is discussed in a later section.

# ANTIARRHYTHMIC THERAPY FOR CORONARY ARTERY DISEASE

## Class I Drugs

A meta-analysis of 59 randomized controlled trials comprising 23,229 patients that investigated the use of quinidine, procainamide, disopyramide, imipramine, moricizine, lidocaine, tocainide, phenytoin, mexiletine, aprindine, encainide, and flecainide after MI showed that mortality was significantly higher in patients receiving class I antiarrhythmic drugs than in patients receiving no antiarrhythmic drugs (odds ratio = 1.14).[26] None of the 59 studies observed a decrease in mortality with class I antiarrhythmic drugs.[26]

In the Cardiac Arrhythmia Suppression Trials I and II, older age also increased the likelihood of adverse effects, including death, in patients after MI receiving encainide, flecainide, or moricizine.[93] Compared with no antiarrhythmic drug, quinidine or procainamide did not reduce mortality in older persons with CAD, normal or abnormal left ventricular ejection fraction, and presence or absence of ventricular tachycardia.[94] On the basis of the available data, persons with CAD should not receive class I antiarrhythmic drugs.

## Sotalol and D-Sotalol

Studies comparing the effect of sotalol with placebo on mortality in patients with complex ventricular arrhythmias have not been done. In the Survival with Oral D-Sotalol (SWORD) trial, 3121 survivors of MI were randomized to D-sotalol or placebo. Mortality was significantly higher at 148-day follow-up in patients treated with D-sotalol (5 percent) than in patients treated with placebo (3.1 percent).[95] On the basis of the available data, older patients with CAD should not be treated with sotalol or D-sotalol.

## Amiodarone

In the European Myocardial Infarction Amiodarone Trial, 1486 survivors of MI with a left ventricular ejection fraction ≤40 percent were randomized to amiodarone or to placebo.[95a] At 2-year follow-up, mortality was similar in the patients treated with amiodarone or placebo. In the Canadian Amiodarone Myocardial Infarction Arrhythmia Trial, 1202 survivors of MI with nonsustained ventricular tachycardia or complex ventricular arrhythmias were randomized to amiodarone or to placebo.[95b] Amiodarone was very effective in suppressing ventricular tachycardia and complex ventricular arrhythmias. However, mortality at 1.8-year follow-up was not significantly different in patients treated with amiodarone or placebo. In addition, 36 percent of patients randomized to amiodarone stopped taking the drug because of adverse effects. On the basis of the available data, amiodarone is not recommended in the treatment of patients with arrhythmias associated with CAD.

## Beta Blockers

Beta blockers have been demonstrated to decrease mortality in patients with non-sustained ventricular tachycardia or complex ventricular arrhythmias after MI with normal or abnormal left ventricular ejection fraction.[32,33,96] On the basis of the available data, beta blockers should be used to treat older persons with CAD and nonsustained ventricular tachycardia or complex ventricular arrhythmias unless there are specific contraindications to their use.

## Automatic Implantable Cardioverter-Defibrillator

If older persons with CAD have life-threatening ventricular tachycardia or ventricular fibrillation that is resistant to antiarrhythmic drugs, an automatic implantable cardioverter-defibrillator should be inserted.[96a] The effect on survival of the automatic implantable cardioverter-defibrillator implanted for ventricular fibrillation or recurrent ventricular tachycardia is similar in older and younger persons.[97]

# ATRIAL FIBRILLATION

The incidence of chronic atrial fibrillation increases with age.[98,99] In a prospective study of 2101 older persons, mean age 81 years, electrocardiography showed that atrial fibrillation was present in 13 percent of persons.[99] Atrial fibrillation was present in 16 percent of 650 older men and in 13 percent of 1451 older women.[99] Atrial fibrillation was present in 5 percent of persons 60 to 70 years of age, in 14 percent of persons 71 to 80 years of age, in 13 percent of persons 81 to 90 years of age, and in 22 percent of persons 91 to 103 years of age.[99] In a prospective study of 1699 unselected older persons, mean age 81 years, with atrial fibrillation (254 persons) or sinus rhythm (1445 persons), persons with atrial fibrillation had a higher prevalence of valvular heart disease, left atrial enlargement, left ventricular hypertrophy, and abnormal left ventricular ejection fraction than persons with sinus rhythm (Table 48-8).[58]

Atrial fibrillation is an independent predictor of new coronary events[92,100] and of new thromboembolic strokes in older persons.[98,99] The 3-year incidence of thromboembolic stroke was 38 percent in older persons with atrial fibrillation and 11 percent in older persons with sinus rhythm.[99] The 5-year incidence of thromboembolic stroke was 72 percent in older persons with atrial fibrillation and 24 percent in older persons with sinus rhythm.[99]

Older persons with atrial fibrillation and a slow ventricular rate due to concomitant atrioventricular nodal disease should not receive a drug that depresses atrioventricular conduction.[91] Persons with atrial fibrillation who have a very fast ventricular rate associated with hypotension, chest pain due to myocardial ischemia, severe CHF, or syncope should undergo immediate direct-current cardioversion.[91] A very fast ventricular rate unassociated with these symptoms should be immediately slowed by intravenous verapamil, diltiazem, or a beta blocker.[91] Digoxin

**TABLE 48-8.** Echocardiographic Findings in 1699 Unselected Older Persons, Mean Age 81 Years, with Atrial Fibrillation (254 Persons) or Sinus Rhythm (1445 Persons)

| Variable | Increased Prevalence in Atrial Fibrillation |
|---|---|
| Mitral annular calcium | 1.7 times |
| Rheumatic mitral stenosis | 17.1 times |
| ≥1 + mitral regurgitation | 2.2 times |
| Valvular aortic stenosis | 2.3 times |
| ≥1 + aortic regurgitation | 2.1 times |
| Left atrial enlargement | 2.9 times |
| Left ventricular hypertrophy | 2.0 times |
| Abnormal left ventricular ejection fraction | 2.5 times |

*Source:* Adapted from Aronow WS, Ahn C, Kronzon I: Echocardiographic findings associated with atrial fibrillation in 1699 patients aged >60 years. *Am J Cardiol* 1995;76:1191–1192, with permission.

should be used to slow a rapid ventricular rate in persons with atrial fibrillation unassociated with increased sympathetic tone, the Wolff-Parkinson-White syndrome, or hypertrophic cardiomyopathy.[91] If a fast ventricular rate associated with atrial fibrillation occurs at rest or during exercise despite oral digoxin, an oral beta blocker, verapamil, or diltiazem should be added to the therapeutic regimen.[91] Oral amiodarone may be used in selected persons with symptomatic life-threatening atrial fibrillation refractory to other drug therapy.[91] Symptomatic older persons in whom a rapid ventricular rate associated with atrial fibrillation cannot be slowed by drug therapy should be referred to a cardiologist for radiofrequency catheter modification of atrioventricular conduction or radiofrequency catheter induction of complete atrioventricular block followed by implantation of a permanent pacemaker.[91]

In addition to ventricular rate control, older persons with atrial fibrillation should be treated with aspirin or warfarin to reduce the incidence of thromboembolic stroke. Table 48-9 lists risk factors for thromboembolic stroke in persons with atrial fibrillation.[63,65,88,98,99,101–106]

In the Stroke Prevention in Atrial Fibrillation III study, high-risk patients with atrial fibrillation were randomized to warfarin to achieve an INR of 2.0 to 3.0 or to aspirin 325 mg/day plus low-dose warfarin to achieve an INR of 1.2 to 1.5.[104] At 1.1-year follow-up, the incidence of ischemic stroke or systemic embolism was reduced from 7.9 percent/year to 1.9 percent/year (76 percent decrease) in those patients treated with warfarin to achieve an INR of 2.0 to 3.0.[104] Nonrandomized data from 312 older nursing home residents found that older persons with atrial fibrillation re-

TABLE 48-9.   Risk Factors for Thromboembolic Stroke in Persons with Atrial Fibrillation

Rheumatic mitral stenosis[101]

Prior arterial thromboembolism[88,99,102–104]

Recent congestive heart failure (within 3 months)[102]

Hypertension[101,102,104]

Echocardiographic left ventricular dysfunction[104,105]

Women older than 75 years[104]

Echocardiographic left ventricular hypertrophy[101]

Age[65,88,98]

Coronary heart disease[65,101,106]

Echocardiographic left atrial enlargement[101,105]

Mitral annular calcium[63,65]

Male sex[88,99]

ceiving oral warfarin to achieve an INR between 2.0 and 3.0 had a 76 percent reduction in new thromboembolic stroke compared with older persons with atrial fibrillation receiving oral aspirin 325 mg/day.[106a]

On the basis of the available data, older persons with chronic or paroxysmal atrial fibrillation who are at high risk for developing thromboembolic stroke and who have no contraindications to anticoagulant therapy, including gait problems or a history of falls, should receive long-term oral warfarin to achieve an INR between 2.0 and 3.0.[104] Because of the potential increased risk of intracranial hemorrhage in persons older than 75 years, those at increased risk for bleeding should be treated with a lower dose of oral warfarin to achieve an INR between 2.0 and 2.5. It is very important that hypertension be controlled. Whenever a prothrombin time is obtained, the blood pressure should also be measured. The physician must be aware of the numerous drugs that potentiate the effect of warfarin, causing an increased prothrombin time and risk of bleeding. Older persons with atrial fibrillation who are at low risk for developing thromboembolic stroke or who are poor candidates for therapy with long-term oral warfarin should be treated with oral aspirin 325 mg/day.

# PACEMAKERS

In a prospective study of 1153 older persons, mean age 82 years, 50 (4.3 percent) had a permanent pacemaker implanted.[107] All 50 persons had an appropriate indication for permanent pacemaker implantation. In a prospective study of 148 older persons, mean age 82 years, with unexplained syncope, 21 persons (14 percent) had pauses greater than 3 s detected by 24-h ambulatory ECGs, requiring pacemaker implantation.[108] Of these 21 older persons, 8 had sinus arrest, 7 had advanced second-degree atrioventricular block, and 6 had atrial fibrillation with a slow ventricular rate which was not drug-induced. At 38-month mean follow-up after permanent pacemaker implantation, 86 percent of these 21 persons had no episodes of recurrent syncope.[108] Table 48-10 lists Class I indications for permanent pacemakers in older persons.[109]

Single-chamber pacemakers should be checked by telephone telemetry or by office visits twice in the first month after implantation, every other month from

#### TABLE 48-10. Class I Indications for Permanent Pacemakers in Older Persons

1. Acquired complete AV block, permanent or intermittent, associated with symptomatic bradycardia, CHF, the necessary use of drugs that suppress escape pacemakers and cause symptomatic bradycardia, pauses ≥3 s, any escape ventricular rate <40 beats/min, post-AV junction ablation, and a confusional state which clears with temporary pacing

2. Acquired second-degree AV block, permanent or intermittent, with symptomatic bradycardia

3. Persistent complete AV block or advanced second-degree AV block after acute MI with associated bundle branch block

4. Transient advanced second-degree AV block after acute MI with associated bundle branch block

5. Bifascicular block with intermittent complete AV block associated with symptomatic bradycardia

6. Bifascicular or trifascicular block with intermittent type II second-degree AV block without symptoms

7. Sinus node dysfunction with symptomatic bradycardia

8. Recurrent syncope provoked by carotid sinus stimulation; minimal carotid sinus pressure induces asystole >3-s duration in the absence of any drug that depresses the sinus node or AV conduction

9. Symptomatic recurrent supraventricular tachycardia when drugs fail to control the arrhythmia

10. Symptomatic recurrent ventricular tachycardia after an automatic defibrillator has been implanted and recurrent ventricular tachycardia is not prevented by drug therapy

AV = atrioventricular; CHF = congestive heart failure; MI = myocardial infarction.

*Source:* Adapted from Gregoratos G, Cheitlin MD, Conill A, et al: ACC/AHA Guidelines for Implantation of Cardiac Pacemakers and Antiarrhythmia Devices: Executive Summary. A Report of the American College of Cardiology/American Heart Association Task Force on Practice Guidelines (Committee on Pacemaker Implantation). *Circulation* 1998; 97:1325–1335.

months 2 to 36 after implantation, and monthly thereafter. Dual-chamber pace-makers should be checked by telephone telemetry or by office visits twice in the first month after implantation, monthly from months 2 to 6 after implantation, every other month from months 7 to 36 after implantation, and monthly thereafter. Threshold checking should be performed yearly.[110]

## REFERENCES

1. Aronow WS, Ahn C: Risk factors for new coronary events in a large cohort of very elderly patients with and without coronary artery disease. *Am J Cardiol* 1996; 77:864–866.
2. Aronow WS: Prevalence of presenting symptoms of recognized acute myocardial infarction and of unrecognized healed myocardial infarction in elderly patients. *Am J Cardiol* 1987; 60:1182.
3. Vokonas PS, Kannel WB: Epidemiology of coronary heart disease in the elderly. In: Tresch DD, Aronow WS (eds): *Cardiovascular Disease in the Elderly Patient,* 2d ed. New York, Marcel Dekker, 1999:139–164.
4. Nadelmann J, Frishman WH, Ooi WL, et al: Prevalence, incidence, and prognosis of recognized and unrecognized myocardial infarction in persons aged 75 years or older: The Bronx Aging Study. *Am J Cardiol* 1990; 66:533–537.
5. Aronow WS, Starling L, Etienne F, et al: Unrecognized Q-wave myocardial infarction in patients older than 64 years in a long-term health-care facility. *Am J Cardiol* 1985; 56:483.
6. Aronow WS: New coronary events at four-year follow-up in elderly patients with recognized or unrecognized myocardial infarction. *Am J Cardiol* 1989; 63:621–622.
7. Siegel D, Kuller L, Lazarus NB, et al: Predictors of cardiovascular events and mortality in the Systolic Hypertension in the Elderly Program pilot project. *Am J Epidemiol* 1987; 126:385–399.
8. LaCroix AZ, Lang J, Scherr P, et al: Smoking and mortality among older men and women in three communities. *N Engl J Med* 1991; 324:1619–1625.
9. Applegate WB: Hypertension in elderly patients. *Ann Intern Med* 1989; 110:901–915.
10. SHEP Cooperative Research Group: Prevention of stroke by antihypertensive drug treatment in older persons with isolated systolic hypertension. Final results of the Systolic Hypertension in the Elderly Program (SHEP). *JAMA* 1991; 265: 3255–3264.
11. Castelli WP, Wilson PWF, Levy D, Anderson K: Cardiovascular disease in the elderly. *Am J Cardiol* 1989; 63:12H–19H.
12. Corti M-C, Guralnik JM, Salive ME, et al: HDL cholesterol predicts coronary heart disease mortality in older persons. *JAMA* 1995; 274:539–544.
13. Hermanson B, Omenn GS, Kronmal RA, Gersh BJ: Beneficial six-year outcome of smoking cessation in older men and women with coronary artery disease. Results from the CASS registry. *N Engl J Med* 1988; 319:1365–1369.
14. Joint National Committee: The Sixth Report of the Joint National Committee on the Detection, Evaluation, and Treatment of High Blood Pressure (JNC VI). *Arch Intern Med* 1997; 157:2413–2444.
15. Amery A, Birkenhager W, Brixko P, et al: Mortality and morbidity results from the European Working Party on Hypertension in Elderly Trial. *Lancet* 1985; 1:1349–1354.

16.  Dahlof B, Lindholm LH, Hansson L, et al: Morbidity and mortality in the Swedish Trial in Old Patients With Hypertension (STOP Hypertension). *Lancet* 1991; 338:1281–1285.

17.  MRC Working Party: Medical Research Council Trial of treatment of hypertension in older adults: Principal results. *Br Med J* 1992; 304:405–412.

18.  Aronow WS: Cardiovascular drug therapy in the elderly. In: Frishman WH, Sonnenblick EH (eds): *Cardiovascular Pharmacotherapeutics.* New York:McGraw-Hill, Inc, 1997:1267–1281.

19.  Scandinavian Simvastatin Survival Study Group: Randomised trial of cholesterol lowering in 4444 patients with coronary heart disease: The Scandinavian Simvastatin Survival Study (4S). *Lancet* 1994; 344:1383–1389.

20.  Sacks FM, Pfeffer MA, Moye LA, et al: The effect of pravastatin on coronary events after myocardial infarction in patients with average cholesterol levels. *N Engl J Med* 1996; 335:1001–1009.

21.  Wenger NK: Physical inactivity as a risk factor for coronary heart disease in the elderly. *Cardiol Elderly* 1994; 2:375–379.

22.  Williams MA, Maresh CM, Aronow WS, et al: The value of early out-patient cardiac exercise programmes for the elderly in comparison with other selected age groups. *Eur Heart J* 1984; 5(suppl E):113–115.

23.  Rich MW: Therapy for acute myocardial infarction. In: Aronow WS, Tresch DD (eds): *Clinics in Geriatric Medicine. Coronary Artery Disease in the Elderly.* Philadelphia: WB Saunders Co., 1996:141–168.

24.  Antiplatelet Trialists' Collaboration: Collaborative overview of randomised trials of antiplatelet therapy—I: Prevention of death, myocardial infarction, and stroke by prolonged antiplatelet therapy in various categories of patients. *Br Med J* 1994; 308:81–106.

25.  Cairns JA, Lewis HD Jr, Meade TW, et al: Antithrombotic agents in coronary artery disease. *Chest* 1995; 108(suppl):380S–400S.

26.  Teo KK, Yusuf S, Furberg CD: Effects of prophylactic antiarrhythmic drug therapy in acute myocardial infarction. An overview of results from randomized controlled trials. *JAMA* 1993; 270:1589–1595.

27.  Hjalmarson A, Elmfeldt D, Herlitz J, et al: Effect on mortality of metoprolol in acute myocardial infarction. *Lancet* 1981; 2:823–827.

28.  Gundersen T, Abrahamsen AM, Kjekshus J, Ronnevik PK: Timolol-related reduction in mortality and reinfarction in patients ages 65–75 years surviving acute myocardial infarction. *Circulation* 1982; 66:1179–1184.

29.  Pedersen TR for the Norwegian Multicentre Study Group: Six-year follow-up of the Norwegian Multicentre Study on Timolol after acute myocardial infarction. *N Engl J Med* 1985; 313:1055–1058.

30.  Beta-Blocker Heart Attack Trial Research Group: A randomized trial of propranolol in patients with acute myocardial infarction. *JAMA* 1982; 247:1707–1714.

31.  Park KC, Forman DE, Wei JY: Utility of beta-blockade treatment for older postinfarction patients. *J Am Geriatr Soc* 1995; 43:751–755.

32.  Aronow WS, Ahn C, Mercando AD, Kronzon I: Effect of propranolol versus no antiarrhythmic drug on sudden cardiac death, total cardiac death, and total death in patients ≥62 years of age with heart disease, complex ventricular arrhythmias, and left ventricular ejection fraction ≥40%. *Am J Cardiol* 1994; 74:267–270.

33.  Kennedy HL, Brooks MM, Barker AH, et al: Beta-blocker therapy in the Cardiac Arrhythmia Suppression Trial. *Am J Cardiol* 1994; 74:674–680.

34.  Aronow WS, Ahn C, Mercando AD, Kronzon I: Decrease of mortality by propranolol

in patients with heart disease and complex ventricular arrhythmias is more an anti-ischemic than an antiarrhythmic effect. *Am J Cardiol* 1994; 74:613–615.

35.  Aronow WS, Ahn C, Mercando AD, Epstein S: Effect of propranolol on circadian variation of ventricular arrhythmias in elderly patients with heart disease and complex ventricular arrhythmias. *Am J Cardiol* 1995; 75:514–516.

36.  Aronow WS, Ahn C, Mercando AD, Epstein S: Effect of propranolol on circadian variation of myocardial ischemia in elderly patients with heart disease and complex ventricular arrhythmias. Am J Cardiol 1995; 75:837–839.

37.  Aronow WS, Ahn C, Mercando AD, Epstein S: Circadian variation of sudden cardiac death or fatal myocardial infarction is abolished by propranolol in patients with heart disease and complex ventricular arrhythmias. *Am J Cardiol* 1994; 74:819–821.

38.  Yusuf S, Wittes J, Probstfield J: Evaluating effects of treatment subgroups of patients within a clinical trial: The case of non-Q-wave myocardial infarction and beta blockers. *Am J Cardiol* 1990; 60:220–222.

39.  Danahy DT, Aronow WS: Hemodynamics and antianginal effects of high dose oral isorbide dinitrate after chronic use. *Circulation* 1977; 56:205–212.

40.  Parker JO, Farrell B, Lahey KA, Moe G: Effect of interval between doses on the development of tolerance to isosorbide dinitrate. *N Engl J Med* 1987; 316:1440–1444.

41.  Pfeffer MA, Braunwald E, Moye LA, et al: Effect of captopril on mortality and morbidity in patients with left ventricular dysfunction after myocardial infarction. Results of the Survival and Ventricular Enlargement Trial. *N Engl J Med* 1992; 327:669–677.

42.  The Acute Infarction Ramipril Efficacy (AIRE) Study Investigators: Effect of ramipril on mortality and morbidity of survivors of acute myocardial infarction with clinical evidence of heart failure. *Lancet* 1993; 342:821–828.

43.  Ambrosioni E, Borghi C, Magnani B, for the Survival of Myocardial Infarction Long-Term Evaluation (SMILE) Study Investigators: The effect of the angiotensin-converting-enzyme inhibitor zofenopril on mortality and morbidity after anterior myocardial infarction. *N Engl J Med* 1995; 332:80–85.

44.  Kober L, Torp-Pedersen C, Carlsen JE, et al: A clinical trial of the angiotensin-converting-enzyme inhibitor trandolapril in patients with left ventricular dysfunction after myocardial infarction. *N Engl J Med* 1995; 333:1670–1676.

45.  Yusuf S, Held P, Furberg C: Update of effects of calcium antagonists in myocardial infarction or angina in light of the second Danish Verapamil Infarction Trial (DAVIT-II) and other recent studies. *Am J Cardiol* 1991; 67:1295–1297.

46.  The Multicenter Diltiazem Postinfarction Trial Research Group: The effect of diltiazem on mortality and reinfarction after myocardial infarction. *N Engl J Med* 1988; 319:385–392.

47.  Danish Study Group on Verapamil in Myocardial Infarction: Trial II-DAVIT II. Effect of verapamil on mortality and major events after acute myocardial infarction. *Am J Cardiol* 1990; 66:779–785.

48.  Grodstein F, Stampfer MJ, Manson JE, et al: Postmenopausal estrogen and progestin use and the risk of cardiovascular disease. *N Engl J Med* 1996; 335:453–461.

48a. Hulley S, Grady D, Bush T, et al: Randomized trial of estrogen plus progestin for secondary prevention of coronary heart disease in postmenopausal women. *JAMA* 1998; 280:605–613.

49.  Aronow WS, Schwartz KS, Koenigsberg M: Correlation of aortic cuspal and aortic root disease with aortic systolic ejection murmurs and with mitral annular calcium in persons older than 62 years in a long-term health care facility. *Am J Cardiol* 1986; 58:651–652.

50. Aronow WS, Schwartz KS, Koenigsberg M: Correlation of murmurs of mitral stenosis and mitral regurgitation with presence or absence of mitral annular calcium in persons older than 62 years in a long-term health care facility. *Am J Cardiol* 1987; 59:181–182.

51. Aronow WS, Kronzon I: Correlation of prevalence and severity of aortic regurgitation detected by pulsed Doppler echocardiography with the murmur of aortic regurgitation in elderly patients in a long-term health care facility. *Am J Cardiol* 1989; 63:128–129.

52. Aronow WS, Ahn C, Kronzon I: Prevalence of echocardiographic findings in 554 men and in 1,243 women aged >60 years in a long-term health care facility. *Am J Cardiol* 1997; 79:379–380.

53. Lindroos M, Kupari M, Heikkila J, Tilvis R: Prevalence of aortic valve abnormalities in the elderly: An echocardiographic study of a random population sample. *J Am Coll Cardiol* 1993; 21:1220–1225.

54. Aronow WS, Kronzon I: Prevalence and severity of valvular aortic stenosis determined by Doppler echocardiography and its association with echocardiographic and electro-cardiographic left ventricular hypertrophy and physical signs of aortic stenosis in elderly patients. *Am J Cardiol* 1991; 67:776–777.

55. Aronow WS, Ahn C, Kronzon I, Nanna M: Prognosis of congestive heart failure in patients aged ≥62 years with unoperated severe valvular aortic stenosis. *Am J Cardiol* 1993; 72:846–848.

56. Aronow WS, Tresch DD, Nanna M: Aortic valve disease in the elderly. In: Tresch DD, Aronow WS (eds): *Cardiovascular Disease in the Elderly Patient,* 2d ed. New York: Marcel Dekker, 1999:345–370.

57. Aronow WS, Ahn C, Kronzon I, Nanna M: Prognosis of patients with heart failure and unoperated severe aortic valvular regurgitation and relation to ejection fraction. *Am J Cardiol* 1994; 74:286–288.

58. Aronow WS, Ahn C, Kronzon I: Echocardiographic findings associated with atrial fibrillation in 1,699 patients aged >60 years. *Am J Cardiol* 1995; 76:1191–1192.

59. Aronow WS, Kronzon I: Correlation of prevalence and severity of mitral regurgitation and mitral stenosis determined by Doppler echocardiography with physical signs of mitral regurgitation and mitral stenosis in 100 patients aged 62 to 100 years with mitral annular calcium. *Am J Cardiol* 1987; 60:1189–1190.

60. Tresch DD: Mitral valvular disease in the elderly. In: Tresch DD, Aronow WS (eds): *Cardiovascular Disease in the Elderly Patient,* 2d ed. New York: Marcel Dekker, 1999: 371–395.

61. Aronow WS, Nair CK: Mitral annular calcium in the elderly. In: Tresch DD, Aronow WS (eds): *Cardiovascular Disease in the Elderly Patient,* 2d ed. New York: Marcel Dekker, 1999:397–415.

62. Nair CK, Thomson W, Ryschon K, et al: Long-term follow-up of patients with echocar-diographically detected mitral annular calcium and comparison with age- and sex-matched control subjects. *Am J Cardiol* 1989; 63:465–470.

63. Aronow WS, Koenigsberg M, Kronzon I, Gutstein H: Association of mitral annular calcium with new thromboembolic stroke and cardiac events at 39-month follow-up in elderly patients. *Am J Cardiol* 1990; 65:1511–1512.

64. Benjamin EJ, Plehn JF, D'Agostino RB, et al: Mitral annular calcification and the risk of stroke in an elderly cohort. *N Engl J Med* 1992; 327:374–379.

65. Boston Area Anticoagulation Trial for Atrial Fibrillation Investigators: The effect of low-dose warfarin on the risk of stroke in patients with nonrheumatic atrial fibrillation. *N Engl J Med* 1990; 323:1505–1511.

66. Aronow WS, Schoenfeld MR, Gutstein H: Frequency of thromboembolic stroke in per-

sons ≥60 years of age with extracranial carotid arterial disease and/or mitral annular calcium. *Am J Cardiol* 1992; 70:123–124.

67. Aronow WS, Kronzon I: Prevalence of hypertrophic cardiomyopathy and its association with mitral annular calcium in elderly patients. *Chest* 1988; 94:1295–1296.

68. Nanna M, Aronow WS: Cardiomyopathies in the elderly. In: Tresch DD, Aronow WS (eds): *Cardiovascular Disease in the Elderly Patient,* 2d ed. New York: Marcel Dekker, 1999:429–452.

69. Aronow WS, Ahn C, Kronzon I: Prognosis of congestive heart failure in elderly patients with normal versus abnormal left ventricular systolic function associated with coronary disease. *Am J Cardiol* 1990; 66:1257–1259.

70. Konstam M, Dracup K, Baker D, et al: *Heart Failure: Management of Patients with Left Ventricular Systolic Dysfunction.* Quick Reference Guide for Clinicians, No. 11, AHCPR Publication No. 94-0613. Rockville, MD, Agency for Health Care Policy and Research, June, 1994, pp. 1–21.

71. Aronow WS, Ahn C, Kronzon I: Normal left ventricular ejection fraction in older persons with congestive heart failure. *Chest* 1998; 113:867–869.

71a. Aronow WS: Echocardiography should be performed in all elderly patients with congestive heart failure. *J Am Geriatr Soc* 1994; 42:1300–1302.

72. Aronow WS: Digoxin or angiotensin converting enzyme inhibitors for congestive heart failure in geriatric patients. Which is the preferred treatment? *Drugs Aging* 1991; 1:98–103.

73. Elkayam U, Amin J, Mehra A, et al: A prospective, randomized, double-blind, crossover study to compare the efficacy and safety of chronic nifedipine therapy with that of isosorbide dinitrate and their combination in the treatment of chronic congestive heart failure. *Circulation* 1990; 82:1954–1961.

74. Garg R, Yusuf S, for the Collaborative Group on ACE Inhibitor Trials: Overview of randomized trials of angiotensin-converting enzyme inhibitors on mortality and morbidity in patients with heart failure. *JAMA* 1995; 273:1450–1456.

75. Aronow WS, Kronzon I: Effect of enalapril on congestive heart failure treated with diuretics in elderly patients with prior myocardial infarction and normal left ventricular ejection fraction. *Am J Cardiol* 1993; 71:602–604.

76. Cohn JN, Archibald DG, Ziesche S, et al: Effect of vasodilator therapy on mortality in chronic congestive heart failure: Results of a Veterans Administration Cooperative Study. *N Engl J Med* 1986; 314:1547–1552.

77. Cohn JN, Johnson G, Veterans Administration Cooperative Study Group: Heart failure with normal ejection fraction: The V-HeFT Study. *Circulation* 1990; 81(suppl III):III-48–III-53.

77a. The Digitalis Investigation Group: The effect of digoxin on mortality and morbidity in patients with heart failure. *N Engl J Med* 1997; 336:525–533.

78. Fleg JL, Gottlieb SH, Lakatta EG: Is digoxin really important in treatment of compensated heart failure? A placebo-controlled crossover study in patients with sinus rhythm. *Am J Med* 1982; 73:244–250.

79. Aronow WS, Starling L, Etienne F: Lack of efficacy of digoxin in treatment of compensated congestive heart failure with third heart sound and sinus rhythm in elderly patients receiving diuretic therapy. *Am J Cardiol* 1986; 58:168–169.

80. Packer M, Bristow MR, Cohn JN, et al: The effect of carvedilol on morbidity and mortality in patients with chronic heart failure. *N Engl J Med* 1996; 334:1349–1355.

81. Aronow WS, Ahn C, Kronzon I: Effect of propranolol versus no propranolol on total mortality plus nonfatal myocardial infarction in older patients with prior myocardial

infarction, congestive heart failure, and left ventricular ejection fraction ≥40% treated with diuretics plus angiotensin-converting-enzyme inhibitors. *Am J Cardiol* 1997; 80:207–209.

81a.    Aronow WS: Update on treatment of congestive heart failure in older persons. *Clin Geriatr Med* 1998; 6(10):18–32.

82.     Packer M, O'Connor CM, Ghali JK, et al: Effect of amlodipine on morbidity and mortality in severe chronic heart failure. *N Engl J Med* 1996; 335:1107–1114.

83.     Cohn JN, Ziesche S, Smith R, et al: Effect of the calcium antagonist felodipine as supplementary vasodilator therapy in patients with chronic heart failure treated with enalapril. V-HeFT III. *Circulation* 1997; 96:856–863.

84.     Setaro JF, Zaret BL, Schulman DS, Soufer R: Usefulness of verapamil for congestive heart failure associated with abnormal left ventricular diastolic filling and normal left ventricular systolic performance. *Am J Cardiol* 1990; 66:981–986.

85.     Aronow WS, Epstein S, Schwartz KS, Koenigsberg M: Correlation of complex ventricular arrhythmias detected by ambulatory electrocardiographic monitoring with echocardiographic left ventricular hypertrophy in persons older than 62 years in a long-term health care facility. *Am J Cardiol* 1987; 60:730–732.

86.     Aronow WS, Epstein S, Mercando AD: Usefulness of complex ventricular arrhythmias detected by 24-hour ambulatory electrocardiogram and by electrocardiograms with one-minute rhythm strips in predicting new coronary events in elderly patients with and without heart disease. *J Cardiovasc Technol* 1991; 10:21–25.

87.     Aronow WS, Epstein S, Schwartz KS, Koenigsberg M: Prevalence of arrhythmias detected by ambulatory electrocardiographic monitoring and of abnormal left ventricular ejection fraction in persons older than 62 years in a long-term health care facility. *Am J Cardiol* 1987; 59:368–369.

88.     Aronow WS, Ahn C, Mercando AD, et al: Correlation of paroxysmal supraventricular tachycardia, atrial fibrillation, and sinus rhythm with incidences of new thromboembolic stroke in 1476 old-old patients. *Aging Clin Exp Res* 1996; 8:32–34.

89.     Fleg JL, Kennedy HL: Long-term prognostic significance of ambulatory electrocardiographic findings in apparently healthy subjects ≥60 years of age. *Am J Cardiol* 1992; 70:748–751.

90.     Aronow WS, Epstein S, Koenigsberg M, Schwartz KS: Usefulness of echocardiographic abnormal left ventricular ejection fraction, paroxysmal ventricular tachycardia, and complex ventricular arrhythmias in predicting new coronary events in patients over 62 years of age. *Am J Cardiol* 1988; 61:1349–1351.

91.     Aronow WS: Optimal management of older patients with atrial fibrillation. *Drugs Aging* 1994; 4:184–193.

92.     Aronow WS, Ahn C, Mercando AD, Epstein S: Correlation of atrial fibrillation, paroxysmal supraventricular tachycardia, and sinus rhythm with incidences of new coronary events in 1359 patients, mean age 81 years, with heart disease. *Am J Cardiol* 1995; 75:182–184.

93.     Akiyama T, Pawitan Y, Campbell WB, et al: Effects of advancing age on the efficacy and side effects of antiarrhythmic drugs in post-myocardial infarction patients with ventricular arrhythmias. *J Am Geriatr Soc* 1992; 40:666–672.

94.     Aronow WS, Mercando AD, Epstein S, Kronzon I: Effect of quinidine or procainamide versus no antiarrhythmic drug on sudden cardiac death, total cardiac death, and total death in elderly patients with heart disease and complex ventricular arrhythmias. *Am J. Cardiol* 1990; 66:423–428.

95.     Waldo AL, Camm AJ, de Ruyter PL, et al: Effect of D-sotalol on mortality in patients

with left ventricular dysfunction after recent and remote myocardial infarction. *Lancet* 1996; 348:7–12.

95a.   Julian DG, Camm AJ, Frangin G, et al: Randomised trial of effect of amiodarone on mortality in patients with left-ventricular dysfunction after recent myocardial infarction: EMIAT. *Lancet* 1997; 349:667–674.

95b.   Cairns JA, Connolly SJ, Roberts R, Gent M, for the Canadian Amiodarone Myocardial Infarction Arrhythmia Trial Investigators: Randomised trial of outcome after myocardial infarction in patients with frequent or repetitive ventricular premature depolarisations: CAMIAT. *Lancet* 1997; 349:675–682.

96.   Friedman LM, Byington RP, Capone RJ, et al for Beta-Blocker Heart Attack Trial Research Group: Effect of propranolol in patients with myocardial infarction and ventricular arrhythmia. *J Am Coll Cardiol* 1986;7:1–8.

96a.   The Antiarrhythmics Versus Implantable Defibrillators (AVID) Investigators: A comparison of antiarrhythmic-drug therapy with implantable defibrillators in patients resuscitated from near-fatal ventricular arrhythmias. *N Engl J Med* 1997; 337:1576–1583.

97.   Tresch DD, Troup PJ, Thakur RK, et al: Comparison of efficacy of automatic implantable cardioverter defibrillator in patients older and younger than 65 years of age. *Am J Med* 1991; 90:717–724.

98.   Wolf PA, Abbott RD, Kannel WB: Atrial fibrillation as an independent risk factor for stroke: The Framingham Study. *Stroke* 1991; 22:983–988.

99.   Aronow WS, Ahn C, Gutstein H: Prevalence of atrial fibrillation and association of atrial fibrillation with prior and new thromboembolic stroke in older patients. *J Am Geriatr Soc* 1996; 44:521–523.

100.   Kannel WB, Abbott RD, Savage DD, McNamara PM: Epidemiologic features of chronic atrial fibrillation. The Framingham Study. *N Engl J Med* 1982; 306:1018–1022.

101.   Aronow WS, Gutstein H, Hsieh FY: Risk factors for thromboembolic stroke in elderly patients with chronic atrial fibrillation. *Am J Cardiol* 1989; 63:366–367.

102.   Stroke Prevention in Atrial Fibrillation Investigators: Predictors of thromboembolism in atrial fibrillation: I. Clinical features of patients at risk. *Ann Intern Med* 1992; 116:1–5.

103.   EAFT (European Atrial Fibrillation Trial) Study Group: Secondary prevention in non-rheumatic atrial fibrillation after transient ischaemic attack or minor stroke. *Lancet* 1993; 342:1255–1262.

104.   Stroke Prevention in Atrial Fibrillation Investigators: Adjusted-dose warfarin versus low-intensity, fixed-dose warfarin plus aspirin for high-risk patients with atrial fibrillation: Stroke Prevention in Atrial Fibrillation III randomised clinical trial. *Lancet* 1996; 348:633–638.

105.   Stroke Prevention in Atrial Fibrillation Investigators: Predictors of thromboembolism in atrial fibrillation: II. Echocardiographic features of patients at risk. *Ann Intern Med* 1992; 116:6–12.

106.   Peterson P, Kastrup J, Helweg-Larsen S, et al: Risk factors for thromboembolic complications in chronic atrial fibrillation. *Arch Intern Med* 1990; 150:819–821.

106a.   Aronow WS, Ahn C, Kronzon I, Gutstein H: Indicence of new thromboembolic stroke in persons 62 years and older with chronic atrial fibrillation heated with warfarin versus aspirin. *J Am Geriatr Soc* 1999; 47:366–368.

107.   Aronow WS: Correlation of arrhythmias and conduction defects on the resting electrocardiogram with new cardiac events in 1,153 elderly patients. *Am J Noninvas Cardiol* 1991; 5:88–90.

108.   Aronow WS, Mercando AD, Epstein S: Prevalence of arrhythmias detected by 24-hour

ambulatory electrocardiography and value of antiarrhythmic therapy in elderly patients with unexplained syncope. *Am J Cardiol* 1992; 70:408–410.

109. Gregoratos G, Cheitlin MD, Conill A, et al: ACC/AHA Guidelines for Implantation of Cardiac Pacemakers and Antiarrhythmia Devices: Executive Summary. A report of the American College of Cardiology/American Heart Association Task Force on Practice Guidelines (Committee on Pacemaker Implantation). *Circulation* 1998; 97:1325–1335.

110. Mercando AD: Bradyarrhythmias and cardiac pacemakers in the elderly. In: Tresch DD, Aronow WS (eds): *Cardiovascular Disease in the Elderly Patient,* 2d ed. New York: Marcel Dekker, 1999:599–615.

THOMAS S. JOHNSTON

# THE HEART AND ENDOCRINE DISEASES

**CHAPTER**

**49**

Endocrinopathies are multisystem disorders caused by hormone excess, hormone deficiency, or hormone resistance. Most endocrine diseases affect the heart. This chapter will review the important cardiac manifestations of endocrine diseases.

## ACROMEGALY

Acromegaly is characterized by chronic excess secretion of growth hormone, usually from a pituitary adenoma. The lower jaw may become prominent and the shoe size may become larger. Carpal tunnel syndrome may develop. Cardiac complications are the main cause of morbidity and mortality in acromegaly. Cardiovascular abnormalities include hypertension, coronary atherosclerotic heart disease, cardiomegaly, congestive heart failure (CHF), and ventricular arrhythmias.[1]

Hypertension affects approximately one-third of patients with acromegaly. Excess growth hormone and the associated blood volume expansion with acromegaly seem to be primarily responsible for the associated hypertension. The hypertension is generally mild and responds to conventional pharmacologic therapy.[2]

The prevalence of coronary artery disease is uncertain, but angina pectoris is not common. The large epicardial arteries are usually normal; however, the small branch vessels often have abnormal wall thickening, possibly contributing to acromegalic heart disease.[1]

Most patients with acromegaly are asymptomatic for years. Initially there is increased contractility of the left ventricle, increased cardiac output, and decreased systemic vascular resistance. Gradually left ventricular hypertrophy and increased myocardial mass develop as a result of the effects of excess growth hormone. Diastolic dysfunction develops as a result of a combination of left ventricular hypertrophy and marked myocardial fibrosis with collagen deposition. As the condition progresses, systolic performance with exercise deteriorates, and dyspnea on exertion develops. If acromegaly is left untreated, myocardial function deteriorates further, and CHF with low cardiac output follows.[1]

Ventricular arrhythmias are common in acromegalic patients and are often life-threatening.[3] Ventricular arrhythmias unfortunately remain a problem after primary treatment of the acromegaly and subsequent reduction of growth hormone levels because of persistent myocardial damage and fibrosis.

Treatment of the cardiovascular complications of acromegaly includes primary management of the pituitary tumor with either surgery or irradiation. Reversibility or partial reversibility of cardiac dysfunction has been shown with octreotide, a drug that suppresses the secretion of growth hormone from the pituitary adenoma.[1,4] Conventional pharmacologic treatment of hypertension, heart failure, and arrhythmias is indicated. Identification and treatment of other cardiovascular risk factors is also important.

# THYROID DISEASES

Thyroid hormone has numerous effects on the cardiovascular system. These changes in the cardiovascular system occur as a result of direct effects of thyroid hormone on the heart and the peripheral vascular system.

## Hypothyroidism

Hypothyroidism is a disorder in which the thyroid gland fails to secrete adequate amounts of thyroid hormone. The patient's voice may become lower-pitched, and the skin may become dry. The outer portions of the eye brows may become thin, and mentation may become slower than usual. The reflexes may show slow relaxation. Hypothyroidism is associated with several cardiac derangements.[5] The most common cardiac abnormalities are pericardial effusions, CHF, and coronary atherosclerosis. The electrocardiogram may reveal bradycardia and low amplitude of QRS complexes.

Pericardial effusions have been reported to complicate hypothyroidism in as many as 30 to 80 percent of untreated patients.[6] Because of modern diagnostic screening tests for thyroid disease, patients rarely present with profound myxedema, and therefore the incidence of pericardial effusion is less than in the past. A recent echocardiographic study of patients with hypothyroidism detected pericardial effusions in only 6 percent of subjects.[7] Because of the slow accumulation of pericardial fluid, cardiac tamponade is rare, even with large effusions. Pericardial effusions usually resolve after treatment with thyroid hormone replacement.

Hypothyroidism may precipitate CHF in patients with underlying cardiac disease. Hypothyroidism is associated with impaired myocardial contractility, increased peripheral vascular resistance, and bradycardia.[6] Though there are case reports, only rarely is hypothyroidism the primary etiology of CHF. Thyroid hormone replacement is expected to improve cardiac performance in hypothyroid patients with heart failure, and therefore current heart failure management guidelines recommend screening for hypothyroidism in all patients with CHF.[8] Before thyroid replacement is initiated, coronary artery disease (CAD) should be excluded, since thyroid replacement can potentially exacerbate myocardial ischemia by increasing heart rate and cardiac workload.

Arrhythmias due to hypothyroidism are uncommon. Sinus bradycardia, atrioventricular block, and rarely torsades de pointes have been reported to be associated with hypothyroidism.[9]

Treatment of hypothyroidism includes thyroid hormone replacement. Because thyroid hormone can precipitate angina as a result of its positive chronotropic and inotropic effects, it should be initiated at low dosages and titrated gradually until the serum thyroid-stimulating hormone level is within the normal range. If worsening angina occurs with thyroid hormone therapy, the dose should be reduced and antianginal therapy intensified. Concurrent treatment of associated abnormalities, such as hyperlipidemia and hypertension, should also be initiated to reduce cardiac risk.

## Hyperthyroidism

Hyperthyroidism, a disease of excess thyroid hormone, is also associated with a variety of cardiac abnormalities. In contrast to those in hypothyroidism, the cardiovascular effects of hyperthyroidism are characterized by high cardiac output, low peripheral vascular resistance, and a hyperdynamic circulatory state.[10] The patient with thyrotoxicosis may have tachycardia, a hyperdynamic precordium, and bounding pulses with warm skin. Atrial tachyarrhythmias and exacerbations of heart failure are common in hyperthyroidism. Fortunately, ventricular arrhythmias are rare.

Thyroid hormones alter cardiac excitability, especially in the atria, and therefore atrial tachyarrhythmias, including premature atrial contractions, supraventricular tachycardia, atrial flutter, and atrial fibrillation, are common manifestations of hyperthyroidism.[9] Atrial fibrillation occurs in up to 25 percent of patients[11] and may be especially rapid because of the associated increased conduction velocity through the atrioventricular node in hyperthyroidism.[12] Atrial fibrillation may be the only obvious clinical manifestation in a significant number of elderly patients with hyperthyroidism. Therefore, all patients with atrial fibrillation should be screened for hyperthyroidism.[13]

Initially, the most important approach is primary control of the hyperthyroidism with appropriate antithyroid drugs, radioactive ablation, or surgery. The initial goal in the treatment of atrial fibrillation is control of the ventricular rate by digitalis glycosides, beta-adrenergic receptor antagonists, or calcium channel antagonists. Because of the hyperadrenergic state, beta-adrenergic receptor antagonists are especially beneficial in this group. In patients with severe obstructive lung disease, however, this class of drugs should be avoided.[14] It is extremely difficult to reduce the heart rate to normal in hyperthyroid patients without risking drug toxicity. Thus, until the euthyroid state is achieved, the target heart rate should be approximately 120 beats per minute. Most patients spontaneously revert to normal sinus rhythm after achieving the euthyroid state, and therefore cardioversion should be deferred. Patients with a history of previous heart disease, patients with a greater than 13-month duration of atrial fibrillation before the euthyroid state is achieved, and patients with atrial fibrillation 3 months after achieving the euthyroid state are unlikely to spontaneously convert to normal sinus rhythm.[15] In these patients, cardioversion should be considered 4 months after the euthyroid state has been achieved. Arterial thromboembolism can complicate thyrotoxic atrial fibrillation, especially when there is associated structural heart disease, such as mitral valvular disease. In recent trials, chronic anticoagulation has had beneficial effects on the rate of thromboembolic complications in atrial fibrillation. A prospective trial evaluating the efficacy of chronic anticoagulation in patients with atrial fibrillation solely due to hyperthyroidism has not been done, however. Clinical judgment is warranted in this situation.

Congestive heart failure associated with hyperthyroidism is usually due to intrinsic heart disease that has been exacerbated by the thyrotoxic state. There are, however, case studies of CHF primarily due to thyrotoxicosis that report normalization of cardiac function after the euthyroid state has been achieved.[16] Standard heart failure treatment with digitalis glycosides, diuretics, angiotensin-converting enzyme (ACE) inhibitors, and beta-adrenergic blockade should be initiated in addition to primary treatment of the hyperthyroid state.

## DIABETES MELLITUS

Cardiovascular disease is responsible for much of the morbidity and mortality associated with diabetes mellitus. Cardiovascular manifestations of diabetes mellitus include coronary atherosclerotic heart disease, cardiomyopathy, CHF, and autonomic neuropathy. As many as one-half of patients with non-insulin-dependent diabetes die of cardiovascular causes.[17]

Diabetes is a strong independent cardiovascular risk factor. In addition, diabetes predisposes to the development of other known cardiac risk factors, such as hypertension and lipid disorders. Though intensive treatment of diabetes delays the onset and progression of diabetic retinopathy, neuropathy, and nephropathy, it has yet to be established that tight glycemic control reduces cardiovascular risk.[18] Strict diabetes control is recommended, however, to reduce the noncardiac complications of diabetes. Current recommendations are to also modify coexisting cardiac risk factors, including hypertension, cigarette smoking, obesity, and lipid disorders.

The extent and severity of coronary *atherosclerotic heart disease* in diabetic patients exceed those in nondiabetic patients.[19] Mortality rates for myocardial infarctions (MIs) are two to four times higher in diabetic men than in nondiabetic men[20] and four to seven times higher in diabetic women.[21] Myocardial ischemia may not be sensed by the patient so angina and even infarction may go undetected by the patient. Congestive heart failure, mortality, recurrent angina, and reinfarction after myocardial infarction are higher in diabetics than in nondiabetics.[20] Heart failure in diabetics after MI is more common and more severe than would be predicted from the size of the infarct alone.[22] Recent advances in the treatment of MI, including thrombolytic therapy, early beta-adrenergic blockade, and aspirin, improve mortality after myocardial infarction, although diabetics (especially women) do worse than nondiabetics.[23] Worse outcomes in diabetic patients are due to more extensive coronary artery disease, higher restenosis rates after percutaneous transluminal coronary angioplasty (PTCA), and poor non-infarct zone ventricular function.

Treatment of coronary heart disease (CHD) in diabetics includes conventional antianginal therapy, such as nitrates, beta-adrenergic blockers, and aspirin. Hypertensive diabetic patients should receive ACE inhibitor therapy to preserve renal function unless contraindicated. Revascularization procedures, such as PTCA and coronary artery bypass graft surgery (CABGS), are often necessary. Unfortunately, survival 5 years after CABGS is less in diabetics than in nondiabetics.[24] Also, diabetes is an independent predictor of coronary lesion progression after CABGS.[25] Diabetic patients initially have high success rates and low complication rates after conventional PTCA. In long-term follow-up after PTCA, however, diabetics have a higher rate of infarction, a greater need for revascularization, and worse 5-year survival. This is probably a result of a higher rate of early restenosis and late progression of coronary artery disease.[26] Diabetic patients with multivessel disease have better survival with CABGS than with multivessel PTCA.[27]

*Autonomic neuropathy* is common in diabetic patients. Diabetic patients often have higher resting heart rates than nondiabetics (as a result of damage to cardiac efferent parasympathetic nerves) and orthostatic hypotension (as a result of peripheral circulatory sympathetic nerve dysfunction). Because of denervation of sympathetic afferent nerves involved in the perception of pain, many diabetics will have silent myocardial ischemia and infarctions.[28] Although many diabetic patients with myocardial ischemia do not have chest discomfort, however, many will have clinically recognizable anginal equivalents, such as dyspnea, nausea, and diaphoresis. Screening for silent myocardial ischemia is important in these patients with known manifestations of diabetic neuropathy elsewhere. Stress electrocardiography with and without imaging and 24-h Holter monitoring (with special ECG leads) can be used to screen these patients. Denervation of cardiac efferent nerves may also play a role in the systolic and diastolic dysfunction seen in some diabetic patients with heart failure.[20]

*Congestive heart failure* is common in patients with diabetes mellitus. The majority of these patients have either coronary atherosclerotic heart disease or hypertension. Many patients with diabetes and heart failure have a primary cardiomyopathy, however. The pathologic features of this primary cardiomyopathy include diffuse subendocardial fibrosis (perhaps due to small vessel CAD) and extensive interstitial deposition of collagen (most likely a metabolic consequence of the diabetes).[20,29,30] Diabetic cardiomyopathy is associated with both systolic and diastolic dysfunction. The severity of the cardiomyopathy is associated with obesity, and weight loss can have a favorable impact on cardiac function. Over a 3-year follow-up period in the SOLVD[31] trial, patients with left ventricular systolic dysfunction and diabetes had more hospitalizations and a higher mortality than did nondiabetic patients with systolic dysfunction. Treatment consists of the standard regimen of diuretics, digoxin, ACE inhibitors, and beta-adrenergic blockers as tolerated.

## CUSHING'S SYNDROME

Cushing's syndrome is characterized by excess serum cortisol and is associated with obesity, hypertension, and glucose intolerance. Hypertension is usually moderate. Patients with Cushing's syndrome are at risk for atherosclerosis because of the associated hypertension, glucose intolerance, hyperinsulinemia, obesity, and elevated plasma lipids. The mortality of patients with Cushing's syndrome is higher than that of the general population, primarily because of the increased risk of cardiovascular disease.[32] In fact, the most common causes of death after bilateral adrenalectomy for Cushing's disease are cardiac and vascular etiologies.[33]

Electrocardiography and echocardiography demonstrate left ventricular hypertrophy in the majority of these patients.[34] This is felt to be primarily due to the effects of long-standing hypertension.

Treatment with standard antihypertensive agents is usually adequate to control blood pressure in patients with cortisol excess. Identification and treatment of other cardiac risk factors is also important.

## HYPERALDOSTERONISM

Hyperaldosteronism is a syndrome associated with hypersecretion of aldosterone. Primary aldosteronism occurs when the primary stimulus to excess production of aldosterone resides within the adrenal gland. This is usually due to an aldosterone-producing adrenal adenoma. In secondary aldosteronism, the stimulus is extraadrenal.

Hypertension is the most common cardiovascular manifestation of hyperaldosteronism. The hypertension is usually diastolic and mild. Hypokalemia is common. Patients with hyperaldosteronism are nonedematous, hypertensive, and often hypokalemic without concurrent diuretic administration.

Electrocardiography and echocardiography demonstrate left ventricular hypertrophy in the majority of these patients.[35] Prominent U waves, premature ventricular contractions, and other cardiac arrhythmias may be seen as a result of the hypokalemia.

When an adrenal adenoma is responsible for the syndrome, surgical excision of the adenoma is the principal treatment. Dietary sodium restriction and the administration of an aldosterone antagonist such as spironolactone may be used to control hypertension and hypokalemia in those patients who either are inoperable or have bilateral adrenal hyperplasia.

### REFERENCES

1. Sacca L, Cittadini A, Fazio S: Growth hormone and the heart. *Endocr Rev* 1994; 15:555–569.

2. Ezzat S, Forster MJ, Berchtold P, et al: Acromegaly: clinical and biochemical features in 500 patients. *Medicine* 1994; 73:233–239.

3. Kahaly G, Olshausen KV, Mohr-Kahaly S, et al: Arrhythmia profile in acromegaly. *Eur Heart J* 1992; 13:51–56.

4. Giustina A, Boni E, Romanelli G, et al: Cardiopulmonary performance during exercise in acromegaly, and the effects of acute suppression of growth hormone hypersecretion with octreotide. *Am J Cardiol* 1995; 75:1042–1047.

5. Klein I, Ojamaa K: Thyroid hormone and the cardiovascular system: from theory to practice (editorial). *J Clin Endocrinol Metab* 1994; 78:1026–1027.

6. Ladenson PW: Recognition and management of cardiovascular disease related to thyroid dysfunction. *Am J Med* 1990; 88:638–641.

7. Kabadi UM, Kumar SP: Pericardial effusion in primary hypothyroidism. *Am Heart J* 1990; 120:1393–1395.

8. ACC/AHA Task Force on Practice Guidelines: Guidelines for the evaluation and management of heart failure. *J Am Coll Cardiol* 1995; 26:1376–1398.

9. Polikar R, Burger AG, Scherrer U, Nicod P: The thyroid and the heart. *Circulation* 1993; 87:1435–1441.

10. Klein I: Thyroid hormone and the cardiovascular system. *Am J Med* 1990; 88:631–637.

11. Woeber KA: Thyrotoxicosis and the heart. *N Engl J Med* 1992; 327:94–97.

12. Slater A, Klein I: Thyroid disease and the heart. *Practical Cardiology* 1991; 17:19–25.

13. Forfar JC, Miller HC, Toft AD: Occult thyrotoxicosis: a correctable cause of "idiopathic" atrial fibrillation. *Am J Cardiol* 1979; 44:9–12.

14. Klein I, Becker DV, Levey GS: Treatment of hyperthyroid disease. *Ann Intern Med* 1994; 121:281–288.

15. Nakazawa HK, Sakurai K, Hamada N, et al: Management of atrial fibrillation in the post-thyrotoxic state. *Am J Med* 1982; 72:903–906.

16. Likoff WB, Levine SA: Thyrotoxicosis as the sole cause of heart failure. *Am J Med Sci* 1943; 206:425–443.

17. Kessler II: Mortality experience of diabetic patients. A twenty-six year follow-up study. *Am J Med* 1971; 51:715–724.

18. The Diabetes Control and Complications Trial Research Group: The effect of intensive treatment of diabetes on the development and progression of long-term complications in insulin-dependent diabetes mellitus. *N Engl J Med* 1993; 329:977–986.

19. Waller BF, Palumbo PJ, Lie JT, Roberts WC: Status of the coronary arteries at necropsy in diabetes mellitus with onset after age 30 years. *Am J Med* 1980; 69:498.

20. Sniderman A, Michel C, Racine N: Commentary. Heart disease in patients with diabetes mellitus. *J Clin Epidemiol* 1992; 45:1357–1370.

21. Rich-Edwards J, Manson JE, Hennekens CH, Buring JE: The primary prevention of coronary heart disease in women. *N Engl J Med* 1995; 332:1758–1766.

22. Stone PH, Muller JE, Hartwell T, et al: The effect of diabetes mellitus on prognosis and serial left ventricular function after acute myocardial infarction: contribution of both coronary disease and diastolic left ventricular dysfunction to the adverse prognosis. *J Am Coll Cardiol* 1989; 14:49–57.

23. Granger CB, Califf RM, Young S, et al: Outcome of patients with diabetes mellitus and acute myocardial infarction treated with thrombolytic agents. *J Am Coll Cardiol* 1993; 21:920–925.

24. Morris JJ, Smith LR, Jones RH, et al: Influence of diabetes and mammary artery grafting on survival after coronary bypass. *Circulation* 1991; 84(suppl III):III-275–III-284.

25. Alderman EL, Corley SD, Fisher LD, et al: Five-year angiographic follow-up of factors

associated with progression of coronary artery disease in the Coronary Artery Surgery Study (CASS). *J Am Coll Cardiol* 1993; 22:1141–1154.

26. Stein B, Weintraub WS, Gebhart S, et al: Influence of diabetes mellitus on late outcome after percutaneous transluminal coronary angioplasty. *Circulation* 1995; 91:979–989.

27. The Bypass Angioplasty Revascularization Investigation (BARI) Investigators: Comparison of coronary bypass surgery with angioplasty in patients with multivessel disease. *N Engl J Med* 1996; 335:217–225.

28. Langer A, Freeman MR, Josse RG, et al: Detection of silent myocardial ischemia in diabetes mellitus. *Am J Cardiol* 1991; 67:1073–1078.

29. Regan TJ, Lyons MM, Ahmed SS, et al: Evidence for cardiomyopathy in familial diabetes mellitus. *J Clin Invest* 1977; 60:885–899.

30. Factor SM, Minase T, Sonnenblick EH: Clinical and morphological features of human hypertensive-diabetic cardiomyopathy. *Am Heart J* 1980; 99:446–457.

31. Schindler DM, Kostis JB, Yusuf S, et al: Diabetes mellitus, a predictor of morbidity and mortality in the Studies of Left Ventricular Dysfunction (SOLVD) trials and registry. *Am J Cardiol* 1996; 77:1017–1020.

32. Etxabe J, Vazquez JA: Morbidity and mortality in Cushing's disease. *Clin Endocrinol* 1994; 40:479.

33. Welbourn RB: Survival and causes of death after adrenalectomy for Cushing's disease. *Surgery* 1985; 97:16–20.

34. Sugihara N, Shimizu M, Kita Y, et al: Cardiac characteristics and postoperative courses in Cushing's syndrome. *Am J Cardiol* 1992; 69:1475–1480.

35. Yoshitomi Y, Nishikimi T, Abe H, et al: Comparison of changes in cardiac structure after treatment in secondary hypertension. *Hypertension* 1996; 27:319–323.

PAUL H. ROBINSON /
PHYLLIS E. KOZARSKY

CHAPTER

# TRAVEL RECOMMENDATIONS FOR PATIENTS WITH HEART DISEASE

# 50

Travel advice for cardiac patients should be tailored to the individual and given by the individual's cardiologist, internist, or individual care provider. This advice will vary greatly, depending upon not only the variety of each patient's specific needs but also the mode and time of travel, the destination, the duration of stay, and specific planned activities. In this chapter, such specific guidance and advice obviously cannot be provided. In a recent article, one of the authors (PK) states: "Prevention of common problems while traveling is both the easiest and hardest thing to do. Most prevention involves the application of common sense, a commodity which unfortunately is often lacking in travelers."[1] Since the authors have over 30 years' experience in clinical cardiology and public health and have traveled frequently both nationally and internationally, writing this chapter should be a simple, straightforward exercise. But the variety and complexity of the problems presented by each individual must be dealt with one-on-one, taking into account the unique characteristics of the patient and the specifics of the travel itinerary. Searching the literature for previous authors' methods of coping with this problem has not been fruitful. The relatively limited number of related articles characteristically address specific cardiac problems in separate travel contexts (e.g., transportation modes, altitude, environmental temperatures, automobile trips, ocean voyages, etc.). This chapter will contain general information that, it is hoped, will provide helpful guidelines that will enable each unique patient to travel wisely, comfortably, and in relative safety.

## CARDIAC FITNESS TO FLY

Approximately 1 billion people worldwide travel by air each year. In the United States, the number traveling annually is expected to double in the next 20 years. Exact statistical information regarding in-flight medical problems is unknown, since reporting of incidents to the U.S. Department of Transportation is not required unless there is a death or a flight is diverted.[2] In recent years, an average of 21 deaths have occurred annually. In a retrospective study of the period from 1971 to 1980, approximately 8000 medical incidents were found to have been reported to the FAA (1 per 35,000 passengers).[3] Chest pain, dyspnea, loss of consciousness, and nausea and vomiting were the most common complaints. In another FAA study, with good documentation, covering the period 1986 to 1988, 50 percent of the 33 in-flight deaths were related to cardiac problems, and 33 percent had no known cause. An FAA study in 1991 documented that there were physicians available in 85 percent of reported in-flight medical problems. U.S. air carriers with passenger seating capacity of 30 or more are required by the FAA to have a basic medical kit, with additional medications such as bronchodilators and antiarrhythmics for international flights. Defibrillators are available on one major carrier fleet and will soon be available on another. These new defibrillators are very compact—just slightly larger than a laptop computer—and are simple enough to use for an inexperienced layperson to operate one. The instructions are simple: When the chest pads are applied and the power is turned on, the computer analyzes the cardiac rhythm, and voice commands instruct the operator. If life-threatening rhythms are interpreted, a countershock is delivered after warning the operator. Some airlines are contracting with physicians who will provide ground-to-air medical support. Although one-half of in-flight emergencies and unscheduled landings are caused by cardiovascular problems, published data about air travel's effects on cardiac patients are sparse.[2] Since symptoms often occur during takeoff or begin on the ground, such factors as stress, exertion, and anxiety may play a significant role, rather than hypoxia. But cardiorespiratory problems certainly can be precipitated by decreased cabin pressure at altitude. Commercial aircraft cruise between 30,000 and 45,000 ft, resulting in cabin pressures of approximately 6000 to 8000 ft. At the latter pressure, the $Pa_{O_2}$ falls to 55 mmHg. Passengers without cardiorespiratory problems, cerebrovascular disease, or anemia usually have no difficulty, but those with possible problems should have appropriate preflight screening.

Such screening guidelines and determinations concerning fitness to fly were developed in 1960 by the American College of Chest Physicians, based on anecdotal reports of in-flight problems. At that time, a patient who sustained a myocardial infarction (MI) was advised not to travel by air for 24 weeks. In 1982 the AMA recommended a 4-week wait. In 1996, after evaluating FAA and other researchers' data, the Aerospace Medical Association Air Transport Medicine Committee published new guidelines and recommendations covering potential cardiovascular complications (Table 50-1) and indications for medical oxygen (Table 50-2). The absence of angina on stress testing is probably a better predictor of tolerance of air travel than a designated arbitrary time after myocardial infarction. After uncomplicated median sternotomy for coronary bypass or valve surgery, a 2-week recuperation period before flying is recommended. A recent survey of 10,000 post-coronary artery bypass graft patients revealed that 40 percent had traveled during the study year, with a very low percentage of cardiac events.[4] No more than a few days' wait is necessary following uncomplicated cardiac catheterization or coronary angioplasty.

**TABLE 50-1.    Cardiovascular Contraindications to Commercial Airline Flights**

1. Uncomplicated myocardial infarction within 3 weeks

2. Complicated myocardial infarction within 6 weeks

3. Unstable angina

4. Congestive heart failure, severe, decompensated

5. Uncontrolled hypertension

6. Coronary artery bypass graft within 2 weeks

7. CVA within 2 weeks

8. Uncontrolled ventricular or supraventricular tachycardia

9. Eisenmenger's syndrome

10. Severe symptomatic valvular heart disease

From Aerospace Medical Association, Air Transport Committee: Medical guidelines for air travel. *Aviat Space Environ Med* 67 (10 suppl): B1–16, 1996, with permission.

# PACEMAKERS AND DEFIBRILLATORS

The great majority of patients with pacemakers or defibrillators should have no problems with airline electronics or security screening. Scanning using a wand or similar device that contains a magnet can temporarily or permanently disable or alter implanted devices. CPI 1600, 1550, and 1625 defibrillators and others can remain nonoperational even after the magnet is removed. If a patient has an implanted cardiac device, it would be safer if no portable security magnetic instruments were used. Such patients should carry a letter from their physician explaining this problem.[5]

**TABLE 50-2. Cardiopulmonary Indications for Medical Oxygen during Commercial Airline Flights**

1. Use of oxygen at baseline altitude

2. $Pa_{O_2} < 70$ mmHg

3. New York Heart Association class III or IV congestive heart failure

4. Unstable angina

5. Cyanotic congenital heart disease

6. Primary pulmonary hypertension

Adapted from Aerospace Medical Association, Air Transport Committee: Medical guidelines for air travel. *Aviat Space Environ Med* 67 (10 suppl): B1–16, 1996; with permission.

**TABLE 50-3. Recommendations for Air Travelers with Cardiac and/or Pulmonary Dysfunction**

1. Carry all medications on board.

2. Be aware of dose intervals while crossing time zones.

3. Carry a recent ECG.

4. Carry a pacemaker card with an ECG.

5. Use airline special services: wheelchair, trolley services, special diet, oxygen, preboarding.

6. Walk through the cabin frequently and perform in-seat range of motion exercises as well as deep-breathing exercises.

7. Avoid alcohol and drink plenty of fluids.

8. Wear support hose.

# SUPPLEMENTAL OXYGEN

Resting arterial blood gas measurement is considered the best predictor of altitude tolerance.[6]

In general, if the $Pa_{O_2}$ is less than 70 mmHg in a normocapneic patient, supplemental $O_2$ is recommended during flight. Observing the patient's ventilation during a stress test or while walking 50 yd or climbing a flight of stairs is a practical way of assessing ventilatory status. A history of prior problems during flight, the altitude of airplanes, and flight duration should be determined. For patients requiring oxygen, the air carrier should be notified in writing at least 3 days prior to departure, with directions for either 2-or 4-L/min flow. Patients cannot use their own oxygen, and charges may be made by the carrier.

Recommendations for patients with cardiac and/or pulmonary problems are found in Table 50-3.

# THROMBOEMBOLISM

Since 10 percent of all acute thromboembolitic events are now estimated to be related to travel, not only cardiac patients but the general population should be advised about measures to reduce this risk. Prolonged immobility, body fluid shifts, dehydration, and popliteal vein compression place even the average passenger at risk. But these factors result in even greater risk of thrombosis and embolism for the cardiac patient, who is usually older, less well conditioned, and on a variety of medications—often including diuretics—and who has multiple comorbid problems, e.g., obesity, diabetes, vascular disease. Patients with any prior history of thrombosis or embolism, even if they are orally anticoagulated, should be considered for a low-molecular-weight heparin regimen if they are taking transcontinental, international flights, or any travel of comparable duration.

## DIVING

Although the number may be low, there are some cardiac patients who will scuba dive on their vacation. Flying too soon after diving may cause decompression sickness (i.e., the bends), which may be accompanied by major organ system dysfunction. If only one dive per day is made, no flying should be done for 12 hs. For additional recommendations, contact the Diver's Alert Network, 1-800-446-2671.

## ALTITUDE SICKNESS

There are also a few cardiac patients who will travel to significantly higher altitudes for business, leisure, snow skiing, hunting, and trekking—often to substantially greater altitudes. Individuals' ability to acclimatize at various altitudes differs greatly and unpredictably. Altitude sickness results from relative hypoxia caused by the decreased atmospheric partial pressure of oxygen. It is divided into three categories:

1. Acute mountain sickness (AMS) is characterized by headache accompanied by at least one of the following: gastrointestinal upset, nausea, vomiting, fatigue, dizziness, or insomnia. Approximately 25 percent of adults traveling from sea level to 8000 ft will have some symptoms of AMS. This percentage reaches 75 percent at 15,000 ft. Although the incidence of AMS decreases with age, it is unrelated to level of fitness or gender. Altitude acclimatization and alleviation of AMS symptoms usually occurs within 48 to 72 h.

2. High-altitude pulmonary edema (HAPE), the most common cause of altitude-related death, can occur within a few hours but may require several days to become significantly symptomatic after rapid ascent from sea level to 8000 ft or higher. A diagnosis of HAPE requires *two* of these symptoms: dyspnea at rest, cough, weakness, decreased exercise tolerance, chest tightness, or congestion, and at least two of these signs: rales, wheezing, tachycardia, tachypnea, or central cyanosis. HAPE is thought to be caused by increased pulmonary vasoconstriction and low hypoxic ventilatory drive. The hyperactive pulmonary vasoconstriction involves only a portion of the vessels, resulting in overperfusion of those that are unaffected; capillary leakage and edema occur in these overperfused vessels, causing increased hypoxia.[7] HAPE occurs more frequently with rapid ascent to altitude, exertion, higher altitude, low ambient temperature, and hypnotic drug intake. Supplemental oxygen is helpful, as is nitric oxide inhalation, but transport to a lower altitude is often necessary.

3. High-altitude cerebral edema (HACE) usually is evident in an individual with both AMS and HAPE when altered level of consciousness occurs. Confusion,

focal neurologic signs, and hallucinations, if untreated, may result in stupor, coma, and death. Intravenous steroids may help, but transport to a lower altitude is mandatory.

At present there are no screening studies that will predict which individuals are susceptible to altitude sickness. Serious problems can usually be prevented by proper acclimatization (Table 50-4). Patients should be advised about acclimatization and recognition of the symptoms of altitude sickness.

## PRE- AND POSTTRAVEL CARE

The cardiac patient's internist, primary care physician, or cardiologist may feel confident in providing medical advice concerning travel but not in providing other general but very important counseling. Various studies have demonstrated that most physicians are inadequately equipped to provide the detailed, destination, and itinerary-specific health advice necessary for successful travel. Thus the specialty of travel medicine has evolved. The International Society of Travel Medicine (ISTM) is made up of over 1300 professionals worldwide who are dedicated to educating health care personnel and the public regarding health care issues. A list of travel clinics is available on the internet at http:www.istm.org. A resources document is being developed by the ISTM to help travel health advisers access the most current data. The ISTM address is P.O. Box 871089. Stone Mountain, GA 30087-0028, telephone 770-736-7060, fax 770-736-6732, or E-mail bcbistm@aol.com.

**TABLE 50-4. Prevention of Acute Mountain Sickness**

I. Nonpharmacologic

   1. Gradual ascent: 1000 ft/day.

   2. Spend a few nights at intermediate altitudes (8000–10,000 ft).

   3. Slowly ascend at > 8000 ft.

   4. Spend an extra night for every 1000 ft, if continuing to ascend.

   5. Climb high, sleep low (1000 ft lower at night).

   6. Avoid alcohol and sedative-hypnotics.

II. Pharmacologic

   1. Acetazolamide   →125–250 mg PO q8h–q12h starting 24 h prior to ascent and continue for first 2 days at altitude.

                                500 mg PO sustained release tab q24h and continue for first 2 days at altitude.

   2. Dexamethasone   →4 mg PO q6h–q12h.

The Centers for Disease Control (CDC) publishes yearly guidelines on health information for international travel. Copies can be ordered by calling the Superintendent of Documents, Government Printing Office in Washington, D.C., at 202-783-3238 and requesting stock # 017.023.00197-3. The CDC's travelers' health hotline is 404-332-4559 and fax 404-332-4565.

## ILLNESS ABROAD

Self-education and physician counseling regarding self-treatment regimens for minor ailments are important. But finding a competent physician may be difficult and frightening. Contacting someone known to friends or family or contacting an embassy for recommendations may be necessary. The International Association for Assistance to Travelers is a Canadian foundation that publishes a booklet listing English-speaking physicians who agree to see travelers. A copy can be obtained by calling 716-754-4883 in New York or 519-836-0102 in Ontario. Travelers should review their health insurance for coverage in other countries. Obtaining trip cancellation insurance and aeromedical evacuation insurance should be considered.

## CONCLUSION

The authors hope that this general overview and guideline for traveling cardiac patients contains sufficient basic information and provides sufficient reference material to enable these patients' physicians to advise and instruct them adequately. Educating patients and demonstrating the need and importance of their participation in their own care and well-being is tantamount to a healthful life and continued safe journeys through it.

## REFERENCES

1. Kozarsky PE: Prevention of common travel infarcts. *Infect Dis Clin North Am* 1998; 12:305–324.
2. Cox GR, Peterson J, Bouchel L, Delmas JJ: Safety of commercial air travel following myocardial infarction. *Aviat Space Environ Med* 1986; 67:976–982.
3. Kay RS: Preventing in-flight medical problems. *Nurse Pract* 1994; 195: 39–46.
4. Hargarten SW, Anderson AJ, Walker J, Barboriak J: Travel of U.S. citizens after coronary artery bypass surgery. *J of Travel Med* 1996; 3:7–10.
5. Leon MN, Lateef M, Fuentes F: Prevention and management of cardiovascular events during travel. *J Travel Med* 1996; 3:227–230.
6. Cottrell JJ: Altitude exposures during aircraft flight: Flying higher. *Chest* 1988; 92:81–84.
7. Hultgren HN: High-altitude pulmonary edema: Current concepts. *Annu Rev Med* 1996; 47:267–284.

JAMES L. LEVENSON

# PSYCHIATRIC CARE OF CARDIAC PATIENTS

CHAPTER

# 51

## DEPRESSION

Major depression is common in the general population (lifetime prevalence about 10 percent), and even more common among cardiac patients, especially post-myocardial infarction (MI), when the prevalence reaches 15 to 20 percent. Depression may precede, coincide with, or follow the development of coronary artery disease (CAD). Even after adjusting for other recognized risk factors, depression is a risk factor for CAD, and CAD is a risk factor for depression. Most of the clinical risk factors for CAD are themselves increased by depression (e.g., smoking, sedentary lifestyle). The social risk factors for CAD are also risks for depression (living alone, low social support, bereavement, life stress, low education, low socioeconomic status). Depression results in increased morbidity and mortality in cardiac patients. A large controlled study of patients following MI demonstrated that depression was associated at 6 months with a relative risk of death of about 4:1 after adjusting for other risk factors.[1] By 18 months, depression during the first 10 days post-MI was associated with a nearly eightfold increase in mortality.[2]

The mechanism(s) by which depression worsens outcome in coronary artery disease have not been clearly established. At the physiologic level, depression has been associated with increased heart rate variability, arrhythmia, and platelet aggregation. At the psychosocial level, depression results in decreases in functional capacity, motivation, and compliance.

While depression is common in cardiac patients, the diagnosis is not always straightforward. Depression already may be present at the time of MI, emerge in the immediate post-MI period, or emerge weeks to months later. The diagnosis of depression in cardiac patients is based on the same criteria used in the physically healthy and is not phenomenologically different from depression seen in general practice. The diagnosis is often missed, however, because classic symptoms of depression are misattributed to a "normal reaction" to MI (or unstable angina, sudden death, cardiac surgery, etc.). The clinician may minimize the mood disturbance, rationalizing that it is natural for the patient to be upset by a cardiac event. Other classic symptoms such as sleep disturbance, diminished interest or pleasure in activities, loss of appetite, fatigue, and difficulty concentrating may be similarly explained away. For most symptoms of depression, it is a matter of degree, i.e., mild and temporary disruptions in mood and functioning may be part of a normal reaction, but not pervasive or persistent symptoms and dysfunction. Suicidal ideation and feelings of worthlessness or excessive or inappropriate guilt are always highly suggestive of depression.

Depression may present differently in particular patients. Depression should always be considered as a possibility in cardiac patients who are noncompliant with medical care and prescriptions; seem unable to change their lifestyle (especially smoking and being sedentary); are unduly pessimistic or irritable; or develop functional incapacity disproportionate to the severity of their cardiac disease. Patients who become extremely anxious after MI, obsessionally ruminating, somatically preoccupied, and hypervigilant for symptoms of cardiac dysfunction often have an agitated depression. Depression with psychomotor retardation should be suspected in cardiac patients who are too passive, asking no questions, not following through with any of what the physician advises, and initiating nothing on their own. A physician's first clue to the presence of depression may be feeling depressed himself or herself during contacts with the patient (depressed mood can be contagious).

False-positive diagnoses of depression also occur. Cardiac disease can mimic some depressive symptoms, and depression's somatic symptoms require more discriminating interpretation. Sleep disturbance is a classic depressive symptom, but in a cardiac patient it actually might be due to orthopnea, paroxysmal dyspnea, or nocturnal angina. Fatigue, anorexia, and weight loss could be due to depression or to low cardiac output. The psychological symptoms of depression (e.g., dysphoric mood, inappropriate guilt, feelings of worthlessness, suicidal ideation) are more specific indicators of its presence in cardiac patients.

For fuller coverage of psychiatric medication in cardiac patients, the reader is referred elsewhere (see Table 51-1).[3,4] Tricyclic antidepressants are currently not considered to be a good first choice in treating depression with coexisting cardiac disease because of their quinidine-like, anticholinergic, and orthostatic properties. While tricyclic antidepressants had been demonstrated to be generally safe in chronic stable heart disease, they fell out of favor after the Cardiac Arrhythmia Suppression Trial unexpectedly showed that class I antiarrhythmics may increase mortality after MI. Tricyclic antidepressants' cardiac effects are responsible for the risk of fatality in overdoses. They will also have additive effects if the patient is already on a type I antiarrhythmic (e.g., quinidine or procainamide). If a patient is already taking a tricyclic antidepressant when cardiac disease develops acutely (e.g., MI), the tricyclic antidepressant should not be abruptly discontinued, as this increases the risk of arrhythmia (presumably through cholinergic rebound). Newer antidepressants, including the selective serotonin reuptake inhibitors (fluoxetine, sertraline, paroxetine, citalopram, fluvoxamine) and others (bupropion, nefazodone, trazodone), rarely cause cardiovascular side effects. It should also be recognized,

TABLE 51-1.   Selected Drugs for Depression in Cardiac Patients

| Drug | Usual Dosage Range (mg/day) | Side Effects |
|---|---|---|
| *Selective serotonin reuptake inhibitors* | | |
| Fluoxetine (Prozac) | 20–60 | Nausea, diarrhea, insomnia, |
| Sertraline (Zoloft) | 50–200 | agitation, headache, |
| Paroxetine (Paxil) | 20–50 | sweating, sexual |
| Fluvoxamine (Luvox) | 100–200 | dysfunction |
| Citalopram (Celexa) | 20–40 | |
| *$5HT_2$ antagonists* | | |
| Trazodone (Desyrel) | 150–400 | Sedation, orthostasis, |
| Nefazodone (Serzone) | 300–500 | priapism (rare), nausea, |
| | | dizziness, restlessness |
| *Serotonin-norepinephrine reuptake inhibitor* | | |
| Venlafaxine (Effexor) | 75–375 | Same as selective serotonin reuptake inhibitors plus mild hypertension |
| *Noradrenergic-dopaminergic antidepressant* | | |
| Bupropion (Wellbutrin, Zyban) | 200–450 | Restlessness, insomnia, nausea, seizures (over 450 mg/day) |
| *Tricyclic Antidepressants* | | |
| Imipramine (Tofranil) | 75–200 | Quinidine-like, anticholinergic, |
| Nortriptyline (Pamelor) | 50–150 | orthostatic, weight gain, |
| Desipramine (Norpramin) | 75–200 | sexual dysfunction |
| *Stimulants* | | |
| Methylphenidate (Ritalin) | 10–30 | Insomnia, restlessness, abuse, palpitations |

however, that the newer the drug, the less experience there has been in patients with significant cardiac disease. Venlafaxine also has little effect on the heart but may cause slight elevation in blood pressure.

Psychostimulants (most often methylphenidate) are another possible option for treating depression in cardiac patients.[5] In low doses (e.g., 5 to 10 mg bid of methylphenidate), they have no cardiovascular effects, including no effect on blood pressure, and no anorexic effects. They are usually more easily tolerated by patients with chronic medical illness, have very few interactions with other drugs, and provide benefits much more quickly than antidepressants. While they provide an excellent short-term option, long-term treatment of depression with stimulants has been little studied. Dependence and abuse can develop, and psychostimulants are contraindicated in most patients with substance abuse or psychosis. Caution is warranted in their use in patients with poorly controlled hypertension or cardiac arrhythmias.

Electroconvulsive therapy, the most acutely effective treatment for severe depression, can be used safely in stable cardiac disease.[6,7] In patients without cardiac disease, evaluation before electroconvulsive therapy routinely includes an ECG and chest x-ray. The extent of cardiac evaluation indicated in patients with heart disease depends on the nature and the status of their disease. Any cardiac risk comes not from the electrical impulse or the resulting seizure, but from both the anesthesia and the parasympathetic and then sympathetic discharges that follow electroconvulsive therapy. Parasympathetic discharge may result in vagally mediated bradycardia, and sympathetic discharge may result in hypertension, tachycardia, and arrhythmias. These autonomic effects are short-lived but significant in magnitude and are prevented or ameliorated via treatment, respectively, with agents like atropine, propanolol, and/or nifedipine. Patients with preexisting bradyarrhythmias are at increased risk for asystole after electroconvulsive therapy, but ensuring adequate anticholinergic premedication usually permits completing the course of electroconvulsive therapy. ST-segment depression is common with electroconvulsive therapy and may represent ischemia secondary to increased myocardial demand.[8] Electroconvulsive therapy thereby occasionally unmasks previously unrecognized CAD and may aggravate known coronary artery disease. However, modifications in technique can render electroconvulsive therapy relatively safe in stable CAD. Recent MI (or unstable angina) is considered a contraindication to electroconvulsive therapy. There are no data on how long a safe waiting period should be after MI, and it is doubtful that there is a single answer that is applicable to all patients. Instead, in each case, the extent of myocardial injury and coronary obstruction and the stability of cardiac function (angina, arrhythmia, ejection fraction) should be weighed against the relative risk of withholding electroconvulsive therapy. Pacemakers are not a contraindication to electroconvulsive therapy; indeed, they eliminate concern about bradyarrhythmias and asystole. Electroconvulsive therapy has been safely used in patients with automatic implantable cardioverter-defibrillators; some authorities advise that the device should be deactivated just before and reactivated after the therapy.[9]

Controlled trials have demonstrated the efficacy of psychotherapy in depression in general. Cognitive-behavioral and interpersonal therapies can be adapted for the depressed cardiac patient to facilitate cardiac rehabilitation; improve compliance with diet, smoking cessation, activity, and medication prescription; and overcome feelings of insecurity, impotence, and being damaged that often follow myocardial infarction. Large randomized controlled trials of antidepressants and psychotherapy in patients with coronary artery disease are underway.

## ANXIETY

Anxiety has long been regarded as a potential precipitant for acute cardiac events, but it has not been as well studied as depression. Like depression, anxiety may arise alongside or following cardiac disease. Anxiety disorders are common in patients with recurrent arrhythmias, especially those who have experienced "sudden death" and receive automatic implantable cardioverter-defibrillators, and also in patients with cardiomyopathy. Anxiety often contributes to delay in seeking medical attention for acute cardiac symptoms, to denial of illness, and to functional incapacity and invalidism. At the physiologic level, anxious mental stress increases silent myocardial ischemia and arrhythmias in patients with coronary artery disease.[10]

Anxiety disorders are now divided into specific subtypes, all of which are common in cardiac patients; these include generalized anxiety, panic attacks, phobias, and posttraumatic stress. Generalized anxiety often takes the form of "anticipatory anxiety," or hypervigilance for any sign of recurrent chest pain, palpitations, etc. Phobic avoidance of real or feared precipitants of cardiac symptoms, e.g., sexual activity, may develop. Posttraumatic stress reactions include flashbacks, intrusive recollection, and nightmares focused on an acute cardiac experience (MI, arrhythmias, aortic balloon pump, cardioverter-defibrillator shock, etc.). Panic attacks may not be easy to distinguish from angina or arrhythmia, since there are many shared symptoms (shortness of breath, palpitations, chest tightness, light-headedness, and autonomic arousal). Panic attacks and paroxysmal atrial tachycardia can be especially difficult to distinguish, since both frequently occur in a young, otherwise healthy, predominantly female population. Making such distinctions is sometimes futile, since panic attacks often follow and become commingled with recurrent cardiac symptoms. There has been a controversial association between panic disorder and mitral valve prolapse, and no convincing etiologic relationship has been established. Most experts consider this to involve mild, nonstructural (nonpathologic) mitral valve prolapse.

Automatic implantable cardioverter-defibrillators can be especially "anxiogenic." Their recipients have already typically had multiple episodes of frightening arrhythmias, including "sudden death," and experienced repeated failures of one antiarrhythmic drug after another. The cardioverter-defibrillator's unpredictable discharge is literally a shocking experience. If the cardioverter-defibrillator discharged in response to recurrent arrhythmia, the patient has been acutely reminded how close he or she remains to a fatal event. If it has erroneously discharged during normal rhythm, the patient may not find it very reassuring to hear that this was "just a little malfunction." Multiple discharges during a short time period are especially psychologically traumatic. This is consistent with the long-standing experimental model for evoking depressive and anxiety syndromes in mammals by administering multiple unpredictable electric shocks.

Benzodiazepines, which have essentially no cardiovascular adverse effects, are safe and effective for the acute treatment of anxiety in cardiac patients (see Table 51-2). For severe acute anxiety, only lorazepam or midazolam can be given intramuscularly (though intramuscular injections are avoided in the cardiac care unit); either of these or diazepam can be given intravenously. For ambulatory patients with anxiety disorders, antidepressants (usually not tricyclic antidepressants for the reasons discussed earlier) are often preferable because there is no risk of dependency or withdrawal. However, the therapeutic effects of antidepressants, for anxiety or depression, are delayed in onset (1 to 6 weeks). Benzodiazepines do provide immediate benefit, and so a common strategy is to prescribe one temporarily until

**TABLE 51-2.  Selected Drugs for Treating Anxiety Disorders in Cardiac Patients**

| Drug | Usual Dosage Range (mg/day) | Side Effects |
|---|---|---|
| *Antidepressants*: | Any agent in Table 51-1 except methylphenidate | |
| Benzodiazepines | | |
| Lorazepam (Ativan) | 1–4 | Sedation, amnesia, ataxia, |
| Alprazolam (Xanax) | 1–4 | dizziness, abuse |
| Clonazepam (Klonopin) | 1–4 | |
| Diazepam (Valium) | 5–40 | |
| Buspirone | | |
| BuSpar | 15–60 | Rare (nausea, headache, dizziness) |

the antidepressant can take effect. A benzodiazepine with an intermediate half-life, such as clonazepam, may be a better choice for chronic therapy than one with a short half-life (alprazolam, lorazepam), since the latter are more likely to result in withdrawal and dependence. Buspirone is another alternative for chronic treatment of the anxious cardiac patient, as it is free of any cardiac side effects and has no risk of withdrawal or addiction. Onset of action is about 1 week, and it must be taken tid. Buspirone is less effective than antidepressants or benzodiazepines for moderate to severe anxiety. Beta blockers reduce peripheral (somatic) manifestations of anxiety, but do not help central (psychological) anxiety, and must be individualized if the patient has congestive heart failure.

Psychotherapy is also effective and often essential in the treatment of anxiety disorders. Relaxation techniques are helpful for most forms of anxiety, and specific techniques can be applied to particular problems (e.g., desensitization for phobic avoidance of exercise-induced tachycardia; biofeedback for stress-induced labile hypertension; cognitive therapy for anxious preoccupation with family history of cardiac disease).

## ATYPICAL CHEST PAIN

Psychopathology commonly occurs in atypical chest pain and also in patients with "typical" angina who have normal or near-normal coronary arteries on cardiac catheterization. Panic disorder, major depression, multiple phobias, somatization disorder, and conversion disorder are frequent causes of atypical chest pain. When chest pain is caused by panic disorder, it typically occurs in brief episodes accompanied by other panic symptoms (see above) in a patient who appears highly anxious. Panic attacks presenting with chest pain are responsible for many emergency room visits and "R/O MI admissions." Chest pain due to major depression is usually more sustained, aching, and accompanied by prominent fatigue and psychomotor retardation (or agitation). Multiple phobias should be suspected when recurrent chest pain occurs as part of exposure to, or in anticipation of, the feared objects or conditions. In somatization disorder, the patient has, in addition to chest pain, multiple unexplained noncardiac physical symptoms over a period of years, often leading to polypharmacy, polyinvestigation, and polysurgery. In conversion disorder, the patient may be incongruously blasé while describing chest pain melodramatically.

When chest pain's presentation is atypical, consideration of a psychiatric etiology should not be delayed until the end of an exhaustive search for a cardiac, pulmonary, or gastrointestinal cause. Psychiatric diagnoses are not diagnoses of exclusion, both in the sense that they are based on positive criteria and in the sense that the presence of an "organic" explanation does not preclude coexisting psychiatric illness.

Thus, in evaluating atypical chest pain, the physician should actively consider the possibility of a psychiatric diagnosis and seek appropriate information in the interview to rule it in or out. Repetitive, excessive evaluations for organic heart disease (e.g., multiple normal catheterizations) not only are inefficient and wasteful but also reinforce psychopathology (e.g., they increase the panic patient's anxiety, the depressed patient's hopelessness, and the somatizing patient's attachment to the sick role). Treatment of psychogenic atypical chest pain should be matched to the particular psychiatric diagnosis. When a definitive psychiatric diagnosis cannot be made, and cardiac or other medical causes are not demonstrable, atypical chest pain may still improve with antidepressant treatment. However, improvement of chest pain following treatment with psychotropic medication does not by itself "prove" a psychiatric etiology, since antidepressants and antianxiety drugs may ameliorate many types of pain.

## COGNITIVE DISORDERS

Cognitive dysfunction may be a reversible or permanent consequence of cardiac disease as a result of hypoxia, poor central nervous system perfusion, or emboli. Low cardiac output does not usually lead to cognitive deficits until the ejection fraction is $\leq 10$ to 15 percent unless the patient also has cerebrovascular disease. If cognitive dysfunction persists after improvement in cardiac output, it is usually irreversible.

Delirium, defined as an acute confusional state with perceptual disturbances (e.g., visual hallucinations) and altered consciousness, is common as a complication of acute heart failure, cardiac surgery, aortic balloon pumps, left ventricular assist devices, and endocarditis. Delirium is more common in the elderly and in patients with preexisting cognitive disorders (especially dementia). Neuropsychiatric complications are common after all major cardiac surgery, including valve replacement, coronary artery bypass graft, and transplantation. Microemboli, time on heart-lung bypass, and preexisting cerebrovascular disease have all been implicated as risk factors. Acute psychosis after cardiac surgery, with delusions, hallucinations, and/or catatonia, typically resolves within 2 weeks. Subtle cognitive deficits may persist much longer.

**TABLE 51-3.**   Selected Drugs for Treating Agitation in Cardiac Patients

| Drug | Usual Parenteral Starting Dose | Side Effects |
|---|---|---|
| *Neuroleptics* <br> Haloperidol (Haldol) | 0.5 mg bid–tid | Dystonia, akathisia, torsades de pointes (rare, high dosage) |
| *Benzodiazepines* <br> Lorazepam (Ativan) | 1 mg bid–tid | Sedation, amnesia, ataxia, dizziness, respiratory depression, hypotension |

The first priority of management is identifying and correcting reversible etiologic factors (e.g., hypoxia, infection, hyponatremia, renal failure, and medication—especially anticholinergic drugs). Environmental interventions, including frequent reorientation, calendars, clocks, familiar objects from home, and night lights, are helpful. Haloperidol is the most commonly used sedative; it can be given orally, intramuscularly, or intravenously (see Table 51-3). It primarily reduces agitation and psychotic symptoms, but it does not reverse the cognitive dysfunction in delirium. Low doses usually suffice (<10 mg/24 h), but on rare occasions patients have required over 1000 mg/24 h. Haloperidol has been the neuroleptic of choice because it is relatively free of the quinidine-like, anticholinergic, and hypotensive effects of antipsychotic drugs like chlorpromazine, although extrapyramidal effects (dystonia, akathisia, cogwheel rigidity) are not uncommon. High-dose intravenous haloperidol has on rare occasions resulted in torsades de pointes, and so extra caution is required when using it in patients with other risk factors for ventricular arrhythmias (prolonged QT interval, alcohol dependence, cardiomyopathy, etc.). Haloperidol can cause T-wave changes on the ECG as well.

# PSYCHIATRIC SIDE EFFECTS OF CARDIAC DRUGS

Nearly all antiarrhythmics have occasionally resulted in psychiatric side effects, most often anxiety, agitation, and psychosis. This was a frequent problem in cardiac care units at the time when all patients admitted with myocardial infarction were placed on lidocaine drips prophylactically. Quinidine can cause confusion and agitation. Digitalis has caused depression, confusion, and psychosis (especially visual hallucinations), even on rare occasions at therapeutic serum levels.

Central nervous system symptoms are the biggest category of side effects of antihypertensives, with depression, insomnia, and reduced libido most common. This is true of beta blockers, clonidine, methyldopa, reserpine, and less frequently ACE inhibitors, calcium channel blockers, and hydralazine. Most diuretics rarely have central nervous system effects themselves, but overdiuresis (hypovolemia, hypokalemia, hyponatremia) commonly causes weakness, confusion, and a depressed appearance. Most inotropic agents (e.g., amrinone, dopamine, dobutamine) do not cross the blood-brain barrier and so have no neuropsychiatric effects. L-dopa does cross, and psychosis, agitation, confusion, and insomnia are common with it. For more details regarding psychiatric side effects, the reader is referred elsewhere.[3]

### REFERENCES

1. Frasure-Smith N, Lesperance F, Talajic M: Depression following myocardial infarction. Impact on 6-month survival. *JAMA* 1993; 270:1819–1825.
2. Frasure-Smith N, Lesperance F, Talajic M: Depression and 18-month prognosis following myocardial infarction. *Circulation* 1995; 91:999–1005.
3. Levenson JL, Dwight M: Cardiovascular disease. In: Stoudemire A, Fogel BS, Greenberg D (eds): *Psychiatric Care of the Medical Patient,* 2d ed. New York, Oxford University Press, 1999 (in press).
4. Stoudemire A, Fogel BS, Gulley LR, Moran MG: Psychopharmacology in the medical patient. In: Stoudemire A, Fogel BS, Greenberg D (eds): *Psychiatric Care of the Medical Patient*, 2d ed. New York, Oxford University Press, 1999 (in press).
5. Masand PS, Tesar GE: Use of stimulants in the medically ill. *Psychiat Clin North Am* 1996; 19:515–548.
6. Rice EH, Sombrotto LB, Markowitz JC, Leon AC: Cardiovascular morbidity in high-risk patients during ECT. *Am J Psychiatry* 1994; 151:1637–1641.
7. Zielinski RJ, Roose SP, Devanand DP, et al: Cardiovascular complications of ECT in depressed patients with cardiac disease. *Am J Psychiatry* 1993; 150:904–909.
8. Messina AG, Paranicas M, Katz B, et al: Effect of electroconvulsive therapy on the electrocardiogram and echocardiogram. *Anesth Analg* 1992; 75:511–514.
9. Pinski SL, Trohman RG: Implantable cardioverter-defibrillators: Implications for the nonelectrophysiologist. *Ann Intern Med* 1995; 122:770–777.
10. Mittleman M, Maclure M: Mental stress during daily life triggers myocardial ischemia. *JAMA* 1997; 277:1558–1559.

# CARDIAC DRUG INTERACTIONS

Frequently, a cardiac patient is placed on a variety of medications (cardiac and non-cardiac) to treat one or more medical conditions. For example, a patient with atrial fibrillation may be on digoxin, amiodarone, and warfarin. That same patient may also be on an angiotensin-converting enzyme (ACE) inhibitor and a diuretic for the treatment of heart failure and on a lipid-lowering medication. Physicians need to recognize adverse drug interactions and be aware of any potential hazard when a new medication is added (or removed if, for example, the patient is on warfarin).

Drug interactions are generally viewed as unpredictable and undesirable. Certain drug interactions, however, can be desirable or advantageous, while others have no clinical consequence. A desirable interaction, for example, might be improved blood pressure control as a result of the additive or synergistic effects obtained when several antihypertensives are combined. The addition of a diuretic to digoxin or an ACE inhibitor may be necessary for the treatment of congestive heart failure and at the same time improve blood pressure control.

While untoward interactions between medications can be subtle and of no clinical significance, some can be serious and life-threatening. It is therefore important to appreciate the general principles that underlie drug interactions. Some medications interact with a large number of others from different categories, making it impossible for a physician to memorize specific interactions.

Drug interactions may involve several mechanisms. Some lead to increased bioavailability of the medication and potentiate its effect, and some make it less available. Such mechanisms are termed pharmacokinetic interactions and include interference with or enhancement of drug absorption, distribution, protein binding, affinity to receptors, liver metabolism, and renal excretion. The effect of such interactions can in some instances be measured by a specific test, such as the international normalized ratio (INR) in the case of warfarin. Other types of interactions are regarded as pharmacodynamic, in which the side effects of two medications become additive or antagonistic. Examples are severe bradycardia caused by a combination of medications with a negative chronotropic effect or excess hypotension caused by a combination of medications that lower blood pressure.

The pharmacokinetic and pharmacodynamic properties of medications and thus the drug interaction potentials can differ substantially among patients. This can be due to a number of reasons, the most important of which are variations in the expression of different cytochrome P450 enzymes. The cytochrome P450 enzymes are a group of enzymes that are found predominantly in the liver but are also present in the brain, gastrointestinal wall, and other tissues. Currently, there are at least 30 related enzymes, which are divided into different families. Cytochrome P450 3A4 has been shown to metabolize the largest number of drugs and constitutes one-third of the P450 in the liver and 70 percent of the enzyme in the gastrointestinal wall. The activity may peak in early life and decrease in older individuals, especially those over the age of 70. Certain drugs may induce the activity of this important enzyme, and others may inhibit its action.

When considering the variable effects of drugs and drug interactions, it is important to recognize the contribution of the patient's age, gender, weight, and current state of health or comorbidities. Other contributing factors such as smoking, alcohol consumption, dietary habits, and the use of over-the-counter or nonprescription medications such as vitamins and herbs or health food items should be assessed.

This chapter will address the most important interactions among the common categories of medications used in patients with cardiovascular diseases. The categories include drugs that affect rhythm, heart rate, blood pressure, congestive heart failure, ischemia, coagulation, and lipids:

- Anticoagulants
- Antiplatelet agents
- Thrombolytics
- Antiarrhythmics
- ACE inhibitors
- Angiotensin II receptor antagonists
- Beta blockers
- Calcium channel blockers
- Nitrates
- Vasodilators
- Diuretics
- Lipid-lowering agents
- Digoxin

## ANTICOAGULANTS[1–5]

Heparin is a frequently used treatment modality in patients admitted to the hospital with unstable angina. It is often coadministered with intravenous nitroglycerin, which can result in reduction of the activated partial thromboplastin time (APTT) and possible rebound after discontinuation of nitroglycerin. Aspirin can enhance the APTT. The anticoagulant effect of heparin can be attenuated by the concomitant use of different drugs, such as digoxin and antihistamines.

The list of medications that can interact with warfarin is very long. This is primarily due to certain properties of the medication, including its cytochrome P450–dependent metabolism and its narrow therapeutic range. It is therefore prudent to check the INR more frequently when an interaction is suspected and to adjust the dose of warfarin accordingly. It is as important to readjust the dose of warfarin in the event that a suspected medication is deleted from the therapeutic regimen.

Medications that are known to enhance the anticoagulant effect of warfarin and therefore increase the INR include a variety of antibiotics, allopurinol, and quinidine. Amiodarone potentiates the effect of warfarin by a mechanism that is not well understood. Because of the extended half-life of amiodarone, its effect on warfarin can last long after it is discontinued. Cimetidine is well known to inhibit the metabolism of several medications, including warfarin. On the other hand, rifampin and the barbiturates increase the rate of warfarin metabolism by inducing hepatic metabolizing enzymes, thus decreasing the INR.

Since warfarin inhibits hepatic synthesis of vitamin K–dependent coagulation factors, drugs that slow the absorption of vitamin K or that reduce the intestinal bacterial flora that produce vitamin K will increase the effect of warfarin.

Examples of drugs that will potentiate the anticoagulant effect of warfarin include metronidazole, Septra, and erythromycin. Drugs that inhibit the anticoagulant effect include cholestyramine, barbiturates, rifampin, griseofulvin, carbamazepine, and penicillin. A complete list of drugs that are known to *increase* or *decrease* the effect of warfarin is available in the *Physicians' Desk Reference* (PDR)[1] under "Coumadin."

# ANTIPLATELET AGENTS[1,6]

In the absence of major contraindications, all patients with coronary artery disease should receive aspirin. The risk of gastrointestinal irritation is increased in patients receiving corticosteroids or nonsteroidal anti-inflammatory drugs (NSAIDs) and who consume excessive amounts of alcohol.

Plavix (clopidogrel bisulfate) is a direct inhibitor of adenosine diphosphate and inhibits platelet aggregation. Its use has increased with intracoronary stenting. It has become customary to use it in combination with aspirin for about 4 weeks following coronary stent implantation. The safety of its concomitant use with aspirin on a chronic basis has not been studied. Plavix does not change the level of coagulation seen with heparin; however, the safety of its combination with either heparin or warfarin has not been established. Care should be taken when Plavix is coadministered with NSAIDs because of the possible potentiation of gastrointestinal bleeding. In vitro studies have shown that high doses of clopidogrel bisulfate can inhibit cytochrome P450 (2C9), but there are no studies that analyze the interaction of Plavix with medications that use this pathway for metabolism, such as warfarin and fluvastatin.

Ticlid (ticlopidine hydrochloride) is another oral agent that inhibits platelet aggregation. In cardiovascular diseases it has been used extensively in the treatment of transient ischemic attacks and with intracoronary stent implantation. Its use has declined in favor of Plavix, however, because of the rare but potentially serious problems with neutropenia and thrombotic thrombocytopenic purpura. The safety of combining ticlopidine with aspirin has not been well studied; therefore, it would be best to avoid the combination of these two antiplatelet agents. Ticlid can increase the levels of drugs that are metabolized by the hepatic microsomal system. Its absorption is somewhat reduced with antacids. The combination of ticlopidine with digoxin causes very little alteration in the therapeutic efficacy of digoxin. Ticlid can result in an increase in the plasma level of theophylline and phenytoin. It is advisable to measure the level of phenytoin in the plasma of patients who are also receiving ticlopidine. No significant drug interactions have been found when ticlopidine was used in combination with calcium antagonists, beta blockers, or diuretics.

## THROMBOLYTICS[1,7]

Care should be taken when coadministering, with thrombolytics, medications that could increase the risk of bleeding such as heparin, warfarin, and antiplatelet agents, which include aspirin, dipyridamole, and the IIb/IIIa platelet receptor antagonists. Also, since the clearance of thrombolytics depends on hepatic blood flow, hypoperfusion of the liver from cardiogenic shock complicating an acute myocardial infarction may increase the risk of drug-drug interactions.

## ANTIARRHYTHMICS[1,2,8]

Quinidine usage in clinical practice has declined dramatically because of quinidine's low safety profile and relatively low efficacy compared to newer antiarrhythmics. Quinidine slows the elimination of digoxin, enhances the effect of warfarin, and potentiates the effect of verapamil (hypotension). The metabolism of quinidine is increased by drugs such as rifampin and slowed by cimetidine. Quinidine has a vasodilating effect as well as a negative inotropic and a vagolytic effect and therefore can interact with drugs that have similar properties.

Quinidine is a potent inhibitor of P450 2D6. This can result in accumulation of susceptible drugs and a decrease in metabolite formation. The inhibition of the P450 2D6–mediated metabolism of propafenone results in elevated plasma concentration and increased beta-adrenergic receptor blockade.

Renal clearance of procainamide decreases with concomitant administration of cimetidine. The plasma concentration level of procainamide can be increased with amiodarone.

Propafenone and quinidine are usually not used together, but when they are, quinidine slows the metabolism of propafenone. The serum level of digoxin is increased with concomitant administration of propafenone. Also, propafenone slows the metabolism of beta blockers such as propranolol and metoprolol, therefore increasing their plasma concentration. Propafenone can increase the prothrombin time in patients on warfarin.

Sotalol is an antiarrhythmic agent with both class II (beta-blocking) and class III (prolongation of action potential) properties. Several drug interactions should be taken into account: Concomitant use of other beta-blocking medications results in an additive effect; similarly, the use of calcium channel blockers with sotalol may have additive effects on atrioventricular (AV) nodal conduction and blood pressure. In general, other antiarrhythmics should be used with caution; in particular, the concomitant use of class Ia and class III medications is not recommended.

In patients receiving digoxin, the proarrhythmic effects of sotalol can be exaggerated. In patients treated for diabetes mellitus, hyperglycemia may occur, requiring adjustment of the insulin or oral hypoglycemic dosages. As with pure beta blockers, the symptoms of hypoglycemia can be masked in diabetic patients receiving sotalol.

Amiodarone has a very long half-life. Therefore, potential drug interactions should be kept in mind after amiodarone is discontinued. Amiodarone has been shown to raise the plasma level of cyclosporine. The level of digitalis can also increase, and that usually necessitates cutting the dose of digitalis in half and following its serum level. Amiodarone's interaction with warfarin is discussed elsewhere in this chapter.

Amiodarone can potentiate bradycardia and should therefore be used cautiously with other medications that can slow the sinoatrial or AV node. It can also prolong the QT interval with type I antiarrhythmics and tricyclic antidepressants.

Amiodarone is a potent inhibitor of the renal elimination and hepatic metabolism of numerous drugs. The dosage of warfarin, quinidine, procainamide, flecainide, and digoxin may need to be reduced with concomitant amiodarone therapy.

# ACE INHIBITORS[1,9-12]

When several antihypertensive medications, such as an ACE inhibitor with a beta blocker and a diuretic, are combined, the risk of hypotension increases because of additive effects. This can be even more pronounced in volume-depleted patients. Potassium-sparing diuretics, potassium supplements, and potassium-containing salt substitutes should be used with caution because of the potassium-retaining properties of the ACE inhibitors. Indomethacin and possibly other NSAIDs can reduce the antihypertensive effect of certain ACE inhibitors such as captopril, especially in patients with low renin hypertension. Coadministration of aspirin was shown not to interfere with the blood pressure–lowering effect of captopril in healthy human subjects. Patients on concomitant lithium and ACE inhibitor therapy should have serum lithium levels monitored frequently because of increased risk of lithium toxicity.

# ANGIOTENSIN II RECEPTOR ANTAGONISTS[1,2]

Losartan has been studied clinically with a number of other medications (warfarin, digoxin, cimetidine, and hydrochlorothiazide), and no appreciable pharmacologic interactions could be demonstrated.

## BETA BLOCKERS[13,14]

In patients with a depressed left ventricular ejection fraction, the addition of a calcium antagonist to a beta blocker can result in further reduction in myocardial contractility and the onset of congestive heart failure. Cimetidine increases blood levels of the beta blockers that are metabolized in the liver, such as metoprolol and atenolol, by decreasing hepatic blood flow. The antihypertensive effect of beta blockers may be reduced by the presence of NSAIDs.

## CALCIUM CHANNEL BLOCKERS[1,2,15,16]

Check for excessive bradycardia and even AV nodal block in patients who are receiving beta blockers and/or digitalis together with a calcium channel blocker such as diltiazem or verapamil. Cimetidine can increase the plasma level of calcium channel blockers. Diltiazem and verapamil can inhibit the hepatic metabolism of certain drugs. Verapamil, for example, increases the plasma level of digoxin, theophylline, quinidine, and prazosin. Diltiazem increases the plasma level of cyclosporine and lovastatin.

## NITRATES[1,2,17,18]

The risk of hypotension is increased with the therapy that is usually used for angina, including nitrates, beta blockers, and calcium channel blockers.

The recent availability of Viagra raises concern regarding patients on nitroglycerin. Viagra (sildenafil citrate) is a selective inhibitor of phosphodiesterase type 5 (PDE 5), which is responsible for degradation of cyclic guanosine monophosphate (cGMP) in the corpus cavernosum. With sexual stimulation, there is local release of nitric oxide, which increases levels of cGMP, causing smooth muscle relaxation and allowing inflow of blood. Similarly, sildenafil leads to increased levels of cGMP, which in the presence of sexual stimulation enhances erection.

PDE 5 is found in human corpus cavernosum smooth muscle but is also found in lower concentrations in other tissues, including vascular smooth muscle. Therefore, Viagra has systemic vasodilatory properties that can result in a transient mild decrease in blood pressure; this is of little clinical significance in most patients. More importantly, Viagra potentiates the hypotensive effects of nitrates, consistent with its actions on the nitric oxide/cGMP pathway.

Coadministration of organic nitrates and Viagra on a regular or intermittent basis is contraindicated. The question of when patients can use nitrates safely after taking Viagra remains unanswered, but it is known that the plasma level of sildenafil at 24 h postdose is very low compared to peak levels.

# VASODILATORS[1,2,17,18]

The combination of hydralazine and monoamine oxidase inhibitors should be used with caution. When used together, hydralazine and diazoxide injections can produce significant hypotension. Hydralazine may increase the plasma levels of metoprolol and propranolol by affecting hepatic blood flow. The concomitant administration of hydralazine and nitrates has been shown to reduce nitrate tolerance.

Orthostatic hypotension is a potential problem with any medication that causes peripheral vasodilatation or volume depletion (diuretics).

# DIURETICS[1,2,17]

Cholestyramine may bind thiazide diuretics and reduce their absorption from the gastrointestinal tract. Combined treatment with steroids and thiazide diuretics may lower the threshold for hypokalemia. The dose of oral hypoglycemics and insulin therapy usually requires adjustment when combined with thiazide diuretics.

Lithium is not metabolized and depends totally on the kidneys for excretion and clearance from the body. Thiazide diuretics lead to depletion of sodium and retention of lithium. Thus, lithium should not be administered with thiazide diuretics, or should be administered with caution, because of the potential for reduced excretion that can result in lithium toxicity. In general, lithium should be avoided with diuretics.

In combination with loop diuretics, potassium-sparing diuretics, or thiazides, NSAIDs may reduce the diuretic efficacy of the medications. In some patients the mechanism is believed to be inhibition of prostaglandin synthesis. There are case reports of reduction in renal clearance, weight gain, and hyperkalemia when furosemide was combined with NSAIDs.

Combining a loop diuretic and a thiazide diuretic produces a positive drug interaction. These drugs produce their diuretic effect on different portions of the renal tubule, and thus their effect is additive, resulting in a greater diuretic response. This can be beneficial in congestive heart failure when the intention is to remove a larger amount of fluid. It can, however, be deleterious and cause hypotension (excessive volume loss) in certain situations.

When given with aminoglycoside antibiotics, loop diuretics such as furosemide can increase the risk of ototoxicity. The risk of ototoxicity also increases when furosemide is combined with ethacrynic acid.

The administration of furosemide and sucralfate should be spaced by at least 2 h because of the potential reduction in the therapeutic effect if the two medications are taken at the same time.

Aldactone (spironolactone) is a potassium-sparing diuretic that has received renewed attention for its beneficial effect in the treatment of congestive heart failure. Hyperkalemia can result from its combination with ACE inhibitors. Spironolactone has been shown to increase the half-life of digoxin. It may potentiate orthostatic hypotension if combined with barbiturates or narcotics.

# LIPID-LOWERING AGENTS[1,19,20]

The risk of myositis and rhabdomyolysis with potential renal failure during therapy with the HMG-CoA reductase inhibitors can be increased when these are combined with cyclosporine, erythromycin, gemfibrozil, or nicotinic acid. However, the benefit of achieving adequate lipid control by combining lipid-lowering medications should be weighed against the small risk of myositis.

Some HMG-CoA reductase inhibitors such as Zocor (simvastatin) and Mevacor (lovastatin) as well as gemfibrozil can increase the effect of warfarin and therefore require close monitoring of the prothrombin time and INR. Pravachol (pravastatin sodium) does not alter the prothrombin time appreciably when used concomitantly with warfarin. Lipitor (atorvastatin calcium), one of the newest synthetic lipid-lowering medications that inhibits HMG-CoA reductase, does not alter the prothrombin time significantly when administered to patients receiving chronic warfarin treatment. It increases the plasma level of digoxin by about 20 percent, however. When Lipitor is used with the antacid Maalox, the plasma concentration is decreased without a definitive alteration in the reduction in low-density lipoprotein cholesterol levels. When Lipitor and erythromycin (an inhibitor of cytochrome P450 3A4) are used concomitantly, the plasma concentration of Lipitor is increased. Mevacor and Zocor are also metabolized by cytochrome P450 3A4. Pravachol (pravastatin) is not metabolized by cytochrome P450 3A4 to a clinically significant extent.

# DIGOXIN[1,2,21,22]

Hypokalemia caused by diuretic therapy may cause digitalis toxicity. The plasma level of digoxin can increase when digoxin is combined with verapamil, amiodarone, propafenone, indomethacin, quinidine, erythromycin, and tetracycline. Certain drugs such as antacids and cholestyramine can decrease absorption of digoxin and therefore lower its serum concentration. Certain anticancer drugs may also reduce intestinal absorption of digoxin and lower its effect.

## REFERENCES

1. *Physicians' Desk Reference* 1999 [www.pdrnet.com].
2. Opie LH: Adverse cardiovascular drug interactions. In: Alexander RW, Schlant RC, Fuster V, et al (eds): *Hurst's The Heart*, 9th ed. New York, McGraw-Hill, 1998: 2371.
3. Harder S, Thurmann P: Clinically important drug interactions with anticoagulants. An update. *Clin Pharmacokinet* 1996; 30:416–444.

4. Doucet J, Chassagne P, Trivalle C, et al: Drug-drug interactions related to hospital admissions in older adults: a prospective study of 1000 patients. *J Am Geriatr Soc* 1996; 44:944–948.

5. Wells PS, Holbrook AM, Crowther NR, Hirsh J: Interactions of warfarin with drugs and food. *Ann Intern Med* 1994; 121:676–683.

6. Wiltink EH: Medication control in hospitals: a practical approach to the problem of drug-drug interactions. *Pharmacy World & Science* 1998; 20:173–177.

7. de Boer A, van Griensven JM: Drug interactions with thrombolytic agents. Current perspectives. *Clin Pharmacokinet* 1995; 28:315–326.

8. Ha HR, Candinas R, Stieger B, et al: Interaction between amiodarone and lidocaine. *J Cardiovasc Pharmacol* 1996; 28:533–539.

9. Boger RH, Bode-Boger SM, Kramme P, et al: Effect of captopril on prostacyclin and nitric oxide formation in healthy human subjects: interaction with low-dose acetylsalicylic acid. *Br J Clin Pharmacol* 1996; 42:721–727.

10. Mignat C, Unger T: ACE inhibitors. Drug interactions of clinical significance. *Drug Safety* 1995; 12:334–347.

11. Di Somma S, Carotenuto A, de Divitiis M, et al: Favourable interaction of calcium antagonist plus ACE inhibitor on cardiac haemodynamics in treating hypertension: rest and effort evaluation. *J Hum Hypertens* 1995; 9:163–168.

12. Shionoiri H: Pharmacokinetic drug interactions with ACE inhibitors. *Clin Pharmacokinet* 1993; 25:20–58.

13. Molina Cuevas V, Arruzazabala ML, Carbajal Quintana D, et al: Effect of policosanol on arterial blood pressure in rats. Study of the pharmacological interaction with nifedipine and propranolol. *Arch Med Res* 1998; 29:21–24.

14. Blaufarb I, Pfeifer TM, Frishman WH: Beta-blockers. Drug interactions of clinical significance. *Drug Safety* 1995; 13:359–370.

15. Azie NE, Brater DC, Becker PA, et al: The interaction of diltiazem with lovastatin and pravastatin. *Clin Pharmacol Ther* 1998; 64:369–377.

16. Rosenthal T, Ezra D: Calcium antagonists. Drug interactions of clinical significance. *Drug Safety* 1995; 13:157–187.

17. Opie LH: Interactions with cardiovascular drugs. *Curr Probl Cardiol* 1993; 18:531–581.

18. Juggi JS, Koenig-Berard E, Vitou P: Vasodilator therapy: interaction of nitrates with angiotensin-converting enzyme inhibitors. *Can J Cardiol* 1991; 7:419–425.

19. von Moltke LL, Greenblatt DJ, Schmider J, et al: Metabolism of drugs by cytochrome P450 3A isoforms. Implications for drug interactions in psychopharmacology. *Clin Pharmacokinet* 1995; 29(suppl 1):33–43; discussion 43–44.

20. Sadowski DC: Drug interactions with antacids. Mechanisms and clinical significance. *Drug Safety* 1994; 11:395–407.

21. Siepmann M, Kleinbloesem C, Kirch W: The interaction of the calcium antagonist RO 40-5967 with digoxin. *Br J Clin Pharmacol* 1995; 39:491–496.

22. Magnani B, Malini PL: Cardiac glycosides. Drug interactions of clinical significance. *Drug Safety* 1995; 12:97–109.

MAHOMED Y. SALAME /
NICOLAS A. F. CHRONOS

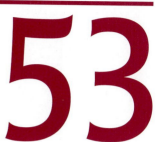

# CHAPTER

# 53

# ANTICOAGULATION AND ANTIPLATELET THERAPY IN HEART DISEASE

There is increasing evidence that the thrombotic process plays a major role in cardiovascular disease. In recent years, there has been a greater understanding of the interrelationship of the coagulation cascade and platelet activation and of their role in cardiovascular pathology.[1] Prior to this, much of antithrombotic therapy had been empiric, with little clinical trial data to support it. Tremendous strides in our understanding of these complex processes have allowed more targeted and effective therapies to be introduced into widespread clinical practice. Thus today, a patient with a prosthetic heart valve should be treated very differently from a patient with unstable angina, as targeted approaches exist for the different types of thrombotic entities.

This chapter examines the important role of antithrombotic therapy in common cardiovascular diseases. A description of the important antithrombotic agents [antiplatelet agents: aspirin, ticlopidine, clopidogrel, and glycoprotein IIb/IIIa (GPIIb/IIIa) inhibitors; and anticoagulation agents: heparin, including low-molecular-weight heparin, and warfarin] is given (Table 53-1). This is followed by a review of the evidence for the use of these agents in the principal areas of thrombosis in heart disease, including acute coronary syndromes, atrial fibrillation, and valvular heart disease, thus giving a framework for the evidence-based usage of these drugs.

## DESCRIPTION OF PRESENT ANTITHROMBOTIC DRUGS

### Antiplatelets

**ASPIRIN.** Until recently, aspirin (acetylsalicylic acid) was the mainstay of antiplatelet therapy at daily doses of 75 to 325 mg; however, it is a relatively weak an-

**TABLE 53-1.   The Commonly Used Antiplatelet and Anticoagulant Agents**

| Antithrombotic Drugs | | |
|---|---|---|
| Antiplatelets | Cyclooxygenase inhibitor: | aspirin |
| | ADP antagonists: | ticlopidine, clopidogrel |
| | GPIIb/IIIa receptor antagonists: | abciximab |
| | | small molecules |
| | | eptifibatide |
| | | tirofiban |
| | | xemilofiban, etc |
| Anticoagulants | Coumadin | Warfarin |
| | Heparin | —unfractionated and low molecular weight |

tiplatelet agent. The documented beneficial coronary effects include the primary prevention of coronary artery disease[2] and improvement of outcome in chronic stable angina,[3,4] unstable angina,[5–7] and acute myocardial infarction (AMI).[8] It also improves the saphenous vein graft patency rate after coronary artery bypass grafting.[9] In the field of percutaneous coronary intervention, preprocedural administration of aspirin reduces the risk of abrupt coronary closure by 50 to 75 percent.[10,11]

It works by irreversibly acetylating and thus inactivating prostaglandin synthetase/cyclooxygenase[12] and results in the decreased formation of thromboxane $A_2$,[13] a potent agonist of platelet aggregation.[14] Platelets, however, are able to undergo aggregation by a number of thromboxane $A_2$–independent pathways [via platelet activators such as thrombin, adenosine diphosphate (ADP), adrenaline, and subendothelial collagen],[15–17] thus limiting the antithrombotic effect of aspirin. A daily dose of 80 mg aspirin is sufficient to produce virtually complete suppression of cyclooxygenase after 2 days, while 160 mg and higher doses will have this effect within 24 h. In addition, aspirin, by inhibiting gastric mucosal prostaglandin E production, has the side effect of gastritis in a significant proportion of patients, resulting in noncompliance. The risk of gastric bleeding is dose-related; it is relatively small at doses of 75 mg/day and progressively increases at doses of 300 to 3600 mg/day.[18–21]

**TICLOPIDINE.**   Ticlopidine, a potent antiplatelet drug, is clinically used in cardiology in patients with unstable angina and in patients undergoing coronary stent implantation. It is effective in inhibiting ADP-induced platelet aggregation even at very high concentrations of ADP.[22] Ticlopidine is normally administered at a dose of 500 mg/day, but several days of therapy are required for optimal efficacy. The antiplatelet effect persists for approximately 72 h following discontinuation of ticlopidine. The drug may produce diarrhea, rash, liver function abnormalities, and, in particular, reversible neutropenia[23] (up to 1 percent of cases) and thrombocytopenia. Leukocyte counts should therefore be monitored in the initial months of therapy.

**CLOPIDOGREL.** Clopidogrel, a thienopyridine compound, is a new analog of ticlopidine that inhibits platelet aggregation[24] by inhibiting the binding of adenosine 5′-diphosphate to its platelet receptor. Clopidogrel does not have the bone marrow suppression problems associated with ticlopidine. A preliminary study in a large group of patients (CARPIE study)[25] has demonstrated its antithrombotic efficacy in the absence of significant neutropenia or hepatic dysfunction. However, clopidogrel has not been evaluated in acute situations.

**GPIIB/IIIA INHIBITORS.** There has been a rapid expansion of trial data on the use of GPIIb/IIIa receptor antagonists across the full spectrum of acute coronary syndromes. This is in part related to a recognition of the limitations of other antiplatelet agents and a better understanding of the mechanisms of platelet activation and aggregation. Because the GPIIb/IIIa platelet receptor is the final common pathway through which all the platelet agonists exhibit their effects on platelet aggregation, this receptor is a promising target for antiplatelet therapy.[26]

The GPIIb/IIIa receptor belongs to the integrin family of adhesion molecules; binds fibrinogen, von Willebrand factor, and vitronectin; and is therefore able to form cross-bridges between adjacent platelets. Platelet activation results in the exposure of the fibrinogen (RGD) binding site of the GPIIb/IIIa receptor on the cell surface.

The GPIIb/IIIa inhibitors are a relatively new class of compound that offers several potential advantages over other currently available therapies. These compounds are relatively specific to platelets; they inhibit platelet aggregation induced by all platelet agonists, while at the same time they do not affect platelet adhesion. Coller et al developed the murine 7E3 monoclonal antibody to the GPIIb/IIIa receptor,[27] and this was further refined to abciximab, a chimeric Fab fragment of the antibody, in order to minimize the immune reaction to the foreign protein.[28] Likewise, a number of peptides and nonpeptides that either contain or mimic the arginine-glycine-asparagine (RGD) necessary for the GPIIb/IIIa receptor–ligand binding have been developed. The small-molecule (either peptidic or nonpeptidic) GPIIb/IIIa inhibitors are designed to avoid antibody-induced disadvantages, such as immunogenicity, and to have rapid onset of action and rapid off rate with cessation of drug delivery.

The intravenous route offers speed of onset of action (which is important in unstable angina requiring hospitalization) and also allows peptides to be administered. Intravenous administration is impractical and expensive for long-term use, however. The intravenous agents include abciximab, tirofiban, and eptifibatide. The current development of orally active GPIIb/IIIa inhibitors, e.g., xemilofiban, sibrafiban, and orbofiban, will allow the strategy of long-term GPIIb/IIIa blockade to be evaluated in thrombotic diseases.

**PERSANTIN.**   Persantin has fallen out of favor as an antiplatelet agent and is therefore considered to be of limited utility in today's clinical practice.

## Anticoagulants

**HEPARIN.**   Unfractionated heparin is a heterogeneous mixture of glycosamino-glycans. It is extracted from beef or pig lung or gut mucosa. The active portion of the molecule is a relatively small component (molecular weight about 5000) containing a pentasaccharide sequence that attaches to antithrombin III. Antithrombin III is a circulating, relatively weak inhibitor of thrombin (factor IIa), activated factor X, and activated factors IX, XI, and XII. When the heparin active site binds to antithrombin III, the inhibitory action is markedly accelerated. Very small fragments of heparin, so long as they contain the high-affinity pentasaccharide sequence, are able to attach to antithrombin III and accelerate inhibition of factor Xa. However, the inhibition of thrombin requires simultaneous binding of heparin to antithrombin III and thrombin, which can be achieved only by heparin fragments of 18 or more polysaccharide residues.

Heparin is effective only parenterally and is administered intravenously (IV) or subcutaneously. After injection, heparin circulates bound to many plasma proteins, several of which may be elevated in inflammatory or malignant disorders (acute-phase reactants), decreasing the anticoagulant effect for a given heparin dose. Heparin kinetics are complex. Initial injection is followed by a phase of rapid elimination as a result of dispersal into the distribution volume and variable protein binding. There is then a phase of more gradual elimination, but the half-life varies depending upon the dose administered and the rate of renal and hepatic elimination. After the usual bolus dose of 75 U/kg, the half-life is approximately 1 h with normal renal and hepatic function. Because the kinetics are unpredictable from patient to patient, and may vary in a given patient depending upon changes in levels of binding proteins, close monitoring of the anticoagulant effect is required in order to ensure optimal dosage. There is evidence that the maintenance of activated partial thromboplastin time (APPT) between 1.5 and 2 is necessary for adequate efficacy, while excessive levels of APPT result in higher bleeding risk.[29]

In general, when states of established thrombosis or embolism exist, heparin is administered in a loading dose of 75 U/kg IV, and maintenance is achieved with continuous IV infusion, initially at 1000 to 1250 U/h. High-dose subcutaneous heparin q12h has been used to achieve an anticoagulant effect. Such treatment is not reliable unless APPTs are monitored and kept in the therapeutic range.[30] Low-dose heparin prophylaxis against venous thrombosis is generally accomplished with subcutaneous heparin 5000 units q8h or 7500 units q12h.

Heparin has several disadvantages. It not only acts to inhibit activated clotting factors, but also appears to activate platelets and increase capillary permeability, enhancing the risk of bleeding at a given level of anticoagulant effect. It is, however, rather ineffective as an inhibitor of fibrin-bound thrombin. Very high doses of heparin are required to inhibit clot-bound thrombin, markedly increasing the risk of bleeding. The unpredictable dose requirements make accurate prediction of a safe initial dosage difficult in acute thrombotic situations and necessitate frequent monitoring and dose adjustments. The requirement for parenteral administration is limiting. Hemorrhagic complications of heparin are relatively infrequent and tend to occur when the APPT is excessively prolonged, a bleeding risk is present, or intermittent rather than continuous heparin administration is employed.[29] Heparin-induced thrombocytopenia may occur; it is usually asymptomatic, but it may be associated with dire clinical consequences, as noted below. It is thought to originate from the formation of an IgG-heparin immune complex that affects the circulating platelets. Its incidence is about 2 percent with therapeutic doses and less with prophylactic doses, and it characteristically appears at 3 to 15 days (mean 10 days) after beginning heparin therapy and resolves within 4 days of discontinuing the drug. The condition may occur within hours if the patient has previously received heparin. Thrombocytopenia may be accompanied paradoxically by venous or arterial thrombosis. Platelet counts should be monitored routinely during heparin therapy. Long-term administration of heparin may cause osteoporosis.

**LOW-MOLECULAR-WEIGHT HEPARIN.** Chemical or enzymatic depolymerization of unfractionated heparin is performed to obtain low-molecular-weight heparin (LMWH) preparations with mean molecular weights ranging from below 4000 to approximately 6500. Their mechanism of antithrombotic action is similar to that of unfractionated heparin in that they bind to antithrombin III and increase the inhibitory effect on several activated coagulation factors. However, the various preparations have different potencies of anti-Xa and antithrombin activity. Shorter fragments containing the essential pentasaccharide are able to bind to antithrombin but lack the required chain length to bind to thrombin at the same time, and thus inhibit only activated factor X. Fragments with molecular weights above 5000 containing the pentasaccharide maintain their property to inhibit factor Xa, but with increasing chain length, they become stronger inhibitors of thrombin.

LMWHs have little or no effect on global tests of blood coagulation such as the activated partial thromboplastin time when used in prophylactic or therapeutic dosages. LMWH treatment has been monitored by measurement of anti-factor Xa activity, but this may not accurately reflect the anticoagulant action because LMWHs also inhibit factor II. The Heptest is a clotting assay that is sensitive to both anti-Xa and anti-IIa activity, as well as to inhibition of the extrinsic pathway by LMWH-stimulated release of tissue factor pathway inhibitor. The plasma thrombin neutralization assay has also been used to measure LMWH and to detect low concentrations to which chromogenic assays are insensitive.[31]

The main clinical advantage of LMWHs is related to their pharmacokinetic properties. While the plasma half-life of unfractionated heparin is nonlinearly dose-related, in part because of the saturable binding to plasma proteins, endothelial cells, and platelets, LMWHs bind far less to these elements and therefore have a plasma half-life two to four times longer, a markedly better bioavailability when injected subcutaneously, and a more predictable and stable dose response. The suitability for the subcutaneous route of delivery; the lower incidence of heparin-induced thrombocytopenia,[32] osteoporosis, and skin necrosis;[33] and the lack of need for routine monitoring of levels make LMWH more suitable for long-term treatment. Neither unfractionated nor low-molecular-weight heparin crosses the placenta, and so both appear to be relatively safe for the fetus, and both can be administered to nursing mothers. In addition to their use in postsurgical and medical prophylaxis of deep vein thrombosis, LMWHs are being used for cardiovascular and cerebrovascular indications.

**WARFARIN.**    Of the many Coumarin derivatives available, sodium warfarin is the principal oral anticoagulant used in North America.[29, 34] The drug is given orally (although parenteral forms are available), is metabolized in the liver by hydroxylation, and is excreted in the urine. Warfarin has relatively rapid absorption. Its action is to inhibit the hepatic synthesis of the vitamin K–dependent factors II, VII, IX, and X, and so its onset of action is gradual and related to the half-lives of these proteins (which range from 5 h for factor VII to 4 days for factor II). Coagulation becomes prolonged as the factors become depleted. Warfarin also suppresses synthesis of the anticoagulant proteins C and S, thus tending to counteract, to some extent, its own overall anticoagulant effect, particularly in the initial phase of treatment.

It is generally recommended that warfarin therapy be initiated with an estimated daily maintenance dose (usually 4 to 5 mg) over 4 to 5 days, thus avoiding a loading dose. If heparin is already being administered, the two therapies are generally overlapped during this initial period, and then the heparin is discontinued. When warfarin is commenced in hospital, there may be some advantage to giving an initial small loading dose, in the range of 10 mg/day, for the first 2 to 3 days. On an outpatient basis, the first International Normalized Ratio (INR) should be measured prior to instituting warfarin. The INR measurement can then be repeated in 3 days, and then done approximately twice weekly for 2 weeks and once weekly for about 2 weeks; after that the intervals may be gradually extended to a maximum of 4 to 8 weeks. The currently employed INR ranges are 2 to 3 for most conditions, although somewhat higher INRs are recommended for mechanical prosthetic heart valves or recurrent systemic embolization. The warfarin itself has a half-life of 36 to 42 h, and therefore the inhibitory effect requires several days to resolve after discontinuing warfarin.

The principal complication of warfarin is hemorrhage, which is more likely to occur with excessive INR prolongation and in patients with bleeding tendencies. The dosage of warfarin required to produce therapeutic prolongation of the INR is highly variable from person to person and often varies from time to time in a given person even when drug compliance is optimal. It is likely that dietary changes resulting from increased vitamin K absorption (i.e., green vegetables) or decreased vitamin K absorption (i.e., fat malabsorption) or perhaps increased catabolism of coagulation factors during febrile illnesses account for some of the variability. Many drugs may influence the INR by altering the metabolism or absorption of warfarin, by altering the synthesis and metabolism of vitamin K and the coagulation factors, or by influencing platelet function. Patients receiving warfarin should not initiate or discontinue any other drug without medical advice. If a change is necessary and the drug is known to enhance or diminish warfarin anticoagulant effects, more frequent INR monitoring is required for a time.

Warfarin crosses the placenta and can produce a characteristic embryopathy during the first trimester, central nervous system abnormalities at any time during the pregnancy, and cerebral hemorrhage at birth.[35] Warfarin should be given to fertile women only when they are practicing reliable contraceptive measures, must be avoided throughout the first trimester, and preferably should be avoided throughout pregnancy. Warfarin also occasionally induces a characteristic skin necrosis that appears to be related to a deficiency of protein C and possibly protein S.[29]

**DIRECT THROMBIN INHIBITORS: HIRUDIN AND HIRULOG.** Hirudin is the first parenteral anticoagulant introduced since the discovery of heparin. It a single peptide chain of 65 amino acids with a molecular weight of approximately 7000 and is the naturally occurring anticoagulant of the leech *Hirudo medicinalis*. R-hirudin, a recombinant form of hirudin, is a potent thrombin-specific inhibitor. The direct thrombin inhibitors have a number of theoretical advantages over heparin: Hirudin does not require antithrombin III as a cofactor; it is not inactivated by antiheparin proteins, e.g., platelet factor 4; and it has no direct effects on platelets and may also inactivate thrombin bound to clot or the subendothelium and thus restrict the further formation of thrombus.[36] Hirudin has a half-life of 2 to 3 h.[37]

Hirulog is a synthetic 20-amino-acid peptide based on the leech-derived compound hirudin. Like hirudin, hirulog is a specific direct inhibitor of free and clot-bound thrombin. Hirulog causes a dose-dependent prolongation of the aPTT and a reduction in plasma fibrinopeptide A levels.

# ACUTE CORONARY SYNDROMES—THE CONSERVATIVE APPROACH

A significant proportion of the population experiences the consequences of acute atherosclerotic plaque rupture, be it spontaneous, as in unstable angina or AMI, or iatrogenic, as in percutaneous transluminal coronary angioplasty (PTCA). At the site of plaque rupture, there is exposure of highly thrombogenic materials,[38] including subendothelial collagen and cholesterol-rich materials that initiate both the activation of platelets and the coagulation cascade, resulting in thrombus formation locally that unfavorably influences the rheology of blood flow to produce even more thrombus.

## Antithrombotic Therapy in Patients with Unstable Angina/Non-Q-Wave MI Who Are Being Treated by Conservative Medical Therapy

**ASPIRIN AND HEPARIN IN UNSTABLE ANGINA/NON-Q-WAVE MI.** The initial large randomized, double-blind clinical trials evaluating aspirin versus placebo in unstable angina/non-Q-wave MI[6,39] focused on the reduction in cardiac death and nonfatal infarction over a 3- to 24-month period. In the Veterans Administration Cooperative Study,[39] 324 mg of aspirin daily for 12 weeks reduced the incidence of death or myocardial infarction by 51 percent (10.1 percent versus 5.0 percent, $p = .001$), with a similar relative reduction in mortality (3.1 percent versus 1.6 percent).

Subsequently, the Theroux study[7] recruited a higher proportion of very unstable patients early in the hospital course, randomized them to aspirin 650 mg daily, heparin, both, or neither, and followed them up over the acute period. Over the mean 6-day follow-up, the incidence of refractory angina was decreased in the heparin-only arm compared to placebo ($p = .002$), while the aspirin-only arm demonstrated a reduction from 23 percent to 17 percent ($p = .217$). Myocardial infarction was significantly reduced in the three treatment arms, from 11.9 percent (placebo) to 3.3 percent (aspirin-only group), 0.8 percent (heparin-only), and 1.6 percent (aspirin plus heparin). There were, however, no significant differences between one treatment arm and another. Other studies have shown a benefit from aspirin at a dose of only 75 mg/day.

The data on heparin are less clear-cut than those for aspirin. Intravenous heparin does appear to reduce cardiac events in this patient group to a similar extent to aspirin in the initial 5 to 7 days of treatment of unstable angina.[7,40] However, reactivation of angina upon stopping heparin is more common in patients treated with heparin without aspirin.[41] A combination of aspirin and heparin appears in most studies to be more effective than either agent alone. Therefore, the combination of aspirin and heparin early in the course of an episode of unstable angina is preferable to aspirin alone, and there appears to be no increase in bleeding risk.

Long-term benefit of aspirin for unstable angina/non-Q-wave MI continues (nonfatal and fatal MI reduced by 52 percent).[7] Indeed, patients on chronic aspirin who are admitted to hospital with unstable angina are less likely to present with non-Q-wave MI than those not on prior aspirin (5 percent versus 14 percent, respectively, $p = .004$).[42] *These data suggest that all patients need to be on long-term aspirin for secondary prevention, provided they can tolerate it.*

**TICLOPIDINE IN PATIENTS WITH UNSTABLE ANGINA/NON-Q-WAVE MI BEING TREATED BY A CONSERVATIVE MEDICAL APPROACH.** In patients with unstable angina who did not receive aspirin, ticlopidine reduced fatal and nonfatal MI by 53 percent. The role of ticlopidine in the conservative treatment of unstable angina is unclear, however, in patients who can take chronic aspirin. It may be an effective alternative to aspirin in patients who are unable to tolerate the latter; however, the risk of neutropenia with chronic use is problematic. Clopidogrel may therefore be a better alternative.

**GPIIB/IIIA INHIBITORS IN THE CONSERVATIVE TREATMENT OF UNSTABLE ANGINA/NON-Q-WAVE MI.** The use of intravenous GPIIb/IIIa inhibitors as part of a pharmacologically based treatment strategy for unstable angina/non-Q-wave MI has been evaluated in four large randomized clinical trials. The results generally show a benefit for the GPIIb/IIIa inhibitors. The pooled analysis from the four trials in over 16,500 patients showed a clear benefit, with a 12 percent reduction in events at 30 days, $p < .01$. The need for heparin in patients with unstable angina treated with GPIIb/IIIa agents is not clearly established. However, in the studies that directly compared GPIIb/IIIa inhibitors with and without heparin, there were fewer events with combination therapy.

**LOW-MOLECULAR-WEIGHT HEPARIN IN UNSTABLE ANGINA/NON-Q-WAVE MI.** These agents appear to be at least as effective as unfractionated heparin. Event rates have been shown to be reduced by the use of LMWH in combination with aspirin. There is also evidence that LMWH may be superior to unfractionated heparin when either is used with aspirin. Thus, LMWH plus aspirin is a suitable and perhaps even preferable alternative to unfractionated heparin plus aspirin in the treatment of unstable angina/non-Q-wave MI.

**WARFARIN IN UNSTABLE ANGINA/NON-Q-WAVE MI.** Several studies have been carried out comparing aspirin against aspirin plus anticoagulant therapy (heparin followed by warfarin) in unstable angina/non-Q-wave MI. On the whole, these trials (including ATACS)[43] have shown additional benefit with combination therapy. The recently published OASIS pilot study[44] demonstrated that long-term treatment with moderate-intensity warfarin (INR 2.0 to 2.5) plus aspirin reduced the rate of recurrent ischemic events in patients with unstable angina, but low-intensity warfarin (INR 1.5) plus aspirin did not. However, there was an excess of minor bleeds in the warfarin group (28.6 percent versus 12.1 percent, $p = .004$). This approach cannot yet be recommended as standard therapy.

**SUMMARY ON THE USE OF ANTITHROMBOTIC THERAPY IN PATIENTS WITH UNSTABLE ANGINA / NON-Q-WAVE MI AND RECEIVING CONSERVATIVE MEDICAL TREATMENT.** The bulk of the evidence suggests that most patients with unstable angina should be treated with both antiplatelet and anticoagulant therapies. Of the antiplatelet agents, aspirin is effective, has the longest clinical experience, and is relatively inexpensive, and so it remains part of standard therapy for acute coronary syndromes. Ticlopidine has been shown to be of benefit in the conservative management of patients (not on aspirin) with unstable angina, and it could therefore be used in those patients who are unable to take aspirin. More recently, GPIIb/IIIa inhibitors in combination with aspirin have been evaluated and have been found to significantly reduce ischemic end points further. With respect to the anticoagulants, direct antithrombins have demonstrated an early but ephemeral clinical benefit. LMWHs appear to be more effective than non-fractionated heparin and are easier and safer to use. A combination of dalteparin and aspirin for at least 6 days could be considered in patients with unstable coronary artery disease (CAD) to reduce the risk of new cardiac events and to allow time for risk stratification and selection of a long-term treatment strategy.

In the future, more potent oral antiplatelet agents such as the oral GPIIb/IIIa inhibitors may have a place in subacute and chronic therapy. Long-term anticoagulation with warfarin at moderate intensity (INR 2.0 to 2.5) in addition to aspirin following acute ischemic syndromes appears to be promising in reducing recurrent ischemic events, and the OASIS-2 trial[45] is aimed at clarifying this.

## Acute Myocardial Infarction

**ASPIRIN IN ACUTE MYOCARDIAL INFARCTION.**   Data from several large trials have shown that aspirin is strikingly effective in the treatment of AMI. Aspirin alone gives a reduction in early mortality of approximately 25 percent, and in combination with thrombolytic agents it gives a reduction of about 40 percent. This early reduction in mortality persists for at least a year when aspirin is continued. Consequently, aspirin therapy for AMI is recommended as soon as possible after the clinical impression of evolving AMI is formed, whether or not thrombolytic therapy is to be given.

**ADJUNCTIVE GPIIB/IIIA INHIBITORS IN PATIENTS WITH AMI UNDERGOING FIBRINOLYTIC THERAPY.**   Over the past decade, the use of fibrinolytic therapy has revolutionized the care of patients with AMI, with much emphasis being placed on the speed of initiating treatment and thus achieving early recanalization. The importance of achieving early recanalization was emphasized by the finding that restoration of effective flow in the infarct-related vessel 90 min after fibrinolytic therapy was associated with a halving of the 30-day mortality compared to no or very low flow. However, even the most efficacious thrombolytic regimens do not give uniformly high flow reperfusion, and there is a relatively high incidence of reocclusion. Thus, alternative adjunctive strategies are being tested. Several pilot trials with GPIIb/IIIa inhibitors and thrombolytic therapy in treatment of AMI have been completed, and larger trials are underway. Preliminary results are encouraging that these antiplatelet drugs will improve reperfusion therapy, but the use of GPIIb/IIIa inhibitors as adjunctive therapy with thrombolytics cannot be recommended at this time.

**CLOPIDOGREL IN AMI.**   In the CAPRIE study[25] of patients with atherosclerotic disease, one of the patient groups included was those with a recent MI (<35 days). Clopidogrel 75 mg once daily was associated with an 8.7 percent relative risk reduction of vascular events compared to aspirin 325 mg once daily in the whole group of patients. Clopidogrel has not been evaluated in the setting of an AMI, however.

**HEPARIN IN AMI.**   The early trials of thrombolysis for acute MI showed that reocclusion of the infarct-related vessel was relatively common. This led to consideration of using heparin as adjunctive therapy to reduce this problem. The potential benefit of this approach appeared to be supported by small angiographic studies in AMI patients. Since the publication of the GUSTO-1 study,[46] which showed that an accelerated tPA regimen followed by intravenous heparin reduced mortality compared to streptokinase plus either subcutaneous or intravenous heparin, it has become standard policy to use intravenous heparin for up to 48 h after tPA infusion for AMI.

**LOW-MOLECULAR-WEIGHT HEPARIN POSTTHROMBOLYSIS FOR AMI.**
At present, there are no reported studies comparing unfractionated heparin and
LMWH post–AMI.

**WARFARIN IN AMI.** Several studies in the prethrombolytic era showed mortality benefit with the long-term use of warfarin in patients who were not on aspirin
and who had had a previous MI (approximately 20 percent reduction). Definitive efficacy of warfarin in this setting has been demonstrated only in the absence of antiplatelet therapy. Warfarin therefore tends to be utilized post-MI in those patients
who are intolerant of aspirin, have left ventricular thrombus or left ventricular
aneurysm, or are prone to atrial fibrillation.

# ADJUNCTIVE ANTITHROMBOTIC THERAPY IN PERCUTANEOUS CORONARY INTERVENTION FOR ACUTE CORONARY SYNDROMES

The prognostic benefit of using antiplatelet therapy in patients with unstable
angina/non-Q-wave MI has been known for some time.[8] In spite of the use of aspirin and heparin, however, the morbidity and mortality of patients in this group
remains a significant problem.[47,48] The hope that an incremental prognostic benefit in patients with unstable angina/non-Q-wave MI could be obtained with
the use of thrombolytic therapy[49] or coronary intervention[50] has not (yet) been
observed.

## Aspirin in Intervention

The administration of preprocedural aspirin results in a 50 to 75 percent reduction
of periprocedural ischemic events with percutaneous coronary intervention.[10,11] Aspirin is routinely started a few days before the elective procedure, or at least just
prior to the procedure in emergency cases, usually at a dose of 325 mg and continued indefinitely. However, the optimal dose, timing, and duration of treatment are
unknown.

## Heparin during PTCA

Heparin is universally used during PTCA, since it reduces the risk of abrupt closure.
However, the optimal dose or activated clotting time (ACT) during the PTCA procedure is not known. Studies on preventing microthrombi during extracorporeal bypass provided early experience and empiric guidance on the level of heparinization
needed for PTCA. Subsequently, a retrospective study of heparin use in patients undergoing PTCA demonstrated that ischemic complications were significantly increased after PTCA when the ACT is less than 250.[51] ACT levels less than 300 and
a diminished ACT response to an initial bolus of heparin (<175 s) have been associated with a higher rate of acute complications after PTCA.[51–54]

In the era of GPIIb/IIIa inhibitors, heparin continues to be used for coronary intervention. EPILOG established the superior safety of a low-dose, weight-adjusted heparin regimen in conjunction with early sheath removal for patients undergoing percutaneous coronary intervention with adjunctive abciximab. The initial heparin bolus was 70 U/kg, followed by the administration of additional boluses as needed to achieve and maintain an ACT of >200 s. Heparin was stopped immediately after the procedure, and the vascular sheath was removed when the ACT reached <175 s, generally 4 to 6 h later. This modification of traditional heparin dosing eliminated the excess bleeding risk in patients treated with abciximab, bringing the incidence of bleeding events down to placebo levels. With confirmation of the safe use of GPIIb/IIIa antagonists in the presence of weight-adjusted heparin in several large trials, the recommendation for their clinical use has come to be based on a weight-adjusted heparin regime. There is a tendency for low-dose heparin to be used as the standard for all percutaneous coronary interventional procedures, as bailout GPIIb/IIIa antagonists may be considered during the procedure. It should be stated, however, that low-dose heparin has not been shown to be safe in PTCA without GPIIb/IIIa inhibitors. The need for heparin when GPIIb/IIIa inhibitors are being used has been demonstrated by the result of the discontinued tirofiban/no heparin arm of the PRISM-PLUS trial.

## Adjunctive GPIIb/IIIa Inhibitors in Percutaneous Coronary Intervention for Unstable Angina

A possible cause for the lack of prognostic benefit from percutaneous coronary intervention in patients with unstable angina could have been the lack of sufficient efficacy of the antiplatelet therapy used in the previous trials. Platelets are able to undergo aggregation through activation of a number of thromboxane $A_2$–independent pathways, thus limiting the antithrombotic effect of aspirin.

The EPIC study[55] was the first large trial to test the hypothesis that blocking the platelet GPIIb/IIIa receptor could prevent postprocedural ischemic complications in "high-risk" patients undergoing PTCA or atherectomy and improve long-term outcome. This was a prospective, randomized, double-blind trial in approximately 2100 patients using the chimeric monoclonal antibody Fab fragment (c7E3 Fab) directed against the GPIIb/IIIa receptor. Patients were considered to be at high risk if they were scheduled to undergo PTCA or atherectomy and had unstable angina with ECG changes despite medical therapy, were undergoing direct or rescue intervention within 12 h of an AMI, or had high-risk lesion angiographic characteristics. Patients were randomized to receive a bolus and infusion of placebo, a bolus of c7E3 Fab and an infusion of placebo, or a bolus and an infusion of c7E3 Fab, and all patients received oral aspirin (325 mg) and intravenous heparin (non-weight-adjusted). The bolus of abciximab was started at least 10 min before the procedure, and the infusion was continued for a 12-h period.

The EPIC subgroup of patients ($n = 489$) with unstable angina or non-Q-wave MI underwent PTCA or atherectomy within 1 h of the initiation of c7E3 Fab administration. Of all the EPIC subgroups, this subgroup had the greatest benefit from the treatment; the 30-day composite end point of death, AMI, or urgent revascularization in the patients randomized to bolus followed by infusion of the drug was reduced by 62 percent (12.5 percent versus 4.8 percent, $p = .012$) when analyzed by intention to treat, and by over 70 percent (13.1 percent versus 3.8 percent, $p = .004$) when the 470 patients who actually received the drug were analyzed and compared to placebo. The corresponding figures for death and MI at 30 days were 11.1 percent versus 0.6 percent, a striking 94 percent relative risk reduction. The 6-month composite end point of death or MI continued to show a significant 88 percent relative risk reduction, 16.6 percent versus 2.0 percent, $p < .001$.[56] This reduction in the event rate at 6 months mainly reflected a decreased need for coronary artery bypass graft (CABG) or repeat percutaneous intervention. Importantly, at 3 years, in the subgroup with highest risk—i.e., those with an evolving MI or unstable angina—there was a significant 60 percent reduction in mortality in the treated group compared to placebo (5.1 percent versus 12.7 percent).[57] The long-term prognostic advantage has been attributed to the prevention of periprocedural MI by abciximab on the basis of a correlation noted between periprocedural creatine kinase rises and risk of late cardiac death.

In view of the clear efficacy seen with the bolus plus infusion of abciximab in the EPIC trial at the expense of a doubling of major bleeding complications when compared to placebo, the EPILOG trial[58] was designed to test the hypothesis that the benefit of abciximab could be extended to patients regarded as being at a "lower risk" of postangioplasty complications and also to evaluate whether the incidence of hemorrhage could be reduced without loss of efficacy by using weight-adjusted heparin (standard or low) dosing.

EPILOG was a prospective double-blind trial in which patients undergoing urgent or elective PTCA were randomized to one of three treatment arms to receive (1) abciximab (bolus plus 12-h infusion) with standard-dose, weight-adjusted heparin 100 U/kg plus bolus doses to achieve an activated coagulation time of $\geq 300$ s; (2) abciximab (bolus plus 12-h infusion) with low-dose, weight-adjusted heparin 70 U/kg plus bolus doses to achieve an activated coagulation time $\geq 200$ s; or (3) placebo with standard-dose, weight-adjusted heparin to achieve an activated coagulation time $\geq 300$ s. The primary end point was death, MI, or urgent revascularization within 30 days of randomization. At the first interim analysis, when 2792 of the planned 4800 patients were enrolled, the trial was terminated by the data safety monitoring board because of the clear superiority of the arms receiving abciximab, the primary composite end point at 30 days being 5.4 percent, 5.2 percent, and 11.7 percent for arms (1), (2), and (3), respectively, with an approximately 55 percent relative reduction for both abciximab arms compared to placebo. The benefits of abciximab were consistent irrespective of age, sex, body weight, and perceived coronary risk.

Although, based on the EPIC results, the EPILOG trial excluded patients who had had either an acute MI or unstable angina with associated electrocardiographic changes within the previous 24 h, the relevance of the EPILOG trial to patients with unstable angina is also discussed, since nearly half the study population had clinical criteria of unstable angina, albeit in the absence of ECG changes. The appropriateness of also considering the EPILOG results in the context of patients with unstable angina and non-Q-wave MI is further supported by the similarity in the results of the placebo arms of the EPIC and EPILOG trials, with the incidence of the composite end point of death, MI, or acute revascularization being around 12 percent for both at 30 days, perhaps indicating the continuing limitations of our current clinical and angiographic criteria for predicting risk. Subgroup analysis of EPILOG reveals that patients who had clinical unstable angina at randomization treated with abciximab plus standard-dose heparin or abciximab plus low-dose heparin had a composite end point at 30 days of 5.0 percent and 4.8 percent, respectively, as compared to 12.2 percent with placebo. The 6-month EPILOG efficacy data similarly showed a significant reduction ($>$40 percent) in the composite end point of death, MI, or *urgent* revascularization in both abciximab arms compared to placebo: approximately 8.3 percent versus 14.7 percent, $p < .001$. However, unlike the EPIC trial, the EPILOG trial showed an attenuation of the risk reduction for the composite end point of death, MI, or *any* revascularization.

The other interventional trials for unstable angina using adjunctive GPIIb/IIIa inhibitors include CAPTURE[59] (abciximab), IMPACT-II[60] (eptifibatide), and RE-STORE[61] (tirofiban). The CAPTURE study differed from the other studies in this group in that the patients had more severe refractory unstable angina and also that the abciximab infusion was started 18 to 24 h before the percutaneous intervention and continued for only 1 h after PTCA. Abciximab resulted in a 29 percent reduction in the composite primary end point at 30 days (11.3 percent versus 15.9 percent, $p = .012$), primarily as a result of a reduction in Q-wave MI ($p = .067$) and non-Q-wave MI ($p = .036$). Subgroup analyses of patients by risk strata showed that the treatment effects were similar to those found from the primary analysis. Of interest, not only was the incidence of MI significantly reduced during intervention and 24 h postintervention (2.6 percent versus 5.5 percent for placebo, a 53 percent reduction, $p = .009$), but the incidence of MI preintervention was also reduced by 71 percent (0.6 percent versus 2.1 percent, $p = .029$), perhaps demonstrating that abciximab stabilized or passivated the plaque. Table 53-2 shows a summary of the interventional trials using adjunctive GPIIb/IIIa. The results of these trials showed clear benefit up to 30 days, similar to EPILOG, but (unlike the results of EPIC) the benefit diminished by 6 months for the composite end point of death, MI, or *any* revascularization.

PRISM-PLUS,[62] although not primarily an interventional trial, is also discussed in this section, as approximately 30 percent of the patients underwent percutaneous coronary intervention. This trial therefore gives us an insight into "real world" use of PTCA after trials of medical therapy for treating unstable angina/non-Q-wave MI. This randomized prospective double-blind trial evaluated tirofiban alone, heparin alone, and tirofiban plus heparin in over 1900 patients with unstable angina/non-Q-wave MI. At 7 days, the combination of heparin and tirofiban significantly reduced the incidence of the composite end point of death, MI, or refractory ischemia by 28 percent (17.9 percent versus 12.9 percent). Although the 475 patients that progressed to receiving percutaneous intervention were not a randomized co-

TABLE 53–2. Efficacy Data of the Use of Adjunctive GP IIb/IIIa Inhibitors in Patients with Coronary Artery Disease Treated with Percutaneous Coronary Intervention

| Trial | | Composite End Point | | | | |
|---|---|---|---|---|---|---|
| | | Treatment, % | Placebo, % | Absolute Reduction, % | Relative Reduction, % | p Value |
| EPIC, 30 days | | 8.3 | 12.8 | 4.5 | 35 | .008 |
| EPIC, 6 months | | 27 | 35.1 | 8.1 | 23 | .001 |
| EPILOG, 30 days | Low-dose heparin | 5.2 | 11.7 | 6.5 | 56 | <.001 |
| | Standard-dose heparin | 5.4 | 11.7 | 6.3 | 54 | <.001 |
| EPILOG, 6 months | Low-dose heparin | 8.4 | 14.7 | 6.3 | 43 | <.001 |
| (death, MI, or *urgent* revascularization) | Standard-dose heparin | 8.3 | 14.7 | 6.4 | 44 | <.001 |
| EPILOG, 6 months | Low-dose heparin | 22.8 | 25.8 | 3.0 | 43 | .07 |
| (death, MI, or *any* revascularization) | Standard-dose heparin | 22.3 | 25.8 | 3.5 | 14 | .04 |
| CAPTURE, 30 days | | 11.3 | 15.9 | 4.6 | 23 | .012 |
| CAPTURE, 6 months | | 30.6 | 30.4 | −0.2 | ~0 | NS |
| RESTORE, 30 days | | 10.3 | 12.3 | 2.0 | 16 | .16 |
| RESTORE, readjudicated 30 days | | 8 | 10.5 | 2.5 | 24 | .052 |
| RESTORE, 6 months | | 24.1 | 27.1 | 3.0 | 11 | .11 |
| IMPACT-II, 30 days | 135/0.5 eptifibatide | 9.2 | 11.4 | 2.2 | 19 | .063 |
| | 135/75 eptifibatide | 9.9 | 11.4 | 1.5 | 13 | .22 |

hort, by 30 days the composite end point occurred in 15.2 percent of the heparin-only group and in 8.8 percent of the tirofiban plus heparin group (*RR* 0.55, confidence interval 0.32–0.94); i.e., patients who underwent angioplasty appeared to derive a 43 percent reduction in the composite end point of death or myocardial infarction from 48 h of pretreatment with tirofiban and heparin.

Similarly, the PURSUIT trial[63] (the largest clinical trial to date of any GPIIb/IIIa inhibitor) did not mandate percutaneous intervention in the protocol, but approximately 60 percent went on to receive it. The trial evaluated bolus plus up to 72 h eptifibatide infusion (96-h infusion if coronary intervention was performed near the end of the 72-h period) versus placebo bolus and infusion in over 10,900 patients presenting with unstable angina or non-Q-wave MI. Although the progression to percutaneous intervention was not subject to randomization, it is interesting to observe the outcomes of patients with unstable angina/non-ST-elevation MI according to whether or not they underwent percutaneous coronary intervention (see Table 53-3).

This finding in the placebo group is in keeping with the results of the VANQWISH trial[50] in that patients receiving aspirin and heparin for unstable angina do not receive incremental benefit from having PTCA. However, in patients receiving eptifibatide, there appears to be a lower incidence of the primary composite end point in those undergoing PTCA. This reopens the debate as to whether percutaneous intervention is preferable to conservative medical management for unstable angina in the new era of GPIIb/IIIa inhibitors.

## GPIIb/IIIa Inhibitors in Patients with AMI Being Treated with Primary Angioplasty or Rescue PTCA

Acute myocardial infarction typically results from the rupture of an atheromatous plaque with consequent platelet activation and localized thrombus formation, resulting in the total occlusion of the coronary artery.[64] Primary angioplasty in centers with rapid patient access to catheterization laboratories has been shown to be superior to fibrinolytic therapy both angiographically and clinically; restoration of effective flow at 90 min post-AMI, which has been shown to be of prognostic benefit,[46] is higher and recurrence of ischemic events lower.[65] However, the incidence of periprocedural adverse events in primary angioplasty in AMI is still significant.[66] Intuitively this is perhaps not surprising, as the procedure of primary angioplasty,

**TABLE 53–3.** The Incidence of the Primary Composite End Point of Death or Myocardial Infarction in Patients in the PURSUIT Trial

|  | Placebo, % | Eptifibatide, % | Absolute Risk Reduction, % | Relative Risk Reduction, % |
|---|---|---|---|---|
| PTCA | 16.7 | 11.6 | 5.1 | 31 |
| No PTCA | 15.6 | 14.5 | 1.1 | 7 |

while relieving the obstruction, merely compresses the thrombus into the vessel wall, and thus the latter is able to act as a nidus for further thrombosis or embolization, resulting in further ischemic events.

Post hoc subgroup analysis of the EPIC study provided early evidence for the possible benefits of GPIIb/IIIa antagonist adjunctive therapy in patients with AMI undergoing primary or rescue PTCA.[56] In the subgroup of patients with AMI ($n$ = 64) in the EPIC study, 42 patients underwent direct PTCA and 22 patients had rescue PTCA. Analysis of the pooled data on the 64 patients revealed an 83 percent reduction in the primary efficacy composite end point of death, reinfarction, or percutaneous or surgical revascularization, 26.1 percent placebo versus 4.5 percent c7E3 bolus and infusion, $p$ = .06. At 6 months, the benefit of abciximab remained, with the composite end point in the abciximab bolus plus infusion arm being 4.5 percent while that with the placebo was 47.8 percent, a relative reduction of 91 percent, $p$ = .002.

In the ReoPro in Acute Myocardial Infarction and Primary PTCA Organization and Randomized Trial (RAPPORT),[67] 483 patients undergoing primary PTCA within 12 h of onset of AMI were randomized to receive placebo or a bolus plus infusion of abciximab started before intervention and continued for 12 h. There was no difference in the incidence of the primary 6-month end point of death, reinfarction, and *any* target vessel revascularization between the treatment and placebo groups (28.1 percent and 28.2 percent). However, when the composite end point of death, reinfarction, and *urgent* target vessel revascularization was used, abciximab was associated with a significant benefit at 7 days (3.3 percent versus 9.9 percent, $p$ = .03), at 30 days (5.8 percent versus 11.2 percent, $p$ = .03), and at 6 months (11.6 percent versus 17.8 percent, $p$ = .05).

Subgroup analysis of the EPISTENT trial[68] showed that patients with AMI who received elective primary stenting had a 30-day composite end point of death, reinfarction, or urgent revascularization of 4.5 percent in the abciximab group versus 9.6 percent with placebo. Similarly, patients with AMI undergoing primary balloon angioplasty had a composite end point of 5.3 percent versus 9.6 percent in the group undergoing primary stenting without adjunctive abciximab.

In the GUSTO-III trial,[46] analysis of 387 patients with AMI undergoing rescue percutaneous coronary intervention following failed fibrinolytic therapy showed that there was a mortality rate at 30 days of 3.7 percent in the 81 patients who received periprocedural abciximab, whereas the mortality rate was 9.8 percent in the 306 patients that did not receive abciximab, $p$ = .04.[46] The use of abciximab was not randomized, however, and patients receiving abciximab were less likely to have had an anterior MI. Nevertheless, this result emphasizes the need for a study on the use of GPIIb/IIIa inhibitors as a rescue therapy in patients with AMI that have failed treatment with fibrinolytic therapy and rescue angioplasty.

On the evidence of the RAPPORT trial and the subgroup analyses of EPIC and EPISTENT, it would appear that the use of abciximab in patients undergoing primary angioplasty or primary stenting for AMI improves clinical outcomes at 30 days. Beyond 30 days, the EPIC subgroup analysis demonstrated a significant benefit, whereas RAPPORT failed to do so. While encouraging, however, the efficacy evidence is based on a relatively small number of patients and needs to be confirmed in larger trials.

**HOW LONG BEFORE PERCUTANEOUS INTERVENTION SHOULD THE GPIIB/IIIA INHIBITOR THERAPY BEGIN?**   The CAPTURE trial demonstrated that starting abciximab 18 to 24 h prior to percutaneous coronary intervention resulted in a reduction of adverse events prior to the intervention. This "passivation" of the culprit lesion may have occurred as a result of the disaggregation of intracoronary thrombus, limiting platelet accumulation to an adherent monolayer on the barotraumatized subendothelial structures. The use of GPIIb/IIIa inhibitors may therefore be beneficial in preventing further adverse thrombotic events in patients with unstable angina while they are waiting for a more definitive coronary intervention. This may have particular relevance to patients in hospitals without immediate access to invasive cardiology or coronary surgery. A treatment paradigm might exist in which patients with unstable angina/non-Q-wave MI receive traditional heparin, aspirin, nitrates, and a GPIIb/IIIa inhibitor for an initial period of time (yet to be determined) and are then triaged to angiography and subsequently to intervention (PTCA or CABG) through use of an ECG exercise test or pharmacological stress single photon emission computed tomography. This might represent a potentially more cost-effective strategy in managing patients with unstable angina/non-Q-wave MI.

## Ticlopidine in Percutaneous Coronary Intervention

The TACT study,[70] a randomized double-blind, placebo-controlled study, demonstrated that ticlopidine (250 mg) reduced periprocedural ischemic events following coronary angioplasty compared to placebo (5.1 percent versus 16.2 percent, $p = .01$). The use of a combination of ticlopidine and aspirin has been shown to be more effective than aspirin alone (STARS)[71] or a combination of aspirin, heparin, and warfarin (STARS, ISAR,[72] FANTASTIC[73]) in reducing cardiac events following coronary stent implantation and has thus become standard practice (Table 53-4). However, there is variation regarding the time for initiating the ticlopidine therapy; some practitioners prefer to start ticlopidine 1 to 3 days before the procedure, while others start it after the procedure. The optimal duration of therapy following stenting is still undefined, although most practitioners continue ticlopidine for 2 to 4 weeks.

## Low-Molecular-Weight Heparin in Coronary Stenting

The ENTICES trial[69] was designed to compare a combination of a LMWH (enoxaparin), ticlopidine, and aspirin with the conventional warfarin anticoagulant treatment in patients who received coronary stents in an effort to decrease stent thrombosis and ischemic clinical events. There were significantly fewer clinical events and vascular complications in the enoxaparin group compared to the group receiving

TABLE 53–4. Results of the Prospective, Randomized Trials of Antiplatelet and Anticoagulant Therapy with Coronary Stenting; 30-Day Outcome

| | Number of Patients | Incidence of Primary End Point, % | p Value* |
|---|---|---|---|
| **ISAR** (*n* = 517) | | | |
| Aspirin + heparin + warfarin | 260 | 6.2 | .01 |
| Aspirin + ticlopidine | 257 | 1.6 | |
| **FANTASTIC** | | | |
| Aspirin + heparin + warfarin | 230 | 4.3 | .03 |
| Aspirin + ticlopidine | 246 | 0.8 | |
| **STARS** (*n* = 1650) | | | |
| Aspirin | 555 | 3.6 | .04 |
| Aspirin + heparin + warfarin | 553 | 2.4 | .02 |
| Aspirin + ticlopidine | 544 | 0.6 | |

* *p* values are for the groups versus aspirin + ticlopidine.

the conventional warfarin anticoagulant regimen. The results of the ATLAST trial[74] comparing aspirin plus ticlopidine with enoxaparin, aspirin, and ticlopidine in a group of patients at high risk undergoing stenting are awaited.

# ANTITHROMBOTIC THERAPY FOR ATRIAL FIBRILLATION, NATIVE VALVULAR HEART DISEASE, AND PROSTHETIC HEART VALVES

## Atrial Fibrillation with Valvular Heart Disease

It is well appreciated that atrial fibrillation in the context of rheumatic mitral valve disease is associated with an increased risk of thromboembolism. In those with rheumatic heart disease, it is usual to give warfarin to reduce the incidence of stroke, although there has been no randomized controlled trial on which to base this approach.

## Nonvalvular Atrial Fibrillation

Nonvalvular atrial fibrillation (NVAF) has a prevalence of about 1 percent in the 60- to 70-year age group, increasing to above 4 percent in persons older than 80 years. The yearly stroke incidence in NVAF patients is 3 to 8 percent, which is five to seven times higher than that in age-matched persons in sinus rhythm. A number of randomized studies, however, have shown that this risk can be reduced by approximately 60 to 70 percent by the use of oral anticoagulants. Multivariate analysis reveals that the independent clinical features associated with atrial fibrillation that increase the risk of strokes include older individuals, previous transient ischemic attack, hypertension, diabetes mellitus, impaired left ventricular function, and left atrial diameter >4.6 cm diameter. With careful control of the INR (2.0 to 3.0), bleeding complications associated with use of these agents can be kept to a minimum. The data on aspirin use in nonrheumatic atrial fibrillation are more limited and less clear. Although one study (SPAF)[75] has shown a benefit with aspirin use, a 42 percent reduction in vascular events with aspirin 325 mg compared to placebo, another trial (the AFASAK[76] study—aspirin 75 mg) failed to find such an effect. The SPAF III study found that in high-risk individuals, variable-dose warfarin optimally controlled to achieve an INR of 2 to 3 was significantly better than a combination of aspirin (325 mg once daily) and fixed low-dose warfarin (INR 1.2 to 1.5). In another group of high-risk individuals (those with recent transient ischemic attack or minor ischemic stroke), warfarin reduced vascular events by 47 percent compared to placebo, while aspirin 300 mg daily was significantly less effective (14 percent reduction compared to placebo).

Overall, patients with nonrheumatic atrial fibrillation who are younger than 75 years of age and lack risk factors can be protected against stroke to a significant extent with aspirin. Younger patients (<75 years) who have risk factors should receive warfarin provided that there are no contraindications to warfarin. Patients older than 75 years appear to benefit from anticoagulation therapy, but this benefit is offset to some extent by the higher risk of bleeding complications. There is a small subgroup of patients with nonrheumatic atrial fibrillation with a low incidence of thromboembolism, the patients with "lone atrial fibrillation." These are younger individuals (<65 years) who have structurally normal hearts on echocardiography and no previous thromboembolic events, diabetes, or hypertension.[77] *Thus, on the basis of present data, aspirin should be advised only for low-risk individuals with lone atrial fibrillation or for patients who are unable or unwilling to take coumarin derivatives.* There are at present no data on the use of the newer antiplatelet or antithrombin agents in atrial fibrillation patients.

## Mechanical Heart Valves

The efficacy of anticoagulant therapy for patients with valvular heart disease has been most clearly demonstrated for individuals with mechanical heart valves. Although large randomized trials of warfarin versus placebo have not been conducted, there is considerable evidence that the thromboembolic rate is unacceptably high if these patients are treated with either antiplatelet therapy alone or no antithrombotic therapy. Initial studies in patients with prosthetic metallic heart valves not treated with warfarin demonstrated an incidence of systemic emboli of approximately 16 to 20 percent by mean follow-up of 3½ years—approximately 4 to 8.7 per

100 patient-years. When aspirin plus dipyridamole was compared to warfarin (INR 1.8 to 2.5) in a prospective randomized trial in patients with metallic heart valve implantation followed by 6 months of warfarin treatment, warfarin was shown to be associated with a lower thromboembolic rate (2.2 per 100 patient-years versus 8.6 per 100 patient-years, $p < .005$). *Even when patients are in sinus rhythm, antiplatelet therapy alone is not sufficient to prevent thrombotic embolism in patients with metallic aortic valve replacement.*

Oral anticoagulation is generally used at higher intensity (INR 2.5 to 4.5) in patients with metallic heart valves.[78] Whether these higher intensities of anticoagulation are superior to lower-intensity therapy for prevention of thromboembolism in these patients is not clear. However, the risk of bleeding with higher-intensity therapy is higher than with low-intensity anticoagulation. In fact, studies that have compared low-intensity anticoagulation (INR 2.0 to 3.0) with higher intensities have found two- to fivefold reductions in bleeding rates.[79]

Despite oral anticoagulation, systemic embolism continues to occur at a rate of approximately 1 to 2 percent per year in individuals with mechanical heart valves. Therefore, a variety of trials have evaluated the combination of antiplatelet and anticoagulant therapy in these patients. Combination therapy of warfarin with high-dose aspirin (approximately 1000 mg per day) produced unacceptable bleeding complications;[80] however, a randomized double-blind, placebo-controlled study[81] that used 100 mg of aspirin plus warfarin (INR 3 to 4.5) documented a 77 percent reduction (8.5 percent versus 1.9 percent per year, $p < .001$) in thromboembolic complications and a reduction in mortality from 7.4 per 100 patient-years to 2.8 per 100 patient-years, $p = .01$, but with a significant increase in *minor* bleeding (35 percent versus 22 percent, $p = .02$).

In summary, patients at high risk for thromboembolism are those with older prosthetic valves and those with a prior history of thromboembolism from a valve. They should be maintained with an INR of 3 to 4.5 or with medium-intensity anticoagulation (INR 2.5 to 3.5) and a platelet inhibitor (aspirin 100 mg/day or dipyridamole 100 mg four times per day). With recently placed prosthetic valves, an INR of 2.5 to 3.5 is recommended.

## Bioprosthetic Heart Valves

In one study,[81] none of the 384 patients in sinus rhythm with a bioprosthetic heart valve had an embolic event, whether they were on warfarin or aspirin, demonstrating the low incidence of thrombotic embolization in this group compared to patients with metallic valves in sinus rhythm. The rate of embolization was increased in patients with tissue valves with concurrent atrial fibrillation, whether they were treated with warfarin (4.6 per 100 patient-years) or aspirin (3.7 per 100 patient-years). A later study[82] showed that patients with a bioprosthetic aortic valve replacement treated with aspirin following 3 months of warfarin treatment had an incidence of embolization of 1.2 per 100 patient-years compared to 5.2 per 100 patient-years in patients not on aspirin after 3 months of warfarin treatment, $p < .02$. A retrospective analysis[83] showed that for patients undergoing tissue valve replacement (aortic or mitral), the incidence of thrombotic emboli diminishes with time and is especially high in the first 90 days. Risk factors for emboli were lack of anticoagulation, mitral valve location, history of thromboembolism, and increasing age. Another retrospective nonrandomized study[84] showed that aspirin is as good as warfarin in preventing thrombotic emboli in patients with either aortic or mitral Carpentier-Edwards tissue valves both in the first 90 days and long-term. *Warfarin (INR 2.0 to 3.0) is therefore recommended for the first 3 months after implantation of a bioprosthetic valve.* However, the use of antithrombotic therapy, e.g., aspirin, beyond 3 months after bioprosthetic valve implantation in patients in sinus rhythm needs evaluating in a prospective randomized trial. Patients with bioprostheses who are in atrial fibrillation or who have had a prior thromboembolism are at high risk and should receive oral anticoagulation indefinitely.

## Native Valvular Heart Disease

Thromboembolic rates are increased in native valvular heart disease, and anticoagulant therapy is particularly indicated if atrial fibrillation is present because of the high risk of systemic embolism. Even in the absence of atrial fibrillation, however, there is still a role for the use of antithrombotic therapy, as in patients with a dilated left atrium, e.g., in mitral stenosis or valvular regurgitation leading to a dilated cardiomyopathy. Definitive studies evaluating anticoagulant therapy in patients with rheumatic mitral stenosis have not been performed. However, cohort studies indicate a lower risk of thromboembolic complications if these patients are treated with anticoagulant therapy. In patients without atrial fibrillation, transesophageal echocardiography may be useful in examining the left auricle for thrombus or "echo contrast." If either of these two echocardiography signs or an enlarged left atrium (>4.5 cm) is present, anticoagulation is recommended. Because of the low incidence of clinically detected systemic embolism in patients in sinus rhythm with aortic valve disease or mitral valve prolapse with a normal left atrial size, anticoagulants are not indicated for these patients (Table 53-5).

## CONCLUSIONS

There clearly are new therapeutic agents available to the practicing physician that make the treatment of the thrombotic risks and complications of cardiovascular disease not only more effective but also clinically more satisfying to manage. Traditional drugs such as Coumadin, heparin, and aspirin still have their role in this management; however, their efficacy can be enhanced or, frequently, they can be replaced by more potent and selective agents. These newer drugs are being used widely, and they can improve the outcomes and morbidity associated with cardiovascular disease.

The continued challenge to the newer antithrombotic agents remains their cost-effectiveness in the setting of decreasing budgets and managed care. Should all interventions be covered with GPIIb/IIIa blockade? There appears to be compelling evidence from EPIC, EPILOG, RESTORE, and PRISM-PLUS that patients pre-

**TABLE 53–5. Antithrombotic Therapy for Valvular Heart Disease and/or Atrial Fibrillation (Provided Drug Not Contraindicated)**

| Condition | Antithrombotic Treatment |
|---|---|
| Chronic AF + valvular heart disease (native or prosthetic) | Warfarin (+ aspirin if further emboli on warfarin), INR 2.5 to 4 |
| Chronic AF + nonvalvular heart disease | Warfarin (aspirin only for lone AF) |
| Valvular heart disease | Warfarin for mitral stenosis,* AF, or previous thrombotic embolus |
| Native or prosthetic: | |
|     Bioprosthesis | Aspirin but warfarin if AF or previous thrombotic embolus |
|     Metallic | Warfarin whether AF or not. Low-dose aspirin added if thrombotic emboli occur despite adequate warfarin treatment |
| Intermittent AF | Optimal treatment is unknown. A pragmatic approach would be to treat these patients according to the above scheme until more data become available |

AF = atrial fibrillation; LA = left atrium.

* LA > 4.5, spontaneous contrast, previous emboli.

senting with acute coronary syndromes benefit from this form of therapy. It should be acknowledged that the predominant influence of these agents is in reducing non-Q-wave MI and large (>2 × normal) CKMB leaks. The significance of the non-Q-wave infarction/CKMB leaks is currently hotly debated. It is probably fair to say that myonecrosis cannot be considered to be a good outcome of intervention, but the reduction of asymptomatic non-Q-wave infarcts by the blanket use of GPIIb/IIIa antagonists could prove to be prohibitively expensive. Research is clearly needed to ascertain the significance of these creatine kinase findings; relate them to the other markers of myonecrosis, including the troponins; and define the medium- and long-term outcome of patients who suffer such ischemic events. Once such data exist, it will be much easier to advocate the widespread use of the newer, more potent antithrombotics and therefore justify the expense.

## REFERENCES

1. Verstraete M, Fuster V: Thrombogenesis and antithrombotic therapy. In: Alexander RW, Schlant RC, Fuster V (eds): *Hurst's The Heart,* 9th ed. New York, McGraw-Hill, 1998: 1501–1552.

2.  Levine MN, Hirsh J, Landefeld S, Raskob G: Hemorrhagic complications of anticoagulant treatment. *Chest* 1992; 102(Suppl 4):352S–363S.

3.  Ridker PM, Manson JE, Gaziano JM, et al: Low-dose aspirin therapy for chronic stable angina. A randomized, placebo-controlled clinical trial. *Ann Intern Med* 1991; (114):835–839.

4.  Chesebro JH, Webster MWI, Smith HC, et al: Antiplatelet therapy in coronary disease progression: reduced infarction and new lesion formation. *Circulation* 1989; 80(Suppl II):II-266.

5.  Lewis HD Jr, Davis JW, Archibald DG, et al: Protective effects of aspirin against acute myocardial infarction and death in men with unstable angina. Results of a Veterans Administration Cooperative Study. *New Engl J Med* 1983; 309:396–403.

6.  Cairns JA, Gent M, Singer J, et al: Aspirin, sulfinpyrazone, or both in unstable angina. Results of a Canadian multicenter trial. *New Engl J Med* 1985; 313:1369–1375.

7.  Theroux P, Ouimet H, McCans J, et al: Aspirin, heparin, or both to treat acute unstable angina. *New Engl J Med* 1988; 319:1105–1111.

8.  Second International Study of Infarct Survival Collaborative Group: Randomised trial of intravenous streptokinase, oral aspirin, both, or neither among 17,187 cases of suspected acute myocardial infarction: ISIS-2. *Lancet* 1988; 2:349–360.

9.  Henderson WG, Goldman S, Copeland JG, et al: Antiplatelet or anticoagulant therapy after coronary artery bypass surgery. A meta-analysis of clinical trials. *Ann Intern Med* 1989; 111:743–750.

10.  Schwartz L, Bourassa MG, Lesperance J, et al: Aspirin and dipyridamole in the prevention of restenosis after percutaneous transluminal coronary angioplasty. *New Engl J Med* 1988; 318:1714–1719.

11.  Mufson L, Black A, Roubin G, et al: A randomised trial of aspirin in PTCA: effect of high vs low dose aspirin on major complications and restenosis. *J Am Coll Cardiol* 1988; 11:236A.

12.  Burch JW, Stanford N, Majerus PW: Inhibition of platelet prostaglandin synthetase by oral aspirin. *J Clin Invest* 1978; 61:314–319.

13.  Patrignani P, Filabozzi P, Patrono C: Selective cumulative inhibition of platelet thromboxane production by low-dose aspirin in healthy subjects. *J Clin Invest* 1982; 69:1366–1372.

14.  Dabaghi SF, Kamat SG, Payne J, et al: Effects of low-dose aspirin on platelet aggregation in the early minutes after ingestion in normal subjects. *Am J Cardiol* 1994; 74:720–723.

15.  Vu T-KH, Hung DT, Wheaton VI, Coughlin SR: Molecular cloning of a functional thrombin receptor reveals a novel proteolytic mechanism of receptor activation. *Cell* 1991; 64:1057–1068.

16.  Greco NJ, Tandon NN, Jackson BW, et al: Identification of a nucleotide binding site on glycoprotein IIb. *J Biol Chem* 1991; 266:13, 627–13,633.

17.  Kobilka BK, Matsui H, Kobilka TS, et al: Cloning, sequencing and expression of the gene coding for the human platelet $\alpha$2-adrenergic receptor. *Science* 1987; 238:650.

18.  Pierson RN, Holt PR, Watson RM, et al: Aspirin and gastrointestinal bleeding: cromate[51] blood loss studies. *Am J Med* 1961; 31:259–265.

19.  Prichard PJ, Kitchingman GK, Hawkey CJ: Gastric mucosal bleeding: what dose of aspirin is safe? *Gut* 1987; 28:A1401.

20.  Prichard PJ, Kitchingman GK, Walt RP, et al: Human gastric mucosal bleeding induced by low dose aspirin, but not warfarin. *Br Med J* 1989; 298:493–496.

21. Hawkey CJ, Somerville KW, Marshall S: Prophylaxis of aspirin-induced gastric mucosal bleeding with ranitidine. *Alimentary Pharmacol Ther* 1988; 2:245–252.

22. McTavish D, Faulds D, Goa KL: Ticlopidine: An updated review of its pharmacology and therapeutic use in platelet-dependent disorders. *Drugs* 1990; 40:238–259.

23. Defreyn G, Bernat A, Delebasse P, Maffrand JP: Pharmacology of ticlopidine: a review. *Semin Thromb Hemos* 1989; 15:159–166.

24. Mills DC, Puri R, Hu CJ, et al: Clopidogrel inhibits the binding of ADP analogues to the receptor mediating inhibition of platelet adenylate cyclase. *Arteriosclerosis & Thrombosis* 1992; 12:430–436.

25. CAPRIE Steering Committee: A randomised, blinded, trial of clopidogrel versus aspirin in patients at risk of ischaemic events (CAPRIE). *Lancet* 1996; 348:1329–1339.

26. Coller BS: Platelets in cardiovascular thrombosis and thrombolysis. In: Fozzard HA, et al., (eds): *The Heart and Cardiovascular System.* New York, Raven Press, 1992:219–273.

27. Coller BS, Peerschke EI, Scudder LE, et al: A murine monoclonal antibody that completely blocks the binding of fibrinogen to platelets produces a thrombasthenic-like state in normal platelets and binds to glycoproteins IIb and/or IIIa. *J Clin Invest* 1983; 72:325–338.

28. Knight DM, Wagner C, Jordan R, et al: The immunogenicity of the 7E3 murine monoclonal Fab antibody fragment variable region is dramatically reduced in humans by substitution of human for murine constant regions. *Mol Immunol* 1995; 32:1271–1281.

29. Hirsh J: Oral anticoagulant drugs. *New Engl J Med* 1991; 324:1865–1875.

30. Meade TW, Mellows S, Brozovic M, et al: Haemostatic function and ischaemic heart disease: principal results of the Northwick Park Heart Study. *Lancet* 1986; 2:533–537.

31. Abbate R, Gori AM, Farsi A, et al: Monitoring of low-molecular-weight heparins in cardiovascular disease. *Am J Cardiol* 1998; 82:33L–36L.

32. Alving BM, Krishnamurti C: Recognition and management of heparin-induced thrombocytopenia (HIT) and thrombosis. *Semin Thromb Hemos* 1997; 23:569–574.

33. Santamaria A, Romani J, Souto JC, et al: Skin necrosis at the injection site induced by low-molecular-weight heparin: case report and review. *Dermatology* 1998; 196:264–265.

34. Hirsh J, Levine MN: Low molecular weight heparin. *Blood* 1992; 79:1–17.

35. Hall JG, Pauli RM, Wilson KM: Maternal and fetal sequelae of anticoagulation during pregnancy. *Am J Med* 1980; 68:122–140.

36. Weitz JI, Hudoba M, Massel D, et al: Clot-bound thrombin is protected from inhibition by heparin-antithrombin III but is susceptible to inactivation by antithrombin III-independent inhibitors. *J Clin Invest* 1990; 86:385–391.

37. Zoldhelyi P, Bichler J, Owen WG, et al: Persistent thrombin generation in humans during specific thrombin inhibition with hirudin. *Circulation* 1994; 90:2671–2678.

38. Badimon L: Models to study thrombotic disorders. *Thromb Haemost* 1997; 78:667–671.

39. Lewis HD Jr, Davis JW, Archibald DG, et al: Protective effects of aspirin against acute myocardial infarction and death in men with unstable angina. Results of a Veterans Administration Cooperative Study. *New Engl J Med* 1983; 309:396–403.

40. Neri Serneri GG, Gensini GF, Poggesi L, et al: Effect of heparin, aspirin, or alteplase in reduction of myocardial ischaemia in refractory unstable angina. *Lancet* 1990; 335:615–618.

41. Theroux P, Waters D, Qiu S, et al: Aspirin versus heparin to prevent myocardial infarction during the acute phase of unstable angina. *Circulation* 1993; 88:2045–2048.

42. Borzak S, Cannon CP, Kraft PL, et al: Effects of prior aspirin and anti-ischemic therapy on outcome of patients with unstable angina. TIMI 7 Investigators. Thrombin Inhibition in Myocardial Ischemia. *Am J Cardiol* 1998; 81:678–681.

43. Cohen M, Adams PC, Parry G, et al and the Antithrombotic Therapy in Acute Coronary Research Group: Combination antithrombotic therapy in unstable rest angina and non-Q-wave infarction in non-prior aspirin users: primary end points analysis from the ATACS trial. *Circulation* 1994; 89:81–88.

44. Anand SS, Yusuf S, Pogue J: Long-term oral anticoagulant therapy in patients with unstable angina or suspected non-Q-wave myocardial infarction: organization to assess strategies for ischemic syndromes (OASIS) pilot study results. *Circulation* 1998; 98: 1064–1070.

45. Organization to Assess Strategies for Ischemic Syndromes (OASIS-2) Investigators: Effects of recombinant hirudin (lepirudin) compared with heparin or death, myocardial infarction, refractory angina, and revascularization procedures in patients with acute myocardial ischaemia without ST elevation: a randomised trial. *Lancet* 1999; 353:(9151):429–438.

46. The GUSTO Angiographic Investigators: The effects of tissue plasminogen activator, streptokinase, or both on coronary-artery patency, ventricular function, and survival after acute myocardial infarction. *New Engl J Med* 1993; 329:1615–1622.

47. van Miltenburg AJM, Simoons ML, Veerhoek RJ, et al: Incidence and follow up of Braunwald subgroups in unstable angina pectoris. *J Am Coll Cardiol* 1995; 25:1286–1292.

48. Braunwald E: Unstable angina: a classification. *Circulation* 1989; 80:410–414.

49. The TIMI IIIB Investigators: Effects of tissue plasminogen activator and a comparison of early invasive and conservative strategies in unstable angina and non-Q-wave myocardial infarction. Results of the TIMI IIIB Trial. *Circulation* 1994; 89:1545–1556.

50. Boden WE, Dai H, on behalf of the VANQWISH Trial Investigators: Long-term outcomes in non-Q-wave infarction patients randomised to an "invasive" versus "conservative" strategy: results of the multicentre VA Non-Q-Wave Infarction Strategies In-hospital (VANQWISH) trial. *Eur Heart J.* 1997; 18(Suppl):351.

51. Ferguson JJ, Dougherty KG, Gaos CM, et al: Relation between procedural activated coagulation time and outcome after percutaneous transluminal coronary angioplasty. *J Am Coll Cardiol* 1994; 23:1061–1065.

52. Ferguson JJ 3d: Conventional antithrombotic approaches. *Am Heart J* 1995; 130:651–657.

53. Dougherty KG, Gaos CM, Bush HS, et al: Activated clotting times and activated partial thromboplastin times in patients undergoing coronary angioplasty who receive bolus doses of heparin. *Cathet Cardiovasc Diagn* 1992; 26:260–263.

54. Narins CR, Hillegass WB Jr, Nelson CL, et al: Relation between activated clotting time during angioplasty and abrupt closure. *Circulation* 1996; 93:667–671.

55. The EPIC Investigators: Use of a monoclonal antibody directed against the platelet glycoprotein IIb/IIIa receptor in high-risk coronary angioplasty. *N Engl J Med* 1994; 330:956–961.

56. Lefkovits J, Ivanhoe RJ, Califf RM, et al, for the EPIC investigators: Effect of platelet glycoprotein IIb/IIIa receptor blockade by a chimeric monoclonal antibody (abciximab) on acute and six-month outcomes after percutaneous transluminal coronary angioplasty (PTCA) for acute myocardial infarction. *Am J Cardiol* 1996; 77:1045–1051.

57. EPIC (Evaluation of Platelet IIb/IIIa Inhibition for Prevention of Ischemic Complication) Investigator Group: Long-term protection from myocardial ischemic events in a randomized trial of brief integrin beta3 blockade with percutaneous coronary intervention. *JAMA* 1997; 278:479–484.

58. The EPILOG Investigators: Platelet glycoprotein IIb/IIIa receptor blockade and low-

dose heparin during percutaneous coronary revascularization. *N Engl J Med* 1997; 336:1689–1696.

59. The CAPTURE Investigators: Randomised placebo-controlled trial of abciximab before and during coronary intervention in refractory unstable angina: the CAPTURE study. *Lancet* 1997; 349:1429–1435.

60. IMPACT-II. Integrilin to Minimize Platelet Aggregation and Coronary Thrombosis-II. Randomised placebo-controlled trial of effect of eptifibatide on complications of percutaneous coronary intervention. Clinical Trial, Phase III. *Lancet* 1997; 349:1422–1428.

61. The RESTORE Investigators: Effects of platelet glycoprotein IIb/IIIa blockade with tirofiban on adverse cardiac events in patients with unstable angina or acute myocardial infarction undergoing coronary angioplasty. *Circulation* 1997; 96:1445–1453.

62. The Platelet Receptor Inhibition in Ischemic Syndrome Management in Patients Limited by Unstable Signs and Symptoms (PRISM-PLUS) Study Investigators: Inhibition of the platelet glycoprotein IIb/IIIa receptor with tirofiban in unstable angina and non-Q-wave myocardial infarction. *N Engl J Med* 1998; 338:1488–1497.

63. The PURSUIT Trial Investigators: Inhibition of platelet glycoprotein IIb/IIIa with eptifibatide in patients with acute coronary syndromes. *New Engl J Med* 1998; 339:436–443.

64. Fuster V: The pathogenesis of coronary artery disease and the acute coronary syndromes. *N Engl J Med* 1992; 326:242–250.

65. Brodie BR, Grines CL, Ivanhoe R, et al: Six-month clinical and angiographic follow-up after direct angioplasty for acute myocardial infarction. *Circulation* 1994; 25:156–162.

66. The Primary Angioplasty in Myocardial Infarction (PAMI) Study Group: A comparison of immediate angioplasty with thrombolytic therapy for acute MI. *N Engl J Med.* 1993; 328:673–679.

67. Brener SJ, Barr LA, Burchenal JE, et al, for the ReoPro and Primary PTCA Organization and Randomized Trial (RAPPORT) Investigators: Randomized, placebo-controlled trial of platelet glycoprotein IIb/IIIa blockade with primary angioplasty for acute myocardial infarction. *Circulation* 1998; 98:734–741.

68. The EPISTENT Investigators: Randomised placebo-controlled and balloon-angioplasty-controlled trial to assess safety of coronary stenting with use of platelet GP IIb/IIIa blockade. *Lancet* 1998; 352:87–91.

69. Zidar JP: Low-molecular-weight heparins in coronary stenting (the ENTICES trial). ENoxaparin and TIClopidine after Elective Stenting. *Am J Cardiol* 1998; 82:29L–32L.

70. Bertrand ME, Allain H, Lablanche JM: Results of a randomised trial of ticlopidine versus placebo for prevention of acute closure and restenosis after coronary angioplasty. The TACT study. *Circulation* 1990; 82(suppl 3):III-190.

71. Leon MB, Baim DS, Popma JJ, et al, for the Stent Anticoagulation Restenosis study (STARS) investigators. *N Engl J Med* 1998; 339:1665–1671.

72. Schuhlen H, Hadamitzky M, Walter H, et al: Major benefit from antiplatelet therapy for patients at high risk for adverse cardiac events after coronary Palmaz-Schatz stent placement: analysis of a prospective risk stratification protocol in the Intracoronary Stenting and Antithrombotic Regimen (ISAR) trial. *Circulation* 1997; 95:2015–2021.

73. Bertrand M, Legrand V, Boland J, et al: Full anticoagulation versus ticlopidine plus aspirin after stent implantation. A randomized multicenter European study: The FANTASTIC trial. *Circulation* 1996; 94:I-685.

74. Aspirin/Ticlopidine vs Low-Molecular Weight Heparin/ASpirin/Ticlopidine High-Risk Stent Trial.–Ongoing.

75. Cowburn P, Cleland JG: SPAF-III results. *Eur Heart J* 1996; 17:1129.

76. Petersen P, Boysen G, Godtfredsen J, et al: Placebo-controlled, randomised trial of war-

farin and aspirin for prevention of thromboembolic complications in chronic atrial fibrillation. The Copenhagen AFASAK study. *Lancet* 1989; 1:175–177.

77.   Kopecky SL, Gersh BJ, McGoon MD, et al: The natural history of lone atrial fibrillation. A population-based study over three decades. *N Engl J Med* 1987; 317:669–674.

78.   Stein B, Fuster V: Invited letter concerning: anticoagulant plus platelet inhibitor therapy in patients with mechanical valve prostheses. *J Thorac Cardiovasc Surg* 1991; 101:557–559.

79.   Hirsh J: Influence of low-intensity warfarin treatment on patients' perceptions of quality of life. *Arch Intern Med* 1991; 151:1921–1922.

80.   Turpie AG, Gent M, Laupacis A, et al: A comparison of aspirin with placebo in patients treated with warfarin after heart-valve replacement. *N Engl J Med* 1993; 329:524–529.

81.   Nunez L, Aguado MG, Celemin D, et al: Aspirin or Coumadin as the drug of choice for valve replacement with porcine bioprosthesis. *Ann Thorac Surg* 1982; 33:354–358.

82.   David TE, Ho WI, Christakis GT: Thromboembolism in patients with aortic porcine bioprostheses. *Ann Thorac Surg* 1985; 40:229–233.

83.   Heras M, Chesebro JH, Fuster V, et al: High risk of thromboemboli early after bioprosthetic cardiac valve replacement. *J Am Coll Cardiol* 1995; 25:1111–1119.

84.   Blair KL, Hatton AC, White WD, et al: Comparison of anticoagulation regimens after Carpentier-Edwards aortic or mitral valve replacement. *Circulation* 1994; 90:II214–II219.

KARA L. JACOBSON/
DAVID P. SCHROEDER/
TERRY A. JACOBSON

# CHAPTER 54

# PATIENT EDUCATION AND COMPLIANCE*

Cardiovascular diseases are responsible for more deaths in the United States each year than any other category of disease. Cardiovascular diseases claimed 959,227 American lives during 1996, amounting to 41.4 percent of all deaths or 1 of every 2.4 deaths.[1] Both behavioral and pharmacologic interventions have been shown not only to restore normal endothelial function but to inhibit the initiation, growth, and rupture of atherosclerotic plaques ("plaque stabilization").[2] Exercise and health education programs in post-myocardial infarction patients have been shown to reduce cardiac and total mortality by 20 percent.[3,4] In order to decrease the prevalence of cardiovascular heart disease, patient education and compliance must be addressed. Cardiac rehabilitation programs and health enhancement programs should be prescribed for all patients with coronary heart disease (CHD).

## HEALTHY PEOPLE 2000

*Healthy People 2000*[5] is the prevention agenda for the entire nation. *Healthy People 2000* is based on the best available scientific knowledge and is used for evidence-based decision making. *Healthy People 2000*'s cardiovascular risk reduction goals for primary care providers include (1) increasing to at least 50 percent the proportion of primary care providers who routinely assess and counsel their patients regarding the frequency, duration, type, and intensity of each patient's physical activity practices; (2) increasing to at least 75 percent the proportion of primary care providers who initiate diet and, if necessary, drug therapy at levels of blood choles-

* The information presented represents the views of the author and not necessarily the views of AETNA U.S. Healthcare or USQA.

terol consistent with current management guidelines for patients with high blood cholesterol; and (3) increasing to at least 75 percent the proportion of primary care providers who routinely advise smoking cessation and provide assistance and follow-up for all of their tobacco-using patients. In order to decrease the prevalence of cardiac disease and move toward *Healthy People 2000* goals, we must more aggressively assess and treat patient behavioral risk factors that are modifiable. The major individual behavioral risk factors leading to CHD include smoking, physical inactivity, dietary fat intake, hypertension, and obesity.

## PATIENT EDUCATION

Lorig has defined patient education as a "set of planned, educational activities designed to improve patients' health behaviors and/or health status."[6] Although changes in patient knowledge may be necessary before patients change behavior, changes in knowledge alone do not necessarily translate into behavior change. Patient education is essentially empowering patients with the necessary skills, motivation, and positive reinforcement for successful long-term behavioral change.

Patients are often poorly informed about cardiovascular disease and often report needing more information about the specific management of their disease, their risk factors, and their required medications.[7] Without a proper patient education component, the medical management plan is incomplete and is unlikely to be complied with. In order to be effective, physicians must educate patients on their disease and the role the patient must play in self-managing the disease. Effective risk factor modification requires the knowledge and skills of a variety of health professionals, including physicians, nurses, health educators, exercise physiologists, and dietitians.

## PROCHASKA'S MODEL OF BEHAVIOR CHANGE

How do we move from changes in patient knowledge to changes in behavior? By understanding a model of behavior change, primary care physicians can be better prepared to provide more effective counseling. There are several models of behavior change, some of which focus on individual behavior changes and some of which focus on the patient's environment. Prochaska's model of the "stages of change"[8] can be applied to any individual behavior change. It states that patients go through various stages in attempting to change a behavior before the change becomes a routine part of everyday life. The stages are summarized in Table 54-1[8] and range from "precontemplation" to "maintenance." There are several tools that can be used to assess a patient's baseline stage and to counsel the patient during the behavior modification process. Most patients with coronary disease present with several risk factors and may be in a different stage of readiness for change for each risk factor. Therefore, stage-specific counseling is recommended. It is important to remember that these behavioral changes do not occur rapidly and that working with patients

**TABLE 54-1.   Prochaska's Stages of Change Model for Patient Health Behavior Change**

*Precontemplation.*   The patient is not even thinking about changing the behavior within the next 6 months.

*Contemplation.*   The patient is considering a behavior change within the next 6 months but not within the next 30 days.

*Preparation.*   The patient has stated that he or she will change his or her behavior in the next 30 days.

*Action.*   The patient has actually implemented the behavior change and contracting has occurred.

*Maintenance.*   The behavior change has been in place for at least 6 months and is being incorporated into patient's lifestyle.

*Relapse.*   Not a specific stage, but something that can occur at any time during the process.

*Source:* Adapted from Prochaska JO, DiClemente C: Stages and processes of self-change in smoking: towards an integrative model of change. *J Consult Clin Psychol* 1983; 5:390–395, with permission.

for months or years is sometimes required before they make these changes. The goal is to move patients forward through the stages of change and to sustain positive changes in health behavior over time.

## Stage-Specific Counseling—Tools Primary Care Physicians Can Use

**PRECONTEMPLATION STAGE.**   It is important that, when counseling patients, physicians base their counsel on the stage of readiness for change that the patient reports. The precontemplator is defined as having no interest in changing his or her health risk behavior within the next 6 months. Specifically, the patient who is defined as a precontemplator responds best to a message that focuses on the health effects of the behavior change. For example, "Quitting smoking will lower your blood pressure and will significantly decrease your chance of having a heart attack. These changes occur just 24 h after your last cigarette."

**CONTEMPLATION STAGE.**   The contemplator is planning on changing his or her behavior within the next 6 months but is not planning on changing it within the next 30 days. Having the patient maintain a diary of cigarettes smoked or a food or physical activity record will allow the patient to better understand his or her behaviors. Focusing on the triggers of the behavior (e.g., stress and reaching for a cigarette) and working toward making small changes over time is recommended. The clinician should tell the patient that during the next follow-up visit, a plan to modify the patient's behavior will be defined and mutually agreed upon by both the patient and the provider.

**PREPARATION STAGE.**   In the preparation stage, the patient is planning to take action to alter the behavior within the next 4 weeks (e.g., the patient can set a "quit date" to occur in the next month). If the patient announces the intended change, she or he will be more likely to commit to action. Helping the patient develop a defined plan for change that is understandable and practical is essential.

**ACTION STAGE.**   This is when the patient begins to modify behavior patterns. The actions are obvious, but actual change requires alteration in the patient's awareness, emotions, and self-image. Counseling the patient in this stage requires extreme support and rewards for initiating the behavior change. A physician-patient contract is useful during the action stage. Written contracts between the physician and the patient are more powerful than oral agreements. Because it is easier to promote a new behavior than to eliminate an old habit, the contract needs to reinforce the patient's new behavior and reward him or her for not reverting to the old behavior pattern. Because contracts can be broken by the patient, emphasis on honesty and the patient's self-esteem is important. An example of how to approach the contract would be to agree on a date when the behavior change will take place, such as the actual "quit date." Contracting should occur within the month. Setting a goal too far in advance is not effective, and the goal will probably be forgotten. If the goal is set too soon, chances are that the patient will not be prepared to make the behavior change.

**MAINTENANCE STAGE.**   In the maintenance stage, the struggle is to prevent relapse for the long term. The patient must consolidate the improvements of the action stage into new lifestyle patterns. Counseling the patient about relapse includes teaching the patient to distinguish between a "slip" and a complete relapse. "Slips" are a normal part of the process, and patients who slip need to identify what led to the slip and, most importantly, need to be encouraged to get back on track. If the trigger that led to a slip is identified and a plan for action to be taken when this trigger occurs again is proposed, a future slip or relapse will be less likely to occur.

# MODIFIABLE RISK FACTORS FOR CORONARY HEART DISEASE

## Smoking

Smoking is the single most preventable cause of death in our society today, and 20 percent of all heart disease deaths can be attributed to smoking (see Chap. 19, Tobacco Abuse—Cardiovascular Effects and Strategies for Cessation).[9] The current Agency for Health Care Policy and Research (AHCPR) guidelines state that all clinicians should routinely assess the smoking status of every patient and offer each patient an effective smoking cessation treatment program. Physicians must ask all patients about their smoking status, advise those of their patients who smoke to quit, assist them in quitting, and arrange follow-up visits.[10] Because of both addictive components of nicotine and the learned habit of smoking, cessation is possibly the most difficult behavior change goal to meet with your patient.

## Physical Inactivity

Physical inactivity is strongly associated with many deaths from cardiovascular disease,[9] and even moderate exercise is beneficial to health (see Chap. 20, Exercise Programs and Post-Myocardial Infarction Rehabilitation Therapy). Less than half of the adult population exercises three or more days per week for at least 20 min, and most older adults do not exercise sufficiently to improve muscle strength and flexibility, which are especially important for their health. The recent Surgeon General's Report (SGR)[11] on Physical Activity is noticeably different from previous exercise guidelines, which emphasized high-intensity physical activity at 85 percent of maximum heart rate three times a week. The new guidelines state that every American should accumulate at least 30 min of *moderate-intensity* physical activity on most days of the week. It is important to note that these guidelines allow for *moderate* activities such as gardening, walking, or heavy housework. Additionally, the recommended level of activity may be reached by *accumulating* the activity in short bouts of 10 min each. Finally, the major physical activity goal is to be active a minimum of 5 days a week. The SGR guidelines represent a more realistic option for most Americans. However, the SGR states that only 30 percent of primary care clinicians routinely provide counseling on physical activity to their patients. In order to assist clinicians, counseling methods and materials that can enable primary care providers to counsel patients to be physically active have been developed. The tool kit is called "P.A.C.E."—*Physician-based Assessment and Counseling for Exercise.*[12] Counseling patients about physical activity is one of the many areas in which primary care providers can influence the lifestyle choices of their patients (see Table 54-2[13]).

## Nutrition Counseling

Although patients express a strong desire for nutritional counseling from primary care providers, fewer than half of all clinicians report regularly providing even basic nutrition assessment and counseling to all patients. As with other types of lifestyle advice, simple, focused interventions can be beneficial to patients. Some of the most important nutrition principles include weight control, reduced total and saturated fat consumption, increased consumption of fruits and vegetables and complex carbohydrates, and the reading of food labels. Table 54-3[13] summarizes general low-fat, low-cholesterol nutrition recommendations for most patients.

**HYPERTENSION.**   Hypertension control based on behavior modification alone can reduce blood pressures to within normal ranges for many years. The value of nonpharmacologic therapy such as weight loss, alcohol reduction, and low-salt diet has been reaffirmed in the recent Joint National Committee Sixth Report guidelines for hypertension. Table 54-4[14] may help guide primary care physicians in the non-

**TABLE 54-2.   Physical Activity**

1. All patients should be asked about their physical activity habits, include both organized sports and exercise and general activities such as housework and walking.

2. An assessment should be made as to whether the patient's activities are sufficient to confer health benefits.

3. Patients who lack physical activity should be assisted in planning or initiating a physical activity program. The plan should be medically safe, enjoyable, convenient, realistic, and structured.

4. Even patients who are unwilling or unable to participate in a regular exercise program should be encouraged to increase the amount of physical activity in their daily lives. Examples include taking the stairs instead of the elevator, getting off the subway or bus one stop early, and doing household chores or yardwork on a regular basis.

5. Nursing and office staff should be involved in monitoring patient progress and providing information and support to patients. Some form of routine follow-up needs to be included.

6. Posters, displays, videotapes, and other resources can be utilized to create an office environment supportive of physical activity.

7. Providers should get adequate physical activity themselves. Studies show that providers who exercise regularly themselves are significantly better at providing exercise counseling to their patients.

*Source:* From The Clinician's Handbook of Preventive Services: *Put Prevention into Practice.* U.S. Department of Health and Human Services, Office of Disease Prevention and Health Promotion, Alexandria, VA, International Medical Pub, 1994.

pharmacologic management of hypertensive patients. Despite better detection and treatment of hypertension, it is estimated that less than 25 percent of patients on antihypertensive medications are controlled, i.e., have blood pressures less than 140/90 mm Hg.[14] The importance of strategies to enhance medication and behavior compliance cannot be emphasized enough. These principles are summarized later under "Compliance."

## Obesity

For patients who are overweight, a diet with fewer total calories and increased levels of physical activity are recommended. The weight loss should not exceed ½ to 1 lb per week. If the weight loss occurs more quickly, it usually is not maintained over time and may lead to other health problems. Behavior therapy and physical activity have been shown to be effective in maintaining weight loss over time. Reduction in caloric intake alone is unlikely to result in long-term weight maintenance.

**TABLE 54-3.  Dietary Fat Intake/Nutrition Counseling**

1. Every patient should be weighed and measured regularly. Patients should be advised of their healthy weight range based on factors such as age, gender, and distribution of body fat.

2. Clinicians should talk with all patients about their dietary habits. Short patient questionnaires can be useful in identifying a need for more in-depth evaluation.

3. Patients should be given basic information about managing a healthy diet. The U.S. Department of Agriculture and the U.S. Department of Health and Human Services recommend the following in *Dietary Guidelines for Americans:*
   - Eat a variety of foods.
   - Maintain a healthy weight.
   - Choose a diet low in total fat (less than 30% of calories), saturated fat (less than 10% of calories), and cholesterol.
   - Choose a diet with plenty of vegetables, fruits, and grains (5 or more servings per day).
   - Use sugars in moderation.
   - Use sodium in moderation.
   - If you drink alcoholic beverages, do so only in moderation (no more than 1 drink daily for women or 2 drinks daily for men).

4. Use of visual aids such as the Food Guide Pyramid can be useful in assisting patients in planning their food choices (see Table 54-6).

5. Clinicians should be familiar with the new food labels and encourage and instruct patients in their use.

6. For patients with borderline or elevated cholesterol levels, the National Cholesterol Education Program (NCEP) recommends that primary care providers instruct patients in the use of a cholesterol-lowering diet. The Step I diet recommended by the NCEP has less than 300 mg per day of cholesterol and 8 to 10 percent of total calories from saturated fatty acids. For patients who fail this behavior modification, the Step II diet is recommended. The Step II diet consists of less than 200 mg per day of cholesterol and less than 7 percent of total calories from saturated fatty acids.

7. It is important to provide follow-up for patients undertaking significant dietary changes. This can include follow-up visits, telephone calls, and postcards. Remind your patients that plateaus and progressions are a normal part of long-term behavior change.

8. Patients with nutritional difficulties should be referred to a registered dietitian. The American Dietetics Association can give you information on how to locate a registered dietitian in your area (1-800-877-1600, ext. 4898).

9. Clinicians who monitor their own diet are more likely to provide good nutrition counseling to their patients.

*Source:* From The Clinician's Handbook of Preventive Services: *Put Prevention into Practice.* U.S. Department of Health and Human Services, Office of Disease Prevention and Health Promotion, Alexandria, VA, International Medical Pub, 1994.

**TABLE 54-4.   Lifestyle Modifications for Hypertension Control**

1.  Lose weight if overweight.

2.  Limit alcohol intake to no more than 2 drinks daily for men and 1 drink daily for women.

3.  Remain physically active 5 days a week with an accumulation of moderate activity for at least 30 min.

4.  Reduce sodium intake to less than 100 mmol per day (<2.3 g of sodium or <6 g of NaCl; 1 teaspoon of salt = 2 g of sodium)

5.  Maintain adequate dietary potassium, calcium, and magnesium intake.

*Source:* From Joint National Committee on Prevention, Detection, Evaluation, and Treatment of High Blood Pressure: The Sixth Report of the Joint National Committee on Prevention, Detection, Evaluation, and Treatment of High Blood Pressure. *Arch Intern Med* 1997; 157:2413–2446, with permission.

# PATIENT EDUCATION COUNSELING FOR THE PRIMARY CARE PHYSICIAN

The primary care physician is often the main and sometimes the only source of health information for most patients,[15] and physicians are the most credible source of health information. Therefore, it is essential that physicians endorse and prescribe specific behavior modifications for their patients. Using advice concerning stopping smoking as an example of physician counseling, the following suggestions offer a brief, effective way for the primary care provider to provide behavior modification counseling to patients:

1.  State your message very clearly to the patient. Personalize the message by linking the message to your patient's specific health concerns. For example, if you were counseling your patient about quitting smoking, you would say: "As your physician, I must tell you that stopping smoking is the single most important thing that you can do for your health and to prevent a heart attack." The incorrect message is: "You really should quit smoking. It's not good for your health." The latter message is not as strong or as personalized.

2.  After having clearly stated your message, give a concrete example of how to perform the behavior change. For smoking counseling, consider the following: "We need to set a 'quit date' for you to stop smoking. Let's pick a date within the next month that you are comfortable with."

3.  Set a realistic goal that you and your patient can agree on. Consider setting a short-term as well as a long-term behavior change goal. Writing down the goal or signing a contract with your patient is effective. In this case, you and your patient can sign a "quit date" contract.

4. Have yourself or someone else in your office follow up with the patient. Another person in your office, such as a nurse or health educator, is ideal. A simple phone call to provide a reminder of the goal and to see how the patient is doing is often effective.[16]

In addition to your own counseling, support from allied health care providers and modifying your office environment may be useful. For suggestions as to ways to make your office environment more supportive and conducive to patient education, see Table 54-5.[13]

# PHYSICIAN BARRIERS TO PREVENTIVE COUNSELING

Although the physician is the best person to provide preventive counseling, there are many barriers that make physician counseling challenging. The most common barriers to counseling include lack of time, lack of training, and reimbursement is-

**TABLE 54-5. Modification of the Office Environment for Optimal Preventive Counseling and Education**

1. The office or clinic environment can be tailored to promote preventive care. Using a variety of venues creates an environment that reinforces healthy behaviors. Pamphlets, posters, and videos need to be visible within the office and available to patients.

2. Short patient questionnaires can be utilized to assess the patient's counseling needs and identify risk factors.

3. Patient's readiness to change health-related behaviors should be assessed. This will assist in focusing the intervention.

4. Nursing and office staff and office systems can help perform and monitor counseling.

5. The clinician and staff should be familiar with the community resources available to them and their patients. Services not provided in the office can then be referred to these sources.

6. Patient behavior change is difficult to achieve; however, it may be more valuable for health than many of the screening tests and immunizations that patients receive. In general, patients value the advice of the clinician. Studies have shown that even brief interventions, such as simple advice to stop smoking, may have a beneficial effect. More counseling tends to be better counseling, but any counseling, no matter how brief, is better than none at all.

*Source:* From The Clinician's Handbook of Preventive Services: *Put Prevention into Practice.* U.S. Department of Health and Human Services, Office of Disease Prevention and Health Promotion, Alexandria, VA, International Medical Pub, 1994.

sues. In order for a physician to provide a brief, effective message to a patient, the minimum time required is 3 to 5 min. Once a physician has initiated the preventive counseling process, it is recommended that he or she then refer the patient to another health professional, such as a nurse, health educator, or dietitian, to complete the counseling process. Physicians are currently not providing enough preventive counseling, and this is not surprising, since few physicians have received any formal training in patient education. Without formal training, physicians have low confidence in their ability to change their patients' behavior and are reluctant to make the attempt. Another barrier to physicians' performing preventive counseling is lack of reimbursement for these services. Both the Joint Commission for the Accreditation of Healthcare Organizations (JCAHO) and the National Commission on Quality Assurance (NCQA) have heightened the importance of physician counseling and now require documentation that physicians provide routine preventive counseling.

## HEALTH EDUCATION BY NONPHYSICIANS

Recently many managed care organizations and large physician group practices have moved to using health educators to help facilitate patient behavioral changes. It is important to recognize a health educator's training and how she or he can be useful within the practice setting. Hiring a health educator is a very cost-effective way to obtain an individual who is trained in behavior modification and patient education. Historically, nurses have performed patient education, but their clinical time may be more valuable and costly. A health educator will not have medical expertise, but she or he can provide you with many diverse, appropriately tailored patient education programs. When searching for a health educator, the authors recommend that you obtain a certified health educator. Certification for health educators is granted by the National Commission on Health Education Credentialing (NCHEC), and is indicated by the initials C.H.E.S. (certified health education specialist). Once certification is obtained, a health educator is considered competent in the following seven areas: (1) assessing individual and health plan (community) needs for health education, (2) planning effective health education programs, (3) implementing health education programs, (4) evaluating the effectiveness of health education programs, (5) coordinating the provision of health education services with other providers, (6) acting as a resources person in health education, and (7) communicating health and health education needs, concerns, and resources.[17]

## COMPLIANCE

The ability or willingness of a patient to adhere to a prescribed treatment regimen is critical, whether the prescription is behavior modification or medication usage. However, a large number of patients do not comply. The problem of noncompliance

can include not filling a prescription or not taking the prescribed medication correctly. In order to improve compliance, the following steps are suggested:

1.  Be certain that patients understand what you have prescribed. Have the patient repeat to you the prescription, including its frequency of dosing and why you have prescribed it. This way, you will know what the patient did and did not understand.
2.  Make counseling culturally appropriate. Information should be presented in a style and format that is sensitive to the culture, values, and traditions of the patient.
3.  Provide information "at a level of comprehension that is consistent with the age and learning skills of the patient, using a dialect and terminology consistent with the patient's language and communication style."[18] Often poor compliance is a direct result of poor patient comprehension or inadequate health literacy. Patients with inadequate health literacy have communication difficulties that may influence compliance. These patients have less understanding about their medical conditions and treatment. Improved patient-physician communication skills and the delivery of a clear and simple message will assist in addressing this problem.[19]
4.  Give the same care and attention to your patients' follow-up visits as you do to an initial patient visit.
5.  During the follow-up visit, discuss any difficulties the patient is having and reinforce the treatment recommendations.
6.  Provide written information that is clear and simple to accompany the verbal message—this will assist the patient in remembering what he or she is to do.
7.  Again, utilize other health professionals to assist you and your patient.

## SUMMARY

Physicians are key in initiating patient education and recommending lifestyle changes for their patients. In order to be most effective, physicians need to understand the continuum of patient behavior change—i.e., a patient's stage of readiness to make a lifestyle change. Because clinician time is often limited, many resources exist to help busy primary care physicians, such as well-developed low-literacy written materials and videos, as well as local community organizations such as the American Heart Association (see Table 54-6). In addition to physicians initiating patient education counseling, allied health care providers (nurses, health educators, and dietitians) are also very important in working with the physician and the patient as a team for the most effective patient care. Organizational and office changes can also promote and facilitate behavior change among patients and demonstrate support for preventive medicine interventions. As managed care continues to guide health care, future quality outcome measures will hinge on evidence of the quality and quantity of physician counseling and its impact on patient outcomes.

**TABLE 54-6.**   Modification of the Office Environment for Optimal Preventive Counseling and Education

| | |
|---|---|
| Pritchett and Hull Associates, Inc.<br>Suite110<br>3440 Oakcliff Road, NE<br>Atlanta, GA 30340-3079<br>1-800-241-4925<br>Web site: http://www.p-h.com | National Heart, Lung, and Blood<br>Institute (NHLBI)<br>National Cholesterol Education<br>  Program<br>National Obesity Program<br>National Physical Activity Program<br>Web site: http://www.nhlbi.nih.gov/ |
| KRAMES/StayWell Communications<br>1100 Grundy Lane<br>San Bruno, CA 94066-3030<br>1-800-333-3032<br>Web site: http://www.krames.com | American Cancer Society<br>1599 Clifton Road<br>Atlanta, GA 30329<br>Web site: http://www.cancer.org<br>1-800-ACS-2345 |
| American Heart Association<br>7272 Greenville Avenue<br>Dallas, TX 75231-4596<br>1-800-242-8721<br>Web site: http://www.amhrt.org | American Lung Association<br>Web site: http://www.lungusa.org/<br>1-800-LUNG-USA (1-800-586-<br>  4872) |
| Pep Up Your Life: A Fitness Book for Se-<br>  niors<br>American Association of Retired Persons<br>Fulfillment Services<br>601 E Street, NW<br>Washington, DC 20049<br>202-434-2277<br>Web site: http://www.aarp.org | Food Guide Pyramid<br>U.S. Department of Agriculture<br>U.S. Government Printing Office<br>Washington, D.C. 20402<br>202-830-3238 |
| ETR Associates<br>PO Box 1830<br>Santa Cruz, CA 95061-1830<br>831-438-4060<br>Web site: http://www.etr.org | National Commission for Health<br>  Education Credentialing<br>  (NCHEC)<br>1-888-NCHC4U; (888) 673-5445<br>610-264-8200<br>944 Marcon Blvd., Suite 310<br>Allentown, PA 18103<br>Web site: http://www.nchec.org/<br>E-mail: nchecckp@fast.net |

## REFERENCES

1. American Heart Association: *Heart and Stroke Statistical Update.* 1999.
2. Pearson, TA: An integrated approach to risk factor modificaion. In: Topol EJ (ed.): *Comprehensive Cardiovascular Medicine.* Philadelphia, Lippincott-Raven, 1998:297–311.
3. O'Connor GT, Buring JE, Yusuf S, et al: An overview of randomized trials of rehabilitation with exercise after myocardial infarction. *Circulation* 1989; 80:234–244.
4. Oldridge NB, Guyatt GH, Fischer ME, Rimm AA: Cardiac rehabilitation after myocardial infarction. Combined experience of randomized clinical trials. *JAMA* 1988; 260:945–950.

5. *Healthy People 2000: National Health Promotion and Disease Prevention Objectives.* Washington, DC, U.S. Department of Health and Human Services, Public Health Service, 1990.

6. Lorig K: *Patient Education: A Practical Approach,* 2d ed. Thousand Oaks, CA, Sage Publications, 1996.

7. Wenger NK: *The Education of the Patient with Cardiac Disease in the Twenty-First Century.* New York, NY, Le Jacq Publishing, 1986.

8. Prochaska JO, DiClemente C: Stages and processes of self-change in smoking: towards an integrative model of change. *J Consult Clin Psychol* 1983; 5:390–395.

9. McGinnis MJ, Foege W: Actual causes of death in the United States. *JAMA* 1993; 270:2207–2212.

10. The Smoking Cessation Clinical Practice Guideline Panel and Staff: The Agency for Health Care Policy and Research Smoking Cessation Clinical Practice Guideline. *JAMA* 1996; 275:1270–1280.

11. U.S. Department of Health and Human Services: *Physical Activity and Health: A Report of the Surgeon General.* Atlanta, GA, U.S. Department of Health and Human Services, Centers for Disease Control and Prevention, National Center For Chronic Disease Prevention and Health Promotion, 1996.

12. *Physician-based Assessment and Counseling for Exercise.* Atlanta, GA, Centers for Disease Control and Prevention, Cardiovascular Health Branch, 1992.

13. The Clinician's Handbook of Preventive Services: *Put Prevention into Practice.* U.S. Department of Health and Human Services, Public Health Service, Office of Disease Prevention and Health Promotion. Alexandria, VA, International Medical Pub, 1994.

14. Joint National Committee on Prevention, Detection, Evaluation, and Treatment of High Blood Pressure: The Sixth Report of the Joint National Committee on Prevention, Detection, Evaluation, and Treatment of High Blood Pressure. *Arch Intern Med* 1997; 157:2413–2446.

15. Williams CL, Bollella M, Wynder E: Preventive cardiology in primary care. *Atherosclerosis* 1994; 108(Suppl):S117–S126.

16. Lando HA, Rolnick S, Klevan D, et al: Telephone support as an adjunct to transdermal nicotine in smoking cessation. *Am J Public Health* 1997; 87:1670–1674.

17. A Competency-Based Framework for Professional Development of Certified Health Education Specialists. The National Commission for Health Education Credentialing, Allentown, PA, 1996.

18. Doak L, Doak C: *Teaching Patients with Low Literacy Skills.* Philadelphia, Lippincott, 1985.

19. Ad Hoc Committee on Health Literacy for the Council on Scientific Affairs, American Medical Association: Health literacy: report of the Council on Scientific Affairs. *JAMA* 1999; 281:552–557.

# INDEX

*Note:* Page numbers followed by the letter *t* indicate tables; page numbers followed by the letter *f* indicate figures.